# Therapeutic Exercise

## Foundations and Techniques

5th Edition

# Therapeutic Exercise

## Foundations and Techniques

### 5th Edition

**CAROLYN KISNER,** PT, MS

*Assistant Professor Emeritus*
The Ohio State University
School of Allied Medical Professions
Physical Therapy Division
Columbus, Ohio

**LYNN ALLEN COLBY,** PT, MS

*Assistant Professor Emeritus*
The Ohio State University
School of Allied Medical Professions
Physical Therapy Division
Columbus, Ohio

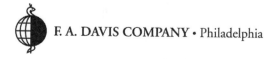

F. A. DAVIS COMPANY • Philadelphia

F. A. Davis Company
1915 Arch Street
Philadelphia, PA 19103
www.fadavis.com

Copyright © 2007 by F. A. Davis Company

Printed in the United States of America

Last digit indicates print number: 10 9 8 7

*Publisher:* Margaret Biblis
*Manager, Content Development:* Deborah J. Thorp
*Developmental Editor:* Jennifer A. Pine
*Art and Design Manager:* Carolyn O'Brien

As new scientific information becomes available through basic and clinical research,
recommended treatments and drug therapies undergo changes. The author(s) and publisher
have done everything possible to make this book accurate, up to date, and in accord with accepted
standards at the time of publication. The author(s), editors, and publisher are not responsible for
errors or omissions or for consequences from application of the book, and make no warranty,
expressed or implied, in regard to the contents of the book. Any practice described in this book
should be applied by the reader in accordance with professional standards of care used in regard
to the unique circumstances that may apply in each situation. The reader is advised always to
check product information (package inserts) for changes and new information regarding dose and
contraindications before administering any drug. Caution is especially urged when using new or
infrequently ordered drugs.

**Library of Congress Cataloging-in-Publication Data**

Kisner, Carolyn.
  Therapeutic exercise : foundations and techniques / Carolyn Kisner, Lynn Allen Colby. — 5th ed.
    p. ; cm.
  Includes bibliographical references and index.
  ISBN-13: 978-0-8036-1584-7
  ISBN-10: 0-8036-1584-1
  1. Exercise therapy—Handbooks, manuals, etc. I. Colby, Lynn Allen. II. Title.
  [DNLM: 1. Exercise Therapy—methods. WB 541 K61t 2007]
  RM725.K53 2007
  615.8′2—dc22                                                    2007007512

# Dedication

*To Jerry and our growing family—as always, your love and support has sustained me through this project.*

*—CK*

*To Rick and my extended family—a source of constant support and joy*

*—LC*

*In memory of our parents—who were supportive throughout our lives*

*To our students—who have taught us so much*

*To our colleagues—who have been helpful and stimulating in our professional growth*

*—LC and CK*

# Preface

You will notice a new "face" with the fifth edition of *Therapeutic Exercise—Foundations and Techniques*. The soft cover, a feature of the first four editions, has been replaced with a hard cover. Each edition of this text has grown in scope and depth to reflect the expanding body of knowledge related to therapeutic exercise. The fifth edition is no exception.

There are many exciting trends in physical therapy which have influenced therapeutic exercise, and thus the content of this edition. These trends include entry-level physical therapist education rapidly progressing toward the Doctor of Physical Therapy degree, basic and clinical research lending evidence for critical analysis and support for therapeutic exercise interventions, and the practice of physical therapy moving toward direct access and autonomy enabling physical therapists with the assistance of physical therapist assistants to provide services to individuals with movement disorders that impair function.

Although there are a number of new features in this edition directed toward the changes in education, clinical practice, and the healthcare environment, this text continues to provide a foundation of concepts, principles, and techniques on which an individualized program of therapeutic exercise can be built. This foundation remains an important component of the text. In addition to principles of exercise and background information on various pathologies and musculoskeletal surgeries, descriptions of exercise interventions and management guidelines are included to assist the reader in the development and progression of individualized and comprehensive therapeutic exercise programs.

Major changes we have made in this fifth edition include:

- A new feature called "Focus on Evidence" appears throughout the text to underscore the importance of evidence-based practice. The reader will find brief descriptions of research that highlight evidence related to various concepts and therapeutic exercise interventions. This feature is in addition to summaries of "outcomes" on selected topics that were added as a feature of the fourth edition and were extensively updated for this edition.

- The content of the text has been expanded to include several new areas and has also been completely reorganized. There are now five major sections. Highlights of each of the sections are as follows.

- Part I, **General Concepts.** We have added a new chapter, "Prevention, Health, and Wellness," by Karen Holtgrefe, DHS, PT, OCS. She has done considerable graduate work and teaches in this area. The content of the chapter describes the importance of these topics in physical therapy practice.

- Part II, **Applied Science of Exercise and Techniques**, covers the basic concepts and principles of therapeutic exercise and foundational techniques. We have added a new chapter, "Exercise for Impaired Balance." This chapter reflects the combined expertise of Anne D. Kloos, PT, PhD, NCS whose doctoral studies, teaching, and research have focused on neural plasticity and neurological physical therapy, and Deborah Givens Heiss, PT, PhD, DPT, OCS whose doctoral studies, teaching, and research have integrated the areas of orthopedic physical therapy and motor control. Their chapter has a rich blend of neurological and orthopedic perspectives to the management of impaired balance.

- Part III, **Principles of Intervention**, was one chapter in previous editions, but to accommodate expanding science and evidence, we divided the content and developed three new chapters. In addition to "Soft Tissue Injury, Repair, and Management" and "Surgical Interventions and Postoperative Management," we added chapters on "Joint, Connective Tissue, and Bone Disorders and Management" (with new information of myofascial pain syndrome and fibromyalgia and expanded information on fracture healing and management) and "Peripheral Nerve Disorders and Management." These chapters provide background information for the practitioner to make sound clinical judgments when developing, implementing, and progressing programs that utilize therapeutic exercise.

- The chapters in Part IV, **Exercise Interventions by Body Region**, have been extensively revised, updated, and expanded. In each of these chapters we feature a table that links physical therapist preferred practice patterns to each of the pathologies and surgeries presented. In addition, the chapters on posture and spinal impairments have been placed before the extremity chapters to emphasize the importance of posture on movement and control of the extremities.

- Lastly, Part V, **Special Areas of Therapeutic Exercise**, contains chapters that expand on areas of practice utilizing therapeutic exercise as a significant component of management, yet have distinct concerns that need to be emphasized. With the important emphasis on women's health, Chapter 23 "Women's Health: Obstetrics and Pelvic Floor" has been expanded by Barbara Settles Huge, BS, PT, Women's

Health Specialist, to provide a background and basic skills for managing women with pelvic floor impairment.

As with previous editions, we hope that our efforts in planning and developing this edition will provide a useful resource for the continued professional growth of students and health practitioners who utilize therapeutic exercise.

**Carolyn Kisner**

**Lynn Allen Colby**

# Acknowledgments

In addition to all of our colleagues who were integral to the development of previous editions, we wish to acknowledge and express our gratitude to the following people for their expertise and contributions to this edition.

Barbara Settles Huge, BS, PT – for her revision of Chapter 23, "Women's Health: Obstetrics and Pelvic Floor."

Karen Holtgrefe, DHS, PT, OCS, for writing the new chapter, "Prevention, Health, and Wellness," for revising the chapter, "Principles of Aerobic Exercise," and for contributing material on fibromyalgia, myofascial pain syndrome, and osteoporosis to Chapter 11.

Anne D. Kloos, PT, PhD, NCS and Deborah Givens Heiss, PT, PhD, DPT, OCS for developing and writing the new chapter, "Exercise for Impaired Balance."

Angie Dolder, PT, MS and the students at The Ohio State University who modeled for the pictures.

A special thank you goes to Berta Steiner of Bermedica Production Ltd, who spearheaded the copyediting and production process.

Once again F.A. Davis has brought their energy and resources to the development of yet another edition of this textbook. We are so grateful for their continued support for more than two decades. As with the fourth edition, Margaret Biblis, Publisher, has brought her vision, keen insight and style to the fifth edition. We also thank Jennifer Pine, our Development Editor, for always moving the project along and keeping us focused, as well as Deborah Thorp, Manager of Content Development for her help and input during our planning stages.

# Contributors

**Terri M. Glenn,** PhD, PT

*Adjunct Faculty*
Doctor of Physical Therapy Program
University of Dayton
Dayton, Ohio


**Deborah Givens Heiss,** PT, PhD, DPT, OCS

*Associate Professor*
Division of Physical Therapy
The Ohio State University
Columbus, Ohio


**Karen Holtgrefe,** DHS, PT, OCS

*Assistant Professor*
College of Mount St. Joseph
Cincinnati, Ohio


**Barbara Settles Huge,** BS, PT

*Women's Health Specialist/Consultant*
BSH Wellness
Adjunct Faculty
Indiana University Physical Therapy Program
Fishers, Indiana


**Anne D. Kloos,** PT, PhD, NCS

*Assistant Professor of Clinical Medicine*
Division of Physical Therapy
The Ohio State University
Columbus, Ohio


**Robert Schrepfer,** MS, PT, MBA

*Former Clinical Director*
The Center for Aquatic Rehabilitation
Associate Director
Bear Stearns Health Care Value Partners
New York, New York

# Brief Contents

# Contents

CHAPTER 7  **Principles of Aerobic Exercise  231**

*Karen Holtgrefe, DHS, PT, OCS*
*Terri M. Glenn, PhD, PT*

# General Concepts

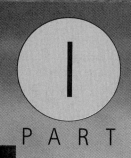

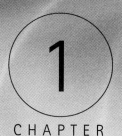

## 1 CHAPTER

# Therapeutic Exercise: Foundational Concepts

Almost everyone, regardless of age, values the ability to function as independently as possible during everyday life. Health-care consumers (patients and clients) typically seek out or are referred for physical therapy services because of physical impairments associated with movement disorders caused by injury, disease, or health-related conditions that interfere with their ability to perform or pursue any number of activities that are necessary or important to them. Physical therapy services may also be sought by individuals who have no impairment but who wish to improve their overall level of fitness or reduce the risk of injury or disease. An individually designed therapeutic exercise program is almost always a fundamental component of the physical therapy services provided. This stands to reason because the ultimate goal of a therapeutic exercise program is the achievement of an optimal level of symptom-free movement during basic to complex physical activities.

To develop and implement effective exercise interventions, a therapist must understand how the many forms of exercise affect tissues of the body and body systems and how those exercise-induced effects have an impact on key aspects of physical function. A therapist must also integrate and apply knowledge of anatomy, physiology, kinesiology, pathology, and the behavioral sciences across the continuum of patient/client management from the initial examination to discharge planning. To develop therapeutic exercise programs that culminate in positive and meaningful functional outcomes for patients and clients, a therapist must understand the relationship between physical function and disability and appreciate how the application of the process of disablement to patient/client management facilitates the provision of effective and efficient health-care services. Finally, a therapist, as a patient/client educator, must know and apply principles of motor learning and motor skill acquisition to exercise instruction and functional training. Therefore, the purpose of this chapter is to present an overview of the scope of therapeutic exercise interventions used by physical therapists. We discuss models of disablement and patient/client management as they relate to therapeutic exercise and explore strategies for teaching and progressing exercises and functional motor skills based on principles of motor learning.

## THERAPEUTIC EXERCISE: IMPACT ON PHYSICAL FUNCTION

Of the many procedures used by physical therapists in the continuum of care of patients and clients, therapeutic exercise takes its place as one of the key elements that lies at the center of programs designed to improve or restore an individual's function or to prevent dysfunction.[2]

### Definition of Therapeutic Exercise

*Therapeutic exercise*[2] is the systematic, planned performance of bodily movements, postures, or physical activities intended to provide a patient/client with the means to

- Remediate or prevent impairments
- Improve, restore, or enhance physical function
- Prevent or reduce health-related risk factors
- Optimize overall health status, fitness, or sense of well-being

Therapeutic exercise programs designed by physical therapists are *individualized* to the unique needs of each patient or client. A *patient* is an individual with impairments and functional limitations diagnosed by a physical therapist who is receiving physical therapy care to improve function and prevent disability.[2] A *client* is an individual without diagnosed dysfunction who engages in physical therapy services to promote health and wellness and to prevent dysfunction.[2] Because the focus of this textbook is on management of individuals with physical impairments and functional limitations, the authors have chosen to use the term "patient" rather than "client" or "patient/client" throughout this text. We believe that all individuals receiving physical therapy services must be active participants rather than passive recipients in the rehabilitation process to learn how to self-manage their health needs.

### Aspects of Physical Function: Definition of Key Terms

The ability to function independently at home, in the workplace, within the community, or during leisure and recreational activities is contingent upon physical as well as psychological and social function. The multidimensional aspects of physical function encompass the diverse yet interrelated areas of performance that are depicted in Figure 1.1. These aspects of function are characterized by the following definitions.

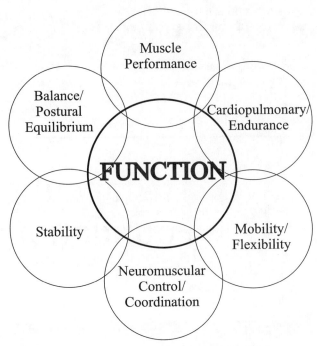

FIGURE 1.1 Interrelated aspects of physical function.

*Balance.* The ability to align body segments against gravity to maintain or move the body (center of mass) within the available base of support without falling; the ability to move the body in equilibrium with gravity via interaction of the sensory and motor systems.[2,66,74,88,124,127,128]

*Cardiopulmonary fitness.* The ability to perform low-intensity, repetitive, total body movements (walking, jogging, cycling, swimming) over an extended period of time[1,81]; a synonymous term is *cardiopulmonary endurance.*

*Coordination.* The correct timing and sequencing of muscle firing combined with the appropriate intensity of muscular contraction leading to the effective initiation, guiding, and grading of movement. It is the basis of smooth, accurate, efficient movement and occurs at a conscious or automatic level.[123,127]

*Flexibility.* The ability to move freely, without restriction; used interchangeably with mobility.

*Mobility.* The ability of structures or segments of the body to move or be moved in order to allow the occurrence of range of motion (ROM) for functional activities (functional ROM).[2,134] Passive mobility is dependent on soft tissue (contractile and noncontractile) extensibility; in addition, active mobility requires neuromuscular activation.

*Muscle performance.* The capacity of muscle to produce tension and do physical work. Muscle performance encompasses strength, power, and muscular endurance.[2]

*Neuromuscular control.* Interaction of the sensory and motor systems that enables synergists, agonists and antagonists, as well as stabilizers and neutralizers to anticipate or respond to proprioceptive and kinesthetic information and, subsequently, to work in correct sequence to create coordinated movement.[72]

***Postural control, postural stability, and equilibrium.*** Used interchangeably with static or dynamic balance.[50,124,127]

***Stability.*** The ability of the neuromuscular system through synergistic muscle actions to hold a proximal or distal body segment in a stationary position or to control a stable base during superimposed movement.[50,127,134] Joint stability is the maintenence of proper alignment of bony partners of a joint by means of passive and dynamic components.[85]

The systems of the body that control each of these aspects of physical function react, adapt, and develop in response to forces and physical stresses (stress = force/area) placed upon tisses that make up body systems.[81,84] Gravity, for example, is a constant force that affects the musculoskeletal, neuromuscular, and circulatory systems. Additional forces, incurred during routine physical activities, help the body maintain a functional level of strength, cardiopulmonary fitness, and mobility. Imposed forces and physical stresses that are excessive can cause acute injuries, such as sprains and fractures, or chronic conditions, such as repetitive stress disorders.[84] The absence of typical forces on the body can also cause degeneration, degradation, or deformity. For example, the absence of normal weight bearing associated with prolonged bed rest or immobilization weakens muscle and bone.[8,20,69,84,108] Prolonged inactivity also leads to decreased efficiency of the circulatory and pulmonary systems.[1]

Impairment of any one or more of the body systems and subsequent impairment of any aspect of physical function, separately or jointly, can result in functional limitation and disability. Therapeutic exercise interventions involve the application of carefully graded physical stresses and forces that are imposed on impaired body systems, specific tissues, or individual structures in a controlled, progressive, safely executed manner to reduce physical impairments and improve function.

## Types of Therapeutic Exercise Intervention

Therapeutic exercise procedures embody a wide variety of activities, actions, and techniques. The techniques selected for an individualized therapeutic exercise program are based on a therapist's determination of the underlying cause or causes of a patient's impairments, functional limitations, or disability. The types of therapeutic exercise interventions presented in this textbook are listed in Box 1.1. Additional exercise interventions are used by therapists for patients with neuromuscular or developmental conditions.[2]

NOTE: Although joint mobilization techniques are often classified as manual therapy procedures, not therapeutic exercise,[2] the authors of this textbook have chosen to include joint mobilization procedures under the broad

---

**BOX 1.1 Therapeutic Exercise Interventions**

- Aerobic conditioning and reconditioning
- Muscle performance exercises: strength, power, and endurance training
- Stretching techniques including muscle-lengthening procedures and joint mobilization techniques
- Neuromuscular control, inhibition, and facilitation techniques and posture awareness training
- Postural control, body mechanics, and stabilization exercises
- Balance exercises and agility training
- Relaxation exercises
- Breathing exercises and ventilatory muscle training
- Task-specific functional training

---

definition of therapeutic exercise to address the full scope of soft tissue stretching techniques.

## Exercise Safety

Regardless of the type of therapeutic exercise interventions in a patient's exercise program, safety is a fundamental consideration in every aspect of the program whether the exercises are performed independently or under a therapist's supervision. Patient safety, of course, is paramount; nonetheless, the safety of the therapist must also be considered, particularly when the therapist is directly involved in the application of an exercise procedure or a manual therapy technique.

Many factors can influence a patient's safety during exercise. Prior to engaging in exercise, a patient's health history and current health status must be explored. A patient unaccustomed to physical exertion may be at risk for the occurrence of an adverse effect from exercise associated with a known or an undiagnosed health condition. Medications can adversely affect a patient's balance and coordination during exercise or cardiopulmonary response to exercise. Therefore, risk factors must be identified and weighed carefully before an exercise program is initiated. Medical clearance from a patient's physician may be indicated before beginning an exercise program.

The environment in which exercises are performed also affects patient safety. Adequate space and a proper support surface for exercise are necessary prerequisites for patient safety. If exercise equipment is used in the clinical setting or at home, to ensure patient safety the equipment must be well maintained and in good working condition, must fit the patient, and must be applied and used properly.

Specific to each exercise in a program, the accuracy with which a patient performs an exercise affects safety, including proper posture or alignment of the body, execution of the correct movement patterns, and performing each exercise with the appropriate intensity, speed, and duration. A patient must be informed of the signs of fatigue, the relationship of fatigue to the risk of injury, and the importance of rest for recovery during and after an exercise routine. When a patient is being directly supervised in a clinical or home setting while learning an exercise program, the therapist can control these variables. However, when a patient is carrying out an exercise program independently at home or at a community fitness facility, patient safety is enhanced and the risk of injury or re-injury is minimized by effective exercise instruction and patient education. Suggestions for effective exercise instruction and patient education are discussed in a later section of this chapter.

As mentioned, therapist safety is also a consideration to avoid work-related injury. For example, when a therapist is using manual resistance during an exercise designed to improve a patient's strength or is applying a stretch force manually to improve a patient's range of motion, the therapist must incorporate principles of proper body mechanics and joint protection into these manual techniques to minimize his or her own risk of injury.

Throughout each of the chapters of this textbook, precautions, contraindications, and safety considerations are addressed for the management of specific pathologies, impairments, and functional limitations and for the use and progression of specific therapeutic exercise interventions.

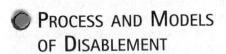

# PROCESS AND MODELS OF DISABLEMENT

It has been said that the physical therapy profession is defined by a body of knowledge and clinical applications that are directed toward the elimination or resolution of disability.[110] Understanding the disabling consequences of disease, injury, and abnormalities of development and how the risk of potential disability can be reduced, therefore, must be fundamental to the provision of effective care and services, which are geared to the restoration of meaningful function for patients and their families, significant others, and caregivers.

## The Disablement Process

### Definition
Disablement is a term that refers to the impact(s) and functional consequences of acute or chronic conditions, such as disease, injury, and congenital or developmental abnormalities, on specific body systems that compromise basic human performance and an individual's ability to meet necessary, customary, expected, and desired societal functions and roles.[60,86,143] Physical therapists most commonly provide care and services to people with *physical* disability. Social, emotional, and cognitive disablement can affect physical function and vice versa and, therefore, should not be disregarded or dismissed.[58,60]

### Implications in Health Care
Knowledge of the process of disablement provides a foundation for health-care professionals to develop an appreciation of the complex relationships among function, disability, and health.[62,132] This knowledge, in turn, provides a theoretical framework upon which practice can be organized and research can be based, thus facilitating effective management and care of patients that is reflected by meaningful functional outcomes.[40,62]

Inherent in the integration and application of knowledge of the disablement process in health-care delivery is an understanding that the process is *not unidirectional*; that is, it is not necessarily unpreventable or irreversible.[14] Furthermore, it is assumed that in most instances, depending on factors such as the severity and duration of the pathological condition, a patient's access to quality health care as well as the motivation and desires of the patient, the progression of the process can indeed be altered and the patient's function improved.[2,14,132,133]

An understanding and application of the disablement process shifts the focus of patient management from strict treatment of a disease or injury to treatment of the *impact* that a disease, injury, or disorder has on a patient's *function* as well as the identification of the underlying causes of the patient's dysfunction. This perspective puts the person, not solely the disease or disorder, at the center of efforts to prevent or halt the progression of disablement by employing interventions that improve a patient's functional abilities while simultaneously reducing or eliminating the causes of disability.[39,132,133]

## Models of Disablement

Several models that depict the process of disablement have been proposed over the past 40 years. The first two schema developed were the Nagi model[86,87] and the International Classification of Impairments, Disabilities, and Handicaps (ICIDH) model for the World Health Organization (WHO).[51] The ICIDH model was revised after its original publication, with adjustments made in the descriptions of the classification criteria of the model based on input from health-care practitioners as they became familiar with the original model.[47] The National Center for Medical Rehabilitation Research (NCMRR) integrated components of the Nagi model with the original ICIDH model to develop its own model.[89] The NCMRR model added interactions of individual risk factors, including physical and social factors, to the disablement process.

Although each of these models uses slightly different terminology, each reflects a spectrum of disablement. Several sources in the literature have discussed or compared and contrasted the terminology and descriptors used in these and other models.[2,39,51,59,60,86,87,89] Despite the variations in these models, each taxonomy reflects the complex *interrelationships* among the following.

- Acute or chronic pathology
- Impairments
- Functional limitations
- Disabilities, handicaps, or societal limitations

The conceptual frameworks of the Nagi, ICIDH, and NCMRR models of disablement, although applied widely

| TABLE 1.1 | Comparison of Terminology of Three Disablement Models | | | |
|---|---|---|---|---|
| Model | Tissue/Cellular Level | Organ/System Level | Personal Level | Societal Level |
| Nagi | Active pathology | Impairment | Functional limitation | Disability |
| ICIDH* | Disease | Impairment | Disability | Handicap |
| ICF† | | Impairment of body structure/function | Activity limitation | Participation restriction |

*International Classification of Impairments, Disabilities, and Handicaps.
†International Classification of Functioning, Disability, and Health.

in clinical practice and research in many health-care professions, have been criticized for their perceived focus on disease and a medical-biological view of disability as well as their lack of attention to the person with a disability.[21] In response to these criticisms, the WHO undertook a broad revision of its conceptual framework and system for classifying disability described in its ICIDH model. Through a comprehensive consensus process over a number of years, the WHO developed the International Classification of Functioning, Disability, and Health (ICF).[52,131-133] This new conceptual model integrates functioning and disability and is characterized as a bio-psycho-social model of disablement that provides a coherent perspective of various aspects of health. The revised model was also designed to place less emphasis on disease and greater emphasis on how people affected by health conditions live.[21,52,132,133] The ICF model consists of the following components of health and health-related influences.

- Impairment of body structure (anatomical) and function (physiological)
- Activity limitation
- Participation restriction
- Impact of contextual factors (environmental and personal) on functioning, disability, and health

The components of the ICF model are compared in Table 1.1 to the Nagi and ICIDH models of disablement.

## Use of Disablement Models and Classifications in Physical Therapy

During the early 1990s physical therapists began to explore the potential use of disablement models and suggested that disablement schema and related terminology provided an appropriate framework for clinical decision making in practice and research.[40,59,120] In addition, practitioners and researchers suggested that consistent use of disablement-related language could be a mechanism to standardize terminology for documentation and communication in the clinical and research settings.[45] The American Physical Therapy Association (APTA) subsequently incorporated an extension of the Nagi disablement model and related terminology into its evolving consensus document, the *Guide to Physical Therapist Practice*[2] (often called the *Guide*), which was developed to reflect "best practice" from the initial examination to the outcomes of intervention. The *Guide* also uses the concept of disablement as a framework for organizing and prioritizing clinical decisions made during the continuum of physical therapy care and services.

To be consistent with the language of the *Guide*, Figure 1.2, which was configured for this textbook, depicts a model of disablement and the potential impacts of therapeutic exercise interventions on the disablement process. The impact of risk factors has also been included in this depiction of the process. Incorporating risk factors into the

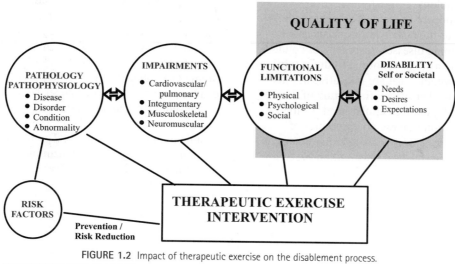

FIGURE 1.2 Impact of therapeutic exercise on the disablement process.

model underscores the assumption that disability can be prevented, eliminated, or reduced if the risk of occurrence or severity of pathology, impairment, or functional limitation is reduced. The model also shows that effective interventions, in particular therapeutic exercise, can have a positive impact on every aspect of the disablement process.

N O T E : Shortly after the second edition of the *Guide* was published, the WHO adopted and disseminated the ICF model of disablement, with its newly developed conceptual framework and system for classifying functioning and disability.[52] Consequently, information about this model and its revised concepts and terminology were not incorporated into the *Guide*, and so the elements of the ICF model are not yet widely used by the physical therapy community. Because physical therapists need to be aware of the changing concepts and language of disablement, it is likely that the next edition of the *Guide* will reflect this information.

By choosing to use a model of disablement as part of the theoretical framework of practice, physical therapists have a responsibility to provide evidence that there are, indeed, links among the elements of the disablement process that can be identified by physical therapy tests and measures. It is also the responsibility of the profession to demonstrate that not only can physical impairments be reduced but functional abilities can be significantly enhanced by physical therapy interventions. This body of evidence has just begun to emerge during the past decade. Examples of some of this evidence are integrated into this chapter and interspersed throughout the textbook.

An overview of the key components of the process of disablement, using language consistent with that in the *Guide*, is presented in the following sections of this chapter, with additional discussion of risk factors and their potential impact on disability. The relationship of the disablement model to patient management and physical therapy interventions, specifically therapeutic exercise, is also discussed.

### Pathology/Pathophysiology

This first major component of the disablement model refers to disruptions of the body's homeostasis as the result of acute or chronic diseases, disorders, or conditions characterized by a set of abnormal findings (clusters of signs and symptoms) that are indicative of alterations or interruptions of structure or function of the body primarily identified at the cellular level.[2,36] Identification and classification of these abnormalities of *anatomical, physiological,* or *psychological* structure or process generally trigger medical intervention based on a medical diagnosis.

Physical therapists in all areas of practice treat patients with a multitude of pathologies. Knowledge of these pathologies (medical diagnoses) is important background information, but it does not tell the therapist how to assess and treat a patient's dysfunction that arises from the pathological condition. Despite an accurate medical diagnosis and a therapist's thorough knowledge of specific pathologies, the experienced therapist knows full well that two patients with the same medical diagnosis, such as rheumatoid arthritis, and the same extent of joint destruction (confirmed radiologically) may have very different severities of impairment and functional limitation and, consequently, very different degrees of disability. This emphasizes the need for physical therapists to always pay close attention to the impact(s) of a particular pathology on function when designing meaningful management strategies to improve functional abilities.

### Impairments

Impairments are the *consequences* of pathological conditions; that is, they are the signs and symptoms that reflect abnormalities at the body system, organ, or tissue level.[2,36,58]

### Types of Impairment

Impairments can be categorized as arising from *anatomical, physiological,* or *psychological* alterations as well as losses or abnormalities of *structure* or *function* of a body system. Physical therapists typically provide care and services to patients with impairments that affect the following systems.

- Musculoskeletal
- Neuromuscular
- Cardiovascular/pulmonary
- Integumentary

Most impairments of these body systems primarily are the result of abnormalities of physiological function or anatomical structure. Some representative examples of physical impairments commonly identified by physical therapists and managed with therapeutic exercise interventions are noted in Box 1.2.

Impairments may arise directly from the pathology *(direct/primary impairments)* or may be the result of pre-existing impairments *(indirect/secondary impairments).* A patient, for example, who has been referred to physical therapy with a medical diagnosis of impingement syndrome or tendinitis of the rotator cuff (pathology) may exhibit primary impairments, such as pain, limited ROM of the shoulder, and weakness of specific shoulder girdle and glenohumeral musculature during the physical therapy examination (Fig. 1.3 A&B). The patient may subsequently develop secondary postural asymmetry because of altered use of the upper extremity.

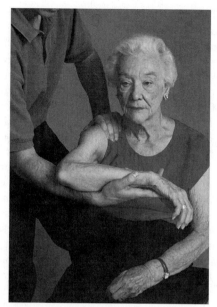

**A**

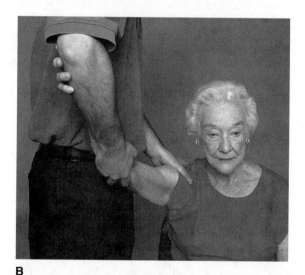
**B**

FIGURE 1.3 (A) Impingement syndrome of the shoulder and associated tendinitis of the rotator cuff (pathology) leading to (B) limited range of shoulder elevation (an impairment) are identified during the examination.

| BOX 1.2 | Common Physical Impairments Managed with Therapeutic Exercise |
|---|---|

**Musculoskeletal**
- Pain
- Muscle weakness/reduced torque production
- Decreased muscular endurance
- Limited range of motion due to
  - Restriction of the joint capsule
  - Restriction of periarticular connective tissue
  - Decreased muscle length
- Joint hypermobility
- Faulty posture
- Muscle length/strength imbalances

**Neuromuscular**
- Pain
- Impaired balance, postural stability, or control
- Incoordination, faulty timing
- Delayed motor development
- Abnormal tone (hypotonia, hypertonia, dystonia)
- Ineffective/inefficient functional movement strategies

**Cardiovascular/Pulmonary**
- Decreased aerobic capacity (cardiopulmonary endurance)
- Impaired circulation (lymphatic, venous, arterial)
- Pain with sustained physical activity (intermittent claudication)

**Integumentary**
- Skin hypomobility (e.g., immobile or adherent scarring)

Furthermore, when an impairment is the result of multiple underlying causes and arises from a combination of primary or secondary impairments, the term *composite impairment* is sometimes used.[120] For example, a patient who sustained a severe inversion sprain of the ankle resulting in a tear of the talofibular ligament and whose ankle was immobilized for several weeks is likely to exhibit a balance impairment of the involved lower extremity after the immobilization order is removed. This composite impairment could be the result of chronic ligamentous laxity and impaired ankle proprioception from the injury or muscle weakness due to immobilization and disuse.

Regardless of the types of impairment exhibited by a patient, a therapist must keep in mind that impairments manifest differently from one patient to another. In addition, not all impairments are necessarily linked to functional limitations or disability. An important key to effective management of a patient's problems is to recognize *functionally relevant impairments,* in other words, impairments that directly contribute to current or future functional limitations and disability. Impairments that can predispose a patient to secondary pathologies or impairments must also be identified.

Equally crucial for the effective management of a patient's dysfunction is the need to analyze and determine, or at least infer and certainly not ignore, the *underlying causes* of the identified physical impairments, particularly those related to impaired movement.[117,118] For example, are biomechanical abnormalities of soft tissues the source of restricted ROM? If so, which soft tissues are restricted, and why are they restricted? This information assists the therapist in the selection of appropriate, effective therapeutic interventions that target the underlying *causes* of the impairments, the impairments themselves, and the resulting functional limitations.

Although most physical therapy interventions, including therapeutic exercise, are designed to correct or reduce physical impairments, such as decreased ROM or strength, poor balance, or limited cardiopulmonary endurance, the focus of treatment must still be on restoration of function and prevention of dysfunction. Elimination or reduction of functionally relevant impairments is certainly necessary during treatment; but from a patient's perspective, *successful outcomes* of treatment are determined by a reduction or resolution of functional limitations or disabilities and the restoration or improvement of function. A therapist cannot simply assume that intervening at the impairment level (e.g., with strengthening or stretching exercises) and subsequently reducing physical impairments (by increasing strength and ROM) necessarily generalizes to remediation of functional limitations and restoration of functional motor abilities for daily living. Mechanisms for integrating correction of physical impairments and restoration of functional abilities through task-specific training are explored in a model of effective patient management later in this chapter.

## Functional Limitations

Functional limitations, the third component of the disablement model, occur at the level of the *whole person.* They are the result of impairments and are characterized by the reduced ability of a person to perform actions or components of motor skills in an efficient or typically expected manner.[2,86,87,89] For example, as shown in Figure 1.4, restricted range of motion (impairment) of the shoulder as the result of shoulder pain can limit a person's ability to reach overhead (functional limitation) while performing, for example, personal grooming or household tasks.

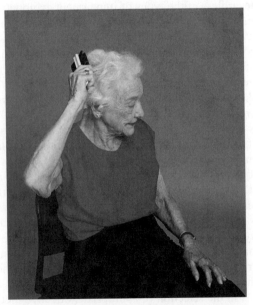

FIGURE 1.4 Limited ability to reach overhead (functional limitation) as the result of impaired shoulder mobility may lead to difficulty performing personal grooming or household tasks independently (disability).

**N O T E :** The term now used by the WHO to denote functional limitation is "ability limitation," as defined in the ICF model of functioning and disability[21,52,131-133] (see Table 1.1).

As previously indicated in Figure 1.2, functional limitations may be *physical, social, or psychological* in nature. The focus of physical therapy interventions is on the management of limitations of physical functioning while respecting the needs of the whole person and recognizing that social and psychological influences can also limit a person's ability to function. In addition, the focus must be on those functional limitations that are most important to the patient and those that are or could be directly causing disability. When impairments cause functional limitations, a person's *quality of life* may begin to deteriorate (see Fig. 1.2). It should also be noted that a single or even several mild impairments often do not cause loss of function. Evidence suggests that the severity and complexity of impairments must reach a critical level, which is different for each person, before degradation of function begins to occur.[95,103]

### Types of Functional Limitations

Functional limitations in the physical domain deal with the performance of sensorimotor tasks, that is, total body actions that are typically *components or elements* of functional activities.[2,89] These activities include basic activities of daily living (ADL), such as bathing, dressing, or feeding, and the more complex tasks known as instrumental activities of daily living (IADL), such as occupational tasks, school-related skills, housekeeping, and recreational activities, or community mobility (driving, using public transportation), just to name a few.

Box 1.3 lists a number of functional limitations that can arise from physical impairments, involve *whole-body movements,* and are necessary component motions of simple to complex daily living skills. Defining functional limi-

| BOX 1.3 | Common Functional Limitations Related to Physical Tasks |
| --- | --- |

Limitation of

- Reaching and grasping
- Lifting and carrying
- Pushing and pulling
- Bending and stooping
- Turning and twisting
- Throwing and catching
- Rolling
- Standing
- Squatting and kneeling
- Standing up and sitting down
- Getting in and out of bed
- Crawling, walking, running
- Ascending and descending stairs
- Hopping and jumping
- Kicking

tations in this way highlights the importance of identifying abnormal or absent component motions of motor skills through task analysis during the physical therapy examination and later integrating task-specific functional motions into a therapeutic exercise program.

NOTE: Not all sources in the literature define functional limitations in this way. For example, some sources[44,45,92] classify all aspects of individual functioning, including basic ADL (personal hygiene and grooming, feeding transfers, locomotion) as functional limitations.

When a person is unable or has only limited ability to perform any of the whole body component motions identified in Box 1.3, decreased independence in ADL and IADL may occur, quality of life may become compromised, and hence, disability may ensue. The following is an example of this relationship between functional limitations and potential disability. To perform a basic home maintenance task (IADL), such as painting a room, a person must be able to grasp a paint brush or roller, climb a ladder, reach overhead, kneel, or stoop down to the floor. If any one of these functional movements is limited, it may not be possible to perform the overall task of painting the room. An essential element of a physical therapy examination and evaluation is the analysis of motor tasks to identify the components of tasks that are difficult for a patient to perform. This analysis helps the therapist determine why a patient is unable to perform specific daily living tasks. This information coupled with identification and measurement of the impairments that are the source of the altered or absent component movement patterns, in turn, is used for treatment planning and selection of interventions to restore function and prevent potential disability.

## Disability

The final category of the disablement continuum is disability, as shown in Figure 1.2. There is a growing body of knowledge suggesting that physical impairments and functional limitations directly contribute to disability.[58,61] Consequently, an approach to patient management that focuses on restoring or improving function may prevent or reduce disability and may have a positive impact on quality of life.

A *disability* is the inability to perform or participate in activities or tasks related to one's self, the home, work, recreation, or the community in a manner or to the extent that the individual or the community as a whole (e.g., family, friends, coworkers) perceive as "normal."[2] This is a broad definition of disability and encompasses *individual functioning* in the context of the environment that includes basic ADL and more complex daily living skills as well as *societal functioning*. These functions, or roles, fall into several categories summarized in Box 1.4.

However, some sources in the literature[44,45,92] classify only difficulty with societal functioning as a disability. Despite the inconsistencies of definitions of disability in the literature, a person's roles or functions in life must be placed in *the context of the physical environment as well as societal expectations*.[40,41] Social expectations or roles

---

| BOX 1.4 | General Categories of Activities Relevant to Disability |
|---|---|

- Self-care
- Mobility in the community
- Occupational tasks
- School-related tasks
- Home management (indoor and outdoor)
- Caring for dependents
- Recreational and leisure activities
- Community responsibilities and service

---

involve interactions with others and participation in activities that are a part of who each of us is. These roles are specific to age, gender, sex, and cultural background.

NOTE: In the ICF model of functioning, disability, and health, the term "participation restriction" is used to denote the problems a person may have fulfilling personal or societal obligations[52,131-133] (see Table 1.1).

Because disability is such a complex process, the extent to which each component of the disablement process affects one's perceived level of disability is not clearly understood. An assumption is made that when impairments and functional limitations are so severe or of such long duration that they cannot be overcome to a degree acceptable to an individual, a family, or society, the perception of "being disabled" occurs.[2,103] The perception of disability is highly dependent on a person's or society's expectations of how or by whom certain roles or tasks *should* be performed.

## Prevention

Understanding the relationships among pathology, impairments, functional limitations, and perceived disability is fundamental to the *prevention* or reduction of disability.[14,39,60] The presence of functional limitations may or may not lead to loss of independence and result in disability. Take, for example, a relatively inactive person with longstanding osteoarthritis of the knees. The inability to get up from the floor or from a low seat (functional limitation) because of limited flexion of the knees and reduced strength of the quadriceps (impairments) could indeed lead to disability in several areas of everyday function. Disability could be expressed by problems in self-care (inability to get in and out of a tub or stand up from a standard height toilet seat), home management (inability to perform selected housekeeping, gardening, or yard maintenance tasks), or community mobility (inability to get into or out of a car or van independently). The perception of disability can be minimized if the patient's functional ROM and strength can be improved with an exercise program and the increased ROM and strength are incorporated into progressively more challenging functional activities or if the physical environment can be altered sufficiently with the use of adaptive equipment and assistive devices.

Adjusting expected roles or tasks within the family may also have a positive impact on the prevention or reduction of disability. Factors within the individual also can have an impact on the prevention, reduction, or progression of disablement. Those factors include level of motivation or willingness to make lifestyle changes and accommodations as well as the ability to understand and cope with an adjusted lifestyle.[143] This example highlights that inherent in any discussion of disability is the assumption that it can be prevented or remediated.[14]

Prevention falls into three categories.[2]

- **Primary prevention:** Activities such as health promotion designed to prevent disease in an at-risk population
- **Secondary prevention:** Early diagnosis and reduction of the severity or duration of existing disease and sequelae
- **Tertiary prevention:** Use of rehabilitation to reduce the degree or limit the progression of existing disability and improve multiple aspects of function in persons with chronic, irreversible disease

Therapeutic exercise, the most frequently implemented physical therapy intervention, has value at all three levels of prevention. For example, the use of resistance exercises and aerobic conditioning exercises in weight-bearing postures is often advocated for the primary and secondary prevention of age-related osteoporosis.[10,20,48,69] However, therapists who work with patients with chronic musculoskeletal or neuromuscular diseases or disorders routinely are involved with tertiary prevention of disability.

### Risk Factors

As shown in Figure 1.2, modifying risk factors through an intervention such as therapeutic exercise is an important tool for reducing or preventing the major components of the disablement process. *Risk factors* related to disablement are influences or characteristics that *predispose* a person to the process of disablement. As such, they exist prior to the onset of the pathology, impairments, functional limitations, or disability.[14,60,143] Some factors that increase the risk of disability are biological characteristics, lifestyle behaviors, psychological characteristics, and the impact of the physical and social environments. Examples of each of these types of risk factor are summarized in Box 1.5.

Some of the risk factors, in particular lifestyle characteristics and behaviors and their impact on the potential for disease or injury, have become reasonably well known because of public service announcements and distribution of educational materials in conjunction with health promotion campaigns, such as *Healthy People 2000*[101] and *Healthy People 2010*.[141] Information on the adverse influences of health-related risk factors, such as a sedentary lifestyle, obesity, and smoking, has been widely disseminated by these public health initiatives. Although the benefits of a healthy lifestyle, which includes regular exercise and physical activity, are well founded and widely documented,[1,101,141] initial outcomes of the previous national campaign, *Healthy People 2000*, suggest

---

| BOX 1.5 | Disablement Risk Factors |
| --- | --- |

**Biological Factors**
- Age, sex, race
- Height/weight relationship
- Congenital abnormalities or disorders (e.g., skeletal deformities, neuromuscular disorders, cardiopulmonary diseases or anomalies)
- Family history of disease; genetic predisposition

**Behavioral/Psychological/Lifestyle Factors**
- Sedentary lifestyle
- Use of tobacco, alcohol, other drugs
- Poor nutrition
- Low level of motivation
- Inadequate coping skills
- Difficulty dealing with change
- Negative affect

**Physical Environment Characteristics**
- Architectural barriers in the home, community, and workplace
- Ergonomic characteristics of the home, work, or school environments

**Socioeconomic Factors**
- Low economic status
- Low level of education
- Inadequate access to healthcare
- Limited family or social support

---

that an increased awareness of risk factors has not translated effectively into dramatic changes in lifestyle behaviors to reduce the risk of disease or injury.[30] This demonstrates that increased knowledge does not necessarily change behavior.

When active pathology exists, the reduction of risk factors by means of *buffers* (interventions aimed at reducing the progression of pathology, impairments, functional limitations, or disability) is appropriate.[60] This focus of intervention is categorized as secondary or tertiary prevention of disability. Initiating a regular exercise program and increasing the level of physical activity on a daily basis or altering the physical environment by removing architectural barriers or using assistive devices for ADL are examples of buffers that can reduce the risk of disability. (Refer to Chapter 2 of this text for in-depth information on prevention, reduction of risk factors, and wellness.)

This summary of the process of disablement has focused on key elements of this complex process. A basic understanding of the process and the various models and classification systems that have been developed over the past four decades provides a conceptual framework for practice and research, establishes a foundation for sound clinical decision making and effective communication, and sets the stage for delivery of effective, efficient, meaningful physical therapy care and services for patients.

## PATIENT MANAGEMENT AND CLINICAL DECISION MAKING: AN INTERACTIVE RELATIONSHIP

An understanding of the disablement process as well as knowledge of the process of making informed clinical decisions based on evidence from the scientific literature are necessary foundations of comprehensive management of patients seeking and receiving physical therapy services. Provision of quality patient care involves the ability to make sound clinical judgments, solve problems that are important to a patient, and apply knowledge of the inter-relationships among pathology, impairment, functional limitation, and disability throughout each phase of man-agement. The primary purpose of this section of the chap-ter is to describe a model of patient management used in physical therapy practice. Inasmuch as clinical reasoning and evidence-based decision making are embedded in each phase of patient management, a brief overview of the con-cepts and processes associated with clinical decision mak-ing and evidence-based practice are presented before exploring a systematic process of patient management in physical therapy. Relevant examples of the clinical deci-sions a therapist must make are highlighted within the context of the patient management model.

### Clinical Decision Making

*Clinical decision making* refers to a dynamic, complex process of reasoning and analytical (critical) thinking that involves making judgments and determinations in the con-text of patient care.[65] One of the many areas of clinical decision making in which a therapist is involved is the selection, implementation, and modification of therapeutic exercise interventions based on the unique needs of each patient or client. To make effective decisions, merging clar-ification and understanding with critical and creative think-ing is necessary.[71] A number of requisite attributes are necessary for making informed, responsible, efficient, and effective clinical decisions.[27,71,79,125] Those requirements are listed in Box 1.6.

There is a substantial body of knowledge in the litera-ture that describes various strategies and models of clinical decision making in the context of patient management by physical therapists.[*] One such model, the Hypothesis-Oriented Algorithm for Clinicians II (HOAC II), describes a series of steps involved in making informed clinical decisions.[112]

The use of clinical decision making in the diagnostic process also has generated extensive discussion in the liter-ature.[†] To assist in and improve the decision-making process, tools known as "clinical prediction rules," first

---

* See references 25, 27, 44, 45, 53, 54, 64, 65, 76, 80, 111, 112, 120, 137.

† See references 10, 13, 24, 27, 38, 40, 59, 76, 109, 117, 137, 140, 149.

---

| BOX 1.6 | Requirements for Skilled Clinical Decision Making During Patient Management |

- Knowledge of pertinent information about the problem(s)
- Prior clinical experience with the same or similar prob-lems
- Ability to recall relevant information
- Cognitive and psychomotor skills to obtain necessary knowledge of an unfamiliar problem
- Ability to integrate new and prior knowledge
- An efficient information-gathering and information-processing style
- Ability to obtain, analyze, and apply evidence from the literature
- Ability to critically organize, categorize, prioritize, and synthesize information
- Ability to recognize clinical patterns
- Ability to form working hypotheses about presenting problems and how they might be solved
- An understanding of the patient's values and goals
- Ability to determine options and make strategic plans
- Use of reflective thinking and self-monitoring strategies to make necessary adjustments

developed in medicine, now are being developed and used by physical therapists.[17] Some clinical prediction rules con-tain predictive factors that help a practitioner establish spe-cific diagnoses or prognoses, whereas others identify subgroupings of patients most likely to benefit from a par-ticular approach to treatment. Among others, prediction tools have been developed to assist in the diagnosis of deep vein thrombosis[106] and ankle fracture after an acute ankle injury,[130] as well as to identify patients with low back pain, who are most likely to respond to stabilization exercises.[49] An additional focus of ongoing study and discussion is the comparison of clinical reasoning of expert versus novice therapists.[28,53,54,57,64,80,107] Key points from studies on each of these topics are addressed throughout this section of the chapter and in later chapters.

Health care continues to move in the direction of physical therapists being the first contact practitioners through whom consumers gain access for services without physician referral. Hence, the need to make sound clinical judgments supported by scientific evidence during each phase of patient management becomes more and more essential for physical therapy practitioners.

### Evidence-Based Practice

Physical therapists who wish to provide high-quality patient care must make informed clinical decisions based on sound clinical reasoning and knowledge of the practice of physical therapy. An understanding and application of the principles of evidence-based practice can guide a clini-cian through the decision-making process during the course of patient care. *Evidence-based practice* is "the conscientious, explicit, and judicious use of current best evidence in making decisions about the care of an individual patient."[115(p. 71)] Evidence-based practice also must involve combining knowledge of evidence from well designed research studies with the expertise of the clinician and the values, goals, and circumstances of the patient.[116]

The process of evidence-based practice involves the following steps.[18,116]

1. Identify a patient problem and convert it into a specific question.
2. Search the literature and collect clinically relevant, scientific studies that contain evidence related to the question.
3. Critically analyze the pertinent evidence found during the literature search and make reflective judgments about the quality of the research and the applicability of the information to the identified patient problem.
4. Integrate the appraisal of the evidence with clinical expertise and experience and the patient's unique circumstances and values to make decisions.
5. Incorporate the findings and decisions into patient management.
6. Assess the outcomes of interventions and ask another question if necessary.

This process enables a practitioner to select and interpret the findings from the evaluation tools used during the examination of the patient and to implement effective treatment procedures that are rooted in sound theory and scientific evidence (rather than anecdotal evidence, opinion, or clinical tradition) to facilitate the best possible outcomes for a patient.

In a survey of physical therapists, all of whom were members of the American Physical Therapy Association, 488 respondents answered questions about their beliefs, attitudes, knowledge, and behavior about evidence-based practice.[63] Results of the survey indicated that the therapists believed that the use of evidence in practice was necessary and that the quality of care for their patients was better when evidence was used to support clinical decisions. However, most thought that carrying out the steps involved in evidence-based practice was time-consuming and seemed incompatible with the demands placed on therapists in a busy clinical setting.

Indeed, it is impractical and inappropriate to suggest that a clinician must search the literature for evidence to support each and every clinical decision that must be made. Despite time constraints in the clinical setting, when determining strategies to solve complex patient problems or when interacting with third-party payers, the "thinking therapist" does have a professional responsibility to seek out evidence that supports the selection and use of specific evaluation and treatment procedures.

One method for staying abreast of current literature is to read one's professional journals regularly. Often a monthly journal contains an article that presents a compilation and review of a number of scientific studies on a particular topic. Evidence-based clinical practice guidelines for management of specific physical conditions also have been developed that address the relative effectiveness of specific treatment strategies and procedures and provide recommendations for management based on a systematic review of current literature.[100,119] Four such clinical practice guidelines that address four musculoskeletal conditions commonly managed by physical therapists—specifically knee pain,[96] low back pain,[97] neck pain,[98] and shoulder pain[99]—were developed by the Philadelphia Panel, a panel of experts from physical therapy and medicine.

If articles that focus on a systematic review of the literature on a specific topic have not been published, a therapist may find it necessary and valuable to perform an individual literature search to identify evidence applicable to a specific patient problem. However, journals exclusively devoted to evidence-based practice are another means to assist the practitioner who wants to identify well conducted research studies from a variety of professional publications without doing an individual search. These journals provide abstracts of research studies that have been critically analyzed and systematically reviewed.

There are also many online database resources that provide systematic reviews of the literature by compiling and critiquing several research articles on a specific patient problem or therapeutic intervention.[5,18,83] One such database is the Cochrane Database of Systematic Reviews (http://www.update-software.com/publications/cochrane/), which reports peer-reviewed summaries of randomized controlled trials. Another database, which can be found on the PEDro website (www.PEDro.fhs.usyd.edu.au/), assesses the quality of randomized clinical trials pertinent to physical therapy and provides systematic reviews and clinical guidelines. Easily accessed online databases such as these streamline the search process and provide a wealth of information from the literature in a concise format.

In support of evidence-based practice, relevant research studies are highlighted or referenced throughout each of the chapters of this text in relationship to the therapeutic exercise interventions, manual therapy techniques, and management guidelines presented and discussed. However, there is also an absence of research findings to support the use of some of the interventions presented. For such procedures, a therapist must rely on clinical expertise and judgment as well as each patient's response to treatment to determine the impact of these interventions on patient outcomes. Examples of how to incorporate the ongoing process of clinical decision making and application of evidence into each phase of patient management is presented in the following discussion of a model for patient management.

## A Patient Management Model

The physical therapy profession has developed a comprehensive approach to patient management designed to guide

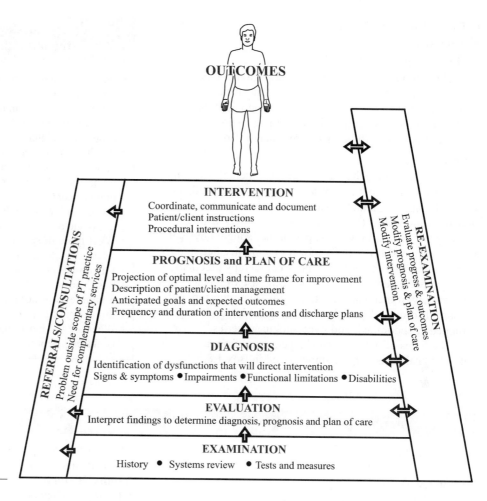

**OUTCOMES**

**INTERVENTION**
Coordinate, communicate and document
Patient/client instructions
Procedural interventions

**PROGNOSIS and PLAN OF CARE**
Projection of optimal level and time frame for improvement
Description of patient/client management
Anticipated goals and expected outcomes
Frequency and duration of interventions and discharge plans

**DIAGNOSIS**
Identification of dysfunctions that will direct intervention
Signs & symptoms ● Impairments ● Functional limitations ● Disabilities

**EVALUATION**
Interpret findings to determine diagnosis, prognosis and plan of care

**EXAMINATION**
History ● Systems review ● Tests and measures

REFERRALS/CONSULTATIONS
Problem outside scope of PT practice
Need for complementary services

RE-EXAMINATION
Evaluate progress & outcomes
Modify prognosis & plan of care
Modify intervention

FIGURE 1.5 A comprehensive outcomes-oriented model of patient management.

a practitioner through a systematic series of steps and decisions for the purpose of helping a patient achieve the highest level of function possible. This model is illustrated in Figure 1.5.

The process of patient management has five basic components.[2,10,33]

● A comprehensive *examination*
● *Evaluation* of data collected
● Determination of a *diagnosis* based on impairments, functional limitations, and disability
● Establishment of a *prognosis* and plan of care based on patient-oriented goals
● Implementation of appropriate *interventions*

The patient management process culminates in the attainment of meaningful, functional *outcomes* by the patient, which then must be re-examined and re-evaluated before a patient's discharge. As the model indicates, the *re-examination* and *re-evaluation* process occurs not only at the conclusion of treatment but throughout each phase of patient management. The ability to make timely decisions and appropriate judgments and to develop or adjust an ongoing series of working hypotheses makes transition from one phase of management to the next occur in an effective, efficient manner.

## Examination

The first component of the patient management model is a comprehensive examination of the patient. *Examination* is the systematic process by which a therapist obtains information about a patient's problem(s) and his or her reasons for seeking physical therapy services. During this initial data collection, the therapist acquires information from a variety of sources. The examination process involves both comprehensive screening and specific diagnostic testing. It is the means by which the therapist gathers sufficient information about the patient's existing or potential problems (pathological conditions, impairments, functional limitations, disabilities) ultimately to formulate a diagnosis and determine whether these problems can be appropriately treated by physical therapy interventions. If treatment of the identified problems does not fall within the scope of physical therapy practice, referral to another health-care practitioner or resource is warranted. The examination is also the means by which baseline measurements of current impairments, functional limitations, and abilities are established as a reference point from which the results of therapeutic interventions can be measured and documented.

There are three distinct elements of a comprehensive examination.[2]

- The patient's health history
- A relevant systems review
- Specific tests and measures

Throughout the examination process, a therapist seeks answers to a number of questions and concurrently makes a series of clinical decisions that shape and guide the examination process. Examples of some questions to be asked and decisions to be made are noted in Box 1.7.

### History

The history is the mechanism by which a therapist obtains an *overview* of current and past information (both subjective and objective) about a patient's present condition(s), general health status (health risk factors and coexisting health problems), and why the patient has sought physical therapy services. It has been shown in a multicenter study that patients seen in outpatient physical therapy practices have extensive health histories including use of medications for a variety of medical conditions (e.g., hypertension, pulmonary disorders, depression) and surgical histories (e.g., orthopedic, abdominal, and gynecologic surgeries.[9]

The types of data that can be generated from a patient's health history are summarized in Box 1.8.[2,10,11]

---

**BOX 1.7   Key Questions to Consider During the Initial Examination**

- What are the most complete and readily available sources for obtaining the patient's history?
- Is there a need to obtain additional information about the patient's presenting pathology or medical diagnosis if one is available?
- Based on initial working hypotheses, which of the patient's signs and symptoms warrant additional testing by physical therapy or by referral to another health-care practitioner?
- Do the patient's problems seem to fall within or outside the scope of physical therapy practice?
- What types of specific tests and measures should be selected to gather data about the patient's impairments, functional limitations, or disability?
- Based on scientific evidence, which diagnostic tests have a high level of accuracy to identify impairments, functional limitations, or disability?
- What are the most important tests to do first? Which could be postponed until a later visit with the patient?

---

**BOX 1.8   Information Generated from the Initial History**

**Demographic Data**
- Age, sex, race, ethnicity
- Primary language
- Education

**Social History**
- Family and caregiver resources
- Cultural background
- Social interactions/support systems

**Occupation/Leisure**
- Current and previous employment
- Job/school-related activities
- Recreational, community activities/tasks

**Growth and Development**
- Developmental history
- Hand and foot dominance

**Living Environment**
- Current living environment
- Expected destination after discharge
- Community accessibility

**General Health Status and Lifestyle Habits and Behaviors: Past/Present (Based on Self or Family Report)**
- Perception of health/disability
- Lifestyle health risks (smoking, substance abuse)
- Diet, exercise, sleep habits

**Medical/Surgical/Psychological History**
**Medications: Current and Past**
**Family History**
- Health risk factors
- Family illnesses

**Cognitive/Social/Emotional Status**
- Orientation, memory
- Communication
- Social/emotional interactions

**Current Conditions/Chief Complaints/Concerns**
- Conditions/reasons physical therapy services sought
- Patient's perceived level of disability
- Patient's needs, goals
- History, onset (date and course), mechanism of injury, pattern and behavior of symptoms
- Family or caregiver needs, goals, perception of patient's problems
- Current or past therapeutic interventions
- Previous outcome of chief complaint(s)

**Functional Status and Activity Level**
- Current/prior functional status: basic ADL and IADL related to self-care and home
- Current/prior functional status in work, school, community-related IADL

**Other Laboratory and Diagnostic Tests**

The therapist determines which aspects of the patient's history are more relevant than others and what data need to be obtained from various sources.

Sources of information about the patient's history include:

- Self-report health history questionnaires filled out prior to or during the initial visit
- Interviews with the patient, family, or other significant individuals involved in patient care
- Review of the medical record
- Reports from the referral source, consultants, or other health-care team members

The extent of information about a patient's health history that is necessary or available may be extensive or limited and may or may not be readily accessible prior to the first contact with the patient. Compare, for example, the information available to the therapist working in an acute care facility who has ready access to a patient's medical record versus the home health therapist who may have only a patient's medical diagnosis or brief surgical history. Regardless of the extent of written reports or medical/surgical history available, reviewing this information prior to the initial contact with the patient helps a therapist prioritize the questions asked and areas explored during the interview with the patient.

The interview is crucial for determining a patient's chief concerns and functional status—past, current, and desired. It also helps a therapist see a patient's problems from the patient's own perspective, specifically with regard to the perception of functional limitations or disability. A patient almost always describes a current problem in terms of functional limitations or disabilities, not the impairment(s). For example, a patient might report, "My elbow really hurts when I pick up something heavy" or "I'm really having trouble playing tennis (or bowling or unloading groceries from the car)." Questions that relate to symptoms (in this case, elbow pain) should identify location, intensity, description, and factors that provoke (aggravate) or alleviate symptoms in a 24-hour period.

Collecting health history data through a self-report questionnaire has been shown to be an accurate source of information from patients seen in an outpatient orthopedic physical therapy practice.[13] In addition, depending on a patient's condition and individual situation, the perceptions of family members, significant others, caregivers, or employers are often as important to the overall picture as the patient's own assessment of the current problems.

While taking a health history, it is useful to group the interview questions into categories to keep the information organized. Gathering and evaluating data simultaneously makes it easier to recognize and identify *patterns or clusters of signs and symptoms* and even to begin to formulate one or more initial, "working" hypotheses, which later will

be supported or rejected. Making these judgments helps organize and structure the examination.[111,112] Experienced therapists tend to form working hypotheses quite early in the examination process, even while reviewing a patient's chart before the initial contact with the patient.[53,54,64,80] This enables a therapist to determine and prioritize which definitive tests and measures should be selected for the later portion of the examination.[54]

**Systems Review**

A brief but relevant screening of the body systems, known as a *systemic review*,[2] is performed during the patient interview as a part of the examination process after organizing and prioritizing data obtained from the health history. The greater the number of health-related risk factors identified during the history, the greater is the importance of the review of systems. The systems typically screened by therapists are the cardiovascular and pulmonary, integumentary, musculoskeletal, and neuromuscular systems, although problems in the gastrointestinal and genitourinary systems may also be relevant.[10,12] This screening process gives a general overview of a patient's cognition, communication, and social/emotional responses. Only limited information on the anatomical and physiological status or function of each system is obtained. Table 1.2 identifies

| TABLE 1.2 | Areas of Screening for the Systems Review |
|---|---|
| **System** | **Screening** |
| Cardiovascular/ pulmonary | Heart rate, respiratory rate, and blood pressure; pain or heaviness in the chest or pulsating pain; lightheadedness; peripheral edema |
| Integumentary | Skin temperature, color, texture, integrity, scars, lumps, growths |
| Musculoskeletal | Height, weight, symmetry, gross ROM, and strength |
| Neuromuscular | General aspects of motor control (balance, locomotion, coordination); sensation, changes in hearing or vision; severe headaches |
| Gastrointestinal/ genitourinary | Heartburn, diarrhea, vomiting, severe abdominal pain, problems swallowing, problems with bladder function, unusual menstrual cycles, pregnancy |
| Cognitive and social/ emotional | Communication abilities (expressive and receptive), cognition, affect, level of arousal, orientation, ability to follow directions or learn, behavioral/emotional stressors and responses |
| General/ miscellaneous | Persistent fatigue, malaise, unexplained weight gain or loss, fever, chills, sweats |

each system and gives examples of customary screening procedures used by physical therapists.

N O T E : Some of this information, such as the patient's psychosocial status, may have been gathered previously while reviewing and taking the patient's history and need not be addressed again.

The purpose of screening each system is to identify any abnormalities or deficits that require further or more specific testing by a therapist or another health-care practitioner.[2,10,12] The systems review serves to identify a patient's symptoms that may have been overlooked during the investigation of the patient's chief symptoms that precipitated the initial visit to therapy.[12] Findings from the systems review coupled with information about a patient's chief complaints secured from the patient's health history enable a therapist to begin to make decisions about the possible causes of a patient's impairments and functional limitations and to distinguish between problems that can and cannot be managed effectively by physical therapy interventions. If a therapist determines that a patient's problems lie outside the scope of physical therapy practice, no additional testing is warranted and referral to another health-care practitioner is appropriate.[2,10,12,38]

### Specific Tests and Measures

Once it is decided that a patient's problems/conditions are most likely amenable to physical therapy intervention, the next determination a therapist must make during the examination process is to decide which aspects of physical function require further investigation through the use of specific tests and measures.

Specific (definitive/diagnostic) tests and measures used by physical therapists provide in-depth information about impairments, functional limitations, and disabilities.[2,32,36] The specificity of these tests enables a therapist to support or refute the working hypotheses formulated while taking the patient's health history and performing the systems review. In addition, the data generated from these definitive tests are the means by which the therapist ascertains the possible *underlying causes* of a patient's impairments and functional limitations. These tests also give the therapist a clearer picture of a patient's current condition(s) and may reveal information about the patient not previously identified during the history and systems review. If treatment is initiated, the results of these specific tests and measures establish *objective baselines* from which changes in a patient's physical status as the result of interventions are measured.

Given the array of specific tests available to a therapist for a comprehensive physical therapy examination, the guidelines summarized in Box 1.9 should be considered when determining which definitive tests and measures need to be selected and administered.[2,32,33,105]

There are more than 20 general categories of specific tests and measures commonly performed by physical therapists.[2,136] Tests are selected and administered to target

---

**BOX 1.9   Guidelines for Selection of Specific Tests and Measures**

- Consider why particular tests are performed and how the interpretation of their results may influence the formulation of a diagnosis.
- Select tests and measures that provide accurate information and are valid and reliable and whose efficacy is supported by evidence generated from sound scientific studies.
- Administer tests that target multiple levels of disablement: impairments, functional limitations, the patient's perceived level of disability.
- Prioritize tests and measures selected to gather in-depth information about key problems identified during the history and systems review.
- Decide whether to administer generic tests or tests that are specific to a particular region of the body.
- Choose tests that provide data specific enough to support or reject working hypotheses formulated during the history and systems review and to determine a diagnosis, prognosis, and plan of care when the data are evaluated.
- Select tests and measures that help determine the types of intervention that most likely are appropriate and effective.
- To complete the examination in a timely manner, avoid collecting more information than is necessary to make informed decisions during the evaluation, diagnosis, and treatment planning phases of management.

---

specific impairments of structures within body systems. Typically, testing involves multiple body systems to identify the scope of a patient's impairments. When examining a patient with chronic knee pain, for example, in addition to performing a thorough musculoskeletal examination it would also be appropriate to administer tests that identify the impact of the patient's knee pain on the neuromuscular system (by assessing balance and proprioception) and the cardiopulmonary system (by assessing aerobic capacity). Because many of the pathological conditions discussed in this textbook involve the musculoskeletal system, some examples of specific tests and measures that identify *musculoskeletal impairments* are noted here. They include but are not limited to:

- Assessment of pain
- Goniometry
- Joint mobility, stability, and integrity tests (including ligamentous testing)
- Tests of muscle performance (manual muscle testing, dynamometry)
- Posture analysis
- Gait analysis
- Assessment of assistive, adaptive, or orthotic devices

N O T E : An outline of a comprehensive and systematic musculoskeletal examination organized to yield data for identification of impairments and functional limitations is described in the Appendix of this textbook.

An in-depth examination of impairments by means of diagnostic tests provides valuable information about the extent and nature of the impairments and is the foundation of the diagnosis(es) made by a physical therapist. A thorough examination of impairments also helps a therapist select the most appropriate types of exercise and other forms of intervention for the treatment plan.

Although specific testing of impairments is crucial, these tests do not tell the therapist how the impairments are affecting the patient's functional capabilities. Therefore, every examination should also include use of instruments that specifically measure *functional limitations and disability.* These tools, often referred to as *functional outcome measures,* are designed to reflect the impact of a patient's pathological condition and resulting impairments on functional abilities and health-related quality of life. These instruments typically supply baseline measurements of subjective information against which changes in a patient's function or a patient's perceived level of disability are documented over the course of treatment. The tests may be generic, covering a wide range of functional abilities, or specific to a particular body region, such as the upper or lower extremities or spine. Generic instruments can be used to assess the global function of patients with a wide array of pathologies and impairments but yield less site-specific data than regional tests of functional abilities or limitations.[105]

The format of functional testing procedures and instruments varies. Some tests gather information by *self-report* (by the patient or family member)[67]; others require *observation and rating of the patient's performance* by a therapist as various functional tasks are carried out. Some instruments measure a patient's ease or difficulty of performing specific physical tasks. Other instruments incorporate temporal (time-based) or spatial (distance-based) criteria, such as measurement of walking speed or distance, in the format.[4] Test scores can also be based on the level of assistance (with assistive devices or by another person) needed to complete a variety of functional tasks.

Indices of disability measure a patient's perception of his or her degree of disability. These self-report instruments usually focus on ADL and IADL, such as the ability or inability to care for one's own needs (physical, social, emotional) or the level of participation in the community that is currently possible, desired, expected, or required. Information gathered with these tools may indicate that the patient requires consultation and possible intervention by other health-care professionals to deal with some of the social or psychological aspects of disability.

N O T E : It is well beyond the scope or purpose of this text to identify and describe the many instruments that measure physical function or disability. The reader is referred to several resources in the literature that provide this information.[4,15,37,75,135]

## Evaluation

Evaluation is a process characterized by the *interpretation of collected data.* The process involves analysis and integration of information to form opinions by means of a series of sound clinical decisions.[2] Although evaluation is depicted as a distinct entity or phase of the patient management model (see Fig. 1.5), some degree of evaluation goes on at every phase of patient management, from examination through outcome. Interpretation of relevant data, one of the more challenging aspects of patient management, is fundamental to the determination of a diagnosis of dysfunction and prognosis of functional outcomes. By pulling together and sorting out subjective and objective data from the examination, a therapist should be able to determine the following.

- A patient's general health status and its impact on current and potential function
- The acuity or chronicity and severity of the current condition(s)
- The extent of impairments of body systems and impact on functional abilities
- A patient's current, overall level of physical function (limitations *and* abilities) compared with the functional abilities needed, expected, or desired by the patient
- The impact of physical dysfunction on social/emotional function
- The impact of the physical environment on a patient's function
- A patient's social support systems and their impact on current, desired, and potential function

The decisions made during the evaluation process may also suggest that additional testing by the therapist or another practitioner is necessary before the therapist can determine a patient's diagnosis and prognosis for positive outcomes from physical therapy interventions. For example, a patient whose chief complaints are related to episodic shoulder pain but who also indicates during the health history that bouts of depression sometimes make it difficult to work or socialize should be referred for a psychological consultation and possible treatment.[10] Results of the psychological evaluation could be quite relevant to the success of the physical therapy intervention.

Addressing the questions posed in Box 1.10 during the evaluation of data derived from the examination enables a therapist to make pertinent clinical decisions that lead to the determination of a diagnosis and prognosis and the selection of potential intervention strategies for the plan of care.

During the evaluation it is particularly useful to ascertain if and to what extent relationships exist among measurements of impairments, functional limitations, and the patient's perceived level of disability. These relationships often are not straightforward. In a study of patients with cervical spine disorders,[48] investigators reported a strong correlation between measurements of impairments (pain, ROM, and cervical muscle strength) and functional limitations (functional axial rotation and lifting capacity) but a relatively weak statistical relationship between measurements of functional limitations and the patient's perceived level of disability as determined by three self-report measures. In another study[138] that compared shoulder ROM with the ability of patients to perform basic self-care activities, a strong correlation was noted between the degree of difficulty of performing these tasks and the extent of shoulder motion limitation. Although the results of these studies to some extent are related to the choice of measurement tools, these findings highlight the complexity of evaluating disability and suggest that identifying the strength or weakness of the links among the levels of disablement may help a therapist more accurately predict a patient's prognosis, with the likelihood of functional improvement the result of treatment. Evaluating these relationships and answering the other questions noted in Box 1.10 lays the foundation for ascertaining a diagnosis and prognosis and developing an effective plan of care.

## Diagnosis

The term *diagnosis* can be used in two ways; it refers to either a *process* or a *category* (label) within a classification system.[40] Both usages of the word are relevant to physical therapy practice. The diagnosis is an essential element of patient management because it directs the physical therapy prognosis (including the plan of care) and interventions.[2,32,117,150]

### Diagnostic Process

The diagnostic process is a complex *sequence* of actions and decisions that begins with: (1) the collection of data (examination); (2) the analysis and interpretation of all relevant data collected, leading to the generation of working hypotheses (evaluation); and (3) organization of data, recognition of clustering of data (a pattern of findings), formation of a diagnostic hypothesis, and subsequent classification of data into categories (impairment-based diagnoses).[2,25,109,118,150]

This process is necessary to develop a prognosis (including a plan of care) and is a prerequisite for treatment.[24,59,109,117,150] Through the diagnostic process a *physical therapist classifies dysfunction* (most often, movement dysfunction), whereas a physician identifies disease.[59,109] For the physical therapist, the diagnostic process focuses on the *consequences* of a disease or health disorder[150] and is a mechanism by which discrepancies and consistencies between a patient's desired level of function and his or her capacity to achieve that level of function are identified.[2]

### Diagnostic Category

A diagnostic classification system recently developed by physical therapists is useful for delineating the knowledge base and scope of practice of physical therapy.[2,24,40,59,109,117,149] The use of a common diagnostic classification scheme not only guides treatment,[49] it fosters clarity of communication in practice and clinical research.[32,59]

A diagnostic category (classification) is a grouping that identifies and describes patterns or clusters of physical findings (signs and symptoms of impairment, functional limitation, and disability). A diagnostic category also describes the impact of a condition on function at the system level (musculoskeletal, neuromuscular, cardiovascular/pulmonary, integumentary) and at the level of the whole person.[2] Within each body system are a number of broad-based diagnostic categories *defined by the primary impairments,* that is, based on clusters of common impairments, exhibited by a patient. Box 1.11 lists the impairment-based diagnostic classifications developed by consensus by physical therapists for the musculoskeletal system.[2] The groupings of impairments exhibited by patients with most of the conditions discussed in this textbook can be classified into at least one of these diagnostic categories.

Patients with different pathologies but similar impairments may be classified by the same diagnostic category. Moreover, it is not uncommon during the diagnostic process for a therapist to identify more than one diagnostic category to describe a patient's impaired function. Complete descriptions of impairment-based diagnostic categories for each body system can be found in the *Guide to Physical Therapist Practice.*[2]

*Preferred practice patterns,* which are identified by the diagnostic categories, represent consensus-based opinions that outline broad patient management guidelines and strategies used by physical therapists for each diagnostic category.[22,42,150] These patterns are *not* designed to indicate a specific pathway of care, such as an exercise protocol for a specific postoperative condition but, rather, are descrip-

---

**BOX 1.10   Key Questions to Consider During the Evaluation and Diagnostic Processes**

- What is the extent, degree, or severity of impairments, functional limitations, or disability?
- What is the stability or progression of dysfunction?
- Is the current condition(s) acute or chronic?
- What actions/events change (relieve or worsen) the patient's signs and symptoms?
- How do preexisting conditions (co-morbidities) affect the current condition?
- How does the information from the patient's medical/surgical history and tests and measures done by other health-care practitioners relate to the findings of the physical therapy examination?
- Have identifiable clusters of findings (i.e., patterns) emerged relevant to the patient's dysfunction?
- Is there an understandable relationship between the patient's extent of impairments and the degree of functional limitation or disability?
- What are the causal factors that seem to be contributing to the patient's impairments, functional limitations, or disability?

<table>
<tr><td>

**BOX 1.11** Diagnostic Classifications for the Musculoskeletal System

</td></tr>
</table>

**BOX 1.11  Diagnostic Classifications for the Musculoskeletal System**

- Primary prevention/risk reduction for skeletal demineralization (pattern 4A)
- Impaired posture (pattern 4B)
- Impaired muscle performance (pattern 4C)
- Impaired joint mobility, motor function, muscle performance, and range of motion (ROM) associated with connective tissue dysfunction (pattern 4D)
- Impaired joint mobility, motor function, muscle performance, and ROM associated with localized inflammation (pattern 4E)
- Impaired joint mobility, motor function, muscle performance, ROM, and reflex integrity associated with spinal disorders (pattern 4F)
- Impaired joint mobility, muscle performance, and ROM associated with fracture (pattern 4G)
- Impaired joint mobility, motor function, muscle performance, and ROM associated with joint arthroplasty (pattern 4H)
- Impaired joint mobility, motor function, muscle performance, and ROM associated with bony or soft tissue surgery (pattern 4I)
- Impaired motor function, muscle performance, ROM, gait, locomotion, and balance associated with amputation (pattern 4J)

**BOX 1.12  Factors That Influence a Patient's Prognosis/Expected Outcomes**

- Complexity, severity, acuity, or chronicity and expected course of the patient's condition(s) (pathology), impairments, and functional limitations
- Patient's general health status and presence of co-morbidities and risk factors
- Patient's and/or family's goals
- Patient's motivation and adherence and responses to previous interventions
- Safety issues and concerns
- Extent of support (physical, emotional, social)

tions of all components of patient management from examination through discharge for which physical therapists are responsible. In other words, the preferred practice patterns describe what it is that physical therapists do. For a detailed description of the suggested procedures for each preferred practice pattern for the musculoskeletal, neuromuscular, cardiovascular/pulmonary, and integumentary systems, refer to the *Guide*.[2]

### Prognosis and Plan of Care

After the initial examination has been completed, data have been evaluated, and an impairment-based diagnosis has been established, a prognosis (see Fig. 1.5), including a plan of care, must be determined before initiating any interventions. A *prognosis* is a prediction of a patient's optimal level of function expected as the result of a course of treatment and the anticipated length of time needed to reach specified functional outcomes.[2] Some factors that influence a patient's prognosis and functional outcomes are noted in Box 1.12.

Determining an accurate prognosis is, indeed, challenging even for experienced therapists. The more complex a patient's problems, the more difficult it is to project the patient's optimal level of function, particularly at the onset of treatment. For example, if an otherwise healthy and fit 70-year-old patient who was just discharged from the hospital after a total knee replacement is referred for home-based physical therapy services, it is relatively easy to predict the time frame that will be needed to prepare the

patient to return to independence in the home and community. In contrast, it may be possible to predict only incremental levels of functional improvement at various stages of rehabilitation for a patient who has sustained multiple fractures and soft tissue injuries as the result of an automobile accident.

In these two examples of establishing prognoses for patients with musculoskeletal conditions, as with most other patient problems, the accuracy of the prognosis is affected in part by the therapist's clinical decision-making ability based on the following.[79]

- Familiarity with the patient's condition including the pathology and the surgical interventions
- Thorough knowledge of the process and time frames of tissue healing
- Experience managing patients with similar pathologies, impairments, and functional limitations
- Knowledge of the efficacy of tests and measures and physical therapy interventions

The *plan of care*, an integral component of the prognosis, delineates the following.[2]

- Anticipated goals
- Expected functional outcomes that are meaningful, utilitarian, sustainable, and measurable
- Extent of improvement predicted and length of time necessary to reach that level
- Specific interventions
- Proposed frequency and duration of interventions
- Specific discharge plans

### Setting Goals and Outcomes in the Plan of Care

Developing a plan of care involves *collaboration* and *negotiation* between the patient (and, when appropriate, the family) and the therapist.[2,56] The *anticipated goals* and *expected outcomes* documented in the plan of care must be patient-centered. That is, the goals and outcomes must be meaningful to the patient. These goals and outcomes must also be measurable and linked to each other. Goals are directed at the reduction or elimination of the physical signs and symptoms of pathology and impairments that seem to be limiting the patient's functional abilities.[2] Outcomes are associated with the amelioration of functional limitations and disability to the greatest extent possible coupled with achieving the optimal level possible of function, general health, and patient satisfaction.[2]

Establishing meaningful, functionally relevant goals and outcomes requires engaging the patient and/or family in the decision-making process from a therapist's first contact with a patient. Patients come to physical therapy not to get stronger or more flexible but, rather, to be able to perform physical activities they enjoy doing or must do in their lives with ease and comfort. Knowing what a patient wants to be able to accomplish as the result of treatment helps a therapist develop and prioritize intervention strategies that target the patient's functional limitations and functionally related impairments. This, in turn, increases the likelihood of successful outcomes from treatment.[93,102] Several resources in the literature identify ways to develop goals and outcomes that are functionally relevant and meaningful to the patient.[3,92,93,102] Some key questions a therapist often asks a patient or the patient's extended support system early in the examination while taking the history that are critical for establishing anticipated goals and expected outcomes in the plan of care are listed in Box 1.13.

An integral aspect of effective goal and outcome setting is explaining to a patient how the pathology and identified impairments are associated with the patient's functional limitations and why specific interventions will be used. Discussing an expected time frame for achieving the negotiated goals and outcomes puts the treatment plan and the patient's perception of progress in a realistic context. This type of information helps a patient and family members set goals that are not just

---

**BOX 1.13    Key Questions to Establish Patient-Centered Goals and Outcomes in the Plan of Care**

- What activities are most important to you at home, school, work, or during your leisure time?
- What activities do you need help with that you would like to be able to do independently?
- Of the activities you are finding difficult to do or cannot do at all at this time, which ones would you like to be able to do better or do again?
- Of the problems you are having, which ones do you want to try to eliminate or minimize first?
- In what areas do you think you have the biggest problems during the activities you would like to do on your own?
- What are your goals for coming to physical therapy?
- What would you like to be able to accomplish through therapy?
- What would make you feel that you were making progress in achieving your goals?
- How soon do you want to reach your goals?

---

meaningful but realistic and attainable. Setting up *short-term and long-term goals,* particularly for patients with severe or complex problems, is also a way to help a patient recognize incremental improvement and progress during treatment.

The plan of care also indicates the optimal level of improvement that will be reflected by the functional outcomes as well as how those outcomes will be measured. An outline of the specific interventions, their frequency and duration of use, and how the interventions are directly related to attaining the stated goals and outcomes must also appear in the plan. Finally, the plan of care concludes with the criteria for discharge. These criteria are addressed following a discussion of elements of intervention in the patient management process.

**N O T E :** Periodic re-examination of a patient and re-evaluation of a patient's response to treatment may necessitate modification of the initial prognosis and plan of care.

### Intervention

*Intervention*, a component of patient management, refers to any *purposeful interaction* a therapist has that directly relates to a patient's care[2] (see Fig. 1.5). There are three broad areas of intervention that occur during the course of patient management.[2]

- Coordination, communication, and documentation
- Procedural interventions
- Patient-related instruction

Each of these areas is an essential aspect of the intervention phase of patient management. Absence of just one of these elements can adversely affect outcomes. For example, inclusion of the most appropriate exercises (procedural intervention) in a treatment program does not lead to a successful outcome if the therapist has not communicated with the necessary parties for an approval or extension of physical therapy services (communication) or if the patient has not learned how to perform the exercises in the program correctly (patient-related instruction). A brief discussion of the three major components of intervention is presented in this section with additional information in the final section of the chapter on exercise instruction, an aspect of patient-related instruction that is most relevant to the focus of this textbook.

**Coordination, Communication, and Documentation**
The physical therapist is the coordinator of physical therapy care and services and must continually communicate verbally and through written documentation with all individuals involved in the care of a patient. This aspect of intervention encompasses many patient-related administrative tasks and professional responsibilities, such as writing reports (evaluations, plans of care, discharge summaries), designing home exercise programs, keeping records, contacting third-party payers, other health care practitioners, or community-based resources, and participating in team conferences.

N O T E : Even during the intervention phase of patient management, a therapist might decide that referral to another practitioner is appropriate and complementary to the physical therapy interventions. This requires coordination and communication with other health-care practitioners. For example, a therapist might refer a patient, who is generally deconditioned from a sedentary lifestyle and who is also obese, to a nutritionist for dietary counseling to complement the physical therapy program designed to improve the patient's aerobic capacity (cardiopulmonary endurance) and general level of fitness.

**Procedural Interventions**

Procedural intervention pertains to the specific procedures used during treatment, such as therapeutic exercise, functional training, or adjunctive modalities (physical agents and electrotherapy). Procedural interventions are identified in the plan of care. Most procedural interventions used by physical therapists, including the many types of therapeutic exercise, are designed to reduce or correct impairments, as depicted in Figure 1.6.

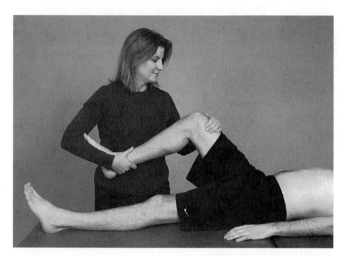

FIGURE 1.6 Manual resistance exercise, a procedural intervention, is a form of therapeutic exercise used during the early stage of rehabilitation if muscle strength or endurance is impaired.

If procedural interventions are to be considered effective, they must result in the reduction or elimination of functional limitations and, whenever possible, reduce the risk of future dysfunction. Moreover, the effectiveness of procedural interventions should be supported by sound evidence, preferably based on prospective, randomized, controlled research studies.

Although the intended outcome of therapeutic exercise programs has always been to enhance a patient's functional capabilities or prevent loss of function, until the past two decades the focus of exercise programs was on the resolution of impairments. Success was measured primarily by the reduction of the identified impairments or improvements in various aspects of physical performance, such as strength, mobility, or balance. It was assumed that if

impairments were resolved, improvements in functional abilities would subsequently follow. Physical therapists now recognize that this assumption is not valid. To reduce functional limitations and improve a patient's health-related quality of life, not only should therapeutic exercise interventions be implemented that correct functionally limiting impairments, but whenever possible exercises should be task-specific; that is, they should be performed using movement patterns that closely match a patient's intended or desired functional activities. In Figure 1.7, strengthening exercises are performed using task-specific lifting patterns.

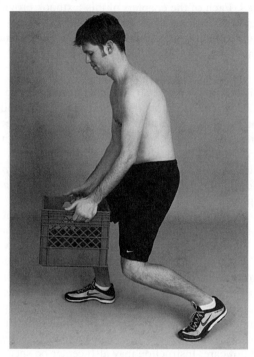

FIGURE 1.7 Task-specific strengthening exercises are carried out by lifting and lowering a weighted crate in preparation for functional tasks at home or work.

Task-specific functional training was investigated in a study of the effects of a resistance exercise program on the stair-climbing ability of ambulatory older women.[19] Rather than having the subjects perform resisted hip and knee extension exercises in nonweight-bearing positions, they trained by ascending and descending stairs while wearing a weighted backpack. This activity not only improved muscle performance (strength and endurance), it directly enhanced the subjects' efficiency in stair climbing during daily activities.

Another way to use therapeutic exercise interventions effectively to improve functional ability is to integrate safe but progressively more challenging functional activities that utilize incremental improvements in strength, endurance, and mobility into a patient's daily routine as early as possible in the treatment program. With this functionally oriented approach to exercise, the activities in the treatment program are specific to and directly support the expected functional outcomes. Selection and use of exercise procedures that target more than one goal or outcome is also an appropriate and efficient way to maximize improvements in a patient's function in the shortest time possible.

Effective use of any procedural intervention must include determining the appropriate *intensity, frequency,* and *duration* of each intervention and periodic re-examination of a patient's responses to the interventions. While implementing therapeutic exercise interventions, a patient's response to exercise is continually monitored to decide when and to what extent to increase the difficulty of the exercise program or when to discontinue specific exercises. Each of the chapters of this textbook provides detailed information on factors that influence selection, application, and progression of therapeutic exercise interventions.

### Patient-Related Instruction

There is no question that physical therapists perceive themselves as patient educators, facilitators of change, and motivators.[16,34,56,73,90] Patient education spans all three domains of learning: cognitive, affective, and psychomotor domains. Education ideally begins during a patient's initial contact with a therapist and involves the therapist *explaining* information, *asking* pertinent questions, and *listening* to the patient or a family member.

*Patient-related instruction*, the third aspect of intervention during the patient management process, is the means by which a therapist helps a patient *learn* how to get better[16] by becoming an active participant in the rehabilitation process. Patient-related instruction may first focus on providing a patient with background information, such as the interrelationships among the primary condition (pathology) and the resulting impairments and functional limitations or explaining the purpose of specific interventions in the plan of care. Instruction may also center on specific aspects of a treatment program, such as teaching a patient, family member, or caregiver a series of exercises to be carried out in a home program, reviewing health and wellness materials, or clarifying directions for safe use of equipment to be used at home.

A therapist must use multiple methods to convey information to a patient or family member, such as one-to-one, therapist-directed instruction, videotaped instruction, or written materials. Each has been shown to have a place in patient education. For instance, it has been shown that patients who were taught exercises by a therapist performed their exercises more accurately in a home program than patients whose sole source of information about their exercises was from reading a brochure.[31] In another study, the effectiveness of three modes of instruction in an exercise program were evaluated. The subjects who received in-person instruction by a therapist or two variations of videotaped instruction performed their exercise program more accurately than subjects who received only written instructions.[104] However, written materials, particularly those with illustrations, can be taken home by a patient and used to reinforce verbal instructions from a therapist or videotaped instructions.

To be an effective patient educator, a therapist must possess an understanding of the process of learning, which most often is directed toward learning or adapting motor skills. As a patient educator, a therapist must also be able to recognize a patient's learning style, implement effective teaching strategies, and motivate a patient to *want* to learn new skills, adhere to an exercise program, or change health-related behaviors.

A therapist's skillful, creative use of all three components of intervention, coupled with vigilant re-examination and re-evaluation of the effectiveness of the interventions selected, paves the way for successful outcomes and a patient's discharge from physical therapy services.

### Outcomes

Simply stated, outcomes are results. Collection and analysis of outcome data related to health-care services is a necessity, not an option.[46] Measurement of out-comes is a means by which quality, efficacy, and cost-effectiveness of services can be assessed. Outcomes are monitored *throughout* an episode of physical therapy care, that is, intermittently during treatment and at the conclusion of treatment.[93] Evaluation of information generated from periodic re-examination and re-evaluation of a patient's response to treatment enables a therapist to ascertain if the anticipated goals and expected outcomes in the plan of care are being met and if the interventions that have been implemented are producing the intended results. It may well be that the goals and outcomes must be adjusted based on the extent of change or lack of change in a patient's function as determined by the level of the interim outcomes. This information also helps the therapist decide if, when, and to what extent to modify the goals, outcomes, and interventions in the patient's plan of care.

There are several broad areas of outcomes commonly assessed by physical therapists during the continuum of patient care. They are listed in Box 1.14.

### Functional Outcomes

The key to the justification of physical therapy services in today's cost-conscious health-care system is the identification and documentation of successful functional outcomes that can be attributed to interventions.[2,4,15,41,135] Functional outcomes must be *meaningful, practical,* and *sustainable.*[135] Outcomes that have an impact on a patient's ability

---

**BOX 1.14   Areas of Outcomes Assessed by Physical Therapists**

- Level of a patient's physical function, including impairments, functional limitations, and perceived disability
- Extent of prevention or reduced risk of occurrence or recurrence of future dysfunction related to pathology, impairments, functional limitations, or disability
- Patient's general health status or level of wellness and fitness
- Degree of patient satisfaction

to function at work, in the home, or in the community in ways that have been identified as important by the patient, family, significant others, caregivers, or employers are considered *meaningful.* If the formulation of anticipated goals and expected outcome has been a collaborative effort between patient and therapist, the outcomes will be meaningful to the patient. The *practical* aspect of functional outcomes implies that improvements in function have been achieved in an efficient and cost-effective manner. Improvements in function that are maintained over time after discharge from treatment (to the extent possible given the nature of the pathology) are considered *sustainable.*

### Measuring the Impact of Physical Therapy Interventions

The expected outcomes identified in a physical therapy plan of care must be *measurable.* More specifically, changes in a patient's status over time must be *quantifiable.* As noted in the previous discussion of the examination component of the patient management model, many of the specific tests and measures used by physical therapists have traditionally measured impairments (i.e., ROM, muscle performance, joint mobility, balance). The reduction of impairments may reflect the impact of interventions on the pathological condition but may or may not translate into improvements in health-related quality of life, such as safety and functional abilities. Hence, there is the need for measurement not only of impairments but also of functional limitations and abilities and a patient's perceived level of disability to assess accurately the outcomes in physical function and the effectiveness of interventions, such as therapeutic exercise.

In response to the need to produce evidence that supports the effectiveness of physical therapy interventions for reducing movement dysfunction, a self-report instrument called OPTIMAL (Outpatient Physical Therapy Improvement in Movement Assessment Log) has been developed for measuring the impact of physical therapy interventions on function and has been tested for validity and reliability.[41] The instrument measures a patient's difficulty with or confidence in performing a series of actions, most of which are related to functional mobility, including moving from lying to sitting and sitting to standing, kneeling, walking, running, and climbing stairs, reaching, and lifting. In addition, to assist the therapist with setting goals for the plan of care, the patient is asked to identify three activities that he or she would like to be able to do without difficulty.

A number of studies that have investigated the benefits of exercise programs for individuals with impaired functional abilities[61,68,114] reflect the trend in research to include an assessment of changes in a patient's health-related quality of life as the result of an intervention. Assessment of outcomes related to the reduction of risks of future injury or further impairment, prevention of further functional limitations or disability, adherence to a home program, or the use of knowledge that promotes optimal health and fitness may also help determine the effectiveness of the services provided. To substantiate that the use of physical therapy

services for prevention is cost-effective, physical therapists are finding that it is important to collect follow-up data that demonstrate a reduced need for future physical therapy services as the result of interventions directed toward prevention and health promotion activities.

Another area of outcome assessment that has become increasingly important in physical therapy practice is that of *patient satisfaction.* An assessment of patient satisfaction during or at the conclusion of treatment can be used as an indicator of quality of care. Patient satisfaction surveys often seek to determine the impact of treatment based on the patient's own assessment of his or her status at the conclusion compared to that at the onset of treatment.[113] Instruments such as the Physical Therapy Outpatient Satisfaction Survey (PTOPS)[113] or the MedRisk Instrument for Measuring Patient Satisfaction with physical therapy (MRPS)[6,7] also measure a patient's perception of many areas of care, including access, the therapist's skills (interpersonal and clinical), and administrative issues such as scheduling and continuity of care. An important quality of patient satisfaction questionnaires is their ability to discriminate among the factors that influence satisfaction. Identification of factors that adversely influence satisfaction may enable the clinician to take steps to modify these factors to maintain an optimal level of services to patients.[7]

### Discharge Planning

Planning for discharge begins early in the rehabilitation process. As previously noted, criteria for discharge are identified in a patient's plan of care. Ongoing assessment of outcomes is the mechanism by which a therapist determines when discharge from care is warranted. A patient is discharged from physical therapy services when the anticipated goals and expected outcomes have been attained.[2] The discharge plan often includes some type of home program, appropriate follow-up, possible referral to community resources, or reinitiation of physical therapy services (an additional episode of care) if the patient's needs change over time and if additional services are approved.

Discontinuation of services is differentiated from discharge.[2] *Discontinuation* refers to the ending of services prior to the achievement of anticipated goals and expected outcomes. Several factors may necessitate discontinuation of services, which may include a decision by a patient to stop services, a change in a patient's medical status such that progress is no longer possible, or the need for further services cannot be justified to the payer.

In conclusion, the patient management model discussed in this section establishes a comprehensive, systematic approach to the provision of effective and efficient physical therapy care and services to patients and clients. The model is a mechanism to demonstrate the interrelationships among the phases of the continuum of patient care set in a conceptual framework of disablement; it is aimed at improving a patient's function and health-related quality of life. The management model also places an emphasis on reducing risk factors for disease, injury, or disability and promoting health and wellness in patients and clients seeking and receiving physical therapy services.

# STRATEGIES FOR EFFECTIVE EXERCISE AND TASK-SPECIFIC INSTRUCTION

As discussed in the previous section of this chapter, patient-related instruction is an essential element of the intervention phase of patient management. As a patient educator, a therapist spends a substantial amount of time teaching patients or their families how to perform exercises correctly and safely. Effective strategies founded on principles of motor learning that are designed to help patients initially learn an exercise program under therapist supervision and then carry it out on an independent basis over a necessary period of time contribute to successful outcomes for the patient. Box 1.15 summarizes some practical suggestions for effective exercise instruction.

## Preparation for Exercise Instruction

When preparing to teach a patient a series of exercises, a therapist should have a plan that will facilitate learning prior to and during exercise interventions. A positive relationship between therapist and patient is a fundamental aspect for creating a motivating environment that fosters learning. A collaborative relationship should be established when the goals for the plan of care are negotiated. This, of course, occurs before exercise instruction begins. Effective exercise instruction is also based on knowing a patient's learning style; that is, if he or she prefers to learn by watching, reading about, or doing an activity. This may not be known early in treatment, so several methods of instruction may be necessary.

---

| BOX 1.15 | Practical Suggestions for Effective Exercise Instruction |
|---|---|

- Select a nondistracting environment for exercise instruction.
- Demonstrate proper performance of an exercise (safe vs. unsafe movements; correct vs. incorrect movements). Then have the patient model your movements.
- If appropriate or feasible, initially guide the patient through the desired movement.
- Use clear and concise verbal and written directions.
- Complement written instructions for a home exercise program with illustrations (sketches) of the exercise.
- Have the patient demonstrate an exercise to you as you supervise and provide feedback.
- Provide specific, action-related feedback rather than general, nondescriptive feedback. For example, explain *why* the exercise was performed correctly or incorrectly.
- Teach an entire exercise program in small increments to allow time for a patient to practice and learn components of the program over several visits.

---

Identifying a patient's attitude toward exercise helps a therapist determine how receptive a patient is likely to be about learning and adhering to an exercise program. Answers to the following questions may help a therapist formulate a strategy for enhancing a patient's motivation to exercise.

- Does the patient believe exercise will lessen symptoms or improve function?
- Is the patient concerned that exercising will be uncomfortable?
- Is the patient accustomed to engaging in regular exercise?

One method for promoting motivation is to design the exercise program so the least complicated or stressful exercises are taught first, thus ensuring early success. Always ending an exercise session with a successful effort also helps maintain a patient's level of motivation. Additional suggestions to enhance motivation and promote adherence to an exercise program are discussed in this section following an overview of the concepts of motor learning and acquisition of simple to complex motor skills.

## Concepts of Motor Learning: A Foundation of Exercise and Task-Specific Instruction

Integration of motor learning principles into exercise instruction optimizes learning an exercise or functional task. An exercise is simply a motor task (a psychomotor skill) that a therapist teaches and a patient is expected to learn.

*Motor learning* is a complex set of internal processes that involves the *relatively permanent* acquisition and retention of a skilled movement or task through practice.[121,122,142,145] In the motor learning literature a differentiation is made between motor performance and motor learning. *Performance* involves acquisition of a skill, whereas *learning* involves both acquisition and retention.[35,121,122] It is thought that motor learning probably modifies the way sensory information in the central nervous system is organized and processed and affects how motor actions are produced. Motor learning is not directly observable; therefore, it must be measured by observation and analysis of how an individual performs a skill.

### Types of Motor Task
There are three basic types of motor tasks: discrete, serial, and continuous.[121,122]

*Discrete task.* A discrete task involves a movement with a recognizable beginning and end. Grasping an object, doing a push-up, or locking a wheelchair are examples of discrete motor tasks. Almost all exercises, such as lifting and lowering a weight or performing a self-stretching maneuver, can be categorized as discrete motor tasks.

*Serial task.* A serial task is composed of a series of discrete movements that are combined in a particular sequence. For example, to eat with a fork, a person must be able to grasp the fork, hold it in the correct position, pierce or scoop up the food, and lift the fork to the mouth. Many functional tasks in the work setting, for instance, are serial tasks with simple as well as complex components. Some serial tasks require specific timing between each segment of the task or momentum during the task. Wheelchair transfers are serial tasks. A patient must learn how to position the chair, lock the chair, possibly remove an armrest, scoot forward in the chair, and then transfer from the chair to another surface. Some transfers require momentum, whereas others do not.

***Continuous task.*** A continuous task involves repetitive, uninterrupted movements that have no distinct beginning and ending. Examples include walking, ascending and descending stairs, and cycling.

Recognizing the type of skilled movements a patient must learn to do helps a therapist decide which instructional strategies will be most beneficial for acquiring specific functional skills. Consider what must be learned in the following motor tasks of an exercise program. To self-stretch the hamstrings, a patient must learn how to position and align his or her body and how much stretch force to apply to perform the stretching maneuver correctly. As flexibility improves, the patient must then learn how to safely control active movements in the newly gained portion of the range during functional activities. This requires muscles to contract with correct intensity at an unaccustomed length. In another scenario, to prevent recurrence of a shoulder impingement syndrome or back pain, a patient may need to learn through posture training how to maintain correct alignment of the trunk during a variety of reaching or lifting tasks that place slightly different demands on the body.

In both of these situations motor learning must occur for the exercise program and functional training to be effective. By viewing exercise interventions from this perspective, it becomes apparent why application of strategies to promote motor learning are an integral component of effective exercise instruction.

### Conditions and Progression of Motor Tasks

If an exercise program is to improve a patient's function, it must include performing and learning a variety of tasks. If a functional training program is to prepare a patient to meet necessary and desired functional goals, it must place demands on a patient under varying conditions. A taxonomy of motor tasks, proposed by Gentile,[35] is a system for analyzing functional activities and a framework for understanding the conditions under which simple to complex motor tasks can be performed. Figure 1.8 depicts these conditions and the dimensions of difficulty of motor tasks.

An understanding of the components of this taxonomy and the interrelationships among its components is a useful framework for a therapist to identify and increase the difficulty of functional activities systematically for a patient with impaired function.

There are four main task dimensions addressed in the taxonomy: (1) the environment in which the task is performed; (2) the intertrial variability of the environment that is imposed on a task; (3) the need for person's body to remain stationary or to move during the task; and (4) the presence or absence of manipulation of objects during the task. Examples of simple to complx everyday activities characteristic of each of the 16 different but interrelated task conditions are shown in Figure 1.9.

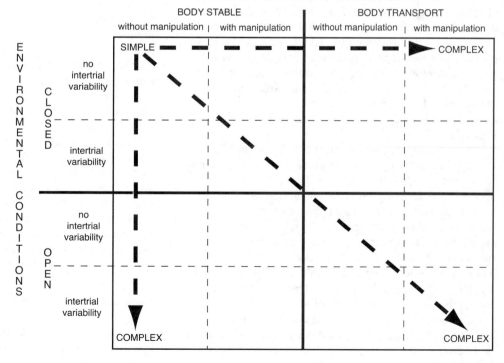

FIGURE 1.8 Taxonomy of motor tasks: dimensions of task difficulty. (From Dennis, JK, McKeough, DM: Mobility. In May, BJ [ed] Home Health and Rehabilitation—Concepts of Care. FA Davis, Philadelphia, 1993, p 147, with permission.)

| | | BODY STABLE | | BODY TRANSPORT | |
|---|---|---|---|---|---|
| | | without manipulation | with manipulation | without manipulation | with manipulation |
| **CLOSED** | without intertrial variability | Maintaining balance in sitting on bed while caregiver combs hair<br><br>Maintaining balance in standing in hallway as caregiver buttons coat | Sitting at the table and eating a meal<br><br>Sitting doing household accounts<br><br>Sitting at desk to write a letter | Rolling over in bed<br><br>Sit <=> stand from bed<br><br>Tub transfers<br><br>Bed <=> bathroom, using same route daily | Carrying a tray of food or drinks from the kitchen to the living room, using the same tray and same route each time |
| | with intertrial variability | Maintaining sitting balance on different chairs in the room e.g., rocker, straight-backed chair, sofa.<br><br>Maintaining standing balance on different surfaces: carpet, wood | Standing in the kitchen unloading a dish-washer<br><br>Sitting on a low stool in the yard, bending over to weed the vegetable garden | Rolling over in a twin bed and a queen bed<br><br>Sit <=> stand from different heights and surfaces<br><br>Up and down curbs of different heights | Carrying a tray of food or drinks from the kitchen to the living room, using different trays and routes each time |
| **OPEN** | without intertrial variability | Maintaining balance in a moving elevator | Rearranging packages while standing in a moving elevator | Walking up or down a moving escalator or a moving sidewalk | Rearranging packages while walking up or down the moving escalator |
| | with intertrial variability | Maintaining sitting or standing balance in a moving bus | Drinking a cocktail on the deck of a cruise ship | Community ambulation<br><br>Walking through a living room where children are playing | Shopping in the supermarket<br><br>Walking a precocious pet on a leash |

FIGURE 1.9 Activities of daily living in the context of the taxonomy of motor tasks. (From Dennis, JK, McKeough, DM: Mobility. In May, BJ [ed] Home Health and Rehabilitation—Concepts of Care, ed 2. FA Davis, Philadelphia, 1999, p 116, with permission.)

***Closed or open environment.*** Environmental conditions of a task address whether objects or people (around the patient) are stationary or moving during the task and if the surface on which the task is performed is fixed or moving. A *closed environment* is one in which objects around the patient and the surface on which the task is performed do not move. When a functional task is performed in this type of environment, the patient's complete attention can be focused on performing the task, and the task can be self-paced. Examples of tasks performed in a closed environment are drinking or eating while sitting in a chair and maintaining an erect turnk, standing at a sink and washing your hands or combing your hair, walking in an empty hallway or in a room where furniture placement is consistent.

A more complex environment is an *open environment*. It is one in which objects, other people, or the support surface are in motion during the task. The movement that occurs in the environment is not under the control of the patient. Tasks that occur in open environments might include maintaining sitting or standing balance on a rocking platform, standing on a moving train or bus, climbing stairs in a crowded stairwell, crossing a street at a busy intersection, or returning a serve in a tennis match or volleyball game. During tasks such as these, the patient must predict the speed and directions of movement of people or objects in the environment or must anticipate the need to make postural or balance adjustments as the support surface moves. Consequently, the patient must pace the per-formance of the tasks to match the imposed environmental conditions.

***Intertrial variability in the environment: absent or present.*** When the environment in which a task is set is unchanging from one performance of a task to the next, intertrial variability is absent. The environmental conditions for the task are predictable; therefore, little attention to the task is required, which often enables a patient to perform two tasks at one time. Some examples of tasks without intertrial variability are practicing safe lifting techniques using a box of the same dimensions and weight, practicing the tasks of standing up and sitting down from just one height or type of chair, or walking on just one type of surface.

A task becomes more complex when there is intertrial variability in the environmental conditions, that is, when the demands change from one attempt or repetition of a task to the next. With such variability, the patient must continually monitor the changing demands of the environment and adapt to the new circumstances by using a variety of movement strategies to complete the task. Lifting and carrying objects of different sizes and weight, climbing stairs of different heights, or walking over varying terrain are tasks with intertial variability.

***Body stable or body transport.*** In addition to environmental conditions, tasks are analyzed from the perspective of the person doing the task. Tasks that involve maintaining the body in a stable (stationary) position, such as maintaining an upright posture, are considered simple tasks, particularly under closed environmental conditions. When the task requirements involve the patient moving from one place to another (body transport), as when rolling, performing a transfer, walking, jumping, or climbing, the task is more complex. When a body transport task is performed in an open environment with intertrial variability, such as walking in a crowded corridor or on different support surfaces, such as grass, gravel, and pavement, the task becomes even more complex and challenging.

*Manipulation of objects: absent or present.* Whether performing a task requires upper extremity manipulation activities also affects the degree of difficulty of the task. When a task is performed without manipulating an object, it is considered less complex than if manipulation is a requirement of the task. Carrying a cup of coffee without spilling it while at home alone and walking from one room to another is a more complex task than walking with hands free. Doing the same task on a busy sidewalk further increases the complexity and difficulty of the task.

In summary, Gentile's taxonomy of motor tasks can be used to analyze the characteristics of functional tasks in the context of the task conditions. The taxonomy provides a framework to structure individual treatment session with a patient or to progress the level of difficulty of motor tasks throughout a functional training program.

### Stages of Motor Learning

There are three stages of motor learning: cognitive, associative, and autonomous.[26,29,35,91,121,122] The characteristics of the learner are different at each stage of learning and consequently affect the type of instructional strategies selected by a therapist in an exercise and functional training program.

#### Cognitive Stage

When learning a skilled movement, a patient first must figure out *what* to do; that is, the patient must learn the goal or purpose and the requirements of the exercise or functional task. Then the patient must learn *how* to do the motor task safely and correctly. At this stage, the patient needs to think about each component or sequence of the skilled movement. The patient often focuses on how his or her body is aligned and how far and with what intensity or speed to move. In other words, the patient tries to get the "feel" of the exercise. Because all of the patient's attention is often directed to the correct performance of the motor task, distractions in the environment, such as a busy, noisy exercise room (an open environment), may initially interfere with learning. During this stage of learning errors in performance are common, but with practice that includes error correction, the patient gradually learns to differentiate correct from incorrect performance, initially with frequent feedback from a therapist and eventually by monitoring his or her own performance (self-evaluation).

#### Associative Stage

The patient makes infrequent errors and concentrates on fine-tuning the motor task during the associative stage of learning. Learning focuses on producing the most consistent and efficient movements. The timing of the movements and the distances moved also may be refined. The patient explores slight variations and modifications of movement strategies while doing the task under different environmental conditions (intertrial variability). The patient also uses problem solving to correct errors when they do occur. At this stage, the patient requires infrequent feedback from the therapist and, instead, begins to anticipate necessary adjustments and make corrections even before errors occur.

#### Autonomous Stage

Movements are automatic in this final stage of learning. The patient does not have to pay attention to the movements in the task, thus making it possible to do other tasks simultaneously. Also, the patient easily adapts to variations in task demands and environmental conditions. Little, if any, instruction goes on in this phase of learning unless the patient encounters a recurrence of symptoms or other problems. In fact, most patients are discharged before reaching this stage of learning.

### Variables That Influence Motor Learning During Exercise Instruction and Functional Training

Motor learning is influenced by many variables, some of which can be manipulated by a therapist during exercise instruction or functional training to facilitate learning. Some of these variables include *pre-practice considerations, practice,* and *feedback.* An understanding of these variables and their impact on motor learning is necessary to develop strategies for successful exercise instruction and functional training. A brief overview of these key variables that influence the acquisition and retention of skilled movements during each stage of motor learning is presented in this section. Because concepts and principles of motor learning encompass an extensive body of knowledge, the reader is referred to several in-depth resources for additional information.[35,91,121,122,142]

#### Pre-Practice Considerations

A number of variables can influence motor learning during an exercise session even before practice begins. A patient's *understanding* of the purpose of an exercise or task, as well as interest in the task, affect skill acquisition and retention. The more meaningful a task is to a patient, the more likely it is that learning will occur. Including tasks the patient identified as important during the initial examination promotes a patient's interest.

*Attention* to the task at hand also affects learning. The ability to focus on the skill to be learned without distracting influences in the environment promotes learning. Instructions given to a patient prior to practice about where his or her attention should be directed during practice may also affect learning. There is evidence in studies of unimpaired individuals that learning is enhanced if a person attends to the outcomes of performing a task rather than to the details of the task itself.[82,148] This finding is addressed in more detail in a later discussion of feedback as it relates to motor learning.

*Demonstration* of a task prior to commencing practice also enhances learning. It is often helpful for a patient to observe another person, usually the therapist or possibly another patient, correctly perform the exercise or functional task and then model those actions. *Pre-practice verbal instructions* that describe the task may also facilitate skill acquisition, but they should be succinct. Extensive information about the task requirements early in the learning process may actually confuse a patient rather than enhance the learning process.

### Practice

Motor learning occurs as the direct result of practice—that is, repeatedly performing a movement or series of movements in a task.[70,121,122] Practice is probably the single most important variable in learning a motor skill. The *amount, type,* and *variability* of practice directly affect the extent of skill acquisition and retention.[91,121,122] In general, the more a patient practices a motor task, the more readily it is learned. In today's health-care environment, most practice of exercises or functional tasks occurs at home, independent of therapist supervision. A therapist often sets the practice conditions for a home program prior to a patient's discharge by providing guidelines on how to increase the difficulty of the newly acquired skills during the later stages of learning.

The type of practice strategy selected also has a significant impact on how readily a motor task is learned.[70,91,121,122,145] Common types of practice are defined in Box 1.16. The type of skill to be learned (discrete, serial, or continuous) and the patient's stage of motor learning determine which practice strategies are more appropriate than others.

***Part versus whole practice.*** *Part practice* has been shown to be most effective in the early stage of learning for acquisition of complex serial skills that have simple and difficult components. Usually it is necessary to practice only the difficult dimensions of a task before practicing the task as a whole. Part practice is less effective than *whole practice* for acquiring continuous skills, such as walking and climbing stairs, or serial tasks in which momentum or timing of the components is the central focus of the learning process. Whole practice is also used for acquisition of discrete tasks, such as an exercise that involves repetitions of a single movement pattern.

***Blocked, random, and random-blocked practice.*** During the initial phase of rehabilitation, practice is usually directed toward learning just a few exercises or tasks. During the cognitive stage of learning a new task, *blocked practice* is the appropriate choice because it rapidly improves performance of skilled movements. A transition to *random* or *random-blocked practice* should be made as soon as possible to introduce variability into the learning process. *Variability* of practice refers to making slight adjustments (variations) in the conditions of a task—for example, by

---

| BOX 1.16 | Types of Practice for Motor Learning |

**Part Versus Whole Practice**
- *Part practice.* A task is broken down into separate dimensions. Individual and usually the more difficult components of the task are practiced. After mastery of the individual segments, they are combined in sequence so the whole task can be practiced
- *Whole practice.* The entire task is performed from beginning to end and is not practiced in separate segments

**Blocked, Random, and Random-Blocked Practice**
- *Blocked practice.* The same task or series of exercises or tasks is performed repeatedly under the same conditions and in a predictable order; for example, the patient may consistently practice walking in the same environment, standing up from the same height chair, or lifting the same size weight or container; therefore, the task does not change from one repetition to the next
- *Random practice.* Slight variations of the same task are carried out in an unpredictable order; for example, a patient could practice standing up from chairs of different heights or styles in a random order; therefore, the task changes with each repetition
- *Random-blocked practice.* Variations of the same task are performed in random order, but each variation of the task is performed more than once; for example, the patient rises from a particular height or style chair, and then repeats the same task a second time before moving on to a different height or style chair

**Physical Versus Mental Practice**
- *Physical practice.* The movements of an exercise or functional task are actually performed
- *Mental practice.* A cognitive rehearsal of how a motor task is to be performed occurs prior to actually doing the task; the terms *visualization* and *imagery* are used synonymously with mental practice

---

varying the support surface or the surroundings where a task is performed.[35,121,122]

Although blocked practice initially improves performance at a faster rate than random practice, random practice leads to better skill retention and generalizability of skills than blocked practice.[91] It is thought that varying tasks just slightly, as is done with random practice, requires more cognitive processing and problem solving than blocked practice and, hence, culminates in greater retention. Random-blocked practice results in faster skill acquisition than random practice and better retention than blocked practice. Because random-blocked practice enables a patient to perform a task at least twice before changing to another variation of the task, this form of practice gives a patient the opportunity to identify and then immediately correct errors in a movement sequence before proceeding to the next variation of the task.[35,121]

***Physical versus mental practice.*** Physical practice has long been a hallmark of exercise instruction and functional training in physical therapy, whereas mental practice (motor imagery) has its roots in sports psychology and sport-related training.[122,129] About two decades ago the applicability of mental practice as a treatment tool in the rehabilitation of patients with movement impairments began to be investigated for its potential.[144] It is thought that mental rehearsal of a motor task reinforces the cognitive component of motor learning, that is, learning what to do when performing a task. Most studies support the finding that physical practice of motor skills by overtly performing the task is superior to mental practice alone for learning motor tasks.[121,122] However, in sports training and rehabilitation, mental practice, when used in conjunction with physical practice, has been shown to enhance motor skill acquisition at a faster rate than use of physical practice alone.[78,91,94]

### Feedback

Second only to practice, feedback is considered the next most important variable that influences learning.[91] *Feedback* is sensory information that is received and processed by the learner during or after performance of a movement or task.[35,91,121,147] There are a number of descriptive terms used to differentiate one type of feedback from another. The terms used to describe feedback are based on the source of feedback (*intrinsic* or *augmented*), the timing or frequency of feedback, and the focus of feed-back (*knowledge of performance* or *knowledge of results*). Box 1.17 defines these terms and other categories of feedback.

Several factors influence the choice of feedback during exercise instruction or functional training and the effectiveness of feedback for skill acquisition (performance) and skill retention (learning). The stage of motor learning has a significant impact on the type, timing, and frequency of feedback used during practice sessions, as does a patient's physical and cognitive status. It has also been suggested that a therapist should encourage a patient to provide input about his or her receptiveness to the type, frequency, and timing of feedback, particularly once the patient has achieved a beginning level of skill acquisition. This participation promotes a sense of self-control in the patient and is thought to have a positive impact on learning.[82]

It is useful to compare the benefits and limitations of several types of feedback because some forms enhance skill acquisition but are less effective than others for achieving skill retention.

***Intrinsic feedback.*** Intrinsic feedback comes from all of the sensory systems of the learner, not from the therapist, and is derived from performing or attempting to perform any movement. Intrinsic feedback is inherent in the movement itself; that is, it occurs naturally during or after a task is performed.[35,91,121] It provides ongoing information about the quality of movement during a task and information

---

**BOX 1.17  Types of Feedback Associated with Motor Learning**

**Knowledge of Performance (KP) Versus Knowledge of Results (KR)**
- *KP.* Either intrinsic feedback sensed during a task or immediate, post-task, augmented feedback (usually verbal) about the *nature* or *quality* of the performance of a motor task
- *KR.* Immediate, post-task, augmented feedback about the *outcome* of a motor task

**Intrinsic Feedback**
- A sensory cue or set of cues that are inherent in the execution of a motor task
- Arises directly from performance of the task
- May immediately follow completion of a task or may occur even before a task has been completed
- Most often involves proprioceptive, kinesthetic, tactile, visual, or auditory cues

**Augmented Feedback**
- Sensory cues from an external source that are supplemental to intrinsic feedback; they are not inherent in the execution of the task
- May arise from a mechanical source or from another person
- Also referred to as extrinsic feedback

**Concurrent Versus Postresponse Feedback**
- *Concurrent.* Occurs during the performance of a task
- *Postresponse (terminal).* Occurs after completion of a task

**Immediate, Delayed, and Summary Feedback**
- *Immediate.* Occurs or is given directly after a task is completed.
- *Delayed.* An interval of time elapses before information is given, which allows time for the learner to reflect on how well or poorly a task was done.
- *Summary.* Information is given about the average performance of several repetitions of a movement or task

**Intermittent Versus Continuous Feedback**
- *Intermittent.* Occurs irregularly, randomly
- *Continuous.* Is ongoing during the course of a task

---

about the outcomes (results) of a task, specifically if the goal of a task was achieved. In everyday life, intrinsic feedback is a continuous source of information that provides knowledge of performance (KP) and knowledge of results (KR) as a person performs routine activities or tries to learn new motor skills.

***Augmented feedback.*** Information about the performance or results of a task that is *supplemental* to intrinsic feedback is known as augmented feedback.[91,121,122,147] It is also referred to as *extrinsic feedback.*[35] Unlike intrinsic feedback, a therapist has control of the type, timing, and frequency of augmented feedback a patient receives during

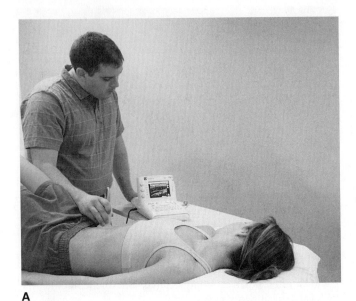

A

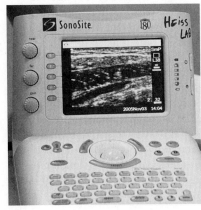

B

FIGURE 1.10  (A, B) An ultrasound imaging unit provides augmented (visual) feedback on the screen during exercise instruction to help the patient learn how to activate the transversus abdominis and internal oblique muscles.

training. Augmented feedback can be provided during or at the conclusion of a task to give information about the quality of the performance (KP) or the quality of the outcome of a task (KR). Although augmented feedback is a commonly used instructional tool to facilitate motor learning in healthy individuals, it is thought to be particularly necessary when teaching motor skills to patients with inadequate or inaccurate intrinsic feedback from impaired sensory systems due to injury or disease.[35,91]

Therapists have many forms of augmented feedback from which to select for exercise instruction and functional training.[35,147] Some examples include *verbal* or *tactile* feedback directly from a therapist who is interacting with a patient during practice, *visual* feedback from mirrors, an ultrasound imaging device (Fig. 1.10), an electromyography (EMG) biofeedback unit, or a videotaped replay of a previous performance.

***Use of knowledge of performance versus knowledge of results.*** Over the past two decades the selection and application of feedback have changed in the clinical setting. Traditionally, a therapist would have a patient focus on sensory information inherent in a motor task (intrinsic feedback) to "get the feel" of movements in the task, such as how it felt to weight shift from side to side while controlling the knees and maintaining standing balance. At the same time the therapist would provide ongoing feedback, usually verbal, about the quality of the patient's posture or knee control during the weight-shifting activity (knowledge of performance). However, research, primarily with nonimpaired subjects, has shown that directing a person's attention to the *outcomes* of movements (knowledge of results)

rather than to the details of the movements themselves enhances learning more effectively.[148]

As therapists have become more familiar with the principles of motor learning, greater emphasis now is placed on providing feedback about the outcomes (results) of performing a task.[147] Going back to the weight-shifting example: To employ knowledge of results a therapist now would have a patient perform weight shifts by reaching for objects placed in various positions just outside the patient's base of support. By giving the patient a target, the task becomes goal-directed as the patient focuses on the intended results of the movement. The patient learns to judge the effectiveness of his or her movements based on feedback received from external cues.[82,148]

***Timing of feedback.*** The timing of augmented feedback also affects learning and should be adjusted during the learning process. During the initial stage of learning, a new exercise or functional task, *concurrent feedback*, using, for example, tactile cues (*manual guidance*), may be necessary for patient safety and may help the patient understand the required movements. However, excessive use of manual guidance during a task does not allow a patient to make "safe mistakes" while figuring out how to perform a movement. As mentioned in the discussion of the stages of motor learning, self-detection and self-correction of errors is absolutely necessary for learning to occur. The key is to use the least amount of concurrent feedback, such as manual guidance, for the shortest time possible so the patient does not become reliant on it to complete a task.[35]

*Immediate, postresponse feedback* is another form of augmented feedback often used during the initial stage of learning. The therapist provides information, often verbally, about the outcome of the task (KR) immediately after each trial. Although immediate feedback may enhance early skill acquisition, it too does not allow time for problem solving by the patient and detection of errors without input from the therapist. Consequently, although initial skill acquisition may occur rather quickly, learning, which includes retention, is delayed.

Use of *delayed feedback* from the therapist after each repetition of a task or exercise or use of *summary feedback* after several trials have been completed gives the patient time for problem solving and self-evaluation of how the task was performed during practice, which in turn promotes retention and generalizability of the learned skills. Although use of delayed or summary feedback may be associated with slower skill acquisition than concurrent or immediate feedback, it is thought that delaying the timing of feedback makes the patient pay attention to intrinsic feedback inherent in the task.[35,121,146]

In a study of nonimpaired individuals, the impact of three forms of augmented feedback (concurrent, immediate postresponse, and summary feedback) was investigated.[146] When subjects practiced a partial weight-bearing activity, those who received concurrent visual feedback (by looking at a scale) achieved the skill more quickly than the subjects who received postresponse feedback (either immediate or summary). However, subjects who received concurrent feedback performed least well on a retention test 2 days after practice ended than the subjects in the two other groups who received postresponse feedback. In addition, summary feedback was found to enhance retention to a greater extent than immediate postresponse feedback.

***Frequency of feedback.*** A basic principle about augmented feedback is that "less is better." *Intermittent* feedback during practice has been shown to promote learning more effectively than *continuous* feedback. Conversely, continuous feedback improves skill acquisition (performance) more quickly during the initial stage of learning than intermittent feeedback.[35] Excessive verbal feedback, for example, provided continuously by a therapist can be distracting and may interrupt a patient's attention to the task.

Although the greatest frequency of feedback is necessary during the cognitive (initial) stage of learning when a patient is first learning how to perform an exercise or a functional task, extended use of any form of augmented feedback can create dependence on the feedback and can be a deterrent to self-detection and correction of errors.[35,121,122] Therefore, it is important to fade (decrease) feedback over time. Use of *summary feedback,* particularly during the associative stage of learning, is an effective strategy to reduce the total amount of feedback given in a practice session. As augmented feedback is reduced, a patient must explore slight modifications of a movement strategy and analyze the results. This promotes problem solving, self-monitoring, and self-correction, all of which

enable a patient to perform tasks independently and safely and to transfer learning to new task conditions.

Box 1.18 summarizes the information discussed in this section with regard to qualities of the learner and effective strategies for exercise instruction and functional training founded on the principles and stages of motor learning.

## Adherence to Exercise

Effective patient-related instruction for a functionally oriented exercise program must include methods to foster *adherence*. This is particularly challenging when an exercise program must be carried out for an extended period of time. Positive outcomes from treatment are contingent not so much on designing the "ideal" exercise program for a patient but, rather, designing a program that a patient or family will actually follow.[55,56,139]

N O T E : Although the terms *adherence* and *compliance* are often used interchangeably by clinicians and in the literature, the term *adherence* has been selected for this discussion because it has a stronger connotation of active involvement of the patient and patient–therapist collaboration. In contrast, *compliance* tends to imply a more passive connotation with respect to a patient's behavior.

### Factors that Influence Adherence to an Exercise Program
Many factors influence adherence to an exercise program.[43,55,56,77,82,90,126,139] These factors can be grouped into three categories: a patient's characteristics, factors related to a patient's health condition or impairments, and program-related variables.

### Characteristics of the Patient
The following patient-related factors can have a positive or negative impact on adherence: understanding the health condition, impairments, or exercise program; level of motivation, attentiveness, memory, and willingness and receptivity to change; degree of fatigue or stress; the patient's self-perception of his or her compatibility with the therapist or the degree of control in the exercise program; socioeconomic and cultural background; the beliefs and attitudes about exercise and the value the patient places on the exercise program; and the patient's access to resources. The patient's age and sex also influence adherence to an exercise program, with men having higher adherence rates than women. The association between age and adherence is less clear.

### Factors Related to the Health Condition or Impairments
The acuity, chronicity, severity, or stability of the primary health condition and related impairments and presence of co-morbidities all have an impact on adherence. Pain is obviously a deterrent to adherence and therefore must be

**BOX 1.18    Qualities of the Learner and Instructional Strategies for the Three Stages of Motor Learning***

### Cognitive Stage
#### Qualities of the Learner
*Must attend only to the task at hand; must think about each step or component; easily distractible; starts to get a "feel" for the exercise; makes errors and alters performance, particularly when given augmented feedback; begins to differentiate correct versus incorrect and safe versus unsafe performance.*

#### Instructional Strategies
- Identify the purpose of the exercise or functional task.
- Demonstrate the movements (modeling).
- Initially, guide or assist the patient through the movements. Reduce this form of feedback as soon as a patient can safely control movements.
- Point out the distance and speed of the movement (how far or fast to move).
- Break complex movements into parts when appropriate.
- Practice only a few motor tasks. Keep repetitions low and alternate tasks to ensure safety and avoid fatigue.
- Provide frequent and explicit positive feedback.
- Use a variety of forms of feedback (verbal, tactile, visual).
- Introduce the concept of self-evaluation and self-correction of movements.
- Allow trial and error to occur within safe limits.

### Associative Stage
#### Qualities of the Learner
*Performs tasks more consistently with fewer errors; executes movements in a well organized manner; refines the movements in the exercise or functional task; detects and self-corrects movement errors when they occur; is less dependent on visual feedback or verbal feedback from the therapist; uses prospective cues and anticipates errors before they occur.*

#### Instructional Strategies
- Emphasize practice of a greater number and variety of movements or tasks.
- Increase the complexity of the exercise or task.
- Emphasize problem solving.
- Avoid manual guidance.
- Vary the sequence of exercise or tasks practiced.
- Allow the patient to practice independently, emphasizing problem solving.
- Introduce simulation of functional tasks into the practice session.
- Decrease the total amount of feedback but increase specificity; allow the learner to perform a full set of exercises or several repetitions of a functional task before providing feedback (summary feedback).
- Delay feedback to give the learner an opportunity to detect errors and self-correct them.
- Increase the level of distraction in the exercise environment.

### Autonomous Stage
#### Qualities of the Learner
*Performs the task consistently and automatically and while doing other tasks; applies the learned movement strategies to increasingly more difficult or new environmental situations; if appropriate, performs the task more quickly or for an extended period of time at a lower energy cost.*

#### Instructional Strategies
- Set up a series of progressively more difficult activities the learner can do independently, such as increasing the speed, distance, and complexity of the exercises or task.
- Suggest ways the learner can vary the original exercise or task and use the task in more challenging situations encountered in everyday activities.
- If the patient is still in therapy, which at most is usually for just a recheck, use little to no feedback unless a potentially unsafe situation arises.

*Adapted from Dennis, JK, McKeough, DM: Mobility. In May, BJ (ed) Home Health and Rehabilitation—Concepts of Care, ed 2. FA Davis, Philadelphia, 1999, pp 121–123, with permission.

minimized in an exercise program. When impairments are severe or long-standing, setting short-term goals that can be regularly achieved fosters adherence to an exercise program that must be followed over a long period of time.

### Program-Related Variables
The complexity and necessary duration of an exercise program, adequacy of instruction and feedback from the therapist, whether the patient has had input into the plan of care, and the continuity of care from an inpatient to a home setting, for example, have an impact on adherence. Programs that address the motivational needs of patients have higher

adherence rates. In the outpatient setting, logistics, such as location and scheduling, the program's atmosphere created by the therapist/exercise instructor, as well as the availability of social support and individualized attention or counseling from personnel are also important factors that foster adherence.

A therapist should expect that most patients will not dutifully adhere to any treatment program, particularly if regular exercise has not been a part of the patient's life prior to the occurrence of disease or injury. The most a therapist can hope to do is implement strategies that foster adherence. Some suggestions from a number of resources in the literature are noted in Box 1.19.[43,55,56,77,82,90,126,139]

| BOX 1.19 | Ways to Foster Adherence to an Exercise Program |
|---|---|

- Explore and try to appreciate the patient's beliefs about exercising or the value the patient places on exercising as a means to "get better."
- Help the patient identify personal benefits derived from adhering to the exercise program.
- Explain the rationale and importance of each exercise and functional activity.
- Identify how specific exercises are designed to meet specific patient-centered goals or functional outcomes.
- Allow and encourage the patient to have input into the nature and scope of the exercise program, the selection and scheduling of practice and feedback, and decisions of when and to what extent exercises are progressively

made more difficult to enhance a patient's sense of self-control.
- Keep the exercise program as brief as possible.
- Identify practical and functionally oriented ways to do selected exercises during everyday tasks.
- Have the patient keep an exercise log.
- If possible, schedule follow-up visit(s) to review or modify exercises.
- Point out specific exercise-related progress.
- Identify barriers to adherence (not enough time in the day to do the exercises; discomfort during the exercises; lack of necessary equipment); then suggest solutions or modify the exercise program.

# INDEPENDENT LEARNING ACTIVITIES

## ● Critical Thinking and Discussion

1. Critically analyze your own, an acquaintance's, or a family member's exercise history. Then identify how a regular regimen of exercise could improve your quality of life or theirs.

2. Research four pathological conditions, diseases, injuries, or disorders that result in primary impairments of the (1) musculoskeletal, (2) neuromuscular, (3) cardiovascular/pulmonary, and (4) integumentary systems. Identify characteristic impairments (signs and symptoms) associated with each pathology and hypothesize what functional limitations and disabilities are most likely to develop.

3. Why is it essential for a physical therapist to understand and be able to articulate (verbally or in written form) the interrelationships among pathology, impairments, functional limitations, and disability?

4. Last month you sprained your ankle (inversion sprain). You had to use crutches for several days, but since then you have been walking independently. Pain and swelling still return after vigorous activity, and your ankle feels unstable on uneven terrain. Using the disablement model as your frame of reference, identify specific functional limitations that would most likely develop in your life as the result of your history and current problems.

5. Using your current knowledge of examination procedures, develop a list of specific tests and measures you would most likely choose to use when examining a patient whose primary impairments affect the (1) musculoskeletal, (2) neuromuscular, (3) cardiovascular and/or pulmonary, and (4) integumentary systems.

6. You have been asked to make recommendations for the adoption of one or more new measurement instruments to be used at your facility for data collection and analy-

sis of functional outcomes. Review the literature on musculoskeletal assessment and identify and summarize key features of five instruments that measure functional limitations associated with musculoskeletal impairments of the extremities, neck, or trunk. In addition, identify and summarize key features of five measurement instruments that assess a patient's perceived level of disability.

7. Three individuals just recently sustained a similar fracture of the hip. All underwent an open reduction with internal fixation. The patients are an otherwise healthy 19-year-old college student who was in an automobile accident and wants to return to campus after discharge from the hospital; a 60-year-old person with a somewhat sedentary lifestyle who plans to return home after postoperative rehabilitation and wishes to return to work in an office as soon as possible; and an 80-year-old individual with severe age-related osteoporosis who has been residing in an assisted living facility for the past year. What issues must be considered when identifying anticipated goals and expected outcomes and determining appropriate interventions in the plans of care for these patients? In what ways would goals and expected outcomes differ for these patients?

8. Identify the key components of the patient management model described in this chapter and discuss how each of those components relates to the potential use of therapeutic exercise interventions.

9. Using the taxonomy of motor tasks discussed in this chapter, identify simple to complex activities that are necessary or important in your daily life. Identify at least three activities that fall within the 16 condition variables described in the taxonomy.

10. You are seeing a patient in the home setting for follow-up of a postoperative exercise program and progression

of functional activities initiated in the hospital. The patient is a 55-year-old computer analyst who had a (L) total knee arthroplasty 10 days ago. You have completed your examination and evaluation. Other than a long-standing history of degenerative arthritis of the (L) knee, the patient has no other significant health-related problems. As you would expect, the patient has pain and limited range of motion of the (L) knee and decreased strength of the (L) lower extremity. The patient is currently ambulating with axillary crutches, weight bearing as tolerated on the (L) lower extremity. (1) Identify the musculoskeletal diagnostic classification (as described in the *Guide to Physical Therapist Practice*[2]) that best describes this patient's impairments. (2) As the patient recovers strength and range of motion, design a series of progressively more challenging functional motor tasks the patient could practice with your supervision or independently at home based on the taxonomy of motor tasks described in this chapter.

# REFERENCES

1. American College of Sports Medicine: ACSM's Guidelines for Exercise Testing and Prescription, ed. 6. Lippincott Williams & Wilkins, Philadelphia, 2000.
2. American Physical Therapy Association: Guide to Physical Therapist Practice, ed. 2. Phys Ther 81:9–744, 2001.
3. Baker, SM, et al: Patient participation in physical therapy goal setting. Phys Ther 81:1118, 2001.
4. Basmajian, J (ed) Physical Rehabilitation Outcome Measures. Canadian Physiotherapy Association in cooperation with Health and Welfare Canada and Canada Communications Group, Toronto, 1994.
5. Beattie, P: Evidence-based practice in outpatient orthopedic physical therapy: using research findings to assist clinical decision making. Orthop Phys Ther Pract 16:27–29, 2004.
6. Beattie, PF, Pinto, MB, Nelson, MK, et al: Patient satisfaction with outpatient physical therapy: instrument validation. Phys Ther 82:557–565, 2002.
7. Beattie, P, Turner, C, Donda, M, et al: MedRisk instrument for measuring patient satisfaction with physical therapy care: a psychometric analysis. J Orthop Sports Phys Ther 35:24–32, 2005.
8. Bloomfield, SA: Changes in musculoskeletal structure and function with prolonged bed rest. Med Sci Sports Exerc 29:197–206, 1997.
9. Boissonnault, WG: Prevalence of comorbid conditions: surgeries and medication use in a physical therapy outpatient population: a multi-centered study. J Orthop Sports Phys Ther 29:506–519, 1999.
10. Boissonnault, WG: Differential diagnosis: taking a step back before stepping forward. PT Magazine Phys Ther 8:46, 2000.
11. Boissonnault, WG: Patient health history including identification of health risk factors. In Boissonnault, WG: Primary Care for the Physical Therapist: Examination and Triage. Elsevier Saunders, St. Louis, 2005, pp 55–65.
12. Boissonnault, WG: Review of systems. In Boissonnault WG (ed) Primary Care for the Physical Therapist: Examination and Triage. Elsevier Saunders, St. Louis, 2005, pp 87–104.
13. Boissonnault, WG, Badke, MB: Collecting health history information: the accuracy of a patient self-administered questionnaire in an orthopedic outpatient setting. Phys Ther 85:531–543, 2005.
14. Brandt, EN Jr, Pope, AM (eds) Enabling America: Assesing the Role of Rehabilitation Science and Engineering. Institute of Medicine, National Academy Press, Washington, DC, 1997, p 62.
15. Charness, AL: Outcomes measurement: intervention versus outcomes. In Cirullo, JA (ed) Orthop Phys Ther Clin North Am 3:147, 1994.
16. Chase, L, et al: Perceptions of physical therapists toward patient education. In Shepard, KF, Jensen, GM (eds) Handbook of Teaching for Physical Therapists. Butterworth Heinemann, Boston, 1997, p 225.
17. Childs, JD, Cleland, JA: Development and application of clinical prediction rules to improve decision making in physical therapist practice. Phys Ther 86(1):122–131, 2006.
18. Cormack, JC: Evidence-based practice....What it is and how to do it? J Orthop Sports Phys Ther 32:484–487, 2002.
19. Cress, ME, et al: Functional training: muscle structure, function and performance in older women. J Orthop Sports Phys Ther 24:4, 1996.
20. Croakin, E: Osteopenia: implications for physical therapists managing patients of all ages. PT Magazine Phys Ther 9:80, 2001.
21. Dahl, TH: International classification of functioning, disability and health: an introduction and discussion of its potential impact on rehabilitation services and research. J Rehabil Med 34:201–204, 2002.
22. Dalton, D: The Guide to Physical Therapist Practice: incorporating preferred practice patterns into orthopedic practice. Orthop Phys Ther Pract 11:15, 1999.
23. Davis, CM: Model for teaching physical therapy diagnosis at the post-entry level. J Phys Ther Educ 9:54, 1995.
24. Dekker, J, et al: Diagnosis and treatment in physical therapy: an investigation of their relationship. Phys Ther 73:568, 1993.
25. DeLitto, A, Snyder-Mackler, L: The diagnostic process: examples in orthopedic physical therapy. Phys Ther 75:203, 1995.
26. Dennis, JK, McKeough, DM: Mobility. In May, BJ (ed) Home Health and Rehabilitation: Concepts of Care, ed 2. FA Davis, Philadelphia, 1999, p 109.
27. Edwards, I, Jones, M, Carr, J, et al: Clinical reasoning strategies in physical therapy. Phys Ther 84:312–330, 2004.
28. Embrey, DG, et al: Clinical decision making by experienced and inexperienced pediatric physical therapists for children with diplegic cerebral palsy. Phys Ther 76:20, 1996.
29. Fitts, PM, Posner, MI: Human Performance. Brooks/Cole, Belmont, CA, 1967.
30. Francis, KT: Status of the year 2000 health goals for physical activity and fitness. Phys Ther 79:405, 1999.
31. Friedrich, M, Cernak, T, Maderbacher, P: The effect of brochure use versus therapist teaching on patients' performing therapeutic exercise and on changes in impairment status. Phys Ther 76:1082, 1996.
32. Fritz, JM, Wainner, RS: Examining diagnostic tests and evidence-based perspective. Phys Ther 81:1546–1564, 2001.
33. Fritz, JM: Evidence-based examination of diagnostic information. In Boissonnault WG (ed) Primary Care for the Physical Therapist: Examination and Triage. Elsevier Saunders, St. Louis, 2005, pp 18–25.
34. Gahimer, JE, Domboldt, E: Amount of patient education in physical therapy practice and perceived effects. Phys Ther 76:1089, 1996.
35. Gentile, AM: Skill acquisition: action, movement, and neuromotor processes. In Carr, J, Shepherd, R (eds) Movement Science: Foundations for Physical Therapy in Rehabilitation. Aspen Publishers, Gaithersburg, MD, 2000, pp 111–187.
36. Giallonardo, L: The Guide to Physical Therapist Practice: an overview for the orthopedic physical therapist. Orthop Phys Ther Pract 10:10, 1998.
37. Goldstein, TS: Functional Rehabilitation in Orthopaedics. Aspen Publishers, Gaithersburg, MD, 1995.
38. Goodman, CC, Snyder, TEK: Differential Diagnosis in Physical Therapy, ed 3. WB Saunders, Philadelphia, 2000.
39. Guccione, A: Arthritis and the process of disablement. Phys Ther 74:408, 1994.
40. Guccione, A: Physical therapy diagnosis and the relationship between impairment and function. Phys Ther 71:449, 1991.
41. Guccione, AA, Mielenz, TJ, DeVellis, RF, et al: Development and testing of a self-report instrument to measure actions: Outpatient Physical Therapy Improvement in Movement Assessment Log (OPTIMAL). Phys Ther 85:515–530, 2005.
42. Hack, LM: History, purpose and structure of part two: preferred practice patterns. PT Magazine Phys Ther 6:72, 1998.
43. Hardman, AE: Physical activity and health: current issues and research needs. Int J Epidemiol 30(5):1193–1197, 2001

44. Harris, BA, Dyrek, DA: A model of orthopedic dysfunction for clinical decision making in physical therapy practice. Phys Ther 69:548, 1989.

45. Harris, BA: Building documentation using a clinical decision making model. In Stewart, DL, Abeln, SH (eds) Documenting Functional Outcomes in Physical Therapy. Mosby-Year Book, St. Louis, 1993, p 81.

46. Hart, DL, Geril, AC, Pfohl, RL: Outcomes process in daily practice. PT Magazine Phys Ther 5:68, 1997.

47. Heerkens, YF, et al: Impairments and disabilities—the difference: proposal for the adjustment of the International Classification of Impairments, Disabilities and Handicaps. Phys Ther 74:430, 1994.

48. Herman, KM, Reese, CS: Relationship among selected measures of impairment, functional limitation and disability in patients with cervical spine disorders. Phys Ther 81:903, 2001.

49. Hicks, GE, Fritz, JM, et al: Preliminary development of a clinical prediction rule for determining which patients with low back pain will respond to a stabilization exercise program. Arch Phys Med Rehabil 86:1753–1762, 2005.

50. Hodges, PW: Motor control. In Kolt, GS, Snyder-Mackler, L (eds) Physical Therapies in Sport and Exercise. Churchill Livingstone, Edinburgh, 2003, pp 107–142.

51. ICIDH: International Classification of Impairments, Disabilities and Handicaps: A Manual of Classification Relating to Consequences of Disease. World Health Organization, Geneva, 1980.

52. International Classification of Functioning, Disability and Health: ICF. World Health Organization, Geneva, 2001.

53. Jensen, GM, Shepard, KF, Hack, LM: The novice versus the experienced clinician: insights into the work of the physical therapist. Phys Ther 70:314, 1990.

54. Jensen, GM, Shepard, KF, Gwyer, J, Hack, LM: Attribute dimensions that distinguish master and novice physical therapy clinicians in orthopedic settings. Phys Ther 72:711, 1992.

55. Jensen, GM, Lorish, C: Promoting patient cooperation with exercise programs: linking research, theory and practice. Arthritis Care Res 7:181, 1994.

56. Jensen, GM, Lorish C, Shepard, KF: Understanding patient receptivity to change: teaching for treatment adherence. In Shepard, KF, Jensen, GM (eds) Handbook of Teaching for Physical Therapists. Butterworth-Heinemann, Boston, 1997, p 241.

57. Jensen, GM, Gwyer J, Shepard KF, Hack, LM: Expert practice in physical therapy. Phys Ther 80:28–43, 2000.

58. Jetle, AM, Branch, LG, Berlin, J: Musculoskeletal impairment and physical disablement among the aged. J Gerontol 45:M203, 1990.

59. Jette, AM: Diagnosis and classification by physical therapists: a special communication. Phys Ther 69:967, 1989.

60. Jette, AM: Physical disablement concepts for physical therapy research and practice. Phys Ther 74:380, 1994.

61. Jette, AM, et al: Exercise—it's never too late: the strong for life program. Am J Public Health 89:66, 1999.

62. Jette, AM: The changing language of disablement [editorial]. Phys Ther 85: 198-199, 2005.

63. Jette, DU, Bacon, K, Batty, C, et al: Evidence-based practice: beliefs, attitudes, knowledge and behaviors of physical therapists. Phys Ther 83:786–805, 2003.

64. Jones, MA: Clinical reasoning in manual therapy. Phys Ther 72:875, 1992.

65. Jones, M, Jensen, G, Rothstein, J: Clinical reasoning in physiotherapy. In Higgs, J, Jones, M (eds) Clinical Reasoning in the Health Professions. Butterworth-Heinemann, Oxford, 1995, p 72.

66. Kauffman, TL, Nashner, LM, Allison, LK: Balance is a critical parameter in orthopedic rehabilitation. Orthop Phys Ther Clin N Am 6:43, 1997.

67. Kelo, MJ: Use of self-report disability measures in daily practice. Orthop Phys Ther Pract 11:22, 1999.

68. Krebs, DE, Jetle, AM, Assmann, SF: Moderate exercise improves gait stability in disabled elders. Arch Phys Med Rehabil 79:1489, 1998.

69. Lane, JN, Riley, EH, Wirgnowicz, PZ: Osteoporosis: diagnosis and treatment. J Bone Joint Surg Am 78:618, 1996.

70. Lee, T, Swanson, L: What is repeated in a repetition: effects of practice conditions on motor skill acquisition. Phys Ther 71:150, 1991.

71. Leighton, RD, Sheldon, MR: Model for teaching clinical decision making in a physical therapy professional curriculum. J Phys Ther Educ 11(Fall):23, 1997.

72. Lephart, S, Swanik, CB, Fu, F: Reestablishing neuromuscular control. In Prentice, WE (ed) Rehabilitation Techniques in Sports Medicine, ed 3. McGraw-Hill, Boston, 1999, p 88.

73. Lorish, C, Gale, JR: Facilitating behavior change: strategies for education and practice. J Phys Ther Educ 13:31, 1999.

74. Lusardi, MM: Mobility and balance in later life. Orthop Phys Ther Clin N Am 6:305, 1997.

75. Magee, DJ: Orthopedic Physical Assessment, ed 4. Saunders, Philadelphia, 2002.

76. Magistro, CM: Clinical decision making in physical therapy: a practitioner's perspective. Phys Ther 69:525, 1989.

77. Mahler, HI, Kulik, JA, Tarazi, RY: Effects of videotape intervention at discharge on diet and exercise compliance after coronary bypass surgery. J Cardiopulm Rehabil 19(3):170–177, 1999.

78. Maring, J: Effects of mental practice on rate of skill acquisition. Phys Ther 70:165, 1990.

79. May, BJ, Dennis, JK: Clinical decision making. In May, BJ (ed) Home Health and Rehabilitation—Concepts of Care, ed 2. FA Davis, Philadelphia, 1999, p 21.

80. May, BJ, Dennis, JK: Expert decision making in physical therapy: a survey of practitioners. Phys Ther 71:190, 1991.

81. McArdle, WD, Katch, FI, Katch, VL: Essentials of Exercise Physiology, ed 2. Lippincott Williams & Wilkins, Philadelphia, 2000.

82. McNevin, NH, Wulf, G, Carlson, C: Effects of attentional focus, self-control and dyad training on motor learning: implications for physical rehabilitation. Phys Ther 80:373, 2000.

83. Miller, PA, McKibbon, KA, Haynes, RB: A quantitative analysis of research publications in physical therapy journals. Phys Ther 83:123–131, 2003.

84. Mueller, MJ, Maluf, KS: Tissue adaptation to physical stress: a proposed "physical stress theory" to guide physical therapist practice, education and research. Phys Ther 82:382–403, 2002.

85. Myers, JB, Ju, Y, Hwang, J, et al: Reflexive muscle activation alterations in shoulders with anterior glenohumeral instability. Am J Sports Med 32(4):1013–1021, 2004.

86. Nagi, S: Some conceptual issues in disability and rehabilitation. In Sussman MB (ed) Sociology and Rehabilitation. American Sociological Association, Washington, DC, 1965, pp 100–113.

87. Nagi, SZ: Disability concepts revisited: implications for prevention. In Pope, AM, Tarlov, AR (eds) Disability in America. National Academy Press Washington, DC, 1991.

88. Nashner, L: Sensory, neuromuscular and biomechanical contributions to human balance. In Duncan, P (ed) Balance. American Physical Therapy Association, Alexandria, VA, 1990, p 5.

89. National Advisory Board on Medical Rehabilitation Research, Draft V: Report and Plan for Medical Rehabilitation Research. National Institutes of Health, Bethesda, MD, 1992.

90. Nemshick, MT: Designing educational interventions for patients and families. In Shepard, KF, Jensen, GM (eds) Handbook of Teaching for Physical Therapists. Butterworth-Heinemann, Boston, 1997, p 303.

91. Nicholson, DE: Teaching psychomotor skills. In Shepard, KF, Jensen, GM (eds) Handbook of Teaching for Physical Therapists. Butterworth-Heinemann, Boston, 1997, p 271.

92. O'Sullivan, SB: Clinical decision making: planning effective treatments. In O'Sullivan, SB, Schmitz, TJ (eds) Physical Rehabilitation: Assessment and Treatment, ed 4. FA Davis, Philadelphia, 2001, p 1.

93. Ozer, MN, Payton, OD, Nelson, CE: Treatment Planning for Rehabilitation: A Patient-Centered Approach. McGraw-Hill, New York, 2000.

94. Page, SJ, Levine, P, Sisto, SA, et al: Mental practice combined with physical practice for upper limb motor deficits in subacute stroke. Phys Ther 81:1455–1462, 2001.

95. Posner, JD, et al: Physical determinants in independence in mature women. Arch Phys Med Rehabil 76:373, 1995.

96. Philadelphia Panel evidence-based clinical practice guidelines on selected rehabilitation interventions for knee pain. Phys Ther 81:1675–1700, 2001.

97. Philadelphia Panel evidence-based clinical practice guidelines on selected rehabilitation interventions for low back pain. Phys Ther 81:1641–1674, 2001.

98. Philadelphia Panel evidence-based clinical practice guidelines on selected rehabilitation interventions for neck pain. Phys Ther 81:1701–1717, 2001.

99. Philadelphia Panel evidence-based clinical practice guidelines on selected rehabilitation interventions for shoulder pain. Phys Ther 81:1719–1730, 2001.

100. Philadelphia Panel evidence-based clinical practice guidelines on selected rehabilitation interventions: overview and methodology. Phys Ther 81:1629–1640, 2001.

101. Public Health Service: Healthy People 2000: National Health Promotion and Disease Prevention Objectives. U.S. Department of Heath and Human Services, Washington, DC, 1991.

102. Randall, KE, McEwen, IR: Writing patient-centered functional goals. Phys Ther 80:1197, 2000.

103. Rantanen, T, et al: Disability, physical activity and muscle strength in older women: the Women's Health and Aging Study. Arch Phys Med Rehabil 80:130, 1999.

104. Reo, JA, Mercer, VS: Effects of live, videotaped or written instruction on learning an upper extremity exercise program. Phys Ther 84:622–633, 2004.

105. Riddle, DL, Stratford, PW: Use of generic vs region-specific functional status measures on patients with cervical spine disorders. Phys Ther 78:951, 1998.

106. Riddle, DL, Hoppener, MR, Kraaijenhagen, RA, et al: Preliminary validation of a clinical assessment for deep vein thrombosis in orthopedic outpatients. Clin Orthop 432:252–257, 2005.

107. Rivett, DA, Higgs, J: Hypothesis generation in the clinical reasoning behavior of manual therapists. J Phys Ther Educ 11:40, 1997.

108. Rose, SJ, Rothstein, JM: Muscle mutability. Part 1. General concepts and adaptations to altered patterns of use. Phys Ther 62:1773, 1982.

109. Rose, SJ: Physical therapy diagnosis: role and function. Phys Ther 69:535, 1989.

110. Rothstein, JM: Disability and our identity [editorial]. Phys Ther 74:374, 1994.

111. Rohstein, JM, Echternach, JL: Hypothesis-oriented algorithm for clinicians: a method for evaluation and treatment planning. Phys Ther 66:1388, 1986.

112. Rothstein JM, Echternach, JL, Riddle, DL: The Hypothesis-Oriented Algorithm for Clinicians II (HOAC II): a guide for patient management. Phys Ther 83:455–470, 2003.

113. Roush, SE, Sonstroen, RJ: Development of the Physical Therapy Outpatient Satisfaction Survey (PTOPS). Phys Ther 79:159, 1999.

114. Ruhland, JL, Shields, RK: The effects of a home exercise program on impairment and health-related quality of life in persons with chronic peripheral neuropathies. Phys Ther 77:1026, 1997.

115. Sackett, DL, Rosenberg, WM, Gray, MJA, et al: Evidence-based medicine: what it is and what it isn't. BMJ 312:71–72, 1996.

116. Sackett, DL, Straus, SE, Richardson, WS, et al: Evidence-Based Medicine: How to Practice and Teach EBM, ed 2. Churchill Livingstone, Edinburgh, 2000.

117. Sahrmann, SA: Diagnosis by physical therapists: a prerequisite for treatment. Phys Ther 68:1703, 1988.

118. Sahrmann, S: Are physical therapists fulfilling their responsibilities as diagnostician [editorial]. J Orthop Sports Phys Ther 35:556–558, 2005.

119. Scalzitti, DA: Evidence-based guidelines: application to clinical practice. Phys Ther 81:1622–1628, 2001.

120. Schenkman, M, Butler, R: A model for multisystem evaluation, interpretation and treatment of individuals with neurologic dysfunction. Phys Ther 69:538, 1989.

121. Schmidt, RA, Lee, TD: Motor Control and Learning: A Behavioral Emphasis, ed 3. Human Kinetics Publishers, Champaign, IL, 1999.

122. Schmidt, RA, Wrisberg, CA: Motor Learning and Performance: A Problem-Based Learning Approach, ed 3. Human Kinetics Publishers, Champaign, IL, 2004.

123. Schmitz, TJ: Coordination assessment. In O'Sullivan, SB, Schmitz, TJ (eds) Physical Rehabilitation: Assessment and Treatment, ed 4. FA Davis, Philadelphia, 2001, p 157.

124. Seyer, MA: Balance deficits: Examination, evaluation, and intervention. In Montgomery PC, Connolly, BH (eds) Clinical Applications for Motor Control. Slack, Thorofare, NJ, 2003, pp 271–306.

125. Seymour, CJ, Dybel, GJ: Developing skillful clinical decision making: evaluation of two classroom teaching strategies. J Phys Ther Educ 10:77, 1996.

126. Shuijs, EM, Kok, GJ, van der Zee, J: Correlates of exercise compliance in physical therapy. Phys Ther 73:771–786, 1993.

127. Shumway-Cook, A, Woollacott, MH: Motor Control: Theory and Practical Applications, ed 2. Lippincott Williams & Wilkins, Philadelphia, 2001.

128. Shumway-Cook, A, et al: The effect of multidimensional exercises on balance, mobility and fall risk in community-dwelling older adults. Phys Ther 77:46, 1997.

129. Sidaway, B, Trzaska, A: Can mental practice increase ankle dorsiflexr torque? Phys Ther 85:1053–1060, 2005.

130. Steill, IG, McKnight, RD, Greenberg, GH, et al: Implementation of the Ottawa ankle rules. JAMA 271:827–832, 1994.

131. Steiner, WA, Ryser, L, Huber, E, et al: Use of the ICF model as a clinical problem-solving tool in physical therapy and rehabilitation medicine. Phys Ther 82:1098–1107, 2002.

132. Stucki, G, Ewert, T, Cieza, A: Value and application of the ICF in rehabilitation medicine. Disabil Rehabil 24:932–938, 2002.

133. Stucki G: International classification of functioning, disability and health (ICF): a promising framework and classification for rehabilitation medicine. Am J Phys Med Rehabil 84(10):733–740, 2005.

134. Sullivan, PE, Markos, PD: Clinical Decision Making in Therapeutic Exercise. Appleton & Lange, Norwalk, CT, 1995.

135. Swanson, G: Functional outcome report: the next generation in physical therapy reporting. In Stewart, DL, Abeln, SH (eds) Documenting Functional Outcomes in Physical Therapy. Mosby-Year Book, St. Louis, 1993, p 101.

136. Task Force for Standards of Measurement in Physical Therapy: standards for tests and measurements in physical therapy practice. Phys Ther 71:589, 1991.

137. Tichenor, CJ, Davidson, J, Jensen, GM: Cases as shared inquiry: model of clinical reasoning. J Phys Ther Educ 9:57, 1995.

138. Triffett, MA: The relationship between motion of the shoulder and the stated ability to perform activities of daily living. J Bone Joint Surg Am 80:41, 1998.

139. Turk, D: Correlates of exercise compliance in physical therapy [commentary]. Phys Ther 73:783, 1993.

140. Umphried, D: Physical therapy differential diagnosis in the clinical setting. J Phys Ther Educ 9:39, 1995.

141. U.S. Department of Health and Human Services, Office of Disease Prevention and Health Promotion: Healthy People 2010. Washington, DC, 1998. Available at www.healthypeople.gov/.

142. Van Sant, AE: Motor control, motor learning and motor development. In Montgomery, PC, Connolly, BH (eds) Clinical Applications for Motor Control. Slack, Thorofare, NJ, 2003, pp 25–52.

143. Verbrugge, L, Jetle, A: The disablement process. Soc Sci Med 38:1, 1994.

144. Warner, L, Mc Neill, ME: Mental imagery and its potential for physical therapy. Phys Ther 68:516–521, 1988.

145. Winstein, C, Sullivan, K: Some distinctions on the motor learning/motor control distinction. Neurol Rep 21:42, 1997.

146. Winstein, C, et al: Learning a partial-weight-bearing skill effectiveness of two forms of feedback. Phys Ther 76:985, 1996.

147. Winstein, C: Knowledge of results and motor learning: implications for physical therapy. Phys Ther 71:140, 1991.

148. Wulf, G, Hob, M, Prinz, W: Instructions for motor learning: differential effects of internal vs. external focus of attention. J Motor Behav 30:169, 1998.

149. Zinny, NJ: Physical therapy management from physical therapy diagnosis: necessary but insufficient. J Phys Ther Educ 9:36, 1995.

150. Zinny, NJ: Diagnostic classification and orthopedic physical therapy practice: what we can learn from medicine. J Orthop Sports Phys Ther 34:105–109, 2004.

# Prevention, Health, and Wellness

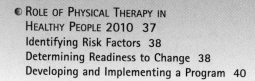

## Karen Holtgrefe, DHS, PT, OCS

In 1979, following the Surgeon General's report on the health of the nation, the U.S. government developed a national prevention agenda. Today the Office of Disease Prevention and Health Promotion in the Department of Health and Human Services oversees this agenda with two overarching goals, 28 focus areas, 467 objectives, and 10 leading health indicators through *Healthy People 2010*.[10,15] The two main goals of Healthy People 2010 are (1) to increase the quality of life and years of healthy living for all individuals of all ages and (2) to eliminate health disparities.

Health, wellness, and health promotion are defined as follows.

● **Health:** general physical, mental, or spiritual condition of the body
● **Wellness:** a state of good health often achieved through healthy lifestyle choices
● **Health promotion:** contributing to the growth and development of health

## ● ROLE OF PHYSICAL THERAPY IN HEALTHY PEOPLE 2010

Two examples of *Healthy People 2010* goals that physical therapists can help address are found in Table 2.1. When assessing the data related to adult physical activity by age group, the percentage of adults participating in moderate physical activity decreases with age. Data from 2003 shows that 42% of adults aged 18 to 24 years meet the objective, whereas only 28% of adults aged 64 to 75 years do.[3] Physical therapists have a unique role in providing

prevention, health, wellness, and fitness activities needed to address these concerns.

Activities designed for health promotion or prevention may take several forms. Examples include screening sessions to identify individuals or groups who would benefit from intervention and specific educational and exercise programs that teach prevention and provide interventions for identified problems. Examples for various prevention activities can be found in Table 2.2. When developing prevention activities, it is important to note that there are three types of prevention.[2]

● **Primary prevention:** preventing a target problem or condition in an individual or in a community at risk; for example, developing fitness programs for children to prevent obesity
● **Secondary prevention:** decreasing the duration and severity of disease; for example, developing resistance programs for individuals with osteoporosis
● **Tertiary prevention:** decreasing the degree of disability and promoting rehabilitation for individuals with chronic or irreversible diseases; for example, developing fitness programs for individuals with spinal cord injury

The *Guide to Physical Therapist Practice*[2] (the *Guide*) describes the various ways to contribute to health and wellness including a prevention/risk reduction item at the beginning of each practice pattern. Primary prevention/risk reduction is identified in the *Guide*[2] for:

● Skeletal demineralization
● Loss of balance and falling
● Cardiovascular/pulmonary disorders
● Integumentary disorders

| TABLE 2.1 | Examples of Healthy People 2010[15] Goals | | | |
|-----------|-------------------------------------------|---|---|---|
| Focus Area | Objective | 2010 Goal (Target) (%) | Baseline (%) | Updated Data 2003 Report (%) |
| Arthritis, osteoporosis, and chronic back pain (focus area #2) | Activity limitations due to chronic back pain* | 25 | 29 | 30 |
| Physical activity and fitness (focus area #22) | Adults ≥ 18 years of age who participate in 30 minutes of moderate physical activity for ≥ 5 days/week† | 50 | 33 | 32 |

*This objective is to reduce the percentage of individuals with restrictions or functional limitations due to back pain.
†This objective is to increase the percentage (number) of adults who participate in physical activity.

## Identifying Risk Factors

When developing specific programs related to health, wellness, and fitness, it is important to conduct pre-participation screenings and risk assessments. The reader is referred to the American College of Sports Medicine (ACSM)[1] for several tools to assess these factors.

### Pre-Participation Screening

Prior to participation in a moderate-intensity exercise program, the individual should be asked several questions as summarized in Box 2.1.[14] Individuals who answer yes to one or more questions should consult with their physician before starting the program.

### Risk Assessment

The participant should be assessed for risk factors associated with specific conditions such as coronary artery disease (CAD) and osteoporosis, as shown in Box 2.2.[1,9] Identification of risk factors guides the therapist when deciding how to proceed. If multiple risk factors, such as those associated with CAD, are identified, a participant may need to be referred to a physician prior to initiating a program. However, if the risk factors are minimal, the therapist would know to monitor and progress the chosen activities

or exercises within established guidelines (see Chapter 7 for guidelines related to aerobic exercise).

An individual with identified risk factors for osteoporosis may require additional screening for balance and strength. The therapist can then develop an appropriate resistance program that reduces the risk of injury during these activities (see Chapter 6 for precautions during resistance training).

## Determining Readiness to Change

Once the pre-participation screenings and risk assessments are completed and specific programs for an individual are developed, it is important to know whether the person is ready to change. There are multiple theories and models related to health promotion interventions that explain how change occurs. Understanding several of these behavioral change theories can help guide the therapist and client toward the desired outcome.

### Behavioral Change Theories

*Social cognitive theory.* The social cognitive theory (SCT) looks at the belief systems of individuals. An individual must believe that he or she can change a particular behavior and that changing that behavior will lead to the desired

| TABLE 2.2 | Prevention Activities | |
|-----------|------------------------|---|
| Screening Risk Assessment | Health Promotion, Wellness, and Fitness | |
| Scoliosis | *Education*: information flyer for parents on identification and treatment for idiopathic scoliosis | |
| Obesity | *Exercise program*: develop exercise/fitness program for overweight teens and adults | |
| Osteoporosis | *Education*: develop community education programs related to osteoporosis (importance of exercise, reducing falls in the home) | |
| | *Exercise programs*: develop resistance and weight-bearing exercise class for individuals with osteoporosis | |
| Falls | *Education*: community program related to reducing falls in the home | |
| | *Exercise programs*: develop exercise program to increase strength, balance, and coordination in older adults | |
| Work site assessment | *Education*: educate company on proper body mechanics, work station redesign | |
| | *Exercise programs*: develop specific exercise programs to reduce work-related problems | |

## BOX 2.1 | Activity Prescreening Questions

1. Have you ever been diagnosed with a heart condition?
2. Have you even been advised that you should only do physical activity under the direction of a physician?
3. Do you experience chest pain when you do physical activity?
4. Have you experienced chest pain during this past month when not physically active?
5. Have you been diagnosed with arthritis or osteoporosis, or experience increased pain in your joints when physically active
6. Are you currently taking prescription drugs for blood pressure or a heart condition?
7. Do you ever lose your balance or lose consciousness?
8. Are you aware of any condition that would prohibit you from doing physical activity?

outcome.[5,8,13] For example, a patient may want to lose weight. In addition to the desire to change the behavior causing the increased weight, the patient needs to believe that he or she is capable of succeeding and that the outcome will improve his or her health. If the patient decides to use exercise to lose weight, clear instructions on how to perform and progress the exercise program must be given. Feedback on performance must then occur to achieve the final outcome of weight reduction.

***Health belief model.*** The health belief model (HBM) is based on several factors.[6,8,11-13] First, an individual must have sufficient concern about developing an illness (perceived threat). Next, the individual needs to believe that by following the health recommendations it is possible to

## BOX 2.2 | Risk Factors for Coronary Artery Disease and Osteoporosis

**Coronary Artery Disease Risk Factors**
• Family history
• Cigarette smoking
• Hypertension
• Hypercholesterolemia
• Impaired fasting glucose level
• Obesity
• Sedentary lifestyle

**Osteoporosis Risk Factors**
• Bone mineral density score of −2.5 or less
• Postmenopausal
• Caucasian or Asian descent
• Family history
• Low body weight
• Little to no physical activity
• Smoking
• Prolonged bed rest
• Prolonged use of corticosteroids

achieve the desired outcome (perceived benefits) at an acceptable cost (perceived barriers). Using the example of losing weight, an individual would have to believe that being overweight puts himself or herself at a greater risk for developing heart disease (perceived threat). This threat may be greater because of a family history. The individual may understand that modifying the diet can help with weight loss but is not sure the best way to proceed. The person may consider joining a weight loss program but may not be sure he or she can afford the weekly fee (perceived barrier). If the perceived threat is sufficiently high, the individual may chose to join the weight loss program to obtain the desired benefit or may chose a different method of weight loss that does not have the same cost.

***Transtheoretical model.*** The transtheoretical model (TTM) looks at the stages required to make changes.[5,6,8,11,12] There are five stages of change.

• Precontemplation: no intention of making any changes within the next 6 months
• Contemplation: intend to make changes within the next 6 months
• Preparation: has begun to take steps toward making the desired change in behavior and plan to make the changes within the next 30 days
• Action: has changed the behavior for less than 6 months
• Maintenance: has changed the behavior for more than 6 months

Knowing what stage patients are in and knowing the beliefs they have regarding the need to change, the physical therapist can assist in planning the intervention, particularly if individuals are not ready to make any changes. It allows the therapist to give information needed at the appropriate time.

 **Focus on Evidence** _____

Using the Health Belief Model (HBM), Jachna and Forbes-Thompson[4] assessed residents of an assisted living facility about their perception of osteoporosis and barriers to treatment. The residents interviewed had very low perceived threats associated with osteoporosis. They considered the condition a normal part of aging with few consequences. They believed it was not life-threatening, was not severe if there was no pain or kyphosis, and was not associated with a risk for fractures. Even though they identified health as being independent in performing activities of daily living, they did not perceive the impact of osteoporosis on themselves and did not understand the benefits of prevention. Additional barriers to intervention included not wanting to take additional medication, cognitive status, and limited knowledge of osteoporosis. The authors recommended specific educational programs, screenings for risk factors of osteoporosis such as bone mineral density tests, and family support in order to increase the perceived threats and susceptibility to osteoporosis, reduce the perceived barriers, and reinforce the benefits of intervention.

## Developing and Implementing a Program

There are several models associated with program planning in health promotion which are beyond the scope of this chapter. Overall several steps can be taken to develop and implement prevention, health, and wellness programs[8] and are summarized in Box 2.3. The following case example illustrates the process.

### ● Case Example: Exercise and Osteoporosis

#### STEP 1: ASSESSING THE NEED

- Gretchen, a physical therapist at ABC Hospital, completed an educational session for a local osteoporosis support group on the most recent research related to resistance training and weight-bearing exercise for increasing bone density.
- The women contacted Gretchen and asked her to develop a resistance training exercise class that included free weights and exercise equipment (as found in a fitness club).

  **NEED:** An exercise class that educates women with osteoporosis about the safe way to perform resistance exercise.

#### STEP 2: SET GOALS AND OBJECTIVES

**Goal**

Develop two education and exercise classes (level 1 and level 2) for women with osteoporosis that emphasize prevention of fractures and proper technique for resistance exercise and weight-bearing activities.

**Objectives**

1. Educate the participants on the effects of resistance training and weight-bearing exercise on bone health.
2. Educate the participants on the indications and contraindications of certain exercises for individuals with osteoporosis.
3. Educate the participants on the correct techniques for resistance exercise including free weights, resistance band and tubing, and exercise machines.
4. Have participates demonstrate the correct technique when performing resistance exercise.
5. Review implications related to posture and body mechanics during daily activities and during exercise.

#### STEP 3: DEVELOP THE INTERVENTION

Gretchen decided to develop two exercise classes: level 1 and level 2. To attend level 2 classes, participants had to complete the level 1 class. The level 1 exercise and education class consisted of four sessions as outlined in Table 2.3.

Gretchen decided to work collaboratively with the Occupational Therapy Department and had them conduct the final class, which emphasized the correct techniques for posture and body mechanics during daily activities. Once the number of classes and general content was de-

---

| BOX 2.3 | Steps to Develop and Implement Prevention, Health, Wellness, and Fitness Programs |

**Step 1: Identify a Need**
- Identify the target audience
  - Children
  - Adults
  - Older adults
  - Industry/business
  - School system
  - Community
  - Specific population (e.g., individuals with Parkinson's disease)

**Step 2: Set Goals and Objectives**
- Identify the *purpose* of the program
- Identify the *goals* to be achieved
  - Screening
  - Education
  - Exercise program
- Identify the *objectives* of the program

**Step 3: Develop the Intervention**
- Screenings: identify valid and reliable right tools to use for the screening
- Education: develop the program including handouts for participants
- Exercise: develop the plan for each class

- Logistics
  - Secure a location for the program
    - Consider parking and access to the facility
  - Determine the time and length of the program
  - Determine the number of people who can attend based on the space
  - Identify who will do the program (self or with assistance)
  - Develop the presentation/program; include handouts for the participants
  - Develop a budget: determine costs and charge to the participants

**Step 4: Implement the Intervention**
- Recognize that even with the best of plans it is important to be adaptable and to be prepared for the unexpected

**Step 5: Evaluate the Results**
- For an educational session, ask the participants to evaluate the program. Consider an additional follow-up assessment.
- For an exercise class, record baseline data and assess progress during the program and at the end.
- Ask participants to evaluate the exercise program.
- Ask for feedback on what could be done to improve the program (e.g., different time, smaller class, longer sessions).

| TABLE 2.3 | Sample: Level 1 Exercise and Educational Class Content for Osteoporosis |
|-----------|------------------------------------------------------------------------|
| **Session** | **Content/Plan** |
| 1 | • Introduction<br>• Discussion about yearly height measurement<br>• Assessment of balance and flexibility of ankles<br>• Review and discussion of good posture<br>• Discussion on benefits of resistance training<br>• Performed exercises: shoulder blade retraction, chin tucks, sit to stand from a chair, pelvic tilt, heel/toe raises |
| 2 | • Brief review and questions related to material from first class<br>• Discussion on prevention of falls<br>• Discussion and demonstration of correct technique for performing strengthening exercises<br>• Performed exercises with resistance band: arms—bilateral horizontal abduction, rhomboids (band in doorway), leg press<br>• Exercise without band—standing hip abduction and step-ups |
| 3 | • Brief review and questions related to previous material<br>• Discussion of types of exercise to avoid (increase stress on vertebral bodies)<br>• Discussion and demonstration on how to lift weights correctly and how to determine starting weight<br>• Discussion on how to increase repetitions and weight during exercise<br>• Performed exercises with and without free weights: overhead press, seated fly, standing hip extension, prone bilateral scapular retraction, prone opposite arm and leg lift, lunges |
| 4 | • Review and questions of previous material<br>• Occupational therapy reviewed various adaptive equipment<br>• Demonstrated correct posture and body mechanics for brushing teeth, making bed, vacuuming<br>• Final questions<br>• Evaluation of program |

cided, Gretchen started planning and developing the program. She:

• Reserved a medium-sized open room in ABC hospital for 4 weeks. The class would take place on Tuesday evenings from 6:00 to 8:30 pm. The room setup was determined to be tables and chairs in the front of the room with open space in the back for exercising. Class would be limited to 20 people.
• Developed the content and objectives for each exercise/education session including handouts for participants. Put all developed material in a binder by week, including a presenter's checklist of what had to be brought to each class.
• Developed a brochure with times and location of the class and sent it to the osteoporosis support group. The cost of the level 1 exercise and education program was $25.00. Interested participants were to call and reserve a spot in the class.

### STEP 4: IMPLEMENT THE PROGRAM
The program had 10 participants and took place as scheduled for 4 weeks.

### STEP 5: EVALUATE THE PROGRAM
Participants were given a course evaluation sheet to complete regarding the location, time, content, and overall sat-

isfaction with the program. In addition, Gretchen evaluated the participants' interest in the proposed level 2 class that would take place in a fitness center with equipment and consist of three classes.

The overall evaluation of the program was positive with a few individuals preferring a different day of the week or time of day for attendance. Altogether, 8 of the 10 participants were interested in participating in the level 2 class.

## Additional Considerations for Developing Prevention, Health, and Wellness Programs

The following are additional points to consider.[7]

◉ The exercise or activity has to be specific to the goals of the individual. An individual training to run a marathon needs to run, not ride a bike. Specific principles and procedures for resistance training and aerobic exercise training can be found in Chapters 6 and 7, respectively.
◉ For children, the program should be fun and less structured but should take place for a specified period of time.
◉ For older adults, the program should start slowly to allow the participants to experience success. Consideration should be given to how the individuals can incorporate the various exercises or activities into their daily

routines. The facility where the program is conducted should be well lit and easily accessible.

● If screenings are conducted, handouts with the results and with follow-up recommendations should be given to the participants.

◉ When making handouts for participants, keep in mind the audience. For children, make them colorful and fun. For older adults, make the print larger. Keep the language simple. Limit the amount of medical terminology used. Write information as clearly as possible.

● Include pictures of exercises whenever possible.

● Consider the time commitment for you and the participants and the cost involved.

Table 2.4 lists issues related to exercise adherence.

| TABLE 2.4 | Issues Affecting Exercise Adherence |
| --- | --- |
| **Poor** | **Good** |
| Poor or limited leadership | Effective leadership |
| Inconvenient time of class or program | Positive reinforcement |
| Injury | Part of regular routine |
| Boredom with exercise | No injury |
| Poor individual commitment | Enjoyment—fun—variety |
| Unaware of any progress being made | Social support from group |
| Poor family support— disapproval | Regular updates on progress |
| | Family approval |

# INDEPENDENT LEARNING ACTIVITIES

## ● Critical Thinking and Discussion

1. In the case example for developing an exercise program for women with osteoporosis, a second class (level 2) was proposed. Develop the level 2 class. Follow the steps outlined for developing and implementing this program including the content of each exercise session, use of fitness equipment for individuals with osteoporosis, and any handouts needed.

2. In this chapter the differences in primary, secondary, and tertiary prevention were reviewed. Describe one screening program and one wellness program (exercise or education) for each of these categories that a physical therapist could provide.

3. In Table 2.1, one of the *Healthy People 2010* goals is to reduce the activity limitations (functional limitations) of individuals with chronic low back pain. Describe the limitations to achieving this goal using one of the behavioral change theories. Identify strategies for obtaining this goal.

4. Using the five steps identified in this chapter, develop a prevention and wellness program for a group of fifth and sixth grade boys and girls (10 to 12 years of age) who have been identified as being at risk for type II diabetes because of obesity and sedentary lifestyle. Refer to Chapter 6 for special considerations when developing exercise programs for children.

# REFERENCES

1. American College of Sports Medicine: ASCM's Guidelines for Exercise Testing and Prescription, ed 7. Lippincott, Williams, & Wilkins, Philadelphia, 2005.
2. American Physical Therapy Association: Guide to Physical Therapist Practice, ed 2. Phys Ther 81:9–744, 2001.
3. Center for Disease Control. Data on Healthy People 2010. Available at: http://wonder.cdc.gov/data2010. Accessed March 2006.
4. Jachna, C, Forbes-Thompson, S: Osteoporosis: health beliefs and barriers to treatment in an assisted living facility. J Gerontol Nurs 31:25–30, 2005.
5. Kosma, M, Cardinal, B, Rintala, P: Motivating individuals with disabilities to be physically active. Quest 54:116–132, 2002.
6. Landry, J, Solmon, M. Self-determination theory as an organizing framework to invesitgate women's physical activity behavior. *Quest* 54:332–354, 2002.
7. McArdle, WD, Katch, FI, Katch VL: Essentials of Exercise Physiology, ed 2. Lippincott Williams & Wilkins, Philadelphia, 1996.
8. McKenzie, J, Neiger, B, Smelter, J: Planning, Implementing and Evaluating Health Promotion Programs, ed 4. Pearson Education, San Francisco, 2005.
9. National Osteoporosis Foundation: Disease Statistics. Available at: http://www.nof.org/osteoporosis/stats.htm/. Accessed February 2003.
10. Office of Disease Prevention and Health Promotion. Steps to a Healthier US. Available at: http://odphp.osophs.dhhs.gov/. Accessed March 2006.
11. Petrocelli, J: Processes and stages of change: counseling with the transtheoretical model of change. J Counsel Dev 80:22–30, 2002.
12. Purdie, N, McCrindle, A: Self-regulation, self-efficacy and health behavior change in older adults. Educ Gerontol 28:379–400, 2002.
13. Rosenstock, I, Strecher, V, Becker M: Social learning theory and the health belief model. Health Educ Q 15:175–183, 1988.
14. Shephard R: PAR-Q, Canadian Home Fitness Test, and Exercise Screening Alternatives. Sports Med 5:185–195, 1988.
15. US Department of Health and Human Services. Healthy People 2010. Available at: www.healthypeople.gov/. Accessed March 2006.

# Applied Science of Exercise and Techniques

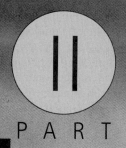

PART **II**

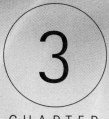

## 3 | Range of Motion

CHAPTER

Range of motion is a basic technique used for the examination of movement and for initiating movement into a program of therapeutic intervention. Movement that is necessary to accomplish functional activities can be viewed, in its simplest form, as muscles or external forces moving bones in various patterns or ranges of motions. When a person moves, the intricate control of the muscle activity that causes or controls the motion comes from the central nervous system. Bones move with respect to each other at the connecting joints. The structure of the joints, as well as the integrity and flexibility of the soft tissues that pass over the joints, affects the amount of motion that can occur between any two bones. The full motion possible is called the **range of motion** (ROM). When moving a segment through its ROM, all structures in the region are affected: muscles, joint surfaces, capsules, ligaments, fasciae, vessels, and nerves. ROM activities are most easily described in terms of joint range and muscle range. To describe joint range, terms such as flexion, extension, abduction, adduction, and rotation are used. Ranges of available joint motion are usually measured with a goniometer and recorded in degrees.[16] Muscle range is related to the functional excursion of muscles.

**Functional excursion** is the distance a muscle is capable of shortening after it has been elongated to its maximum.[26] In some cases the functional excursion, or range of a muscle, is directly influenced by the joint it crosses. For example, the range for the brachialis muscle is limited by the range available at the elbow joint. This is true of one-joint muscles (muscles with their proximal and distal attachments on the bones on either side of one joint). For two-joint or multijoint muscles (those muscles that cross over two or more joints), their range goes beyond the limits of any one joint they cross. An example of a two-joint muscle functioning at the elbow is the biceps brachii muscle. If it contracts and moves the elbow into flexion and the forearm into supination while simultaneously moving the shoulder into flexion, it shortens to a point known as *active insufficiency,* where it can shorten no more. This is one end of its range. The muscle is lengthened full range by extending the elbow, pronating the forearm, and simultaneously extending the shoulder. When fully elongated it is in a position known as *passive insufficiency.* Two-joint or multijoint muscles normally function in the midportion of their functional excursion, where ideal length-tension relations exist.[26]

To maintain normal ROM, the segments must be moved through their available ranges periodically, whether it is the available joint range or muscle range. It is recognized that many factors can lead to decreased ROM, such as systemic, joint, neurological, or muscular diseases; surgical or traumatic insults; or simply inactivity or immobilization for any reason. Therapeutically, ROM activities are administered to maintain joint and soft tissue mobility to minimize loss of tissue flexibility and contracture formation.[6] Extensive research by Salter has provided evidence of the benefits of movement on the healing of tissues in various pathological conditions in both the laboratory and clinical settings.[20-25]

The principles of ROM described in this chapter do not encompass stretching to increase range. Principles and techniques of stretching and joint mobilization for treating impaired mobility are described in Chapters 4 and 5.

## TYPES OF ROM EXERCISES

- **Passive ROM.** Passive ROM (PROM) is movement of a segment within the unrestricted ROM that is produced entirely by an *external force*; there is little to or no voluntary muscle contraction. The external force may be from gravity, a machine, another individual, or another part of the individual's own body.[8] PROM and passive stretching are not synonymous (see Chapter 4 for definitions and descriptions of passive stretching).
- **Active ROM.** Active ROM (AROM) is movement of a segment within the unrestricted ROM that is produced by active contraction of the *muscles* crossing that joint.
- **Active-Assistive ROM.** Active-assistive ROM (A-AROM) is a type of AROM in which assistance is provided manually or mechanically by an outside force because the prime mover muscles need assistance to complete the motion.

## INDICATIONS AND GOALS FOR ROM

### Passive ROM

#### Indications for PROM

- In the region where there is acute, inflamed tissue, passive motion is beneficial; active motion would be detrimental to the healing process. Inflammation after injury or surgery usually lasts 2 to 6 days.
- When a patient is not able to or not supposed to actively move a segment or segments of the body, as when comatose, paralyzed, or on complete bed rest, movement is provided by an external source.

#### Goals for PROM

The primary goal for PROM is to decrease the complications that would occur with immobilization, such as cartilage degeneration, adhesion and contracture formation, and sluggish circulation.[8,20,25] Specifically, the goals are to:

- Maintain joint and connective tissue mobility
- Minimize the effects of the formation of contractures
- Maintain mechanical elasticity of muscle
- Assist circulation and vascular dynamics
- Enhance synovial movement for cartilage nutrition and diffusion of materials in the joint
- Decrease or inhibit pain
- Assist with the healing process after injury or surgery
- Help maintain the patient's awareness of movement

#### Other Uses for PROM

- When a therapist is examining inert structures, PROM is used to determine limitations of motion, to determine joint stability, and to determine muscle and other soft tissue elasticity.
- When a therapist is teaching an active exercise program, PROM is used to demonstrate the desired motion.
- When a therapist is preparing a patient for stretching, PROM is often used preceding the passive stretching techniques.

### Active and Active-Assistive ROM

#### Indications for AROM

- Whenever a patient is able to contract the muscles actively and move a segment with or without assistance, AROM is used.
- When a patient has weak musculature and is unable to move a joint through the desired range (usually against gravity), A-AROM is used to provide enough assistance to the muscles in a carefully controlled manner so the muscle can function at its maximum level and be progressively strengthened. Once patients gain control of their ROM, they are progressed to manual or mechanical resistance exercises to improve muscle performance for a return to functional activities (see Chapter 6).
- AROM can be used for aerobic conditioning programs (see Chapter 7).

- When a segment of the body is immobilized for a period of time, AROM is used on the regions above and below the immobilized segment to maintain the areas in as normal a condition as possible and to prepare for new activities, such as walking with crutches.

### Goals for AROM

If there is no inflammation or contraindication to active motion, the same goals of PROM can be met with AROM. In addition, there are physiological benefits that result from active muscle contraction and motor learning from voluntary muscle control. Specific goals are to:

- Maintain physiological elasticity and contractility of the participating muscles
- Provide sensory feedback from the contracting muscles
- Provide a stimulus for bone and joint tissue integrity
- Increase circulation and prevent thrombus formation
- Develop coordination and motor skills for functional activities

 ## LIMITATIONS OF ROM EXERCISES

### Limitations of Passive Motion

True passive, relaxed ROM may be difficult to obtain when muscle is innervated and the patient is conscious. Passive motion *does not:*

- Prevent muscle atrophy
- Increase strength or endurance
- Assist circulation to the extent that active, voluntary muscle contraction does

### Limitations of Active ROM

For strong muscles, active ROM *does not* maintain or increase strength. It also *does not* develop skill or coordination except in the movement patterns used.

 ## PRECAUTIONS AND CONTRA-INDICATIONS TO ROM EXERCISES

Although both PROM and AROM are contraindicated under any circumstance when motion to a part is disruptive to the healing process (Box 3.1), complete immobility leads to adhesion and contracture formation, sluggish circulation, and a prolonged recovery time. In light of research by Salter[22] and others,[14] early, continuous PROM within a pain-free range has been shown to be beneficial to the healing and early recovery of many soft tissue and joint lesions (discussed later in the chapter). Historically, ROM has been contraindicated immediately after acute tears, fractures, and surgery; but because the benefits of controlled motion have demonstrated decreased pain and an increased rate of recovery, early controlled motion is used so long as the patient's tolerance is monitored.

---

> **BOX 3.1** **Summary of Precautions and Contraindications to Range of Motion Exercises**
>
> ROM should not be done when motion is disruptive to the healing process.
>
> - Carefully controlled motion within the limits of pain-free motion during early phases of healing has been shown to benefit healing and early recovery.
> - Signs of too much or the wrong motion include increased pain and inflammation.
>
> ROM should not be done when patient response or the condition is life-threatening.
>
> - PROM may be carefully initiated to major joints and AROM to ankles and feet to minimize venous stasis and thrombus formation.
> - After myocardial infarction, coronary artery bypass surgery, or percutaneous transluminal coronary angioplasty, AROM of upper extremities and limited walking are usually tolerated under careful monitoring of symptoms.

NOTE: ROM is not synonymous with stretching. For precautions and contraindications to passive and active stretching techniques, see Chapters 4 and 5.

It is imperative that the therapist recognizes the value as well as potential abuse of motion and stays within the range, speed, and tolerance of the patient during the acute recovery stage.[8] Additional trauma to the part is contraindicated. Signs of too much or the wrong motion include increased pain and increased inflammation (greater swelling, heat, and redness). See Chapter 10 for principles of when to use the various types of passive and active motion therapeutically.

Usually, AROM of the upper extremities and limited walking near the bed are tolerated as early exercises after myocardial infarction, coronary artery bypass surgery, and percutaneous transluminal coronary angioplasty.[7,10] Careful monitoring of symptoms, perceived exertion, and blood pressure is necessary. If the patient's response or the condition is life-threatening, PROM may be carefully initiated to the major joints along with some AROM to the ankles and feet to avoid venous stasis and thrombus formation. Individualized activities are initiated and progress gradually as the patient tolerates.[7,10]

 ## PRINCIPLES AND PROCEDURES FOR APPLYING ROM TECHNIQUES

### Examination, Evaluation, and Treatment Planning

1. Examine and evaluate the patient's impairments and level of function, determine any precautions and prognosis, and plan the intervention.

2. Determine the ability of the patient to participate in the ROM activity and whether PROM, A-AROM, or AROM can meet the immediate goals.
3. Determine the amount of motion that can be safely applied for the condition of the tissues and health of the individual.
4. Decide what patterns can best meet the goals. ROM techniques may be performed in the
    a. *Anatomic planes of motion*: frontal, sagittal, transverse
    b. *Muscle range of elongation*: antagonistic to the line of pull of the muscle
    c. *Combined patterns*: diagonal motions or movements that incorporate several planes of motion
    d. *Functional patterns*: motions used in activities of daily living (ADL)
5. Monitor the patient's general condition and responses during and after the examination and intervention; note any change in vital signs, any change in the warmth and color of the segment, and any change in the ROM, pain, or quality of movement.
6. Document and communicate findings and intervention.
7. Re-evaluate and modify the intervention as necessary.

## Patient Preparation

1. Communicate with the patient. Describe the plan and method of intervention to meet the goals.
2. Free the region from restrictive clothing, linen, splints, and dressings. Drape the patient as necessary.
3. Position the patient in a comfortable position with proper body alignment and stabilization but that also allows you to move the segment through the available ROM.
4. Position yourself so proper body mechanics can be used.

## Application of Techniques

1. To control movement, grasp the extremity around the joints. If the joints are painful, modify the grip, still providing support necessary for control.
2. Support areas of poor structural integrity, such as a hypermobile joint, recent fracture site, or paralyzed limb segment.
3. Move the segment through its complete pain-free range to the point of tissue resistance. Do not force beyond the available range. If you force motion, it becomes a stretching technique.
4. Perform the motions smoothly and rhythmically, with 5 to 10 repetitions. The number of repetitions depends on the objectives of the program and the patient's condition and response to the treatment.

## Application of PROM

1. During PROM the force for movement is external, being provided by a therapist or mechanical device. When appropriate, a patient may provide the force and be taught to move the part with a normal extremity.

2. No active resistance or assistance is given by the patient's muscles that cross the joint. If the muscles contract, it becomes an active exercise.
3. The motion is carried out within the free ROM, that is, the range that is available without forced motion or pain.

## Application of AROM

1. Demonstrate the motion desired using PROM; then ask the patient to perform the motion. Have your hands in position to assist or guide the patient if needed.
2. Provide assistance only as needed for smooth motion. When there is weakness, assistance may be required only at the beginning or the end of the ROM, or when the effect of gravity has the greatest moment arm (torque).
3. The motion is performed within the available ROM.

##  ROM TECHNIQUES

The descriptions of positions and ROM techniques in this section may be used for PROM as well as A-AROM and AROM. When making the transition from PROM to AROM, gravity has a significant impact especially in individuals with weak musculature. When the segment moves up against gravity, it may be necessary to provide assistance to the patient. However, when moving parallel to the ground (gravity eliminated or gravity neutral), the part may need only to be supported while the muscles take the part through the range. When the part moves downward, with gravity causing the motion, muscles antagonist to the motion become active and may need assistance in controlling the descent of the part. The therapist must be aware of these effects and modify the patient's position if needed to meet desired goals for A-AROM and AROM. Principles and techniques for progression to manual and mechanical resistance ROM to develop strength are described in Chapter 6.

The following descriptions are, for the most part, with the patient in the supine position. Alternate positions for many motions are possible and, for some motions, necessary. For efficiency, perform all motions possible in one position; then change the patient's position and perform all appropriate motions in that position, progressing the treatment with minimal turning of the patient. Individual body types or environmental limitations might necessitate variations of the suggested hand placements. Use of good body mechanics by the therapist while applying proper stabilization and motion to the patient to accomplish the goals and avoid injury to weakened structures is the primary consideration.

**NOTE:** The term *upper or top hand* means the hand of the therapist that is toward the patient's head; *bottom or lower hand* refers to the hand toward the patient's foot. Antagonistic ROMs are grouped together for ease of application.

# Upper Extremity

## Shoulder: Flexion and Extension (Fig. 3.1)

**Hand Placement and Procedure**

- Grasp the patient's arm under the elbow with your lower hand.
- With the top hand, cross over and grasp the wrist and palm of the patient's hand.
- Lift the arm through the available range and return.

**N O T E :** For normal motion, the scapula should be free to rotate upward as the shoulder flexes. If motion of only the glenohumeral joint is desired, the scapula is stabilized as described in the chapter on stretching (see Chapter 4).

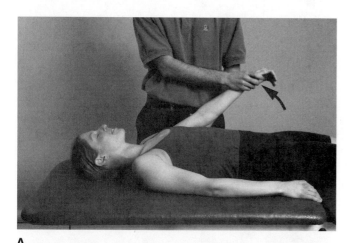

**A**

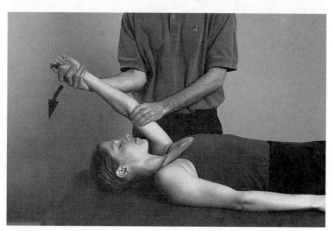

**B**

FIGURE 3.1 Hand placement and positions for (*A*) initiating and (*B*) completing shoulder flexion.

## Shoulder: Extension (Hyperextension) (Fig. 3.2)

**Alternate Positions**

Extension past zero is possible if the patient's shoulder is at the edge of the bed when supine or if the patient is positioned side-lying, prone, or sitting.

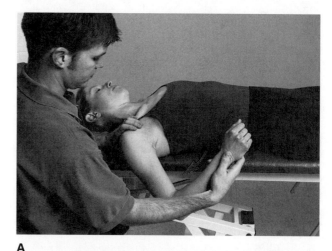

**A**

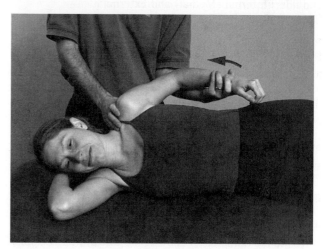

**B**

FIGURE 3.2 Hyperextension of the shoulder (*A*) with the patient at the edge of the bed and (*B*) with the patient side-lying.

## Shoulder: Abduction and Adduction (Fig. 3.3)

**Hand Placement and Procedure**

Use the same hand placement as with flexion, but move the arm out to the side. The elbow may be flexed.

**N O T E :** To reach full range of abduction, there must be external rotation of the humerus and upward rotation of the scapula.

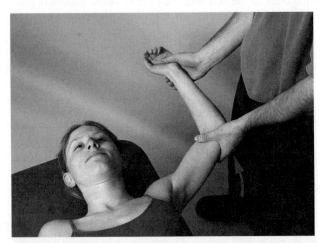

FIGURE 3.3 Abduction of the shoulder with the elbow flexed.

## Shoulder: Internal (Medial) and External (Lateral) Rotation (Fig. 3.4)

### Patient Position

If possible, the arm is abducted to 90°, the elbow is flexed to 90°, and the forearm is held in neutral position. Rotation may also be performed with the patient's arm at the side of the thorax, but full internal rotation is not possible in this position.

### Hand Placement and Procedure

- Grasp the hand and the wrist with your index finger between the patient's thumb and index finger.
- Place your thumb and the rest of your fingers on either side of the patient's wrist, thereby stabilizing the wrist.
- With the other hand, stabilize the elbow.
- Rotate the humerus by moving the forearm like a spoke on a wheel.

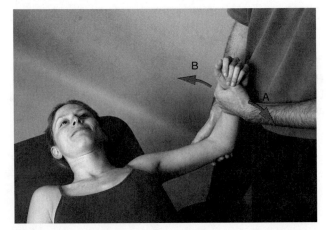

FIGURE 3.4 The 90/90 position for initiating (A) internal and (B) external rotation of the shoulder.

## Shoulder: Horizontal Abduction (Extension) and Adduction (Flexion) (Fig. 3.5)

### Patient Position

The patient's shoulder must be at the edge of the table to reach full horizontal abduction. Begin with the arm either flexed or abducted 90°.

### Hand Placement and Procedure

Hand placement is the same as with flexion, but turn your body and face the patient's head as you move the patient's arm out to the side and then across the body.

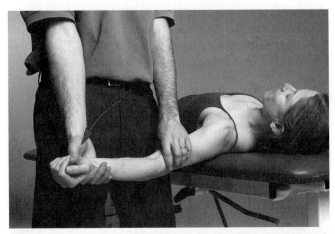

A

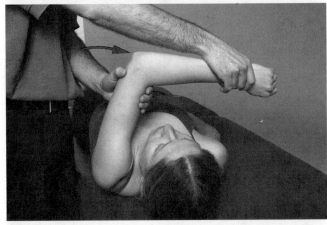

B

FIGURE 3.5 Horizontal (A) abduction and (B) adduction of the shoulder.

## Scapula: Elevation/Depression, Protraction/Retraction, and Upward/Downward Rotation (Fig. 3.6)

### Alternate Positions

The patient should be prone, with his or her arm at the side, or side-lying, with the patient facing the therapist and the patient's arm draped over the therapist's bottom arm (see Fig. 3.6B).

## Hand Placement and Procedure

- Cup the top hand over the acromion process and place the other hand around the inferior angle of the scapula.
- For elevation, depression, protraction, and retraction, the clavicle also moves as the scapular motions are directed at the acromion process.
- For rotation, direct the scapular motions at the inferior angle of the scapula while simultaneously pushing the acromion in the opposite direction to create a force couple turning effect.

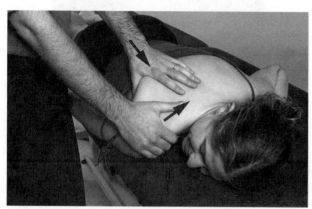

**A**

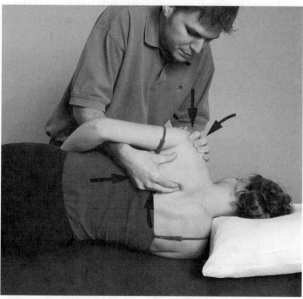

**B**

**FIGURE 3.6** ROM of the scapula with the patient (A) prone and with the patient (B) side-lying.

## Elbow: Flexion and Extension (Fig. 3.7)

### Hand Placement and Procedure
Hand placement is the same as with shoulder flexion except the motion occurs at the elbow as it is flexed and extended.

**N O T E :** Control forearm supination and pronation with your fingers around the distal forearm. Perform elbow flexion and extension with the forearm pronated as well as supinated. The scapula should not tip forward when the elbow extends, as it disguises the true range.

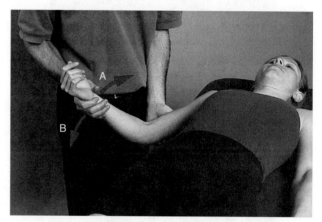

**FIGURE 3.7** Elbow flexion and extension with the forearm supinated.

## Elongation of Two-Joint Biceps Brachii Muscle

### Patient Position
To extend the shoulder beyond zero, position the patient's shoulder at the edge of the table when supine or position the patient prone lying, sitting, or standing.

### Hand Placement and Procedure

- First pronate the patient's forearm by grasping the wrist and extend the elbow while supporting it.
- Then extend (hyperextended) the shoulder to the point of tissue resistance in the anterior arm region. At this point, full available lengthening of the two-joint muscle is reached.

## Elongation of Two-Joint Long Head of the Triceps Brachii Muscle (Fig. 3.8)

### Alternate Positions
When near-normal range of the triceps brachii muscle is available, the patient must be sitting or standing to reach the full ROM. With marked limitation in muscle range, ROM can be performed in the supine position.

### Hand Placement and Procedure

- First, fully flex the patient's elbow with one hand on the distal forearm.
- Then flex the shoulder by lifting up on the humerus with the other hand under the elbow.
- Full available range is reached when discomfort is experienced in the posterior arm region.

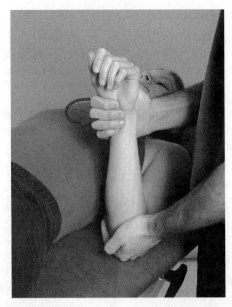

FIGURE 3.9 Pronation of the forearm.

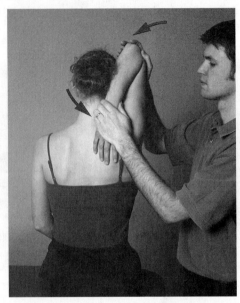

FIGURE 3.8 End ROM for the long head of the triceps brachii muscle.

### Forearm: Pronation and Supination (Fig. 3.9)

### Hand Placement and Procedure

- Grasp the patient's wrist, supporting the hand with the index finger and placing the thumb and the rest of the fingers on either side of the distal forearm.
- Stabilize the elbow with the other hand.
- The motion is a rolling of the radius around the ulna at the distal radius.

### Alternate Hand Placement
Sandwich the patient's distal forearm between the palms of both hands.

N O T E : Pronation and supination should be performed with the elbow both flexed and extended.

P R E C A U T I O N : Do not stress the wrist by twisting the hand; control the pronation and supination motion by moving the radius around the ulna.

### Wrist: Flexion (Palmar Flexion) and Extension (Dorsiflexion); Radial (Abduction) and Ulnar (Adduction) Deviation (Fig. 3.10)

### Hand Placement and Procedure
For all wrist motions, grasp the patient's hand just distal to the joint with one hand and stabilize the forearm with your other hand.

N O T E : The range of the extrinsic muscles to the fingers affect the range at the wrist if tension is placed on them. To obtain full range of the wrist joint, allow the fingers to move freely as you move the wrist.

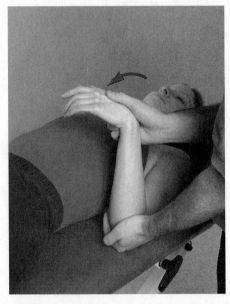

FIGURE 3.10 ROM at the wrist. Shown is wrist flexion; note that the fingers are free to move in response to passive tension in the extrinsic tendons.

## Hand: Cupping and Flattening the Arch of the Hand at the Carpometacarpal and Intermetacarpal Joints (Fig. 3.11)

### Hand Placement and Procedure

● Face the patient's hand; place the fingers of both of your hands in the palms of the patient's hand and your thenar eminences on the posterior aspect.
● Roll the metacarpals palmarward to increase the arch, and dorsalward to flatten it.

### Alternate Hand Placement

One hand is placed on the posterior aspect of the patient's hand, with the fingers and thumb cupping the metacarpals.

N O T E : Extension and abduction of the thumb at the carpometacarpal joint are important for maintaining the web space for functional movement of the hand. Isolated flexion-extension and abduction-adduction ROM of this joint should be performed by moving the first metacarpal while stabilizing the trapezium.

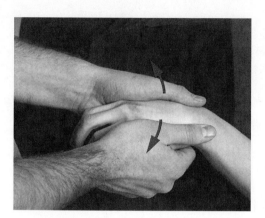

FIGURE 3.11 ROM to the arch of the hand.

## Joints of the Thumb and Fingers: Flexion and Extension and Abduction and Adduction (Fig. 3.12)

The joints of the thumbs and fingers include the metacarpophalangeal and interphalangeal joints.

### Hand Placement and Procedure

● Depending on the position of the patient, stabilize the forearm and hand on the bed or table or against your body.
● Move each joint of the patient's hand individually by stabilizing the proximal bone with the index finger and thumb of one hand and moving the distal bone with the index finger and thumb of the other hand.

### Alternate Procedure

Several joints can be moved simultaneously if proper stabilization is provided. Example: To move all the metacarpophalangeal joints of digits 2 through 5, stabilize the metacarpals with one hand and move all the proximal phalanges with the other hand.

N O T E : To accomplish full joint ROM, do not place tension on the extrinsic muscles going to the fingers. Tension on the muscles can be relieved by altering the wrist position as the fingers are moved.

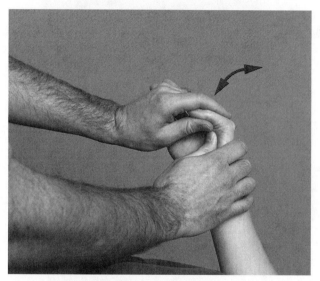

FIGURE 3.12 ROM to the metacarpophalangeal joint of the thumb.

## Elongation of Extrinsic Muscles of the Wrist and Hand: Flexor and Extensor Digitorum Muscles (Fig. 3.13)

### General Technique

To minimize compression of the small joints of the fingers, begin the motion with the distalmost joint. Elongate the muscles over one joint at a time, stabilize that joint, then elongate the muscle over the next joint until the multijoint muscles are at maximum length. This is particularly critical is there is restricted flexibility in the extrinsic musculature.

### Hand Placement and Procedure

● First move the distal interphalangeal joint and stabilize it; then move the proximal interphalangeal joint.
● Hold both these joints at the end of their range; then move the metacarpophalangeal joint to the end of the available range.
● Stabilize all the finger joints and begin to extend the wrist. When the patient feels discomfort in the forearm, the muscles are fully elongated.

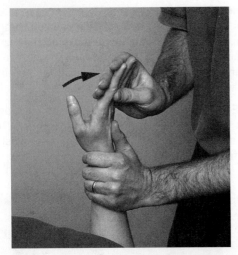

A

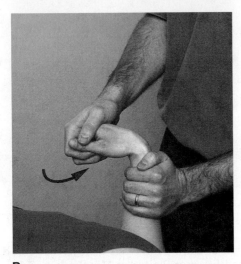

B

FIGURE 3.13 End of range for the (A) extrinsic finger flexors and (B) extensors.

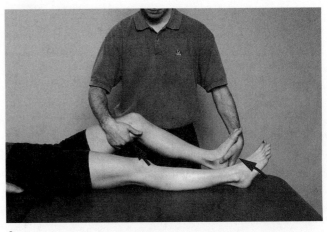

A

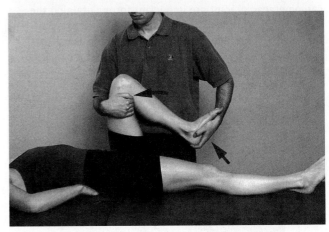

B

FIGURE 3.14 (A) Initiating and (B) completing combined hip and knee flexion.

## Lower Extremity

### Combined Hip and Knee: Flexion and Extension (Fig. 3.14)

**Hand Placement and Procedure**

● Support and lift the patient's leg with the palm and fingers of the top hand under the patient's knee and the lower hand under the heel.
● As the knee flexes full range, swing the fingers to the side of the thigh.

**N O T E :** To reach full range of hip flexion, the knee must also be flexed to release tension on the hamstring muscle group. To reach full range of knee flexion, the hip must be flexed to release tension on the rectus femoris muscle.

### Hip: Extension (Hyperextension) (Fig. 3.15)

**Alternate Positions**

Prone or side-lying must be used if the patient has near-normal or normal motion.

**Hand Placement and Procedure**

● If the patient is prone, lift the thigh with the bottom hand under the patient's knee; stabilize the pelvis with the top hand or arm.
● If the patient is side-lying, bring the bottom hand under the thigh and place the hand on the anterior surface; stabilize the pelvis with the top hand. For full range of hip extension, do not flex the knee full range, as the two-joint rectus femoris would then restrict the range.

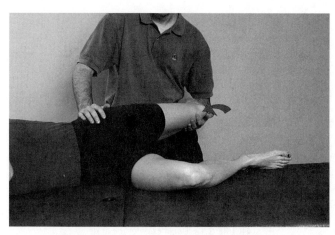

FIGURE 3.15 Hip extension with the patient side-lying.

## Elongation of the Two-Joint Hamstring Muscle Group (Fig. 3.16)

**Hand Placement and Procedure**

- Place the lower hand under the patient's heel and the upper hand across the anterior aspect of the patient's knee.
- Keep the knee in extension as the hip is flexed.
- If the knee requires support, cradle the patient's leg in your lower arm with your elbow flexed under the calf and your hand across the anterior aspect of the patient's knee. The other hand provides support or stabilization where needed.

**Variation**

If the hamstrings are so tight as to limit the knee from going into extension, the available range of the muscle is reached simply by extending the knee as far as the muscle allows and not moving the hip.

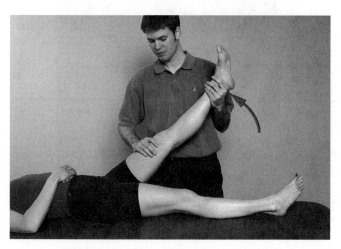

FIGURE 3.16 ROM to the hamstring muscle group.

## Elongation of the Two-Joint Rectus Femoris Muscle

**Alternate Positions**

The patient is supine, with knee flexed over the edge of the treatment table, or prone.

**Hand Placement and Procedure**

- When supine, stabilize the lumbar spine by flexing the hip and knee of the opposite lower extremity and placing the foot on the treatment table (hook lying).
- When prone, stabilize the pelvis with the top hand (see Fig. 4.31)
- Flex the patient's knee until tissue resistance is felt in the anterior thigh, which means the full available range is reached.

## Hip: Abduction and Adduction (Fig. 3.17)

**Hand Placement and Procedure**

- Support the patient's leg with the upper hand under the knee and the lower hand under the ankle.
- For full range of adduction, the opposite leg needs to be in a partially abducted position.
- Keep the patient's hip and knee in extension and neutral to rotation as abduction and adduction are performed.

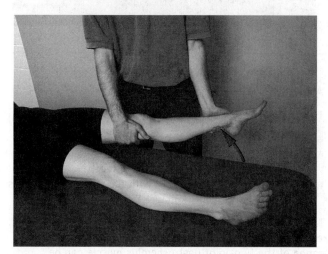

FIGURE 3.17 Abduction of the hip, maintaining the hip in extension and neutral to rotation.

## Hip: Internal (Medial) and External (Lateral) Rotation

**Hand Placement and Procedure with the Hip and Knee Extended**

- Grasp just proximal to the patient's knee with the top hand and just proximal to the ankle with the bottom hand.
- Roll the thigh inward and outward.

### Hand Placement and Procedure for Rotation With the Hip and Knee Flexed (Fig. 3.18)

- Flex the patient's hip and knee to 90°; support the knee with the top hand.
- If the knee is unstable, cradle the thigh and support the proximal calf and knee with the bottom hand.
- Rotate the femur by moving the leg like a pendulum.
- This hand placement provides some support to the knee but should be used with caution if there is knee instability.

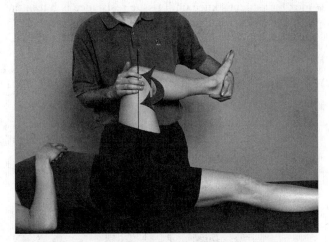

FIGURE 3.18 Rotation of the hip with the hip positioned in 90° of flexion.

### Ankle: Dorsiflexion (Fig. 3.19)

#### Hand Placement and Procedure

- Stabilize around the malleoli with the top hand.
- Cup the patient's heel with the bottom hand and place the forearm along the bottom of the foot.
- Pull the calcaneus distalward with the thumb and fingers while pushing upward with the forearm.

N O T E : If the knee is flexed, full range of the ankle joint can be obtained. If the knee is extended, the lengthened range of the two-joint gastrocnemius muscle can be obtained, but the gastrocnemius limits full range of dorsiflexion. Apply dorsiflexion in both positions of the knee to provide range to both the joint and the muscle.

### Ankle: Plantarflexion

#### Hand Placement and Procedure

- Support the heel with the bottom hand.
- Place the top hand on the dorsum of the foot and push it into plantarflexion.

N O T E : In bed-bound patients, the ankle tends to assume a plantarflexed position from the weight of the blankets and the pull of gravity, so this motion may not need to be performed.

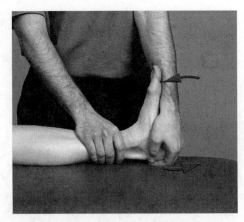

FIGURE 3.19 Dorsiflexion of the ankle.

### Subtalar (Lower Ankle) Joint: Inversion and Eversion (Fig. 3.20)

#### Hand Placement and Procedure

- Using the bottom hand, place the thumb medial and the fingers lateral to the joint on either side of the heel.
- Turn the heel inward and outward.

N O T E : Supination of the foot may be combined with inversion, and pronation may be combined with eversion.

### Transverse Tarsal Joint

#### Hand Placement and Procedure

- Stabilize the patient's talus and calcaneus with one hand.
- With the other hand, grasp around the navicular and cuboid.
- Gently rotate the midfoot by lifting and lowering the arch.

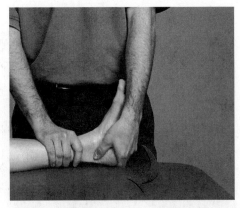

FIGURE 3.20 Inversion of the subtalar joint.

### Joints of the Toes: Flexion and Extension and Abduction and Adduction (Metatarsophalangeal and Interphalangeal Joints) (Fig. 3.21)

**Hand Placement and Procedure**

- Stabilize the bone proximal to the joint that is to be moved with one hand, and move the distal bone with the other hand.
- The technique is the same as for ROM of the fingers.

**Alternate Procedure**
Several joints of the toes can be moved simultaneously if care is taken not to stress any structure.

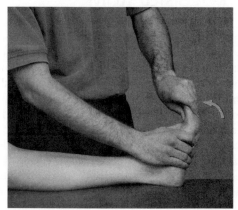

FIGURE 3.21 Extension of the metatarsophalangeal joint of the large toe.

## Cervical Spine

**Position of Therapist and Hand Placement**
Standing at the end of the treatment table, securely grasp the patient's head by placing both hands under the occipital region.

### Flexion (Forward Bending) (Fig. 3.22A)

**Procedure**

- Lift the head as though it were nodding (chin towards larynx) to flex the head on the neck.
- Once full nodding is complete, continue to flex the cervical spine and lift the head toward the sternum.

### Extension (Backward Bending or Hyperextension)

**Procedure**
Tip the head backward.

N O T E : If the patient is supine, only the head and upper cervical spine can be extended; the head must clear the end of the table to extend the entire cervical spine. The patient may also be prone or sitting.

### Lateral Flexion (Side Bending) and Rotation (Fig. 3.22B)

**Procedure**
Maintain the cervical spine neutral to flexion and extension as you direct the head and neck into side bending (approximate the ear toward the shoulder) and rotation (rotate from side to side).

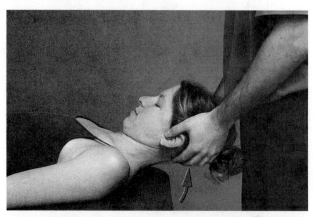

A

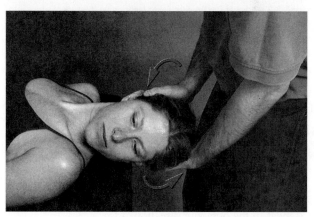

B

FIGURE 3.22 Cervical (A) flexion and (B) rotation.

## Lumbar Spine

### Flexion (Fig. 3.23)

**Hand Placement and Procedure**

- Bring both of the patient's knees to the chest by lifting under the knees (hip and knee flexion).
- Flexion of the spine occurs as the hips are flexed full range and the pelvis starts to rotate posteriorly.
- Greater range of flexion can be obtained by lifting under the patient's sacrum with the lower hand.

### Extension

**Alternate Position**
The patient is prone.

## Hand Placement and Procedure

With hands under the thighs, lift the thighs upward until the pelvis rotates anteriorly and the lumbar spine extends.

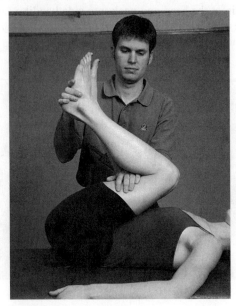

FIGURE 3.23 Lumbar flexion is achieved by bringing the patient's hips into flexion until the pelvis rotates posteriorly.

## Rotation (Fig. 3.24)

**Alternate Position**
The patient is hook-lying.

**Hand Placement and Procedure**

- Push both of the patient's knees laterally in one direction until the pelvis on the opposite side comes up off the treatment table.
- Stabilize the patient's thorax with the top hand.
- Repeat in the opposite direction.

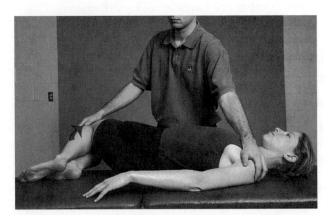

FIGURE 3.24 Rotation of the lumbar spine results when the thorax is stabilized and the pelvis lifts off the table as far as allowed.

## Combined Patterns of Motion

Effective and efficient ROM can be administered by combining several joint motions that transect several planes resulting in oblique or diagonal patterns. For example, wrist flexion may be combined with ulnar deviation, or shoulder flexion may be combined with abduction and lateral rotation so movement follows functional patterns. Proprioceptive neuromuscular facilitation (PNF) patterns of movement follow specific guidelines and may be effectively used for PROM, A-AROM, or AROM techniques (see Chapter 6 for descriptions of these patterns).

# ● SELF–ASSISTED ROM

Patient involvement in self-care should begin as soon as the individual is able to understand and learn what to do. Even with weakness or paralysis, the patient can learn how to move the involved part and be instructed in the importance of movement within safe parameters. After surgery or traumatic injury, self-assisted ROM (S-AROM) is used to protect the healing tissues when more intensive muscle contraction is contraindicated. A variety of devices as well as use of a normal extremity may be used to meet the goals of PROM or A-AROM. Incorporation of S-AROM then becomes a part of the home exercise program (Box 3.2).

---

**BOX 3.2    Self-Assisted Range of Motion Techniques**

**Forms of Self-Assisted ROM**
- Manual
- Equipment
  - Wand or T-bar
  - Finger ladder, wall climbing, ball rolling
  - Pulleys
  - Skate board/powder board
  - Reciprocal exercise devices

**Guidelines for Teaching Self-Assisted ROM**
- Educate the patient on the value of the motion.
- Teach the patient correct body alignment and stabilization.
- Observe patient performance and correct any substitute or unsafe motions.
- If equipment is used, be sure all hazards are eliminated for application to be safe.
- Provide drawings and clear guidelines for number of repetitions and frequency.

Review the exercises at a follow-up session. Modify or progress the exercise program based on the patient response and treatment plan for meeting the outcome goals.

## Self-Assistance

With cases of unilateral weakness or paralysis, or during early stages of recovery after trauma or surgery, the patient can be taught to use the uninvolved extremity to move the involved extremity through ranges of motion. These exercises may be done supine, sitting, or standing. The effects of gravity change with patient positioning, so when lifting the part against gravity, gravity provides a resistive force against the prime motion and therefore the prime mover requires assistance. When the extremity moves downward, gravity causes the motion; and the antagonists need assistance to control the motion eccentrically.

### Arm and Forearm

Instruct the patient to reach across the body with the uninvolved (or assisting) extremity and grasp the involved extremity around the wrist, supporting the wrist and hand (Fig. 3.25).

- ***Shoulder flexion and extension.*** The patient lifts the involved extremity over the head and returns it to the side (Fig. 3.25).

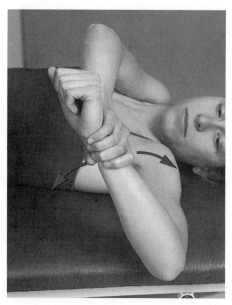

FIGURE 3.26 Arm position of patient for giving self-assisted ROM to internal and external rotation of shoulder.

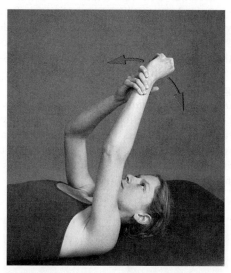

FIGURE 3.25 Patient giving self-assisted ROM to shoulder flexion and extension. Horizontal abduction and adduction can be applied with the same hand placement.

- ***Shoulder horizontal abduction and adduction.*** Beginning with the arm abducted 90°, the patient pulls the extremity across the chest and returns it out to the side.
- ***Shoulder rotation.*** Beginning with the arm at the patient's side in slight abduction or abducted 90° and elbow flexed 90°, the patient rotates the forearm with the uninvolved extremity (Fig. 3.26). It is important to emphasize rotating the humerus, not merely flexing and extending the elbow.

- ***Elbow flexion and extension.*** The patient bends the elbow until the hand is near the shoulder and then moves the hand down toward the side of the leg.
- ***Pronation and supination of the forearm.*** Beginning with the forearm resting across the body, the patient rotates the radius around the ulna; emphasize to the patient not to twist the hand at the wrist joint.

### Wrist and Hand

The patient moves the uninvolved fingers to the dorsum of the hand and the thumb into the palm of the hand.

- ***Wrist flexion and extension and radial and ulnar deviation.*** The patient moves the wrist in all directions, applying no pressure against the fingers (Fig. 3.27).

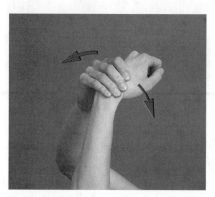

FIGURE 3.27 Patient applying self-assisted wrist flexion and extension, with no pressure against the fingers.

• *Finger flexion and extension.* The patient uses the uninvolved thumb to extend the involved fingers and cups the normal fingers over the dorsum of the involved fingers to flex them (Fig. 3.28).

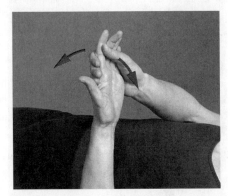

FIGURE 3.28 Patient applying self-assisted finger flexion and extension.

• *Thumb flexion with opposition and extension with reposition.* The patient cups the uninvolved fingers around the radial border of the thenar eminence of the involved thumb and places the uninvolved thumb along the palmar surface of the involved thumb to extend it (Fig. 3.29). To flex and oppose the thumb, the patient cups the normal hand around the dorsal surface of the involved hand and pushes the first metacarpal toward the little finger.

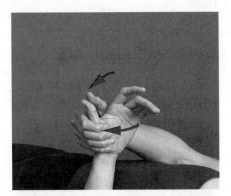

FIGURE 3.29 Patient applying self-assisted thumb extension.

## Hip and Knee

• *Hip and knee flexion.* With the patient supine, instruct the patient to initiate the motion by lifting up the involved knee with a strap or belt under the involved knee (Fig. 3.30). The patient can then grasp the knee with one or both hands to bring the knee up toward the chest to complete the range. With the patient sitting, he or she may lift the thigh with the hands and flex the knee to the end of its available range.

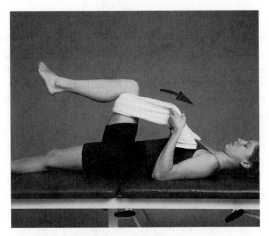

FIGURE 3.30 Self-assisted flexion of the hip.

• *Hip abduction and adduction.* It is difficult for the weak patient to assist the lower extremities into abduction and adduction when supine owing to the weight of the leg and he friction of the bed surface. It is necessary, though, for the individual to move a weak lower extremity from side to side for bed mobility. To practice this functional activity as an exercise, instruct the patient to slide the normal foot from the knee down to the ankle and then move the involved extremity from side to side. S-AROM can be performed sitting by using the hands to assist moving the thigh outward and inward.

• *Combined hip abduction with external rotation.* The patient is sitting on the floor or on a bed with the back supported and the involved hip and knee flexed and foot resting on the surface. The knee is moved outward (toward the table/bed) and back inward, with assistance from the upper extremity (Fig. 3.31).

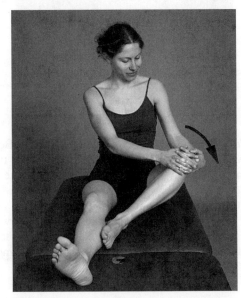

FIGURE 3.31 Self-assisted hip abduction and external rotation.

## Ankle and Toes

 The patient sits with the involved extremity crossed over the uninvolved one so the distal leg rests on the normal knee. The uninvolved hand moves the involved ankle into dorsiflexion, plantarflexion, inversion, and eversion, and toe flexion and extension (Fig. 3.32).

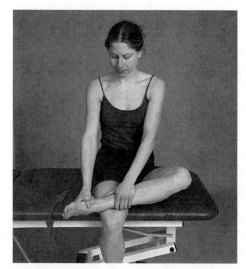

FIGURE 3.32 Position of patient and hand placement for self-assisted ankle and toe motions; shown is inversion and eversion.

## Wand (T–Bar) Exercises

When a patient has voluntary muscle control in an involved upper extremity but needs guidance or motivation to complete the ROM in the shoulder or elbow, a wand (dowel rod, cane, wooden stick, T-bar, or similar object) can be used to provide assistance (Fig. 3.33).

The choice of position is based on the patient's level of function. Most of the techniques can be performed supine if maximum protection is needed. Sitting or standing requires greater control. Choice of position is also guided by the effects of gravity on the weak muscles. Initially, guide the patient through the proper motion for each activity to ensure that he or she does not use substitute motions. The patient grasps the wand with both hands, and the normal extremity guides and controls the motions.

 **Shoulder flexion and return.** The wand is grasped with the hands a shoulder-width apart. The wand is lifted forward and upward through the available range, with the elbows kept in extension if possible (Fig. 3.33A). Scapulohumeral motion should be smooth; do not allow scapular elevation or trunk movement.
 **Shoulder horizontal abduction and adduction.** The wand is lifted to 90° shoulder flexion. Keeping the elbows extended, the patient pushes and pulls the wand back and forth across the chest through the available range (Fig. 3.33B). Do not allow trunk rotation.
 **Shoulder internal and external rotation.** The patient's arms are at the sides, and the elbows are flexed 90°. Rotation of the arms is accomplished by moving the

wand from side to side across the trunk while maintaining the elbows at the side (Fig. 3.33C). The rotation should occur in the humerus; do not allow elbow flexion and extension. To prevent substitute motions as well as provide a slight distraction force to the glenohumeral joint, a small towel roll may be placed in the axilla with instruction to the patient to "keep the roll in place."

### Alternate Position
The patient's shoulders are abducted 90° and the elbows flexed 90°. For external rotation, the wand is moved toward the patient's head; for internal rotation, the wand is moved toward the waistline.

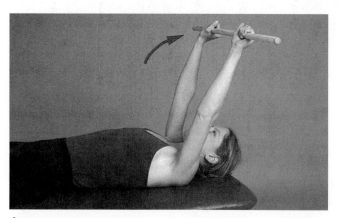

A

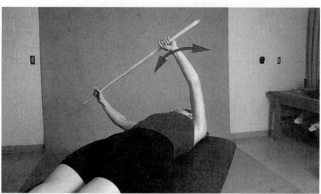

B

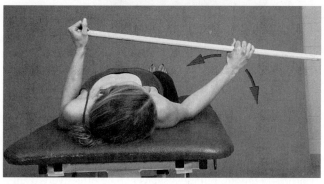

C

FIGURE 3.33 Patient using a wand for self-assisted shoulder (A) flexion, (B) horizontal abduction/adduction (C) rotation.

● *Elbow flexion and extension.* The patient's forearms may be pronated or supinated; the hands grasp the wand a shoulder-width apart. Instruct the patient to flex and extend the elbows.

● *Shoulder hyperextension.* The patient may be standing or prone. He or she places the wand behind the buttocks, grasps the wand with hands a shoulder-width apart, and then lifts the wand backward away from the trunk. The patient should avoid trunk motion.

● *Variations and combinations of movements.* For example, the patient begins with the wand behind the buttocks and then moves the wand up the back to achieve scapular winging, shoulder internal rotation, and elbow flexion.

## Wall Climbing

Wall climbing (or use of a device such as a finger ladder) can provide the patient with objective reinforcement and, therefore, motivation for performing shoulder ROM. Wall markings may also be used to provide visual feedback for the height reached. The arm may be moved into flexion or abduction (Fig. 3.34). The patient steps closer to the wall as the arm is elevated.

**P R E C A U T I O N :** The patient must be taught the proper motions and not allowed to substitute with trunk side bending, toe raising, or shoulder shrugging.

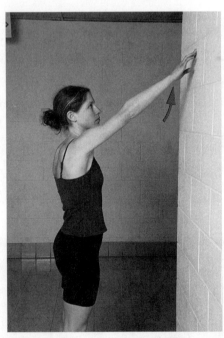

FIGURE 3.34 Wall climbing for shoulder elevation.

## Overhead Pulleys

If properly taught, pulley systems can be effectively used to assist an involved extremity in performing ROM. The pulley has been demonstrated to utilize significantly more muscle activity than therapist-assisted ROM and continu-

ous passive motion machines (described later in the chapter), so this form of assistance should be used only when muscle activity is desired.[5]

For home use, a single pulley may be attached to a strap that is held in place by closing the strap in a door. A pulley may also be attached to an overhead bar or affixed to the ceiling. The patient should be set up so the pulley is directly over the joint that is moving or so the line of pull is effectively moving the extremity and not just compressing the joint surfaces together. The patient may be sitting, standing, or supine.

### Shoulder ROM (Fig. 3.35)

Instruct the patient to hold one handle in each hand and, with the normal hand, pull the rope and lift the involved extremity forward (flexion), out to the side (abduction), or in the plane of the scapula (scaption is 30° forward of the frontal plane). The patient should not shrug the shoulder (scapular elevation) or lean the trunk. Guide and instruct the patient so there is smooth motion.

**P R E C A U T I O N :** Assistive pulley activities for the shoulder are easily misused by the patient, resulting in compression of the humerus against the acromion process. Continual compression leads to pain and decreased function. Proper patient selection and appropriate instruction can avoid this problem. If a patient cannot learn to use the pulley with proper shoulder mechanics, these exercises should not be performed. Discontinue this activity if there is increased pain or decreased mobility.

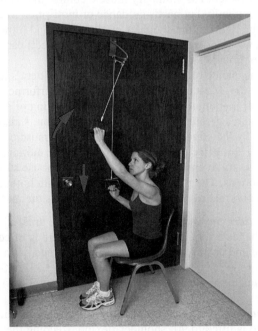

FIGURE 3.35 Use of overhead pulleys to assist shoulder elevation.

### Elbow Flexion

With the arm stabilized along the side of the trunk, the patient lifts the forearm and bends the elbow.

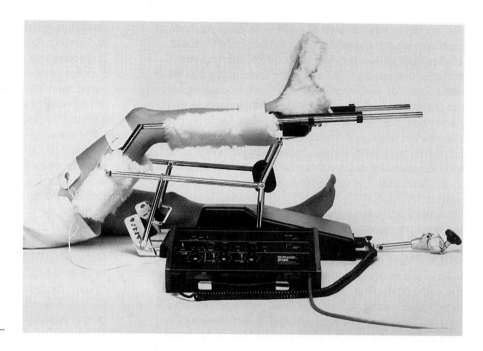

**FIGURE 3.36** CM-100 Continuous Motion Device. (Courtesy of Empi, St. Paul, MN.)

## Skate Board/Powder Board

Use of a friction-free surface may encourage movement without the resistance of gravity or friction. If available, a skate with rollers may be used. Other methods include using powder on the surface or placing a towel under the extremity so it can slide along the smooth surface of the board. Any motion can be done, but most common are abduction/adduction of the hip while supine and horizontal abduction/adduction of the shoulder while sitting.

## Reciprocal Exercise Unit

Several devices, such as a bicycle, upper body, or lower body ergometer, or a reciprocal exercise unit can be set up to provide some flexion and extension to an involved extremity using the strength of the normal extremity. Movable devices are available that can be attached to a patient's bed, wheelchair, or standard chair. The circumference of motion as well as excursion of the extremities can be adjusted. A reciprocal exercise unit has additional exercise benefits in that it can be used for reciprocal patterning, endurance training, and strengthening by changing the parameters of the exercise and monitoring the heart rate and fatigue. (See Chapter 3 for principles of resistance exercise and Chapter 6 for principles of aerobic exercise.)

##  CONTINUOUS PASSIVE MOTION

*Continuous passive motion* (CPM) refers to passive motion performed by a mechanical device that moves a joint slowly and continuously through a controlled ROM. The mechanical devices that exist for nearly every joint in the body (Fig. 3.36) were developed as a result of

the research by Robert Salter, who demonstrated that continual passive motion has beneficial healing effects on diseased or injured joint structures and soft tissues in animal and clinical studies.[20-25] Since the development of CPM, many studies have been done to determine the parameters of application; but because the devices are used for many conditions, and studies have used various protocols with varying research designs, no definitive delineation has been established.[3,13,17]

## Benefits of CPM

CPM has been reported to be effective in lessening the negative effects of joint immobilization in conditions such as arthritis, contractures, and intra-articular fractures; it has also improved the recovery rate and ROM after a variety of surgical procedures.[13,17,20-25,27] Basic research and clinical studies reported by Salter have demonstrated the effectiveness of CPM in a number of areas.

- Prevents development of adhesions and contractures and thus joint stiffness
- Provides a stimulating effect on the healing of tendons and ligaments
- Enhances healing of incisions over the moving joint
- Increases synovial fluid lubrication of the joint and thus increases the rate of intra-articular cartilage healing and regeneration
- Prevents the degrading effects of immobilization
- Provides a quicker return of ROM
- Decreases postoperative pain

### ⦿ Focus on Evidence _____

Recent studies have compared short- and long-term outcomes of CPM use after various types of surgery using various parameters as well as CPM with other methods of early movement and positioning.[1,4,5,11,12,17-19,28,30] Some studies have shown no significant difference between patients undergoing CPM and those undergoing PROM or other forms of early motion.[4,11,12,19,29] Many studies support the short-term benefits of CPM use after surgery in that patients gain ROM more quickly and therefore may experience earlier discharge from the hospital when CPM is used compared with other forms of intervention. However, long-term functional gains are reported to be no different from those in patients who underwent other forms of early motion.[3,28,30]

Some studies have identified detrimental effects, such as the need for greater analgesic intervention and increased postoperative blood drainage, when using CPM[18,29] in contrast to claims that CPM decreases postoperative pain and postoperative complications.[21-25,27] Cost-effectiveness of the CPM equipment, patient compliance, utilization and supervision of equipment by trained personnel, length of hospital stay, speed of recovery, and determination of appropriate patient populations become issues to consider when making the choice of whether or not to utilize CPM devices.[12,15]

## General Guidelines for CPM

General guidelines for CPM are as follows.[2,3,9,13,14,20,25]

1. The device may be applied to the involved extremity immediately after surgery while the patient is still under anesthesia or as soon as possible if bulky dressings prevent early motion.
2. The arc of motion for the joint is determined. Often a low arc of 20° to 30° is used initially and progressed 10° to 15° per day as tolerated. The portion of the range used initially is based on the range available and patient tolerance. One study looked at accelerating the range of knee flexion after total knee arthroplasty and found that a greater range and earlier discharge was attained for that group of patients,[30] although there was no difference between the groups at 4 weeks.
3. The rate of motion is determined; usually 1 cycle/45 sec or 2 min is well tolerated.
4. The amount of time on the CPM machine varies for different protocols: anywhere from continuous for 24 hours to continuous for 1 hour three times a day.[9,14,25] The longer periods of time per day reportedly result in a shorter hospital stay, fewer postoperative complications, and greater ROM at discharge,[9] although no significant difference was found in a study comparing CPM for 5 hr/day with CPM for 20 hr/day.[2] A recent study compared short-duration CPM (3 to 5 hr/day) with long duration CPM (10 to 12 hr/day) and found that patient compliance and the most gained range occurred with a CPM duration of 4 to 8 hours.[3]
5. Physical therapy treatments are usually initiated during periods when the patient is not on CPM, including active-assistive and muscle-setting exercises. It is important that patients learn to use and develop motor control of the ROM as motion improves.
6. The duration minimum for CPM is usually less than 1 week or when a satisfactory range of motion is reached. Because CPM devices are portable, home use is possible in cases where the therapist or physician deems additional time would be beneficial. In these cases, the patient, a family member, or a caregiver is instructed in proper application.
7. CPM machines are designed to be adjustable, easily controlled, versatile, and portable. Some are battery operated (with rechargeable batteries) to allow the individual to wear the device for up to 8 hours while functioning with daily activities.

# ROM THROUGH FUNCTIONAL PATTERNS

To accomplish motion through functional patterns, first determine what pattern of movement is desired and then move the extremity through that pattern using manual assistance, mechanical assistance if it is appropriate, or self-assistance from the patient. Functional patterning can be beneficial in initiating the teaching of ADL and instrumental activities of daily living (IADL) as well as in instructing patients with visual impairments in functional activities. Utilizing functional patterns helps the patient recognize the purpose and value of ROM exercises and develop motor patterns that can be used in daily activities as strength and endurance improves. Box 3.3 identifies some examples and the basic motions that are utilized. When the patient no longer requires assistance to perform the pattern safely and correctly, the activity is incorporated into his or her daily activities so motor learning is reinforced and the motion becomes functional.

## BOX 3.3 Functional Range of Motion Activities

Early ROM training for functional upper extremity and neck patterns may include activities such as

- Grasping an eating utensil; utilizing finger extension and flexion
- Eating (hand to mouth); utilizing elbow flexion and forearm supination and some shoulder flexion, abduction, and lateral rotation
- Reaching to various shelf heights; utilizing shoulder flexion and elbow extension
- Brushing or combing back of hair; utilizing shoulder abduction and lateral rotation, elbow flexion, and cervical rotation
- Holding a phone to the ear; shoulder lateral rotation, forearm supination, and cervical side bend
- Donning or doffing a shirt or jacket; utilizing shoulder extension, lateral rotation, elbow flexion and extension

- Reaching out a car window to an ATM machine; utilizing shoulder abduction, lateral rotation, elbow extension, and some lateral bending of the trunk

Early ROM training for functional lower extremity and trunk patterns may include activities such as

- Going from supine to sitting at the side of a bed; utilizing hip abduction and adduction followed by hip and knee flexion
- Standing up/sitting down and walking; utilizing hip and knee flexion and extension, ankle dorsi and plantar flexion and some hip rotation
- Putting on socks and shoes; utilizing hip external rotation and abduction, knee flexion and ankle dorsi and plantar flexion, and trunk flexion

# INDEPENDENT LEARNING ACTIVITIES

## ● Critical Thinking and Discussion

1. Analyze a variety of functional activities, such as grooming, dressing, and bathing, and determine the functional ranges needed to perform each task.
2. Look at the effects of gravity or other forces on the ROM for each activity in #1. If you had a patient who was unable to do the activity because of an inability to control the range needed, determine how you would establish an exercise program to begin preparing the individual to develop the desired function.

## ● Laboratory Practice

1. Perform PROM of the upper and lower extremities with your partner placed in the following positions: prone, side-lying, sitting.
   a. What are the advantages and disadvantages of each of the positions for some of the ranges, such as shoulder and hip extension, knee flexion with the hip extended, rotation of the hip?
   b. Progress the PROM to A-AROM and AROM and determine the effects of gravity and the effort required in these positions compared to that in the supine position.
2. Compare the ROMs of the hip, knee, and ankle when each of the two joint muscles is elongated over its respective joint versus when each of the muscles is slack.

# REFERENCES

1. Alfredson, H, Lorentzon, R: Superior results with continuous passive motion compared to active motion after periosteal transplantation: a retrospective study of human patella cartilage defect treatment. Knee Surg Sports Traumatol Arthrosc 7(4):232, 1999.
2. Basso, DM, Knapp, L: Comparison of two continuous passive motion protocols for patients with total knee implants. Phys Ther 67:360, 1987.
3. Chiarello, CM, Gunersen, L, O'Halloran, T: The effect of continuous passive motion duration and increment on range of motion in total knee arthroplasty patients. J Orthop Sports Phys Ther 25(2):119, 1997.
4. Denis, M, Moffet, H, Caron, F, et al: Effectiveness of continuous passive motion and conventional physical therapy after total knee arthroplasty: a randomized clinical trial. Phys Ther 86(2):174–185, 2006.
5. Dockery, ML, Wright, TW, LaStayo, P: Electromyography of the shoulder: an analysis of passive modes of exercise. Orthopedics 11:1181, 1998.
6. Donatelli, R, Owens-Burckhart, H: Effects of immobilization on the extensibility of periarticular connective tissue. J Orthop Sports Phys Ther 3:67, 1981.
7. Fletcher, GF, et al: Exercise Standards: A Statement for Health Professionals. American Heart Association, Dallas, 1991.
8. Frank, C, et al: Physiology and therapeutic value of passive joint motion. Clin Orthop 185:113, 1984.
9. Gose, J: Continuous passive motion in the postoperative treatment of patients with total knee replacement. Phys Ther 67:39, 1987.
10. Guidelines for Exercise Testing and Prescription, ed 4. American College of Sports Medicine, Lea & Febiger, Philadelphia, 1991.
11. Kumar, PJ, McPherson, EJ, et al: Rehabilitation after total knee arthroplasty: a comparison of 2 rehabilitation techniques. Clin Orthop 331:93, 1996.
12. LaStayo, PC, Wright T, et al: Continuous passive motion after repair of the rotator cuff: a prospective outcome study. J Bone Joint Surg Am 80(7):1002, 1998.
13. LaStayo, PC: Continuous passive motion for the upper extremity. In Hunter, JM, MacKin, EJ, Callahan AD (eds) Rehabilitation of the Hand: Surgery and Therapy, ed 4. Mosby, St/ Louis, 1995.
14. McCarthy, MR, et al: The clinical use of continuous passive motion in physical therapy. J Orthop Sports Phys Ther 15:132, 1992.

15. Nadler, SF, Malanga, GA, Jimmerman, JR: Continuous passive motion in the rehabilitation setting: a retrospective study. Am J Phys Med Rehabil 72(3):162, 1993.

16. Norkin, CC, White, DJ: Measurement of Joint Motion: A Guide to Goniometry, ed 3. FA Davis, Philadelphia, 2003.

17. O'Driscoll, SW, Giori, NJ: Continuous passive motion (CPM) theory and principles of clinical application. J Rehabil Res Dev 37(2):179, 2000.

18. Pope, RO, Corcoran, S, et al: Continuous passive motion after primary total knee arthroplasty: does it offer any benefits? J Bone Joint Surg Br 79(6):914, 1997.

19. Rosen, MA, Jackson, DW, Atwell, EA: The efficacy of continuous passive motion in the rehabilitation of anterior cruciate ligament reconstructions. Am J Sports Med 20(2):122, 1992.

20. Salter, RB: History of rest and motion and the scientific basis for early continuous passive motion. Hand Clin 12(1):1, 1996.

21. Salter, RB, Simmens, DF, Malcolm, BW: The biological effects of continuous passive motion on the healing of full thickness defects in articular cartilage. J Bone Joint Surg Am 62:1232, 1980.

22. Salter, RB: The prevention of arthritis through the preservation of cartilage. J Can Assoc Radiol 31:5, 1981.

23. Salter, RB, Bell, RS, Keely, FW: The protective effect of continuous passive motion on living cartilage in acute septic arthritis. Clin Orthop 159:223, 1981.

24. Salter, RB: Textbook of Disorders and Injuries of the Musculoskeletal System, ed 3. Williams & Wilkins, Baltimore, 1999.

25. Salter, RB, et al: Clinical application of basic research on continuous passive motion for disorders and injuries of synovial joints. J Orthop Res 1:325, 1984.

26. Smith, LK, Weiss, EL, Lehmkuhl, LD: Brunnstrom's Clinical Kinesiology, ed 5. FA Davis, Philadelphia, 1996.

27. Stap, LJ, Woodfin, PM: Continuous passive motion in the treatment of knee flexion contractures: a case report. Phys Ther 66:1720, 1986.

28. Wasilewski, SA, Woods, LC, et al: Value of continuous passive motion in total knee arthroplasty. Orthopedics 13(3):291, 1990.

29. Witherow, GE, Bollen, SR, Pinczewski, LA: The use of continuous passive motion after arthroscopically assisted anterior cruciate ligament reconstruction: help or hindrance? Knee Surg Sports Traumatol Arthrosc 1(2):68, 1993.

30. Yashar, AA, Venn Watson, E, et al: Continuous passive motion with accelerated flexion after total knee arthroplasty. Clin Orthop 345:38, 1997.

# Stretching for Impaired Mobility

The term *mobility* can be described based on two different but interrelated parameters. It is often defined as the ability of structures or segments of the body to move or be moved to allow the presence of range of motion for functional activities *(functional ROM)*.[1,134] It can also be defined as the ability of an individual to initiate, control, or sustain active movements of the body to perform simple to complex motor skills *(functional mobility)*.[38,118,134] Mobility, as it relates to functional ROM, is associated with joint integrity as well as the *flexibility* (i.e., *extensibility* of soft tissues that cross or surround joints—muscles, tendons, fascia, joint capsules, ligaments, nerves, blood vessels, skin), which are necessary for unrestricted, pain-free movements of the body during functional tasks of daily living. The ROM needed for the performance of functional activities does not necessarily mean full or "normal" ROM.

Sufficient mobility of soft tissues and ROM of joints must be supported by a requisite level of muscle strength and endurance and neuromuscular control to allow the body to accommodate to imposed stresses placed upon it during functional movement and thus to enable an individual to be functionally mobile. Furthermore, soft tissue mobility, neuromuscular control, and muscular endurance and strength consistent with demand are thought to be an important factor in the prevention of injury or reinjury of the musculoskeletal system.[69,74,75,80,159]

*Hypomobility* (restricted motion) caused by adaptive shortening of soft tissues can occur as the result of many disorders or situations. Factors include (1) prolonged immobilization of a body segment, (2) sedentary lifestyle, (3) postural malalignment and muscle imbalances, (4) impaired muscle performance (weakness) associated with an array of musculoskeletal or neuromuscular disorders, (5) tissue trauma resulting in inflammation and pain, and (6) congenital or acquired deformities. Any factor that limits mobility, that is, causes decreased extensibility of soft tissues, may also impair muscular performance.[60,85] Hypomobility, in turn, can lead to functional limitations and disability in a person's life.[8,18]

Just as strength and endurance exercises are essential interventions to improve impaired muscle performance or prevent injury, when restricted mobility adversely affects function and increases the risk of injury, stretching interventions become an integral component of the individualized rehabilitation program. Stretching exercises are also thought to be an important element of fitness and conditioning programs designed to promote wellness and reduce the risk of injury and reinjury. *Stretching* is a general term used to describe any therapeutic maneuver designed to *increase* the extensibility of soft tissues, thereby improving flexibility by elongating (lengthening) structures that have adaptively shortened and have become hypomobile over time.[7,71,154]

Only through a systematic examination, evaluation, and diagnosis of a patient's presenting problems can a therapist determine what structures are restricting motion and if, when, and what types of stretching procedures are indicated. Early in the rehabilitation process manual stretching and joint mobilization, which involve direct, "hands-on" intervention by a practitioner, may be the most appropriate techniques. Later, self-stretching exercises performed independently by a patient after careful instruction and close supervision may be a more suitable intervention. In some situations the use of mechanical stretching devices are indicated, particularly when manual therapies have been ineffective. Regardless of the types of stretching procedures selected for an exercise program, if the gain in ROM is to become permanent it must be complemented by an appropriate level of strength and endurance and used on a regular basis in functional activities.

The stretching interventions described in this chapter are designed to elongate the contractile and noncontractile components of muscle.-tendon units and periarticular structures. The efficacy of these interventions is explored throughout the chapter. In addition to the stretching procedures for the extremities illustrated in this chapter, self-stretching exercises for each region of the body are described and illustrated in Chapters 16 through 22. Joint mobilization and manipulation procedures of extremity joints are described and illustrated in Chapter 5.

## ⬤ DEFINITIONS OF TERMS RELATED TO MOBILITY AND STRETCHING

### Flexibility

*Flexibility* is the ability to move a single joint or series of joints smoothly and easily through an unrestricted, pain-free ROM.[85,105] Muscle length in conjunction with joint integrity and the extensibility of periarticular soft tissues determine flexibility.[1] Flexibility is related to the extensibility of musculotendinous units that cross a joint, based on their ability to relax or deform and yield to a stretch force. The arthrokinematics of the moving joint (the ability of the joint surfaces to roll and slide) as well as the ability of periarticular connective tissues to deform also affect joint ROM and an individual's overall flexibility.

### Dynamic and Passive Flexibility

*Dynamic flexibility.* This form of flexibility, also referred to as active mobility or active ROM, is the degree to which an active muscle contraction moves a body segment through the available ROM of a joint. It is dependent on the degree to which a joint can be moved by a muscle contraction and the amount of tissue resistance met during the active movement.

*Passive flexibility.* This aspect of flexibility, also referred to as passive mobility or passive ROM, is the degree to which a joint can be passively moved through the available ROM and is dependent on the extensibility of muscles and connective tissues that cross and surround a joint. Passive flexibility is a prerequisite for but does not ensure dynamic flexibility.

### Hypomobility

*Hypomobility* refers to decreased mobility or restricted motion. A wide range of pathological processes can restrict movement and impair mobility. There are many factors that may contribute to hypomobility and stiffness of soft tissues, the potential loss of ROM, and the development of contractures. These factors are summarized in Table 4.1.

### Contracture

Restricted motion can range from mild muscle shortening to irreversible contractures. *Contracture* is defined as the adaptive shortening of the muscle-tendon unit and other soft tissues that cross or surround a joint that results in significant resistance to passive or active stretch and limitation of ROM, and it may compromise functional abilities.[10,33,49,85,110]

There is no clear delineation of how much limtation of motion from loss of soft tissue extensibility must exist to designate the limitation of motion as a contracture. In one reference,[85] contracture is defined as an almost complete loss of motion, whereas the term *shortness* is used to denote partial loss of motion. The same resource discourages the use of the term *tightness* to describe restricted motion due to adaptive shortening orf soft tissue despite its common usage in the clinical and fitness settings to describe mild muscle shortening. However, another resource[71] uses the term *muscle tightness* to denote adaptive shortening of the contractile and noncontractile elements of muscle.

| TABLE 4.1 | Factors That Contribute to Restricted Motion |
|---|---|
| **Contributing Factors** | **Examples** |
| Prolonged immobilization | |
|   Extrinsic | Fractures, osteotomy, soft tissue trauma or repair |
|     Casts and splints | |
|     Skeletal traction | |
|   Intrinsic | |
|     Pain | Microtrauma or macrotrauma; degenerative diseases |
|     Joint inflammation and effusion | Joint diseases or trauma |
|     Muscle, tendon, or fascial disorders | Myositis, tendonitis, fasciitis |
|     Skin disorders | Burns, skin grafts, scleroderma |
|     Bony block | Osteophytes, ankylosis, surgical fusion |
|     Vascular disorders | Peripheral lymphedema |
| Sedentary lifestyle and habitual faulty or asymmetrical postures | Confinement to bed or a wheelchair; prolonged positioning associated with occupation or work environment |
| Paralysis, tonal abnormalities, and muscle imbalances | Neuromuscular disorders and diseases: CNS or PNS dysfunction (spasticity, rigidity, flaccidity, weakness, muscle guarding, spasm) |
| Postural malalignment: congenital or acquired | Scoliosis, kyphosis |

## Designation of Contractures by Location

Contractures are described by identifying the action of the shortened muscle. If a patient has shortened elbow flexors and cannot fully extend the elbow, he or she is said to have an elbow flexion contracture. When a patient cannot fully abduct the leg because of shortened adductors of the hip, he or she is said to have an adduction contracture of the hip.

## Contracture Versus Contraction

The terms *contracture* and *contraction* (the process of tension developing in a muscle during shortening or lengthening) are *not* synonymous and should not be used interchangeably.

## Types of Contracture

One way to clarify what is meant by the term *contracture* is to describe contractures by the pathological changes in the different types of soft tissues involved.[32]

### Myostatic Contracture

In a myostatic (myogenic) contracture, although the musculotendinous unit has adaptively shortened and there is a significant loss of ROM, there is no specific muscle pathology present.[32] From a morphological perspective, although there may be a reduction in the number of sarcomere units in series, there is no decrease in individual sarcomere length. Myostatic contractures can be resolved in a relatively short time with stretching exercises.[32,49]

### Pseudomyostatic Contracture

Impaired mobility and limited ROM may also be the result of hypertonicity (i.e., spasticity or rigidity) associated with a central nervous system lesion such as a cerebral vascular accident, a spinal cord injury, or traumatic brain injury.[32,49] Muscle spasm or guarding and pain may also

cause a pseudomyostatic contracture. In both situations the involved muscles appear to be in a constant state of contraction, giving rise to excessive resistance to passive stretch. Hence, the term *pseudomyostatic contracture or apparent* contracture is used. If inhibition procedures to reduce muscle tension temporarily are applied, full, passive elongation of the apparently shortened muscle is then possible.[24]

### Arthrogenic and Periarticular Contractures

An arthrogenic contracture is the result of intra-articular pathology. These changes may include adhesions, synovial proliferation, joint effusion, irregularities in articular cartilage, or osteophyte formation.[49] A periarticular contracture develops when connective tissues that cross or attach to a joint or the joint capsule lose mobility, thus restricting normal arthrokinematic motion.

### Fibrotic Contracture and Irreversible Contracture

Fibrous changes in the connective tissue of muscle and periarticular structures can cause adherence of these tissues and subsequent development of a fibrotic contracture. Although it is possible to stretch a fibrotic contracture and eventually increase ROM, it is often difficult to re-establish optimal tissue length.[33]

Permanent loss of extensibility of soft tissues that cannot be reversed by nonsurgical intervention may occur when normal muscle tissue and organized connective tissue are replaced with a large amount of relatively nonextensible, fibrotic adhesions and scar tissue[33] or even heterotopic bone. These changes can occur after long periods of immobilization of tissues in a shortened position or after tissue trauma and the subsequent inflammatory response. The longer a fibrotic contracture exists or the greater the replacement of normal muscle and connective tissue with nonextensible adhesions and scar tissue or bone, the more difficult it becomes to regain optimal mobility of soft tissues and the more likely it is that the contracture will become irreversible.[33,66,144]

## Interventions to Increase Mobility of Soft Tissues

Many therapeutic interventions have been designed to improve the mobility of soft tissues and consequently increase ROM and flexibility. Stretching and mobilization are general terms that describe any therapeutic maneuver that increases the extensibility of restricted soft tissues. There are situations in which stretching interventions are approriate and safe; however, there are also instances when stretching should not be implemented. Boxes 4.1 and 4.2 list indications and contraindications for the use of stretching interventions.

The following are terms that describe a number of procedures designed to increase soft tissue and joint mobility, only some of which are addressed in depth in this chapter.

### Manual or Mechanical/Passive or Assisted Stretching

A sustained or intermittent external, end-range stretch force, applied with overpressure and by manual contact or a mechanical device, elongates a shortened muscle-tendon unit and periarticular connective tissues by moving a restricted joint just past the available ROM. If the patient is as relaxed as possible, it is called *passive stretching*. If the patient assists in moving the joint through a greater range, it is called *assisted stretching.*

### Self-Stretching

Any stretching exercise that is carried out independently by a patient after instruction and supervision by a therapist is referred to as *self-stretching*. The terms self-stretching and *flexibility exercises* are often used interchangeably. However, some practitioners prefer to limit the definition of flexibility exercises to ROM exercises that are part of a general conditioning and fitness program carried out by individuals without mobility impairment. *Active stretching* is another term sometimes used to denote self-stretching procedures. However, stretching exercises that incorporate inhibition or facilitation techniques into stretching maneuvers have also been referred to as active stretching.[158]

### Neuromuscular Facilitation and Inhibition Techniques

Neuromuscular facilitation and inhibition procedures are purported to relax tension in shortened muscles reflexively prior to or during muscle elongation. Because the use of inhibition techniques to assist with muscle elongation is associated with an approach to exercise known as proprioceptive neuromuscular facilitation (PNF),[134,147] many clinicians and some authors refer to these combined inhibition/muscle lengthening procedures as *PNF stretching,*[19,71,110] active inhibition,[71] active stretching,[158] or facilitated stretching.[119] Stretching procedures based on principles of PNF are discussed in a later section of this chapter.

### Muscle Energy Techniques

Muscle energy techniques are manipulative procedures that have evolved out of osteopathic medicine and are designed to lengthen muscle and fascia and to mobilize joints.[22,26,46,109,157] The procedures employ voluntary muscle contractions by the patient in a precisely controlled direction and intensity against a counterforce applied by the practitioner. Because principles of neuromuscular inhibition are incorporated into this approach, another term used to describe these techniques is *postisometric relaxation.*

### Joint Mobilization/Manipulation

Joint mobilization/manipulation methods are manual therapy techniques specifically applied to joint structures and are used to stretch capsular restrictions or reposition a subluxed or dislocated joint.[82,104] Basic techniques for the extremity joints are described and illustrated in detail in Chapter 5. Mobilization with movement techniques for the extremities are described and illustrated throughout the regional chapters (see Chapters 17 to 22).

## Soft Tissue Mobilization and Manipulation

Soft tissue mobilization/manipulation techniques are designed to improve muscle extensibility and involve the application of specific and progressive manual forces (e.g., by means of sustained manual pressure or slow, deep stroking) to effect change in the myofascial structures that can bind soft tissues and impair mobility. Techniques, including *friction massage*,[71,137] *myofascial release*,[21,65,97,137] *acupressure*,[71,137,146] and *trigger point therapy*,[97,137,146] are designed to improve tissue mobility by mobilizing and manipulating connective tissue that binds soft tissues. Although they are useful adjuncts to manual stretching procedures, specific techniques are not described in this textbook.

## Neural Tissue Mobilization (Neuromeningeal Mobilization)

After trauma or surgical procedures, adhesions or scar tissue may form around the meninges and nerve roots or at the site of injury at the plexus or peripheral nerves. Tension placed on the adhesions or scar tissue leads to pain or neurological symptoms. After tests to determine neural tissue mobility are conducted, the neural pathway is mobilized through selective procedures.[20,71,104] These maneuvers are described in Chapter 13.

## Selective Stretching

*Selective stretching* is a process whereby the overall function of a patient may be improved by applying stretching techniques selectively to some muscles and joints but allowing limitation of motion to develop in other muscles or joints. When determining which muscles to stretch and which to allow to become slightly shortened, the therapist must always keep in mind the functional needs of the patient and the importance of maintaining a balance between mobility and stability for maximum functional performance.

The decision to allow restrictions to develop in selected musculotendon units and joints is usually made in patients with permanent paralysis. For example:

- In a patient with spinal cord injury, stability of the trunk is necessary for independence in sitting. With thoracic and cervical lesions, the patient does not have active control of the back extensors. If the hamstrings are routinely stretched to improve or maintain their extensibility and moderate hypomobility is allowed to develop in the extensors of the low back, this enables a patient to lean into the slightly shortened structures and have some trunk stability for long-term sitting. However, the patient must still have enough flexibility for independence in dressing and transfers. Too much limitation of motion in the low back can decrease function.
- Allowing slight hypomobility to develop in the long flexors of the fingers while maintaining flexibility of the wrist enables the patient with spinal cord injury who lacks innervation of the intrinsic finger muscles to develop grasp ability through a tenodesis action.

## Overstretching and Hypermobility

*Overstretching* is a stretch well beyond the normal length of muscle and ROM of a joint and the surrounding soft tissues,[85] resulting in *hypermobility* (excessive mobility).

- Creating selective hypermobility by overstretching may be necessary for certain healthy individuals with normal strength and stability participating in sports that require extensive flexibility.
- Overstretching becomes detrimental and creates joint *instability* when the supporting structures of a joint and the strength of the muscles around a joint are insufficient and cannot hold a joint in a stable, functional position during activities. Instability of a joint often causes pain and may predispose a person to musculoskeletal injury.

## ● PROPERTIES OF SOFT TISSUE—RESPONSE TO IMMOBILIZATION AND STRETCH

The ability of the body to move freely, that is, without restrictions and with control during functional activities, is dependent on the passive mobility of soft tissues as well as active neuromuscular control. Motion is necessary for the health of tissues in the body.[111] As mentioned previously, the soft tissues that can become restricted and impair mobility are muscles with their contractile and noncontractile elements and various types of connective tissue (tendons, ligaments, joint capsules, fascia, skin). For the most part, decreased extensibility of connective tissue, not the contractile elements of muscle tissue, is the primary cause of restricted ROM in both healthy individuals and patients with impaired mobility as the result of injury, disease, or surgery.

Morphological adaptations of tissues often accompany immobilization. Each type of soft tissue has unique properties that affect its response to immobilization and its ability to regain extensibility after immobilization. When stretching procedures are applied to these soft tissues, the direction, velocity, intensity (magnitude), duration, and frequency of the stretch force as well as tissue temperature affect the responses of the various types of soft tissue.

Mechanical characteristics of contractile and noncontractile soft tissue and the neurophysiological properties of contractile tissue affect tissue lengthening. Most of the information on the biomechanical, biochemical, and neurophysiological responses of soft tissues to immobilization and remobilization is derived from animal studies; and as such, the exact physiological mechanism by which stretching procedures produce an increase in the extensibility of human tissues is still unclear. Despite this, an understanding of the properties of these tissues and their responses to immobilization and stretch is the basis for selecting and applying the safest, most effective stretching procedures in a therapeutic exercise program for patients with impaired mobility.

When soft tissue is stretched, elastic, viscoelastic, or plastic changes occur. *Elasticity* is the ability of soft tissue to return to its prestretch resting length directly after a short-duration stretch force has been removed.[36,92,94,130] *Viscoelasticity* is a time-dependent property of soft tissue that initially resists deformation, such as a change in length, of the tissue when a stretch force is first applied. If a stretch force is sustained, viscoelasticity allows a change in the length of the tissue and then enables the tissue to return gradually to its prestretch state after the stretch force has been removed.[102,103,140] *Plasticity* is the tendency of soft tissue to assume a new and greater length after the stretch force has been removed.[54,127,144] Both contractile and noncontractile tissues have elastic and plastic qualities; however, only connective tissues, not the contractile elements of muscle, have viscoelastic properites.

## Mechanical Properties of Contractile Tissue

Muscle is composed of both contractile and noncontractile connective tissues. The contractile elements of muscle (Fig. 4.1) give it the characteristics of contractility and irritability.

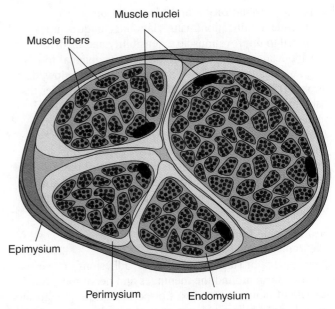

FIGURE 4.2 Muscular connective tissue. Cross-sectional view of the connective tissue in a muscle shows how the perimysium is continuous with the outer layer of epimysium. *(From Levangie and Norkin,[92] p. 93, with permission.)*

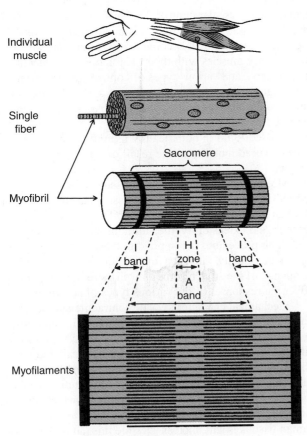

FIGURE 4.1 Structure of skeletal muscle.

The noncontractile connective tissue in and around muscle (Fig. 4.2) has the same properties as all connective tissue, including the ability to resist deforming forces.[92,102,103] The connective tissue structures, which act as a "harness" of a muscle, are the *endomysium,* which is the innermost layer that separates individual muscle fibers and myofibrils; the *perimysium,* which encases fiber burrelles; and the *epimysium,* which is the enveloping fascial sheath around the entire muscle. It is the connective tissue framework of muscle that is the primary source of a muscle's resistance to passive elongation.[33,92,113] When contractures develop, adhesions in and between collagen fibers resist and restrict movement.[33]

### Contractile Elements of Muscle

Individual muscles are composed of many *muscle fibers* that lie in parallel with one another. A single muscle fiber is made up of many *myofibrils*. Each myofibril is composed of even smaller structures called *sarcomeres,* which lie in series within a myofibril. The sarcomere is the contractile unit of the myofibril and is composed of overlapping *myofilaments* of actin and myosin that form cross-bridges. The sarcomere gives a muscle its ability to contract and relax. When a motor unit stimulates a muscle to contract, the actin-myosin filaments slide together, and the muscle actively shortens. When a muscle relaxes, the cross-bridges slide apart slightly, and the muscle returns to its resting length (Fig. 4.3).

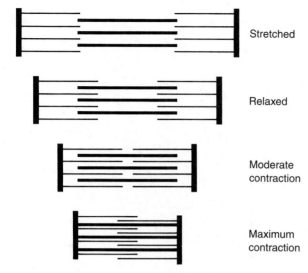

FIGURE 4.3 A model of myofilament sliding. Elongation and shortening of the sarcomere, the contractile unit of muscle.

## Mechanical Response of the Contractile Unit to Stretch and Immobilization

There are a number of changes that occur over time in the anatomical structure and physiological function of the contractile units (sarcomeres) in muscle if a muscle is stretched during an exercise or if it is immobilized in either a lengthened or shortened position for an extended period of time and then remobilized. A discussion of these changes follows. Of course, the noncontractile structures in and around muscle also affect a muscle's response to stretch and immobilization.[31,140] Those responses and adaptations are discussed later in the chapter.

### Response to Stretch

When a muscle is stretched and elongates, the stretch force is transmitted to the muscle fibers via connective tissue (endomysium and perimysium) in and around the fibers. It is hypothesized that molecular interactions link these noncontractile elements to the contractile unit of muscle, the sarcomere.[36]

During passive stretch both longitudinal and lateral force transduction occurs.[36] When initial lengthening occurs in the series elastic (connective tissue) component, tension rises sharply. After a point, there is mechanical disruption (influenced by neural and biochemical changes) of the cross-bridges as the filaments slide apart, leading to abrupt lengthening of the sarcomeres,[36,52,94] sometimes referred to as *sarcomere give*.[52] When the stretch force is released, the individual sarcomeres return to their resting length[36,94] (see Fig. 4.3). As noted previously, the tendency of muscle to return to its resting length after short-term stretch is called elasticity.[92,130] If more permanent (plastic) length increases are to occur, the stretch

force must be maintained over an extended period of time.[36]

### Response to Immobilization and Remobilization

*Morphological changes.* If a muscle is immobilized for a prolonged period of time, the muscle is not used during functional activities, and consequently the physical stresses placed on the muscle are substantially diminshed. This results in decay of contractile protein in the immobilized muscle, a decrease in muscle fiber diameter, a decrease in the number of myofibrils, and a decrease in intramuscular capillary density, the outcome of which is muscle *atrophy* and *weakness* (decreased muscle force).[11,17,32,60,61,64,81,84, 91,111,131,141] As the immobilized muscle atrophies, an increase in fibrous and fatty tissue in muscle also occurs.[111]

The composition of muscle affects its response to immobilization, with atrophy occurring more quickly and more extensively in tonic (slow-twitch) postural muscle fibers than in phasic (fast-twitch) fibers.[94] The duration and position of immobilization also affect the extent of atrophy and loss of strength and power. The longer the duration of immobilization, the greater is the atrophy of muscle and loss of functional strength. Atrophy can begin within as little as a few days to a week.[83,84,141] Not only is there a decrease in the cross-sectional size of muscle fibers over time, an even more significant deterioration in motor unit recruitment occurs as reflected by electromyographic activity.[94] Both compromise the force-producing capabilities of the muscle.

*Immobilization in a shortened position.* When a muscle is immobilized in a shortened position for several weeks, which is often necessary after a fracture or surgical repair of a muscle tear or tendon rupture, there is a reduction in the length of the muscle and its fibers and in the number of sarcomeres in series within myofibrils as the result of *sarcomere absorption*.[56,81,135,138,155] This absorption occurs at a faster rate than the muscle's ability to regenerate sarcomeres in an attempt to restore itself. The decrease in the overall length of the muscle fibers and their in-series sarcomeres, in turn, contributes to muscle atrophy and weakness. It has also been suggested that a muscle immobilized in a shortened position atrophies and weakens at a faster rate than if it is held in a lengthened position over time.[17]

There is a shift to the left in the length–tension curve of a shortened muscle, which decreases the muscle's capacity to produce maximum tension at its normal resting length as it contracts.[60] The increased proportion of fibrous tissue and subcutaneous fat in muscle that occurs with immobilization contributes to the decreased extensibility of the shortened muscle but may also serve to protect the weakened muscle when it stretches.[33,61]

***Immobilization in a lengthened position.*** Sometimes a muscle is immobilized in a position of maximum available length for a prolonged period of time. This occurs with the application of a series of positional casts (serial casts)[76] or the use of a dynamic splint to stretch a long-standing contracture and increase ROM.[10,68,106] There is some evidence from animal studies[135,138,155] to suggest that if a muscle is held in a lengthened position for an extended time period, it adapts by increasing the number of sarcomeres in series (*myofibrillogenesis*[36]) to maintain the greatest functional overlap of actin and myosin filaments. This may lead to a relatively permanent (plastic) form of muscle lengthening if the newly gained length is used on a regular basis in functional activities.

The minimum time frame necessary for a stretched muscle (fiber) to become a longer muscle (fiber) by adding sarcomeres in series is not known. In animal studies that have reported increased muscle length as the result of myofibrillogenesis, the stretched muscle was continuously immobilized in a lengthened position for several weeks.[135,138,155] There is speculation that this same process contributes to gains in ROM associated with use of serial casts[76] and dynamic splints[68,106] and possibly as the result of stretching exercises.[36]

The adaptation of the contractile units of muscle (an increase or decrease in the number of sarcomeres) to prolonged positioning in either lengthened or shortened positions is transient, lasting only 3 to 5 weeks if the muscle resumes its preimmobilization use and degree of lengthening for functional activities.[84,135] In clinical situations, this underscores the need for patients to use full-range motions during a variety of functional activities to maintain the full available ROM.

## Neurophysiological Properties of Contractile Tissue

The neurophysiological properites of the muscle-tendon unit also influence a muscle's response to stretch and the effectiveness of stretching interventions to elongate muscle. In particular, two sensory organs of muscle-tendon units, the *muscle spindle* and the *Golgi tendon organ*, are mechanoreceptors that convey information to the central nervous system about what is occurring in a muscle-tendon unit and affect a muscle's response to stretch.

### Muscle Spindle

The muscle spindle is the major sensory organ of muscle and is senstive to quick and sustained (tonic) stretch (Fig. 4.4). The main function of muscle spindles is to receive and convey information about changes in the length of a muscle and the velocity of the length changes.

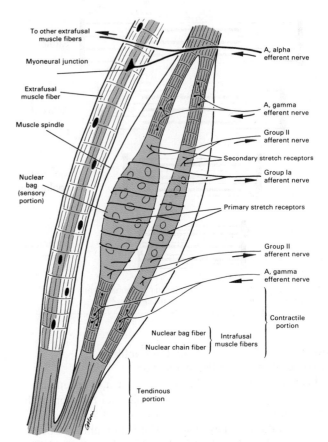

**FIGURE 4.4** Muscle spindle. Diagram shows intrafusal and extrafusal muscle fibers. The muscle spindle acts as a stretch receptor. *(From Lemkuhl, LD, Smith, LK: Brunnstrom's Clinical Kinesiology, ed 4. FA Davis, Philadelphia, 1983, p 97, with permission.)*

Muscle spindles are small, encapsulated receptors composed of afferent sensory fiber endings, efferent motor fiber endings, and specialized muscle fibers called *intrafusal fibers*. Intrafusal muscle fibers are bundled together and lie between and parallel to extrafusal muscle fibers that make up the main body of a skeletal muscle.[61,77,98,120] Because intrafusal muscle fibers connect at their ends to extrafusal muscle fibers, when a muscle is stretched, intrafusal fibers are also stretched. Only the ends (polar regions), not the central portion (equatorial region), of an intrafusal fiber is contractile. Consequently, when an intrafusal muscle fiber is stimulated and contracts, it lengthens the central portion. Small-diameter motor neurons, known as *gamma* motor neurons, innervate the contractile polar regions of intrafusal muscle fibers and adjust the sensitivity of muscle spindles. Large-diameter *alpha* motor neurons innervate extrafusal fibers.

There are two general types of intrafusal fiber: *nuclear bag fibers* and *nuclear chain fibers*, so named because of the arrangement of their nuclei in the central portions of the fibers. Primary (type Ia fiber) afferent endings, which arise from nuclear bag fibers, sense and cause muscle to respond to both quick and sustained (tonic) stretch. However, secondary (type II) afferents from the nuclear chain fibers are sensitive only to tonic stretch. Primary and secondary fibers synapse on the alpha or gamma motoneurons, which when stimulated cause excitation of their own extrafusal and intrafusal fibers, respectively. There are essentially two ways to stimulate these sensory fibers by means of stretch; one is by overall lengthening of the muscle, and the other is by stimulating contraction of intrafusal fibers via the gamma efferent neural pathways.

### Golgi Tendon Organ

The Golgi tendon organ (GTO) is a sensory organ located near the musculotendinous junctions of extrafusal muscle fibers. The function of a GTO is to monitor changes in tension of muscle-tendon units. These encapsulated nerve endings are woven among collagen strands of a tendon and transmit sensory information via Ib fibers. These sensory organs are sensitive to even slight changes of tension on a muscle-tendon unit as the result of passive stretch of a muscle or with active muscle contractions during normal movement.

When tension develops in a muscle, the GTO fires, inhibits alpha motoneuron activity, and decreases tension in the muscle-tendon unit being stretched.[61,77,120] With respect to the neuromuscular system, *inhibition* is a state of decreased neuronal activity and altered synaptic potential, which reflexively diminishes the capacity of a muscle to contract.[74,77,98]

Originally, the GTO was thought to fire and inhibit muscle activation only in the presence of high levels of muscle tension as a protective mechanism. However, the GTO has since been shown to have a low threshold for firing (fires easily) so it can continuously monitor and adjust the force of active muscle contractions during movement or the tension in muscle during passive stretch.[53,120]

### Neurophysiological Response of Muscle to Stretch

When a stretch force is applied to a muscle-tendon unit either quickly or over a prolonged period of time, the primary and secondary afferents of intrafusal muscle fibers sense the length changes and activate extrafusal muscle fibers via alpha motor neurons in the spinal cord, thus activating the stretch reflex and increasing (facilitating) tension in the muscle being stretched. The increased tension causes resistance to lengthening and, in turn, is thought to compromise the effectiveness of the stretching procedure. When the stretch reflex is activated in a muscle being lengthened, decreased activity (inhibition) in the muscle on the opposite side of the joint, referred to as *reciprocal inhibition*, may also occur.[98,147] However, this phenomenon has been documented only in studies using animal models. To minimize activation of the stretch reflex and the subsequent increase in muscle tension and reflexive resistance to muscle lengthening during stretching procedures, a slowly applied, low-intensity, prolonged stretch is considered prefereable to a quickly applied, short-duration stretch.

In contrast, the GTO, as it monitors tension in the muscle fibers being stretched, has an inhibitory impact on the level of muscle tension in the muscle-tendon unit in which it lies, particularly if the stretch force is prolonged. This effect is called *autogenic inhibition*.[61,92,98,120] Inhibition of the contractile components of muscle by the GTO contributes to reflexive muscle relaxation during a stretching maneuver, enabling a muscle to be elongated against less muscle tension. It is thought that if a low-intensity, slow stretch force is applied to muscle, the stretch reflex is less likely to be activated as the GTO fires and inhibits tension in the muscle, allowing the parallel elastic component (the sarcomeres) of the muscle to remain relaxed and to lengthen.

That being said, improvement in muscle extensibility attributed to stretching procedures are more likely due to tensile stresses placed on the noncontractile connective tissue in and around muscle than to inhibition of the contractile elements of muscle.[102,103,140] A discussion of the effects of stretching on noncontractile soft tissue follows.

## Mechanical Properties of Noncontractile Soft Tissue

Noncontractile soft tissue permeates the entire body and is organized into various types of connective tissue to support the structures of the body. Ligaments, tendons, joint capsules, fasciae, noncontractile tissue in muscles (see Fig. 4.2), and skin have connective tissue characteristics that can lead to the development of adhesions and contractures and thus affect the flexibility of the tissues crossing joints. When these tissues restrict ROM and require stretching, it is important to understand how they respond to the intensity and duration of stretch forces and to recognize that the only way to increase the extensibility of connective tissue is to remodel its basic architecture.[33]

### Composition of Connective Tissue

Connective tissue is composed of three types of fiber: collagen, elastin and reticulin, and nonfibrous ground substance.[30,66,144]

***Collagen fibers.*** Collagen fibers are responsible for the strength and stiffness of tissue and resist tensile deformation. Tropocollagen crystals form the building blocks of collagen microfibrils. Each additional level of composition of the fibers is arranged in an organized relationship and dimension (Fig. 4.5). There are six classes with 19 types[31] of collagen; the fibers of tendons and ligaments mostly contain type I collagen, which is highly resistant to tension.[144] As collagen fibers develop and mature, they bind together, initially with unstable hydrogen bonding, which then converts to stable covalent bonding. The stronger the bonds, the greater is the mechanical stability of the tissue. Tissue with a greater proportion of collagen provides greater stability.

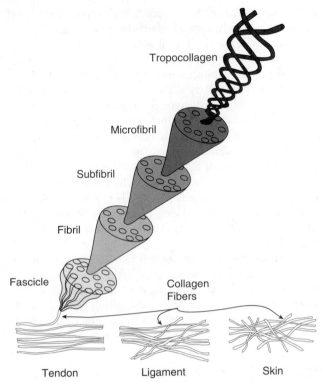

**FIGURE 4.5** Composition of collagen fibers showing the aggregation of tropocollagen crystals as the building blocks of collagen. Organization of the fibers in connective tissue is related to the function of the tissue. Tissues with parallel fiber orientation, such as tendons, are able to withstand greater tensile loads than tissue such as skin, where the fiber orientation appears more random.

***Elastin fibers.*** Elastin fibers provide extensibility. They show a great deal of elongation with small loads and fail abruptly without deformation at higher loads. Tissues with greater amounts of elastin have greater flexibility.

***Reticulin fibers.*** Reticulin fibers provide tissue with bulk.

***Ground substance.*** Ground substance is made up of proteoglycans (PGs) and glycoproteins. The PGs function to hydrate the matrix, stabilize the collagen networks, and resist compressive forces. (This is most important in cartilage and intervertebral discs.) The type and amount of PGs are proportional to the types of compressive and tensile stress the tissue undergoes.[60] The glycoproteins provide linkage between the matrix components and between the cells and matrix opponents. In essence, the ground substance is mostly an organic gel containing water that reduces friction between fibers, transports nutrients and metabolites, and may help prevent excessive cross-linking between fibers by maintaining space between fibers.[41,144]

## Mechanical Behavior of Noncontractile Tissue

The mechanical behavior of the various noncontractile tissues is determined by the proportion of collagen and elastin fibers and by the structural orientation of the fibers. The proportion of proteoglycans (PGs) also influences the mechanical properties of connective tissue. Those high in

collagen and low in PGs are designed to resist high tensile loads; those tissues that withstand greater compressive loads have greater concentrations of PGs.[60]

Collagen is the structural element that absorbs most of the tensile stress. Collagen fibers elongate quickly under light loads (wavy fibers align and straighten). With increased loads, tension in the fibers increases, and the fibers stiffen. The fibers strongly resist the tensile force, but with continued loading the bonds between collagen fibers begin to break. When a substantial number of bonds are broken, the fibers fail. When tensile forces are applied the maximum elongation of collagen is less than 10%, whereas elastin may lengthen 150% and return to its original configuration. Collagen is five times as strong as elastin. The alignment of collagen fibers in various tissues reflects the tensile forces acting on that tissue (see Fig. 4.5).

- In tendons, collagen fibers are parallel and can resist the greatest tensile load. They transmit forces to the bone created by the muscle.
- In skin, collagen fibers are random and weakest in resisting tension.
- In ligaments, joint capsules, and fasciae, the collagen fibers vary between the two extremes, and they resist multidirectional forces. Ligaments that resist major joint stresses have a more parallel orientation of collagen fibers and a larger cross-sectional area.[116]

## Interpreting Mechanical Behavior of Connective Tissue: The Stress–Strain Curve

The stress–strain curve illustrates the mechanical strength of structures (Fig. 4.6) and is used to interpret what is happening to connective tissue under stress loads.[30,93,142,144,166]

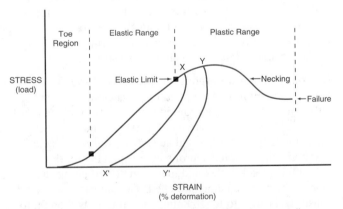

**FIGURE 4.6** Stress–strain curve. When stressed, initially the wavy collagen fibers straighten (toe region). With additional stress, recoverable deformation occurs in the elastic range. Once the elastic limit is reached, sequential failure of the collagen fibers and tissue occurs in the plastic range, resulting in release of heat (hysteresis) and new length when the stress is released. The length from the stress point (X) results in a new length when released (X'); the heat released is represented by the area under the curve between these two points (hysteresis loop). (Y to Y' represents additional length from additional stress with more heat released.) Necking is the region in which there is considerable weakening of the tissue and less force is needed for deformation. Total failure quickly follows even under smaller loads.

## Stress and Strain

*Stress* is force per unit area. Mechanical stress is the internal reaction or resistance to an external load. There are three kinds of stress.

- *Tension*: a force applied perpendicular to the cross-sectional area of the tissue in a direction away from the tissue. A stretching force is a tension stress.
- *Compression*: a force applied perpendicular to the cross-sectional area of the tissue in a direction toward the tissue. Muscle contraction and loading of a joint during weight bearing cause compression stresses in joints.
- *Shear*: a force applied parallel to the cross-sectional area of the tissue.
- *Strain*: the amount of deformation or lengthening that occurs when a load (stress) or stretch force is applied.

### Regions of the Stress-Strain Curve

*Toe region.* That area of the stress–strain curve where there is considerable deformation without the use of much force is called the toe region. This is the range where most functional activity normally occurs. Collagen fibers at rest are wavy and are situated in a three-dimensional matrix, so some distensibility in the tissue occurs by straightening and aligning the fibers.

*Elastic range/linear phase.* Strain is directly proportional to the ability of tissue to resist the force. This occurs when tissue is taken to the end of its ROM, and gentle stretch is applied. With stress in this phase the collagen fibers line up with the applied force, the bonds between fibers and between the surrounding matrix are strained, some microfailure between the collagen bonds begins, and some water may be displaced from the ground substance. There is complete recovery from this deformation, and the tissue returns to its original size and shape when the load is released if the stress is not maintained for any length of time (see the following discussion on creep and stress-relaxation for prolonged stretch).

*Elastic limit.* The point beyond which the tissue does not return to its original shape and size is the elastic limit.

*Plastic range.* The range beyond the elastic limit extending to the point of rupture is the plastic range. Tissue strained in this range has permanent deformation when the stress is released. In this range there is sequential failure of the bonds between collagen fibrils and eventually of collagen fibers. Heat is released and absorbed in the tissue. Because collagen is crystalline, individual fibers do not stretch but, instead, rupture. In the plastic range it is the rupturing of fibers that results in increased length.

*Ultimate strength.* The greatest load the tissue can sustain is its ultimate strength. Once this load is reached, there is increased strain (deformation) without an increase in stress required. The *region of necking* is reached in which there is considerable weakening of the tissue, and it rapidly fails. The therapist must be cognizant of the tissue feel when stretching because as the tissue begins necking, if the stress is maintained, there could be complete tearing of the tissue. Experimentally, maximum tensile deformation of isolated collagen fibers prior to failure is 7% to 8%. Whole ligaments may withstand strain of 20% to 40%.[116]

*Failure.* Rupture of the integrity of the tissue is called failure.

*Structural stiffness.* Tissues with greater stiffness have a higher slope in the elastic region of the curve, indicating that there is less elastic deformation with greater stress. Contractures and scar tissue have greater stiffness, probably because of a greater degree of bonding between collagen fibers and their surrounding matrix.

### Connective Tissue Responses to Loads

*Creep.* When a load is applied for an extended period of time, the tissue elongates, resulting in permanent deformation (Fig. 4.7A). It is related to the viscosity of the tissue and is therefore time-dependent. The amount of deformation depends on the amount of force and the rate at which the force is applied. Low-magnitude loads, usually in the elastic range and applied for long periods, increase the deformation of connective tissue and allow gradual rearrangement of collagen fiber bonds (remodeling) and redistribution of water to surrounding tissues.[33,94,140,142] Increasing the temperature of the part increases the creep and therefore the distensibility of the tissue.[89,150,153] Complete recovery from creep may occur over time, but not as rapidly as a single strain. Patient reaction dictates the time a specific load is tolerated.

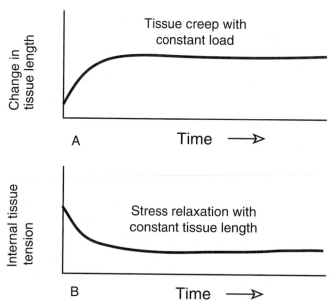

FIGURE 4.7 Tissue response to prolonged stretch forces as a result of viscoelastic properties. (*A*) Effects of creep. A constant load, applied over time, results in increased tissue length until equilibrium is reached. (*B*) Effects of stress–relaxation. A load applied with the tissue kept at a constant length results in decreased internal tension in the tissue until equilibrium is reached.

*Stress-relaxation.* When a force (load) is applied to stretch a tissue and the length of the tissue is kept constant, after the initial creep there is a decrease in the force required to maintain that length, and the tension in the tissue decreases[33] (Fig. 4.7B). This, like creep, is related to the viscoelastic qualities of the connective tissue and redistribution of the water content. Stress-relaxation is the underlying principle used in prolonged stretching procedures where the stretch position is maintained for several hours or days. Recovery (i.e., no change) versus permanent changes in length is dependent on the amount of deformation and the length of time the deformation is maintained.[33]

*Cyclic loading and connective tissue fatigue.* Repetitive loading of tissue increases heat production and may cause failure below the yield point. The greater the applied load, the fewer number of cycles needed for failure. This principle can be used for stretching by applying repetitive (cyclic) loads at a submaximal level on successive days. The intensity of the load is determined by the patient's tolerance. A minimum load is required for this failure. Below the minimum load an apparently infinite number of cycles do not cause failure. This is the *endurance limit.* Examples of connective tissue fatigue from cyclic loading are stress fractures and overuse syndromes, neither of which is desired as a result of stretching. Therefore, periodically, time is allowed between bouts of cyclic stretching to allow for remodeling and healing in the new range.

## Summary of Mechanical Principles for Stretching Connective Tissue

● Connective tissue deformation (stretch) occurs to different degrees at different intensities of force. It requires breaking of collagen bonds and realignment of the fibers for there to be permanent elongation or increased flexibility. Failure of tissue begins as microfailure of fibrils and fibers before complete failure of the tissue occurs. Complete tissue failure can occur as a single maximal event (acute tear from a traumatic injury or manipulation that exceeds the failure point) or from repetitive submaximal stress (fatigue or stress failure from cyclic loading). Microfailure (needed for permanent lengthening) also occurs with creep, stress-relaxation, and controlled cyclic loading.

● Healing and adaptive remodeling capabilities allow the tissue to respond to repetitive and sustained loads if time is allowed between bouts. This is important for increasing both flexibility and tensile strength of the tissue. If healing and remodeling time is not allowed, a breakdown of tissue (failure) occurs as in overuse syndromes and stress fractures. Intensive stretching is usually not done every day in order to allow time for healing. If the inflammation from the microruptures is excessive, additional scar tissue is laid down, which could become more restrictive.[33]

● It is imperative that the individual use any newly gained range to allow the remodeling of tissue and to train the muscle to control the new range, or the tissue eventually returns to its shortened length.

## Changes in Collagen Affecting Stress–Strain Response

### Effects of Immobilization
There is weakening of the tissue because of collagen turnover and weak bonding between the new, nonstressed fibers. There is also adhesion formation because of greater cross-linking between disorganized collagen fibers and because of decreased effectiveness of the ground substance maintaining space and lubrication between the fibers.[41,142] The rate of return to normal tensile strength is slow. For example, after 8 weeks of immobilization, the anterior cruciate ligament in monkeys failed at 61% of maximum load; after 5 months of reconditioning, it failed at 79%; after 12 months of reconditioning, it failed at 91%.[114,115] There was also a reduction in energy absorbed and an increase in compliance (decreased stiffness) prior to failure following immobilization. Partial and near-complete recovery followed the same 5-month and 12-month pattern.[115]

### Effects of Inactivity (Decrease of Normal Activity)
There is a decrease in the size and amount of collagen fibers, resulting in weakening of the tissue. There is a proportional increase in the predominance of elastin fibers, resulting in increased compliance. Recovery takes about 5 months of regular cyclic loading. Physical activity has a beneficial effect on the strength of connective tissue.

### Effects of Age
There is a decrease in the maximum tensile strength and the elastic modulus, and the rate of adaptation to stress is slower.[116] There is an increased tendency for overuse syndromes, fatigue failures, and tears with stretching.[166]

### Effects of Corticosteroids
There is a long-lasting deleterious effect on the mechanical properties of collagen with a decrease in tensile strength.[166] There is fibrocyte death next to the injection site with delay in reappearance up to 15 weeks.[116]

### Effects of Injury
Excessive tensile loading can lead to rupture of ligaments and tendons at musculotendinous junctions. Healing follows a predictable pattern (see Chapter 10), with bridging of the rupture site with newly synthesized type III collagen. This is structurally weaker than mature type I collagen. Remodeling progresses, and eventually collagen matures to type I. Remodeling usually begins about 3 weeks postinjury and continues for several months to a year, depending on the size of the connective tissue structure and magnitude of the tear.[60]

---

**BOX 4.3** Determinants of Stretching Interventions

- *Alignment:* positioning a limb or the body such that the stretch force is directed to the appropriate muscle group
- *Stabilization:* fixation of one site of attachment of the muscle as the stretch force is applied to the other bony attachment
- *Intensity of stretch:* magnitude of the stretch force applied
- *Duration of stretch:* length of time the stretch force is applied during a stretch cycle
- *Speed of stretch:* speed of initial application of the stretch force
- *Frequency of stretch:* number of stretching sessions per day or per week
- *Mode of stretch:* form or manner in which the stretch force is applied (static, ballistic, cyclic); degree of patient participation (passive, assisted, active); or the source of the stretch force (manual, mechanical, self)

---

**BOX 4.4** Types of Stretching

- Static stretching
- Cyclic/intermittent stretching
- Ballistic stretching
- Proprioceptive neuromuscular facilitation stretching procedures (PNF stretching)
- Manual stretching
- Mechanical stretching
- Self-stretching
- Passive stretching
- Active stretching

---

 **DETERMINANTS, TYPES, AND EFFECTS OF STRETCHING INTERVENTIONS**

As with other forms of therapeutic exercise, such as strengthening exercises and endurance training, there are a number of essential elements that determine the effectiveness of stretching interventions. The elements (determinants) of stretching, all of which are interrelated, include *alignment* and *stabilization* of the body during stretching; the *intensity (magnitude), duration, speed, frequency,* and *mode* of stretch; and the integration of neuromuscular inhibition or facilitation and functional activities into stretching programs. By manipulating the determinants of stretching interventions, which are defined in Box 4.3, a therapist has many options from which to choose when designing stretching programs that are safe and effective and meet many patients' needs, functional goals, and capabilities. Each of these determinants is discussed in this section of the chapter.

There are four broad categories of stretching exercises: static stretching, cyclic stretching, ballistic stretching, and stretching techniques based on the principles of proprioceptive neuromuscular facilitation.[19,35,44,72,165] Each of these approaches to stretching can be carried out in various manners—that is, manually or mechanically, passively or actively, and by a therapist or independently by a patient—giving rise to many terms that are used in the literature to describe stretching interventions. The stretching interventions listed in Box 4.4 are defined and discussed in this section.

Extensive evidence from numerous research studies has shown that stretching interventions can improve flexi-bility and increase ROM, but recommended protocols vary substantially. Some of this research is highlighted in this section. Injury prevention or risk reduction, prevention or reduction of postexercise muscle soreness, and enhanced physical performance also are effects that have been attributed to stretching interventions. However, the evidence to support these claims, for the most part, is mixed.[58,59,70,121]

**● Focus on Evidence** _____

Many of the investigations comparing the intensity, duration, frequency, and mode of stretching have been carried out with healthy, young adults as subjects. The findings and recommendations of these studies are difficult to generalize and apply to patients with long-standing contractures or other forms of tissue restriction. Therefore, many decisions, particularly those related to the type, intensity, duration, and frequency of stretching, must continue to be based on a balance of scientific evidence and sound clinical judgments by the therapist.

---

## Alignment and Stabilization

Just as appropriate alignment and effective stabilization are fundamental components of muscle testing and goniometry as well as ROM and strengthening exercises, they are also essential elements of effective stretching.

### Alignment
Proper alignment or positioning of the patient and the specific muscles and joints to be stretched is necessary for patient comfort and stability during stretching. Alignment influences the amount of tension present in soft tissue and consequently affects the ROM available in joints. Alignment of the muscles and joint to be stretched as well as the alignment of the trunk and adjacent joints must all be considered. For example, to stretch the rectus femoris (a muscle that crosses two joints) effectively, as the knee is flexed and the hip extended, the lumbar spine and pelvis should be aligned in a neutral position. The pelvis should not tilt anteriorly nor should the low back hyperextend; the hip should not abduct or remain flexed (Fig. 4.8). When a

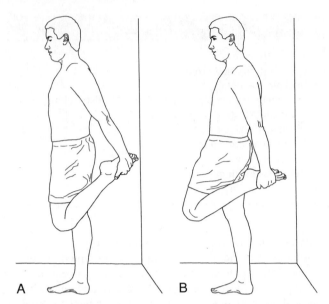

FIGURE 4.8 (A) Correct alignment when stretching the rectus femoris: the lumbar spine, pelvis, and hip are held in a neutral position as the knee is flexed. (B) Incorrect position of the hip in flexion. In addition, avoid anterior pelvic tilt, hyperextension of the lumbar spine, and abduction of the hip.

patient is self-stretching to increase shoulder flexion, the trunk should be erect, not slumped (Fig. 4.9B).

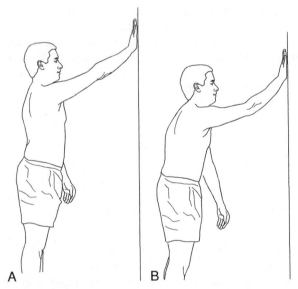

FIGURE 4.9 (A) Correct alignment when stretching to increase shoulder flexion: the cervical and thoracic spine is erect. (B) Incorrect alignment: forward head and rounded spine.

**N O T E :** Throughout this and later chapters, recommendations for appropriate alignment and positioning during stretching procedures are identified. If it is impossible for a patient to be placed in or assume the recommended postures because of discomfort, restrictions of motion of adjacent joints, inadequate neuromuscular control, or cardiopulmonary capacity, the therapist must critically analyze the situation to determine an alternative position.

## Stabilization

To achieve an effective stretch of a specific muscle or muscle group and associated periarticular structures, it is imperative to stabilize (fixate) either the proximal or distal attachment site of the muscle-tendon unit being elongated. Either site may be stabilized, but for manual stretching it is common for a therapist to stabilize the proximal attachment and move the distal segment, as shown in Figure 4.10A.

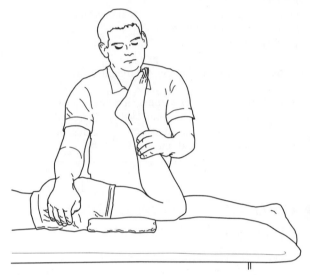

FIGURE 4.10 (A) The proximal attachment (femur and pelvis) of the muscle being stretched (the quadriceps) is stabilized as the distal segment is moved to increase knee flexion.

For self-stretching procedures, a stationary object, such as a chair or a doorframe, or active muscle contractions by the patient may provide stabilization of one segment as the other segment moves. During self-stretching, it is often the distal attachment that is stabilized as the proximal segment moves (Fig. 4.10B).

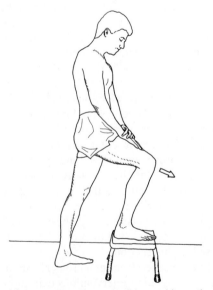

FIGURE 4.10 (B) During this self-stretch of the quadriceps, the distal segment (tibia) is stabilized through the foot as the patient moves the proximal segment (femur) by lunging forward.

Stabilization of multiple segments of a patient's body also helps maintain the proper alignment necessary for an effective stretch. For example, when stretching the iliopsoas, the pelvis and lumbar spine must maintain a neutral position as the hip is extended to avoid stress to the low back region. Sources of stabilization include manual contacts, body weight, or a firm surface such as a table, wall, or floor.

## Intensity of Stretch

The intensity (magnitude) of a stretch force is determined by the load placed on soft tissue to elongate it. There is general agreement among clinicians and researchers that stretching should be applied at a *low intensity* by means of a *low load*.[10,12,28,44,72,89,96,100,165] Low-intensity stretching in comparison to high-intensity stretching makes the stretching maneuver more comfortable for the patient and minimizes voluntary or involuntary muscle guarding so a patient can either remain relaxed or assist with the stretching maneuver.

Low-intensity stretching (coupled with a long duration of stretch) results in optimal rates of improvement in ROM without exposing tissues, possibly weakened by immobilization, to excessive loads and potential injury.[89,96,100] Low-intensity stretching has also been shown to elongate dense connective tissue, a significant component of chronic contractures, more effectively and with less soft tissue damage and post-exercise soreness than a high-intensity stretch.[2]

## Duration of Stretch

One of the most important decisions a therapist must make when selecting and implementing a stretching intervention (stretching exercises or use of a mechanical stretching device) is to determine the duration of stretch that is expected to be safe, effective, practical, and efficient for each situation.

The duration of stretch refers to the period of time a stretch force is applied and shortened tissues are held in a lengthened position. Duration most often refers to how long a *single cycle* of stretch is applied. If more than one repetition of stretch (*stretch cycle*) is carried out during a treatment session (which is most often the case), the cumulative time of all the stretch cycles is also considered an aspect of duration.

In general, the shorter the duration of a single stretch cycle, the greater the number of repetitions applied during a stretching session. Any number of combinations have been studied. For example, in a study by Cipriani et al.,[25] two repetitions of 30-second hamstring stretches were found to be equally effective compared to six repetitions of 10-second stretches. However, Roberts and Wilson[124] found that over the course of a 5-week period three 15-second hamstring stretches each day yielded significantly greater stretch-induced gains in ROM than nine daily 5-second stretches.

Despite numerous studies, there continues to be a lack of agreement on the "ideal" combination of the duration of a single cycle and the number of repetitions of stretch that should be applied in a daily stretching program to achieve the greatest and most sustained stretch-induced gains in ROM. The duration of stretch must be put in context with other stretching parameters, including intensity, frequency, and mode of stretch. Key findings from several studies are summarized in Box 4.5 on the following page.

Numerous descriptors are used to differentiate between a long-duration versus a short-duration stretch. Terms such as *static, sustained, maintained,* and *prolonged* are all used to describe a long-duration stretch, whereas terms such as *cyclic, intermittent,* or *ballistic* are used to characterize a short-duration stretch. There is no specific time period assigned to any of these descriptors, nor is there a time frame that distinguishes a long-duration from a short-duration stretch.

### Static Stretching

*Static stretching** is a commonly used method of stretching in which soft tissues are elongated just past the point of tissue resistance and then held in the lengthened position with a sustained stretch force over a period of time. Other terms used interchangeably are sustained, maintained, or prolonged stretching. The duration of static stretch is predetermined prior to stretching or is based on the patient's tolerance and response during the stretching procedure.

In research studies the term "static stretching" has been linked to durations of a single stretch cycle ranging from as few as 5 seconds to 5 minutes per repetition when either a manual stretch or self-stretching procedure is employed.[†] If a mechanical device provides the static stretch, the time frame can range from almost an hour to several days or weeks.[15,68,76,79,96,100,106] (See additional information on mechanical stretching later in this section.)

 **Focus on Evidence** _____

In a systematic review of the literature (28 studies) on hamstring stretching,[35] a 30-second manual or self-stretching procedure performed for one or more repetitions was the most frequently used duration per repetition of stretch in static stretching programs. A 30-second stretch per repetition was also identified as the median duration of stretch in a review of the literature of studies on calf muscle stretching.[163]

_____

Static stretching is well accepted as an effective form of stretching to increase flexibility[19,35,44,71,72] and has been considered a safer form of stretching than ballistic stretching (described in the next section on speed of stretch) for many years.[39] Research has shown that tension created in muscle during static stretching is approximately half that created during ballistic stretching.[148] This is consistent with

_____
* See references 4,5,6,13,14,25,35,39,40,50,55,58,86,95,101,112,124, 126,133,151,161,163.
† See references 4,5,6,12,13,14,25,50,96,124,126,151,161,163.

## BOX 4.5    Intensity, Duration, Frequency, and Mode of Stretch—Interrelationships and Impact on Stretching Outcomes

- There is an inverse relationship between intensity and duration as well as between intensity and frequency of stretch.
  - The lower the intensity of stretch, the longer the time the patient will tolerate stretching and the soft tissues can be held in a lengthened position.
  - The higher the intensity, the less frequently the stretching intervention can be applied to allow time for tissue healing and resolution of residual muscle soreness.
- A low-load (low-intensity), long-duration stretch is considered the safest form of stretch and yields the most significant, elastic deformation and long-term, plastic changes in soft tissues.[89]
- Manual stretching and self-stretching in hypomobile but healthy subjects[4–6,13,25,50] and prolonged mechanical stretching in patients with chronic contractures[15,76,79,96,107] yield significant stretch-induced gains in ROM.
- In the well elderly, stretch cycles of 15, 30, and 60 seconds applied to the hamstrings for four repetitions have all been shown to produce significant gains in ROM with the greatest and longest-lasting improvements occurring with the use of 60-second stretch cycles.[50]
- In healthy young and/or middle-age adults
  - Stretch durations of 15, 30, 45, or 60 seconds or 2 minutes to lower extremity musculature produced significant gains in ROM.[4,5,25,40,101,156]
  - Stretch cycles of 30- and 60-second duration applied to the hamstrings for one repetition daily are both more effective than one repetition daily of a 15-second stretch cycle but are equally effective when compared to each other.[4]

- Two repetitions daily of a 30-second static stretch of the hamstrings yield significant gains in hamstring flexibility similar to those seen with six repetitions of 10-second static stretches daily.[25]
- Static stretches of the hip adductors for 15 seconds or 2 minutes produce equal improvements in ROM.[101]
- There seems to be no additional benefit to holding each stretch cycle beyond 60 seconds.[5,87]
- Three cycles of 30-second and 1-minute stretches are no more effective for improving ROM than one cycle of each duration of stretch.[5]
- When the total duration of stretch is equal, cyclic stretching is equally effective and possibly more comfortable than static stretching.[132]
- In patients with chronic, fibrotic contractures:
  - Common durations of manual stretching or self-stretching may not be effective.[96,112]
  - Use of prolonged static stretch with splints or casts is more effective.[15,79,96,107]
- Frequency of stretching needs to occur a minimum of two times per week[58] for healthy hypomobile individuals, but more frequent stretching is necessary for patients with soft tissue pathology to achieve gains in ROM.
- Although stretch-induced gains in ROM often persist for several weeks to a month in healthy adults after cessation of a stretching program, permanent improvement in mobility can be achieved only by use of the newly gained ROM in functional activities and/or with a maintenance stretching program.[156]

---

our understanding of the viscoelastic properties of connective tissue, which lies in and around muscles, as well as the neurophysiological properties of the contractile elements of muscle. As discussed in the previous section of this chapter, noncontractile soft tissues are known to yield more readily to a low-intensity, continuously applied stretch force, as used in static stretching.

Furthermore, during static stretching it is thought that the GTO, which monitors tension created by stretch of a muscle-tendon unit, may contribute to muscle elongation by overriding any facilitative impulses from the primary afferents of the muscle spindle (Ia afferent fibers) and may contribute to muscle relaxation by inhibiting tension in the contractile units of the muscle being stretched. For these reasons clinicians believe that static stretching, if applied at a low intensity, generates less tissue trauma and less post-exercise muscle soreness than ballistic stretching.

### Static Progressive Stretching

Static progressive stretching is another term that describes how static stretch is applied for maximum effectiveness. The shortened soft tissues are held in a comfortably length-

ened position until a degree of relaxation is felt by the patient or therapist. Then the shortened tissues are incrementally lengthened even further and again held in the new end-range position for an additional duration of time.[15,79,112] This approach involves continuous displacement of a limb by varying the stretch force (stretch load). This approach to stretching capitalizes on the stress-relaxation properties of soft tissue[107,112,131] (see Fig. 4.7B).

Most studies that have explored the merits of static *progressive* stretching have examined the effectiveness of a dynamic orthosis (see Fig. 4.13, below), which allows the patient to control the degree of displacement of the limb.[15,79] Manual stretching and self-stretching procedures are also routinely applied in this manner.

### Cyclic (Intermittent) Stretching

A relatively short-duration stretch force that is repeatedly but gradually applied, released, and then reapplied is described as a cyclic (intermittent) stretch.[12,48,108,132] Cyclic stretching, by its very nature, is applied for multiple repetitions (stretch cycles) during a single treatment session. With cyclic stretching the end-range stretch force is applied at a *slow* velocity, in a controlled manner, and at relatively low intensity. For these reasons, cyclic stretching is *not* synonymous with ballistic stretching, which is characterized by high-velocity movements.

The differentiation between cyclic stretching and static stretching based on the duration that each stretch is applied is not clearly defined in the literature. According to some authors, for cyclic stretching each cycle of stretch is held between 5 and 10 seconds.[48,132] However, investigtors in other studies refer to stretching that involves 5- and 10-second stretch cycles as static stretching.[25,124] There is also no consensus on the optimal number of repetitions of cyclic stretching during a treatment session. Rather, this determination is often based on the patient's response to stretching.

Based on clinical experience, some therapists hold the opinion that appropriately applied, end-range cyclic stretching is as effective and more comfortable for a patient than a static stretch of comparable intensity, particularly if the static stretch is appled continuously for more than 30 seconds. There is some evidence to support this opinion. Although there have been few studies on cyclic or intermittent stretching (aside from those on ballistic stretching), cyclic loading has been shown to increase flexibility as or more effectively than static stretching.[108,132]

 **Focus on Evidence** _____

In a study of nonimpaired young adults, 60 seconds of cyclic stretching of calf muscles caused tissues to yield at slightly lower loads than one 60-second, two 30-second, or four 15-second static stretches, possibly due to decreased muscle stiffness.[108] In another study that compared cyclic and static stretching,[132] the authors speculated that heat production might occur because of the movement inherent in cyclic stretching and cause soft tissues to yield more readily to stretch. The authors of the latter study also concluded that cyclic stretching was more comfortable than a prolonged static stretch.

_____

## Speed of Stretch

### Importance of a Slowly Applied Stretch
To ensure optimal muscle relaxation and prevent injury to tissues, the speed of stretch should be *slow*.[39,55,58,126,127] The stretch force should be applied and released *gradually*. A slowly applied stretch is less likely to increase tensile stresses on connective tissues[95,102,103] or to activate the stretch reflex and increase tension in the contractile structures of the muscle being stretched.[98,120] Remember, the Ia fibers of the muscle spindle are sensitive to the *velocity* of muscle lengthening. A stretch force applied at a low velocity is also easier for the therapist or patient to control and is therefore safer than a high-velocity stretch. In addition, a slow rate stretch affects the viscoelastic properties of connective tissue, making them more compliant.

### Ballistic Stretching
A *rapid, forceful* intermittent stretch—that is, a high-speed *and* high-intensity stretch—is commonly called *ballistic*

*stretching.*[5-7,19,44,87,126,165] It is characterized by the use of quick, bouncing movements that create momentum to carry the body segment through the ROM to stretch shortened structures. Although both static stretching and ballistic stretching have been shown to improve flexibility equally, ballistic stretching is thought to cause greater trauma to stretched tissues and greater residual muscle soreness than static stretching.[152]

Consequently, although ballistic stretching has been shown to increase ROM safely in young, healthy subjects participating in a conditioning program,[67] it is, for the most part, not recommended for elderly or sedentary individuals or patients with musculoskeletal pathology or chronic contractures. The rationale for this recommendation is[33]:

● Tissues, weakened by immobilization or disuse, are easily injured.
● Dense connective tissue found in chronic contractures does not yield easily with high-intensity, short-duration stretch; rather, it becomes more brittle and tears more readily.

### High-Velocity Stretching in Conditioning Programs and Advanced-Phase Rehabilitation
Although somewhat controversial, certain practitioners and authors believe there are situations when high-velocity stretching is appropriate for carefully selected individuals.[19,44] For example, a highly trained athlete involved in a sport such as gymnastics that requires significant dynamic flexibility may need to incorporate high-velocity stretching in a conditioning program. Also, a young, active patient in the final phase of rehabilitation who wishes to return to high-demand, recreational activities after a musculoskeletal injury may need to perform carefully progressed, high-velocity stretching activities prior to beginning plyometric training or simulated, sport-specific exercises or drills.

If high-velocity stretching is employed, rapid, but *low-load (low-intensity)* stretches are recommemded, paying close attention to effective stabilization. The following self-stretching sequence, referred to as a Progressive Velocity Flexibility Program, has been suggested for a safe transition and progression from static stretching to ballistic stretching to improve dynamic flexibility.[165]

● Static stretching → Slow, short end-range stretching → Slow, full-range stretching → Fast, short end-range stretching → Fast, full-range stretching.
● The stretch force is initiated by having the patient actively contract the muscle group opposite the muscle and connective tissues to be stretched.

## Frequency of Stretch

Frequency of stretching refers to the *number of bouts (sessions) per day or per week* a patient carries out a stretching regimen.[5,58] The recommended frequency of stretching is often based on the underlying cause of impaired mobility, the quality and level of healing of tissues, the chronicity and severity of a contracture, as well as a patient's age, use of corticosteroids, and previous response to stretching. Because few studies have attempted to determine the optimal frequency of stretching within a day or a week,[5,58] it is not possible to draw evidence-based guidelines from the literature. As with decisions on the most appropriate number of repetitions of stretch in an exercise session, most suggestions are based on opinion. Frequency on a weekly basis ranges from two to five sessions, allowing time for rest between sessions for tissue healing and to minimize postexercise soreness. Ultimately, the decision is based on the clinical discretion of the therapist and the response and needs of the patient.

A therapist must be aware of any breakdown of tissues with repetitive stretch. A fine balance between collagen tissue breakdown and repair is needed to allow an increase in soft tissue lengthening. If there is excessive frequency of loading, tissue breakdown exceeds repair; and ultimate tissue failure is a possibility. In addition, if there is progressive loss of ROM over time rather than a gain in range, continued low-grade inflammation from repetitive stress can cause excessive collagen formation and hypertrophic scarring.

## Mode of Stretch

The mode of stretch refers to the form of stretch or the manner in which stretching exercises are carried out. Mode of stretch can be defined by who or what is applying the stretch force or whether the patient is actively participating in the stretching maneuver. Categories include but are not limited to *manual* and *mechanical stretching* or *self-stretching* as well as *passive, assisted,* or *active stretching*. Regardless of the form of stretching selected and implemented, it is imperative that the shortened muscle remains relaxed and that the restricted connective tissues yield as easily as possible to the stretch. To accomplish this, stretching procedures should be preceded by either low-intensity active exercise or therapeutic heat to warm up the tissues that are to be lengthened.

There is no best form of stretching. What is important is that the therapist and patient have many modes of stretching from which to choose. Box 4.6 lists some questions a therapist needs to answer to determine which forms of stretching are most appropriate and most effective for each patient at different stages of a rehabilitation program.

### Manual Stretching

During manual stretching a therapist or other trained practitioner or caregiver applies an external force to move the involved body segment *slightly beyond* the point of tissue resistance and available ROM. The therapist manually controls the site of stabilization as well as the direction, speed, intensity, and duration of stretch. As with ROM exercises (described in Chapter 3), manual stretching can be performed *passively, with assistance from the patient,* or even *independently by the patient.*

N O T E : Remember, stretching and ROM exercises are not synonymous terms. Stretching takes soft tissue structures

---

**BOX 4.6  Considerations for Selecting Methods of Stretching**

- Based on the results of your examination, what tissues are involved and impairing mobility?
- Is there evidence of pain or inflammation?
- How long has the hypomobility existed?
- What is the stage of healing of restricted tissues?
- What form(s) of stretching have been implemented previously? How did the patient respond?
- Are there any underlying diseases, disorders, or deformities that might affect the choice of stretching procedures?
- Does the patient have the ability to actively participate in, assist with, or independently perform the exercises? Consider the patient's physical capabilities, age, ability to cooperate, or ability to follow and remember instructions.
- Is assistance from a therapist or caregiver necessary to execute the stretching procedures and appropriate stabilization? If so, what is the size and strength of the therapist or the caregiver who is assisting the patient with a stretching program?

---

*beyond* their available length to *increase* ROM. ROM exercises stay within the limits of tissue extensibility to *maintain* the available length of tissues. Figures 4.16 through 4.36 of this chapter depict manual stretching techniques of the extremities.

Manual stretching usually employs a controlled, end-range, static, progressive stretch applied at an intensity consistent with the patient's comfort level, held for 15 to 60 seconds and repeated for at least several repetitions. When compared to mechanical stretching, manual stretching could be categorized as a high-intensity, short-duration stretch.[96]

Despite widespread use in the clinical setting, the effectiveness of manual passive stretching for increasing the extensibility of range-limiting muscle-tendon units is debatable. Some investigators[40,101,136] have found that manual passive stretching increases muscle length and ROM in nonimpaired subjects. However, the short duration of stretch that typically occurs with manual stretching may be why other investigators have reported that the effect of a manual passive stretching program is negligible,[62] especially in the presence of long-standing contractures associated with tissue pathology.[96]

The following are points to consider about the use of manual stretching.

- Manual stretching may be most appropriate in the early stages of a stretching program when a therapist wants to determine how a patient responds to varying intensities or durations of stretch and when optimal stabilization is most critical.
- Manual stretching performed *passively* is an appropriate choice for a therapist or caregiver if a patient cannot perform self-stretching owing to a lack of neuromuscular control of the body segment to be stretched.

- If a patient has control of the body segment to be stretched, it is often helpful to ask the patient to assist the therapist with the manual stretching maneuver, particularly if the patient is apprehensive and is having difficulty relaxing. For example, if the patient concentrically contracts the muscle opposite the short muscle and assists with joint movement, the range-limiting muscle tends to relax reflexively, thus decreasing muscle tension interfering with elongation. This is one of several stretching procedures based on proprioceptive neuromuscular facilitation techniques that are discussed later in this chapter.

- Using procedures and hand placements similar to those described for self-ROM exercises (see Chapter 3), a patient can also independently lengthen range-limiting muscles and periarticular tissues with manual stretching. As such, this form of stretching is usually referred to as *self-stretching* and is discussed in more detail as the next topic in this section.

N O T E : Specific guidelines for the application of manual stretching, as well as descriptions and illustrations of manual stretching techniques for the extremities are presented in later sections of this chapter.

### Self-Stretching

Self-stretching (also referred to as *flexibility exercises* or *active stretching*) is a type of stretching procedure a patient carries out independently after careful instruction and supervised practice. Self-stretching enables a patient to maintain or increase the ROM gained as the result of direct intervention by a therapist. This form of stretching is often an integral component of a home exercise program and is necessary for long-term self-management of many musculoskeletal and neuromuscular disorders.

Teaching a patient to carry out self-stretching procedures *correctly* and *safely* is fundamental for preventing reinjury or future dysfunction. Proper alignment of the body or body segments is critical for effective self-stretching. Sufficient stabilization of either the proximal or distal attachment of a shortened muscle is necessary but can be difficult to achieve with self-stretching. Every effort should be made to see that restricted structures are stretched specifically and that adjacent structures are not overstretched.

The guidelines for the intensity, speed, duration, and frequency of stretch that apply to manual stretching are also appropriate for self-stretching procedures. Static stretching with a 30- to 60-second duration per repetition is considered the safest type of stretching for a self-stretching program.

Self-stretching exercises can be carried out in several ways.

- Using positions for self-ROM exercises described in Chapter 3, a patient can passively move the distal segment of a restricted joint with one or both hands to elongate a shortened muscle while stabilizing the proximal segment (Fig. 4.11A).

- If the distal attachment of a shortened muscle is fixed (stabilized) on a support surface, body weight can be used as the source of the stretch force to elongate the shortened muscle-tendon unit (Fig. 4.11B).

- Neuromuscular inhibition, using PNF stretching techniques, can be integrated into self-stretching procedures to promote relaxation in the muscle that is being elongated.

- Low-intensity acitve stretching (referred to by some as *dynamic ROM*[6]), using repeated, short-duration, end-range active muscle contractions of the muscle opposite the shortened muscle is another form of self-stretching exercise.[6,151,158]

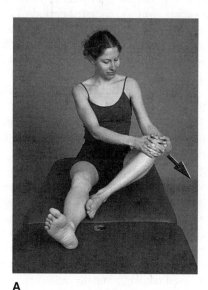

**A**

FIGURE 4.11 (*A*) When manually self-stretching the adductors and internal rotators of the hip, the patient moves the distal segment (femur) while stabilizing the proximal segment (pelvis) with body weight.

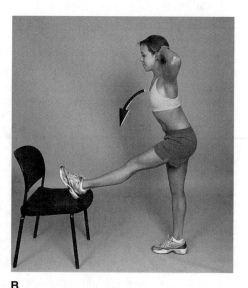

**B**

FIGURE 4.11 (*B*) When self-stretching the hamstrings, the distal segment (tibia) is stabilized through the foot on the surface of a chair as the patient bends forward and moves the proximal segment. The weight of the upper body is the source of the stretch force.

## Mechanical Stretching

There are many ways to use equipment to stretch shortened tissues and increase ROM. The equipment can be as simple as a cuff weight or weight-pulley system or as sophisticated as some adjustable orthoses or automated stretching machines.* These mechanical stretching devices provide either a constant load with variable displacement or constant displacement with variable loads. Studies[15,79] about the efficacy of these two categories of mechanical stretching devices base their effectiveness on the soft tissue properties of either creep or stress-relaxation, which occur within a short period of time, as well as plastic deformation, which occurs over an extended period of time.

It is often the responsibility of a therapist to recommend the type of stretching device that is most suitable and teach a patient how to safely use the equipment and monitor its use in the home setting. A therapist may also be involved in the fabrication of serial casts or splints.

Mechanical stretching devices apply a very low-intensity stretch force (low load) over a prolonged period of time to create relatively permanent lengthening of soft tissues, presumably due to plastic deformation.

N O T E : Be cautious of studies or product information that report "permanent" lengthening as the result of use of mechanical stretching devices. Permanent may mean that length increases were maintained for as little as a few days or a week after use of a stretching device has been discontinued. Long-term follow-up may indicate that tissues have returned to their shortened state if the newly gained motion has not been used regularly in daily activities.

Each of the following forms of mechanical stretching has been shown to be effective, particularly in reducing long-standing contractures.

● An effective stretch load applied with a cuff weight (Fig. 4.12) can be as low as a few pounds.[96]

---

* See references 10, 15, 79, 89, 91, 96, 100, 106, 127, 131, 132, 149, 150.

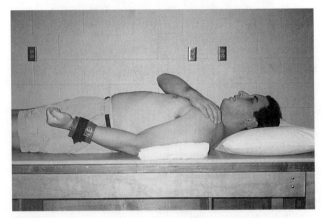

FIGURE 4.12 Low-load mechanical stretch with a cuff weight and self-stabilization of the proximal humerus to stretch the elbow flexors and increase end-range elbow extension.

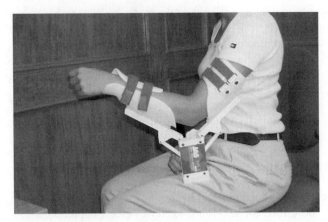

FIGURE 4.13 JAS orthosis is a patient-directed device that applies a static progressive stretch. (Courtesy of Joint Active Systems, Effingham, IL.)

● Some devices, such as the Joint Active Systems™ adjustable orthosis (Fig. 4.13), allow a patient to control and adjust the load (stretch force) during a stretching session.[15,79]
● With other devices the load is preset prior to the application of the splint, and the load remains constant while the splint is in place.[68]

### Duration of Mechanical Stretch

Mechanical stretching involves a substantially longer overall duration of stretch than is practical with manual stretching or self-stretching exercises. The duration of mechanical stretch reported in the literature ranges from 15 to 30 minutes[15,79] to as long as 8 to 10 hours at a time[68] or continuous throughout the day except for time out of the device for hygiene and exercise.[10] Serial casts are worn for days or weeks at a time before being removed and then reapplied.[76] The time frame is dependent on the type of device employed, the cause and severity of impairment, and patient tolerance. The longer durations of stretch are required for patients with chronic contractures as the result of neurological or musculoskeletal disorders than for healthy subjects with only mild hypomobility.[15,76,79,96,100,107,112]

###  Focus on Evidence

Light and colleagues[96] studied nonambulatory, elderly nursing home residents with long-standing bilateral knee flexion contractures and compared the effects of mechanical and manual stretching. Over a 4-week period twice-daily stretching sessions occurred 5 days per week. Low-intensity, prolonged mechanical stretching (a 5- to 12-lb poundstretch force applied by a weight-pulley system for 1 hour each session) was applied to one knee, and manual passive stretching was applied to the other knee by a therapist (three repetitions of 1-minute static stretches per stretching session). At the conclusion of the study, the mechanical stretching procedure was found to be considerably more effective than the manual stretching procedure for increasing knee extension. The patients also reported that the prolonged mechanical stretch was more comfortable than the manual stretching procedure, which tended to be applied at a higher intensity. The investigators recognized that the total duration of mechanical stretch (40 hours) was substantially longer over the course of the study than the total duration of manual stretch (2 hours) but believed that the manual stretching sessions were typical and practical in the clinical setting.

## Proprioceptive Neuromuscular Facilitation Stretching Techniques

Proprioceptive neuromuscular facilitation techniques used for stretching (*PNF stretching*),[19,29,72,117,165] also referred to as *active stretching*[158] or *facilitative stretching*,[119] integrate active muscle contractions into stretching maneuvers purportedly to facilitate or inhibit muscle activation and to increase the likelihood that the muscle to be lengthened remains as relaxed as posssible as it is stretched. It is believed that when muscle fibers are reflexively inhibited through autogenic or reciprocal inhibition, there is less resistance to elongation by the contractile elements of the muscle.[134,147] However, inhibition techniques are designed to relax only the contractile structures of muscle, not the connective tissue in and around shortened muscles.

N O T E : The PNF stretching techniques described in this section require normal innervation and voluntary control of either the shortened muscle or the muscle on the opposite side of the joint. As such, these techniques cannot be used effectively in patients with paralysis or spasticity resulting from neuromuscular diseases or injury. Furthermore, because PNF stretching procedures are designed to affect the contractile elements of muscle, not noncontractile connective tissues, they are more appropriate when muscle spasm limits motion and less appropriate for stretching fibrotic contractures.

The PNF stretching techniques, most of which have been adapted from the PNF techniques originally described by Knott and Voss,[134,147] have been used for many years in the clinical setting as an adjunct to manual stretching or self-stretching. Although the efficacy of the neurophysiological principles on which PNF was founded has come into question, the results of numerous studies have demonstrated that the various PNF stretching techniques effectively increase flexibility and ROM.[6,48,117,126,133,136,158,162] However, there is no consensus on whether one PNF technique is consistently superior to another or whether PNF stretching is more, less, or equally effective as static stretching.

### Types of PNF Stretching

There are several types of PNF stretching procedures. They include:

- Hold–relax (HR) or contract–relax (CR)
- Agonist contraction (AC)
- Hold–relax with agonist contraction (HR-AC).

With classic PNF, these techniques are performed with combined muscle groups acting in diagonal patterns[134,147] but have been modified in a number of studies and resources[6,27,65,74,117,158] by stretching in anatomical planes or opposite the line of pull of a specific muscle group. (For a description of the PNF diagonal patterns, refer to Chapter 6.)

#### Hold–Relax and Contract–Relax

With the hold–relax (HR) procedure,[27,74,119,134] the range-limiting muscle is first lengthened to the point of limitation or to the extent that is comfortable for the patient. The patient then performs a *prestretch, end-range, isometric contraction* (for 5 to 10 seconds) followed by voluntary relaxation of the tight muscle. The limb is then passively moved into the new range as the range-limiting muscle is elongated. A sequence for using the HR technique to stretch shortened pectoralis major muscles bilaterally and increase horizontal abduction of the shoulders is illustrated in Figure 4.14.

N O T E : In the clinical setting and in a number of investigations the terms contract–relax (CR) and hold–relax (HR) are often used interchangably. However, it should be noted that for classic PNF the techniques are not identical. Although both techniques are performed in diagonal patterns, for the CR technique the rotators of the limb are allowed to contract concentrically whereas all other muscle groups contract isometrically during the prestretch contraction of the restricting muscles.[134,147] For the HR technique, the prestretch contraction is isometric in all muscles of the diagonal pattern.

Practitioners in the clinical and athletic training settings have reported that the HR and CR techniques appear to make passive elongation of muscles more comfortable for a patient than manual passive stretching.[74] It has been assumed that the sustained, prestretch contraction is followed by reflexive relaxation accompanied by a decrease in electromyographic (EMG) activity in the range-limiting muscle, possibly as the result of autogenic inhibition.[99,119] This assumption has been challenged in one study but supported in a later study. In the earlier study,[45] a postcontraction sensory discharge (increased EMG activity) was identified in the muscle to be stretched, suggesting that there was lingering tension in the muscle after the prestretch isometric contraction and that the muscle to be stretched was not effectively relaxed. In the later study, no postcontraction elevation in EMG activity was found with the use of the HR or CR techniques.[28] Consequently, clinicians must evaluate the effectiveness of the HR and CR

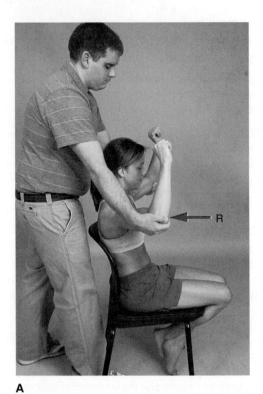

**A**

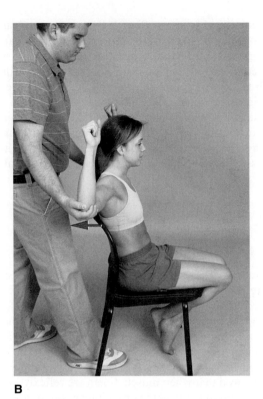

**B**

FIGURE 4.14 Hold–relax (HR) procedure to stretch the pectoralis major muscles bilaterally. (*A*) The therapist horizontally abducts the shoulders bilaterally to a comfortable position. The patient isometrically contracts the pectoralis major muscles against the therapist's resistance for 5 to 10 seconds.

FIGURE 4.14 (*B*) The patient relaxes, and the therapist passively lengthens the pectoralis major muscles by horizontally abducting the shoulders into the newly gained range. After a 10-second rest with the muscle maintained in a comfortably lengthened position, the entire sequence is repeated.

techniques and determine their effectiveness with individual patients.

PRECAUTION: It is not necessary for the patient to perform a maximal isometric contraction of the tight muscle prior to stretch. Multiple repetitions of maximal prestretch isometric contractions have been shown to result in an acute increase in arterial blood pressure, most notably after the third repetition.[29] To minimize the adverse effects of the Valsalva maneuver (elevation in blood pressure), have the patient breathe regularly while performing submaximal (low-intensity) isometric contractions held for 5 to 10 seconds with each repetition of the stretchimg procedure. A submaximal contraction is also easier for the therapist to control if the patient is strong.

**Agonist Contraction**
Another PNF stretching technique is the *agonist contraction* (AC) procedure. This term has been used by several authors[19,24,28,74] but can be misunderstood. The "agonist" refers to the muscle *opposite* the range-limiting muscle. "Antagonist," therefore, refers to the range-limiting muscle.[24] Think of it as the short muscle (the antagonist) preventing the full movement of the prime mover (the agonist). *Dynamic range of motion* (DROM)[6] and *active stretching*[158] are terms that have been used to describe the AC procedure.

To perform the AC procedure the patient *concentrically contracts (shortens) the muscle opposite the range-limiting muscle* and then holds the end-range position for

at least several seconds.[19,28,74] The movement of the limb is independently controlled by the patient and is deliberate and slow, not ballistic. In most instances the shortening contraction is performed without the addition of resistance. For example, if the hip flexors are tight, the patient can perform end-rage, prone leg lifts by contracting the hip extensors concentrically; the end-range contraction is held for a number of seconds. After a brief rest period, the patent repeats the procedure.

It has been suggested that when the agonist is activated and contracts concentrically, the antagonist (the range-limiting muscle) is reciprocally inhibited, allowing it to relax and lengthen more easily.[119,124,147] However, the theoretical mechanism of receiprocal inhibition has been substantiated only in animal studies, not in studies of humans.[120]

 **Focus on Evidence** _____

Several studies have evaluated the effectiveness of the agonist contraction procedure for improving flexibility and ROM. Two studies compared the effect of the AC procedure, referred to as DROM, to static stretching of the hamstrings of healthy subjects who participated in 6-week stretching programs. In one study[151] DROM was found to be as effective as static stretching, but in the other study[6] one daily repetition of a 30-second static stretch was almost three times as effective in increasing hamstring flexibility as six repetitions daily (with a 5-second, end-range hold) of DROM.

In a study of young adults with hypomobile hip flexors and periodic lumbar or lower-quarter pain, investigators compared "active stretching" using the AC procedure to static passive stretching.[158] Both techniques resulted in increased hip extension with no significant difference between the active and passive stretching groups.

In addition to the results of studies on the the AC stretching procedure, clinicians have observed the following.

- The AC technique seems to be especially effective when significant muscle guarding restricts muscle lengthening and joint movement and is less effective in reducing chronic contractures.
- This technique is also useful when a patient cannot generate a strong, pain-free contraction of the range-limiting muscle, which must be done during the HR procedure.
- This technique is also useful for initiating neuromuscular control in the newly gained range to re-establish dynamic flexibility.
- The AC technique is least effective if a patient has close to normal flexibility.

PRECAUTIONS: Avoid full-range, balllistic movements when performing concentric contractions of the agonist muscle group. Rest after each repetition to avoid muscle cramping when the agonist is contracting in the very shortened portion of its range.

### Hold–Relax with Agonist Contraction

The HR-AC stretching technique combines the HR and AC procedures. The HR-AC technique is also referred to as the slow reversal hold–relax technique.[134,147] To perform the HR-AC procedure, move the limb to the point that tissue resistance is felt in the tight (range-limiting) muscle; then have the patient perform a resisted, prestretch isometric contraction of the range-limiting muscle *followed* by relaxation of that muscle and an immediate concentric contraction of the muscle *opposite* the tight muscle.[28,50,119,134,147]

For example, to stretch knee flexors, extend the patient's knee to a comfortable position and then have the patient perform an isometric contraction of the knee flexors against resistance for 5 to 10 seconds. Tell the patient to relax the knee flexors and then actively extend the knee as far as possible, holding the newly gained range for several seconds.

 **Focus on Evidence** _____

Studies comparing two PNF stretching procedures produced differing results. In one study,[48] the HR-AC technique produced a greater increase in ankle dorsiflexion range than did the HR technique. Both PNF techniques produced a greater increase in range of ankle dorsiflexion than did manual passive stretching. However, in another study, there was no significant difference between the use of the HR and HR-AC techniques.[74]

PRECAUTIONS: Follow the same precautions as described for both the HR and AC procedures.

## Integration of Function into Stretching

### Importance of Strength and Muscle Endurance

As previously discussed, the strength of soft tissue is altered when it is immoblized for a period of time.[23,60,111] The magnitude of peak tension produced by muscle decreases, and the tensile strength of noncontractile tissues decreases. A muscle group that has been overstretched because its opposing muscle group has been in a shortened state for an extended period of time also becomes weak.[85] Therefore, it is critical to begin low-load resistance exercises to improve muscle performance (strength and endurance) as early as possible in a stretching program.

Initially, it is important to place emphasis on developing neuromuscular control and strength of the agonist, the muscle group opposite the muscle that is being stretched. For example, if the elbow flexors are the range-limiting muscle group, emphasize contraction of the elbow extensors in the gained range. Complement stretching the hamstrings to reduce a knee flexion contracture by using the quadriceps in the new range. Early use of the agonist enables the patient to elongate the hypomobile structures actively and use the recently gained ROM.

As ROM approaches a "normal," or functional, level, the muscles that were shortened and then stretched must also be strengthened to maintain an appropriate balance of strength between agonists and antagonists throughout the ROM. Manual and mechanical resistance exercises are effective ways to load and strengthen muscles, but functional weight-bearing activities, such as those mentioned below also strengthen antigravity muscle groups.

### Use of Increased Mobility for Functional Activities

As mentioned previously, gains in flexibility and ROM achieved as the result of a stretching program are transient, lasting only about 4 weeks after cessation of stretching.[156] The most effective means of achieving *permanent* increases in ROM and reducing functional limitations is to integrate functional activities into a stretching program to use the gained range on a regular basis. Use of functional activities to maintain mobility lends diversity and interest to a stretching program.

Active movements should be within the pain-free ROM. Examples of movements of the upper or lower extremities or spine that are components of daily activities include reaching, grasping, turning, twisting, bending, pushing, pulling, and squatting to name just a few. As soon as even small increases in tissue extensibility and ROM have been achieved, have the patient use the gained range by performing motions that *simulate* functional activities. Later have the patient use all of the available ROM while actually doing specific functional tasks.

Functional movements that are practiced should complement the stretching program. For example, if a patient

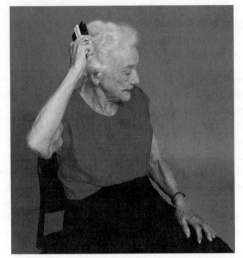

**A**

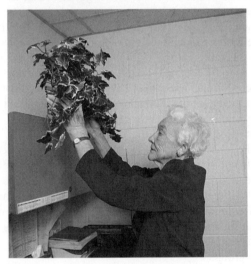

**B**

FIGURE 4.15  (A, B) Stretching-induced gains in ROM are used during daily activities.

has been performing stretching exercises to increase shoulder mobility, have the patient fully use the available ROM by reaching as far as possible behind the back and overhead when grooming or dressing or by reaching for or placing objects on a high shelf (Fig. 4.15). Gradually increase the weight of objects placed on or removed from a shelf to strengthen shoulder musculature simultaneously.

If the focus of a stretching program has been to increase knee flexion after removal of a long-leg cast, emphasize flexing both knees before standing up from a chair or when stooping to pick up an object from the floor. These weight-bearing activities also strengthen the quadriceps that became weak while the leg was immobilized and the quadricepts was held in a shortened position.

# PROCEDURAL GUIDELINES FOR APPLICATION OF STRETCHING INTERVENTIONS

The following guidelines are central to the development and implementation of stretching interventions. The results of an examination and evaluation of a patient's status determine the need for and types of stretching procedures that will be most effective in a patient's plan of care. This section identifies general guidelines to be addressed before, during, and after stretching procedures as well as guidelines specific to the application of manual stretching. Special considerations for teaching self-stretching exercises and using mechanical stretching devices are listed in Boxes 4.7 and 4.8.

## Examination and Evaluation of the Patient

- Carefully review the patient's history and perform a thorough systems review.
- Select and perform appropriate tests and measurements. Determine the ROM available in involved and adjacent joints and if either active or passive mobility is impaired.
- Determine if hypomobility is related to other impairments and if it is causing functional limitations or disability.
- Ascertain if, and if so, which soft tissues are the source of the impaired mobility. In particular, differentiate between joint capsule, periarticular noncontractile tissue, and muscle length restrictions as the cause of limited ROM. Be sure to assess joint play and fascial mobility.
- Evaluate the irritability of the involved tissues and determine their stage of healing. When moving the patient's extremities or spine, pay close attention to the patient's reaction to movements. This not only helps identify the stage of healing of involved tissues, it helps determine the probable dosage (such as intensity and duration) of stretch that stays within the patient's comfort range.
- Assess the underlying strength of muscles in which there is limitation of motion and realistically consider the value of stretching the range-limiting structures. An individual must have the capability of developing adequate strength to control and safely use the new ROM.
- Be sure to determine what outcome goals (i.e., functional improvements) the patient is seeking to achieve as the result of the intervention program and determine if those goals are realistic.
- Analyze the impact of any factors that could adversely affect the projected outcomes of the stretching program.

| BOX 4.7 | Special Considerations for Teaching Self-Stretching Exercises |

- Be sure to carefully teach the patient all elements of self-stretching procedures, including appropriate alignment and stabilization, intensity, duration, and frequency of stretching. Because many self-stretching exercises are performed using a portion of the body weight as the stretch force (by moving the body over a fixed distal segment), emphasize the importance of performing a slow, sustained stretch, not a ballistic stretch that creates momentum and may lengthen but can potentially injure hypomobile soft tissues.
- Make sure that the patient is taught to carry out stretching exercises on a firm, stable, comfortable surface to maintain proper alignment.
- Supervise the patient and make suggestions or corrections to be certain the patient performs each exercise using safe biomechanics that protect joints and ligaments, especially at the end of the ROM. Pay particular attention to maintaining postural alignment and effective stabilization. For example, while self-stretching the hamstrings in a long-sitting position or while standing with one leg resting on a table, be sure that the patient knows to keep the thoraco-

lumbar segments of the spine in extension and to bend forward at the hips to prevent posterior pelvic tilt and overstretch of the low back.
- Emphasize the importance of warming up the tissues with low-intensity, rhythmic activities, such as cycling, prior to stretching. Stretching should not be the first activity in an exercise routine because cold tissue is more brittle and more easily torn.
- If appropriate and possible, teach the patient how to incorporate neuromuscular inhibition techniques independently, such as the hold–relax (HR) procedure, into selected stretching exercises.
- Provide written instructions with illustrations to which the patient can refer when independently performing the self-stretching exercises.
- Demonstrate how items commonly found around the house, such as a towel, belt, broomstick, or homemade weight, can be used to assist with stretching activities.
- Emphasize the importance of using the gained ROM during appropriately progressed functional activities.

| BOX 4.8 | Special Considerations for Use of Mechanical Stretching Devices |

- Become thoroughly familiar with the manufacturer's product information.
- Become familiar with stretching protocols recommended by the manufacturer; seek out research studies that provide evidence of the efficacy of the equipment or protocols.
- Determine if modifying a suggested protocol is warranted to meet your patient's needs. For example, should the suggested intensity of stretch or recommended wearing time (duration and frequency) be modified?
- Check the fit of a device before sending it home with a patient. Teach the patient how to apply and safely adjust the device and how to maintain it in good working order. Be sure that the patient knows who to contact if the equipment appears to be defective.
- Teach the patient where and how to inspect the skin to detect areas of excessive pressure from the stretching device and potential skin irritation.
- If the mechanical stretching device is "homemade," such as a cuff weight, check to see if the equipment is safe and effective.
- Have the patient keep a daily record of using the stretching device.
- Re-examine and re-evaluate the patient and equipment periodically to determine the effectiveness of the mechanical stretching program and to modify and progress the program as necessary.
- Be sure the patient complements the use of mechanical stretching with active exercises.

## Preparation for Stretching

- Review the goals and desired outcomes of the stretching program with the patient. Obtain the patient's consent to initiate treatment.
- Select the stretching techniques that will be most effective and efficient.
- Warm up the soft tissues to be stretched by the application of local heat or by active, low-intensity exercises. Warming up tight structures may increase their extensibility and may decrease the risk of injury from stretching.
- Have the patient assume a comfortable, stable position that allows the correct plane of motion for the stretching procedure. *The direction of stretch is exactly opposite the direction of the joint or muscle restriction.*
- Explain the procedure to the patient and be certain he or she understands.
- Free the area to be stretched of any restrictive clothing, bandages, or splints.
- Explain to the patient that it is important to be as relaxed as possible or assist when requested. Also explain that the stretching procedures are geared to his or her tolerance level.

## Application of Manual Stretching Procedures

- Move the extremity slowly through the free range to the point of tissue restriction.
- Grasp the areas proximal and distal to the joint in which motion is to occur. The grasp should be firm but not uncomfortable for the patient. Use padding, if necessary, in areas with minimal subcutaneous tissue, reduced sen-

sation, or over a bony surface. Use the broad surfaces of your hands to apply all forces.

- Firmly stabilize the proximal segment (manually or with equipment) and move the distal segment.
- To stretch a multijoint muscle, stabilize either the proximal or distal segment to which the range-limiting muscle attaches. Stretch the muscle over one joint at a time and then over all joints simultaneously until the optimal length of soft tissues is achieved. To minimize compressive forces in small joints, stretch the distal joints first and proceed proximally.
- Consider incorporating a prestretch, isometric contraction of the range-limiting muscle (the hold–relax procedure) to relax the muscle reflexively prior to stretching it.
- To avoid joint compression during the stretching procedure, apply gentle (grade I) distraction to the moving joint.
- Apply a low-intensity stretch in a slow, sustained manner. Remember, the direction of the stretching movement is directly opposite the line of pull of the range-limiting muscle. Ask the patient to assist you with the stretch or apply a passive stretch to lengthen the tissues. Take the hypomobile soft tissues to the point of firm tissue resistance and then move just beyond that point. The force must be enough to place tension on soft tissue structures but not so great as to cause pain or injure the structures. The patient should experience a *pulling sensation*, but not pain, in the structures being stretched. When stretching adhesions of a tendon within its sheath, the patient may experience a "stinging" sensation.
- Maintain the stretched position for 30 seconds or longer. During this time, the tension in the tissues should slowly decrease. When tension decreases, move the extremity or joint a little farther to progressively lengthen the hypomobile tissues.
- Gradually release the stretch force and allow the patient and therapist to rest momentarily while maintaining the range-limiting tissues in a comfortably elongated position. Then repeat the sequence several times.
- If the patient does not seem to tolerate a sustained stretch, use several very slow, gentle, intermittent stretches with the muscle in a lengthened position.
- If deemed appropriate, apply selected soft tissue mobilization procedures, such as fascial massage or cross-fiber friction massage, at or near the sites of adhesion during the stretching maneuver.

N O T E : Do not attempt to gain the full range in one or two treatment sessions. Resolving mobility impairment is a slow, gradual process. It may take several weeks of stretching to see significant results.

## After Stretching

- Apply cold to the soft tissues that have been stretched and allow these structures to cool in a lengthened position. Cold may minimize poststretch muscle soreness that can occur as the result of microtrauma during stretching. When soft tissues are cooled in a lengthened

position, increases in ROM are more readily maintained.[77,107]

- Regardless of the type of stretching intervention used, have the patient perform active ROM and strengthening exercises through the gained range immediately after stretching. With your supervision and feedback, have the patient use the gained range by performing simulated functional movement patterns that are part of daily living, occupational, or recreational tasks.
- Develop a balance in strength in the antagonistic muscles in the new range so there is adequate neuromuscular control and stability as flexibility increases.

# ● PRECAUTIONS FOR STRETCHING

There are a number of general precautions that apply to all forms of stretching interventions. In addition, some special precautions must be taken when advising patients about stretching exercises that are part of community-based fitness programs or commercially available exercise products marketed to the general public.

## General Precautions

- Do not passively force a joint beyond its normal ROM. Remember, normal (typical) ROM varies among individuals. In adults, flexibility is greater in women than in men.[164] When treating older adults, be aware of age-related changes in flexibility.

 **Focus on Evidence.**_____

Some studies suggest that flexibility decreases with age, particularly when coupled with decreased activity levels.[2,3,95] However, the results of a study of more than 200 adults ages 20 to 79 who regularly exercised demonstrated that hamstring length did not significantly decrease with age.[164]

---

- Use extra caution in patients with known or suspected osteoporosis due to disease, prolonged bed rest, age, or prolonged use of steroids.
- Protect newly united fractures; be certain there is appropriate stabilization between the fracture site and the joint in which the motion takes place.
- Avoid vigorous stretching of muscles and connective tissues that have been immobilized for an extended period of time. Connective tissues, such as tendons and ligaments, lose their tensile strength after prolonged immobilization. High-intensity short-duration stretching procedures tend to cause more trauma and resulting weakness of soft tissues than low-intensity, long-duration stretch.
- Progress the dosage (intensity, duration, and frequency) of stretching interventions gradually to minimize soft tissue trauma and postexercise muscle soreness. If a patient

experiences joint pain or muscle soreness lasting more than 24 hours after stretching, too much force has been used during stretching, causing an an inflammatory response. This, in turn, causes increased scar tissue formation. Patients should experience no more residual discomfort than a transitory feeling of tenderness.

◉ Avoid stretching edematous tissue, as it is more susceptible to injury than normal tissue. Continued irritation of edematous tissue usually causes increased pain and edema.

◉ Avoid overstretching weak muscles, particularly those that support body structures in relation to gravity.

## Special Precautions for Mass-Market Flexibility Programs

In an effort to develop and maintain a desired level of fitness, many people, young and old, participate in physical conditioning programs at home or in the community. Flexibility (self-stretching) exercises are an integral component of these programs. As a result, individuals frequently learn self-stretching procedures in fitness classes or from popular videos or television programs. Although much of the information in these resources is usually safe and accurate, there may be some errors and potential problems in flexibility programs designed for the mass market.

### Common Errors and Potential Problems

*Nonselective or poorly balanced stretching activities.* General flexibility programs may include stretching regions of the body that are already mobile or even hypermobile but may neglect regions that are tight from faulty posture or inactivity. For example, in the sedentary population, some degree of hypomobility tends to develop in the hip flexors, trunk flexors, shoulder extensors and internal rotators, and scapular protractors from sitting in a slumped posture. Yet many commercially available flexibility routines overemphasize exercises that stretch posterior muscle groups, already overstretched, and fail to include exercises to stretch the tight anterior structures. Consequently, faulty postures may worsen rather than improve.

*Insufficient warm-up.* Individuals involved in flexibility programs often fail to warm up prior to stretching.

*Ineffective stabilization.* Programs often lack effective methods of self-stabilization. Therefore, an exercise may fail to stretch the intended tight structures and may transfer the stretch force to structures that are already mobile or even hypermobile.

*Use of ballistic stretching.* Although a less common problem than in the past, some exercise routines still demonstrate stretches using ballistic maneuvers. Because this form of stretching is not well controlled, it increases the likelihood of postexercise muscle soreness and significant injury to soft tissues.

*Excessive intensity.* The phrase *"no pain, no gain"* is often used inappropriately as the guideline for intensity

of stretch. An effective flexibility routine should be progressed gradually and should not cause pain or excessive stress to tissues.

*Abnormal biomechanics.* Some popular stretching exercises do not respect the biomechanics of the region. For example, the "hurdler's" stretch is designed to stretch unilaterally the hamstrings of one lower extremity and the quadriceps of the opposite extremity but imposes unsafe stresses on the medial capsule and ligaments of the flexed knee.

*Insufficient information about age-related differences.* One flexibility program does not fit all age groups. As a result of the normal aging process, mobility of connective tissues diminishes.[2,3,81] Consequently, elderly individuals, whose physical activity level has diminished with age, typically exhibit less flexibility than young adults. Even an adolescent after a growth spurt temporarily exhibits restricted flexibility, particularly in two-joint muscle groups. Flexibility programs marketed to the general public may not be sensitive to these normal, age-related differences in flexibility and may foster unrealistic expectations.

### Strategies for Risk Reduction

◉ Whenever possible, assess the appropriateness and safety of exercises in a "prepackaged" flexibility program.

◉ If a patient you are treating is participating in a community-based fitness class, review the exercises in the program and determine their appropriateness and safety for your patient.

◉ Stay up-to-date on current exercise programs, products, and trends by monitoring the content and safety and your patient's use of home exercise videotapes.

◉ Determine whether a class or video is geared for individuals of the same age or with similar pathological conditions.

◉ Eliminate or modify those exercises that are inconsistent with the intervention plan you have developed for your patient.

◉ See that the flexibility program maintains a balance of mobility between antagonistic muscle groups and emphasizes stretching those muscle groups that often become shortened with age, faulty posture, or sedentary lifestyle.

◉ Teach your patient basic principles of self-stretching and how to apply those principles to select safe and appropriate stretching exercises and to avoid those that perpetuate impairments or have no value.

◉ Make sure your patient understands the importance of warming up prior to stretching. Give suggestions on how to warm up before stretching.

◉ Be certain that the patient knows how to provide effective self-stabilization to isolate stretch to specific muscle groups.

◉ Teach your patient how to determine the appropriate intensity of stretch; be sure your patient knows that, at most, postexercise muscle soreness should be mild and last no more than 24 hours.

# ADJUNCTS TO STRETCHING INTERVENTIONS

Interventions that promote general or local relaxation can complement a stretching program. Therapists managing patients with impairments, including chronic pain, muscle guarding, or imbalances, and restricted mobility may find it useful to integrate relaxation exercises into a patient's plan of care. Superficial or deep heat, massage, biofeedback, and joint traction also are useful adjuncts to stretching procedures.

## Relaxation Training

*Relaxation training*, using methods of general relaxation (total body relaxation), has been used for many years by a variety of practitioners[47,51,78,128,145,160] to help patients learn to relieve or reduce pain, muscle tension, anxiety or stress, and associated physical impairments including tension headaches, high blood pressure, and respiratory distress. Volumes have been written by health professionals from many disciplines on topics such as chronic pain management, progressive relaxation, biofeedback, stress and anxiety management, and imagery. A brief overview of techniques is presented in this section.

### Common Elements of Relaxation Training

Relaxation training involves a reduction in muscle tension in the entire body or the region that is painful or restricted by *conscious* effort and thought. Training occcurs in a quiet environment with low lighting and soothing music or an auditory cue on which the patient may focus. The patient performs deep breathing exercises or visualizes a peaceful scene. When giving instructions the therapist uses a soft tone of voice.

### Examples of Approaches to Relaxation Training

*Autogenic training.* This approach, advocated by Schultz and colleagues,[47,128] involves conscious relaxation through autosuggestion and a progression of exercises as well as meditation.

*Progressive relaxation.* This technique, developed by Jacobson,[78] uses systematic, distal to proximal progression of voluntary contraction and relaxation of muscles. It is sometimes incorporated into childbirth education.

*Awareness through movement.* The system of therapy developed by Feldenkrais[51] combines sensory awareness, movements of the limbs and trunk, deep breathing, conscious relaxation procedures, and self-massage to alter muscle imbalances and abnormal postural alignment to remediate muscle tension and pain.

### Sequence for Progressive Relaxation Techniques

- Place the patient in a quiet area and in a comfortable position, and be sure that restrictive clothing is loosened.
- Have the patient breathe in a deep, relaxed manner.

---

| BOX 4.9 | Indicators of Relaxation |

- Decreased muscle tension
- Lowered heart and respiratory rates and blood pressure
- Increased skin temperature in the extremities associated with vasodilation
- Constricted pupils
- Little to no body movement
- Eyes closed and flat facial expression
- Jaw and hands relaxed with palms open
- Decreased distractability

- Ask the patient to contract the distal musculature in the hands or feet voluntarily for several (5 to 7) seconds and then consciously relax those muscles for 20 to 30 seconds.
- Suggest that the patient try to feel a sense of heaviness in the hands or feet and a sense of warmth in the muscles just relaxed.
- Progress to a more proximal area of the body and have the patient actively contract and actively relax the more proximal musculature. Eventually have the patient isometrically contract and consciously relax the entire extremity.
- Suggest to the patient that he or she should feel a sense of relaxation and warmth throughout the entire limb and eventually throughout the whole body.

### Indicators of Relaxation

There are a number of physiological, behavioral, cognitive, and emotional responses that occur during total body relaxation.[145] These key indicators are summarized in Box 4.9.

## Heat

Warming up prior to stretching is a common practice in rehabilitation and fitness programs.[109] It is well documented in human and animal studies that as intramuscular temperature increases the extensibility of contractile and noncontractile soft tissues likewise increases. In addition, as the temperature of muscle increases, the amount of force required and the time the stretch force must be applied decrease.[89-91,93,125,150,153] There is also a decrease in the rate of firing of the type II efferents from the muscle spindles and an increase in the sensitivity of the GTO, which makes it more likely to fire.[53] In turn, it is believed that when tissues relax and more easily lengthen, stretching is associated with less muscle guarding and is more comfortable for the patient.[89-91] It has also been suggested that warming up prior to exercise reduces postexercise muscle sorenesss and the risk of injury to soft tissues.[165] However, not all of these assumptions about the clinical application of heat are well supported by evidence.[70,121]

PRECAUTION: Although stretching is often thought of as a warm-up activity performed prior to vigorous exercise, an appropriate warm-up must also occur in preparation for stretching.

## Methods of Warm-up

Superficial heat (hot packs, paraffin) or deep-heating modalities (ultrasound, shortwave diathermy) provide different mechanisms to heat tissues.[110,123] These thermal agents are used primarily to heat small areas such as individual joints, muscle groups, or tendons and may be applied prior to or during the stretching procedure.[42,43,87,125] There is no consensus whether heating modalities should be applied prior to or during the stretching procedure.

Low-intensity, active exercises, which generally increase circulation and core body temperature, also have been used as a mechanism to warm up large muscle groups prior to stretching.[40,57,73,87,129] Some common warm-up exercises are a brief walk, nonfatiguing cycling on a stationary bicycle, use of a stair-stepping machine, active heel raises, or a few minutes of active arm exercises.

## Effectiveness of Warm-up Methods

The use of heat alone (a thermal agent or warm-up exercises) without stretching has been shown to have either little or no effect on improving muscle flexibility.[16,40,67,132] Although a body of knowledge indicates that heat combined with stretching produces greater long-term gains in tissue length than stretching alone,[42,43,90] the results of other studies have shown comparable improvement in ROM with no significant differences between conditions.[40,57,67,87,139]

N O T E : The application of cold prior to stretching (cryostretching) compared to heat has been studied.[122,139] Advocates suggest its use to decrease muscle tone and make the muscle less sensitive during stretch in healthy subjects[63] and in patients with spasticity or rigidity secondary to upper motor neuron lesions.[147] The use of cold immediately after soft tissue injury effectively decreases pain and muscle spasm.[88,90,122] However, once soft tissue healing and scar formation begin, cold makes healing tissues less extensible and more susceptible to microtrauma during stretching.[33,88,90,93] Cooling soft tissues in a lengthened position *after* stretching has been shown to promote more lasting increases in soft tissue length and minimize poststretch muscle soreness.[91,127]

To summarize, the authors of this text recommend that cold be applied to injured soft tissues during the first 24 to 48 hours after injury to minimize swelling, muscle spasm, and pain. Remember, stretching is contraindicated in the presence of inflammation that occurs during the acute phase of tissue healing (see Chapter 10). When inflammation subsides and stretching is indicated, the authors advocate warming soft tissues prior to or during a stretching maneuver. After stretching, cold should be applied to soft tissues held in a lengthened position to minimize poststretch muscle soreness and to promote longer-lasting gains in ROM.

## Massage

### Massage for Relaxation

Local muscle relaxation can be enhanced by massage, particularly with light or deep stroking techniques.[37,137] In some approaches to stress and anxiety or pain management, self-massage, using light stroking techniques (effleurage), is performed during the relaxation process.[51] In sports and conditioning programs,[9,137] massage has been used for general relaxation purposes or to enhance recovery after strenuous physical activity, although the efficacy of the latter is not well founded.[143] Because massage has been shown to increase circulation to muscles and decrease muscle spasm, it is a useful adjunct to stretching exercises.

### Soft Tissue Mobilization Techniques

Another broad category of massage is soft tissue mobilization. Although soft tissue mobilization and manipulation techniques involve various forms of deep massage, the primary purpose of these techniques is not relaxation but, rather, increasing the mobility of adherent or shortened connective tissues including fascia, tendons, and ligaments.[21]

There are many techniques and explanations as to their effects on connective tissues, including the mechanical effects of stress and strain. Stresses are applied long enough for creep and stress-relaxation of tissues to occur. With *myofascial massage*,[21,97] stretch forces are applied across fascial planes or between muscle and septae. With *friction massage*,[34,71,137] deep circular or cross-fiber massage is applied to break up adhesions or minimize rough surfaces between tendons and their synovial sheaths. Friction massage is also used to increase the mobility of scar tissue in muscle as it heals. Theoretically, it applies stresses to scar tissue as it matures to align collagen fibers along the lines of stress for normal mobility. These forms of connective tissue massage as well as many other approaches and techniques of soft tissue mobilization are useful interventions for patients with restricted mobility.

## Biofeedback

Biofeedback is another tool to help a patient learn and practice the process of relaxation. A patient, if properly trained, can electronically monitor and learn to reduce the amount of tension in muscles, as well as heart rate and blood pressure, through biofeedback instrumentation.[47,145] Through visual or auditory feedback, a patient can begin to sense or feel what muscle relaxation is. By reducing muscle tension, pain can be decreased and flexibility increased.

N O T E : Biofeedback is also a useful means to help a patient learn how to activate a muscle, rather than relax it, such as when learning how to perform quadriceps setting exercises after knee surgery.

## Joint Traction or Oscillation

Slight manual distraction of joint surfaces prior to or in conjunction with joint mobilization or muscle-tendon stretching techniques can be used to inhibit joint pain and spasm of muscles around a joint (see Chapter 5).[34,71,82] Pendular motions of a joint use the weight of the limb to distract the joint surfaces and simultaneously oscillate and relax the limb. The joint may be further distracted by adding a 1- or 2-lb weight to the extremity, which causes a stretch force on joint tissues.

# ⊙ MANUAL STRETCHING TECHNIQUES IN ANATOMICAL PLANES OF MOTION

As with the ROM exercises described in Chapter 3, the manual stretching techniques in this section are described with the patient in a *supine* position. Alternate patient positions such as prone or sitting are indicated for some motions and are noted when necessary. Manual stretching procedures in an aquatic environment are described in Chapter 9.

Effective manual stretching techniques require adequate stabilization of the patient and sufficient strength and good body mechanics of the therapist. Depending on the size (height and weight) of the therapist and the patient, modifications in the patient's position and suggested hand placements for stretching or stabilization may have to be made by the therapist.

Each description of a stretching technique is identified by the anatomical plane of motion that is to be increased followed by a notation of the muscle group being stretched. Limitations in functional ROM usually are caused by shortening of multiple muscle groups and periarticular structures, and they affect movement in combined (as well as anatomical) planes of motion. In this situation, however, stretching multiple muscle groups simultaneously using diagonal patterns (i.e., $D_1$ and $D_2$ flexion and extension of the upper or lower extremities as described in Chapter 6) is *not* recommended and therefore is not described in this chapter. The authors believe that combined, diagonal patterns are appropriate for maintaining available ROM with passive and active exercises and increasing strength in multiple muscle groups but are ineffective for *isolating* a stretch force to specific muscles or muscle groups of the extremities that are shortened and restricting ROM. Special considerations for each region being stretched are also noted in this section.

Prolonged passive stretching techniques using mechanical equipment are applied using the same points of stabilization as manual stretching. The stretch force is applied at a lower intensity and is applied over a much longer period than with manual stretching. The stretch force is provided by weights or splints rather than the strength or endurance of a therapist. The patient is stabilized with belts, straps, or counterweights.

N O T E :  Manual stretching procedures for the musculature of the cervical, thoracic, and lumbar spine may be found in Chapter 16. Selected self-stretching techniques of the extremities and spine that a patient can do without assistance from a therapist are not described in this chapter.

These exercises are for each joint of the extremities may be found in Chapters 16 through 22.

## Upper Extremity Stretching

### The Shoulder: Special Considerations
Many muscles involved with shoulder motion attach to the scapula rather than the thorax. Therefore, when most muscles of the shoulder girdle are stretched, it is imperative to stabilize the scapula. Without scapular stabilization the stretch force is transmitted to the muscles that normally stabilize the scapula during movement of the arm. This subjects these muscles to possible overstretching and disguises the true ROM of the glenohumeral joint.

Remember:

⊙ When the scapula is stabilized and not allowed to abduct or upwardly rotate, only 120° of shoulder flexion and abduction can occur at the glenohumeral joint.
⊙ The humerus must be externally rotated to gain full ROM of abduction.
⊙ Muscles most apt to become shortened are those that *prevent* full shoulder flexion, abduction, and external rotation. It is rare to find restrictions in structures that prevent shoulder adduction and extension to neutral.

### Flexion of the Shoulder
*To increase flexion of the shoulder* (to stretch the shoulder extensors) (Fig. 4.16).

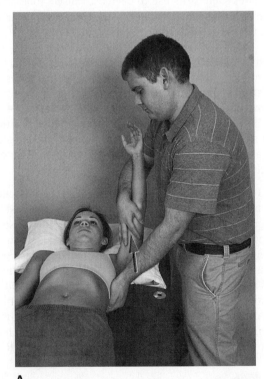

**A**

FIGURE 4.16  (A) Hand placement and stabilization of the scapula to stretch the teres major and increase shoulder flexion.

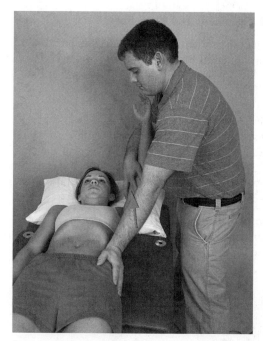

**B**

FIGURE 4.16 (*B*) Hand placement and stabilization of the pelvis to stretch the latissimus dorsi and increase shoulder flexion.

### Hand Placement and Procedure

- Grasp the posterior aspect of the distal humerus, just above the elbow.
- Stabilize the axillary border of the scapula to stretch the teres major, or stabilize the lateral aspect of the thorax and superior aspect of the pelvis to stretch the latissimus dorsi.
- Move the patient's arm into full shoulder flexion to elongate the shoulder extensors.

### Hyperextension of the Shoulder

*To increase hyperextension of the shoulder* (to stretch the shoulder flexors) (Fig. 4.17).

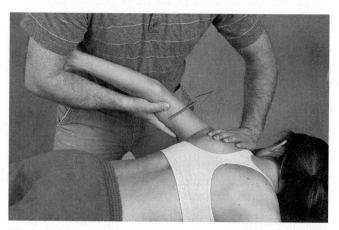

FIGURE 4.17 Hand placement and stabilization of the scapula to increase extension of the shoulder beyond neutral.

### Patient Position

Place the patient in a prone position.

### Hand Placement and Procedure

- Support the forearm and grasp the distal humerus.
- Stabilize the posterior aspect of the scapula to prevent substitute movements.
- Move the patient's arm into full hyperextension of the shoulder to elongate the shoulder flexors.

### Abduction of the Shoulder

*To increase abduction of the shoulder* (to stretch the adductors) (Fig. 4.18).

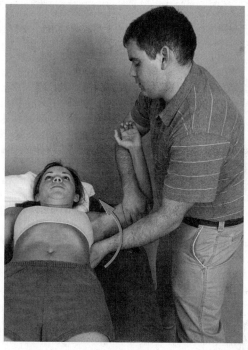

FIGURE 4.18 Hand placement and stabilization of the scapula for the stretching procedure to increase shoulder abduction.

### Hand Placement and Procedure

- With the elbow flexed to 90°, grasp the distal humerus.
- Stabilize the axillary border of the scapula.
- Move the patient into full shoulder abduction to lengthen the adductors of the shoulder.

### Adduction of the Shoulder

To *increase adduction of the shoulder* (to stretch the abductors). It is rare when a patient is unable to adduct the shoulder fully to 0° (so the upper arm is at the patient's side). Even if a patient has worn an abduction splint after a soft tissue or joint injury of the shoulder, when he or she is upright the constant pull of gravity elongates the shoulder abductors so the patient can adduct to a neutral position.

### External Rotation of the Shoulder

To *increase external rotation of the shoulder* (stretch the internal rotators) (Fig. 4.19).

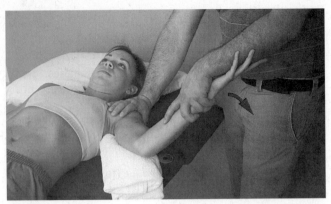

FIGURE 4.19 Shoulder position (slightly abducted and flexed) and hand placement at the mid to proximal forearm to increase external rotation of the shoulder. A folded towel is placed under the distal humerus to maintain the shoulder in slight flexion. The table stabilizes the scapula.

### Hand Placement and Procedure

- Abduct the shoulder to a comfortable position—initially 30° or 45° and later to 90° if the glenohumeral (GH) joint is stable—or place the arm at the patient's side.
- Flex the elbow to 90° so the forearm can be used as a lever.
- Grasp the volar surface of the mid-forearm with one hand.
- Stabilization of the scapula is provided by the table on which the patient is lying.
- Externally rotate the patient's shoulder by moving the patient's forearm closer to the table. This fully lengthens the internal rotators.

P R E C A U T I O N :  Because it is necessary to apply the stretch forces across the intermediate elbow joint when elongating the internal and external rotators of the shoulder, be sure the elbow joint is stable and pain-free. In addition, keep the intensity of the stretch force very low, particularly in patients with osteoporosis.

### Internal Rotation of the Shoulder

*To increase internal rotation of the shoulder* (stretch the external rotators) (Fig. 4.20).

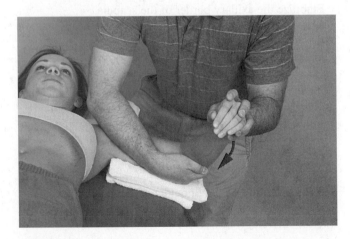

FIGURE 4.20 Hand placement and stabilization of the shoulder to increase internal rotation of the shoulder.

### Hand Placement and Procedure

- Abduct the shoulder to a comfortable position that allows internal rotation to occur without the thorax blocking the motion (initially to 45° and eventually to 90°).
- Flex the elbow to 90° so the forearm can be used as a lever.
- Grasp the dorsal surface of the midforearm with one hand, and stabilize the anterior aspect of the shoulder and support the elbow with your other forearm and hand.
- Move the patient's arm into internal rotation to lengthen the external rotators of the shoulder.

### Horizontal Abduction of the Shoulder

*To increase horizontal abduction of the shoulder* (stretch the pectoralis muscles) (Fig. 4.21).

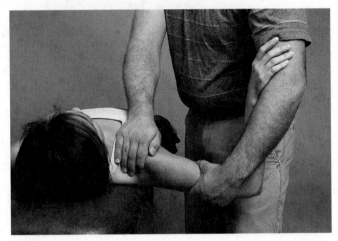

FIGURE 4.21 Hand placement and stabilization of the anterior aspect of the shoulder and chest to increase horizontal abduction of the shoulder past neutral (to stretch the pectoralis major).

### Patient Position

To reach full horizontal abduction in the supine position, the patient's shoulder must be at the edge of the table. Begin with the shoulder in 60° to 90° of abduction. The patient's elbow may also be flexed.

### Hand Placement and Procedure

- Grasp the anterior aspect of the distal humerus.
- Stabilize the anterior aspect of the shoulder.
- Move the patient's arm below the edge of the table into full horizontal abduction to stretch the horizontal adductors.

N O T E :  The horizontal adductors are usually tight bilaterally. Stretching techniques can be applied bilaterally by the therapist, or a bilateral self-stretch can be done by the patient by using a corner or wand (see Figs. 17.30 through 17.32).

### Scapular Mobility

To have full shoulder motion, a patient must have normal scapular mobility. (See scapular mobilization techniques in Chapter 5.)

## The Elbow and Forearm: Special Considerations

Several muscles that cross the elbow, such as the biceps brachii and brachioradialis, also influence supination and pronation of the forearm. Therefore, when stretching the elbow flexors and extensors, the techniques should be performed with the forearm pronated as well as supinated.

### Elbow Flexion

*To increase elbow flexion* (stretch the one-joint elbow extensors).

#### Hand Placement and Procedure

- Grasp the distal forearm just proximal to the wrist.
- With the arm at the patient's side supported on the table, stabilize the proximal humerus.
- Flex the patient's elbow just past the point of tissue resistance to lengthen the elbow extensors.

*To increase elbow flexion with the shoulder flexed* (stretch the long head of the triceps) (Fig. 4.22).

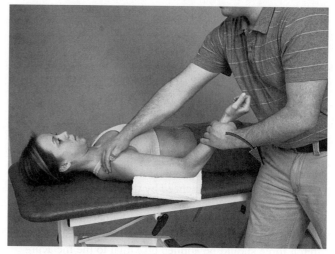

FIGURE 4.23 Hand placement and stabilization of the scapula and proximal humerus for stretching procedures to increase elbow extension.

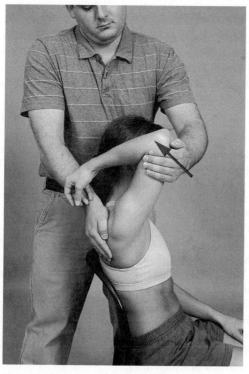

FIGURE 4.22 Hand placement and stabilization to increase elbow flexion with shoulder flexion (to stretch the long head of the triceps brachii).

#### Patient Position, Hand Placement, and Procedure

- With the patient sitting or lying supine with the arm at the edge of the table, flex the patient's shoulder as far as possible.
- While maintaining shoulder flexion, grasp the distal forearm and flex the elbow as far as possible.

### Elbow Extension

*To increase elbow extension* (to stretch the elbow flexors) (Fig. 4.23).

#### Hand Placement and Procedure

- Grasp the distal forearm.
- With the upper arm at the patient's side supported on the table. stabilize the scapula and anterior aspect of the proximal humerus.
- Extend the elbow just past the point of tissue resistance to lengthen the elbow flexors.

N O T E : Be sure to do this with the forearm in supination, pronation, and neutral position to stretch each of the elbow flexors.

*To increase elbow extension with the shoulder extended* (stretch the long head of the biceps).

#### Patient Position, Hand Placement, and Procedure

- With the patient lying supine close to the side of the table, stabilize the anterior aspect of the shoulder or with the patient lying prone, stabilize the scapula.
- Pronate the forearm, extend the elbow, and then extend the shoulder.

P R E C A U T I O N : It has been reported that heterotopic ossification (the appearance of ectopic bone in the soft tissues around a joint) can develop around the elbow after traumatic or burn injuries.[46] It is believed that *vigorous, forcible* passive stretching of the elbow flexors may increase the risk of this condition developing. Passive or assisted stretching, therefore, should be applied very gently and gradually in the elbow region. Use of active stretching, such as agonist contraction, might also be considered.

### Supination or Pronation of the Forearm

*To increase supination or pronation of the forearm.*

#### Hand Placement and Procedure

- With the patient's humerus supported on the table and the elbow flexed to 90°, grasp the distal forearm.
- Stabilize the humerus.

- Supinate or pronate the forearm just beyond the point of tissue resistance.
- Be sure the stretch force is applied to the radius rotating around the ulna. Do not twist the hand, thereby avoiding stress to the wrist articulations.
- Repeat the procedure with the elbow extended. Be sure to stabilize the humerus to prevent internal or external rotation of the shoulder.

### The Wrist and Hand: Special Considerations
The extrinsic muscles of the fingers cross the wrist joint and therefore may influence the ROM of the wrist. Wrist motion may also be influenced by the position of the elbow and forearm because the wrist flexors and extensors attach proximally on the epicondyles of the humerus.

When stretching the musculature of the wrist, the stretch force should be applied proximal to the metacarpophalangeal (MCP) joints, and the fingers should be relaxed.

### Patient Position
When stretching the muscles of the wrist and hand, have the patient sit in a chair adjacent to you with the forearm supported on a table to stabilize the forearm effectively.

### Wrist Flexion
*To increase wrist flexion.*

### Hand Placement and Procedure

- The forearm may be supinated, in midposition, or pronated.
- Stabilize the forearm against the table and grasp the dorsal aspect of the patient's hand.
- To elongate the wrist extensors, flex the patient's wrist and allow the fingers to extend passively.
- To further elongate the wrist extensors, extend the patient's elbow.

### Wrist Extension
*To increase wrist extension* (Fig. 4.24).

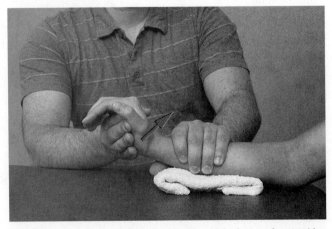

FIGURE 4.24 Hand placement and stabilization of the forearm for stretching procedure to increase extension of the wrist.

### Hand Placement and Procedure

- Pronate the forearm or place it in midposition, and grasp the patient at the palmar aspect of the hand. If there is a severe wrist flexion contracture, it may be necessary to place the patient's hand over the edge of the treatment table.
- Stabilize the forearm against the table.
- To lengthen the wrist flexors, extend the patient's wrist, allowing the fingers to flex passively.

### Radial Deviation
*To increase radial deviation.*

### Hand Placement and Procedure

- Grasp the ulnar aspect of the hand along the fifth metacarpal.
- Hold the wrist in midposition.
- Stabilize the forearm.
- Radially deviate the wrist to lengthen the ulnar deviators of the wrist.

### Ulnar Deviation
*To increase ulnar deviation.*

### Hand Placement and Procedure

- Grasp the radial aspect of the hand along the second metacarpal, not the thumb.
- Stabilize the forearm.
- Deviate the wrist ulnarly to lengthen the radial deviators.

### The Digits: Special Considerations
The complexity of the relationships among the joint structures and the intrinsic and multijoint extrinsic muscles of the digits requires careful examination and evaluation of the factors that contribute to loss of function in the hand because of limitation of motion. The therapist must determine if a limitation is from restriction of joints, decreased muscle flexibility, or adhesions of tendons or ligaments. The digits should always be stretched individually, not simultaneously. If an extrinsic muscle limits motion, lengthen it over one joint while stabilizing the other joints. Then hold the lengthened position and stretch it over the second joint, and so forth, until normal length is obtained. As noted in Chapter 3, begin the motion with the most distal joint to minimize shearing and compressive stresses to the surfaces of the small joints of the digits. Specific methods of intervention for dealing with adhesions of tendons are described in Chapter 19.

### CMC Joint of the Thumb
*To increase flexion, extension, abduction, or adduction of the carpometacarpal (CMC) joint of the thumb.*

### Hand Placement and Procedure

- Stabilize the trapezium with your thumb and index finger.
- Grasp the first metacarpal (not the first phalanx) with your other thumb and index finger.
- Move the first metacarpal in the desired direction to increase CMC flexion, extension, abduction, and adduction.

### MCP Joints of the Digits

*To increase flexion, extension, abduction, or adduction of the MCP joints of the digits.*

#### Hand Placement and Procedure

● Stabilize the metacarpal with your thumb and index finger.
● Grasp the proximal phalanx with your other thumb and index finger.
● Keep the wrist in midposition.
● Move the MCP joint in the desired direction for stretch.
● Allow the interphalangeal (IP) joints to flex or extend passively.

### PIP and DIP Joints

*To increase flexion or extension of the proximal (PIP) and distal (DIP) interphalangeal joints.*

#### Hand Placement and Procedure

● Grasp the middle or distal phalanx with your thumb and finger.
● Stabilize the proximal or middle phalanx with your other thumb and finger.
● Move the PIP or DIP joint in the desired direction for stretch.

### Stretching Specific Extrinsic and Intrinsic Muscles of the Fingers

Elongation of extrinsic and intrinsic muscles of the hand is described in Chapter 3. To stretch these muscles beyond their available range, the same hand placement and stabilization are used as with passive ROM. The only difference in technique is that the therapist moves each segment into the stretch range.

## Lower Extremity Stretching

### The Hip: Special Considerations

Because muscles of the hip attach to the pelvis or lumbar spine, the pelvis must always be stabilized when lengthening muscles about the hip. If the pelvis is not stabilized, the stretch force is transferred to the lumbar spine, in which unwanted compensatory motion then occurs.

### Flexion of the Hip

*To increase flexion of the hip with the knee flexed (stretch the gluteus maximus).*

#### Hand Placement and Procedure

● Flex the hip and knee simultaneously.
● Stabilize the opposite femur in extension to prevent posterior tilt of the pelvis.
● Move the patient's hip and knee into full flexion to lengthen the one-joint hip extensor.

### Flexion of the Hip with Knee Extension

*To increase flexion of the hip with the knee extended (stretch the hamstrings) (Fig. 4.25).*

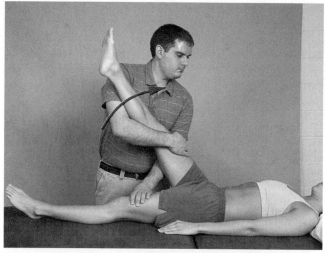

A

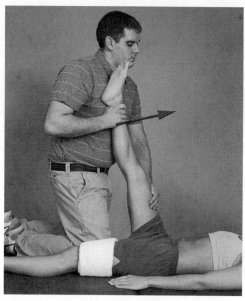

B

FIGURE 4.25 (*A, B*) Hand placement and stabilization of the opposite femur to stabilize the pelvis and low back for stretching procedures to increase hip flexion with knee extension (stretch the hamstrings) with the therapist standing by the side of the table or kneeling on the table.

#### Hand Placement and Procedure

● With the patient's knee fully extended, support the patient's lower leg with your arm or shoulder.
● Stabilize the opposite extremity along the anterior aspect of the thigh with your other hand or a belt or with the assistance of another person.
● With the knee at 0° extension, and the hip in neutral rotation, flex the hip as far as possible.

N O T E : Externally rotate the hip prior to hip flexion to isolate the stretch force to the medial hamstrings and internally rotate the hip to isolate the stretch force to the lateral hamstrings.

## Alternate Therapist Position

Kneel on the mat and place the patient's heel or distal tibia against your shoulder. Place both of your hands along the anterior aspect of the distal thigh to keep the knee extended. The opposite extremity is stabilized in extension by a belt or towel around the distal thigh and held in place by the therapist's knee.

### Extension of the Hip

*To increase hip extension* (to stretch the iliopsoas) (Fig. 4.26).

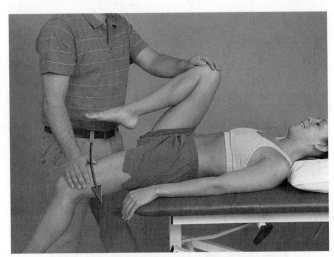

FIGURE 4.26 Hand placement and stabilization of the pelvis to increase extension of the hip (stretch the iliopsoas) with the patient lying supine. Flexing the knee when in this position also elongates the rectus femoris.

### Patient Position

Have the patient close to the edge of the treatment table so the hip being stretched can be extended beyond neutral. The opposite hip and knee are flexed toward the patient's chest to stabilize the pelvis and spine.

### Hand Placement and Procedure

- Stabilize the opposite leg against the patient's chest with one hand, or if possible have the patient assist by grasping around the thigh and holding it to the chest to prevent an anterior tilt of the pelvis during stretching.
- Move the hip to be stretched into extension or hyperextension by placing downward pressure on the anterior aspect of the distal thigh with your other hand. Allow the knee to extend so the two-joint rectus femoris does not restrict the range.

## Alternate Position

The patient can lie prone (Fig. 4.27).

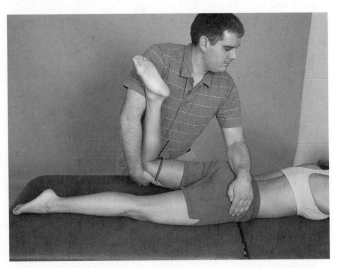

FIGURE 4.27 Hand placement and stabilization to increase hyperextension of the hip with the patient lying prone.

### Hand Placement and Procedure

- Support and grasp the anterior aspect of the patient's distal femur.
- Stabilize the patient's buttocks to prevent movement of the pelvis.
- Extend the patient's hip by lifting the femur off the table.

### Extension of the Hip with Knee Flexion

*To increase hip extension and knee flexion simultaneously* (stretch the rectus femoris).

### Patient Position

Use either of the positions previously described for increasing hip extension in the supine or prone positions (see Figs. 4.26 and 4.27).

### Hand Placement and Procedure

- With the hip held in full extension on the side to be stretched, move your hand to the distal tibia and gently flex the knee of that extremity as far as possible.
- Do not allow the hip to abduct or rotate.

### Abduction of the Hip

*To increase abduction of the hip* (stretch the adductors) (Fig. 4.28).

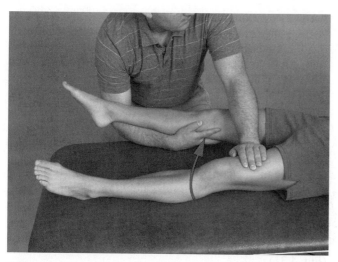

FIGURE 4.28 Hand placement and stabilization of the opposite extremity (or pelvis) for the stretching procedure to increase abduction of the hip.

### Hand Placement and Procedure

- Support the distal thigh with your arm and forearm.
- Stabilize the pelvis by placing pressure on the opposite anterior iliac crest or by maintaining the opposite lower extremity in slight abduction.
- Abduct the hip as far as possible to stretch the adductors.

N O T E : You may apply your stretch force cautiously at the medial malleolus only if the knee is stable and pain-free. This creates a great deal of stress to the medial supporting structures of the knee and is generally not recommended by the authors.

### Adduction of the Hip
*To increase adduction of the hip* [stretch the tensor fasciae latae and iliotibial (IT) band] (Fig. 4.29).

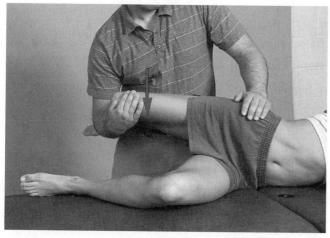

FIGURE 4.29 Patient positioned side-lying. Hand placement and procedure to stretch the tensor fasciae latae and IT band.

### Patient Position
Place the patient in a side-lying position with the hip to be stretched uppermost. Flex the bottom hip and knee to stabilize the patient.

### Hand Placement and Procedure

- Stabilize the pelvis at the iliac crest with your proximal hand.
- Flex the knee and extend the patient's hip to neutral or into slight hyperextension, if possible.
- Let the patient's hip adduct with gravity and apply an additional stretch force with your other hand to the lateral aspect of the distal femur to further adduct the hip.

N O T E : If the patient's hip cannot be extended to neutral, the hip flexors must be stretched before the tensor fasciae latae can be stretched.

### External Rotation of the Hip
*To increase external rotation of the hip* (stretch the internal rotators) (Fig. 4.30A).

### Patient Position
Place the patient in a prone position, hips extended and knee flexed to 90°.

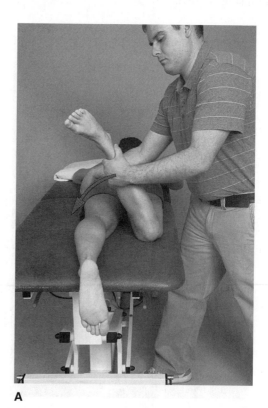

**A**

FIGURE 4.30 (*A*) Hand placement and stabilization of the pelvis to increase external rotation of the hip.

### Hand Placement and Procedure

● Grasp the distal tibia of the extremity to be stretched.
● Stabilize the pelvis by applying pressure with your other hand across the buttocks.
● Apply pressure to the lateral malleolus or lateral aspect of the tibia, and externally rotate the hip as far as possible.

### Alternate Position and Procedure

Sitting at the edge of a table with hips and knees flexed to 90°.
● Stabilize the pelvis by applying pressure to the iliac crest with one hand.
● Apply the stretch force to the lateral malleolus or lateral aspect of the lower leg, and externally rotate the hip.

N O T E : When you apply the stretch force against the lower leg in this manner, thus crossing the knee joint, the knee must be stable and pain-free. If the knee is not stable, it is possible to apply the stretch force by grasping the distal thigh, but the leverage is poor and there is a tendency to twist the skin.

### Internal Rotation of the Hip

*To increase internal rotation of the hip* (stretch the external rotators) (Fig. 4.30B).

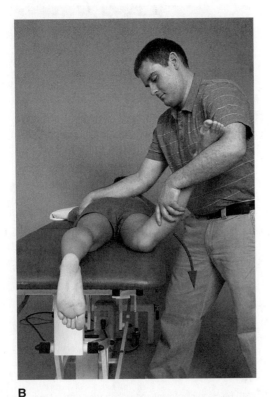

**B**

FIGURE 4.30 (continued) (*B*) Hand placement and stabilization of the pelvis to increase internal rotation of the hip with the patient prone.

### Patient Position and Stabilization

Position the patient the same as when increasing external rotation, described previously.

### Hand Placement and Procedure

Apply pressure to the medial malleolus or medial aspect of the tibia, and internally rotate the hip as far as possible.

### The Knee: Special Considerations

The position of the hip during stretching influences the flexibility of the flexors and extensors of the knee. The flexibility of the hamstrings and the rectus femoris must be examined and evaluated separately from the one-joint muscles that affect knee motion.

### Knee Flexion

*To increase knee flexion* (stretch the knee extensors) (Fig. 4.31).

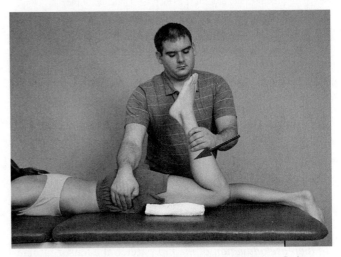

FIGURE 4.31 Hand placement and stabilization to increase knee flexion (stretch the rectus femoris and quadriceps) with the patient lying prone.

### Patient Position

Have the patient assume a prone position.

### Hand Placement and Procedure

● Stabilize the pelvis by applying downward pressure across the buttocks.
● Grasp the anterior aspect of the distal tibia, and flex the patient's knee.

P R E C A U T I O N : Place a rolled towel under the thigh just above the knee to prevent compression of the patella against the table during the stretch. Stretching the knee extensors too vigorously in the prone position can traumatize the knee joint and cause swelling.

### Alternate Position and Procedure

● Have the patient sit with the thigh supported on the treatment table and leg flexed over the edge as far as possible.

● Stabilize the anterior aspect of the proximal femur with one hand.
● Apply the stretch force to the anterior aspect of the distal tibia and flex the patient's knee as far as possible.

N O T E : This position is useful when working in the 0° to 100° range of knee flexion. The prone position is best for increasing knee flexion from 90° to 135°.

## Knee Extension
*To increase knee extension in the midrange* (stretch the knee flexors) (Fig. 4.32).

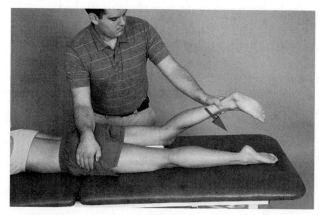
FIGURE 4.32 Hand placement and stabilization to increase mid-range knee extension with the patient lying prone.

### Patient Position
Place the patient in a prone position and put a small, rolled towel under the patient's distal femur, just above the patella.

### Hand Placement and Procedure
● Grasp the distal tibia with one hand and stabilize the buttocks to prevent hip flexion with the other hand.
● Slowly extend the knee to stretch the knee flexors.

## End-Range Knee Extension
*To increase end-range knee extension* (Fig. 4.33).

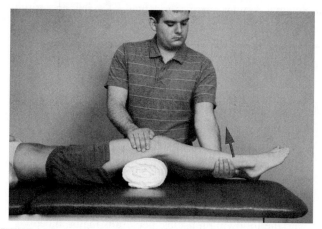
FIGURE 4.33 Hand placement and stabilization to increase terminal knee extension.

### Patient Position
Patient assumes a supine position.

### Hand Placement and Procedure
● Grasp the distal tibia of the knee to be stretched.
● Stabilize the hip by placing your hand or forearm across the anterior thigh. This prevents hip flexion during stretching.
● Apply the stretch force to the posterior aspect of the distal tibia, and extend the patient's knee.

### The Ankle and Foot: Special Considerations
The ankle and foot are composed of multiple joints. Consider the mobility of these joints (see Chapter 5) as well as the multijoint muscles that cross these joints when increasing ROM of the ankle and foot.

### Dorsiflexion of the Ankle
*To increase dorsiflexion of the ankle with the knee extended* (stretch the gastrocnemius muscle) (Fig. 4.34).

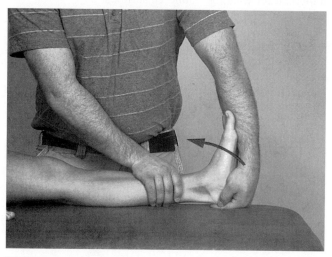
FIGURE 4.34 Hand placement and procedure to increase dorsiflexion of the ankle with the knee extended (stretching the gastrocnemius).

### Hand Placement and Procedure
● Grasp the patient's heel (calcaneus) with one hand, maintain the subtalar joint in a neutral position, and place your forearm along the plantar surface of the foot.
● Stabilize the anterior aspect of the tibia with your other hand.
● Dorsiflex the talocrural joint of the ankle by pulling the calcaneus in an inferior direction with your thumb and fingers while gently applying pressure in a superior direction just proximal to the heads of the metatarsals with your forearm.

*To increase dorsiflexion of the ankle with the knee flexed* (stretch the soleus muscle). To eliminate the effect of the two-joint gastrocnemius muscle, the knee must be flexed. Hand placement, stabilization, and stretch force are the same as when stretching the gastrocnemius.

PRECAUTION: When stretching the gastrocnemius or soleus muscles, avoid placing too much pressure against the heads of the metatarsals and stretching the long arch of the foot. Overstretching the long arch of the foot can cause a flat foot or a rocker-bottom foot.

### Plantarflexion of the Ankle

*To increase plantarflexion of the ankle.*

#### Hand Placement and Procedure

- Support the posterior aspect of the distal tibia with one hand.
- Grasp the foot along the tarsal and metatarsal areas.
- Apply the stretch force to the anterior aspect of the foot, and plantarflex the foot as far as possible.

### Inversion and Eversion of the Ankle

*To increase inversion and eversion of the ankle.* Inversion and eversion of the ankle occur at the subtalar joint as a component of pronation and supination. Mobility of the subtalar joint (with appropriate strength) is particularly important for walking on uneven surfaces.

#### Hand Placement and Procedure

- Stabilize the talus by grasping just distal to the malleoli with one hand.
- Grasp the calcaneus with your other hand, and move it medially and laterally at the subtalar joint.

### Stretching Specific Muscles of the Ankle and Foot

#### Hand Placement and Procedure

- Stabilize the distal tibia with your proximal hand.
- Grasp around the foot with your other hand and align the

motion and force opposite the line of pull of the tendons. Apply the stretch force against the bone to which the muscle attaches distally.

- To stretch the tibialis anterior (which inverts and dorsiflexes the ankle): Grasp the dorsal aspect of the foot across the tarsals and metatarsals and plantarflex and abduct the foot.
- To stretch the tibialis posterior (which plantarflexes and inverts the foot): Grasp the plantar surface of the foot around the tarsals and metatarsals and dorsiflex and abduct the foot.
- To stretch the peroneals (which evert the foot): Grasp the lateral aspect of the foot at the tarsals and metatarsals and invert the foot.

### Flexion and Extension of the Toes

*To increase flexion and extension of the toes.* It is best to stretch any musculature that limits motion in the toes individually. With one hand, stabilize the bone proximal to the restricted joint, and with the other hand move the phalanx in the desired direction.

## Neck and Trunk

Stretching techniques to increase mobility in the cervical, thoracic, and lumbar spine may be found in Chapter 16.

## Self-Stretching Techniques

Examples of self-stretching techniques, performed independently by the patient after appropriate instruction, may be found in Chapters 17 through 22 (upper and lower extremities) and Chapter 16 (neck and trunk).

---

# INDEPENDENT LEARNING ACTIVITIES

## ● Critical Thinking and Discussion

1. What physical findings from an examination of a patient would lead you to decide that stretching exercises were an appropriate intervention?
2. Discuss the advantages and disadvantages of various stretching exercises, specifically manual stretching, self-stretching, and mechanical stretching. Under what circumstances would one form be a more appropriate choice than another?
3. Discuss how the effectiveness of a program of stretching activities is influenced by the responses of contractile and noncontractile soft tissues to stretch. Consider such factors as intensity, speed, duration, and frequency of stretch.
4. Discuss how your approach to and application of stretching would differ when developing stretching exercises for a healthy young adult with limited mobility in the (a) shoulder, (b) knee, or (c) ankle in contrast to an elderly individual with osteoporosis and limited motion in the same regions.

5. Explain the procedures for and rationale behind each of the following types of neuromuscular inhibition: HR, HR-AC, CR, and AC. Under what circumstances would you choose one technique over another?
6. Select a popular exercise videotape. Review and critique the flexibility exercises on the tape. Was there a balance in the flexibility exercises in the program? Were the exercises executed safely and correctly? Were the exercises appropriate for the target population?

## ● Laboratory Practice

1. Manually stretch as many major muscle groups of the upper and lower extremities as is *safe* and *practical* with the patient in prone-lying, side-lying, or seated positions.
2. While considering individual muscle actions and lines of pull, demonstrate how to specifically and fully elongate the following muscles: pectoralis major, biceps brachii, brachioradialis, brachialis, triceps, extensor or flexor carpi ulnaris or radialis, flexor digitorum superfi-

cialis or profundus, rectus femoris versus the iliopsoas, gastrocnemius versus soleus, and the tibialis anterior and posterior.

3. Teach your partner how to stretch major muscle groups of the upper and lower extremities using either body weight or a cuff weight as the stretch force. Be sure to include effective stabilization procedures for these stretching techniques whenever possible.

4. Using either the hold-relax or contract-relax and the hold-relax agonist contraction neuromuscular inhibition techniques, elongate at least two major muscle groups at the shoulder, elbow, wrist, hip, knee, and ankle. Be sure to position, align, and stabilize your partner properly.

5. Design an effective and efficient series of self-stretching exercises that a person who works at a desk most of the day should incorporate into a daily home fitness routine. Demonstrate and teach each self-stretching exercise to your laboratory partner.

6. Identify a recreational/sport activity that your partner enjoys (i.e., tennis, golf, cycling, jogging, etc.) and design and demonstrate a program of self-stretching exercises to prepare your partner for the activity and reduce the risk of injury.

7. Design a program of progressive relaxation exercises for total body relaxation. Then implement the relaxation training sequence with your partner.

# REFERENCES

1. American Physical Therapy Association: Guide to Physical Therapist Practice, ed 2. Phys Ther 81(1):1–768, 2001.
2. Amundsen, LR: The effect of aging and exercise on joint mobility. Orthop Phys Ther Clin North Am 2:241, 1993.
3. Amundsen, LR: Effects of age on joints and ligaments. In Kauffman, TL (ed): Geriatric Rehabilitation Manual. Churchill Livingstone, New York, 1999, pp 14–16.
4. Bandy, WB, Irion, JM: The effects of time on static stretch on the flexibility of the hamstring muscles. Phys Ther 74:845–850, 1994.
5. Bandy, W, Irion, J, Briggler, M: The effect of time and frequency of static stretch on flexibility of the hamstring muscle. Phys Ther 77:1090–1096, 1997.
6. Bandy, W, Irion, J, Briggler, M: The effect of static stretch and dynamic range of motion training on the flexibility of the hamstring muscles. J Orthop Sports Phys Ther 27(4):295–300, 1998.
7. Beaulieu, JA: Developing a stretching program. Physician Sportsmed 9:59, 1981.
8. Beissner, KL, Collins JE, Holmes H: Muscle force and range of motion as predictors of function in older adults. Phys Ther 80:556–563, 2000.
9. Benjamin, PJ, Lamp, SP: Understanding Sports Massage. Human Kinetics, Champaign, IL, 1996.
10. Blanton, S, Grissom, SP, Riolo, L: Use of a static adjustable ankle-foot orthosis following tibial nerve block to reduce plantar-flexion contracture in an individual with brain injury. Phys Ther 82(11):1087–1097, 2002.
11. Bloomfield, SA: Changes in musculoskeletal structure and function with prolonged bed rest. Med Sci Sports Exerc 29:197–206, 1997.
12. Bohannon, RW: Effect of repeated eight minute muscle loading on the angle of straight leg raising. Phys Ther 64:491, 1984.
13. Bohannon, RW, Larkin, PA: Passive ankle dorsiflexion increases in patients after a regimen of tilt table: wedge board standing. Phys Ther 65:1676, 1985.
14. Bohannon, R, Tiberio, D, Zito, M: Effect of 5 minutes of stretch on ankle dorsiflexion range of motion. J Phys Ther Sci 6:2–8, 1994.
15. Bonutti, PM, et al: Static progressive stretch to re-establish elbow range of motion. Clin Orthop 303:128, 1994.
16. Boone, L, Ingersoll, CD, Cordova, ML: Passive hip flexion does not increase during or following ultrasound treatment of the hamstring muscle. Sports Med Training Rehab 9(3):189–198, 2000.
17. Booth, FW: Physiologic and biochemical effects of immobilization on muscle. Clin Orthop 219:5, 1987.
18. Brach, J, Van Swearingen, JM: Physical impairment and disability: relationship to performance of activities of daily living in community-dwelling older men. Phys Ther 82:752–761, 2002.
19. Brody, LT: Impaired joint mobility and range of motion. In Hall, CM, Brody, LT (eds): Therapeutic Exercise–Moving Toward Function, ed 2. Lippincott Williams & Wilkins, Philadelphia, 2005, pp 113–148.
20. Butler, DS: Mobilization of the Nervous System. Churchill Livingstone, Melbourne, 1991.
21. Cantu, RI, Grodin, AJ: Myofascial Manipulation: Theory and Clinical Application, ed 2. Aspen, Gaithersburg, MD, 2001.
22. Chaitow, L: Muscle Energy Techniques. Churchill Livingstone, New York, 1996.
23. Chandler, JM: Understanding the relationship between strength and mobility in frail elder persons: a review of the literature. Top Geriatr Rehabil 11:20, 1996.
24. Cherry, D: Review of physical therapy alternatives for reducing muscle contracture. Phys Ther 60:877, 1980.
25. Cipriani, D, Abel, B, Purrwitz, D: A comparison of two stretching protocols on hip range of motion: implications for total daily stretch duration. J Strength Cond Res 17:274–278, 2003.
26. Clark, MA: Muscle energy techniques in rehabilitation. In Prentice, WE, Voight, ML (eds): Techniques in Musculoskeletal Rehabilitation. McGraw-Hill, New York, 2001, pp 215–223.
27. Clark, S, Christiansen A, Hellman DF, et al: Effects of ipsilateral anterior thigh soft tissue stretching on passive unilateral straight leg raise. J Orthop Sports Phys Ther 29(1):4–9, 1999.
28. Condon, SN, Hutton, RS: Soleus muscle electromyographic activity and ankle dorsiflexion range of motion during four stretching procedures. Phys Ther 67:24, 1987.
29. Cornelius, WL, Jensen, RL, Odell, ME: Effects of PNF stretching phases on acute arterial blood pressure. J Appl Physiol 20:222–229, 1995.
30. Cornwall, M: Biomechanics of non-contractile tissue: a review. Phys Ther 64:1869, 1984.
31. Culav, EM, Clark, CH, Merrilees, MJ: Connective tissue matrix composition and its relevance to physical therapy. J Orthop Sports Phys Ther 79:308–319, 1999.
32. Cummings, GS, Crutchfeld, CA, Barnes. MR: Soft Tissue Changes in Contractures, vol 1. Stokesville, Atlanta, 1983.
33. Cummings, GS, Tillman, LJ: Remodeling of dense connective tissue in normal adult tissues. In Currier, DP, Nelson, RM (eds): Dynamics of Human Biologic Tissues. FA Davis, Philadelphia, 1992, p 45.
34. Cyriax, J: Textbook of Orthopedic Medicine: Treatment by Manipulation, ed 11. WB Saunders, Philadelphia, 1984.
35. Decoster, LC, Cleland, J, Altieri, C, Russell, P: The effect of hamstring stretching on range of motion: a systematic literature review. J Orthop Sports Phys Ther 35:377–387, 2005.
36. DeDeyne, PG: Application of passive stretch and its implications for muscle fibers. Phys Ther 81(2):819–827, 2001.
37. DeDomenico, G, Wood, EC: Beard's Massage, ed 4: WB Saunders, Philadelphia, 1997.
38. Dennis, JK, McKeough, DM: Mobility. In May, BJ (ed): Home Health and Rehabilitation: Concepts of Care. FA Davis, Philadelphia, 1999, pp 109–143.
39. De Vries, HA: Evaluation of static stretching procedures for improvement of flexibility. Res Q 33:222–229, 1962.
40. De Weiger, VC, Gorniak, GC, Shamus, E: The effect of static stretch and warm-up exercise on hamstring length over the course of 24 hours. J Orthop Sports Phys Ther 33(12):727–732, 2003.

41. Donatelli, R, Owens-Burkhart, H: Effects of immobilization on the extensibility of periarticular connective tissue. J Orthop Sports Phys Ther 3:67, 1981.

42. Draper, DO, Richard, MD: Rate of temperature decay in human muscle following 3 MHz ultrasound: the stretching window revealed J Athletic Training 30:304–307, 1996.

43. Draper, DO, Castro, JL, Feland, B, et al: Shortwave diathermy and prolonged stretching increase hamstring flexibility more than prolonged stretching alone. J Orthop Sports Phys Ther 34(1):13–20, 2004.

44. Dutton, M: Orthopedic Examination, Evaluation, and Intervention. McGraw-Hill, New York, 2004.

45. Eldred, E, Hulton, RS, Smith, JL: Nature of persisting changes in afferent discharge from muscle following its contraction. Prog Brain Res 44:157, 1976.

46. Ellerin, BE, Helfet, D, Parikh, S, et al: Current therapy in the management of heterotopic ossification of the elbow: a review with case studies. Am J Phys Med Rehabil 78(3):259–271, 1999.

47. Engel, JM: Relaxation and related techniques. In Hertling, D, Kessler, RM: Management of Common Musculoskeletal Disorders, ed 4. Lippincott Williams and Wilkins, Philadelphia, 2006, pp 261–266.

48. Etnyre, BR, Abraham, LD: Gains in range of ankle dorsiflexion using three popular stretching techniques. Am J Phys Med 65:189–196, 1986.

49. Euhardy, R: Contracture. In Kauffman, TL (ed): Geriatric Rehabilitation Manual. Churchill-Livingstone, New York, 1999, pp 77–80.

50. Feland, JB, et al: The effect of duration of stretching of the hamstring muscle group for increasing range of motion in people aged 65 years or older. Phys Ther 81:1110, 2001.

51. Feldenkrais, M: Awareness Through Movement. Harper & Row, New York, 1985.

52. Flitney, FW, Hirst, DG: Cross bridge detachment and sarcomere "give" during stretch of active frog's muscle. J Physiol 276:449, 1978.

53. Fukami, Y, Wilkinson, RS: Responses of isolated golgi tendon organs of the cat. J Physiol 265:673–689, 1977.

54. Fung, YC: Biomechanics: Mechanical Properties of Living Tissue, ed 2. Springer-Verlag, New York, 1993.

55. Gajdosik, RL: Effects of static stretching on the maximal length and resistance to passive stretch of short hamstring muscles. J Orthop Sports Phys Ther 14(6):250–255, 1991.

56. Garrett, W, Tridball, J: Myotendinous junction: structure, function and failure. In Woo, SL-Y, Buchwalter, JA (eds): Injury and Repair of the Musculoskeletal Soft Tissues. American Academy of Orthopedic Surgeons, Park Ridge, IL, 1988.

57. Gillette, TM, et al: Relationship of body core temperature and warm-up to knee range of motion. J Orthop Sports Phys Ther 13(3):126–131, 1991.

58. Godges, JJ, et al: The effects of two stretching procedures on hip range of motion and gait economy. J Orthop Sports Phys Ther 10(9):350–356, 1989.

59. Godges, JJ, MacRae, PG, Engelke, KA: Effects of exercise on hip range of motion, trunk muscle performance and gait economy. Phys Ther 73:468–477, 1993.

60. Gossman, M, Sahrmann, S, Rose, S: Review of length-associated changes in muscle. Phys Ther 62:1799, 1982.

61. Guyton, AC, Hall, JE: Textbook of Muscle Physiology, ed 10. WB Saunders, Philadelphia, 2000.

62. Halbertsma, JPK, Mulder, I, Goeken, LNH, et al: Repeated passive stretching: acute effect on the passive muscle moment and extensibility of short hamstrings. Arch Phys Med Rehabil 80:407–414, 1999.

63. Halkovich, LR, et al; Effect of Fluori-Methane® spray on passive hip flexion. Phys Ther 61:185–189, 1981.

64. Hansen, M: Pathophysiology: Foundations of Disease and Clinical Intervention. WB Saunders, Philadelphia, 1998.

65. Hanten, WP, Chandler, SD: The effect of myofascial release leg pull and sagittal plane isometric contract-relax technique on passive straight-leg raise angle. J Orthop Sports Phys Ther 20:138–144, 1994.

66. Hardy, MA: The biology of scar formation. Phys Ther 69:1015, 1989.

67. Henricson, AS, et al: The effect of heat and stretching on range of hip motion. J Orthop Sports Phys Ther 6(2):110–115, 1984.

68. Hepburn, G, Crivelli, K: Use of elbow Dynasplint for reduction of elbow flexion contracture: a case study. J Orthop Sports Phys Ther 5:269, 1984.

69. Herbert, LA: Preventative stretching exercises for the workplace. Orthop Phys Ther Pract 11:11, 1999.

70. Herbert, RD, Gabriel, M: Effects of stretching before and after exercising on muscle soreness and risk of injury: systematic review. BMJ 325:468–472, 2002.

71. Hertling, D, Kessler, RM: Introduction to manual therapy. In Hertling, D, Kessler, RM (eds): Management of Common Musculoskeletal Disorders, ed 4. Lippincott Williams & Wilkins, Philadelphia, 2006, pp 112–132.

72. Hertling, D: Soft tissue manipulations. In Hertling, D, Kessler, RM (eds): Management of Common Musculoskeletal Disorders, ed 4. Lippincott Williams & Wilkins, Philadelphia, 2006, pp 179–259.

73. Hubley, CL, Korzey, JW, Stansih, WD: The effects of static stretching exercise and stationary cycling on range of motion at the hip joint. J Orthop Sports Phys Ther 6(2):104–109, 1984.

74. Hulton, RS: Nueromuscular basis of stretching exercise. In Komi, PV (ed): Strength and Power in Sports. Blackwell Scientific, Boston, 1992, pp 29–38.

75. Isernbagen, SJ: Industrial physical therapy. In Malone, TK, McPoil, T, Nitz, AJ (eds): Orthopedic and Sports Physical Therapy, ed 3. Mosby-Year Book, St. Louis, 1997, pp 597–610.

76. Ito, CS: Conservative management of joint deformities and dynamic posturing. Orthop Phys Ther Clin N Am 2(1):25–38, 1993.

77. Iyer, MB, Mitz, AR, Winstein, C: Motor 1: lower centers. In Cohen, H (ed): Neuroscience for Rehabilitation. Lippincott Williams & Wilkins, Philadelphia, 1999, pp 209–242.

78. Jacobson, E: Progressive Relaxation. University of Chicago Press, Chicago, 1929.

79. Jansen, CM, et al: Treatment of a knee contracture using a knee orthosis incorporating stress-relaxation techniques. Phys Ther 76(2):182–186, 1996.

80. Johnagen, S, Nemeth, G, Grikkson, F: Hamstring injuries in sprinters: the role of concentric and eccentric muscle strength and flexibility. Am J Sports Med 22:262–266, 1994.

81. Jokl P, Konstadt, S: The effect of limb immobilization on muscle function and protein composition. Clin Orthop 174:222, 1983.

82. Kaltenborn, FM: The Kaltenborn Method of Examination and Treatment, Vol 1: The Extremities, ed 5. Olaf Norlis Bokhandel, Oslo, 1999.

83. Kannus, P, et al: The effects of training, immobilization and remobilization on musculoskeletal tissue. I. Training and immobilization. Scand J Med Sci Sports 2:100–118, 1992.

84. Kannus, P, et al: The effects of training, immobilization and remobilization on musculoskeletal tissue. II. Remobilization and prevention of immobilization atrophy. Scand J Med Sci Sports 2:164–176, 1992.

85. Kendall, F, McCreary, EK, Provance, PG, et al: Muscles, Testing and Function: With Posture and Pain, ed 5. Lippincott Williams & Wilkins, Philadelphia, 2005.

86. Kirch, RF, Weiss, PL, Dannenbaum, RM, Kearney, RE: Effect of maintained stretch on the range of motion of the human anklejoint. Clin Biomech 10:166–168, 1995.

87. Knight, CA, Rutledge, CR, Cox, ME, et al: Effect of superficial heat, deep heat, and active exercise warm-up on the extensibility of the plantar flexors. Phys Ther 81(6):1206–1214, 2001.

88. Knight, KL: Cryotherapy: Theory, Technique and Physiology. Chattanooga Corp., Chattanooga, TN, 1989.

89. Kottke, FJ, Pauley, DL, Park, RA: The rationale for prolonged stretching for correction of shortening of connective tissue. Arch Phys Med Rehabil 47:345–352, 1966.

90. Lehmann, JF, DeLateur, BJ: Therapeutic heat. In Lehmann, JF (ed): Therapeutic Heat and Cold, ed 4. Williams & Wilkins, Baltimore, 1990.

91. Lentell, G, et al: The use of thermal agents to influence the effectiveness of a low-load prolonged stretch. J Orthop Sports Phys Ther 16(5):200–207, 1992.

92. Levangie, PK, Norkin, CC: Joint Structure and Function: A Comprehensive Analysis, ed 3. FA Davis, Philadelphia, 2001.

93. Leveau, B: Basic biomechanics in sports and orthopedic therapy. In Gould, J, Davies, G (eds): Orthopedic and Sports Physical Therapy. CV Mosby, St. Louis, 1985.

94. Lieber, RL, Boodine-Fowler, SC: Skeletal muscle mechanisms: implications for rehabilitation. Phys Ther 73:844–856, 1993.
95. Liebesman, JL, Cafarelli, E: Physiology of range of motion in human joints: a critical review. Crit Rev Phys Rehabil Med 6:131–160, 1994.
96. Light, KE, Nuzik,S, Personius, W, Barstrom, A: Low-load prolonged stretch vs. high-load brief stretch in treating knee contractures. Phys Ther 64(3):330–333, 1984.
97. Liston, C: Specialized systems of massage. In De Domenico, G, Wood, EC (eds): Beard's Massage, ed 4. WB Saunders, Philadelphia, 1997, pp 163–171.
98. Lundy-Ekman, L: Neuroscience: Fundamentals for Rehabilitation, ed 2. WB Saunders, Philadelphia, 2002.
99. Macefield, G, Hagbath, KE, Gorman, R, et al: Decline in spindle support to alpha motoneurons during sustained voluntary contractions. J Physiol 440:497–512, 1991.
100. MacKay-Lyons, M: Low-load prolonged stretch in treatment of elbow flexion contractures secondary to head trauma: a case report. Phys Ther 69:292–296, 1989.
101. Madding, SW, et al: Effect of duration of passive stretch on hip abduction range of motion. J Orthop Sports Phys Ther 8:409–416, 1987.
102. Magnusson, SP, Simonsen, EB, Aagaard, P, et al: Biomechanical responses to repeated stretches in human hamstring muscle in vivo. Am J Sports Med 24:622–628, 1996.
103. Magnusson, SP, Simonsen, EB, Asgaard, P, et al: A mechanism for altered flexibility in human skeletal muscle. J Physicol 497:291–298, 1996.
104. Maitland, GD: Vertebral Manipulation (ed 5). Butterworth, London, 1986.
105. McClure, M: Exercise and training for spinal patients. Part B. Flexibility training. In Basmajian, JV, Nyberg, R (eds): Rational Manual Therapies. Williams & Wilkins, Baltimore, 1993, p 359.
106. McClure, PW, Blackburn, LG, Dusold, C: The use of splints in the treatment of stiffness: biologie ranoncle and an algorithm for making clinical decisions. Phys Ther 74:1101–1107, 1994.
107. McHugh MP, Magnuson, SP, Gleim, GW, Nicholas JA: Viscoelastic stress relaxation in human skeletal muscle. Med Sci Sports Exerc 24:1375–1381, 1992.
108. McNair, PJ, Dombroski, EW, Hewson, DH, et al: Stretching at the ankle joint: viscoelastic responses to hold and continuous passive motion. Med Sci Sports Exerc 33:354–358, 2001.
109. Mitchell, FL: Elements of muscle energy techniques. In Basmagian, JV, Nyberg, R (eds): Rational Manual Therapies. Williams & Wilkins, Baltimore, 1993.
110. Monroe, LG: Motion restrictions. In Cameron, MH (ed): Physical Agents in Rehabilitation, ed 2. WB Saunders, Philadelphia, 2003, pp 111–128.
111. Mueller, MJ, Maluf, KS: Tissue adaptation to physical stress: a proposed "physical stress theory" to guide physical therapist practice, education, and research. Phys Ther 82(4):383–403.
112. Muir, IW, Chesworth, BM, Vandervoort, AA: Effect of a static calf-stretching exercise on resistive torque during passive ankle dorsiflexion in healthy subjects. J Orthop Sports Phys Ther 29:107–113, 1999.
113. Neuman, DA: Kinesiology of the Musculoskeletal System: Foundations for Physical Rehabilitation. Mosby, St. Louis, 2002.
114. Noyes, FR, et al: Biomechanics of ligament failure. J Bone Joint Surg Am 56:1406, 1974.
115. Noyes, FR: Functional properties of knee ligaments and alterations induced by immobilization. Clin Orthop 123:210, 1977.
116. Noyes, FR, Keller, CS, Grood, ES, Butler, DL: Advances in understanding of knee ligament injury, repair and rehabilitation. Med Sci Sports Exerc 16:427, 1984.
117. Ostering LR, Robertson, R, Troxel, R, Hansen, R: Differential response to proprioceptive neuromuscular facilitation (PNF) stretch technique. Med Sci Sports Exerc 22:106–111, 1990.
118. O'Sullivan, SB: Assessment of motor function. In O'Sullivan, SB, Schmitz, TJ (eds): Physical Rehabilitation: Assessment and Treatment, ed 4. FA Davis, Philadelphia, 2001, pp 197–198.
119. O'Sullivan, SB: Strategies to improve motor control and motor learning. In O'Sullivan, SB, Schmitz, TJ (eds): Physical Rehabilitation:
Assessment and Treatment, ed 4. FA Davis, Philadelphia, 2001, pp 363–411.
120. Pearson, K, Gordon, J: Spinal reflexes. In Kandel, ER, Schwartz, JH, Jessell, TM (eds): Principles of Neural Science, ed 4. McGraw-Hill, New York, 2000, pp 713–736.
121. Pope, RP, Herbert, RD, Kirwan, JD, Graham, BJ: A randomized trial of pre-exercise stretching for prevention of lower limb injury. Med Sci Sports Exerc 32:271–277, 2000.
122. Prentice, WE: An electromyographic analysis of the effectiveness of heat or cold and stretching for inducing relaxation in an injured muscle. J Orthop Sports Phys Ther 3:133–140, 1982.
123. Rennie, GA, Michlovitz, SL: Biophysical principles of heating and superficial heating agents. In Michlovitz, SL (ed): Thermal Agents in Rehabilitation. FA Davis, Philadelphia, 1996.
124. Roberts, JM, Wilson, K: Effect of Stretching duration on active and passive range of motion in the lower extremity. Br J Sports Med 33:259–263, 1999.
125. Rose, S, Draper, DO, et al: The stretching window, part two: rate of thermal decay in deep muscle following 1 MHz ultrasound. J Athletic Training 31:139–143, 1996.
126. Sady, SP, Wortman, M, Blanke, D: Flexibility training: ballistic, static or proprioceptive neuromuscular facilitation. Arch Phys Med Rehabil 63:261, 1982.
127. Sapega, A, et al: Biophysical factors in range of motion exercises. Physician Sportsmed 9:57, 1981.
128. Schultz, JH, Luthe, W: Autogenic Training: A Psychophysiologic Approach in Psychotherapy. Grune & Stratton, New York, 1959.
129. Smith, CA: The warm-up procedure: to stretch or not to stretch; a brief review. J Orthop Sports Phys Ther 19(1):12–17, 1994.
130. Smith, LK, Weiss, EL, Lehmkuhl, LD: Brunnstrom's Clinical Kinesiology, ed 5: FA Davis, Philadelphia, 1995.
131. Sotoberg, GL: Skeletal muscle function. In Currier, DP, Nelson, RM (eds): Dynamics of Human Biologic Tissues. FA Davis, Philadelphia, 1992, p 74.
132. Starring, DT, et al: Comparison of cyclic and sustained passive stretching using a mechanical device to increase resting length of hamstring muscles. Phys Ther 68:314, 1988.
133. Sullivan, MK, Dejulia, JJ, Worrell, TW: Effect of pelvic position and stretching method on hamstring muscle flexibility. Med Sci Sports Exerc 24:1383–1389, 1992.
134. Sullivan, PE, Markos, PD: Clinical Decision Making in Therapeutic Exercise. Appleton & Lange, Norwalk, CT, 1995.
135. Tabary, JC, et al: Physiological and structural changes in the cat soleus muscle due to immobilization at different lengths by plaster casts. J Physiol (Lond) 224:231–244, 1972.
136. Tannigawa, M: Comparison of the hold-relax procedure and passive mobilization on increasing muscle length. Phys Ther 52:725, 1972.
137. Tappan, FM, Benjamin, PJ: Tappan's Handbook of Healing Massage Techniques. Appleton & Lange, Stamford CT, 1998.
138. Tardieu, C, et al: Adaptation of connective tissue length to immobilization in the lengthened and shortened position in cat soleus muscle. J Physiol (Paris) 78:214, 1982.
139. Taylor, BF, Waring, CA, Brashear, TA: The effects of therapeutic heat or cold followed by static stretch on hamstring muscle length. J Orthop Sports Phys Ther 21:283–286, 1995.
140. Taylor, D, Dalton, J, Seaber, A, Garrett, W: Viscoelastic properties of muscle-tendon units: the biomechanical effects of stretching. Am J Sports Med 18(3):300–309, 1990.
141. Thompson, LV: Skeletal muscle adaptations with age, inactivity, and therapeutic exercise. J Orthop Sports Phys Ther 32(2):33–57, 2002
142. Threlkeld, AJ: The effects of manual therapy on connective tissue. Phys Ther 72:893, 1992.
143. Tiidus, PM: Manual massage and recovery of muscle function following exercise: a literature review. J Orthop Sports Phys Ther 25:107–112, 1997.
144. Tillman, LJ, Cummings, GS: Biologic mechanisms of connective tissue mutability. In Currier, DP, Nelson, RM (eds): Dynamics of Human Biologic Tissues. FA Davis, Philadelphia, 1992, p 1.
145. Townsend, MC: Psychiatric Mental Health Nursing: Concepts of Care, ed 3. FA Davis, Philadelphia, 2000.

146. Travell, JG, Simons, DG: Myofascial Pain and Dysfunction Trigger Point Manuals, Vol. 2. Williams & Wilkins, Baltimore, 1992.

147. Voss, DE, Ionla, MK, Myers, BJ: Proprioceptive Neuromuscular Facilitation, ed 3. Harper & Row, Philadelphia, 1985.

148. Walker, SM: Delay of twitch relaxation induced by stress and stress relaxation. J Appl Physiol 16:801, 1961.

149. Warren, CG, Lehmann, JF, Koblanski, JN: Heat and stretch procedures: an evaluation using rat tail tendon. Arch Phys Med Rehabil 57:122, 1976.

150. Warren, CG, Lehmann, JF, Koblanski, JN: Elongation of rat tail tendon: effect of load and temperature. Arch Phys Med Rehabil 51:481, 1970.

151. Webright, WG, Randolph, BJ, Perin, DH: Comparison of nonballistic active knee extension in neural slump position and static stretch techniques on hamstring flexibility. J Orthop Sports Phys Ther 26:7–13, 1997.

152. Wessel, J, Wan, A: Effect of stretching on intensity of delayed-onset muscle soreness. J Sports Med 2: 83–87, 1994.

153. Wessling, KC, Derane, DA, Hylton, CR: Effect of static stretch vs. static stretch and ultrasound combined on triceps surae muscle extensibility in healthy women. Phys Ther 67:674–679, 1987.

154. Wilkinson, A: Stretching the truth: a review of the literature on muscle stretching. Aust J Physiother 38:283–287, 1992.

155. Williams, PE, Goldspink, G: Changes in sarcomere length and physiological properties in immobilized muscle. J Anat 127:459–468, 1978.

156. Willy, RW, Kyle, BA, Moore, SA, Chleboun, GS: Effect of cessation and resumption of static hamstring muscle stretching on joint range of motion. J Orthop Sports Phys Ther 31:138–144, 2001.

157. Wilson, E, Payton, O, Donegan-Shoaf, L, Dec, K: Muscle energy techniques in patients with acute low back pain: a pilot clinical trial. J Orthop Sports Phys Ther 33(9):502–512, 2003.

158. Winters, MV, Blake, CG, Trost, JS, et al: Passive versus active stretching of hip flexor muscles in subjects with limited hip extension: a randomized clinical trial. Phys Ther 84(9):800–807, 2004.

159. Witvrouw, E, Danneels, L, Asselman, P, et al: Muscle flexibility as a risk factor for developing muscle injuries in male professional soccer players: a prospective study. Am J Sports Med 31:41–46, 2003.

160. Wolpe, J: Psychotherapy by Reciprocal Inhibition. Stanford University Press, Stanford, CA, 1958.

161. Worrell, T, McCullough, M, Pfeiffer, A: Effect of foot position on gastrocnemius/soleus stretching in subjects with normal flexibility. J Orthop Sports Phys Ther 19:352–356, 1994.

162. Worrell, TW, Smith, TL, Winegardner, J: Effect of hamstring stretching on hamstring muscle performance. J Orthop Sports Phys Ther 20:154–159, 1994.

163. Youdas, JW, Krause, DA, Egan, KS, et al: The effect of static stretching of the calf muscle-tendon unit on active ankle dorsiflecion range of motion. J Orthop Sports Phys Ther 33(7):408–417, 2003.

164. Youdas, JW, Krause, DA, Hollman, JH, et al: The influence of gender and age on hamstring muscle length in healthy adults. J Orthop Sports Phys Ther 35(4):246–252. 2005.

165. Zachazewski, JE: Flexibility in sports. In Sanders, B (ed): Sports Physical Therapy. Appleton & Lange, Norwalk, CT, 1990, pp 201–229.

166. Zarins, B: Soft tissue injury and repair: biomechanical aspects. Int J Sports Med 3:9, 1982.

# Peripheral Joint Mobilization

Joint mobilization refers to manual therapy techniques that are used to modulate pain and treat joint dysfunctions that limit range of motion (ROM) by specifically addressing the altered mechanics of the joint. The altered joint mechanics may be due to pain and muscle guarding, joint effusion, contractures or adhesions in the joint capsules or supporting ligaments, or malalignment or subluxation of the bony surfaces. Joint mobilization stretching techniques differ from other forms of passive or self-stretching (described in Chapter 4) in that they specifically address restricted capsular tissue by replicating normal joint mechanics while minimizing abnormal compressive stresses on the articular cartilage in the joint.[14,27]

To use joint mobilization for treatment effectively, the practitioner must know and be able to examine the anatomy, arthrokinematics, and pathology of the neuromusculoskeletal system and to recognize when the techniques are indicated or when other techniques would be more effective for regaining lost motion. Indiscriminate use of joint mobilization techniques, when not indicated, could lead to potential harm to the patient's joints. We assume that prior to learning the joint mobilization techniques presented here the student or therapist has had (or will be concurrently taking) a course in orthopedic examination and evaluation and therefore will be able to choose appropriate, safe techniques for treating the patient's functional limitation. The reader is referred to several resources for additional study of evaluation procedures.[5,14,16,17] When indicated, joint mobilization is a safe, effective means of restoring or maintaining joint play within a joint and can also be used for treating pain.[14]

## DEFINITIONS OF TERMS

### Mobilization/Manipulation

Mobilization and manipulation are two words that have come to have the same meaning[18] and are therefore interchangeable. They are passive, skilled manual therapy techniques applied to joints and related soft tissues at varying speeds and amplitudes using physiological or accessory motions for therapeutic purposes.[2] The varying speeds and amplitudes could range from a small-amplitude force applied at high velocity to a large-amplitude force applied at slow velocity; that is, there is a continuum of intensities and speeds at which the technique could be applied.[2]

### Self-Mobilization (Auto-mobilization)

Self-mobilization refers to self-stretching techniques that specifically use joint traction or glides that direct the stretch force to the joint capsule. Self-mobilization techniques are described in the chapters on specific regions of the body.

### Mobilization with Movement

Mobilization with movement (MWM) is the concurrent application of sustained accessory mobilization applied by a therapist and an active physiological movement to end range applied by the patient. Passive end-of-range overpressure, or stretching, is then delivered without pain as a barrier. The techniques are always applied in a pain-free direction and are described as correcting joint tracking from a positional fault.[20,21] Brian Mulligan of New Zealand originally described these techniques.[21]

### Physiological Movements

Physiological movements are movements the patient can do voluntarily (e.g., the classic or traditional movements, such as flexion, abduction, and rotation). The term *osteokinematics* is used when these motions of the bones are described.

### Accessory Movements

Accessory movements are movements in the joint and surrounding tissues that are necessary for normal ROM but that cannot be actively performed by the patient.[22] Terms that relate to accessory movements are component motions and joint play.

- *Component motions* are those motions that accompany active motion but are not under voluntary control. The

term is often used synonymously with accessory movement. For example, motions such as upward rotation of the scapula and rotation of the clavicle, which occur with shoulder flexion, and rotation of the fibula, which occurs with ankle motions, are component motions.
- *Joint play* describes the motions that occur between the joint surfaces and also the distensibility or "give" in the joint capsule, which allows the bones to move. The movements are necessary for normal joint functioning through the ROM and can be demonstrated passively, but they cannot be performed actively by the patient.[25] The movements include distraction, sliding, compression, rolling, and spinning of the joint surfaces. The term *arthrokinematics* is used when these motions of the bone surfaces within the joint are described.

NOTE: Procedures to distract or slide the joint surfaces to decrease pain or restore joint play are the fundamental joint mobilization techniques described in this text.

### Thrust

Thrust is a high-velocity, short-amplitude motion such that the patient cannot prevent the motion.[17,25] The motion is performed at the end of the pathological limit of the joint and is intended to alter positional relationships, snap adhesions, or stimulate joint receptors.[25] Pathological limit means the end of the available ROM when there is restriction.

### Manipulation Under Anesthesia

Manipulation under anesthesia is a medical procedure used to restore full ROM by breaking adhesions around a joint while the patient is anesthetized. The technique may be a rapid thrust or a passive stretch using physiological or accessory movements.

### Muscle Energy

Muscle energy techniques use active contraction of deep muscles that attach near the joint and whose line of pull can cause the desired accessory motion. The technique requires the therapist to provide stabilization to the segment on which the distal aspect of the muscle attaches. A command for an isometric contraction of the muscle is given that causes accessory movement of the joint. These techniques are not described in this text.

## BASIC CONCEPTS OF JOINT MOTION: ARTHROKINEMATICS

### Joint Shapes

The type of motion occurring between bony partners in a joint is influenced by the shape of the joint surfaces. The shape may be described as *ovoid* or *sellar*.[14,29]

- In ovoid joints one surface is convex, the other is concave (Fig. 5.1A).
- In sellar joints, one surface is concave in one direction and convex in the other, with the opposing surface convex and concave, respectively; similar to a horseback rider being in complementary opposition to the shape of a saddle (Fig. 5.1B).

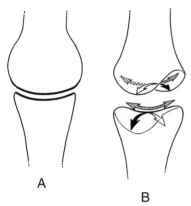

FIGURE 5.1 (A) With ovoid joints, one surface is convex, and the other is concave. (B) With sellar joints, one surface is concave in one direction and convex in the other, with the opposing surface convex and concave, respectively.

## Types of Motion

As a bony lever moves about an axis of motion, there is also movement of the bone surface on the opposing bone surface in the joint.

- The movement of the bony lever is called *swing* and is classically described as flexion, extension, abduction, adduction, and rotation. The amount of movement can be measured in degrees with a goniometer and is called ROM.
- Motion of the bone surfaces in the joint is a variable combination of *rolling* and *sliding*, or *spinning*.[14,23,29] These accessory motions allow greater angulation of the bone as it swings. For the rolling, sliding, or spinning to occur, there must be adequate capsule laxity or joint play.

### Roll

Characteristics of one bone rolling on another (Fig. 5.2) are as follows.

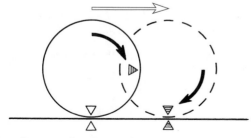

FIGURE 5.2 Representation of one surface rolling on another. New points on one surface meet new points on the opposing surface.

- The surfaces are incongruent.
- New points on one surface meet new points on the opposing surface.
- Rolling results in angular motion of the bone (swing).
- Rolling is always in the same direction as the swinging bone motion whether the surface is convex (Fig. 5.3A) or concave (Fig. 5.3B).
- Rolling, if it occurs alone, causes compression of the surfaces on the side to which the bone is swinging and separation on the other side. Passive stretching using bone angulation alone may cause stressful compressive forces to portions of the joint surface, potentially leading to joint damage.
- In normally functioning joints, pure rolling does not occur alone but in combination with joint sliding and spinning.

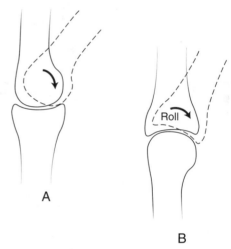

FIGURE 5.3 Rolling is always in the same direction as bone motion, whether the moving bone is (A) convex or (B) concave.

### Slide/Translation

Characteristics of one bone sliding (translating) across another include the following.

- For a pure slide, the surfaces must be congruent, either flat (Fig. 5.4A) or curved (Fig. 5.4B).
- The same point on one surface comes into contact with the new points on the opposing surface.

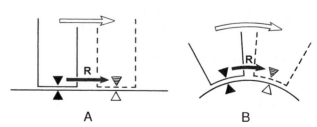

FIGURE 5.4 Representation of one surface sliding on another, whether (A) flat or (B) curved. The same point on one surface comes into contact with new points on the opposing surface.

● Pure sliding does not occur in joints because the surfaces are not completely congruent.
● The direction in which sliding occurs depends on whether the moving surface is concave or convex. Sliding is in the opposite direction of the angular movement of the bone if the moving joint surface is convex (Fig. 5.5A). Sliding is in the same direction as the angular movement of the bone if the moving surface is concave (Fig. 5.5B).

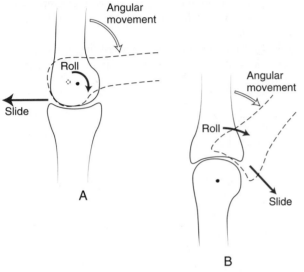

**A**

**B**

FIGURE 5.5 Representation of the concave-convex rule. (*A*) If the surface of the moving bone is convex, sliding is in the direction opposite to that of the angular movement of the bone. (*B*) If the surface of the moving bone is concave, sliding is in the same direction as the angular movement of the bone.

N O T E : This mechanical relationship is known as the *convex-concave rule* and is the basis for determining the direction of the mobilizing force when joint mobilization gliding techniques are used.[14]

● **Focus on Evidence**

Several studies[10,11,13] have examined the translational movement of the humeral head with shoulder motions and have documented translations opposite to what is predicted by the convex-concave rule. Hsu et al.[12] proposed that this apparent contradiction to the convex-concave rule is the result of asymmetrical tightening of the shoulder joint capsule during movement resulting in translation of the moving bone opposite to the direction of capsular tightening. They documented that stretching the tight capsule with translations that affect the restricting tissues leads to greater ROM in cadaver shoulder joints.

## Combined Roll–Sliding in a Joint

● The more congruent the joint surfaces are, the more sliding there is of one bony partner on the other with movement.
● The more incongruent the joint surfaces are, the more rolling there is of one bony partner on the other with movement.
● When muscles actively contract to move a bone, some of the muscles may cause or control the sliding movement of the joint surfaces. For example, the caudal sliding motion of the humeral head during shoulder abduction is caused by the rotator cuff muscles, and the posterior sliding of the tibia during knee flexion is caused by the hamstring muscles. If this function is lost, the resulting abnormal joint mechanics may cause microtrauma and joint dysfunction.
● The joint mobilization techniques described in this chapter use the sliding component of joint motion to restore joint play and reverse joint hypomobility. Rolling (passive angular stretching) is not used to stretch tight joint capsules because it causes joint compression.

N O T E : When the therapist passively moves the articulating surface using the slide component of joint motion, the technique is called translatoric glide, translation, or simply glide.[14] It is used to control pain when applied gently or to stretch the capsule when applied with a stretch force.

## Spin

Characteristics of one bone spinning on another include the following.

● There is rotation of a segment about a stationary mechanical axis (Fig. 5.6).
● The same point on the moving surface creates an arc of a circle as the bone spins.

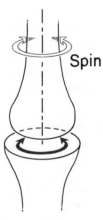

FIGURE 5.6 Representation of spinning. There is rotation of a segment about a stationary mechanical axis.

- Spinning rarely occurs alone in joints but in combination with rolling and sliding.
- Three examples of spin occurring in joints of the body are the shoulder with flexion/extension, the hip with flexion/extension, and the radiohumeral joint with pronation/supination (Fig. 5.7).

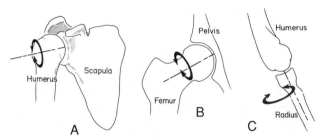

**FIGURE 5.7**  Examples of joint spin location in the body. (*A*) Humerus with flexion/extension. (*B*) Femur with flexion/extension. (*C*) Head of the radius with pronation/supination.

## Passive-Angular Stretching Versus Joint-Glide Stretching

Passive-angular stretching procedures,[27] as when the bony lever is used to stretch a tight joint capsule, may cause increased pain or joint trauma because:

- The use of a lever significantly magnifies the force at the joint.
- The force causes excessive joint compression in the direction of the rolling bone (see Fig. 5.3).
- The roll without a slide does not replicate normal joint mechanics.

Joint glide (mobilization) stretching procedures, as when the translatoric slide component of the bones is used to stretch a tight capsule, are safer and more selective because:

- The force is applied close to the joint surface and controlled at an intensity compatible with the pathology.
- The direction of the force replicates the sliding component of the joint mechanics and does not compress the cartilage.
- The amplitude of the motion is small yet specific to the restricted or adherent portion of the capsule or ligaments. Thus, the forces are selectively applied to the desired tissue.

## Other Accessory Motions that Affect the Joint

### Compression

Compression is the decrease in the joint space between bony partners.

- Compression normally occurs in the extremity and spinal joints when weight bearing.
- Some compression occurs as muscles contract, which provides stability to the joints.
- As one bone rolls on the other (see Fig. 5.3), some compression also occurs on the side to which the bone is angulating.
- Normal intermittent compressive loads help move synovial fluid and thus help maintain cartilage health.
- Abnormally high compression loads may lead to articular cartilage changes and deterioration.[23]

### Traction/Distraction

Traction and distraction are not synonymous. Traction is a longitudinal pull. Distraction is a separation, or pulling apart.

- Separation of the joint surfaces (distraction) does not always occur when a traction force is applied to the long axis of a bone. For example, if traction is applied to the shaft of the humerus, it results in a glide of the joint surface (Fig. 5.8A). Distraction of the glenohumeral joint requires a pull at right angles to the glenoid fossa (Fig. 5.8B).
- For clarity, whenever there is pulling on the long axis of a bone, the term *long-axis traction* is used. Whenever the surfaces are to be pulled apart, the term *distraction, joint traction,* or *joint separation* is used.

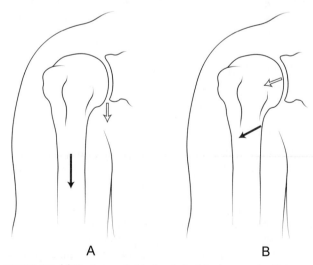

**FIGURE 5.8**  (*A*) Traction applied to the shaft of the humerus results in caudal gliding of the joint surface. (*B*) Distraction of the glenohumeral joint requires separation at right angles to the glenoid fossa.

N O T E : For joint mobilization techniques, distraction is used to control or relieve pain when applied gently or to stretch the capsule when applied with a stretch force. A slight distraction force is used when applying gliding techniques.

## Effects of Joint Motion

Joint motion stimulates biological activity by moving synovial fluid, which brings nutrients to the avascular articular cartilage of the joint surfaces and intra-articular fibrocartilage of the menisci.[23] Atrophy of the articular cartilage begins soon after immobilization is imposed on joints.[1,7,8]

Extensibility and tensile strength of the articular and periarticular tissues are maintained with joint motion. With immobilization there is fibrofatty proliferation, which causes intra-articular adhesions as well as biochemical changes in tendon, ligament, and joint capsule tissue, which in turn causes joint contractures and ligamentous weakening.[1]

Afferent nerve impulses from joint receptors transmit information to the central nervous system and therefore provide awareness of position and motion. With injury or joint degeneration, there is a potential decrease in an important source of proprioceptive feedback that may affect an individual's balance response.[30] Joint motion provides sensory input relative to[32,33]:

- Static position and sense of speed of movement (type I receptors found in the superficial joint capsule)
- Change of speed of movement (type II receptors found in deep layers of the joint capsule and articular fat pads)
- Sense of direction of movement (type I and III receptors; type III found in joint ligaments)
- Regulation of muscle tone (type I, II, and III receptors)
- Nociceptive stimuli (type IV receptors found in the fibrous capsule, ligaments, articular fat pads, periosteum, and walls of blood vessels)

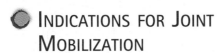

# INDICATIONS FOR JOINT MOBILIZATION

## Pain, Muscle Guarding, and Spasm

Painful joints, reflex muscle guarding, and muscle spasm can be treated with *gentle joint-play* techniques to stimulate neurophysiological and mechanical effects.[17]

### Neurophysiological Effects
Small-amplitude oscillatory and distraction movements are used to stimulate the mechanoreceptors that may inhibit the transmission of nociceptive stimuli at the spinal cord or brain stem levels.[25,29]

### Mechanical Effects
Small-amplitude distraction or gliding movements of the joint are used to cause synovial fluid motion, which is the vehicle for bringing nutrients to the avascular portions of the articular cartilage (and intra-articular fibrocartilage

when present). Gentle joint-play techniques help maintain nutrient exchange and thus prevent the painful and degenerating effects of stasis when a joint is swollen or painful and cannot move through the ROM.

N O T E : The small-amplitude joint techniques used to treat pain, muscle guarding, or muscle spasm should not place stretch on the reactive tissues (see sections on Contraindications and Precautions).

## Reversible Joint Hypomobility

Reversible joint hypomobility can be treated with *progressively vigorous joint-play stretching* techniques to elongate hypomobile capsular and ligamentous connective tissue. Sustained or oscillatory stretch forces are used to distend the shortened tissue mechanically.[14,17]

## Positional Faults/Subluxations

Malposition of one bony partner with respect to its opposing surface may result in limited motion or pain. This can occur with a traumatic injury, after periods of immobility, or with muscle imbalances. The malpositioning may be perpetuated with maladapted neuromuscular control across the joint so whenever attempting active ROM there is faulty tracking of the joint surfaces resulting in pain or limited motion. MWM techniques attempt to realign the bony partners while the person actively moves the joint through its ROM.[21] Manipulations are used to reposition an obvious subluxation, such as a pulled elbow or capitate-lunate subluxation.

## Progressive Limitation

Diseases that progressively limit movement can be treated with joint-play techniques to maintain available motion or retard progressive mechanical restrictions. The dosage of distraction or glide is dictated by the patient's response to treatment and the state of the disease.

## Functional Immobility

When a patient cannot functionally move a joint for a period of time, the joint can be treated with nonstretch gliding or distraction techniques to maintain available joint play and prevent the degenerating and restricting effects of immobility.

 **Focus on Evidence** _____

DiFabio[6] summarized evidence on the effectiveness of manual therapy (primarily mobilization and manipulation) on patients with somatic pain syndromes in the low back region and concluded that there was significantly greater improvement in patients receiving manual therapy than in controls. Boissonnault et al.[4] cited several studies that demonstrated the effectiveness of manual therapy interventions (defined as "a continuum of skilled passive movements to the joints and/or related soft tissues that are applied at varying speeds and amplitudes") in patients with not only low back pain but also shoulder impingement, knee osteoarthritis, and cervical pain. However, there is a lack of randomized, controlled studies on the effects of mobilization/manipulation for all the peripheral joints. Case studies that describe patient selection and/or interventions using joint mobilization/manipulation techniques are identified in various chapters in this text (see Chapters 15, 17 to 22).

# LIMITATIONS OF JOINT MOBILIZATION TECHNIQUES

Mobilization techniques cannot change the disease process of disorders such as rheumatoid arthritis or the inflammatory process of injury. In these cases, treatment is directed toward minimizing pain, maintaining available joint play, and reducing the effects of any mechanical limitations (see Chapter 11).

The skill of the therapist affects the outcome. The techniques described in this text are relatively safe if directions are followed and precautions are heeded; but if these techniques are used indiscriminately on patients not properly examined and screened for such maneuvers or if they are applied too vigorously for the condition, joint trauma or hypermobility may result.

# CONTRAINDICATIONS AND PRECAUTIONS

The only true contraindications to stretching techniques are hypermobility, joint effusion, and inflammation.

## Hypermobility

- The joints of patients with potential necrosis of the ligaments or capsule should not be stretched.
- Patients with painful hypermobile joints may benefit from gentle joint-play techniques if kept within the limits of motion. Stretching is not done.

## Joint Effusion

There may be joint swelling (effusion) due to trauma or disease. Rapid swelling of a joint usually indicates bleeding in the joint and may occur with trauma or diseases such as hemophilia. Medical intervention is required for aspiration of the blood to minimize its necrotizing effect on the articular cartilage. Slow swelling (more than 4 hours) usually indicates serous effusion (a buildup of excess synovial fluid) or edema in the joint due to mild trauma, irritation, or a disease such as arthritis.

- Do not stretch a swollen joint with mobilization or passive stretching techniques. The capsule is already on a stretch by being distended to accommodate the extra fluid. The limited motion is from the extra fluid and muscle response to pain, not from shortened fibers.
- Gentle oscillating motions that do not stress or stretch the capsule may help block the transmission of a pain stimulus so it is not perceived and may also help improve fluid flow while maintaining available joint play.
- If the patient's response to gentle techniques results in increased pain or joint irritability, the techniques were applied too vigorously or should not have been done with the current state of pathology.

### Inflammation

Whenever inflammation is present, stretching increases pain and muscle guarding and results in greater tissue damage. Gentle oscillating or distraction motions may temporarily inhibit the pain response. See Chapter 10 for an appropriate approach to treatment when inflammation is present.

### Conditions Requiring Special Precautions for Stretching

In most cases, joint mobilization techniques are safer than passive angular stretching, in which the bony lever is used to stretch tight tissue and joint compression results. Mobilization may be used with extreme care in the following conditions if the signs and the patient's response are favorable.

- Malignancy
- Bone disease detectable on radiographs
- Unhealed fracture (depends on the site of the fracture and stabilization provided)
- Excessive pain (determine the cause of pain and modify treatment accordingly)
- Hypermobility in associated joints (associated joints must be properly stabilized so the mobilization force is not transmitted to them)
- Total joint replacements (the mechanism of the replacement is self-limiting, and therefore the mobilization gliding techniques may be inappropriate)
- Newly formed or weakened connective tissue such as immediately after injury, surgery, or disuse or when the patient is taking certain medications such as corticosteroids (gentle progressive techniques within the tolerance of the tissue help align the developing fibrils, but forceful techniques are destructive)
- Systemic connective tissue diseases such as rheumatoid arthritis, in which the disease weakens the connective tissue (gentle techniques may benefit restricted tissue, but forceful techniques may rupture tissue and result in instabilities)

- Elderly individuals with weakened connective tissue and diminished circulation (gentle techniques within the tolerance of the tissue may be beneficial to increase mobility)

# PROCEDURES FOR APPLYING PASSIVE JOINT MOBILIZATION TECHNIQUES

## Examination and Evaluation

If the patient has limited or painful motion, examine and decide which tissues are limiting function and the state of pathology. Determine whether treatment should be directed primarily toward relieving pain or stretching a joint or soft tissue limitation.[5,17]

### Quality of pain
The quality of pain when testing the ROM helps determine the stage of recovery and the dosage of techniques used for treatment (see Fig. 10.2).

- If pain is experienced *before* tissue limitation—such as the pain that occurs with muscle guarding after an acute injury or during the active stage of a disease—gentle pain-inhibiting joint techniques may be used. The same techniques can also help maintain joint play (see next section on Grades or Dosages of Movement). Stretching under these circumstances is contraindicated.
- If pain is experienced *concurrently* with tissue limitation—such as the pain and limitation that occur when damaged tissue begins to heal—the limitation is treated cautiously. Gentle stretching techniques specific to the tight structure are used to improve movement gradually yet not exacerbate the pain by reinjuring the tissue.
- If pain is experienced *after* tissue limitation is met because of stretching of tight capsular or periarticular tissue, the stiff joint can be aggressively stretched with joint-play techniques and the periarticular tissue with the stretching techniques described in Chapter 4.

### Capsular Restriction
The joint capsule is limiting motion and should respond to mobilization techniques if the following signs are present.

- The passive ROM for that joint is limited in a capsular pattern (these patterns are described for each peripheral joint under the respective sections on joint problems in Chapters 17 through 22).
- There is a firm capsular end-feel when overpressure is applied to the tissues limiting the range.
- There is decreased joint-play movement when mobility tests (articulations) are performed.
- An adhered or contracted ligament is limiting motion if there is decreased joint play and pain when the fibers of

the ligament are stressed; ligaments often respond to joint mobilization techniques if applied specific to their line of stress.

### Subluxation or Dislocation
Subluxation or dislocation of one bony part on another and loose intra-articular structures that block normal motion may respond to thrust techniques. Some of the simpler manipulations are described in appropriate sections in this text. Others require more advanced training and are beyond the scope of this book.

## Grades or Dosages of Movement

Two systems of grading dosages for mobilization are used.[14,17]

### Graded Oscillation Techniques (Fig. 5.9)

**Dosages**
- **Grade I:** Small-amplitude rhythmic oscillations are performed at the beginning of the range.
- **Grade II:** Large-amplitude rhythmic oscillations are performed within the range, not reaching the limit.
- **Grade III:** Large-amplitude rhythmic oscillations are performed up to the limit of the available motion and are stressed into the tissue resistance.
- **Grade IV:** Small-amplitude rhythmic oscillations are performed at the limit of the available motion and stressed into the tissue resistance.
- **Grade V:** A small-amplitude, high-velocity thrust technique is performed to snap adhesions at the limit of the available motion. Thrust techniques used for this purpose require advanced training and are beyond the scope of this book.

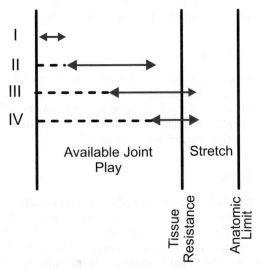

FIGURE 5.9 Representation of graded oscillation techniques. *(Adapted from Maitland.[17])*

## Uses

- Grades I and II are primarily used for treating joints limited by pain. The oscillations may have an inhibitory effect on the perception of painful stimuli by repetitively stimulating mechanoreceptors that block nociceptive pathways at the spinal cord or brain stem levels.[25,34] These nonstretch motions help move synovial fluid to improve nutrition to the cartilage.
- Grades III and IV are primarily used as stretching maneuvers.

## Techniques

The oscillations may be performed using physiological (osteokinematic) motions or joint-play (arthrokinematic) techniques.

### Sustained Translatory Joint–Play Techniques (Fig. 5.10)

#### Dosages

- **Grade I (loosen):** Small-amplitude distraction is applied where no stress is placed on the capsule. It equalizes cohesive forces, muscle tension, and atmospheric pressure acting on the joint.
- **Grade II (tighten):** Enough distraction or glide is applied to tighten the tissues around the joint. Kaltenborn[14] called this "taking up the slack."
- **Grade III (stretch):** A distraction or glide is applied with an amplitude large enough to place stretch on the joint capsule and surrounding periarticular structures.

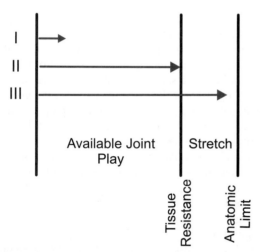

FIGURE 5.10 Representation of sustained translatory joint-play techniques. *(Adapted from Kaltenborn.[14])*

## Uses

- Grade I distraction is used with all gliding motions and may be used for relief of pain.
- Grade II distraction is used for the initial treatment to determine how sensitive the joint is. Once the joint reaction is known, the treatment dosage is increased or decreased accordingly.

- Gentle grade II distraction applied intermittently may be used to inhibit pain. Grade II glides may be used to maintain joint play when ROM is not allowed.
- Grade III distractions or glides are used to stretch the joint structures and thus increase joint play.

## Techniques

This grading system describes only joint-play techniques that separate (distract) or glide/translate (slide) the joint surfaces.

## Comparison

When using either grading system, dosages I and II are low intensity and so do not cause a stretch force on the joint capsule or surrounding tissue, although, by definition, sustained grade II techniques take up the slack of the tissues whereas grade II oscillation techniques stay within the slack. Grades III and IV oscillations and grade III sustained stretch techniques are similar in intensity in that they all are applied with a stretch force at the limit of motion. The differences are related to the rhythm or speed of repetition of the stretch force.

- For clarity and consistency, when referring to dosages in this text, the notation *graded oscillations* means to use the dosages as described in the section on graded oscillation techniques. The notation *sustained grade* means to use the dosages as described in the section on sustained translatory joint-play techniques.
- The choice of using oscillating or sustained techniques depends on the patient's response.
  - When dealing with managing pain, either grade I or II oscillation techniques or slow intermittent grade I or II sustained joint distraction techniques are recommended; the patient's response dictates the intensity and frequency of the joint-play technique.
  - When dealing with loss of joint play and thus decreased functional range, sustained techniques applied in a cyclic manner are recommended; the longer the stretch force can be maintained, the greater the creep and plastic deformation of the connective tissue.
  - When attempting to maintain available range by using joint-play techniques, either grade II oscillating or sustained grade II techniques can be used.

## Positioning and Stabilization

- The patient and the extremity to be treated should be positioned so the patient can relax. To relax the muscles crossing the joint, techniques of inhibition (see Chapter 4) may be appropriately used prior to or between joint mobilization techniques.
- Examination of joint play and the first treatment are initially performed in the resting position for that joint so the greatest capsule laxity is possible. In some cases, the position to use is the one in which the joint is least

painful. With progression of treatment, the joint is positioned at or near the end of the available range prior to application of the mobilization force. This places the restricting tissue in its most lengthened position where the stretch force can be more specific and effective.[12]

◉ Firmly and comfortably stabilize one joint partner, usually the proximal bone. A belt, one of the therapist's hands, or an assistant holding the part may provide stabilization. Appropriate stabilization prevents unwanted stress to surrounding tissues and joints and makes the stretch force more specific and effective.

## Treatment Force and Direction of Movement

◉ The treatment force (either gentle or strong) is applied as close to the opposing joint surface as possible. The larger the contact surface, the more comfortable is the patient with the procedure. For example, instead of forcing with your thumb, use the flat surface of your hand.

◉ The direction of movement during treatment is either parallel or perpendicular to the treatment plane. *Treatment plane* was described by Kaltenborn[14] as a plane perpendicular to a line running from the axis of rotation to the middle of the concave articular surface. The plane is in the concave partner, so its position is determined by the position of the concave bone (Fig. 5.11).

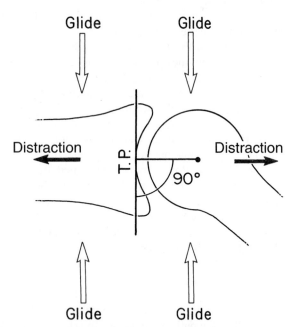

FIGURE 5.11 Treatment plane (T.P.) is at right angles to a line drawn from the axis of rotation to the center of the concave articulating surface and lies in the concave surface. Joint traction (distraction) is applied perpendicular to and glides parallel to the treatment plane.

◉ Distraction techniques are applied perpendicular to the treatment plane. The entire bone is moved so the joint surfaces are separated.

◉ Gliding techniques are applied parallel to the treatment plane. The direction of gliding is easily determined by using the convex-concave rule (described earlier in the chapter). If the surface of the moving bony partner is convex, the treatment glide should be opposite to the direction in which the bone swings. If the surface of the moving bony partner is concave, the treatment glide should be in the same direction (see Fig. 5.5).

◉ The entire bone is moved so there is gliding of one joint surface on the other. The bone should not be used as a lever; it should have no arcing motion (swing), which would cause rolling and thus compression of the joint surfaces.

## Initiation and Progression of Treatment (Fig. 5.12)

1. The initial treatment is the same whether treating to decrease pain or increase joint play. The purpose is to determine joint reactivity before proceeding. Use a sustained grade II distraction of the joint surfaces with the joint held in resting position or the position of greatest relaxation.[14] Note the immediate joint response relative to irritability and range.

2. The next day, evaluate joint response or have the patient report the response at the next visit.
   • If there is increased pain and sensitivity, reduce the amplitude of treatment to grade I oscillations.
   • If the joint is the same or better, perform either of the following: Repeat the same maneuver if the goal of treatment is to maintain joint play, or progress the maneuver to stretching techniques if the goal of treatment is to increase joint play.

3. To maintain joint play by using gliding techniques when ROM techniques are contraindicated or not possible for a period of time, use sustained grade II or grade II oscillation techniques.

4. To progress the stretch technique, move the bone to the end of the available ROM, then apply a sustained grade III distraction or glide technique. Progressions include prepositioning the bone at the end of the available range and rotating it prior to applying grade III distraction or glide techniques. The direction of the glide and rotation is dictated by the joint mechanics. For example, laterally rotate the humerus as shoulder abduction is progressed; medially rotate the tibia as knee flexion is progressed.

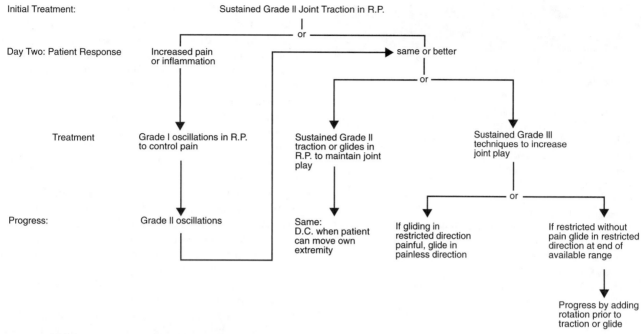

FIGURE 5.12 Initiation and progression of treatment.

## Focus on Evidence

A cadavaric study demonstrated improvement in gleno-humeral abduction ROM when dorsal and ventral translational glides were applied at the end of the range but not when applied in the resting position.[12]

5. Hints
- Warm the tissue around the joint prior to stretching. Modalities, massage, or gentle muscle contractions increase the circulation and warm the tissues.
- Muscle relaxation techniques and oscillation techniques may inhibit muscle guarding and should be alternated with the stretching techniques, if necessary.
- When using grade III gliding techniques, a grade I distraction should be used with it. A grade II or III distraction should not be used with a grade III glide to avoid excessive trauma to the joint.
- If gliding in the restricted direction is too painful, begin gliding mobilizations in the painless direction. Progress to gliding in the restricted direction when mobility improves a little and it is not painful.
- When applying stretching techniques, move the bony partner through the available range of joint play first, that is, "take up the slack." When tissue resistance is felt, apply the stretch force against the restriction.
- Incorporate MWM techniques (described later in the chapter) as part of the total approach to treatment.

## Speed, Rhythm, and Duration of Movements

### Oscillations
- Grades I and IV are usually rapid oscillations, like manual vibrations.
- Grades II and III are smooth, regular oscillations at 2 or 3 per second for 1 to 2 minutes.
- Vary the speed of oscillations for different effects such as low amplitude and high speed to inhibit pain or slow speed to relax muscle guarding.

### Sustained
- For painful joints, apply intermittent distraction for 7 to 10 seconds with a few seconds of rest in between for several cycles. Note the response and either repeat or discontinue.
- For restricted joints, apply a minimum of a 6-second stretch force followed by partial release (to grade I or II), then repeat with slow, intermittent stretches at 3- to 4-second intervals.

## Patient Response

- Stretching maneuvers usually cause soreness. Perform the maneuvers on alternate days to allow the soreness to decrease and tissue healing to occur between stretching sessions. The patient should perform ROM into any newly gained range during this time. If there is increased pain after 24 hours, the dosage (amplitude) or duration of treatment was too vigorous. Decrease the dosage or duration until the pain is under control.
- The patient's joint and ROM should be reassessed after treatment and again before the next treatment. Alterations in treatment are dictated by the joint response.

## Total Program

Mobilization techniques are one part of a total treatment program when there is decreased function. If muscles or connective tissues are also limiting motion, inhibition and

| BOX 5.1 | Suggested Sequence of Treatment to Gain and Reinforce Functional Mobility |
|---|---|

1. Warm the tissues.
2. Relax the muscles.
   - Hold-relax inhibition technique
   - Grade I or II joint oscillation techniques
3. Joint mobilization stretches.
   - Position and dosage for level of tissue tolerance
4. Passive stretch periarticular tissues.
5. Patient actively uses new range.
   - Reciprocal inhibition
   - Active ROM
   - Functional activities
6. Maintain new range; patient instruction.
   - Self-stretching
   - Auto-mobilization
   - Active, resistive ROM
   - Functional activities using the new range

passive stretching techniques are alternated with joint mobilization during the same treatment session. Therapy should also include appropriate ROM, strengthening, and functional exercises so the client learns effective control and use of the gained mobility (Box 5.1).

## MOBILIZATION WITH MOVEMENT: PRINCIPLES OF APPLICATION

Brian Mulligan's concept of mobilization with movement (MWM) is the natural continuance of progression in the development of manual therapy from active self-stretching exercises, to therapist-applied passive physiological movement, to passive accessory mobilization techniques.[20] Mobilization with movement is the concurrent application of pain-free accessory mobilization with active and/or passive physiological movement.[21] Passive end-range overpressure or stretching is then applied without pain as a barrier. These techniques are applicable when:

- No contraindication for manual therapy exists (described earlier in the chapter).
- A full orthopedic scanning examination has been completed, and evaluation of the results indicate local musculoskeletal pathology.[5]
- A specific biomechanical analysis reveals localized loss of movement and/or pain associated with function.[17]
- No pain is produced during or immediately after application of the technique.[19]

### Principles of MWM in Clinical Practice

- One or more *comparable signs* are identified during the examination.[17] A comparable sign is a positive test sign that can be repeated after a therapeutic maneuver to

determine the effectiveness of the maneuver. For example, a comparable sign may include loss of joint play movement, loss of ROM, or pain associated with movement during specific functional activities such as lateral elbow pain with resisted wrist extension, painful restriction of ankle dorsiflexion, or pain with overhead reaching.

- A passive joint mobilization is applied as described in the previous section following the principles of Kaltenborn.[14] This accessory glide or distraction performed parallel or perpendicular to the treatment plane must be pain-free.[21]
- Utilizing knowledge of joint anatomy and mechanics, a sense of tissue tension, and sound clinical reasoning, the therapist investigates various combinations of parallel or perpendicular accessory glides to find the pain-free direction and grade of accessory movement. This may be a glide, spin, distraction, or combination of movements.
- While the therapist sustains the pain-free accessory mobilization, the patient is requested to perform the comparable sign. The comparable sign should now be significantly improved; that is, there should be increased ROM, and the motion should *be free of the original pain.*[21]
- The therapist must continuously monitor the patient's reaction to ensure no pain is produced. Failure to improve the comparable sign would indicate that the therapist has not found the correct direction of accessory mobilization or the grade of movement or that the technique is not indicated.
- The previously restricted and/or painful motion or activity is repeated 6 to 10 times by the patient while the therapist continues to maintain the appropriate accessory mobilization. Further gains are expected with repetition during a treatment session, particularly when *pain-free* passive overpressure is applied to achieve end-range loading.

### Pain as the Guide

Successful MWM techniques should render the comparable sign painless while significantly improving function during the application of the technique. Self-treatment is often possible using MWM principles with sports-type adhesive tape and/or the patient providing the mobilization component of the MWM concurrent with the active physiological movement.[9] Having restored articular function with MWMs, the therapist progresses the client through the ensuing rehabilitation sequences of the recovery of muscular power, endurance, and neural control. Sustained improvements are necessary to justify ongoing intervention.

### Techniques

Techniques applicable to the extremity joints are described throughout this text in the treatment sections for various conditions (see Chapters 17 through 22).

## Theoretical Framework

Mulligan postulated a positional fault model to explain the results gained through his concept. Alternately, inappropriate joint tracking mechanisms due to an altered instantaneous axis of rotation and neurophysiological response models have also been considered.[9,19,20,22] For further details of the application of the Mulligan concept as it applies to the spine and extremities, refer to *Manual Therapy, "NAGS," "SNAGS," "MWMs," Etc.*[21]

 **Focus on Evidence** _____

Early research on the MWM approach confirms its benefits; however, the mechanism by which it affects the musculoskeletal system, whether mechanical or physiological, has yet to be fully determined.[3,15,24,26,28,31] A study by Paungmail et al.[26] measured a significant reduction in pain, increased grip strength, and increased sympathetic nervous system response immediately following MWM for chronic lateral epicondylalgia compared with a placebo intervention, results that were similar to studies of spinal manipulation. They interpreted this to imply that there is a multisystem response to manipulation whether the spine or the elbow is manipulated.

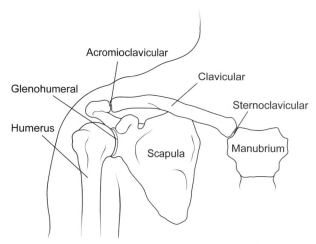

FIGURE 5.13 Bones and joints of the shoulder girdle complex.

## PERIPHERAL JOINT MOBILIZATION TECHNIQUES

The following are suggested joint distraction and gliding techniques for use by entry-level therapists and those attempting to gain a foundation in joint mobilization. A variety of adaptations can be made from these techniques. Some adaptations are described in the respective chapters where specific impairments and interventions are discussed (see Chapters 17 through 22). The distraction and glide techniques should be applied with respect to the dosage, frequency, progression, precautions, and procedures as described in the previous sections.

N O T E : Terms such as proximal hand, distal hand, lateral hand, or other descriptive terms indicate that the therapist should use the hand that is more proximal, distal, or lateral to the patient or the patient's extremity.

## Shoulder Girdle Complex (Fig. 5.13)

N O T E : To gain full elevation of the humerus, the accessory and component motions of clavicular elevation and rotation, scapular rotation, and external rotation of the humerus as well as adequate joint play anteriorly and inferiorly are necessary. The clavicular and scapular techniques are described following the glenohumeral joint techniques. For a review of the mechanics of the shoulder complex, see Chapter 17.

### Glenohumeral Joint

The concave glenoid fossa receives the convex humeral head.

### Resting Position

The shoulder is abducted 55°, horizontally adducted 30°, and rotated so the forearm is in the horizontal plane.

### Treatment Plane

The treatment plane is in the glenoid fossa and moves with the scapula.

### Stabilization

Fixate the scapula with a belt or have an assistant help.

### Glenohumeral Distraction (Fig. 5.14)

### Indications

Testing; initial treatment (sustained grade II); pain control (grade I or II oscillations); general mobility (sustained grade III).

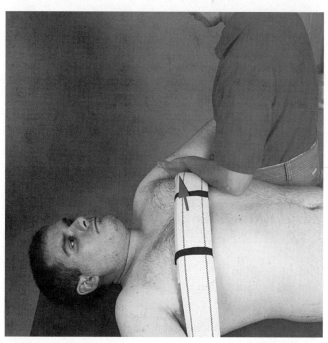

FIGURE 5.14 Glenohumeral joint: distraction in resting position. Note that the force is perpendicular to the treatment plane in the glenoid fossa.

### Patient Position

Supine, with arm in the resting position. Support the forearm between your trunk and elbow.

### Hand Placement

- Use the hand nearer the part being treated (e.g., left hand if treating the patient's left shoulder) and place it in the patient's axilla with your thumb just distal to the joint margin anteriorly and fingers posteriorly.
- Your other hand supports the humerus from the lateral surface.

### Mobilizing Force

With the hand in the axilla, move the humerus laterally.

N O T E : The entire arm moves in a translatoric motion away from the plane of the glenoid fossa. Distractions may be performed with the humerus in any position (see Figs. 5.17, 5.19, and 17.20). You must be aware of the amount of scapular rotation and adjust the distraction force against the humerus so it is perpendicular to the plane of the glenoid fossa.

### Glenohumeral Caudal Glide, Resting Position (Fig. 5.15)

### Indications

To increase abduction (sustained grade III); to reposition the humeral head if superiorly positioned.

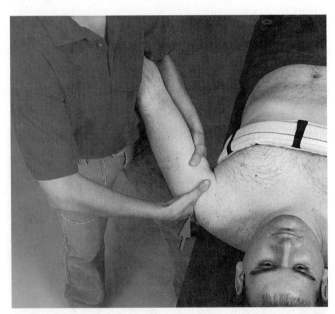

FIGURE 5.15 Glenohumeral joint: caudal glide in the resting position. Note that the distraction force is applied by the hand in the axilla, and the caudal glide force is from the hand superior to the humeral head.

### Patient Position

Same as for distraction.

### Hand Placement

- Place one hand in the patient's axilla to provide a grade I distraction.
- The web space of your other hand is placed just distal to the acromion process.

### Mobilizing Force

With the superiorly placed hand, glide the humerus in an inferior direction.

### GH Caudal Glide: Alternate

### Hand Placement

Same as for distraction (see Fig. 5.14).

### Mobilizing Force

The force comes from the hand around the arm, pulling caudally as you shift your body weight inferiorly.

N O T E : This glide is also called long-axis traction.

### Glenohumeral Caudal Glide Progression (Fig. 5.16)

### Indication

To increase abduction.

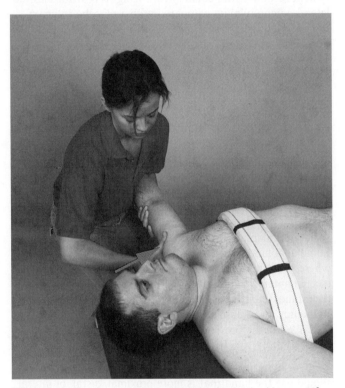

FIGURE 5.16 Glenohumeral joint: caudal glide with the shoulder near 90°.

### Patient Position

- Supine or sitting, with the arm abducted to the end of its available range.
- External rotation of the humerus should be added to the end-range position as the arm approaches and goes beyond 90°.

### Therapist Position and Hand Placement

- With the patient supine, stand facing the patient's feet and stabilize the patient's arm against your trunk with the hand farthest from the patient. Slight lateral motion of your trunk provides grade I distraction. With the patient sitting, face the patient and cradle the distal humerus with the hand closest to the patient; this hand provides a grade I distraction.

- Place the web space of your other hand just distal to the acromion process on the proximal humerus.

### Mobilizing Force

With the hand on the proximal humerus, glide the humerus in an inferior direction.

### Glenohumeral Elevation Progression (Fig. 5.17)

### Indication

To increase elevation beyond 90° of abduction.

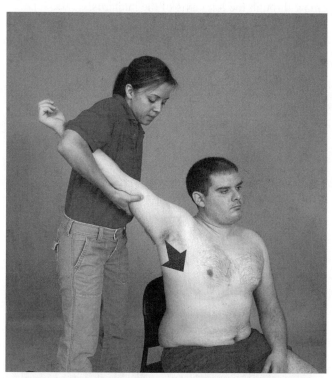

FIGURE 5.17 Glenohumeral joint: elevation progression in the sitting position. This is used when the range is greater than 90°. Note the externally rotated position of the humerus; pressure against the head of the humerus is toward the axilla.

### Patient Position

Supine or sitting, with the arm abducted and externally rotated to the end of its available range.

### Therapist Position and Hand Placement

- Hand placement is the same as for caudal glide progression.
- Adjust your body position so the hand applying the mobilizing force is aligned with the treatment plane.
- With the hand grasping the elbow, apply a grade I distraction force.

### Mobilizing Force

- With the hand on the proximal humerus, glide the humerus in a progressively anterior direction against the inferior folds of the capsule in the axilla.
- The direction of force with respect to the patient's body depends on the amount of upward rotation and protraction of the scapula.

### Glenohumeral Posterior Glide, Resting Position (Fig. 5.18)

### Indications

To increase flexion; to increase internal rotation.

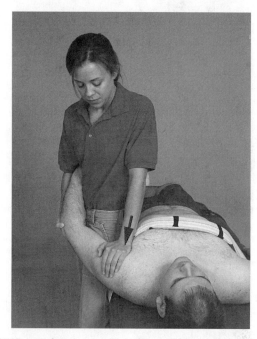

FIGURE 5.18 Glenohumeral joint: posterior glide in the resting position.

### Patient Position

Supine, with the arm in resting position.

### Therapist Position and Hand Placement

- Stand with your back to the patient, between the patient's trunk and arm.
- Support the arm against your trunk, grasping the distal humerus with your lateral hand. This position provides grade I distraction to the joint.
- Place the lateral border of your top hand just distal to the anterior margin of the joint, with your fingers pointing superiorly. This hand gives the mobilizing force.

### Mobilizing Force

Glide the humeral head posteriorly by moving the entire arm as you bend your knees.

## Glenohumeral Posterior Glide Progression (Fig. 5.19)

### Indications

To increase posterior gliding when flexion approaches 90°; to increase horizontal adduction.

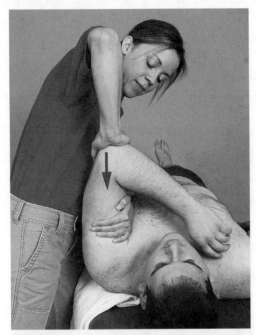

A

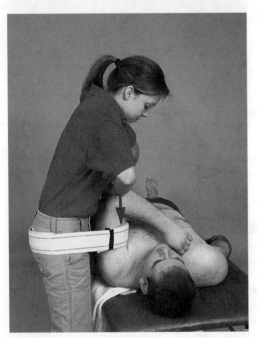

B

FIGURE 5.19 Glenohumeral joint: posterior glide progression. One hand (A) or a belt (B) is used to exert a grade 1 distraction force.

### Patient Position

Supine, with the arm flexed to 90° and internally rotated and with the elbow flexed. The arm may also be placed in horizontal adduction.

### Hand Placement

- Place padding under the scapula for stabilization.
- Place one hand across the proximal surface of the humerus to apply a grade I distraction.
- Place your other hand over the patient's elbow.
- A belt placed around your pelvis and the patient's humerus may be used to apply the distraction force.

### Mobilizing Force

Glide the humerus posteriorly by pushing down at the elbow through the long axis of the humerus.

## Glenohumeral Anterior Glide, Resting Position (Fig. 5.20)

### Indications

To increase extension; to increase external rotation.

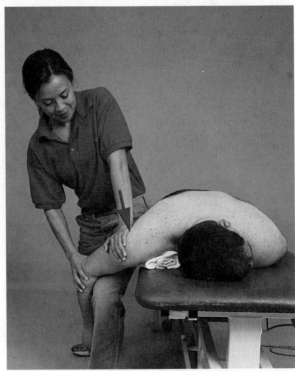

FIGURE 5.20 Glenohumeral joint: anterior glide in the resting position.

### Patient Position

Prone, with the arm in resting position over the edge of the treatment table, supported on your thigh. Stabilize the acromion with padding. Supine position may also be used.

## Therapist Position and Hand Placement

● Stand facing the top of the table with the leg closer to the table in a forward stride position.
● Support the patient's arm against your thigh with your outside hand; the arm positioned on your thigh provides a grade I distraction.
● Place the ulnar border of your other hand just distal to the posterior angle of the acromion process, with your fingers pointing superiorly; this hand gives the mobilizing force.

## Mobilizing Force

Glide the humeral head in an anterior and slightly medial direction. Bend both knees so the entire arm moves anteriorly.

PRECAUTION: Do not lift the arm at the elbow and thereby cause angulation of the humerus: Such angulation could lead to anterior subluxation or dislocation of the humeral head. Do not use this position to progress external rotation. Placing the shoulder in 90° abduction with external rotation and applying an anterior glide may cause anterior subluxation of the humeral head.

## Glenohumeral External Rotation Progressions (Fig. 5.21)

### Indication

To increase external rotation.

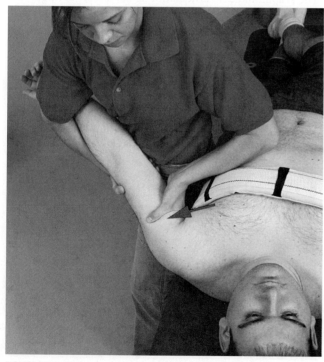

FIGURE 5.21 Glenohumeral joint: distraction for external rotation progression. Note that the humerus is positioned in the resting position with maximum external rotation prior to the application of distraction stretch force.

## Techniques

Because of the danger of subluxation when applying an anterior glide with the humerus externally rotated, use a distraction progression or elevation progression to gain range.

● Distraction progression: Begin with the shoulder in resting position; externally rotate the humerus to end range and then apply a grade III distraction perpendicular to the treatment plane in the glenoid fossa.
● Elevation progression (see Fig. 5.17). This technique incorporates end-range external rotation.

## Acromioclavicular Joint: Anterior Glide (Fig. 5.22)

### Indication

To increase mobility of the joint.

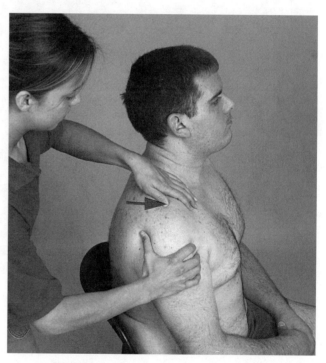

FIGURE 5.22 Acromioclavicular joint: anterior glide.

### Stabilization

Fixate the scapula with your more lateral hand around the acromion process.

### Patient Position

Sitting or prone.

### Hand Placement

● With the patient sitting, stand behind the patient and stabilize the acromion process with the fingers of your lateral hand.
● The thumb of your other hand pushes downward through the upper trapezius and is placed posteriorly on the clavicle, just medial to the joint space.
● With the patient prone, stabilize the acromion with a towel roll under the shoulder.

## Mobilizing Force
Your thumb pushes the clavicle anteriorly.

## Sternoclavicular Joint
The proximal articulating surface of the clavicle is convex superiorly/inferiorly and concave anteriorly/posteriorly.

### Patient Position and Stabilization
Supine; the thorax provides stability to the sternum.

## Sternoclavicular Posterior Glide and Superior Glide (Fig. 5.23)

### Indications
Posterior glide to increase retraction; superior glide to increase depression of the clavicle.

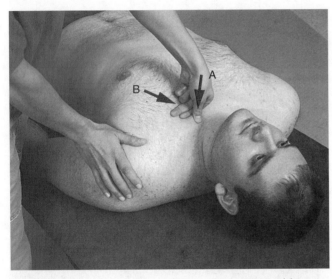

**FIGURE 5.23** Sternoclavicular joint: posterior and superior glides. (*A*) Press down with the thumb for posterior glide. (*B*) Press upward with the index finger for superior glide.

### Hand Placement
- Place your thumb on the anterior surface of the proximal end of the clavicle.
- Flex your index finger and place the middle phalanx along the caudal surface of the clavicle to support the thumb.

### Mobilizing Force
- Posterior glide: Push with your thumb in a posterior direction.
- Superior glide: Push with your index finger in a superior direction

## Sternoclavicular Anterior Glide and Caudal (Inferior) Glide (Fig. 5.24)

### Indications
Anterior glide to increase protraction; caudal glide to increase elevation of the clavicle.

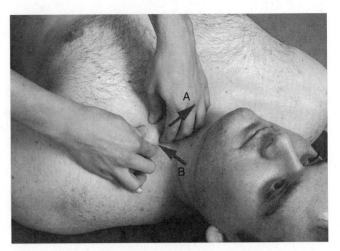

**FIGURE 5.24** Sternoclavicular joint: anterior and inferior glides. (*A*) Pull the clavicle upward for an anterior glide. (*B*) Press caudalward with the curled fingers for an inferior glide.

### Hand Placement
Your fingers are placed superiorly and thumb inferiorly around the clavicle.

### Mobilizing Force
- The fingers and thumb lift the clavicle anteriorly for an anterior glide.
- The fingers press inferiorly for a caudal glide.

## Scapulothoracic Mobilization (Fig. 5.25)
The scapulothoracic articulation is not a true joint, but the soft tissue is stretched to obtain normal shoulder girdle mobility.

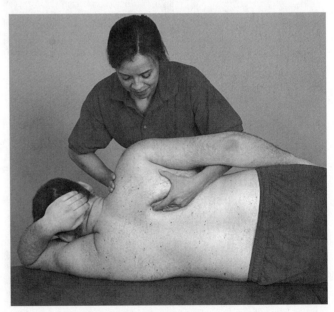

**FIGURE 5.25** Scapulothoracic articulation: elevation, depression, protraction, retraction, upward and downward rotations, and winging.

## Indications

To increase scapular motions of elevation, depression, protraction, retraction, rotation, upward and downward rotations, and winging.

## Patient Position

● If there is considerable restriction in mobility, begin prone and progress to side-lying, with the patient facing you.
● Support the weight of the patient's arm by draping it over your inferior arm and allowing it to hang so the scapular muscles are relaxed.

## Hand Placement

● Place your superior hand across the acromion process to control the direction of motion.
● With the fingers of your inferior hand, scoop under the medial border and inferior angle of the scapula.

## Mobilizing Force

Move the scapula in the desired direction by lifting from the inferior angle or by pushing on the acromion process.

## Elbow and Forearm Complex (Fig. 5.26)

N O T E : The elbow and forearm complex consists of four joints: humeroulnar, humeroradial, proximal radioulnar and distal radioulnar. For full elbow flexion and extension, accessory motions of varus and valgus (with radial and ulnar glides) are necessary. The techniques for each of the joints as well as accessory motions are described in this section. For a review of the joint mechanics, see Chapter 18.

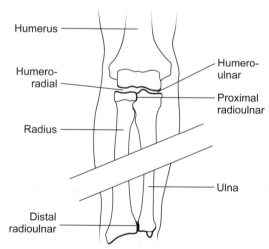

FIGURE 5.26 Bones and joints of the elbow complex.

## Humeroulnar Articulation

The convex trochlea articulates with the concave olecranon fossa.

## Resting Position

Elbow is flexed 70°, and forearm is supinated 10°.

## Treatment Plane

The treatment plane is in the olecranon fossa, angled approximately 45° from the long axis of the ulna (Fig. 5.27).

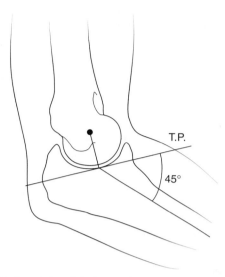

FIGURE 5.27 Lateral view of the humeroulnar joint, depicting the treatment plane (T.P.).

## Stabilization

Fixate the humerus against the treatment table with a belt or use an assistant to hold it. The patient may roll onto his or her side and fixate the humerus with the contralateral hand if muscle relaxation can be maintained around the elbow joint being mobilized.

### Humeroulnar Distraction and Progression (Fig. 5.28A)

#### Indications

Testing; initial treatment (sustained grade II); pain control (grade I or II oscillation); to increase flexion or extension (grade III or IV).

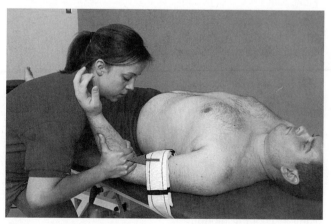

A

FIGURE 5.28 Humeroulnar joint: (A) distraction and

### Patient Position

Supine, with the elbow over the edge of the treatment table or supported with padding just proximal to the olecranon process. Rest the patient's wrist against your shoulder, allowing the elbow to be in resting position for the initial treatment. To stretch into either flexion or extension, position the joint at the end of its available range.

### Hand Placement

When in the resting position or at end-range flexion, place the fingers of your medial hand over the proximal ulna on the volar surface; reinforce it with your other hand. When at end-range extension, stand and place the base of your proximal hand over the proximal portion of the ulna and support the distal forearm with your other hand.

### Mobilizing Force

Force against the proximal ulna at a 45° angle to the shaft of the bone.

### Humeroulnar Distal Glide (Fig. 5.28B)

#### Indication

To increase flexion.

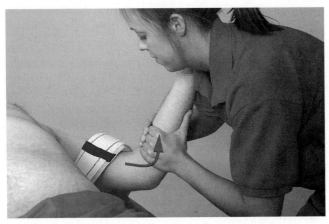

**B**

FIGURE 5.28 (continued) (B) distraction with distal glide (scoop motion).

### Patient Position and Hand Placement

Supine, with the elbow over the edge of the treatment table. Begin with the elbow in resting position. Progress by positioning it at the end range of flexion. Place the fingers of your medial hand over the proximal ulna on the volar surface; reinforce it with your other hand.

### Mobilizing Force

First apply a distraction force to the joint at a 45° angle to the ulna, then while maintaining the distraction, direct the force in a distal direction along the long axis of the ulna using a scooping motion.

### Humeroulnar Radial Glide

#### Indication

To increase varus. This is an accessory motion of the joint that accompanies elbow flexion and is therefore used to progress flexion.

#### Patient Position

- Side-lying on the arm to be mobilized, with the shoulder laterally rotated and the humerus supported on the table.
- Begin with the elbow in resting position; progress to end-range flexion.

#### Hand Placement

Place the base of your proximal hand just distal to the elbow; support the distal forearm with your other hand.

#### Mobilizing Force

Force against the ulna in a radial direction.

### Humeroulnar Ulnar Glide

#### Indication

To increase valgus. This is an accessory motion of the joint that accompanies elbow extension and is therefore used to progress extension.

#### Patient Position

- Same as for radial glide except a block or wedge is placed under the proximal forearm for stabilization (using distal stabilization).
- Initially, the elbow is placed in resting position and is progressed to end-range extension.

#### Mobilizing Force

Force against the distal humerus in a radial direction, causing the ulna to glide ulnarly.

### Humeroradial Articulation

The convex capitulum articulates with the concave radial head (see Fig. 5.26).

#### Resting Position

Elbow is extended, and forearm is supinated to the end of the available range.

#### Treatment Plane

The treatment plane is in the concave radial head perpendicular to the long axis of the radius.

#### Stabilization

Fixate the humerus with one of your hands.

### Humeroradial Distraction (Fig. 5.29)

#### Indications

To increase mobility of the humeroradial joint; to manipulate a pushed elbow (proximal displacement of the radius).

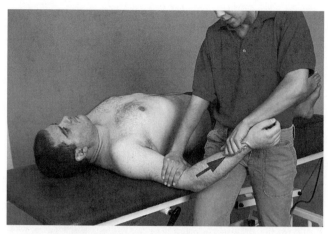

FIGURE 5.29 Humeroradial joint: distraction.

**Patient Position**
Supine or sitting, with the arm resting on the treatment table.

**Therapist Position and Hand Placement**

⦿ Position yourself on the ulnar side of the patient's forearm so you are between the patient's hip and upper extremity.
⦿ Stabilize the patient's humerus with your superior hand.
⦿ Grasp around the distal radius with the fingers and thenar eminence of your inferior hand. Be sure your are not grasping around the distal ulna.

**Mobilizing Force**
Pull the radius distally (long-axis traction causes joint traction).

## Humeroradial Dorsal/Volar Glides (Fig. 5.30)

**Indications**
Dorsal glide head of the radius to increase elbow extension; volar glide to increase flexion.

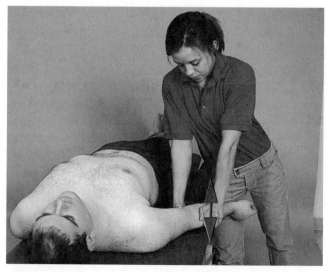

FIGURE 5.30 Humeroradial joint: dorsal and volar glides. This may also be done sitting, as in Figure 5.32, with the elbow positioned in extension and the humerus stabilized by the proximal hand (rather than the ulna).

**Patient Position**
Supine or sitting with the elbow extended and supinated to the end of the available range.

**Hand Placement**

⦿ Stabilize the humerus with your hand that is on the medial side of the patient's arm.
⦿ Place the palmar surface of your lateral hand on the volar aspect and your fingers on the dorsal aspect of the radial head.

**Mobilizing Force**

⦿ Move the radial head dorsally with the palm of your hand or volarly with your fingers.
⦿ If a stronger force is needed for the volar glide, realign your body and push with the base of your hand against the dorsal surface in a volar direction.

## Humeroradial Compression (Fig. 5.31)

**Indication**
To reduce a pulled elbow subluxation.

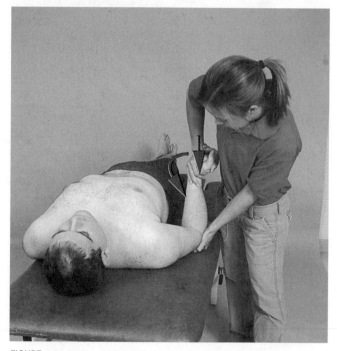

FIGURE 5.31 Humeroradial joint: compression manipulation. This is a quick thrust with simultaneous supination and compression of the radius.

**Patient Position**
Sitting or supine.

**Hand Placement**

⦿ Approach the patient right hand to right hand, or left hand to left hand. Stabilize the elbow posteriorly with the other hand. If supine, the stabilizing hand is under the elbow supported on the treatment table.
⦿ Place your thenar eminence against the patient's thenar eminence (locking thumbs).

**Mobilizing Force**
Simultaneously, extend the patient's wrist, push against the thenar eminence, and compress the long axis of the radius while supinating the forearm.

N O T E : To replace an acute subluxation, a quick motion (thrust) is used.

**Proximal Radioulnar Joint, Dorsal/Volar Glides (Fig. 5.32)**
The convex rim of the radial head articulates with the concave radial notch on the ulna (see Fig. 5.26).

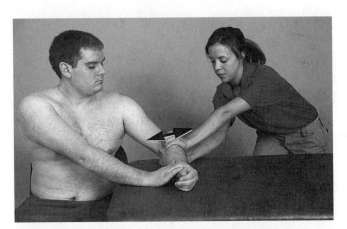

FIGURE 5.32 Proximal radioulnar joint: dorsal and volar glides.

**Resting Position**
The elbow is flexed 70° and the forearm supinated 35°.

**Treatment Plane**
The treatment plane is in the radial notch of the ulna, parallel to the long axis of the ulna.

**Stabilization**
Proximal ulna is stabilized.

**Indications**
Dorsal glide to increase pronation; volar glide to increase supination.

**Patient Position**

- Sitting or supine, with the elbow and forearm in resting position.
- Progress by placing the forearm at the limit of the range of pronation prior to administering the dorsal glide or at the limit of the range of supination prior to administering the volar glide.

**Hand Placement**

- Fixate the ulna with your medial hand around the medial aspect of the forearm.
- Place your other hand around the head of the radius with the fingers on the volar surface and the palm on the dorsal surface.

**Mobilizing Force**

- Force the radial head volarly by pushing with your palm or dorsally by pulling with your fingers.
- If a stronger force is needed for the dorsal glide, move around to the other side of the patient, switch hands, and push from the volar surface with the base of your hand against the radial head.

**Distal Radioulnar Joint, Dorsal/Volar Glides (Fig. 5.33)**
The concave ulnar notch of the radius articulates with the convex head of the ulna.

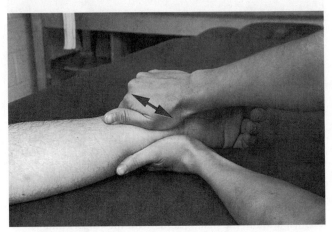

FIGURE 5.33 Distal radioulnar joint: dorsal and volar glides.

**Resting Position**
The resting position is with the forearm supinated 10°.

**Treatment Plane**
The treatment plane is the articulating surface of the radius, parallel to the long axis of the radius.

**Stabilization**
Distal ulna.

**Indications**
Dorsal glide to increase supination; volar glide to increase pronation.

**Patient Position**
Sitting, with the forearm on the treatment table. Begin in the resting position and progress to end-range pronation or supination.

**Hand Placement**
Stabilize the distal ulna by placing the fingers of one hand on the dorsal surface and the thenar eminence and thumb on the volar surface. Place your other hand in the same manner around the distal radius.

**Mobilizing Force**
Glide the distal radius dorsally or volarly parallel to the ulna.

## Wrist Complex (Fig. 5.34)

N O T E : When mobilizing the wrist, begin with general distractions and glides that include the proximal row and distal row of carpals as a group. For full ROM, individual carpal mobilizations/manipulations may be necessary. They are described following the general mobilizations. For a review of the mechanics of the wrist complex, see Chapter 19.

### Radiocarpal Joint

The concave distal radius articulates with the convex proximal row of carpals, which is composed of the scaphoid, lunate, and triquetrum.

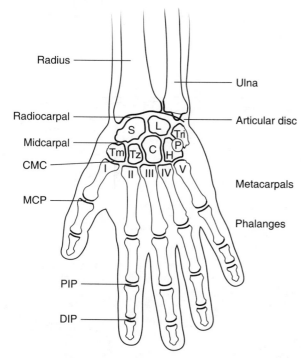

FIGURE 5.34 Bones and joints of the wrist and hand.

### Resting Position

The resting position is a straight line through the radius and third metacarpal with slight ulnar deviation.

### Treatment Plane

The treatment plane is in the articulating surface of the radius perpendicular to the long axis of the radius.

### Stabilization

Distal radius and ulna.

### Radiocarpal Distraction (Fig. 5.35)

### Indications

Testing; initial treatment; pain control; general mobility of the wrist.

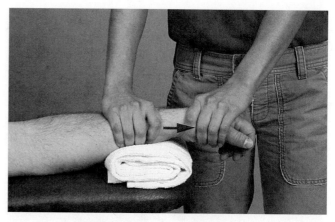

FIGURE 5.35 Wrist joint: general distraction.

### Patient Position

Sitting, with the forearm supported on the treatment table, wrist over the edge of the table.

### Hand Placement

- With the hand closest to the patient, grasp around the styloid processes and fixate the radius and ulna against the table.
- Grasp around the distal row of carpals with your other hand.

### Mobilizing Force

Pull in a distal direction with respect to the arm.

### Radiocarpal Joint, General Glides, and Progression

### Indications

Dorsal glide to increase flexion (Fig. 5.36A); volar glide to increase extension (Fig. 5.36B); radial glide to increase

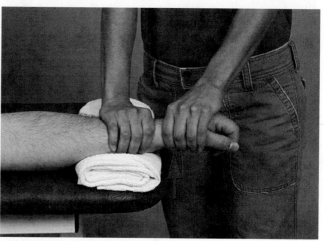

A

FIGURE 5.36 Wrist joint: general mobilization. (A) Dorsal glide.

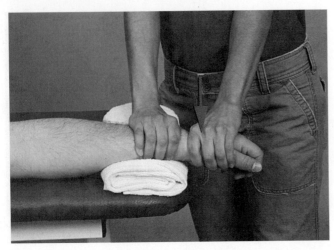

**B**

FIGURE 5.36  (continued) (*B*) Volar glide.

ulnar deviation; ulnar glide to increase radial deviation (Fig. 5.37).

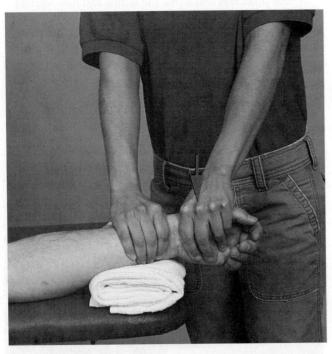

FIGURE 5.37  Wrist joint: general mobilization—ulnar glide.

### Patient Position and Hand Placement
Sitting with forearm resting on the table in pronation for the dorsal and volar techniques and in mid-range position

for the radial and ulnar techniques. Progress by moving the wrist to the end of the available range and glide in the defined direction. Specific carpal gliding techniques described in the next sections are used to increase mobility at isolated articulations.

### Mobilizing Force
The mobilizing force comes from the hand around the distal row of carpals.

### Specific Carpal Gliding (Figs. 5.38, 5.39)

N O T E :  Specific techniques to mobilize individual carpal bones may be necessary to gain full ROM of the wrist. Specific biomechanics of the radiocarpal and intercarpal joints are described in Chapter 19. To glide one carpal on another or on the radius, utilize the following guidelines:

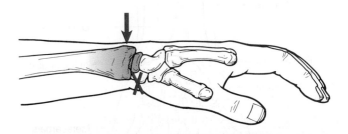

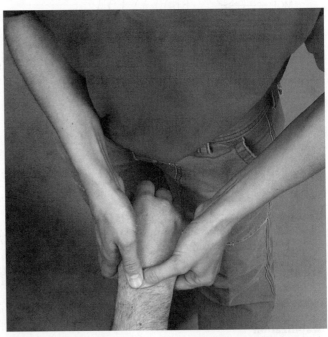

FIGURE 5.38  Specific carpal mobilizations: stabilization of the distal bone and volar glide of the proximal bone. Shown is stabilization of the scaphoid and lunate with the index fingers and a volar glide to the radius with the thumbs to increase wrist flexion.

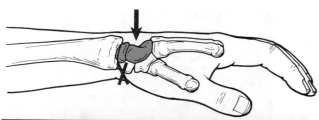

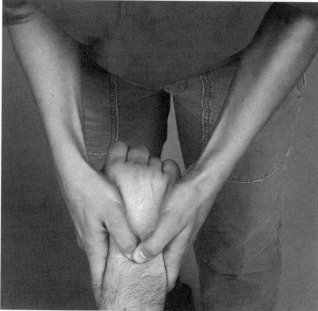

FIGURE 5.39 Specific carpal mobilizations: stabilization of the proximal bone and volar guide of the distal bone. Shown is stabilization of the lunate with the index fingers and volar glide to the capitate with the thumbs to increase extension.

## Patient and Therapist Positions

- The patient sits.
- You stand and grasp the patient's hand so the elbow hangs unsupported.
- The weight of the arm provides slight distraction to the joint (grade I), so you then need only to apply the glides.

## Hand Placement

Identify the specific articulation to be mobilized and place your index fingers on the volar surface of the bone to be stabilized. Place the overlapping thumbs on the dorsal surface of the bone to be mobilized. The rest of your fingers hold the patient's hand so it is relaxed.

- To increase *extension*, the stabilizing index fingers are placed under the bone that is *concave* (on the volar surface), and the mobilizing thumbs are overlapped on the dorsal surface of the bone that is *convex*.
- To increase *flexion*, the stabilizing index fingers are placed under the bone that is *convex* (on the volar surface), and the mobilizing thumbs are overlapped on the dorsal surface of the bone that is *concave*.

## Mobilizing Force

- In each case, the force comes from the overlapping thumbs on the dorsal surface.

- By mobilizing from the dorsal surface, pressure against the nerves, blood vessels, and tendons in the carpal tunnel and Guyon's canal is minimized, and a stronger mobilizing force can be used without pain.

**Indications**
To increase flexion.

- Glide the concave radius volarly on the stabilized scaphoid.
- Glide the concave radius volarly on the stabilized lunate (see Fig. 5.38).
- Glide the concave trapezium-trapezoid unit volarly on the stabilized scaphoid.
- Glide the concave lunate volarly on the stabilized capitate.
- Glide the concave triquetrum volarly on the stabilized hamate.

    To increase extension.

- Glide convex scaphoid volarly on the stabilized radius.
- Glide convex lunate volarly on the stabilized radius.
- Glide convex scaphoid volarly on the stabilized trapezium-trapezoid unit.
- Glide convex capitate volarly on the stabilized lunate (see Fig. 5.39).
- Glide convex hamate volarly on the stabilized triquetrum.

### Ulnar–Meniscal Triquetral Articulation

**Indications**
To unlock the articular disk, which may block motions of the wrist or forearm; apply a glide of the ulna volarly on a fixed triquetrum (see Fig. 19.7).

## Hand and Finger Joints

### Carpometacarpal and Intermetacarpal Joints of Digits II–V: Distraction (Fig. 5.40)

**Indication**
To increase mobility of the hand.

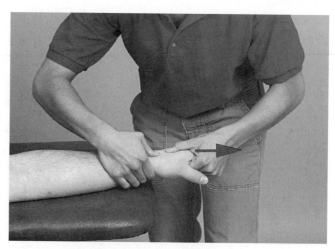

FIGURE 5.40 Carpometacarpal joint: distraction.

## Stabilization and Hand Placement
Stabilize the respective carpal with thumb and index finger of one hand. With your other hand, grasp around the proximal portion of a metacarpal.

## Mobilizing Force
Apply long-axis traction to the metacarpal to separate the joint surfaces.

### Carpometacarpal and Intermetacarpal: Volar Glide

## Indication
To increase mobility of the arch of the hand.

## Stabilization and Hand Placement
Stabilize the carpals with the thumb and index finger of one hand; place the thenar eminence of your other hand along the dorsal aspect of the metacarpals to provide the mobilization force.

## Mobilizing Force
Glide the proximal portion of the metacarpal volar ward. See also the stretching technique for cupping and flattening the arch of the hand described in Chapter 4.

### Carpometacarpal Joint of the Thumb
The CMC of the thumb is a saddle joint. The trapezium is concave, and the proximal metacarpal is convex for abduction/adduction. The trapezium is convex, and the proximal metacarpal is concave for flexion/extension.

## Resting Position
The resting position is midway between flexion and extension and between abduction and adduction.

## Stabilization
Fixate the trapezium with the hand that is closer to the patient.

## Treatment Plane
The treatment plane is in the trapezium for abduction-adduction and in the proximal metacarpal for flexion-extension.

### Carpometacarpal Distraction (Thumb)

## Indications
Testing; initial treatment; pain control; general mobility.

## Patient Position
The patient is positioned with forearm and hand resting on the treatment table.

## Hand Placement
- Fixate the trapezium with the hand that is closer to the patient.
- Grasp the patient's metacarpal by wrapping your fingers around it (similar to Fig. 6.41A).

## Mobilizing Force
Apply long-axis traction to separate the joint surfaces.

### Carpometacarpal Glides (Thumb) (Fig. 5.41)

## Indications
Ulnar glide to increase flexion; radial glide to increase extension; dorsal glide to increase abduction; volar glide to increase adduction.

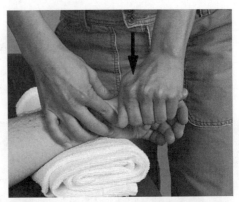

A

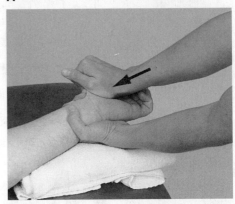

B

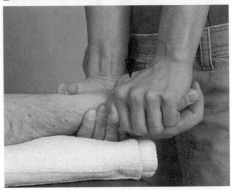

C

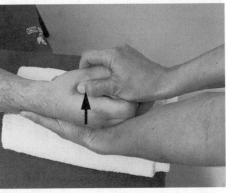

D

**FIGURE 5.41** Carpometacarpal joint of the thumb. (*A*) Ulnar glide to increase flexion. (*B*) Radial glide to increase extension. (*C*) Dorsal glide to increase abduction. (*D*) Volar glide to increase adduction. Note that the thumb of the therapist is placed in the web space between the index and thumb of the patient's hand to apply a volar glide.

## Patient Position and Hand Placement

- The trapezium is stabilized by grasping it directly or by wrapping your fingers around the distal row of carpals.
- Place the thenar eminence of your other hand against the base of the patient's first metacarpal on the side opposite the desired glide. For example, as pictured in Fig. 5.41A, the surface of the thenar eminence is on the radial side of the metacarpal to cause an ulnar glide.

### Mobilizing Force

The force comes from your thenar eminence against the base of the metacarpal. Adjust your body position to line up the force as illustrated in Figure 5.41A–D.

### Metacarpophalangeal and Interphalangeal Joints of the Fingers

In all cases, the distal end of the proximal articulating surface is convex, and the proximal end of the distal articulating surface is concave.

NOTE: Because all the articulating surfaces are the same for the digits, all techniques are applied in the same manner to each joint.

### Resting Position

The resting position is in light flexion for all joints.

### Treatment Plane

The treatment plane is in the distal articulating surface.

### Stabilization

Rest the forearm and hand on the treatment table; fixate the proximal articulating surface with the fingers of one hand.

### Metacarpophalangeal and Interphalangeal Distraction (Fig. 5.42)

### Indications

Testing; initial treatment; pain control; general mobility.

### Hand Placement

Use your proximal hand to stabilize the proximal bone; wrap the fingers and thumb of your other hand around the distal bone close to the joint.

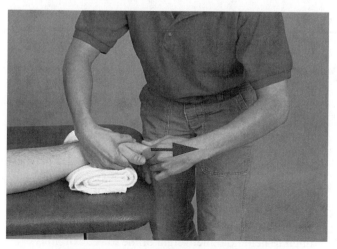

FIGURE 5.42 Metacarpophalangeal joint: distraction.

### Mobilizing Force

Apply long-axis traction to separate the joint surface.

### Metacarpophalangeal and Interphalangeal Glides and Progression

### Indications

Volar glide to increase flexion (Fig. 5.43); dorsal glide to increase extension; radial or ulnar glide (depending on finger) to increase abduction or adduction.

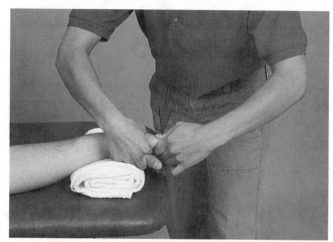

FIGURE 5.43 Metacarpophalangeal joint: volar glide.

### Mobilizing Force

The glide force is applied by the thumb against the proximal end of the bone to be moved. Progress by taking the joint to the end of its available range and applying slight distraction and the glide force. Rotation may be added prior to applying the gliding force.

## Hip Joint (Fig. 5.44)

The concave acetabulum receives the convex femoral head. Biomechanics of the hip joint are reviewed in Chapter 20.

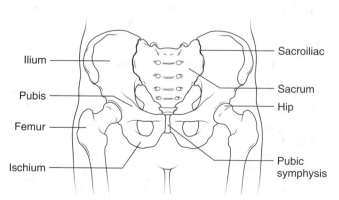

FIGURE 5.44 Bones and joints of the pelvis and hip.

## Resting Position
The resting position is hip flexion 30°, abduction 30°, and slight external rotation.

## Stabilization
Fixate the pelvis to the treatment table with belts.

## Hip Distraction of the Weight-Bearing Surface, Caudal Glide (Fig. 5.45)

N O T E : Because of the deep configuration of this joint, traction applied perpendicular to the treatment plane causes lateral glide of the superior, weight-bearing surface. To obtain separation of the weight-bearing surface, caudal glide is used.

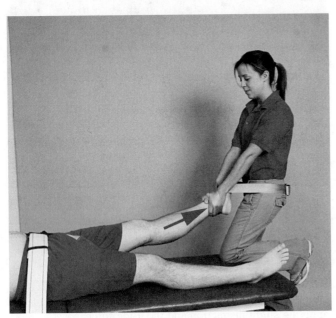

FIGURE 5.45 Hip joint: distraction of the weight-bearing surface.

## Indications
Testing; initial treatment; pain control; general mobility.

## Patient Position
Supine, with the hip in resting position and the knee extended.

P R E C A U T I O N : In the presence of knee dysfunction, this position should not be used; see alternate position following.

## Therapist Position and Hand Placement
Stand at the end of the treatment table; place a belt around your trunk, then cross the belt over the patient's foot and around the ankle. Place your hands proximal to the malleoli, under the belt. The belt allows you to use your body weight to apply the mobilizing force.

## Mobilizing Force
Long-axis traction is applied by pulling on the leg as you lean backward.

## Alternate Position for Hip Caudal Glide

## Indication
To apply distraction to the weight-bearing surface of the hip joint when there is knee dysfunction.

## Patient Position
Supine, with the hip and knee flexed.

## Therapist Position and Hand Placement
Wrap your hands around the epicondyles of the femur and distal thigh. Do not compress the patella.

## Mobilizing Force
The force comes from your hands and is applied in a caudal direction as you lean backward.

## Hip Posterior Glide (Fig. 5.46)

## Indications
To increase flexion; to increase internal rotation.

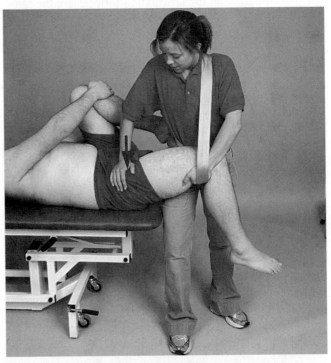

FIGURE 5.46 Hip joint: posterior glide.

## Patient Position
- Supine, with hips at the end of the table.
- The patient helps stabilize the pelvis and lumbar spine by flexing the opposite hip and holding the thigh against the chest with the hands.
- Initially, the hip to be mobilized is in resting position; progress to the end of the range.

## Therapist Position and Hand Placement
- Stand on the medial side of the patient's thigh.
- Place a belt around your shoulder and under the patient's thigh to help hold the weight of the lower extremity.

● Place your distal hand under the belt and distal thigh. Place your proximal hand on the anterior surface of the proximal thigh.

**Mobilizing Force**

Keep your elbows extended and flex your knees; apply the force through your proximal hand in a posterior direction.

### Hip Anterior Glide (Fig. 5.47)

**Indications**

To increase extension; to increase external rotation.

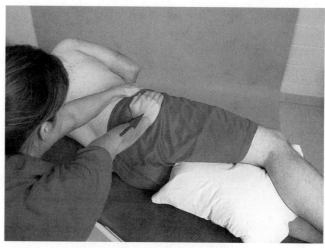

**B**

FIGURE 5.47 (*B*) side-lying.

● Push against the posterior aspect of the greater trochanter in an anterior direction with your caudal hand.

### Knee and Leg (Fig. 5.48)

**Tibiofemoral Articulation**

The concave tibial plateaus articulate on the convex femoral condyles. Biomechanics of the knee joint are described in Chapter 21.

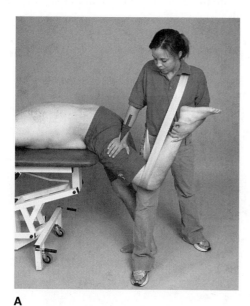

**A**

FIGURE 5.47 Hip joint: anterior glide (*A*) prone

**Patient Position**

Prone, with the trunk resting on the table and hips over the edge. The opposite foot is on the floor.

**Therapist Position and Hand Placement**

● Stand on the medial side of the patient's thigh.
● Place a belt around your shoulder and the patient's thigh to help support the weight of the leg.
● With your distal hand, hold the patient's leg.
● Place your proximal hand posteriorly on the proximal thigh just below the buttock.

**Mobilizing Force**

Keep your elbow extended and flex your knees; apply the force through your proximal hand in an anterior direction.

**Alternate Position (Fig. 5.47B)**

● Position the patient side-lying with the thigh comfortably flexed and supported by pillows.
● Stand posterior to the patient and stabilize the pelvis across the anterior superior iliac spine with your cranial hand.

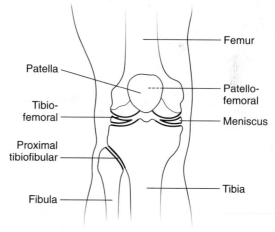

FIGURE 5.48 Bones and joints of the knee and leg.

**Resting Position**

The resting position is 25° flexion.

**Treatment Plane**

The treatment plane is along the surface of the tibial plateaus; therefore, it moves with the tibia as the knee angle changes.

**Stabilization**

In most cases, the femur is stabilized with a belt or by the table.

## Tibiofemoral Distraction, Long–Axis Traction (Fig. 5.49)

### Indications
Testing; initial treatment; pain control; general mobility.

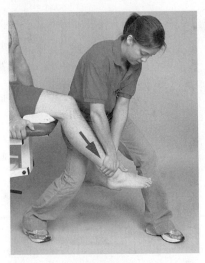

**A**

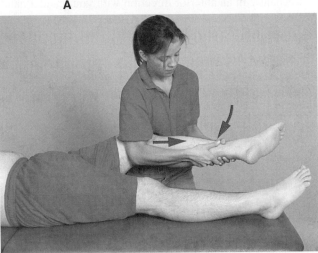

**B**

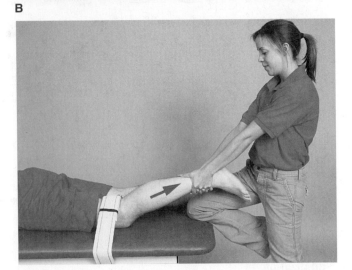

**C**

FIGURE 5.49 Tibiofemoral joint: distraction (A) sitting, (B) supine, and (C) prone.

### Patient Position
- Sitting, supine, or prone, beginning with the knee in the resting position.
- Progress to positioning the knee at the limit of the range of flexion or extension.
- Rotation of the tibia may be added prior to applying the traction force. Use internal rotation at end-range flexion and external rotation at end-range extention.

### Hand Placement
Grasp around the distal leg, proximal to the malleoli with both hands.

### Mobilizing Force
Pull on the long axis of the tibia to separate the joint surfaces.

## Tibiofemoral Posterior Glide (Fig. 5.50)

### Indications
Testing; to increase flexion.

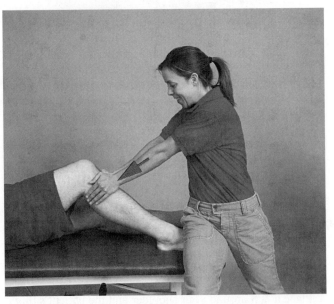

FIGURE 5.50 Tibiofemoral joint: posterior glide (drawer).

### Patient Position
Supine, with the foot resting on the table. The position for the drawer test can be used to mobilize the tibia either anteriorly or posteriorly, although no grade I distraction can be applied with the glides.

### Therapist Position and Hand Placement
Sit on the table with your thigh fixating the patient's foot. With both hands, grasp around the tibia, fingers pointing posteriorly and thumbs anteriorly.

### Mobilizing Force
Extend your elbows and lean your body weight forward; push the tibia posteriorly with your thumbs.

## Tibiofemoral Posterior Glide: Alternate Positions and Progression (Fig. 5.51)

### Indication
To increase flexion.

### Patient Position

- Sitting, with the knee flexed over the edge of the treatment table, beginning in the resting position (Fig. 5.51). Progress to near 90° flexion with the tibia positioned in internal rotation.
- Once the knee flexes past 90°, position the patient prone; place a small rolled towel proximal to the patella to minimize compression forces against the patella during the mobilization.

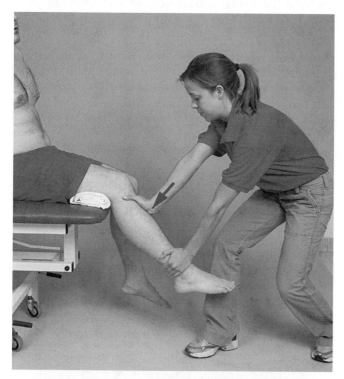

FIGURE 5.51 Tibiofemoral joint: posterior glide, sitting.

### Therapist Position and Hand Placement

- When in resting position, stand on the medial side of the patient's leg. Hold the distal leg with your distal hand and place the palm of your proximal hand along the anterior border of the tibial plateaus.
- When near 90° sit on a low stool; stabilize the leg between your knees and place one hand on the anterior border of the tibial plateaus.
- When prone, stabilize the femur with one hand and place the other hand along the border of the tibial plateaus.

### Mobilizing Force

- Extend your elbow and lean your body weight onto the tibia, gliding it posteriorly.

- When progressing with medial rotation of the tibia at the end of the range of flexion, the force is applied in a posterior direction against the medial side of the tibia.

## Tibiofemoral Anterior Glide (Fig. 5.52)

### Indication
To increase extension.

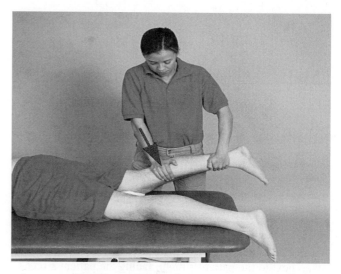

FIGURE 5.52 Tibiofemoral joint: anterior glide.

### Patient Position

- Prone, beginning with the knee in resting position; progress to the end of the available range.
- The tibia may also be positioned in lateral rotation.
- Place a small pad under the distal femur to prevent patellar compression.

### Hand Placement
Grasp the distal tibia with the hand that is closer to it and place the palm of the proximal hand on the posterior aspect of the proximal tibia.

### Mobilizing Force
Force with the hand on the proximal tibia in an anterior direction. The force may be directed to the lateral or medial tibial plateau to isolate one side of the joint.

### Alternate Position

- If the patient cannot be positioned prone, position him or her supine with a fixation pad under the tibia.
- The mobilizing force is placed against the femur in a posterior direction.

N O T E : The drawer test position can also be used. The mobilizing force comes from the fingers on the posterior tibia as you lean backward (see Fig. 5.50).

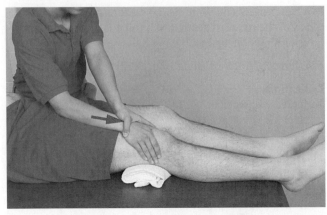

FIGURE 5.53  Patellofemoral joint: distal glide.

## Patellofemoral Joint, Distal Glide (Fig. 5.53)

**Indication**
To increase patellar mobility for knee flexion.

**Patient Position**
Supine, with knee extended; progress to positioning the knee at the end of the available range in flexion.

**Hand Placement**
Stand next to the patient's thigh, facing the patient's feet. Place the web space of the hand that is closer to the thigh around the superior border of the patella. Use the other hand for reinforcement.

**Mobilizing Force**
Glide the patella in a caudal direction, parallel to the femur.

P R E C A U T I O N :  Do not compress the patella into the femoral condyles while performing this technique.

## Patellofemoral Medial–Lateral Glide (Fig. 5.54)

**Indication**
To increase patellar mobility.

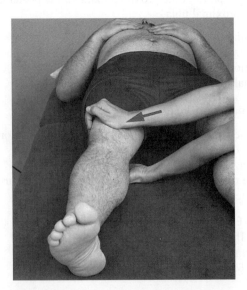

FIGURE 5.54  Patellofemoral joint: lateral glide.

**Patient Position**
Supine with the knee extended. Side-lying may be used to apply a medial glide (see Fig. 21.3)

**Hand Placement**
Place the heel of your hand along either the medial or lateral aspect of the patella. Stand on the opposite side of the table to position your hand along the medial border and on the same side of the table to position your hand along the lateral border. Place the other hand under the femur to stabilize it.

**Mobilizing Force**
Glide the patella in a medial or lateral direction, against the restriction.

## Proximal Tibiofibular Articulation: Anterior (Ventral) Glide (Fig. 5.55)

**Indications**
To increase movement of the fibular head; to reposition a posteriorly positioned head.

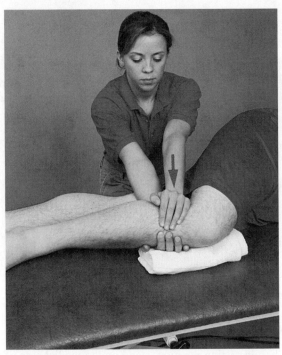

FIGURE 5.55  Proximal tibiofibular joint: anterior glide.

**Patient Position**

- Side-lying, with the trunk and hips rotated partially toward prone.
- The top leg is flexed forward so the knee and lower leg are resting on the table or supported on a pillow.

**Therapist Position and Hand Placement**

- Stand behind the patient, placing one of your hands under the tibia to stabilize it.
- Place the base of your other hand posterior to the head of the fibula, wrapping your fingers anteriorly.

**Mobilizing Force**
The force comes from the heel of your hand against the posterior aspect of the fibular head, in an anterior-lateral direction.

### Distal Tibiofibular Articulation: Anterior (Ventral) or Posterior (Dorsal) Glide (Fig. 5.56)

**Indication**
To increase mobility of the mortise when it is restricting ankle dorsiflexion.

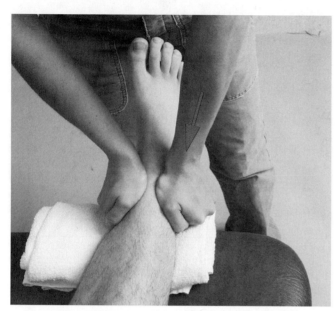

FIGURE 5.56 Distal tibiofibular articulation: posterior glide.

**Patient Position**
Supine or prone.

**Hand Placement**
Working from the end of the table, place the fingers of the more medial hand under the tibia and the thumb over the tibia to stabilize it. Place the base of your other hand over the lateral malleolus, with the fingers underneath.

**Mobilizing Force**
Press against the fibula in an anterior direction when prone and in a posterior direction when supine.

## Ankle and Foot Joints (Fig. 5.57)

Biomechanics of the ankle and foot are summarized in Chapter 22.

### Talocrural Joint (Upper Ankle Joint)
The convex talus articulates with the concave mortise made up of the tibia and fibula.

**Resting Position**
The resting position is 10° plantarflexion.

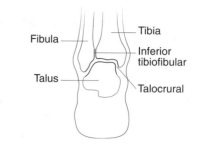
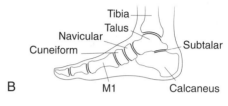
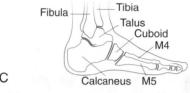

FIGURE 5.57 (A) Anterior view of the bones and joints of the lower leg and ankle. (B) Medial view. (C) Lateral view of the bones and joint relationships of the ankle and foot.

**Treatment Plane**
The treatment plane is in the mortise, in an anterior-posterior direction with respect to the leg.

**Stabilization**
The tibia is strapped or held against the table.

### Talocrural Distraction (Fig. 5.58)

**Indications**
Testing; initial treatment; pain control; general mobility.

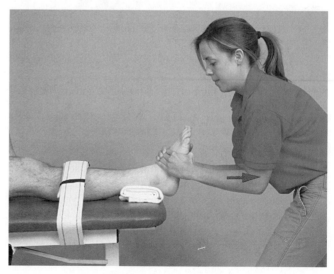

FIGURE 5.58 Talocrural joint: distraction.

## Patient Position

Supine, with the lower extremity extended. Begin with the ankle in resting position. Progress to the end of the available range of dorsiflexion or plantarflexion.

## Therapist Position and Hand Placement

- Stand at the end of the table; wrap the fingers of both hands over the dorsum of the patient's foot, just distal to the mortise.
- Place your thumbs on the plantar surface of the foot to hold it in resting position.

## Mobilization Force

Pull the foot away from the long axis of the leg in a distal direction by leaning backward.

## Talocrural Dorsal (Posterior) Glide (Fig. 5.59)

### Indication

To increase dorsiflexion.

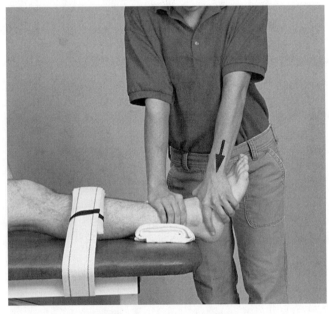

FIGURE 5.59 Talocrural joint: posterior glide.

## Patient Position

Supine, with the leg supported on the table and the heel over the edge.

## Therapist Position and Hand Placement

- Stand to the side of the patient.
- Stabilize the leg with your cranial hand or use a belt to secure the leg to the table.
- Place the palmar aspect of the web space of your other hand over the talus just distal to the mortise.
- Wrap your fingers and thumb around the foot to maintain the ankle in resting position. Grade I distraction force is applied in a caudal direction.

## Mobilizing Force

Glide the talus posteriorly with respect to the tibia by pushing against the talus.

## Talocrural Ventral (Anterior) Glide (Fig. 5.60)

### Indication

To increase plantarflexion.

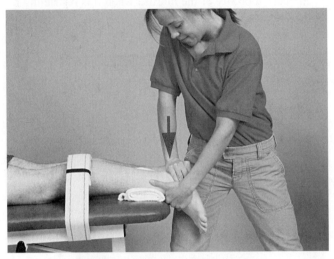

FIGURE 5.60 Talocrural joint: anterior glide.

## Patient Position

Prone, with the foot over the edge of the table.

## Therapist Position and Hand Placement

- Working from the end of the table, place your lateral hand across the dorsum of the foot to apply a grade I distraction.
- Place the web space of your other hand just distal to the mortise on the posterior aspect of the talus and calcaneus.

## Mobilizing Force

Push against the calcaneus in an anterior direction (with respect to the tibia); this glides the talus anteriorly.

## Alternate Position

- Patient is supine. Stabilize the distal leg anterior to the mortise with your proximal hand.
- The distal hand cups under the calcaneus.
- When you pull against the calcaneus in an anterior direction, the talus glides anteriorly.

## Subtalar Joint (Talocalcaneal), Posterior Compartment

The calcaneus is convex, articulating with a concave talus in the posterior compartment.

## Resting Position

The resting position is midway between inversion and eversion.

## Treatment Plane
The treatment plane is in the talus, parallel to the sole of the foot.

## Subtalar Distraction (Fig. 5.61)

### Indications
Testing; initial treatment; pain control; general mobility for inversion/eversion.

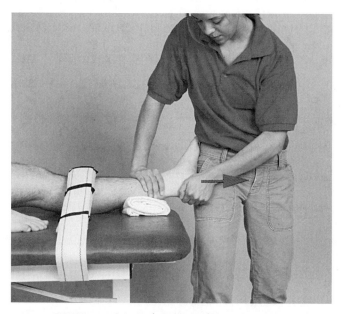

FIGURE 5.61  Subtalar (talocalcaneal) joint: distraction.

## Patient and Therapist Positions

- The patient is placed in a supine position, with the leg supported on the table and heel over the edge.
- The hip is externally rotated so the talocrural joint can be stabilized in dorsiflexion with pressure from your thigh against the plantar surface of the patient's forefoot.

## Hand Placement
The distal hand grasps around the calcaneus from the posterior aspect of the foot. The other hand fixes the talus and malleoli against the table.

## Mobilizing Force
Pull the calcaneus distally with respect to the long axis of the leg.

## Subtalar Medial Glide or Lateral Glide (Fig. 5.62)

### Indications
Medial glide to increase eversion; lateral glide to increase inversion.

### Patient Position
The patient is side-lying or prone, with the leg supported on the table or with a towel roll.

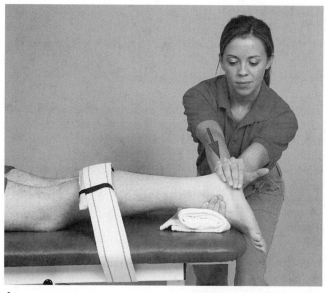

**A**

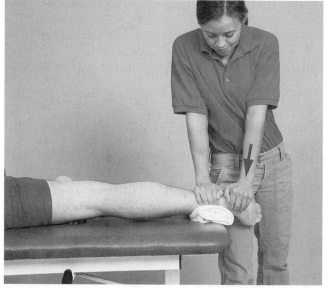

**B**

FIGURE 5.62  Subtalar joint: lateral glide: (A) prone and (B) side-lying.

## Therapist Position and Hand Placement

- Align your shoulder and arm parallel to the bottom of the foot.
- Stabilize the talus with your proximal hand.
- Place the base of the distal hand on the side of the calcaneus medially to cause a lateral glide and laterally to cause a medial glide.
- Wrap the fingers around the plantar surface.

## Mobilizing Force
Apply a grade I distraction force in a caudal direction, then push with the base of your hand against the side of the calcaneus parallel to the planter surface of the heel.

## Alternate Position

Same as the position for distraction, moving the calcaneus in the medial or a lateral direction with the base of the hand.

## Intertarsal and Tarsometatarsal Joints

When moving in a dorsal-plantar direction with respect to the foot, all of the articulating surfaces are concave and convex in the same direction. For example, the proximal articulating surface is convex and the distal articulating surface is concave. The technique for mobilizing each joint is the same. The hand placement is adjusted to stabilize the proximal bone partner so the distal bone partner can be moved.

## Intertarsal and Tarsometatarsal Plantar Glide (Fig. 5.63)

### Indication

To increase plantarflexion accessory motions (necessary for supination).

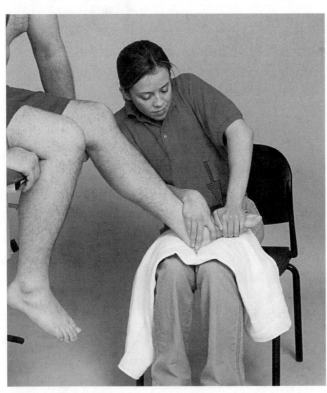

FIGURE 5.63 Plantar glide of a distal tarsal bone on a stabilized proximal bone. Shown is the cuneiform bone on the navicular.

### Patient Position

Supine, with hip and knee flexed, or sitting, with knee flexed over the edge of the table and heel resting on your lap.

### Stabilization

Fixate the more proximal bone with your index finger on the plantar surface of the bone.

## Hand Placement

- To mobilize the tarsal joints along the medial aspect of the foot, position yourself on the lateral side of the foot. Place the proximal hand on the dorsum of the foot with the fingers pointing medially so the index finger can be wrapped around and placed under the bone to be stabilized.
- Place your thenar eminence of the distal hand over the dorsal surface of the bone to be moved and wrap the fingers around the plantar surface.
- To mobilize the lateral tarsal joints, position yourself on the medial side of the foot, point your fingers laterally, and position your hands around the bones as just described.

### Mobilizing Force

Push the distal bone in a plantar direction from the dorsum of the foot.

## Intertarsal and Tarsometatarsal Dorsal Glide (Fig. 5.64)

### Indication

To increase the dorsal gliding accessory motion (necessary for pronation).

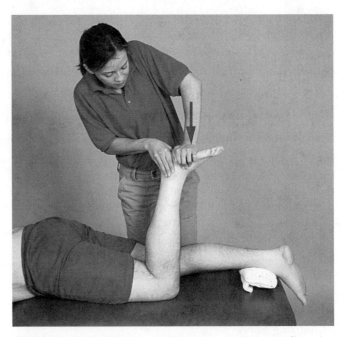

FIGURE 5.64 Dorsal gliding of a distal tarsal on a proximal tarsal. Shown is the cuboid bone on the calcaneus.

### Patient Position

Prone, with knee flexed.

### Stabilization

Fixate the more proximal bone.

### Hand Placement

- To mobilize the lateral tarsal joints (e.g., cuboid on calcaneus), position yourself on the medial side of the patient's leg and wrap your fingers around the lateral side of the foot (as in Fig. 5.64).

● To mobilize the medial bones (e.g., navicular on talus), position yourself on the lateral side of the patient's leg and wrap your fingers around the medial aspect of the foot.

● Place your second metacarpophalangeal joint against the bone to be moved.

**Mobilizing Force**
Push from the plantar surface in a dorsal direction.

**Alternate Technique**
Same position and hand placements as for plantar glides, except the distal bone is stabilized and the proximal bone

is forced in a plantar direction. This is a relative motion of the distal bone moving in a dorsal direction.

### Intermetatarsal, Metatarsophalangeal, and Interphalangeal Joints

The intermetatarsal, metatarsophalangeal, and interphalangeal joints of the toes are stabilized and mobilized in the same manner as the fingers. In each case, the articulating surface of the proximal bone is convex, and the articulating surface of the distal bone is concave. It is easiest to stabilize the proximal bone and glide the surface of the distal bone either plantarward for flexion, dorsalward for extension, and medially or laterally for adduction and abduction.

---

## INDEPENDENT LEARNING ACTIVITIES

### ● Critical Thinking and Discussion

1. An individual is immobilized in a cast for 4 to 6 weeks following a fracture. In general, what structures lose their elasticity, and what restrictions do you feel when testing range of motion, joint play, and flexibility?

2. Describe the normal arthrokinematic relationships for the extremity joints and define the location of the treatment plane for each joint.

3. Using the information from item 1, define a specific fracture, such as a Colle's fracture of the distal forearm. Identify what techniques are necessary to gain joint mobility and range of motion in the related joints such as the wrist, forearm, and elbow joints, connective tissues, and muscles. Practice using each of the techniques.

4. Explain the rationale for using passive joint techniques to treat patients with limitations because of pain and muscle guarding or to treat patients with restricted capsular or ligamentous tissue. What is the difference in the way the techniques are applied in each case?

5. Describe how joint mobilization techniques fit into the total plan of therapeutic intervention for patients with impaired joint mobility.

6. Explain the difference between passive joint mobilization techniques and mobilization with movement techniques.

### ● Laboratory Practice

With a partner, practice mobilizing each joint in the upper and lower extremities.

*Precaution:* Do not practice on an individual with a hypermobile or unstable joint.

1. Begin with the joint in its resting position and apply distraction techniques at each intensity (sustained grades I, II, and III) to develop a feel for "very gentle," "taking up the slack," and "stretch." Do not apply a vigorous stretch to someone with a normal joint. Be sure to use appropriate stabilization.

2. With the joint in its resting position, practice all appropriate glides for that joint. Be sure to use a grade I distraction with each gliding technique. Vary the techniques between sustained and oscillation.

3. Practice progressing each technique by taking the joint to a point that you determine to be the "end of the range" and:
   • Apply a distraction technique with the extremity in that position.
   • Apply the appropriate glide at that range (be sure to apply a grade I distraction with each glide).
   • Add rotation (e.g., external rotation for shoulder abduction) and then apply the appropriate glide.

---

## REFERENCES

1. Akeson, WH, et al: Effects of immobilization on joints. Clin Orthop 219:28, 1987.
2. American Physical Therapy Association. Guide to physical therapist practice, ed 2. Phys Ther 81:9–746, 2001.
3. Backstrom, KM: Mobilization with movement as an adjunct intervention in a patient with complicated DeQuervain's tenosynovitis: a case report. J Orthop Sports Phys Ther 32(3):86–97, 2002.
4. Boissonnault, W, Bryan, JM, Fox, KJ: Joint manipulation curricula in physical therapist professional degree programs. J Orthop Sports Phys Ther 34(4):171–181, 2004.
5. Cyriax, J: Textbook of Orthopaedic Medicine. Vol I. The Diagnosis of Soft Tissue Lesions, ed 8. Bailliere & Tindall, London, 1982.
6. DiFabio, RP: Efficacy of manual therapy. Phys Ther 72:853–864, 1992.
7. Donatelli, R, Owens-Burkhart, H: Effects of immobilization on the extensibility of periarticular connective tissue. J Orthop Sports Phys Ther 3:67, 1981.
8. Enneking, WF, Horowitz, M: The intra-articular effects of immobilization on the human knee. J Bone Joint Surg Am 54:978, 1972.
9. Exelby, L: Mobilizations with movement, a personal view. Physiotherapy 81(12):724, 1995.
10. Harryman, DT, Sidles, JA, et al: Translation of the humeral head on the glenoid with passive glenohumeral motion. J Bone Joint Surg Am 72:1334–1343, 1990.
11. Howell, SM, Galinat, BJ, et al: Normal and abnormal mechanics of

the glenohumeral jont in the horizontal plane. J Bone Joint Surg Am 70:227–232, 1988.

12. Hsu, AT, Hedman, T, Chang, TH, et al: Changes in abduction and rotation range of motion in response to simulated dorsal and ventral translational mobilization of the glenohumeral joint. Phys Ther 82(6):544–556, 2002.

13. Itoi, E, Motzkin, NE, et al: Contribution of axial arm rotation to the humeral head translation. Am J Sports Med 22:499–503, 1994.

14. Kaltenborn, FM: The Kaltenborn Method of Joint Examination and Treatment. Vol I. The Extremities, ed 5. Olaf Norlis Bokhandel, Oslo, 1999.

15. Kavanagh, J: Is there a positional fault at the inferior tibiofibular joint in patients with acute or chronic ankle sprains compared to normals? Manual Ther 4(1):19, 1999.

16. Magee, DJ: Orthopedic Physical Assessment, ed 3. WB Saunders, Philadelphia, 1997.

17. Maitland, GD: Peripheral Manipulation, ed 3. Butterworth-Heinemann, Boston, 1991.

18. McDavitt, S: Practice affairs corner; a revision for the Guide to Physical Therapist Practice; mobilization or manipulation? Yes! That is my final answer! Orthop Phys Ther Pract 12(4), 2000.15.

19. Meadows, J: Orthopedic Differential Diagnosis in Physical Therapy: A Case Study Approach. McGraw-Hill, Toronto, 1999.

20. Miller, J: The Mulligan concept—the next step in the evolution of manual therapy. Orthop Division Rev 2:9, 1999.

21. Mulligan, BR: Manual Therapy "NAGS," "SNAGS," "MWM'S: Etc., ed 4. Plane View Press, Wellington, 1999.

22. Mulligan, BR: Mobilizations with movement (MWM'S). J Manual Manipulative Ther 1(4):154, 1993.

23. Norkin, C, Levangie, P: Joint Structure and Function: A Comprehensive Analysis, ed 2. FA Davis, Philadelphia, 1992.

24. O'Brien, T, Vincenzino, B: A study of the effects of Mulligan's mobilization with movement of lateral ankle pain using a case study design. Manual Ther 3(2):78, 1998.

25. Paris, SV: Mobilization of the spine. Phys Ther 59:998, 1979.

26. Paungmali, A, O'Leary, S, et al: Hypoalgesic and sympathoexcitatory effects of mobilization with movement for lateral epicondylalgia. Phys Ther 83(4):374–383, 2003.

27. Smith, LK, Weiss, EL, Lehmkuhl, LD: Brunnstrom's Clinical Kinesiology, ed 5. FA Davis, Philadelphia, 1996.

28. Vincenzino, B, Wright, A: Effects of a novel manipulative physiotherapy technique on tennis elbow: a single case study. Manual Ther 1(1):30, 1995.

29. Warwick, R, Williams, S (eds): Arthrology. In Gray's Anatomy, 35th British ed. WB Saunders, Philadelphia, 1973.

30. Wegener, L, Kisner, C, Nichols, D: Static and dynamic balance responses in persons with bilateral knee osteoarthritis. J Orthop Sports Phys Ther 25:13, 1997.

31. Wilson, E. Mobilizations with movement and adverse neutral tension: an exploration of possible links. Manipulative Phys Ther 27(1):40, 1995.

32. Wyke, B: The neurology of joints. Ann R Coll Surg 41:25, 1967.

33. Wyke, B: Articular neurology: a review. Physiotherapy March:94, 1972.

34. Wyke, B: Neurological aspects of pain for the physical therapy clinician. Physical Therapy Forum 1982. Lecture presented at Columbus, Ohio, 1982.

# Resistance Exercise For Impaired Muscle Performance

*Muscle performance* refers to the capacity of a muscle to do work (force × distance).[10] Despite the simplicity of the definition, muscle performance is a complex component of functional movement and is influenced by all of the body systems. Factors that affect muscle performance include the morphological qualities of muscle; neurological, biochemical, and biomechanical influences; and metabolic, cardiovascular, respiratory, cognitive, and emotional function. For a person to anticipate, respond to, and control the forces applied to the body and carry out the physical demands of everyday life in a safe and efficient manner, the body's muscles must be able to produce, sustain, and regulate muscle tension to meet these demands.

The key elements of muscle performance are *strength*, *power*, and *endurance*.[10] If any one or more of these areas of muscle performance is impaired, functional limitations and disability or increased risk of dysfunction may ensue. Many factors, such as injury, disease, immobilization, disuse, and inactivity, may result in impaired muscle performance, leading to weakness and muscle atrophy.[193,207,231] When deficits in muscle performance place a person at risk for injury or hinder function, the use of resistance exercise is an appropriate therapeutic intervention to improve the integrated use of strength, power, and muscular endurance during functional movements, reduce the risk of injury or reinjury, and enhance physical performance.

*Resistance exercise* is any form of active exercise in which dynamic or static muscle contraction is resisted by an outside force applied manually or mechanically.[103,250] Resistance exercise, also referred to as *resistance training*,[8,9,32,168] is an essential element of rehabilitation programs for persons with impaired function and an integral component of conditioning programs for those who wish to promote or maintain health and physical well-being, potentially enhance performance of motor skills, and prevent or reduce the risk of injury and disease.[8,105,118]

A comprehensive examination and evaluation of a patient or client is the basis on which a therapist determines whether a program of resistance exercise is warranted and can improve a person's current level of function or prevent potential dysfunction. Many factors influence how appropriate, effective, or safe resistance training is and how the exercises are designed, implemented, and progressed. Factors such as the underlying pathology, the extent and severity of muscle performance impairments, the presence of other deficits, the stage of tissue healing after injury or surgery, and a patient's or client's age, overall level of fitness, and the ability to cooperate and learn all must be considered. Once a program of resistance exercise is developed and prescribed to meet specific functional goals and outcomes, direct intervention by a therapist initially to implement the exercise program or to begin to teach and supervise the prescribed exercises for a smooth transition to an independent, home-based program is imperative.

This chapter provides a foundation of information on resistance exercise, identifies the determinants of resistance training programs, summarizes the principles and guidelines for application of manual and mechanical resistance exercise, and addresses a variety of regimens for resistance training. It also addresses the scientific evidence, when available, of the relationship between improvements in muscle performance and enhanced functional abilities. The specific techniques described and illustrated in this chapter focus on manual resistance exercise for the extremities, primarily used during the early phase of rehabilitation. Additional exercises performed independently by a patient or client using resistance equipment are described and illustrated in Chapters 17 to 22. The use of resistance exercise for spinal conditions is presented in Chapter 16.

## ⬤ MUSCLE PERFORMANCE AND RESISTANCE EXERCISE—DEFINITIONS AND GUIDING PRINCIPLES

The three elements of muscle performance[10]—strength, power, and endurance—can be enhanced by some form of resistance exercise. To what extent each of these elements is altered by exercise depends on how the principles of resistance training are applied and how factors such as the intensity, frequency, and duration of exercise are manipulated. Because the physical demands of work, recreation and everyday living usually involve all three aspects of muscle performance, most resistance training programs seek to achieve a balance of strength, power, and muscular endurance to suit an individual's needs and goals. In addition to having a positive impact on muscle performance, resistance training can produce many other benefits.[8,9] These potential benefits are listed in Box 6.1. After a brief

---

**BOX 6.1    Potential Benefits of Resistance Exercise**

- Enhanced muscle performance: restoration, improvement or maintenance of muscle strength, power, and endurance
- Increased strength of connective tissues: tendons, ligaments, intramuscular connective tissue
- Greater bone mineral density or less bone demineralization
- Decreased stress on joints during physical activity
- Reduced risk of soft tissue injury during physical activity
- Possible improvement in capacity to repair and heal damaged soft tissues due to positive impact on tissue remodeling
- Possible improvement in balance
- Enhanced physical performance during daily living, occupational, and recreational activities
- Positive changes in body composition: ↑ lean muscle mass or ↓ body fat
- Enhanced feeling of physical well-being
- Possible improvement in perception of disability and quality of life

description of the three elements of muscle performance, guiding principles of exercise prescription and training are discussed in this section.

## Strength

*Muscle strength* is a broad term that refers to the ability of contractile tissue to produce tension and a resultant force based on the demands placed on the muscle.[184,193,233] More specifically, muscle strength is the greatest measurable force that can be exerted by a muscle or muscle group to overcome resistance during a *single* maximum effort.[10] *Functional strength* relates to the ability of the neuromuscular system to produce, reduce, or control forces, contemplated or imposed, during functional activities, in a smooth, coordinated manner.[39,219] Insufficient muscular strength can contribute to major functional losses of even the most basic activities of daily living.

*Strength training.* The development of muscle strength is an integral component of most rehabilitation or conditioning programs for individuals of all ages and all ability levels.[8,91,226] *Strength training (strengthening exercise)* is defined as a systematic procedure of a muscle or muscle group lifting, lowering, or controlling heavy loads (resistance) for a relatively low number of repetitions or over a short period of time.[30,32,103] The most common adaptation to heavy resistance exercise is an increase in the maximum force-producing capacity of muscle, that is, an increase in muscle strength, primarily as the result of neural adaptations and an increase in muscle fiber size.[9,121,193]

## Power

*Muscle power*, another aspect of muscle performance, is related to the strength and speed of movement and is defined as the work (force × distance) produced by a muscle per unit of time (force × distance/time).[10,184,193,201,237] In other words, it is the *rate* of performing work. The rate at which a muscle contracts and produces a resultant force and the relationship of force and velocity are factors that affect muscle power.[30,201] Because work can be produced over a very brief or an extended period of time, power can be expressed by either a single burst of high-intensity activity (such as lifting a heavy piece of luggage onto an overhead rack or performing a high jump) or by repeated bursts of less intense muscle activity (such as climbing a flight of stairs). The terms *anaerobic power* and *aerobic power,* respectively, are sometimes used to differentiate these two aspects of power.[193,237]

*Power training.* Many motor skills in our lives are composed of movements that are explosive and involve both strength and speed. Therefore, re-establishing muscle power may be an important priority in a rehabilitation program. Muscle strength is a necessary foundation for developing muscle power. Power can be enhanced by either

increasing the work a muscle must perform during a specified period of time or reducing the amount of time required to produce a given force. The greater the intensity of the exercise and the shorter the time period taken to generate force, the greater is the muscle power.[201,237] For power training regimens, such as *plyometric training* or *stretch-shortening drills* the speed of movement is the variable that is most often manipulated.[19,20,284,286,302]

## Endurance

Endurance is a broad term that refers to the ability to perform low-intensity, repetitive, or sustained activities over a prolonged period of time. *Cardiopulmonary endurance (total body endurance)* is associated with repetitive, dynamic motor activities such as walking, cycling, swimming, or upper extremity ergometry, which involve use of the large muscles of the body.[8,32] This aspect of endurance is explored in Chapter 7.

*Muscle endurance* (sometimes referred to as *local endurance*) is the ability of a muscle to contract repeatedly against a load (resistance), generate and sustain tension, and resist fatigue over an extended period of time.[8,10,14,32,233] The term *aerobic power* is sometimes used interchangeably with muscle endurance.[237] Maintenance of balance and proper alignment of the body segments requires sustained control (endurance) by the postural muscles. In fact, almost all daily living tasks require some degree of muscle and cardiopulmonary endurance.

Although strength and muscle endurance, as elements of muscle performance, are associated, they do not always correlate well with each other. Just because a muscle group is strong, it does not preclude the possibility that muscular endurance is impaired. For example, an individual in the workplace who is strong has no difficulty lifting a 10-pound object several times—but does the worker have sufficient muscle endurance in the upper extremities and the stabilizing muscles of the trunk and lower extremities to lift 10-pound objects several hundred times during the course of a day's work without excessive fatigue or potential injury?

*Endurance training. Endurance training (endurance exercise)* is characterized by having a muscle contract and lift or lower a light load for many repetitions or sustain a muscle contraction for an extended period of time.[9,32,193,264] The key elements of endurance training are low-intensity muscle contractions, a large number of repetitions, and a prolonged time period. Unlike strength training, muscles adapt to endurance training by increases in their oxidative and metabolic capacities, which allows better delivery and use of oxygen. For many patients with impaired muscle performance, endurance training has a more positive impact on improving function than strength training. In addition, using low levels of resistance in an exercise program minimizes adverse forces on joints, produces less irritation to soft tissues, and is more comfortable than heavy resistance training.

## Overload Principle

### Description

A guiding principle of exercise prescription that has been one of the foundations on which the use of resistance exercise to improve muscle performance is based is the *overload principle.* Simply stated, if muscle performance is to improve, a load that exceeds the metabolic capacity of the muscle must be applied; that is, the muscle must be challenged to perform at a level greater than that to which it is accustomed.[8,9,129,193,207] If the demands remain constant after the muscle has adapted, the level of muscle performance can be maintained but not increased.

### Application of the Overload Principle

The overload principle focuses on the *progressive* loading of muscle by manipulating, for example, the intensity or volume of exercise. *Intensity* of resistance exercise refers to how much weight (resistance) is imposed on the muscle, whereas *volume* encompasses variables such as repetitions, sets, or frequency of exercise, any one or more of which can be gradually adjusted to increase the demands on the muscle.

- In a strength training program, the *amount of resistance* applied to the muscle is incrementally and progressively increased.
- For endurance training, more emphasis is placed on increasing the *time* a muscle contraction is sustained or the *number of repetitions* performed than on increasing resistance.

PRECAUTION: To ensure safety, the extent and progression of overload must always be applied in the context of the underlying pathology, age of the patient, stage of tissue healing, fatigue, and the overall abilities and goals of the patient. The muscle and related body systems must be given time to *adapt* to the demands of an increased load or repetitions before the load or number of repetitions is again increased.

## SAID Principle

The SAID principle (specific adaptation to imposed demands)[193] suggests that a framework of specificity is a necessary foundation on which exercise programs should be built. This principle applies to all body systems and is an extension of Wolff's law (body systems adapt over time to the stresses placed on them). The SAID principle helps therapists determine the exercise prescription and which parameters of exercise should be selected to create specific training effects that best meet specific functional needs and goals.

### Specificity of Training

*Specificity of training,* also referred to as *specificity of exercise,* is a widely accepted concept suggesting that the adaptive effects of training, such as improvement of strength, power, and endurance, are highly specific to the training method employed.[32,81] Whenever possible, exercises incorporated in a program should mimic the anticipated function. For example, if the desired functional activity requires greater muscular endurance than strength, the intensity and duration of exercises should be geared to improve muscular endurance.

Specificity of training should also be considered relative to mode (type) and velocity of exercise[23,80,200,206,224] as well as patient or limb position (joint angle)[49,161,162,293] and the movement pattern during exercise. For example, if the desired functional outcome is the ability to ascend and descend stairs, exercise should be performed eccentrically and concentrically in a weight-bearing pattern and progressed to the desired speed. Regardless of the simplicity or complexity of the motor task to be learned, task-specific practice must always be emphasized. It has been suggested that the basis of specificity of training is related to morphological and metabolic changes in muscle as well as neural adaptations to the training stimulus associated with motor learning.[218]

### Transfer of Training

In contrast to the SAID principle, carryover of training effects from one variation of exercise or task to another has also been reported. This phenomenon is called *transfer of training, overflow,* or *cross-training.* Transfer of training has been reported to occur on a *very limited* basis with respect to the velocity of training[143,200,278] and the type or mode of exercise.[80] It has also been suggested that a cross-training effect can occur from an exercised limb to a nonexercised, contralateral limb in a resistance training program.[67,291,292]

A program of exercises designed to develop muscle strength has also been shown to improve muscular endurance at least moderately. In contrast, endurance training has little to no cross-training effect on strength.[16,81,103] Strength training at one speed of exercise has been shown to provide some improvement in strength at higher or lower speeds of exercise. However, the overflow effects are substantially less than the training effects resulting from specificity of training.

Despite the evidence that a small degree of transfer of training does occur in resistance exercise programs, most studies support the importance of designing an exercise program that most closely replicates the desired functional activities. As many variables as possible in the exercise program should match the requirements and demands placed on a patient during specific functional activities.

## Reversibility Principle

Adaptive changes in the body's systems, such as increased strength or endurance, in response to a resistance exercise program are transient unless training-induced improvements are regularly used for functional activities or unless an individual participates in a maintenance program of resistance exercises.[8,42,90,193]

*Detraining,* reflected by a reduction in muscle performance, begins within a week or two after the cessation of resistance exercises and continues until training effects are lost.[168,208] For this reason, it is imperative that gains in strength and endurance are incorporated into daily activities as early as possible in a rehabilitation program. It is also advisable for patients to participate in a maintenance program of resistance exercises as an integral component of a lifelong fitness program.

## SKELETAL MUSCLE FUNCTION AND ADAPTATION TO RESISTANCE EXERCISE

Knowledge of the factors that influence the force-producing capacity of normal muscle during an active contraction is fundamental to understanding how the neuromuscular system adapts as the result of resistance training. This knowledge, in turn, provides a basis on which a therapist is able to make sound clinical decisions when designing a resistance exercise program for patients with weakness and functional limitations as the result of injury or disease or to enhance physical performance and prevent or reduce the risk of injury in healthy individuals.

### Factors that Influence Tension Generation in Normal Skeletal Muscle

NOTE: For a brief review of the structure of skeletal muscle, refer to Chapter 4 of this textbook. For in-depth information on muscle structure and function, numerous resources are available.[121,184,193,250,254]

Diverse but interrelated factors affect the tension-generating capacity of *normal* skeletal muscle necessary to control the body and perform motor tasks. Determinants and correlates include morphological, biomechanical, neurological, metabolic, and biochemical factors. All contribute to the *magnitude, duration,* and *speed* of force production as well as how resistant or susceptible a muscle is to fatigue. Properties of muscle itself as well as key neural factors and their impact on tension generation during an active muscle contraction are summarized in Table 6.1.[121,166,184,193,254]

Additional factors such as the energy stores available to muscle, the influence of fatigue and recovery from exercise, and a person's age, gender, and psychological/cognitive status, as well as many other factors, affect a muscle's ability to develop and sustain tension. A therapist must recognize that these factors affect a patient's performance during exercise and the potential outcomes of the exercise program.

#### Energy Stores and Blood Supply
Muscle needs adequate sources of energy (fuel) to contract, generate tension, and resist fatigue. The predominant fiber type found in the muscle and the adequacy of blood supply, which transports oxygen and nutrients to muscle and removes waste products, affect the tension-producing capacity of a muscle and its resistance to fatigue.[166] The three main energy systems (ATP-PC system, anaerobic/glycolytic/lactic acid system, aerobic system) are reviewed in Chapter 7.

| TABLE 6.1 | Determinants and Correlates that Affect Tension Generation of Skeletal Muscle |
|---|---|
| **Factor** | **Influence** |
| Cross-section and size of the muscle (includes muscle fiber number and size) | The larger the muscle diameter, the greater its tension-producing capacity |
| Fiber arrangement and fiber length (also relates to cross-sectional diameter of the muscle) | Short fibers with pinnate and multipinnate design in high force producing muscles (ex. quadriceps, gastrocnemius, deltoid, biceps brachii) |
| | Long parallel design in muscles with high rate of shortening but less force production (ex. sartorius, lumbricals) |
| Fiber-type distribution of muscle: type I (tonic, slow-twitch) and type IIA & IIB (phasic, fast-twitch) | High percentage of type I fibers: low force production, slow rate of maximum force development, resistant to fatigue |
| | High percentage of type IIA and IIB fibers: rapid high force production; rapid fatigue |
| Length-tension relationship of muscle at time of contraction | Muscle produces greatest tension when it is near or at the physiological resting position at the time of contraction |
| Recruitment of motor units | The greater the number and synchronization of motor units firing, the greater the force production |
| Frequency of firing of motor units | The higher the frequency of firing, the greater the tension |
| Type of muscle contraction | Force output from greatest to least: eccentric, isometric, concentric muscle contraction |
| Speed of muscle contraction (force-velocity relationship) | Concentric contraction: ↑ speed → ↓ tension. Eccentric contraction: ↑ speed → ↑ tension |

## Fatigue

Fatigue is a complex phenomenon that affects muscle performance and must be considered in a resistance training program. Fatigue has a variety of definitions that are based on the type of fatigue being addressed.

***Muscle (local) fatigue.*** Most relevant to resistance exercise is the phenomenon of skeletal muscle fatigue. Muscle (local) fatigue—the diminished response of muscle to a repeated stimulus—is reflected in a progressive decrement in the amplitude of motor unit potentials.[121,193] This occurs during exercise when a muscle repeatedly contracts statically or dynamically against an imposed load.[61,166]

This *acute* physiological response to exercise is *normal* and *reversible*. It is characterized by a gradual decline in the force-producing capacity of the neuromuscular system, that is, a *temporary* state of exhaustion (failure), leading to a decrease in muscle strength.[54,61,257]

The diminished response of the muscle is caused by a combination of factors, which include:

- Disturbances in the contractile mechanism of the muscle itself because of a decrease in energy stores, insufficient oxygen, and a build-up of $H^+$
- Inhibitory (protective) influences from the central nervous system
- Possibly a decrease in the conduction of impulses at the myoneural junction, particularly in fast-twitch fibers

The fiber-type distribution of a muscle, which can be divided into two broad categories (type I and type II), affects how resistant it is to fatigue.[121,184,193,233] Type II (phasic, fast-twitch) muscle fibers are further divided into two additional classifications (types IIA and IIB) based on contractile and fatigue characteristics. Some resources subdivide type II fibers into three classifications.[240] In general, type II fibers generate a great amount of tension within a short period of time, with type IIB being geared toward anaerobic metabolic activity and having a tendency to fatigue more quickly than type IIA fibers. Type I (tonic, slow-twitch) muscle fibers generate a low level of muscle tension but can sustain the contraction for a long time. These fibers are geared toward aerobic metabolism, as are type IIA fibers. However, type I fibers are more resistant to fatigue than type IIA. Table 6.2 compares the characteristics of muscle fiber types.[121,184,193]

Because different muscles are composed of varying proportions of tonic and phasic fibers, their function becomes specialized. For example, a heavy distribution of type I (tonic) fibers is found in postural muscles, which allows muscles such as the soleus to sustain a low level of tension for extended periods of time to hold the body erect against gravity or stabilize against repetitive loads. On

the other end of the fatigue spectrum, muscles with a large distribution of type IIB (phasic) fibers, such as the gastrocnemius or biceps brachii, produce a great burst of tension to enable a person to lift the entire body weight or to lift, lower, push, or pull a heavy load but fatigue quickly.

Clinical signs of muscular fatigue during exercise are summarized in Box 6.2. When these signs and symptoms develop during resistance exercise, it is time to decrease the load on the exercising muscle or stop the exercise and shift to another muscle group to allow time for the fatigued muscle to rest and recover.

***Cardiopulmonary (general) fatigue.*** This type of fatigue is the diminished response of an individual (the entire body) as the result of prolonged physical activity, such as walking, jogging, cycling, or repetitive lifting or digging. It is related to the body's ability to use oxygen efficiently. Cardiopulmonary fatigue associated with endurance training is probably caused by a combination of the following factors.[22,61,114]

| TABLE 6.2 | Muscle Fiber Types and Resistance to Fatigue | | |
|---|---|---|---|
| **Characteristics** | **Type I** | **Type IIA** | **Type IIB** |
| Resistance to fatigue | High | Intermediate | Low |
| Capillary density | High | High | Low |
| Energy system | Aerobic | Aerobic | Anerobic |
| Diameter | Small | Intermediate | Large |
| Twitch rate | Slow | Fast | Fast |
| Maximum muscle-shortening velocity | Slow | Fast | Fast |

| BOX 6.2 | Signs and Symptoms of Muscle Fatigue |
|---|---|

- An uncomfortable sensation in the muscle, even pain and cramping
- Tremulousness in the contracting muscle
- Active movements jerky, not smooth
- Inability to complete the movement pattern through the full range of available motion during dynamic exercise against the same level of resistance
- Use of substitute motions—that is, incorrect movement patterns—to complete the movement pattern
- Inability to continue low-intensity physical activity
- Decline in peak torque during isokinetic testing

- Decrease in blood sugar (glucose) levels
- Decrease in glycogen stores in muscle and liver
- Depletion of potassium, especially in the elderly patient

***Threshold for fatigue.*** Threshold for fatigue is the level of exercise that cannot be sustained indefinitely.[22] A patient's threshold for fatigue could be noted as the length of time a contraction is maintained or the number of repetitions of an exercise that initially can be performed. This sets a baseline from which adaptive changes in physical performance can be measured.

***Factors that influence fatigue.*** Factors that influence fatigue are diverse. A patient's health status, diet, or lifestyle (sedentary or active) all influence fatigue. In patients with neuromuscular, cardiopulmonary, oncologic, inflammatory, or psychological disorders, the onset of fatigue is often abnormal.[4,54,98] For instance, it may occur abruptly, more rapidly, or at predictable intervals.

It is advisable for a therapist to become familiar with the patterns of fatigue associated with different diseases and medications. In multiple sclerosis, for example, the patient usually awakens rested and functions well during the early morning. By mid-afternoon, however, the patient reaches a peak of fatigue and becomes notably weak. Then by early evening the fatigue diminishes, and strength returns. Patients with cardiac, peripheral vascular, and pulmonary diseases, as well as patients with cancer undergoing chemotherapy or radiation therapy, all have deficits that compromise the oxygen transport system. Therefore, these patients fatigue more readily and require a longer period of time for recovery from exercise.[4,98]

Environmental factors, such as outside or room temperature, air quality, and altitude, also influence how quickly the onset of fatigue occurs and how much time is required for recovery from exercise.[14,169,193]

### Recovery from Exercise
Adequate time for recovery from fatiguing exercise must be built into every resistance training program. This applies to both intrasession and intersession recovery. After vigorous exercise, the body must be given time to restore itself to a state that existed prior to the exhaustive exercise. Recovery from acute exercise, where the force-producing capacity of muscle returns to 90% to 95% of the pre-exercise capacity, usually takes 3 to 4 minutes, with the greatest proportion of recovery occurring in the first minute.[48,61,246]

Changes that occur in muscle during recovery are:

- Oxygen stores are replenished in muscles.
- Energy stores are replenished.

- Lactic acid is removed from skeletal muscle and blood within approximately 1 hour after exercise.
- Glycogen is replaced over several days.

 **Focus on Evidence**

It has been known for some time that if light exercise is performed during the recovery period (*active recovery*), recovery from exercise occurs more rapidly than with total rest (*passive recovery*).[27,48,61,113,246] Faster recovery with light exercise is probably the result of neural as well as circulatory influences.[48,61,246]

PRECAUTIONS: Only if a patient is allowed adequate time to recover from fatigue after each exercise session does long-term muscle performance (strength, power, or endurance) improve.[27,113] If a sufficient rest interval is not a recurring component of a resistance exercise program, a patient's performance plateaus or deteriorates. Evidence of overtraining or overwork weakness may become apparent (see additional discussion in a later section of this chapter). It has also been shown that fatigued muscles are more susceptible to acute strains.[191]

### Age
Muscle performance changes throughout the life span. Whether the goal of a resistance training program is to remediate impairments and functional limitations or enhance fitness and performance of physical activities, an understanding of "typical" changes in muscle performance and response to exercise during each phase of life from early childhood through the advanced years of life is necessary to prescribe effective, safe resistance exercises for individuals of all ages. Key aspects of how muscle performance changes throughout life are discussed in this section and summarized in Box 6.3.

#### Early Childhood and Preadolescence
In absolute terms, muscle performance (specifically strength), which in part is related to the development of muscle mass, increases *linearly* with chronological age in both boys and girls from birth through early and middle childhood to puberty.[192,265,298] Muscle endurance also increases linearly during the childhood years.[298] Muscle fiber number is essentially determined prior to or shortly after birth,[242] although there is speculation that fiber number may continue to increase into early childhood.[298] The rate of fiber growth (increase in cross-sectional area) is relatively consistent from birth to puberty. Change in fiber type distribution is relatively complete by the age of 1, shifting from a predominance of type II fibers to

---

**BOX 6.3    Summary of Age-Related Changes in Muscle and Muscle Performance**

Infancy, Early Childhood, and Preadolescence
- At birth, muscle accounts for about 25% of body weight.
- Total number of muscle fibers is established prior to or early during infancy.
- Postnatal changes in distribution of type I and type II fibers in muscle are relatively complete by the end of the first year of life.
- Muscle fiber size and muscle mass increase linearly from infancy to puberty.
- Muscle strength and muscle endurance increase linearly with chronological age in boys and girls throughout childhood until puberty.
- Muscle mass (absolute and relative) and muscle strength is just slightly greater (approximately 10%) in boys than girls from early childhood to puberty.
- Training-induced strength gains occur equally in both sexes during childhood without evidence of hypertrophy until puberty.

Puberty
- Rapid acceleration in muscle fiber size and muscle mass, especially in boys. During puberty, muscle mass increases more than 30% per year.
- Rapid increase in muscle strength in both sexes.
- Marked difference in strength levels develops in boys and girls.
- In boys, muscle mass and body height and weight peak before muscle strength; in girls, strength peaks before body weight.
- Relative strength gains as the result of resistance training are comparable between the sexes, with significantly greater muscle hypertrophy in boys.

Young and Middle Adulthood
- Muscle mass peaks in women between 16 and 20 years of age; muscle mass in men peaks between 18 and 25 years of age.
- Decreases in muscle mass occur as early as 25 years of age.
- Muscle mass constitutes approximately 40% of total body weight during early adulthood, with men having slightly more muscle mass than women.

- Strength continues to develop into the second decade, especially in men.
- Muscle strength and endurance reach a peak during the second decade, earlier for women than men.
- By sometime in the third decade, strength declines between 8% and 10% per decade through the fifth or sixth decade.
- Strength and muscle endurance deteriorate less rapidly in physically active versus sedentary adults.
- Improvements in strength and endurance are possible with only a modest increase in physical activity.

Late Adulthood
- Rate of decline of muscle strength accelerates to 15% to 20% per decade during the sixth and seventh decades and increases to 30% per decade thereafter.
- Loss of muscle mass continues; by the eighth decade, skeletal muscle mass has decreased by 50% compared to peak muscle mass during young adulthood.
- Muscle fiber size (cross-sectional area), type I and type II fiber numbers, and the number of alpha motoneurons all decrease. Preferential atrophy of type II muscle fibers occurs.
- Decrease in the speed of muscle contractions and peak power.
- Gradual but progressive decrease in endurance and maximum oxygen uptake.
- Loss of flexibility reduces the force-producing capacity of muscle.
- Minimal decline in performance of functional skills during the sixth decade.
- Significant deterioration in functional abilities by the eighth decade associated with a decline in muscular endurance.
- With a resistance training program, a significant improvement in muscle strength, power, and endurance is possible during late adulthood.
- Evidence of the impact of resistance training on the level of performance of functional motor skills is mixed but promising.

---

a more balanced distribution of type I and type II fibers.[298]

Throughout childhood, boys have slightly greater absolute and relative muscle mass (kilograms of muscle per kilogram of body weight) than girls, with boys approximately 10% stronger than girls from early childhood to puberty.[192] This difference may be associated with differences in relative muscle mass, although social expectations, especially by mid-childhood, also may contribute to the observed difference in muscle strength.

There is no question that an appropriately designed resistance exercise program can improve muscle strength in children above and beyond gains attributable to typical growth and development. A review of the literature[91] cited many studies that support this statement. However, there is concern that children who participate in resistance training may be at risk for injuries, such as an epiphyseal fracture or avulsion fracture, because the musculoskeletal system is immature.[26,103,107,271] The American Academy of Pediatrics[6] and the American College of Sports Medicine[314] support youth participation in resistance training programs if they are designed appropriately and carefully supervised (Fig. 6.1). With this in mind, two important questions need to be addressed: (1) At what point during childhood is a resistance training program appropriate? (2) What constitutes a safe training program?

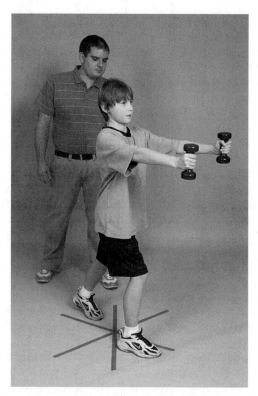

FIGURE 6.1 Resistance training, if initiated during the preadolescent years, should be performed using body weight or light weights and carefully supervised.

There is general consensus that during the toddler, preschool, and even the early elementary school years, free play and organized but age-appropriate physical activities are effective methods to promote fitness and improve muscle performance, rather than structured resistance training programs. The emphasis throughout most or all of the first decade of life should be on recreation and learning motor skills.[283]

However, there is lack of agreement on when and under what circumstances resistance training is an appropriate form of exercise. During the past two decades it has become popular for older (preadolescent) boys and girls to participate in resistance training programs, in theory, to enhance athletic performance and reduce the risk of sport-related injury. In addition, prepubescent children who sustain injuries during everyday activities may require rehabilitation that may include resistance exercises. Consequently, an understanding of the effects of exercise in this age group founded on current research must be the basis for establishing a safe program with realistic goals.

### ⦿ Focus on Evidence_____

In the preadolescent age group many studies have shown that improvements in strength and muscular endurance occur on a relative basis similar to training-induced gains in young adults.[26,92,93,148] It is also important to point out that, although only a few studies have looked at the effects of detraining in children, when training ceases strength levels gradually return to a pretraining level, as occurs in adults.[90] This suggests that some maintenance level of training could be useful in children as with adults.[91]

In addition, although evidence to suggest that a structured resistance training program for children (in addition to a general sports conditioning program) reduces injuries or enhances sports performance is inconclusive,[6] other health-related benefits have been noted, including increased cardiopulmonary fitness, decreased blood lipids levels, and improved psychological well-being.[26,90,148] These findings suggest that participation in a resistance training program during the later childhood (preadolescent) years may, indeed, be of value if the program is performed at an appropriate level (low loads and repetitions) and is closely supervised.[6,271]

### Adolescence

At puberty, as hormonal levels change, there is rapid acceleration in the development of muscle strength, especially in boys. During this phase of development, typical strength levels become markedly different in boys and girls, which in part are caused by hormonal differences between the sexes. Longitudinal studies[33,192] of adolescent boys indicate that strength increases about 30% per year between ages 10 and 16, with muscle mass peaking before muscle strength. In adolescent girls, peak strength develops before peak weight.[95] Overall, during the adolescent years, muscle mass increases more than 5-fold in boys and approximately 3.5-fold in girls.[33,192] Although most longitudinal studies of growth stop at age 18, strength continues to develop, particularly in males, well into the second and even into the third decade of life.[292]

As with prepubescent children, resistance training during puberty also results in significant strength gains. During puberty these gains average 30% to 40% above that which is expected as the result of normal growth and maturation.[91] Benefits of strength training noted during puberty are similar to those noted in prepubescent children.[90,93]

### Young and Middle Adulthood

Although data on typical strength and endurance levels during the second through the fifth decades of life are more often from studies of men than women, a few generalizations can be made that seem to apply to both sexes.[186] Strength reaches a maximal level earlier in women than men, with women reaching a peak during the second decade and in most men by age 30. Strength then declines approximately 1% per year,[298] or 8% per decade.[109] This decline in strength appears to be minor until about age 50[283] and tends to occur at a later age or slower rate in active adults versus those who are sedentary.[111,298] The potential for improving muscle performance with a resistance training program (Fig. 6.2 A&B) or by participation in even moderately demanding activities several times a week is high during this phase of life. Guidelines for young and middle-aged adults participating in resistance training have been published by the American College of Sports Medicine (ACSM).[8]

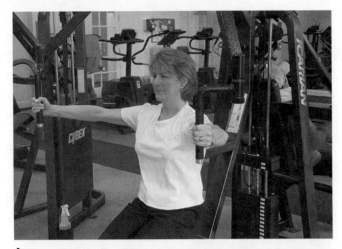

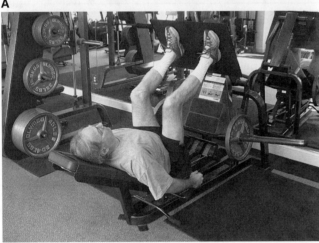

FIGURE 6.2 Conditioning and fitness programs for active young and middle-age adults include resistance training with a balance of (A) upper extremity and (B) lower extremity strengthening exercises.

## Late Adulthood

The rate of decline in the tension-generating capacity of muscle in most cases accelerates to approximately 15% to 20% per decade in men and women in their sixties and seventies, and it increases to 30% per decade thereafter.[111,186] However, the rate of decline may be significantly less (only 0.3% decrease per year) in elderly men and women who maintain a high level of physical activity.[119] These disparate findings and others suggest that loss of muscle strength during the advanced years may be due, in part, to progressively greater inactivity and disuse.[35] Loss of muscle strength during late adulthood, particularly during the eighties and beyond, is associated with a gradual increase in functional limitations as well as an increase in the frequency of falling.[35]

The decline in muscle strength and endurance in the elderly is associated with many factors in addition to progressive disuse and inactivity. It is difficult to determine if these factors are causes or effects of age-related deterioration in strength. Neuromuscular factors include a decrease in muscle mass (atrophy), decrease in the number of type I and II muscle fibers with a corresponding increase in con-

nective tissue in muscle, a decrease in the cross-sectional size of muscle, selective atrophy of type II fibers, and change in the length–tension relationship of muscle associated with loss of flexibility, more so than deficits in motor unit activation and firing rate.[35,109,141,240,276,283,304] The decline in the number of motor units appears to begin after age 60.[141] All of these changes have an impact on strength and physical performance.

In addition to decreases in muscle strength, declines in speed of muscle contraction, muscle endurance, and the ability to recover from muscular fatigue occur with advanced age.[141,276] The time needed to produce the same absolute and relative levels of torque output and the time necessary to achieve relaxation after a voluntary contraction are lengthened in the elderly compared to younger adults.[109] Consequently, as velocity of movement declines, so does the ability to generate muscle power during activities that require quick responses, such as rising from a low chair or adjusting one's balance to prevent a fall.

Information on changes in muscle endurance with aging is limited. There is some evidence to suggest that the ability to sustain low-intensity muscular effort also declines with age, in part because of reduced blood supply and capillary density in muscle, decreased mitochondrial density, changes in enzymatic activity level, and decreased glucose transport.[109] As a result, muscle fatigue may tend to occur more readily in the elderly. In the healthy and active (community-dwelling) elderly population, the decline in muscle endurance appears to be minimal well into the seventies.[141]

During the past few decades, as the health care community and the public have become more aware of the benefits of resistance training during late adulthood, more and more older adults are participating in fitness programs that include resistance exercises (Fig. 6.3). ACSM has also pub-

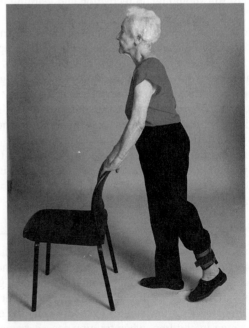

FIGURE 6.3 Incorporating resistance training into a fitness program has many benefits for older adults.

lished guidelines for resistance training for healthy adults over 60 to 65 years of age.[8]

 **Focus on Evidence**_____

A review of the literature indicates that when healthy or frail elderly individuals participate in a resistance training program of appropriate duration and intensity, muscle strength and endurance increase.* Some of these studies have also measured pretraining and post-training levels of functional abilities, such as balance, stair climbing, walking speed, and chair rise. The effect of strength and endurance training on functional abilities is promising but still inconclusive, with most but not all[35] investigations demonstrating a positive impact.[3,36,43,97,145,179,226,270] This disparity of outcomes among investigations underscores the point that resistance training has a direct impact on muscle performance but only an indirect impact on functional performance, a more complex variable. Studies of elderly individuals have also shown that if resistance training is discontinued, detraining gradually occurs; and subsequently strength and functional capabilities deteriorate close to pretraining levels.[42,179] In summary, evidence indicates that the decline in muscle strength and functional abilities that occurs during late adulthood can be slowed or at least partially reversed with a resistance training program. However, as in other age groups, if these training-induced improvements are to be maintained, some degree of resistance training must be continued.[304]

---

### Psychological and Cognitive Factors

An array of psychological factors can positively or negatively influence muscle performance and how easily, vigorously, or cautiously a person moves. Just as injury and disease adversely affect muscle performance, so can one's mental status. For example, fear of pain, injury, or reinjury, depression related to physical illness, or impaired attention or memory as the result of age, head injury, or the side effects of medication can adversely affect the ability to develop or sustain sufficient muscle tension for execution or acquisition of functional motor tasks. In contrast, psychological factors can also positively influence physical performance.

The principles and methods employed to maximize motor performance and learning as functions of effective patient education are discussed in Chapter 1. These principles and methods should be applied in a resistance training program to develop a requisite level of muscle strength, power, and endurance for functional activities. The following interrelated psychological factors as well as other aspects of motor learning may influence muscle performance and the effectiveness of a resistance training program.

#### Attention

A patient must be able to focus on a given task (exercise) to learn how to perform it correctly. Attention involves the ability to process relevant data while screening out irrele-

vant information from the environment and to respond to internal cues from the body. Both are necessary when first learning an exercise and later when carrying out an exercise program independently. Attention to form and technique during resistance training is necessary for patient safety and optimal long-term training effects.

#### Motivation and Feedback

If a resistance exercise program is to be effective, a patient must be willing to put forth and maintain sufficient effort and adhere to an exercise program over time to improve muscle performance for functional activities. Use of activities that are meaningful and are perceived as having potential usefulness or periodically modifying an exercise routine help maintain a patient's interest in resistance training. Charting or graphing a patient's strength gains, for example, also helps sustain motivation. Incorporating gains in muscle performance into functional activities as early as possible in a resistance exercise program puts improvements in strength to practical use, thereby making those improvements meaningful.

The importance of feedback for learning an exercise or a motor skill is discussed in Chapter 1. In addition, feedback can have a positive impact on a patient's motivation and subsequent adherence to an exercise program. For example, some computerized equipment, such as isokinetic dynamometers, provide visual or auditory signals that let the patient know if each muscle contraction during a particular exercise is in a zone that causes a training effect. Documenting improvements over time, such as the amount of weight (exercise load) used during various exercises or changes in walking distance or speed, also provides positive feedback to sustain a patient's motivation in a resistance exercise program.

## Physiological Adaptations to Resistance Exercise

The use of resistance exercise in rehabilitation and conditioning programs has a substantial impact on all systems of the body. Resistance training is equally important for patients with impaired muscle performance and individuals who wish to improve or maintain their level of fitness, enhance performance, or reduce the risk of injury. When body systems are exposed to a greater than usual but appropriate level of resistance in an exercise program, they initially react with a number of *acute* physiological responses[166] and then later adapt. That is, body systems accommodate over time to the newly imposed physical demands.[8,121,172,193] Training-induced adaptations to resistance exercise, known as *chronic* physiological responses, that affect muscle performance are summarized in Table 6.3 and discussed in this section. Key differences in adaptations from strength training versus endurance training are noted.

Adaptations to overload create changes in muscle performance and, in part, determine the effectiveness of a resistance training program. The time course for these adaptations to occur varies from one individual to another

---

* See references 35, 36, 43, 120, 145, 179, 203, 213, 248, 267, 270, 304

| TABLE 6.3 | Physiological Adaptations to Resistance Exercise | |
|---|---|---|
| **Variable** | **Strength Training Adaptations** | **Endurance Training Adaptations** |
| Skeletal muscle structure | Hypertrophy of muscle fibers; greater in type II fibers<br>Hyperplasia (possibly) of muscle fibers<br>Fiber type composition: remodeling of type IIB to type IIA; no change in type I to type II distribution (i.e., no conversion)<br>Capillary bed density: ↓ or no change<br>Mitochondrial density and volume: ↓ | Hypertrophy: minimal or no change<br><br><br><br><br>Capillary bed density: ↑<br>Mitochondrial density and volume: ↑ |
| Neural system | Motor unit recruitment: ↑ # motor units firing<br>Rate of firing: ↑ (↓ twitch contraction time)<br>Synchronization of firing: ↑ | |
| Metabolic system | ATP and CP storage: ↑<br>Myoglobin storage: ↑<br>Stored triglycerides: not known | ATP and CP storage: ↑<br>Myoglobin storage: ↑<br>Stored triglycerides: ↑ |
| Enzymes | Creatine phosphokinase: ↑<br>Myokinase: ↑ | Similar ↑<br>Similar ↑ |
| Body composition | Lean body (fat-free) mass: ↑ % body fat: ↓ | Lean body (fat-free) mass: no change % body fat: ↓ |
| Connective tissue | Tensile strength of tendons, ligaments, and connective tissue in muscle: ↑<br>Bone: ↑ bone mineral density; no change or possible ↑ in bone mass | Tensile strength of tendons, ligaments, and connective tissue in muscle: ↑<br>Bone: ↑ mineralization with weight-bearing activities |

and is dependent on a person's health status and previous level of participation in a resistance exercise program.[9]

## Neural Adaptations

It is well accepted that in a resistance training program the initial, rapid gain in the tension-generating capacity of skeletal muscle is largely attributed to neural responses, not adaptive changes in muscle itself.[204,234,235] This is reflected by an increase in electromyographic (EMG) activity during the first 4 to 8 weeks of training with little to no evidence of muscle fiber hypertrophy. It is also possible that increased neural activity is the source of additional gains in strength late in a resistance training program even after muscle hypertrophy has reached a plateau.[193]

Neural adaptations are attributed to motor learning and improved coordination[168,169,172,193] and include *increased recruitment* in the number of motor units firing as well as an *increased rate and synchronization* of firing.[168,224,234,235] It is speculated that these changes are caused by a decrease in the inhibitory function of the central nervous system (CNS), decreased sensitivity of the Golgi tendon organ (GTO), or changes at the myoneural junction of the motor unit.[172,234,235]

## Skeletal Muscle Adaptations

### Hypertrophy

As noted previously, the tension-producing capacity of muscle is directly related to the physiological cross-sectional area of the individual muscle fibers. *Hypertrophy* is an increase in the size (bulk) of an individual muscle fiber caused by an increase in myofibrillar volume.[207,276]

After an extended period of moderate- to high-intensity resistance training, usually by 4 to 8 weeks[1,172,295] but possibly as early as 2 to 3 weeks with very high-intensity resistance training,[259] hypertrophy becomes an increasingly important adaptation that accounts for strength gains in muscle.

Although the mechanism of hypertrophy is complex and the stimulus for growth is not clearly understood, hypertrophy of skeletal muscle appears to be the result of an increase in protein (actin and myosin) synthesis and a decrease in protein degradation. Hypertrophy is also associated with biochemical changes that stimulate uptake of amino acids.[168,193,207,276]

The greatest increases in protein synthesis and therefore hypertrophy are associated with high-volume, moderate-resistance exercise performed eccentrically.[168] In addition, it is the type IIB muscle fibers that appear to increase in size most readily with resistance training.[172,193]

### Hyperplasia

Although the topic has been debated for many years and evidence of the phenomenon is sparse, there is some thought that a portion of the increase in muscle size that occurs with heavy resistance training is caused by *hyperplasia*, an increase in the *number* of muscle fibers. It has been suggested that this increase in fiber number, observed in laboratory animals,[116,117] is the result of longitudinal splitting of fibers.[12,140,198] It has been postulated that fiber splitting occurs when individual muscle fibers increase in size to a point where they are inefficient, then subsequently split to form two distinct fibers.[116]

Critics of the concept of hyperplasia suggest that evidence of fiber splitting may actually be caused by inappropriate tissue preparation in the laboratory.[115] The general opinion in the literature is that hyperplasia either does not occur; or if it does occur to a slight degree, its impact is insignificant.[189] In a recent review article it was the authors' opinion that if hyperplasia is a valid finding, it probably accounts for a very small proportion (less than 5%) of the increase in muscle size that occurs with resistance training.[169]

### Muscle Fiber Type Adaptation

As previously mentioned, type II (phasic) muscle fibers preferentially hypertrophy with heavy resistance training. In addition, a substantial degree of plasticity exists in muscle fibers with respect to contractile and metabolic properties.[240] Transformation of type IIB to type IIA is common with endurance training,[240] as well as during the early weeks of heavy resistance training,[259] making the type II fibers more fatigue-resistant. There is some evidence that demonstrates type I to type II fiber type conversion in the denervated limbs of laboratory animals,[216,311] in humans with spinal cord injury, and after an extended period of weightlessness associated with space flight.[240] However, there is little to no evidence of type II to type I conversion under training conditions in rehabilitation or fitness programs.[193,240]

### Vascular and Metabolic Adaptations

Adaptations of the cardiovascular and respiratory systems as the result of low-intensity, high-volume resistance training are discussed in Chapter 7. Opposite to what occurs with endurance training, when muscles hypertrophy with high-intensity, low-volume training, capillary bed density actually decreases because of an increase in the number of myofilaments per fiber.[172] Athletes who participate in heavy resistance training actually have fewer capillaries per muscle fiber than endurance athletes and even untrained individuals.[154,274] Other changes associated with metabolism, such as a decrease in mitochondrial density, also occur with high-intensity resistance training.[168,172] This is associated with reduced oxidative capacity of muscle.

### Adaptations of Connective Tissues

Although the evidence is limited, it appears that the tensile strength of tendons and ligaments as well as bone increases with resistance training designed to improve the strength or power of muscles.[45,263,286,312]

### Tendons, Ligaments, and Connective Tissue in Muscle

Strength improvement in tendons probably occurs at the musculotendinous junction, whereas increased ligament strength may occur at the ligament–bone interface. It is believed that tendon and ligament tensile strength increases in response to resistance training to support the adaptive strength and size changes in muscle.[312] The connective tissue in muscle (around muscle fibers) also thickens, giving more support to the enlarged fibers.[193] Consequently, strong ligaments and tendons may be less prone to injury.

It is also thought that noncontractile soft tissue strength may develop more rapidly with eccentric resistance training than with other types of resistance exercises.[262,263]

### Bone

Numerous sources indicate there is a high correlation between muscle strength and the level of physical activity across the life span with bone mineral density.[239,243] Consequently, physical activities and exercises, particularly those performed in weight-bearing positions, are typically recommended to minimize or prevent age-related bone loss.[225] They are also prescribed to reduce the risk of fractures or improve bone density when osteopenia or osteoporosis is already present.[52,112,239]

 **Focus on Evidence**

Although the evidence from prospective studies is limited and mixed, resistance exercises performed with adequate intensity and with site-specific loading through weight bearing of the bony area to be tested has been shown to increase or maintain bone mineral density.[156,160,175,197,210] In contrast, a number of studies in young, healthy women[230] and postmenopausal women[227,247] have reported that there was no significant increase in bone mineral density with resistance training. However, the resistance exercises in these studies were not combined with site-specific weight bearing. In addition, the intensity of the weight training programs may not have been high enough to have an impact on bone density.[175,239] The time course of the exercise program also may not have been long enough. It has been suggested that it may take as long as 9 months to a year of exercise for detectable and significant increases in bone mass to occur.[243] In the spine, although studies to date have not shown that resistance training prevents spinal fractures, there is some evidence to suggest that the strength of the back extensors closely correlates with bone mineral density of the spine.[247]

---

Research continues to determine the most effective forms of exercise to enhance bone density and prevent age-related bone loss and fractures. For additional information on prevention and management of osteoporosis, refer to Chapter 11.

##  DETERMINANTS OF RESISTANCE EXERCISE

Many elements (variables) determine whether a resistance exercise program is appropriate, effective, and safe. This holds true when resistance training is a part of a rehabilitation program for individuals with known or potential impairments in muscle performance or when it is incorporated into a general conditioning program to improve the level of fitness of healthy individuals.

Each of the interrelated elements discussed in this section should be addressed to improve one or more aspects of

BOX 6.4 | Determinants of a Resistance Exercise Program

- *Alignment* of segments of the body during exercise
- *Stabilization* of proximal or distal joints to prevent substitution
- *Intensity:* the exercise load (level of resistance)
- *Volume:* the total number of repetitions and sets in an exercise session multiplied by the resistance used
- *Exercise order:* the sequence in which muscle groups are exercised during an exercise session
- *Frequency:* the number of exercise sessions per day or per week
- *Rest interval:* time allotted for recuperation between sets and sessions of exercise
- *Duration:* total time frame of a resistance training program
- *Mode* of exercise: type of muscle contraction, position of the patient, form (source) of resistance, arc of movement, or the primary energy system utilized
- *Velocity* of exercise
- *Periodization:* variation of intensity and volume during specific periods of resistance training
- *Integration of exercises into functional activities:* use of resistance exercises that approximate or replicate functional demands

muscle performance and achieve desired functional outcomes. Appropriate *alignment* and *stabilization* are always basic elements of any exercise designed to improve muscle performance. A suitable *dosage* of exercise must also be determined. In resistance training, dosage includes *intensity, volume, frequency,* and *duration* of exercise and *rest interval.* Each factor is a mechanism by which the muscle can be progressively overloaded to improve muscle performance. The *velocity* of exercise and the *mode* of exercise must also be considered. These elements are summarized in Box 6.4.

Consistent with the SAID principle discussed in the first section of this chapter, these elements of resistance exercise must be specific to the patient's desired functional goals. Other factors, such as the underlying cause or causes of the deficits in muscle performance, the extent of impairment, and the patient's age, medical history, mental status, and social situation also affect the design and implementation of a resistance exercise program.

## Alignment and Stabilization

Just as correct alignment and effective stabilization are basic elements of manual muscle testing and dynamometry, they are also crucial in resistance exercise. To strengthen a specific muscle or muscle group effectively and avoid substitute motions, appropriate positioning of the body and alignment of a limb or body segment are essential. *Substitute motions* are compensatory movement patterns caused by muscle action of a stronger adjacent agonist or a muscle

group that normally serves as a stabilizer (fixator).[158] If the principles of alignment and stabilization for manual muscle testing[137,158] are applied whenever possible during resistance exercise, substitute motions can usually be avoided.

### Alignment

***Alignment and muscle action.*** Proper alignment is determined by the direction of muscle fibers and the line of pull of the muscle to be strengthened. The patient or a body segment must be positioned so the direction of movement of a limb or segment of the body replicates the action of the muscle or muscle groups to be strengthened. For example, to strengthen the gluteus medius, the hip must remain slightly extended, not flexed; and the pelvis must be rotated slightly forward as the patient abducts the lower extremity against the applied resistance. If the hip is flexed as the leg abducts, the adjacent tensor fasciae latae becomes the prime mover and is strengthened.

***Alignment and gravity.*** The alignment or position of the patient or the limb with respect to gravity may also be important during some forms of resistance exercises, particularly if body weight or free weights (dumbbells, barbells, cuff weights) are the source of resistance. The patient or limb should be positioned so the muscle being strengthened acts against the resistance of gravity and the weight. This, of course, is contingent on the comfort and mobility of the patient.

Staying with the example of strengthening the gluteus medius, if a cuff weight is placed around the lower leg, the patient must assume the side-lying position so abduction occurs through the full ROM against gravity and the additional resistance of the cuff weight. If the patient rolls toward the supine position, the resistance force is applied primarily to the hip flexors, not the abductors.

### Stabilization

Stabilization refers to holding down a body segment or holding the body steady.[158] To maintain appropriate alignment, ensure the correct muscle action and movement pattern, and avoid unwanted substitute motions during resistance exercise, effective stabilization is imperative. Exercising on a *stable surface,* such as a firm treatment table, helps hold the body steady. *Body weight* may also provide a source of stability during exercise, particularly in the horizontal position. It is most common to stabilize the proximal attachment of the muscle being strengthened, but sometimes the distal attachment is stabilized as the muscle contracts.

Stabilization can be achieved externally or internally.

- *External stabilization* can be applied manually by the therapist or sometimes by the patient with equipment, such as belts and straps, or by a firm support surface, such as the back of a chair or the surface of the treatment table.
- *Internal stabilization* is achieved by an isometric contraction of an adjacent muscle group that does not enter into the movement pattern but holds the body segment of the proximal attachment of the muscle being strength-

ened firmly in place. For example, when performing a bilateral straight leg raise, the abdominals contract to stabilize the pelvis and lumbar spine as the hip flexors raise the legs. This form of stabilization is effective only if the fixating muscle group is strong enough or not fatigued.

## Intensity

The *intensity* of exercise in a resistance training program is the amount of resistance (weight) imposed on the contracting muscle during each repetition of an exercise. The amount of resistance is also referred to as the *exercise load* (training load), that is, the extent to which the muscle is loaded or how much weight is lifted, lowered, or held.

Remember, consistent with the overload principle, to improve muscle performance the muscle must be loaded to an extent greater than loads usually incurred. One way to overload a muscle progressively is to gradually increase the amount of resistance used in the exercise program.[9,103,169] The intensity of exercise and the degree to which the muscle is overloaded is also dependent on the volume, frequency, and order of exercise or the length of rest intervals.

### Submaximal Versus Maximal Exercise Loads

Many factors, including the goals and expected functional outcomes of the exercise program, the cause of deficits in muscle performance, the extent of impairment, the stage of healing of injured tissues, the patient's age, general health, and fitness level, and other factors determine whether the exercise is carried out against submaximal or maximal muscle loading. In general, the level of resistance is often lower in rehabilitation programs for persons with impairments than in conditioning programs for healthy individuals.

***Submaximal loading.*** Exercise at moderate to low intensities is indicated:

- At the beginning of an exercise program to evaluate the patient's response to resistance exercise, especially after extended periods of inactivity
- In the early stages of soft tissue healing when injured tissues must be protected
- After periods of immobilization when the articular cartilage is not able to withstand large compressive forces or when bone demineralization may have occurred, increasing the risk of pathological fracture
- For most children or older adults
- When the goal of exercise is to improve muscle endurance
- To warm up and cool down prior to and after a session of exercise
- During slow-velocity isokinetic training to minimize compressive forces on joints

***Near maximal or maximal loading.*** High-intensity exercise is indicated:

- When the goal of exercise is to increase muscle strength and power and possibly increase muscle size

- For otherwise healthy adults in the *advanced phase* of a *rehabilitation* program after a musculoskeletal injury in preparation for returning to high-demand occupational or recreational activities
- In a conditioning program for individuals with no known pathology
- For individuals training for competitive weight lifting or body building

PRECAUTION: The intensity of exercise should never be so great as to cause pain. As the intensity of exercise increases and a patient exerts a maximum or near-maximum effort, cardiovascular risks substantially increase. A patient needs to be continually reminded to incorporate rhythmic breathing into each repetition of an exercise to minimize these risks.

### Initial Level of Resistance (Load) and Documentation of Training Effects

It is always challenging to estimate how much resistance to apply manually or how much weight a patient should use during resistance exercises to improve muscle strength particularly at the beginning of a strengthening program. With manual resistance exercise the decision is entirely subjective, based on the therapist's judgment during exercise. In an exercise program using mechanical resistance the determination can be made quantitatively.

**Repetition Maximum**

One method of measuring the effectiveness of a resistance exercise program and calculating an appropriate exercise load for training is to determine a repetition maximum. This term was first reported decades ago by DeLorme in his investigations of an approach to resistance training called progressive resistive exercise (PRE).[63-65] A *repetition maximum* (RM) is defined as the greatest amount of weight (load) a muscle can move through the available range of motion (ROM) a specific number of times.

***Use of a repetition maximum.*** There are two main reasons for determining a repetition maximum: (1) to document a baseline measurement of the dynamic strength of a muscle or muscle group against which exercise-induced improvements in strength can be compared and (2) to identify an exercise load (amount of weight) to be used during exercise for a specified number of repetitions. DeLorme reported use of a 1 RM (the greatest amount of weight a subject can lift through the available ROM just one time) as the baseline measurement of a subject's maximum effort but used a 10 RM (the amount of weight that could be lifted and lowered exactly 10 times) during training.[64,65]

In the clinical setting, a practical, time-saving way to establish a baseline RM for a particular muscle group is for a therapist to select a specific amount of resistance (weight) and document how many repetitions can be completed through the full range before the muscle begins to fatigue. Remember, a sign of fatigue is the inability to complete the available ROM against the applied resistance.

Despite criticism that establishing a 1 RM involves some trial and error, it is a frequently used method for

| BOX 6.5 | Percentage of Body Weight as an Initial Exercise Load |
|---|---|

- Universal bench press: 30% body weight
- Universal leg extension: 20% body weight
- Universal leg curl: 10% to 15% body weight
- Universal leg press: 50% body weight

measuring muscle strength in research studies and has been shown to be a safe and reliable measurement tool with healthy young adults and athletes[103,169] as well as active older adults prior to beginning conditioning programs.[203,213,270,281]

PRECAUTION: Use of a 1 RM as a baseline measurement of dynamic strength is inappropriate for some patient populations because it requires one maximum effort. It is not safe for patients, for example, with joint impairments, patients who are recovering from or who are at risk for soft tissue injury, or patients with known or at risk for osteoporosis or cardiovascular pathology.

**Alternative Methods of Determining Baseline Strength and a Beginning Exercise Load**
Cable tensiometry[193] and isokinetic or handheld dynamometry[55] are alternatives to a repetition maximum for establishing a baseline measurement of strength. A percentage of body weight also has been proposed to estimate how much resistance (load) should be used in a strengthening program.[236] Some examples for different exercises are listed in Box 6.5. The percentages indicated are meant as guidelines for the advanced stage of rehabilitation and are based on 10 repetitions of each exercise at the beginning of an exercise program. Percentages vary for different muscle groups.

**Training Zone**
After establishing the baseline RM, the amount of resistance (exercise load) to be used at the initiation of resistance training is often calculated as a *percentage* of a 1 RM for a particular muscle group. At the beginning of an exercise program the percentage necessary to achieve training-induced adaptations in strength is low (30% to 40%) for sedentary, untrained individuals or very high (80% to 95%) for those already highly trained. For healthy but untrained adults, a typical training zone usually falls between 60% and 70% of an RM.[9] The lower percentage of this range is safer at the beginning of a program to enable an individual to focus on learning exercise form and technique.

Exercising at a low to moderate percentage of the established RM is also recommended for children and the elderly.[8,286] For patients with significant deficits in muscle strength or to train for muscular endurance, using a low load, possibly at the 30% to 50% level, is safe yet challenging.

## Volume

In resistance training the *volume* of exercise is the summation of the total number of repetitions and sets of a particular exercise during a single exercise session multiplied by the resistance used.[9,169] The same combination of repetitions and sets is not and should not be used for all muscle groups.

There is an inverse relationship between the number of repetitions performed and the intensity of the resistance. The higher the intensity (load), the lower the number of repetitions that are possible; and conversely, the lower the load, the greater the number of repetitions possible. Therefore, the exercise load directly dictates how many repetitions and sets are possible.

### Repetitions and Sets

*Repetitions.* The number of *repetitions* in a dynamic exercise program refers to the number of times a particular movement is repeated. More specifically, it is the number of muscle contractions performed to move the limb through a series of continuous and complete excursions against a specific exercise load.

If the RM designation is used, the number of repetitions at a specific exercise load is reflected in the designation. For example, 10 repetitions at a particular exercise load is a 10 RM. If a 1 RM has been established as a baseline level of strength, a percentage of the 1 RM used as the exercise load influences the number of repetitions a patient is able to perform. The "average," untrained adult, when exercising with a load that is equivalent to 75% of the 1 RM, is able to complete approximately 10 repetitions before needing to rest.[16,193] At 60% intensity about 15 repetitions are possible, and at 90% intensity only 4 or 5 repetitions are usually possible.

For practical reasons, after a beginning exercise load is selected, the target number of repetitions performed for each exercise before a brief rest is often within a range rather than an exact number of repetitions. For example, a patient might be able to complete between 8 and 10 repetitions against a specified load before resting. This is sometimes referred to as a *RM zone*[193]; it gives the patient a goal but builds in some flexibility.

The number of repetitions selected depends on the patient's status and whether the goal of the exercise is to improve muscle strength or endurance. No optimal number for strength training or endurance training has been identified. Training effects (greater strength) have been reported employing 2 to 3 RM to 15 RM.[16,170]

*Sets.* A predetermined number of repetitions grouped together is known as a set or bout. After each set of a specified number of repetitions, there is a brief interval of rest. For example, during a single exercise session to strengthen a particular muscle group, a patient might be directed to lift a load 8 to 10 times, rest, and then lift the load 8 to 10 more times. That would be two sets of an 8 to 10 RM

As with repetitions, there is no optimal number of sets per exercise session. As few as one set and as many as six sets have yielded positive training effects.[9] Single-set exercises at low intensities are most common in the very early phases of a resistance exercise program or in a maintenance program. Multiple-set exercises are used to progress the program and have been shown to be superior to single-set regimens in advanced training.[170]

### Training to Improve Strength or Endurance: Impact of Exercise Load and Repetitions

Overall, because many variations of intensity and volume cause positive training-induced adaptations in muscle performance, there is a substantial amount of latitude for selecting an exercise load/repetition and set scheme for each exercise. The question is: Is the goal to improve strength, muscular endurance, or both?

#### To Improve Muscle Strength

In DeLorme's early studies[63-65] three sets of a 10 RM performed for 10 repetitions over the training period led to gains in strength. Current recommendations are to use an exercise load that causes fatigue after 6 to 12 repetitions for two to three sets (6 to 12 RM).[103] When fatigue no longer occurs after the target number of repetitions has been completed, the level of resistance is increased to once again overload the muscle.

#### To Improve Muscle Endurance

Training to improve local endurance involves performing many repetitions of an exercise against a submaximal load.[32,264] For example, as many as three to five sets of 40 to 50 or more repetitions against a low amount of weight or a light grade of elastic resistance might be used. When increasing the number of repetitions or sets becomes inefficient, the load can be increased slightly.

Endurance training can also be accomplished by maintaining an isometric muscle contraction for incrementally longer periods of time. Because endurance training is performed against very low levels of resistance, it can and should be initiated very early in a rehabilitation program without risk of injury to healing tissues. Remember, when injured muscles are immobilized, type I (slow twitch) fibers atrophy at a faster rate than type II (fast twitch) fibers.[207,231] This underscores the need for early initiation of endurance training.

### Exercise Order

The sequence in which exercises are performed during an exercise session has an impact on muscle fatigue and the adaptive training effects. When multiple muscle groups are exercised in a single session, as is often the case in rehabilitation or conditioning programs, large muscle groups should be exercised before small muscle groups and multijoint muscles before single-joint muscles.[9,103,168] In addition, after an appropriate warm-up, higher intensity exercises should be performed before lower intensity exercises.[9]

### Frequency

*Frequency* in a resistance exercise program refers to the number of exercise sessions per day or per week.[236] As with other aspects of dosage, frequency is dependent on other determinants, such as intensity and volume as well as the patient's goals, general health status, previous participation in a resistance exercise program, and response to training. The greater the intensity and volume of exercise, the more time is needed between exercise sessions to recover from the temporarily fatiguing effects of exercise. A common cause of a decline in performance from overtraining (see discussion later in the chapter) is excessive frequency, inadequate rest, and progressive fatigue. Some forms of exercise should be performed less frequently than others because they require greater recovery time. High-intensity eccentric exercise, for example, is associated with greater microtrauma to soft tissues and a higher incidence of delayed-onset muscle soreness than other modes of exercise.[13,108,212] Therefore, rest intervals between exercise sessions are longer and the frequency of exercise is less than with other forms of exercise.

Although an optimal frequency per week has not been determined, a few generalizations can be made. Initially in an exercise program, so long as the intensity and number of repetitions are low, short sessions of exercises sometimes can be performed on a daily basis several times per day. This frequency is often indicated for early postsurgical patients when the operated limb is immobilized and the extent of exercise is limited to low-intensity isometric (setting) exercises to prevent or minimize atrophy. As the intensity and volume of exercise increases, every other day or up to five exercise sessions per week is common.[8,103,168] Frequency is again reduced for a maintenance program, usually to two times per week. With prepubescent children[314] and the very elderly,[8] frequency is usually limited to two to three sessions per week. Highly trained athletes involved in body building, power lifting, and weight lifting who know their own response to exercise often train at a high intensity and volume up to 6 days per week.[170]

### Duration

Exercise *duration* is the total number of weeks or months during which a resistance exercise program is carried out. Depending on the cause of an impairment in muscle performance, some patients require only a month or two of training to return to the desired level of function or activity, whereas others need to continue the exercise program for a lifetime to maintain optimal function.

As noted earlier in the chapter, strength gains, observed early in a resistance training program (after 2 to 3 weeks) are the result of neural adaptation. For significant changes to occur in muscle, such as hypertrophy or increased vascularization, at least 6 to 12 weeks of resistance training is required.[1,8,193]

## Rest Interval (Recovery Period)

### Purpose of Rest Intervals

Rest is a critical element of a resistance training program and is necessary to allow time for the body to recuperate from the acute effects of exercise associated with muscle fatigue or to offset adverse responses, such as exercise-induced, delayed-onset muscle soreness. Only with an appropriate balance of progressive loading and adequate rest intervals can muscle performance improve. Therefore, rest between sets of exercise and between exercise sessions must be addressed.

### Integration of Rest into Exercise

Rest intervals for each exercising muscle group are dependent on the intensity and volume of exercise. In general, the higher the intensity of exercise the longer the rest interval. For moderate-intensity resistance training, a 2- to 3-minute rest period after each set is recommended. A shorter rest interval is adequate after low-intensity exercise; longer rest intervals (4 to 5 minutes) are appropriate with high-intensity resistance training, particularly when exercising large, multijoint muscles, such as the hamstrings, which tend to fatigue rapidly.[9,61] While the muscle group that was just exercised is resting, resistance exercises can be performed by another muscle group in the same extremity or by the same muscle group in the opposite extremity.

Patients with pathological conditions that make them more susceptible to fatigue, as well as children and the elderly, should rest at least 3 minutes between sets by performing an unresisted exercise, such as low-intensity cycling, or performing the same exercise with the opposite extremity. Remember, active recovery is more efficient than passive recovery for neutralizing the effects of muscle fatigue.[61]

Rest between exercise sessions must also be considered. When strength training is initiated at moderate intensities (typically in the intermediate phase of a rehabilitation program after soft tissue injury) a 48-hour rest interval between exercise sessions (that is, training every other day) allows the patient adequate time for recovery.

## Mode of Exercise

The *mode* of exercise in a resistance exercise program refers to the form of exercise, the type of muscle contraction that occurs, and the manner in which the exercise is carried out. For example, a patient may perform an exercise dynamically or statically or in a weight-bearing or non-weight-bearing position. Mode of exercise also encompasses the form of resistance, that is, how the exercise load is applied. Resistance can be applied manually or mechanically.

As with other determinants of resistance training, the modes of exercise selected are based on a multitude of factors already highlighted throughout this section. A brief overview of the various modes of exercise is presented in this section. An in-depth explanation and analysis of each of these types of exercise can be found in the next section of the chapter and in Chapter 7.

### Type of Muscle Contraction

Figure 6.4 depicts the types of muscle contraction that may be performed in a resistance exercise program and their relationships to each other and to muscle performance.[184,250]

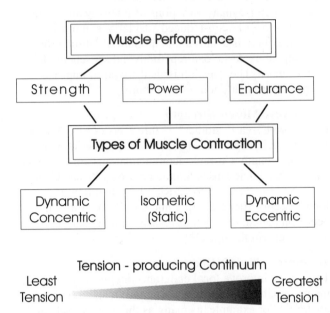

FIGURE 6.4 Types of muscle contractions: their relationships to muscle performance and their tension-generating capacities.

- *Isometric* (static) or *dynamic* muscle contractions are two broad categories of exercise.
- Dynamic resistance exercises can be performed using *concentric* (shortening) or *eccentric* (lengthening) contractions, or both.
- When the velocity of limb movement is held consistent by a rate-controlling device, the term *isokinetic* contraction is sometimes used.[250] An alternative perspective is that this is simply a dynamic (shortening or lengthening) contraction that occurs under controlled conditions.[184]

### Position for Exercise: Weight–Bearing or Non–Weight–Bearing

The patient's body position or the position of a limb in non-weight-bearing or weight-bearing positions also alters the mode of exercise. When a non-weight-bearing position is assumed and the distal segment (foot or hand) moves freely during exercise, the term *open-chain* exercise is often used. When a weight-bearing position is assumed and the body moves over a fixed distal segment, the term *closed-chain* exercise is commonly used.[184,250] Concepts associated with this approach to classifying exercises and definitions of this terminology are addressed later in the chapter.

## Forms of Resistance

- *Manual* resistance and *mechanical* resistance are the two broad methods by which resistance can be applied.
- A *constant* or *variable* load can be imposed using mechanical resistance (e.g., free weights or weight machines).
- *Accommodating* resistance[138] can be implemented by use of an isokinetic dynamometer that controls the velocity of active movement during exercise.
- *Body weight* or partial body weight is also a source of resistance if the exercise occurs in an antigravity position. Although an exercise performed against only the resistance of the weight of a body segment (and no additional external resistance) is defined as an active rather than an active-resistive exercise, a substantial amount of resistance from the weight of the body can be imposed on contracting muscles by altering a patient's position. For example, progressive loads can be placed on upper extremity musculature during push-ups by starting with wall push-ups while standing, progressing to push-ups while leaning against a countertop, push-ups in a horizontal position (Fig. 6.5), and finally push-ups from a head-down position on an incline board.

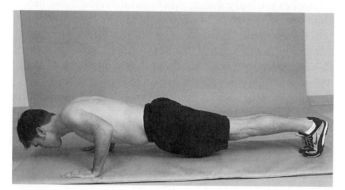

FIGURE 6.5 Body weight serves as the source of resistance during a push-up.

### Energy Systems

Modes of exercise can also be classified by the energy systems used during the exercise. *Anaerobic* exercise involves high-intensity (near-maximal) exercise carried out for a very few number of repetitions because muscles rapidly fatigue. Strengthening exercises fall into this category. *Aerobic* exercise is associated with low-intensity, repetitive exercise of large muscle groups performed over an extended period of time. This mode of exercise primarily increases muscular and cardiopulmonary endurance (refer to Chapter 7 for an in-depth explanation).

### Range of Movement: Short–Arc or Full–Arc Exercise

Resistance through the full, available range of movement *(full-arc exercise)* is necessary to develop strength through the ROM. Sometimes resistance exercises are executed through only a portion of the available range. This is known as *short-arc exercise.* This form of exercise is used to avoid a painful arc of motion or a portion of the range where the joint is unstable or to protect healing tissues after injury or surgery.

### Mode of Exercise and Application to Function

Mode-specific training is essential if a resistance training program is to have a positive impact on function. When tissue healing allows, the type of muscle contractions performed or the position in which an exercise is carried out should mimic the desired functional activity.[206]

## Velocity of Exercise

The velocity at which a muscle contracts significantly affects the tension that the muscle produces and subsequently affects muscular strength and power.[217] The velocity of exercise is frequently manipulated in a resistance training program to prepare the patient for a variety of functional activities that occur across a range of slow to fast velocities.

### Force–Velocity Relationship

The force-velocity relationship is different during concentric and eccentric muscle contractions, as depicted in Figure 6.6.

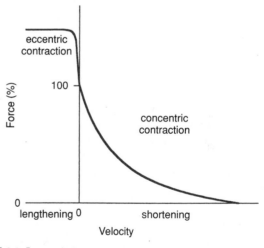

FIGURE 6.6 Force–velocity curve for concentric and eccentric exercise. *(From Levangie, PK, Norkin, CC: Joint Structure and Function—A Comprehensive Analysis, ed. 3. FA Davis, Philadelphia, 2001, p 97, with permission.)*

### Concentric Muscle Contraction

As the velocity of muscle *shortening* increases, the force the muscle can generate *decreases*. EMG activity and torque decrease as a muscle shortens at faster contractile velocities, possibly because the muscle may not have sufficient time to develop peak tension.[50,184,250,303]

### Eccentric Muscle Contraction

Findings are less consistent for eccentric than concentric muscle actions. During an eccentric contraction, as the velocity of active muscle *lengthening* increases, force production in the muscle initially also *increases* but then *quickly levels off.*[34,62,184,250] The initial increase in force production may be a protective response of the muscle when it is first overloaded. It is thought that this increase may be important for shock absorption or rapid deceleration of a limb during quick changes of direction.[78,250] The rise in tension may also be caused by stretch of the non-contractile tissue in muscle.[62] In contrast, other research indicates that eccentric force production is essentially unaffected by velocity and remains constant at slow and fast velocities.[50,122]

### Application to Resistance Training

A range of slow to fast exercise velocities has a place in an exercise program. Resistance training with free weights is safe and effective only at slow to medium velocities of limb movement so the patient can maintain control of the moving weight. Because many functional activities involve reasonably fast velocities of limb movement, training at only slow velocities is inadequate. The development of the isokinetic dynamometer during the late 1960s[138,199] gave clinicians a tool to implement resistance training at fast as well as slow velocities. In recent years, some variable-resistance exercise units (pneumatic and hydraulic) as well as elastic resistance products also have afforded additional options for safely training at fast velocities.

*Speed-specific training* is fundamental to a successful rehabilitation program. Results of numerous studies since the 1970s have shown that training-induced strength gains in a resistance exercise program primarily occur at the training speeds,[23,80,149,200] with limited transfer of training (physiological overflow) to other speeds of movement.[143,278] Accordingly, training velocities for resistance exercises should be geared to match or approach the demands of the desired functional activities.[55,149]

Isokinetic training, using *velocity spectrum rehabilitation* regimens, and *plyometric training,* also known as *stretch-shortening drills*, often emphasize high-speed training. These approaches to exercise are discussed later in the chapter.

### Periodization

Periodization, also known as *periodized training*, is an approach to resistance training that builds *systematic varia-* tion in exercise intensity and repetitions, sets, or frequency at regular intervals over a specified period of time.[102] This approach to training was developed for highly trained athletes preparing for competitive weight-lifting or power-lifting events. The concept was designed to prevent over-training and psychological staleness prior to competition and to optimize performance during competition.[102]

In preparation for competition, the training calendar is broken down into cycles, or phases, that sometimes extend over an entire year. The idea is to prepare for a "peak" performance at the time of competition. Different types of exercises at varying intensities, volume, frequency, and rest intervals are performed over a specific time period. Table 6.4 summarizes the characteristics of each cycle.

Although periodized training is commonly implemented prior to a competitive event, evidence to support the efficacy of periodization is limited.[102,170,193] Despite this, periodized training has also been used on a limited basis in the clinical setting for injured athletes during the advanced stage of rehabilitation.[96]

## Integration of Function

### Balance of Stability and Active Mobility

Control of the body during functional movement and the ability to perform functional tasks require a balance of active movement superimposed over a stable background of neuromuscular control. Sufficient performance of agonist and antagonist muscles about a joint contributes to the dynamic stability of individual joints. For example, a person must be able to hold the trunk erect and stabilize the spine while lifting a heavy object. Stability is also necessary to control quick changes of direction during functional movements. Hence, a resistance exercise program must address the static strength as well as the dynamic strength of the trunk and extremities.

### Balance of Strength, Power, and Endurance

Functional tasks related to daily living, occupational, and recreational activities require many combinations of muscle strength, power, and endurance. Various motor tasks require slow and controlled movements, rapid movements, repeated movements, and long-term positioning. Analysis of the tasks a patient would like to be able to do provides

| TABLE 6.4 | Characteristics of Periodized Training | |
| --- | --- | --- |
| **Period of Training** | **Intensity of Exercise** | **Volume and Frequency of Exercise** |
| Preparation | Lower loads | High number of reps and sets<br>More exercises per session<br>More frequent exercise sessions per day and per week |
| Competition | Higher loads (peaking just prior to competition) | Decreased reps and sets<br>Fewer exercises per session<br>Less frequent exercise sessions per day per week |
| Recuperation | Gradual decrease in exercise loads | Additional decrease in reps, sets, number of exercises, and frequency |

the framework for a task-specific resistance exercise program.

### Task–Specific Movement Patterns During Resistance Exercise

There is a place in a resistance exercise program for strengthening isolated muscle groups as well as strengthening muscles in combined patterns. Applying resistance during exercise in anatomical planes, diagonal patterns, and combined task-specific movement patterns should be integral components of a carefully progressed resistance exercise program. Use of simulated functional movements under controlled, supervised conditions is a means to return a patient safely to independent functional activities.[206] Pushing, pulling, lifting, and holding activities, for example, can first be done against a low level of resistance for a limited number of repetitions. Over time, a patient can gradually return to using the same movements during functional activities in an unsupervised work or home setting. The key to successful self-management is to teach a patient how to judge the speed, level, and duration of tension generation in muscle as well as the appropriate timing that is necessary to perform a motor task safely.

 ## TYPES OF RESISTANCE EXERCISE

The types of exercise selected for a resistance training program are contingent on many factors, including the cause and extent of primary and secondary impairments. Deficits in muscle performance, the stage of tissue healing, the condition of joints and their tolerance to compression and movement, the general abilities (physical and cognitive) of the patient, the availability of equipment, and of course the patient's goals and the intended functional outcomes of the program must be considered. A therapist has an array of exercises from which to choose to design a resistance exercise program to meet the individual needs of each patient. There is no one best form or type of resistance training. Prior to selecting specific types of resistance exercise for a patient's rehabilitation program, a therapist may want to consider the questions listed in Box 6.6.

Application of the SAID principle based on the concept of specificity of training is key to making sound exercise decisions. In addition to selecting the appropriate types of exercise, a therapist must also make decisions about the intensity, volume, order, frequency, rest interval, and other factors discussed in the previous section of this chapter to progress selected resistance exercises effectively. Table 6.5 summarizes general guidelines for progression of exercise.

The types of exercise presented in this section are static (isometric) and dynamic, concentric and eccentric, isokinetic, and open-chain and closed-chain exercise, as well as manual and mechanical and constant and variable resistance exercises. The benefits, limitations, and applications of each of these forms of resistance exercise are

analyzed and discussed. When available, supporting evidence from the scientific literature is summarized. Specific regimens or systems of resistance training, such as progressive resistive exercise (PRE), circuit weight training, velocity spectrum rehabilitation, and plyometric training, are addressed in a later section of the chapter.

### Manual and Mechanical Resistance Exercise

From a broad perspective a load can be applied to a contracting muscle in two ways: manually or mechanically. The benefits and limitations of these two forms of resistance training are summarized in Boxes 6.13 and 6.14 (later in the chapter).

#### Manual Resistance Exercise

Manual resistance exercise is a type of active-resistive exercise in which resistance is provided by a therapist or other health professional. A patient can be taught how to apply self-resistance to selected muscle groups. Although the amount of resistance cannot be measured quantitatively, this technique is useful in the early stages of an exercise program when the muscle to be strengthened is weak and can overcome only minimal to moderate resistance. It is also useful when the range of joint movements needs to be

**TABLE: 6.5   Progression of a Resistance Training Program: Factors for Consideration**

| Factors | Progression |
|---|---|
| Intensity (exercise load) | Submaximal → maximal (or near-maximal) intensity<br>Low load → high load |
| Body position (nonweight- or weight-bearing) | Variable: depending on pathology and impairments, weight-bearing restrictions (pain, swelling, instability) and goals of the rehabilitation program |
| Repetitions and sets | Low volume → high volume |
| Frequency | Variable: depends on intensity and volume of exercise |
| Type of muscle contraction | Static → dynamic<br>Concentric and eccentric: variable progression |
| Range of motion | Short arc → full arc<br>Stable portion of range → unstable portion of range |
| Plane of movement | Uniplanar → multiplanar |
| Speed of movement | Slow → fast velocities |
| Neuromuscular control | Proximal → distal control |
| Functional movement patterns | Simple → complex<br>Single joint → multijoint<br>Proximal control → distal control |

carefully controlled. The amount of resistance given is limited only by the strength of the therapist.

N O T E : Techniques for application of manual resistance exercises in anatomical planes and diagonal patterns are presented in later sections of the chapter.

## Mechanical Resistance Exercise

Mechanical resistance exercise is a form of active-resistive exercise in which resistance is applied through the use of equipment or mechanical apparatus. The amount of resistance can be measured quantitatively and incrementally progressed over time. It is also useful when the amount of resistance necessary is greater than what the therapist can apply manually.

N O T E : Systems and regimens of resistance training that use mechanical resistance and advantages and disadvantages of various types of mechanical resistance equipment are addressed later in the chapter.

## Isometric Exercise (Static Exercise)

*Isometric exercise* is a static form of exercise in which a muscle contracts and produces force without an appreciable change in the length of the muscle and without visible joint motion.[139,184,250,254] Although there is no mechanical work done (force × distance), a measurable amount of tension and force output are produced by the muscle. Sources of resistance for isometric exercise include holding against a force applied manually, holding a weight in a particular position, maintaining a position against the resistance of body weight, or pushing or pulling an immovable object.

During the 1950s and 1960s, isometric resistance training became popular as an alternative to dynamic resistance exercise and initially was thought to be a more effective and efficient method of muscle strengthening.[132,185] Based on the early research it was reported that isometric strength gains of 5% per week occurred when healthy subjects performed a single, near-maximal isometric contraction everyday over a 6-week period.[132] Although replications of this study refuted some of the original findings, particularly the rapid rate of strength gain, additional studies during the 1960s showed that *repetitive* isometric contractions (a set of 20 per day) held for 6 seconds each against near-maximal resistance consistently improved isometric strength.[185] A cross-exercise effect (a limited increase in strength of the contralateral, unexercised muscle group), as the result of transfer of training, has also been observed with maximum isometric training.[67] Each of these early investigations concluded that isometric training was a viable means of improving muscle strength.

### Rationale for Use of Isometric Exercise

The need for static strength and endurance is apparent in almost all aspects of control of the body during functional activities. Loss of static muscle strength occurs rapidly with immobilization and disuse, with estimates from 8% per week[188] to as much as 5% per day.[209]

Functional demands often involve the need to hold a position against either a high level of resistance for a short period of time or a low level of resistance over a prolonged period of time. Of these two aspects of static muscle performance, it has been suggested that muscular endurance plays a more important role than muscle strength in maintaining sufficient postural stability and in preventing injury during daily living tasks.[193] For example, the postural muscles of the trunk and lower extremities must contract isometrically to hold the body erect against gravity and provide a background of stability for balance and functional movements in an upright position.[218,269] Dynamic stabili-

## BOX 6.7 Isometric Exercise: Rationale and Indications

- To prevent or minimize muscle atrophy when joint movement is not possible owing to external immobilization (casts, splints, skeletal traction)
- To activate muscles (facilitate muscle firing) to begin to re-establish neuromuscular control but protect healing tissues when joint movement is not advisable after soft tissue injury or surgery
- To develop postural or joint stability
- To improve muscle strength when use of dynamic resistance exercise could compromise joint integrity or cause joint pain
- To develop static muscle strength at particular points in the ROM consistent with specific task-related needs

ty of joints is achieved by activating and maintaining a low level of co-contraction, that is, concurrent isometric contractions of antagonist muscles that surround joints.[196] The importance of isometric strength and endurance in the elbow, wrist, and finger musculature, for example, is apparent when a person holds and carries a heavy object for an extended period of time.

With these examples in mind, there can be no doubt that isometric exercises are an important part of a rehabilitation program designed to improve functional abilities. The rationale and indications for isometric exercise in rehabilitation are summarized in Box 6.7.

### Types of Isometric Exercise

Several forms of isometric exercise with varying degrees of resistance and intensity of muscle contractions serve different purposes during successive phases of rehabilitation. All but one type (muscle setting) incorporate some form of significant resistance and therefore are used to improve static strength or develop sustained muscular control (endurance). Because no appreciable resistance is applied, muscle setting technically is not a form of resistance exercise but is included in this discussion to show a continuum of isometric exercise that can be used for multifaceted goals in a rehabilitation program.

*Muscle-setting exercises.* Setting exercises involve low-intensity isometric contractions performed against little to no resistance. They are used to decrease muscle pain and spasm and to promote relaxation and circulation after injury to soft tissues during the *acute* stage of healing. Two common examples of muscle setting are of the quadriceps and gluteal muscles.

Because muscle setting is performed against no appreciable resistance, it does not improve muscle strength except in very weak muscles. However, setting exercises can retard muscle atrophy and maintain mobility between muscle fibers when immobilization of a muscle is necessary to protect healing tissues during the very early phase of rehabilitation.

*Stabilization exercises.* This form of isometric exercise is used to develop a submaximal but sustained level of co-contraction to improve postural stability or dynamic stability of a joint by means of mid-range isometric contractions against resistance in antigravity positions and in weight-bearing postures if weight bearing is permissible.[196] Body weight or manual resistance often are the sources of resistance. Variations terms are used to describe stabilization exercises. They include *rhythmic stabilization* and *alternating isometrics*, two techniques associated with proprioceptive neuromuscular facilitation (PNF) described later in the chapter.[269,296] Stabilization exercises that focus on trunk/postural control include *dynamic, core, and segmental stabilization* exercises, described in Chapter 16.[37,228]

*Multiple-angle isometrics.* This term refers to a system of isometric exercise where resistance is applied, manually or mechanically, at multiple joint positions within the available ROM.[55] This approach is used when the goal of exercise is to improve strength throughout the ROM when joint motion is permissible but dynamic resistance exercise is painful or inadvisable.

### Characteristics and Effects of Isometric Training

Effective use of isometric exercise in a resistance training program is founded on an understanding of its characteristics and its limitations.

*Intensity of muscle contraction.* The amount of tension that can be generated during an isometric muscle contraction depends in part on joint position and the length of the muscle at the time of contraction.[139,293] It is sufficient to use an exercise intensity (load) of 60% to 80% of a muscle's force-developing capacity to improve strength.[162,293] Therefore, the amount of resistance against which the muscle is able to hold varies and needs to be adjusted at different points in the range. Resistance must be progressively increased to continue to overload the muscle as it becomes stronger.

*Duration of muscle activation.* To achieve adaptive changes in static muscle performance, an isometric contraction should be held for 6 seconds and no more than 10 seconds because muscle fatigue develops rapidly. This allows sufficient time for peak tension to develop and for metabolic changes to occur in the muscle.[132,193] A 10-second contraction allows a 2-second rise time, a 6-second hold time, and a 2-second fall time.[55]

*Repetitive contractions.* Use of repetitive contractions, held for 6 to 10 seconds each, decreases muscle cramping and increases the effectiveness of the isometric regimen.[55,185]

*Joint angle and mode specificity.* Gains in muscle strength occur only at or closely adjacent to the training angle.[161,162,293] Physiological overflow is minimal, occurring no more than 10° in either direction in the ROM from the training angle.[162] Therefore, when performing multiple-angle isometrics, resistance at four to six points in the ROM is usually recommended. Isometric resistance training is also mode-specific. It increases static strength but has little to no impact on dynamic strength (concentric or eccentric).[172]

PRECAUTIONS: To avoid potential injury to the contracting muscle, apply and release the resistance gradually. This helps to grade the muscle tension and ensures that the muscle contraction is pain-free. It also minimizes the risk of uncontrolled joint movement.

Breath-holding commonly occurs during isometric exercise, particularly when performed against substantial resistance. This is likely to cause a pressor response as the result of the Valsalva maneuver, causing a rapid increase in blood pressure.[94] Rhythmic breathing, emphasizing exhalation during the contraction, should always be performed during isometric exercise to minimize this response.

CONTRAINDICATION: High-intensity isometric exercises may be contraindicated for patients with a history of cardiac or vascular disorders.

## Dynamic Exercise—Concentric and Eccentric

A dynamic muscle contraction causes joint movement and excursion of a body segment as the muscle contracts and shortens (concentric contraction) or lengthens under tension (eccentric contraction). As represented in Figure 6.7, the term *concentric exercise* refers to a form of dynamic muscle loading where tension in a muscle develops and physical shortening of the muscle occurs as an external force (resistance) is overcome, as when lifting a weight. In contrast, *eccentric exercise* involves dynamic loading of a muscle beyond its force-producing capacity, causing physical lengthening of the muscle as it attempts to control the load, as when lowering a weight.[62]

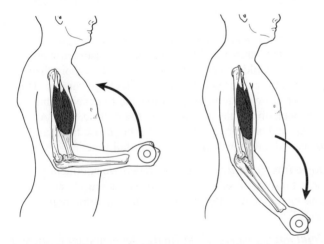

FIGURE 6.7 (A) Concentric and (B) eccentric strengthening of the elbow flexors occurs as a weight is lifted and lowered.

During concentric and eccentric exercise, resistance can be applied in several ways: (1) constant resistance, such as body weight, a free weight, or a simple weight-

pulley system; (2) a weight machine that provides variable resistance; or (3) an isokinetic device that controls the velocity of limb movement.

NOTE: Although the term *isotonic* (meaning equal tension) has been used for many years to describe a resisted, dynamic muscle contraction, application of this terminology is incorrect. In fact, when a body segment moves through its available range, the tension that the muscle is capable of generating *varies* through the range as the muscle shortens or lengthens. This is due to the changing length–tension relationship of the muscle and the changing torque of the load.[184,250] Therefore, in this textbook "isotonic" is not used to describe dynamic resistance exercise.

### Rationale for Use of Concentric and Eccentric Exercise

Both concentric and eccentric exercise have distinct value in rehabilitation and conditioning programs. Concentric muscle contractions accelerate body segments, whereas eccentric contractions decelerate body segments (e.g., during sudden changes of direction or momentum). Eccentric contractions also act as a source of shock absorption during high-impact activities.[62,176,254]

A combination of concentric and eccentric muscle action is evident in countless tasks of daily life, such as walking up and down inclines, ascending and descending stairs, rising from a chair and sitting back down, or picking up or setting down an object. Hence, it is advisable to incorporate a variety of concentric and eccentric resistance exercises in a rehabilitation progression for patients with impaired muscle performance to improve muscle strength, power, or endurance and to meet necessary functional demands.

Eccentric training, in particular, is thought to be an essential component of a rehabilitation or conditioning program to reduce the risk of musculoskeletal injury or reinjury during activities that involve high-intensity deceleration and quick changes of direction.[176,258] Although chronic muscle-tendon disorders are commonly associated with activities that involve repetitive, eccentric muscle contractions, the progressive use of eccentric resistance training is advocated during the advanced stage of rehabilitaion, and its efficacy is supported by evidence.[176]

Regimens of exercise that emphasize eccentric loading, such as *plyometric training (stretch-shortening drills)* or fast-velocity, eccentric isokinetic training (both of which are discussed later in the chapter), are often used to prepare a patient for high-demand sports or work-related activities. In addition, high-intensity, eccentric exercise is thought to improve physical performance, especially sport-related performance.[9,176]

### Characteristics and Effects of Concentric and Eccentric Exercise

*Exercise load.* A maximum concentric contraction produces less force than a maximum eccentric contraction under the same conditions (see Fig. 6.6). In other words, greater loads can be lowered than lifted. This difference in the magnitude of loads that can be controlled by concentric versus eccentric muscle contractions may be associated with the contributions of the contractile and noncontractile components of muscle. When a load is lowered, the force exerted by the load is controlled not only by the active, contractile components of muscle but also by the connective tissue in and around the muscle. In contrast, when a weight is lifted, only the contractile components of the muscle lift the load.[62]

With a concentric contraction, greater numbers of motor units must be recruited to control the same load compared to an eccentric contraction, suggesting that concentric exercise has less mechanical efficiency than eccentric exercise.[62,78] Consequently, it requires more effort by a patient to control the same load during concentric exercise than during eccentric exercise. As a result, maximum resistance during the concentric phase of an exercise does not provide a maximum load during the eccentric phase. Although not practical, for maximum resistance during the eccentric phase, an additional load must be applied.

Although greater loads can be used for eccentric training than for concentric training, the relative adaptive gains in eccentric and concentric strength appear to be similar at the conclusion of an concentric or eccentric exercise program. It has been suggested that the higher incidence of delayed-onset muscle soreness associated with high-intensity eccentric exercise may influence the outcome of these two modes of training.[62,80,108]

NOTE: Given that eccentric exercise requires recruitment of fewer motor units to control a load than concentric exercise, when a muscle is very weak—less than a fair (3/5) muscle grade—active eccentric muscle contractions against no external resistance (other than gravity) can be used to generate active muscle contractions and develop a beginning level of strength and neuromuscular control. In other words, in the presence of substantial muscle weakness, it may be easier to control lowering a limb against gravity than lifting the limb.

PRECAUTIONS: There is greater stress on the cardiovascular system (i.e., increased heart rate and arterial blood pressure) during eccentric exercise than during concentric exercise,[62] possibly because greater loads can be used for eccentric training. This underscores the need for rhythmic breathing during high-intensity exercise. (Refer to a later section of this chapter for additional information on cardiovascular precautions.)

*Velocity of exercise.* The velocity at which concentric or eccentric exercises are performed directly affects the force-generating capacity of the neuromuscular unit.[50,78,217] At slow velocities with a maximum load, an eccentric contraction generates greater tension than a concentric contraction. At slow velocities, therefore, a greater load (weight) can be lowered (with control) than lifted. As the velocity of exercise increases, concentric contraction tension rapidly and consistently decreases, whereas eccentric contraction forces increase slightly but then rapidly reach a plateau under maximum load conditions (see Fig. 6.6).

NOTE: A common error made by some weightlifters during high-intensity resistance training is to assume that if a weight is lifted quickly (concentric contraction) and lowered slowly (eccentric contraction), the slow eccentric contraction generates greater tension. In fact, if the load is constant, less tension is generated during the eccentric phase. The only way to develop greater tension is to increase the weight of the applied load during the eccentric phase of each exercise cycle. This usually requires assistance from an exercise partner to help lift the load during each concentric contraction. This is a highly intense form of exercise and should be undertaken only by healthy individuals training for high-demand sports or weightlifting competition. This technique is not appropriate for individuals recovering from musculoskeletal injuries.

*Energy expenditure.* Eccentric exercise consumes less oxygen and energy stores than concentric exercise against similar loads.[38] Therefore, the use of eccentric activities such as downhill running may improve muscular endurance more efficiently than similar concentric activities because muscle fatigue occurs less quickly with eccentric exercise.[62,193]

*Mode specificity.* Opinions and results of studies vary on whether the effects of training with concentric and eccentric contractions in the exercised muscle group are mode-specific. Although there is substantial evidence to support specificity of training,[11,23,80,206,280] there is also some evidence to suggest that training in one mode leads to strength gains, though less significant, in the other mode.[86,241] Because transfer of training is quite limited, selection of exercises that simulate the functional movements needed by a patient is a prudent choice.

*Cross-training effect.* Concentric[291] and eccentric[292] training has been shown to cause a *cross-training effect,* that is, a slight increase in strength in the same muscle group of the opposite, unexercised extremity. This effect, sometimes referred to as *cross-exercise,* also occurs with high-intensity exercise that involves a combination of concentric and eccentric contractions (lifting and lowering a weight). This effect in the unexercised muscle group may be caused by repeated contractions of the unexercised extremity in an attempt to stabilize the body during high-effort exercise. Although cross-training is an interesting phenomenon, there is no evidence to suggest that a cross-training effect has a positive impact on a patient's functional capabilities.

*Exercise-induced muscle soreness.* Repeated and rapidly progressed eccentric muscle contractions against resistance are associated with a significantly higher incidence and severity of delayed-onset muscle soreness (DOMS) than resisted concentric exercise.[13,40,108,212] Why DOMS occurs more readily with eccentric exercise is speculative, possibly the result of greater damage to muscle and connective tissue when heavy loads are controlled and lowered.[13,40] It should be noted that there is at least limited evidence to suggest that if the intensity and volume of concentric and eccentric exercise are equal, there is no significant difference in the degree of DOMS after exercise.[100]

## Dynamic Exercise—Constant and Variable Resistance

The most common system of resistance training used with dynamic exercise against constant or variable resistance is *progressive resistance exercise* (PRE). A later section of the chapter, which covers systems of training using mechanical resistance, addresses PRE.

### Dynamic Constant External Resistance Exercise

Dynamic constant external resistance (DCER) exercise is a form of resistance training where a limb moves through a ROM against a *constant external load,* provided by free weights such as a handheld or cuff weight, torque arm units (Fig. 6.8), weight machines, or pulley systems.[193] This terminology (DCER exercise) is used in lieu of the term "isotonic exercise" because although the imposed load (weight) does not change the torque imposed by the weight and the tension generated by the muscle do change throughout the range of movement.[184,250] If the load is less than the torque generated by the muscle, the muscle contracts concentrically and accelerates the load; if the load exceeds the muscle's torque production, the muscle contracts eccentrically to decelerate the load.

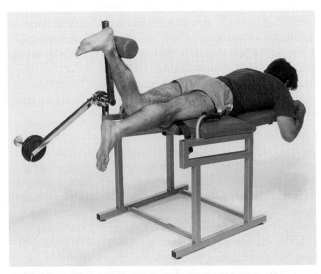

FIGURE 6.8 N–K Exercise Unit with torque arm and interchangeable weights provides constant external resistance. *(Courtesy of N-K Products Company, Soquel, CA.)*

DCER exercise has an inherent limitation. When lifting or lowering a constant load, the contracting muscle is challenged maximally at only one point in the ROM where the maximum torque of the resistance matches the maximum torque output of the muscle. A therapist needs to be aware of the changing torque of the exercise and the changing length–tension relationship of the muscle and modify body position and resistance accordingly to match where in the range the maximum load needs to be applied. Despite this limitation, constant external resistance has been and continues to be an effective form of muscle load-

ing for training-induced improvements in muscle performance; and it is a mainstay of resistance exercise programs.

### Variable–Resistance Exercise

Variable-resistance exercise, a form of dynamic exercise, addresses the primary limitation of dynamic exercise against a constant external load (DCER exercises). Specially designed resistance equipment imposes varying levels of resistance to the contracting muscles to load the muscles more effectively at multiple points in the ROM. The resistance is altered throughout the range by means of a weight-cable system that moves over an asymmetrically shaped cam, by a lever arm system, or by hydraulic or pneumatic mechanisms.[251] How effectively these machines vary the resistance to match muscle torque curves is questionable.

Dynamic exercise with elastic resistance products (bands and tubing) can also be thought of in the broadest sense as a variable-resistance exercise because of the inherent properties of the material and its response to stretch.[146,152,245] Furthermore, when dynamic exercise is performed against manual resistance, a skilled therapist can vary the load applied to the contracting muscle throughout the ROM. The therapist adjusts the resistance based on the patient's response so the muscle is appropriately loaded at all portions of the range.

### Special Considerations for DCER and Variable–Resistance Exercise

During either DCER or the variable-resistance exercise, the velocity and excursion of limb movement is controlled exclusively by the patient (with the exception of manual resistance exercise and performing exercises on units that have range-limiting devices). Exercises must be performed at a relatively *slow velocity* to avoid momentum and uncontrolled movements, which could jeopardize the safety of the patient.

N O T E : Hydraulic and pneumatic variable-resistance equipment and elastic resistance products do allow safe, high-velocity resistance training. Because most daily living and occupational activities occur at moderate to fast velocities, the training-induced improvements in muscle strength that occur only at slow velocities may not prepare the patient for activities that require rapid bursts of strength or quick changes of direction.

## Isokinetic Exercise

*Isokinetic exercise* is a form of dynamic exercise in which the velocity of muscle shortening or lengthening and the angular limb velocity is predetermined and held constant by a rate-limiting device known as an isokinetic dynamometer (Fig. 6.9).[55,84,138,199] The term *isokinetic* refers to movement that occurs at an equal (constant) velocity. Unlike DCER exercise where a specific weight (amount of resistance) is selected and superimposed on the contracting muscle, in isokinetic resistance training the *velocity* of limb movement, not the load, is manipulated. The force encountered by the muscle depends on the extent of force applied to the equipment.[5,138]

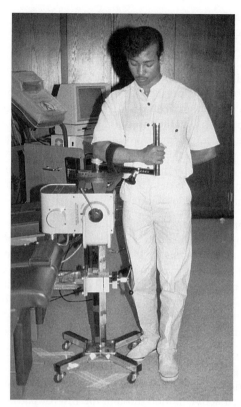

**FIGURE 6.9** Isokinetic strengthening of the internal and external rotators of the shoulder with the arm at the side to protect a potentially unstable gleno-humeral joint.

Isokinetic exercise is also called *accommodating resistance exercise.*[138] Theoretically, if an individual is putting forth a maximum effort during each repetition of exercise, the contracting muscle produces variable but *maximum* force output, consistent with the muscle's variable tension-generating capabilities at all portions in the range of movement, not at only one small portion of the range as occurs with DCER training. Although early advocates of isokinetic training suggested it was superior to resistance training with free weights or weight-pulley systems, this claim has not been well supported by evidence. Today, use of isokinetic training is regarded as one of many tools that can be integrated into the later stages of rehabilitation.[5]

## Characteristics of Isokinetic Training

A brief overview of the key characteristics of isokinetic exercise are addressed in this section. For more detailed information on isokinetic testing and training, a number of resources are available.[5,55,57,82,84,123]

***Constant velocity.*** Fundamental to the concept of isokinetic exercise is that the velocity of muscle shortening or lengthening is preset and controlled by the unit and remains constant throughout the ROM.

***Range and selection of training velocities.*** Isokinetic training affords a wide range of exercise velocities in rehabilitation from very slow to fast velocities. Current dynamometers manipulate the speed of limb movement

| TABLE 6.6 | Classification of Velocity of Training in Concentric Isokinetic Exercises* |
|---|---|
| **Classification** | **Angular Velocity** |
| Isometric | 0°/sec |
| Slow | 30°–60°/sec |
| Medium | 60°–180°/sec |
| Fast | 180°–360°/sec and above** |

*Training velocities tend to be substantially slower for eccentric training, ranging from 30° to 120°/sec with most eccentric training usually initiated between 60° and 120°/sec.

**Although isokinetic equipment offers speed settings up to 500°/sec, training at velocities above 300°–360°/sec is not frequently used because the patient must accelerate the limb to the predetermined setting before "catching" the machine, that is, before meeting resistance from the unit.

from 0°/sec up to 500°/sec. As shown in Table 6.6, these training velocities are classified as slow, medium, and fast. This range theoretically provides a mechanism by which a patient can prepare for the demands of functional activities that occur at a range of velocities of limb movement.

Selection of training velocities should be as specific as possible to the demands of the anticipated functional tasks. The faster training velocities appear to be similar to or approaching the velocities of limb movements inherent in some functional motor skills such as walking or lifting.[5,308] For example, the average angular velocity of the lower extremity during walking has been calculated at 230° to 240°/sec.[5,55,57,308] Nevertheless, the velocity of limb movements during many functional activities far exceeds the fastest training velocities available.

The training velocities selected may also be based on the mode of exercise (concentric or eccentric) to be performed. As noted in Table 6.6, the range of training velocities advocated for concentric exercise is substantially greater than for eccentric training.[5,84,123]

***Reciprocal versus isolated muscle training.*** Use of reciprocal training of agonist and antagonist muscles emphasizing quick reversals of motion is possible on an isokinetic dynamometer. For example, the training parameter can be set so the patient performs concentric contraction of the quadriceps followed by concentric contraction of the hamstrings. An alternative approach is to target the same muscle in a concentric mode, followed by an eccentric mode, thus strengthening only one muscle group at a time.[307] Both of these approaches have merit.

***Specificity of training.*** Isokinetic training for the most part is *speed-specific,*[23,123,149] with only limited evidence of significant overflow from one training speed to another.[143,278] Evidence of mode-specificity (concentric vs. eccentric) with isokinetic exercise is less clear.* Because isokinetic exercise tends to be speed-specific, patients typi-

---

* See references 11, 84, 122, 206, 241.

cally train at several medium and fast velocities (between 90° and 360°/sec) using a system of training known as *velocity spectrum rehabilitation*.[5,55,57,84] (This approach to isokinetic training is discussed later in the chapter.)

***Compressive forces on joints.*** During concentric exercise, as force output decreases, the compressive forces across the moving joint are less at faster angular velocities than at slow velocities.[5,55,82,84]

***Accommodation to fatigue.*** Because the resistance encountered is directly proportional to the force applied to the resistance arm of the isokinetic unit, as the contracting muscle fatigues, a patient is still able to perform additional repetitions even though the force output of the muscle temporarily diminishes.

***Accommodation to a painful arc.*** If a patient experiences transient pain at some portion of the arc of motion during isokinetic exercise, this form of training accommodates for the painful arc. The patient simply pushes less vigorously against the resistance arm to move without pain through that portion of the range. If a patient needs to stop a resisted motion because of sudden onset of pain, the resistance is eliminated as soon as the patient stops pushing against the torque arm of the dynamometer.

### Training Effects and Carryover to Function
Numerous studies have shown that isokinetic training is effective for improving one or more of the parameters of muscle performance.[11,23,84,143,194,206,241] In contrast, only a limited number of studies have investigated the relationship between isokinetic training and improvement in the performance of functional skills. Two such studies indicated that the use of high-velocity concentric and eccentric isokinetic training was associated with enhanced performance (increased velocity of serving in tennis and throwing a ball).[86,202]

Several factors inherent in the design of most types of isokinetic equipment may limit the extent to which isokinetic training carries over to improvements in functional performance. Although isokinetic training affords a spectrum of velocities for training, the velocity of limb movement during many daily living and sport-related activities far exceeds the maximum velocity settings available on isokinetic equipment. In addition, limb movements during most functional tasks occur at multiple velocities, not at a constant velocity, depending on the conditions of the task.

Furthermore, isokinetic exercise usually isolates a single muscle or opposite muscle groups, involves movement of a single joint, is uniplanar, and does not involve weight bearing. Although isolation of a single muscle can be beneficial in remediating strength deficits in specific muscle groups, most functional activities require contractions of multiple muscle groups and movement of multiple joints in several planes of motion, some in weight-bearing positions. However, it is important to note that some of these limitations can be addressed by adapting the setup of the equipment to allow multiaxis movements in diagonal planes or

multijoint resisted movements with the addition of an attachment for closed-chain training.

### Special Considerations for Isokinetic Training

#### Availability of Equipment
From a pragmatic perspective, one limitation of isokinetic exercise is that a patient can incorporate this form of exercise into a rehabilitation program ***only*** by going to a facility where the equipment is available. In addition, a patient must be given assistance to set up the equipment and often requires supervision during exercise. These considerations contribute to high costs for the patient enrolled in a long-term rehabilitation program.

#### Appropriate Setup
The setups recommended in the product manuals often must be altered to ensure that the exercise occurs in a position that is safe for a particular joint. For example, even though a manufacturer may describe a 90°/90° position of the shoulder and elbow for strengthening the shoulder rotators, exercising with the arm at the side may be a safer, more comfortable position (see Fig. 6.9).

#### Initiation and Progression of Isokinetic Training During Rehabilitation
Isokinetic training is begun in the later stages of rehabilitation, when active motion through the full (or partial) ROM is pain-free. Suggested guidelines for implementation and progression are summarized in Box 6.8.[5,55,57,84,123]

## Open–Chain and Closed–Chain Exercise

### Background
Functional motor skills are composed of an array of movements carried out in various positions in the environment.

---

**BOX 6.8    Progression of Isokinetic Training for Rehabilitation**

- Initially to keep resistance low, submaximal isokinetic exercise is implemented before isokinetic exercise with maximal effort.
- Short-arc movements are used before full-arc motions, when necessary, to avoid movement in an unstable or painful portion of the range. This is accomplished by a mechanical range-limiting device or with a computerized dynamometer.
- Slow to medium training velocities (60°–180°/sec) are incorporated into the exercise program before progressing to faster velocities.
- Maximal concentric contractions at various velocities are performed before introducing eccentric isokinetic exercises for the following reasons.
  - Concentric isokinetic exercise is easier to learn and is fully under the control of the patient.
  - During eccentric isokinetic exercise the velocity of movement of the resistance arm is robotically controlled by the dynamometer, not the patient.

The cornerstone of a *functionally relevant* therapeutic exercise program is the inclusion of task-specific movements and postural control associated with the necessary, expected, and desired functional demands in a patient's life.

In the clinical setting and in the rehabilitation literature, functional activities and exercises are commonly categorized as having weight-bearing or non-weight-bearing characteristics. Another frequently used method of classifying movements and exercises is based on "open or closed kinetic chain" and "open or closed kinematic chain" concepts. These concepts, which were introduced during the 1950s and 1960s in the human biomechanics and kinesiology literature by Steindler[260] and Brunnstrom,[31] respectively, were put forth to describe how segments (structures) and motions of the body are linked and how muscle recruitment changes during different types of movement and in response to different loading conditions in the environment.

In his analysis of human motion, Steindler[260] proposed that the term "open kinetic chain" applies to completely unrestricted movement in space of a peripheral segment of the body, as in waving the hand or swinging the leg. In contrast, he suggested that during closed kinetic chain movements the peripheral segment meets with "considerable external resistance." He stated that if the terminal segment remains fixed, the encountered resistance moves the proximal segments over the stationary distal segments. He also noted that in a closed kinetic chain motion in one joint is accompanied by motions of adjacent joints that occur in reasonably predictable patterns.

Both Steindler and Brunnstrom pointed out that the action of a muscle changes when the distal segment is free to move versus when it is fixed in place. For example, in an open chain the tibialis posterior muscle functions to invert and plantarflex the foot and ankle. In contrast, during the stance phase of gait (during loading), when the foot is planted on the ground the tibialis posterior contracts to decelerate pronation of the subtalar joint and to supinate the foot to rotate the lower leg externally during the mid and terminal stance.

During the late 1980s and early 1990s, clinicians and researchers in rehabilitation, who were becoming familiar with the open and closed kinetic (or kinematic) chain approach to classifying human motion, began to describe exercises based on these concepts.[220,279]

### Controversy and Inconsistency in Use of Open-Chain and Closed-Chain Terminology
Although use of open- and closed-chain terminology is now prevalent in the clinical setting and in the rehabilitation literature, as investigators have discussed and applied open- and closed-chain concepts to exercise a lack of consensus has emerged about how, or even if, this terminology should be used and what constitutes an open-chain versus a closed-chain exercise.[24,71,72,125,253,299,301]

One source of inconsistency is whether weight bearing is an inherent component of closed kinetic chain motions. Steindler[260] did not specify that weight bearing must occur

for a motion to be categorized as closed kinetic chain, but many of his examples of closed-chain movements, particularly in the lower extremities, involved weight bearing. In the current literature, descriptions of a closed kinetic chain often do[59,101] but sometimes do not[128,253] include weight bearing as a necessary element. One author suggested that all weight-bearing exercises involve some elements of closed-chain motions, but not all closed-chain exercises are performed in weight-bearing positions.[253]

Another point of ambiguity is whether the distal segment must be absolutely fixed to a surface and not moving to be classified as a closed-chain motion. Steindler[260] described this as one of the conditions of a closed-chain motion. However, another condition in his description of closed kinetic chain motions is that if the "considerable external resistance" is overcome it results in movement of the peripheral segment. Examples Steindler cited were pushing a cart away from the body and lifting a load. Consequently, some investigators classify a bench press exercise, a seated or reclining leg press exercise, or cycling as closed-chain exercises because they involve pushing motions and axial loading.[24,58] If these exercises fit under the closed-chain umbrella, does an exercise in which the distal segment slides across the support surface also qualify as a closed-chain motion? Opinion is divided.

Lifting a handheld weight or pushing against the force arm of an isokinetic dynamometer are consistently cited in the literature as examples of open-chain exercises.* Although there is no axial loading in these exercises, considering Steindler's condition for closed-chain motion just discussed, should these exercises more correctly be classified as closed-chain rather than open-chain exercises in that the distal segment is overcoming considerable external resistance? Again, there is no consensus.

Given the complexity of human movement, it is not surprising that a single classification system cannot adequately group the multitude of movements found in functional activities and therapeutic exercise interventions.

### Alternatives to Open-Chain and Closed-Chain Terminology
To address the unresolved issues associated with open-chain and closed-chain terminology, several authors have offered alternative or additional terms to classify exercises. One suggestion is to use the terms *distally fixated* and *nondistally fixated* in lieu of closed chain and open chain.[205] Another suggestion is to add a category dubbed *partial kinetic chain*[299,301] to describe exercises in which the distal segment (hand or foot) meets resistance but is not absolutely stationary, such as using a leg press machine, bicycle, stepping machine, or slide board. The term closed kinetic chain is then reserved for instances when the terminal segment does not move.

To avoid use of the open- or closed-chain concepts, another classification system categorizes exercises as either *joint isolation exercises* (movement of only one joint segment) or *kinetic chain exercises* (simultaneous movement

---

* See references 58, 59, 87, 101, 128, 229, 261, 299, 305.

of multiple segments that are linked).[159,220] Boundaries of movement of the peripheral segment (movable or stationary) or loading conditions (weight bearing or nonweight bearing) are not parameters of this terminology. However, other, more complex classification systems do take these conditions into account.[72,183]

Although these alternative terms have been put forth, open- and closed-chain terminology continues to be widely used in the clinical setting and in the literature.[†] Therefore, despite the many inconsistencies and shortcomings of the kinetic or kinematic chain terminology, and recognizing that many exercises and functional activities often involve a combination of open- and closed-chain motions or do not fit either open- or closed-chain definitions, the authors of this textbook have chosen to continue to use open- and closed-chain terminology to describe exercises.

### Characteristics of Open-Chain and Closed-Chain Exercises

The following operational definitions and characteristics of open- and closed-chain exercises are presented for clarity and as the basis for the discussion of open- and closed-chain exercises described throughout this textbook. The parameters of the definitions are those most frequently noted in the current literature. Common characteristics of open- and closed-chain exercises are compared in Table 6.7.

**Open-Chain Exercises**

Open-chain exercises involve motions in which the distal segment (hand or foot) is free to move in space, without necessarily causing simultaneous motions at adjacent joints.[58,85,87,101,159] Limb movement only occurs *distal* to the moving joint. Muscle activation occurs in the muscles that cross the moving joint. For example, during knee flex-

_____
[†]See references 25, 30, 58, 59, 75, 84, 85, 125, 128, 150, 178, 195, 266, 305.

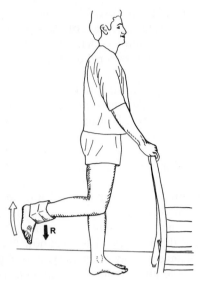

**FIGURE 6.10** Open-chain resisted knee flexion.

ion in an open-chain exercise (Fig. 6.10), the action of the hamstrings is independent of recruitment of other hip or ankle musculature. Open-chain exercises also are typically performed in non-weight-bearing positions.[59,101,310] In addition, during resistance training, the exercise load (resistance) is applied to the moving distal segment.

**Closed-Chain Exercises**

Closed-chain exercises involve motions in which the body moves on a distal segment that is fixed or stabilized on a support surface.[58,85,87,101,128,159,253,299] Movement at one joint causes simultaneous motions at distal as well as proximal joints in a relatively predictable manner. For example, when a patient is performing a bilateral short-arc squatting motion (mini-squat) (Fig. 6.11) and then returning to an erect position, as the knees flex and extend, the

| TABLE 6.7 Characteristics of Open-Chain and Closed-Chain Exercises | |
|---|---|
| **Open-Chain Exercises** | **Closed-Chain Exercises** |
| Distal segment moves in space | Distal segment remains in contact with or stationary (fixed in place) on support surface |
| Independent joint movement; no predictable joint motion in adjacent joints | Interdependent joint movements; relatively predictable movement patterns in adjacent joints |
| Movement of body segments only distal to the moving joint | Movement of body segments may occur distal and/or proximal to the moving joint |
| Muscle activation occurs predominantly in the prime mover and is isolated to muscles of the moving joint | Muscle activation occurs in multiple muscle groups, both distal and proximal to the moving joint |
| Typically performed in non weight-bearing positions | Typically but not always performed in weight-bearing positions |
| Resistance is applied to the moving distal segment | Resistance is applied simultaneously to multiple moving segments |
| Use of external rotary loading | Use of axial loading |
| External stabilization (manually or with equipment) usually required | Internal stabilization by means of muscle action, joint compression, and congruency and postural control |

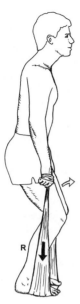

FIGURE 6.11 Bilateral closed-chain resisted hip and knee extension.

hips and ankles move in a predictable pattern along with the knees.

Closed-chain exercises are primarily performed in weight-bearing positions.[58,86,101,128,310] Examples in the upper extremities include balance activities in quadruped, sitting press-ups, wall push-offs, or prone push-ups; examples in the lower extremities include lunges, squats, step-up or step-down exercises, or heel rises to name a few.

N O T E : In this textbook, as in some other publications,[85,87,128,266] inclusive in the scope of closed-chain exercises are *weight-bearing activities* where the distal segment *moves but remains in contact with the support surface,* as when using a bicycle, cross-country ski machine, or stair-stepping machine. In the upper extremities a few non-weight-bearing activities qualify as closed-chain exercises, such as pull-ups on a trapeze in bed or chin-ups at an overhead bar.

### Rationale for Use of Open–Chain and Closed–Chain Exercises

The rationale for selecting open- or closed-chain exercises is based on the goals of an individualized rehabilitation program and a critical analysis of the potential benefits and limitations inherent in either form of exercise.[60] Because functional activities involve many combinations and considerable variations of open- and closed-chain motions, inclusion and integration of task-specific open-chain and closed-chain exercises into a rehabilitation or conditioning program is both appropriate and prudent.

 **Focus on Evidence**_____

Although often suggested, there is no evidence to support the global assumption that closed-chain exercises are "more functional" than open-chain exercises. A review of the literature by Davies[56] indicated there is a substantial body of evidence that both open- and closed-chain exercises are effective for reducing deficits in muscle performance

in the upper and lower extremities. However, of the studies reviewed, very few randomized, controlled trials demonstrated that these improvements in muscle performance were associated with a reduction of functional limitations or improvement in physical performance.

_____

A summary of the benefits and limitations of open- and closed-chain exercises and the rationale for their use follows. Whenever possible, presumed benefits and limitations or comparisons of both forms of exercise are analyzed in light of existing scientific evidence. Some of the reported benefits and limitations are supported by evidence, whereas others are often founded on opinion or anecdotal reports. Evidence is presented as available.

N O T E : Most reports and investigations comparing or analyzing closed- or open-chain exercises have focused on the knee, in particular the anterior cruciate ligament (ACL) or patellofemoral joint. Far fewer articles have addressed the application or impact of open- and closed-chain exercises on the upper extremities.

### Isolation of Muscle Groups

Open-chain testing and training identifies strength deficits and improves muscle performance of individual muscles or muscle groups more effectively than closed-chain exercises. The possible occurrence of substitute motions that compensate for and mask strength deficits of individual muscles is greater with closed-chain exercise than open-chain exercise.

 **Focus on Evidence**_____

In a study of the effectiveness of a closed-chain-*only* resistance training program after ACL reconstruction, residual muscle weakness of the quadriceps femoris was identified.[252] The investigators suggested that this residual strength deficit, which altered gait, might have been avoided with the inclusion of open-chain quadriceps training in the postoperative rehabilitation program.

_____

### Control of Movements

During open-chain resisted exercises a greater level of control is possible with a *single* moving joint than with multiple moving joints as occurs during closed-chain training. With open-chain exercises stabilization is usually applied externally by a therapist's manual contacts or with belts or straps. In contrast, during closed-chain exercises the patient most often uses muscular stabilization to control joints or structures proximal and distal to the targeted joint. The greater levels of control afforded by open-chain training are particularly advantageous during the early phases of rehabilitation.

### Joint Approximation

Almost all muscle contractions have a compressive component that approximates the joint surfaces and provides stability to the joint whether in open- or closed-chain situations.[184,250] Joint approximation also occurs during weight bearing and is associated with lower levels of shear forces at a moving joint. This has been demonstrated at the knee (decreased anterior or posterior tibiofemoral translation)[309,310] and possibly at the glenohumeral joint.[289] The joint approximation that occurs with the axial loading and weight bearing during closed-chain exercises is thought to cause an increase in joint congruency, which in turn contributes to stability.[58,85]

### Co-activation and Dynamic Stabilization

Because most closed-chain exercises are performed in weight-bearing positions, it has been assumed and commonly reported in the neurorehabilitation literature that closed-chain exercises stimulate joint and muscle mechanoreceptors, facilitate co-activation of agonists and antagonists (co-contraction), and consequently promote dynamic stability.[268,269,287] During a standing squat, for example, the quadriceps and hamstrings are thought to contract concurrently to control the knee and hip, respectively. In studies of lower extremity closed-chain exercises and activity of the knee musculature, this assumption has been both supported[29,46,256,300] and refuted.[88]

In the upper extremity, closed-chain exercises in weight-bearing positions are also thought to cause co-activation of the scapular and glenohumeral stabilizers and, therefore, to improve dynamic stability of the shoulder complex.[85,299] The assumption seems plausible, but evidence of co-contraction of muscles of the shoulder girdle during weight-bearing exercises, such as a prone push-up or a press-up in a chair, is just beginning to emerge,[177] making it difficult for clinicians to draw conclusions or make evidence-based decisions at this time.

There is also some thought that co-activation (co-contraction) of agonist and antagonist muscle groups may occur with selected open-chain exercises. Exercise interventions, such as alternating isometrics associated with PNF,[268,269,287] some stretch-shortening drills performed in non-weight-bearing positions,[302] use of a BodyBlade® (see Fig. 6.55), and high-velocity isokinetic training, may stimulate co-activation of muscle groups to promote dynamic stability. However, evidence of this possibility is limited.

In several studies of open-chain, high-velocity, concentric isokinetic training of knee musculature,[17,77,124] co-activation of agonist and antagonist muscle groups was noted briefly at the end the range of knee extension. Investigators speculated that the knee flexors fired and contracted eccentrically at the end of the range of knee extension to decelerate the limb just before contact was made with the ROM stop. However in another study, there was no evidence of co-activation of knee musculature or decreased anterior tibial translation with maximum-effort, slow-velocity (60°/sec), open-chain training.[174]

P R E C A U T I O N : High-load, open-chain exercise may have an adverse effect on unstable, injured, or recently repaired joints, as demonstrated in the ACL-deficient knee.[88,150,300,309]

### Proprioception, Kinesthesia, Neuromuscular Control, and Balance

Conscious awareness of joint position or movement is one of the foundations of motor learning during the early phase of training for neuromuscular control of functional movements. After soft tissue or joint injury, proprioception and kinesthesia are disrupted and alter neuromuscular control. Re-establishing the effective, efficient use of sensory information to initiate and control movement is a high priority in rehabilitation. Studies of the ACL-reconstructed knee have shown that proprioception and kinesthesia do improve after rehabilitation.[18,180]

It is thought that closed-chain training provides greater proprioceptive and kinesthetic feedback than open-chain training. Theoretically, because multiple muscle groups that cross multiple joints are activated during closed-chain exercise, more sensory receptors in more muscles and intra-articular and extra-articular structures are activated to control motion than during open-chain exercises. The weight-bearing element (axial loading) of closed-chain exercises, which causes joint approximation, is believed to stimulate mechanoreceptors in muscles and in and around joints to enhance sensory input for the control of movement.*

 **Focus on Evidence**_____

Despite the assumption that joint position or movement sense is enhanced to a greater extent under closed-chain than open-chain conditions, the evidence is mixed. The results of one study[181] indicated that in patients with unstable shoulders kinesthesia improved to a greater extent with a program of closed-chain and open-chain exercises compared to a program of only open-chain exercises. In contrast, in a comparison of the ability to detect knee position during closed-chain versus open-chain conditions, no significant difference was reported.[273]

---

Finally, closed-chain positioning is the obvious choice to improve balance and postural control in the upright position. Balance training is believed to be an essential element of the comprehensive rehabilitation of patients after musculoskeletal injuries or surgery, particularly in the lower extremities, to restore functional abilities and prevent reinjury.[155] Activities and parameters to challenge the body's balance mechanisms are discussed in Chapter 8.

### Carryover to Function and Injury Prevention

As already noted, there is ample evidence to demonstrate that both open- and closed-chain exercises effectively improve muscle strength, power, and endurance.[56,58,59] Evidence also suggests that if there is a comparable level of loading (amount of resistance) applied to a muscle group, EMG activity is similar regardless of whether open-chain or closed-chain exercise is performed.[24,72]

That being said, and consistent with the principle of motor learning and task-specific training, exercises should be incorporated into a rehabilitation program that simulate

---

* See references 128, 180, 181, 182, 183, 229, 253, 300.

the desired functions if the selected exercises are to have the most positive impact on function.[58,125,253,299] Studies of lower extremity functional tasks and open- and closed-chain exercises support specificity of training.

 **Focus on Evidence**

In a study of older women, stair-climbing abilities improved to a greater extent in participants who performed lower extremity strengthening exercises while standing (closed-chain exercises) and wearing a weighted backpack than those who performed traditional (open-chain) resistance exercises.[49] In another study, squatting exercises while standing, a closed-chain exercise, were shown to enhance performance of a jumping task more effectively than open-chain isokinetic knee extension exercises.[15] Closed-chain training, specifically a program of jumping activities, also has been shown to decrease landing forces through the knees and reduce the risk of knee injuries in female athletes.[133]

### Implementation and Progression of Open- and Closed-Chain Exercises

Principles and general guidelines for the implementation and progression of open-chain and closed-chain exercises are similar with respect to variables such as intensity, volume, frequency, and rest intervals. These variables were discussed earlier in the chapter. Relevant features of closed-chain exercises and guidelines for progression are summarized in Table 6.8.

### Introduction of Open-Chain Training

Because open-chain training typically is performed in non-weight-bearing postures, it may be the only option when weight bearing is contraindicated or must be significantly restricted or when unloading in a closed-chain position is not possible. Soft tissue pain and swelling or restricted motion of any segment of the chain may also necessitate the use of open-chain exercises at adjacent joints. After a fracture of the tibia, for example, the lower extremity usually is immobilized in a long leg cast, and weight bearing is restricted for at least a few weeks. During this period, hip strengthening exercises in an open chain manner can still be initiated and gradually progressed until partial weight bearing and closed-chain activities are permissible.

Any activity that involves open-chain motions can easily be replicated with open-chain exercises, first by developing isolated control and strength of the weak musculature and then by combining motions to simulate functional patterns.

### Closed-Chain Exercises and Weight-Bearing Restrictions—Use of Unloading

If weight bearing must be restricted, a safe alternative to open-chain exercises may be to perform closed-chain exer-

| TABLE 6.8 | Parameters and Progression of Closed-Chain Exercises |
|---|---|
| **Parameters** | **Progression** |
| % Body weight | Partial → full weight-bearing |
| | (LE: aquatic exercise, parallel bars, overhead harnessing; UE: wall push-up → modified prone push-up → prone push-up) |
| | Full weight bearing + additional weight |
| | (weighted vest or belt, handheld or cuff weights, elastic resistance) |
| Base of support | Wide → narrow |
| | Bilateral → unilateral |
| | Fixed on support surface → sliding on support surface |
| Support surface | Stable → unstable/moving |
| | (LE: floor → rocker board, wobble board, sideboard, treadmill) |
| | (UE: floor, table or wall → rocker or side board, ball) |
| | Rigid → soft |
| | (Floor, table → carpet, foam) |
| | Height: ground level → increasing height |
| | (Low step → high step) |
| Balance | With external support → no external support |
| | Eyes open → eyes closed |
| Exclusion of limb movement | Small → large ranges |
| | Short-arc → full-arc (if appropriate) |
| Plane or direction of movement | Uniplanar → multiplanar |
| | Anterior → posterior → diagonal |
| | (forward walking → retrowalking; forward step-up → backward step-up) |
| | Sagittal → frontal or transverse |
| | (forward-backward sliding → side to side sliding; forward or backward step-up → lateral step-up) |
| Speed of movement or directional changes | Slow → fast |

cises while partial weight bearing on the involved extremity. This is simple to achieve in the upper extremity; but in the lower extremity, because the patient is in an upright position during closed-chain exercises, axial loading in one or both lower extremities must be reduced.

Use of aquatic exercises, as described in Chapter 9, or decreasing the percentage of body weight borne on the involved lower extremity in parallel bars are both feasible unloading strategies even though each has limitations. It is difficult to control the extent of weight bearing when performing closed-chain exercises in parallel bars. In addition, lower limb movements while standing in the parallel bars or in water tend to be slower than what typically occurs during functional tasks. An alternative is the use of a harnessing system to unload the lower extremities.[157] This system enables a patient to perform a variety of closed-chain exercises and to begin ambulation on a treadmill at functional speeds early in rehabilitation.

### Progression of Closed-Chain Exercises

The parameters and suggestions for progression of closed-chain activities noted in Table 6.8 are not all-inclusive and are flexible. As a rehabilitation program progresses, plyometric training (discussed later in the chapter) and agility drills, more advanced forms of closed-chain training, can be introduced.[60,87] The selection and progression of activities should always be based on the discretion of the therapist and the patient's functional needs and response to exercise interventions.

## GENERAL PRINCIPLES OF RESISTANCE TRAINING

The principles of resistance training presented in this section apply to the use of both manual and mechanical resistance exercises for persons of all ages, but these principles are not "set in stone." There are many instances when they may or should be modified based on the judgment of the therapist. Additional guidelines specific to the application of manual resistance exercise, proprioceptive neuromuscular facilitation, and mechanical resistance exercise are addressed in later sections of this chapter.

### Examination and Evaluation

As with all forms of therapeutic exercise, a comprehensive examination and evaluation is the cornerstone of an individualized resistance training program. Therefore, prior to initiating any form of resistance exercise:

- Perform a thorough examination of the patient, including a health history, systems review, and selected tests and measurements.
  - Determine qualitative and quantitative baselines of strength, muscular endurance, ROM, and overall level of functional performance against which progress can be measured.
  - Implement testing procedures, such as manual muscle testing, determination of a repetition maximum,

dynamometry, goniometry, quantitative functional performance tests, and assessment of the patient's perceived level of disability.
- Interpret the findings to determine if the use of resistance exercise is appropriate or inappropriate at this time. Some questions that may need to be answered are noted in Box 6.9. Be sure to identify the most functionally relevant impairments, the goals the patient is seeking to achieve and the expected functional outcomes of the exercise program.
- Establish how resistance training will be integrated into the plan of care with other therapeutic exercise interventions, such as stretching, joint mobilization techniques, balance training, and cardiopulmonary conditioning exercises.
- Re-evaluate periodically to document progress and determine if and how the dosage of exercises (intensity, volume, frequency, rest) and the types of resistance exercise should be adjusted to continue to challenge the patient.

---

**BOX 6.9  Is Resistance Training Appropriate? Questions to Consider**

- Were deficits in muscle performance identified? If so, do these deficits appear to be contributing to limitations of functional abilities that you have observed or the patient or family has reported?
- Could identified deficits cause future impairment of function?
- What is the irritability and current stage of healing of involved tissues?
- Is there evidence of tissue swelling?
- Is there pain? (At rest or with movement? At what portion of the ROM? In what tissues?)
- Are there other deficits (such as impaired mobility, balance, sensation, coordination, or cognition) that are adversely affecting much of the performance?
- What are the patient's goals or desired functional outcomes? Are they realistic in light of the findings of the examination?
- Given the patient's current status, are resistance exercises indicated? Contraindicated?
- Can the identified deficits in muscle performance be eliminated or minimized with resistance exercises?
- If a decision is made to prescribe resistance exercises in the treatment plan, what resistance exercises are expected to be most effective?
- Should one area of muscle performance be emphasized over another?
- Will the patient require supervision or assistance over the course of the exercise program or can the program be carried out independently?
- What is the expected frequency and duration of the resistance training program? Will a maintenance program be necessary?
- Are there any precautions specific to the patient's physical status, general health, or age that may warrant special consideration?

## Preparation for Resistance Exercises

● Select and prescribe the forms of resistance exercise that are appropriate and expected to be effective, such as whether to implement manual or mechanical resistance exercises, or both.
● If implementing mechanical resistance exercise, determine what equipment is needed and available.
● Review the anticipated goals and expected functional outcomes.
● Explain the exercise plan and procedures. Be sure that the patient and/or family understands and gives consent.
● Have the patient wear nonrestrictive clothing and supportive shoes appropriate for exercise. If the patient is wearing a hospital gown, use a sheet to drape for modesty.
● If possible, select a firm but comfortable support surface for exercise.
● Demonstrate each exercise and the desired movement pattern.

## Application of Resistance Exercises

N O T E : These general guidelines apply to the use of *dynamic* exercises against manual *or* mechanical resistance. In addition to these guidelines, refer to special considerations and guidelines unique to the application of manual and mechanical resistance exercises in the sections of this chapter that follow.

### Warm Up

Prior to initiating resistance exercises, warm up with light, repetitive, dynamic, site-specific movements without applying resistance. For example, prior to lower extremity resistance exercises, have the patient walk on a treadmill, if possible, for 5 to 10 minutes followed by flexibility exercises for the trunk and lower extremities.

### Placement of Resistance

● Resistance is typically applied to the distal end of the segment in which the muscle to be strengthened attaches. Distal placement of resistance generates the greatest amount of external torque with the least amount of manual or mechanical resistance (load). For example, to strengthen the anterior deltoid, resistance is applied to the distal humerus as the patient flexes the shoulder (Fig. 6.12).
● Resistance may be applied across an intermediate joint if that joint is stable and pain-free and if there is adequate muscle strength supporting the joint. For example, to strengthen the anterior deltoid using mechanical resistance, a handheld weight is a common source of resistance.
● Revise the placement of resistance if pressure from the load is uncomfortable.

### Direction of Resistance

During *concentric* exercise resistance is applied in the direction *directly opposite* to the desired motion, whereas during *eccentric* exercise resistance is applied in the *same* direction as the desired motion (see Fig. 6.12).

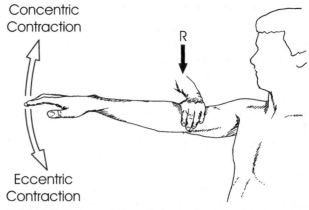

**FIGURE 6.12** Resistance (R) is applied to the distal end of the segment being strengthened. Resistance is applied in the *direction opposite* to that of limb movement to resist a concentric muscle contraction and in the *same direction* as limb movement to resist an eccentric contraction.

### Stabilization

Stabilization is necessary to avoid unwanted, substitute motions.

● For non-weight-bearing resisted exercises, external stabilization of a segment is usually applied at the proximal attachment of the muscle to be strengthened. In the case of the biceps brachii muscle, for example, stabilization should occur at the anterior shoulder as elbow flexion is resisted (Fig. 6.13). Equipment such as belts or straps are effective sources of external stabilization.
● During multijoint resisted exercises in weight-bearing postures, the patient must use muscle control (internal stabilization) to hold nonmoving segments in alignment.

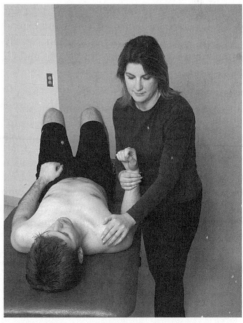

**FIGURE 6.13** Stabilization is applied at the proximal attachment of the muscle being strengthened. In this figure the proximal humerus and scapula are stabilized as elbow flexion is resisted.

### Intensity of Exercise/Amount of Resistance

N O T E : The intensity of the exercise (submaximal to near-maximal) must be consistent with the intended goals of resistance training and the type of muscle contraction as well as other aspects of dosage.

- Initially, have the patient practice the movement pattern against a minimal load to learn the correct pattern and the exercise technique.
- Have the patient exert a forceful but controlled and pain-free effort. The level of resistance should be such that movements are smooth and nonballistic or tremulous.
- Adjust the alignment, stabilization, or the amount of resistance if the patient is unable to complete the available ROM, muscular tremor develops, or substitute motions occur.

### Volume/Number of Repetitions and Sets and Rest Intervals

- In general, for most adults, use 8 to 12 repetitions of a specific motion against a moderate exercise load. This volume induces typical acute and chronic responses; that is, muscular fatigue and adaptive gains in muscular strength, respectively.
- Decrease the amount of resistance if the patient cannot complete 8 to 12 repetitions.
- After a brief rest, perform additional repetitions: a second set of 8 to 12 repetitions, if possible.
- For progressive overloading, initially increase the number of repetitions or sets; at a later point in the exercise program, gradually increase the resistance.

### Verbal or Written Instructions

When teaching an exercise using mechanical resistance or when applying manual resistance, use simple instructions that are easily understood. Do not use medical terminology or jargon. For example, tell the patient to "Bend and straighten your elbow" rather than "Flex and extend your elbow." Be sure that descriptions of resistance exercises to be performed in a home program are written and clearly illustrated.

### Monitoring the Patient

Assess the patient's responses before, during, and after exercise. It may be advisable to monitor the patient's vital signs. Adhere to relevant precautions discussed in the next section of the chapter.

### Cool Down

Cool down after a series of resistance exercises with rhythmic, unresisted movements, such as arm swinging, walking, or cycling. Gentle stretching is also appropriate after resistance exercise.

## PRECAUTIONS FOR RESISTANCE EXERCISE

Regardless of the goals of a resistance exercise program and the types of exercises prescribed and implemented,

---

| BOX 6.10 | General Precautions During Resistance Training |

- Keep the ambient temperature of the exercise setting comfortable for vigorous exercise. Select clothing for exercise that facilitates heat dissipation and does not impede sweat evaporation.
- Caution the patient that pain should *not* occur *during* exercise.
- Do not initiate resistance training at a maximal level of resistance, particularly with eccentric exercise to minimize delayed-onset muscle soreness (DOMS). Use light to moderate exercise during the recovery period.
- Avoid use of heavy resistance during exercise for children, older adults, and patients with osteoporosis.
- Do not apply resistance across an unstable joint or distal to a fracture site that is not completely healed.
- Have the patient avoid breath-holding during resisted exercises to prevent the Valsalva maneuver; emphasize exhalation during exertion.
- Avoid uncontrolled, ballistic movements as they compromise safety and effectiveness.
- Prevent incorrect or substitute motions by adequate stabilization and an appropriate level of resistance.
- Avoid exercises that place excessive, unintended secondary stress on the back.
- Be aware of medications a patient is using that can alter acute and chronic responses to exercise.
- Avoid cumulative fatigue due to excessive frequency of exercise and the effects of overtraining or overwork by incorporating adequate rest intervals between exercise sessions to allow adequate time for recovery after exercise.
- Discontinue exercises if the patient experiences pain, dizziness, or unusual or precipitous shortness of breath.

---

the exercises must not only be effective but *safe*. The therapist's interpretation of the examination's findings determine the exercise prescription. Awareness of precautions maximizes patient safety. General precautions for resistance training are summarized in Box 6.10.

Additional information about several of these precautions is presented in this section. Special considerations and precautions for children and older adults who participate in weight-training programs are addressed later in the chapter.

### Valsalva Maneuver

The Valsalva maneuver (phenomenon), which is defined as an expiratory effort against a closed glottis, must be avoided during resistance exercise. The Valsalva maneuver is characterized by the following sequence. A deep inspiration is followed by closure of the glottis and contraction of the abdominal muscles. This increases intra-abdominal and intrathoracic pressures, which in turn forces blood from the heart, causing an abrupt, temporary increase in arterial blood pressure.[151]

During exercise the Valsalva phenomenon occurs most often with *high-effort* isometric[94] and dynamic[187] muscle contractions. It has been shown that the rise in blood pressure induced by an isometric muscle contraction is proportional to the percentage of maximum voluntary force exerted.[187] During isokinetic (concentric) testing, if a patient exerts maximum effort at increasing velocities, the rise in blood pressure appears to be the same at all velocities of movement despite the fact that the force output of the muscle decreases.[76] Although occurrence of the Valsalva phenomenon more often is thought to be associated with isometric[94,151] and eccentric[62] resistance exercise, a recent study[187] indicated that the rise in blood pressure appears to be based more on extent of effort—not strictly on the mode of muscle contraction.

### At-Risk Patients

The risk of complications from a rapid rise in blood pressure is particularly high in patients with a history of coronary artery disease, myocardial infarction, cerebrovascular disorders, or hypertension. Also at risk are patients who have had neurosurgery or eye surgery or who have intervertebral disc pathology. High-risk patients must be monitored closely.

N O T E : Although resistance training is often recommended for individuals with a history of or who have a high risk for cardiovascular disorders,[7,8] it is important to distinguish those individuals for whom resistance training is or is not safe and appropriate. In addition to communicating with a patient's physician, guidelines are available to assist with this screening process.[7,8]

### Prevention During Resistance Exercise

- Caution the patient about breath-holding.
- Ask the patient to breathe rhythmically, count, or talk during exercise.
- Have the patient exhale with each resisted effort.
- Be certain that high-risk patients avoid high-intensity resistance exercises.

## Substitute Motions

If too much resistance is applied to a contracting muscle during exercise, substitute motions can occur. When muscles are weak because of fatigue, paralysis, or pain, a patient may attempt to carry out the desired movements that the weak muscles normally perform by any means possible.[158] For example, if the deltoid or supraspinatus muscles are weak or abduction of the arm is painful, a patient elevates the scapula (shrugs the shoulder) and laterally flexes the trunk to the opposite side to elevate the arm. It may appear that the patient is abducting the arm, but in fact that is not the case. To avoid substitute motions during exercise, an appropriate amount of resistance must be applied, and correct stabilization must be used with manual contacts, equipment, or by means of muscular (internal) stabilization by the patient.

## Overtraining and Overwork

Exercise programs in which heavy resistance is applied or exhaustive training is performed repeatedly must be progressed cautiously to avoid a problem known as overtraining or overwork. These terms refer to deterioration in muscle performance and physical capabilities (either temporary or permanent) that can occur in healthy individuals or in patients with certain neuromuscular disorders.

In most instances, the uncomfortable sensation associated with acute muscle fatigue induces an individual to cease exercising. This is not necessarily the case in highly motivated athletes who are said to be *overreaching* in their training program[110] or in patients who may not adequately sense fatigue because of impaired sensation associated with a neuromuscular disorder.[219]

### Overtraining

The term *overtraining* is commonly used to describe a decline in physical performance in healthy individuals participating in high-intensity, high-volume strength and endurance training programs.[14,110,173] The terms *chronic fatigue, staleness,* and *burnout* are also used to describe this phenomenon. When overtraining occurs, the individual progressively fatigues more quickly and requires more time to recover from strenuous exercise because of physiological and psychological factors.

Overtraining is brought on by inadequate rest intervals between exercise sessions, too rapid progression of exercises, and inadequate diet and fluid intake. Fortunately, in healthy individuals, overtraining is a preventable, reversible phenomenon that can be resolved by tapering the training program for a period of time by periodically decreasing the volume and frequency of exercise (periodization).[110,168,170,173]

### Overwork

The term *overwork*, sometimes called *overwork weakness*, refers to progressive deterioration of strength in muscles already weakened by nonprogressive neuromuscular disease.[219] This phenomenon was first observed more than 50 years ago in patients recovering from polio who were actively involved in rehabilitation.[21] In many instances the decrement in strength that was noted was permanent or prolonged. More recently, overwork weakness has been reported in patients with other nonprogressive neuromuscular diseases, such as Guillain-Barré syndrome.[54] Postpolio syndrome is also thought to be related to long-term overuse of weak muscles.[98]

*Overwork weakness* has been produced in laboratory animals,[130] which provides some insight to its cause. When strenuous exercise was initiated soon after a peripheral nerve lesion, the return of functional motor strength was retarded. It was suggested that this could be caused by excessive protein breakdown in the denervated muscle.

Prevention is the key to dealing with overwork weakness. Patients in resistance exercise programs who have impaired neuromuscular function or a systemic, metabolic, or inflammatory disease that increases susceptibility to muscle fatigue must be monitored closely, progressed slowly and cautiously, and re-evaluated frequently to determine their response to resistance training. These patients should not exercise to exhaustion and should be given longer and more frequent rest intervals during and between exercise sessions.[4,54]

## Exercise-Induced Muscle Soreness

Almost every individual unaccustomed to exercise who begins a resistance training program, particularly one that includes eccentric exercise, experiences muscle soreness. Exercise-induced muscle soreness falls into two categories: acute and delayed onset.

### Acute Muscle Soreness

Acute muscle soreness develops during or directly after strenuous exercise performed to the point of muscle exhaustion.[41] This response occurs as a muscle becomes fatigued during acute exercise because of the lack of adequate blood flow and oxygen (ischemia) and a temporary buildup of metabolites, such as lactic acid and potassium, in the exercised muscle.[41,166] The sensation is characterized as a feeling of burning or aching in the muscle. It is thought that the noxious metabolic waste products may stimulate free nerve endings and cause pain. The muscle pain experienced during intense exercise is transient and subsides quickly after exercise when adequate blood flow and oxygen are restored to the muscle. An appropriate cool-down period of low-intensity exercise (active recovery) can facilitate this process.[48]

### Delayed-Onset Muscle Soreness

After vigorous and unaccustomed resistance training or any form of muscular overexertion, delayed-onset muscle soreness (DOMS), which is noticeable in the muscle belly or at the myotendinous junction,[70,104,144] begins to develop approximately 12 to 24 hours after the cessation of exercise. As was already pointed out in the discussion of concentric and eccentric exercise in this chapter, high-intensity eccentric muscle contractions consistently cause the most severe DOMS symptoms.[13,62,78,100,104,215] Box 6.11 lists the signs and symptoms over the time course of DOMS.[*] The DOMS sensation usually intensifies and peaks 24 to 48 hours after exercise. Although the time course varies, the signs and symptoms, which can last up to 10 to 14 days, gradually dissipate.[13,78,100]

**Etiology of DOMS.** Despite years of research dating back to the early 1900s,[142] the underlying mechanism of tissue damage associated with DOMS is still unclear.[40] Several theories have been proposed, and some have subsequently been refuted. Early investigators proposed the *metabolic waste accumulation theory,* which suggested that both acute and delayed-onset muscle soreness was caused by a buildup of lactic acid in muscle after exercise. Although

---

[*] See references 13, 40, 41, 70, 84, 104, 126, 144.

---

| BOX 6.11 | Delayed-Onset Muscle Soreness: Clinical Signs and Symptoms |
|---|---|

- Muscle soreness and aching beginning 12 to 24 hours after exercise and peaking at 48 to 72 hours
- Tenderness with palpation throughout the involved muscle belly or at the myotendinous junction
- Increased soreness with passive lengthening or active contraction of the involved muscle
- Local edema and warmth
- Muscle stiffness reflected by spontaneous muscle shortening[66] before the onset of pain
- Decreased ROM during the time course of muscle soreness
- Decreased muscle strength prior to onset of muscle soreness that persists for up to 1 to 2 weeks after soreness has remitted[38,117,229]

---

this is a source of muscle pain with acute exercise, this theory has been disproved as a cause of DOMS.[288] Multiple studies have shown that it requires only about 1 hour of recovery after exercise to exhaustion to remove almost all lactic acid from skeletal muscle and blood.[104]

The *muscle spasm theory* also was proposed as the cause of DOMS, suggesting that a feedback cycle of pain caused by ischemia and a buildup of metabolic waste products during exercise led to muscle spasm.[69] This, it was hypothesized, caused the DOMS sensation and an ongoing reflex pain–spasm cycle that lasted for several days after exercise. The muscle spasm theory has been discounted in subsequent research that showed no increase in EMG activity and therefore no evidence of spasm in muscles with delayed soreness.[2]

Although studies on the specific etiology of DOMS continue, current research seems to suggest that DOMS is linked to some form of contraction-induced, mechanical disruption (microtrauma) of muscle fibers and/or connective tissue in and around muscle that results in degeneration of the tissue.[40,108] Evidence of tissue damage such as elevated blood serum levels of creatine kinase, is present for several days after exercise and is accompanied by inflammation and edema.[2,106,108]

The temporary loss of strength and the perception of soreness or aching associated with DOMS appear to occur independently and follow different time courses. Strength deficits develop prior to the onset of soreness and persist after soreness has remitted.[66,212] Thus, force production deficits appear to be the result of muscle damage, possibly myofibrillar damage at the Z bands,[40,211] which directly affects the structural integrity of the contractile units of muscle, not neuromuscular inhibition as the result of pain.[211,212]

**Prevention and treatment of DOMS.** Prevention and treatment of DOMS at the initiation of an exercise program after a short or long period of inactivity has been either ineffective or, at best, marginally successful. It is a commonly held opinion in clinical and fitness settings that the initial onset of DOMS can be prevented or at least kept to a minimum by progressing the intensity and volume of exercise *gradually*,[44,78] by performing low-intensity warm-up and cool-down activities,[68,78,193,249] or by gently stretching the exercised muscles before and after strenuous exercise.[68,249] Although these techniques are regularly advocated and employed, little to no evidence in the literature supports their efficacy in the prevention of DOMS.

There is some evidence to suggest that the use of repetitive concentric exercise prior to DOMS-inducing eccentric exercise does not entirely prevent but reduces the severity of muscle soreness and other markers of muscle damage.[214] Paradoxically, the best prevention of DOMS appears to be a regular routine of exercise, particularly eccentric exercise, after an initial episode of DOMS has developed and remitted.[40,41,44,172] It may well be that with repeated bouts of the same level of eccentric exercise or activity that caused the initial episode of DOMS the muscle adapts to the physical stress, resulting in the prevention of additional episodes of DOMS.[40,176]

Effective treatment of DOMS once it has occurred is continually being sought because, to date, the efficacy of DOMS treatment has been mixed. Evidence shows that continuation of a training program that has induced DOMS does not worsen the muscle damage or slow the recovery process.[40,215] Light, high-speed (isokinetic), concentric exercise has been reported to reduce muscle soreness and hasten the remediation of strength deficits associated with DOMS,[126] but other reports suggest no significant improvement in strength or relief of muscle soreness with light exercise.[74,290]

The value of therapeutic modalities and massage techniques is also questionable. Electrical stimulation to reduce soreness has been reported to be effective[66] and ineffective.[290] Although cryotherapy (cold water immersion) after vigorous eccentric exercise reduces signs of muscle damage (creatine kinase activity), it has been reported to have no effect on the perpetuation of muscle tenderness or strength deficit.[89] There is also no significant evidence that postexercise massage, despite its widespread use in sports settings, reduces the signs and symptoms of DOMS.[153,277,290]

In a prospective study[167,171] of DOMS that was induced by maximal eccentric exercise, the use of a compression sleeve over the exercised muscle group resulted in no increase in circumferential measurements of the upper arm (which could suggest prevention of soft tissue swelling), more rapid reduction in the perception of muscle soreness, and more rapid amelioration of deficits in peak torque than recovery from DOMS without the use of compression. Finally, topical salicylate creams, which provide an analgesic effect, may also reduce the severity of and hasten the recovery from DOMS-related symptoms.[134] In summary, although some interventions for the treatment of DOMS appear to have potential, a definitive treatment has yet to be determined.

## Pathological Fracture

When a patient with known (or at high risk for) osteoporosis or osteopenia participates in a resistance exercise program, the risk of pathological fracture must be addressed. *Osteoporosis,* which is discussed in greater detail in Chapter 11, is a systemic skeletal disease characterized by reduced mineralized bone mass that is associated with an imbalance between bone resorption and bone formation, leading to fragility of bones. In addition to the loss of bone mass, there is also narrowing of the bone shaft and widening of the medullary canal.[28,83,175,243]

The changes in bone associated with osteoporosis make the bone less able to withstand physical stress. Consequently, bones become highly susceptible to pathological fracture. A *pathological fracture* (fragility fracture) is a fracture of bone already weakened by disease that occurs as the result of minor stress to the skeletal system.[28,83,112,190,210] Pathological fractures most commonly occur in the vertebrae, hips, wrists, and ribs.[83,175] Therefore, to design and implement a safe exercise program, a therapist needs to know if a patient has a history of osteoporosis and, as such, an increased risk of pathological fracture. If there is no known history of osteoporosis, the therapist must be able to recognize those factors that place a patient at risk for osteoporosis.[28,51,52,83,112,175,190] As noted in Chapter 11, postmenopausal women, for example, are at high risk for primary (type I) osteoporosis. Secondary (type II) osteoporosis is associated with prolonged immobilization or disuse, restricted weight bearing, or extended use of certain medications, such as systemic corticosteroids or immunosuppressants.

### Prevention of Pathological Fracture
As noted earlier in the chapter, evidence of the positive osteogenic effects of resistance exercise is promising but not yet clear. Despite this, resistance exercises have become an essential element of rehabilitation and conditioning programs for patients with known, or who are at risk for, osteoporosis.[51,225,239,243] Therefore, patients who are at risk for pathological fracture often engage in resistance training.[210]

Successful, safe resistance training for these patients imposes enough load (greater than what regularly occurs with activities of daily living) to achieve the goals of the exercise program (which include increasing bone density as well as improving muscle performance and functional abilities) but not too heavy a load that could cause a pathological fracture. Precautions to prevent or reduce the risk of pathological fracture are summarized in Box 6.12.[51,112,210,225,239,243]

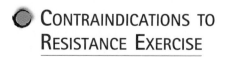

## CONTRAINDICATIONS TO RESISTANCE EXERCISE

There are only a few instances when resistance exercises are contraindicated. Resistance training is most often con-

## BOX 6.12    Precautions to Reduce the Risk of Pathological Fracture During Exercise

- Avoid high-intensity (high-load), high-volume weight training. Depending on the severity of osteoporosis, begin weight training at low intensities; initially, perform only one set of several exercises and keep the intensity low for the first 6 to 8 weeks.
- Progress intensity and volume (repetitions) gradually; eventually work up to three or four sets of each exercise at moderate levels of intensity, if appropriate.
- Avoid high-impact activities such as jumping or hopping. Perform most strengthening exercises in weight-bearing postures that involve low impact to no impact, such as lunges or step-ups/step-downs against additional resistance (hand-held weights, a weighted vest, or elastic resistance).
- Avoid high-velocity movements of the spine or extremities.
- Avoid trunk flexion with rotation and end-range resisted flexion of the spine that could place excessive loading on the anterior portion of the vertebrae, potentially resulting in anterior compression fracture, wedging of the vertebral body, and loss of height.
- Avoid lower extremity weight-bearing activities that involve torsional movements of the hips, particularly if there is evidence of osteoporosis of the proximal femur.
- To avoid loss of balance or falling during lower extremity exercises while standing, have the patient hold onto a stable surface such as a countertop for balance. If the patient is at high risk for falling or has a history of falls, perform exercises in a chair to provide weight bearing through the spine.
- In group exercise classes keep participant/instructor ratios low; for patients at high risk for falling or with a history of previous fracture, consider direct supervision on a one-to-one basis from another trained person.

traindicated during periods of acute inflammation and with some acute diseases and disorders.[32] By carefully selecting the appropriate mode of exercise (static vs. dynamic; weight-bearing vs. non-weight-bearing) and keeping the initial intensity of the exercise at a very low to moderate level, adverse effects from resistance training can be avoided.

## Pain

If a patient experiences severe joint or muscle pain during active-free (unresisted) movements, dynamic resistance exercises should not be initiated. During testing, if a patient experiences acute muscle pain during a resisted isometric contraction, resistance exercises (static or dynamic) should not be initiated. If a patient experiences pain that cannot be eliminated by reducing the resistance, the exercise should be stopped.

## Inflammation

Dynamic and static resistance training is absolutely contraindicated in the presence of inflammatory neuromuscular disease. For example, in patients with acute anterior horn cell disease (Guillain-Barré) or inflammatory muscle disease (polymyositis, dermatomyositis) resistance exercises may actually cause irreversible deterioration of strength as the result of damage to muscle. *Dynamic* resistance exercises are contraindicated in the presence of acute inflammation of a joint. The use of dynamic resisted exercise can irritate the joint and cause more inflammation. Gentle setting (static) exercises against negligible resistance are appropriate.

## Severe Cardiopulmonary Disease

Severe cardiac or respiratory diseases or disorders associated with acute symptoms contraindicate resistance training. For example, patients with severe coronary artery disease, carditis, or cardiac myopathy should not participate in vigorous physical activities, including a resistance training program.[7,8] Resistance training should be postponed for up to 12 weeks after myocardial infarction or coronary artery bypass graft surgery or until the patient has clearance from a physician.[32]

##  MANUAL RESISTANCE EXERCISE

### Definition and Use

*Manual resistance exercise* is a form of active resistive exercise in which the resistance force is applied by the therapist to either a dynamic or a static muscular contraction.

- When joint motion is permissible, resistance is usually applied throughout the available ROM as the muscle contracts and shortens or lengthens under tension.
- Exercise is carried out in the anatomical planes of motion, in diagonal patterns associated with proprioceptive neuromuscular facilitation (PNF) techniques,[165,287] or in combined patterns of movement that simulate functional activities.
- A specific muscle may also be strengthened by resisting the action of that muscle, as described in manual muscle-testing procedures.[137,158]
- In rehabilitation programs, manual resistance exercise, which may be preceded by active-assisted and active exercise, is part of the continuum of active exercises available to a therapist for the improvement or restoration of muscular strength and endurance.

There are many advantages to the use of manual resistance exercises, but there are also disadvantages and limitations to this form of resistance exercises. These issues are summarized in Box 6.13.

BOX 6.13 Manual Resistance Exercise:
Advantages and Disadvantages

### Advantages

- Most effective during the early stages of rehabilitation when muscles are weak (4/5 or less).
- Effective form of exercise for transition from assisted to mechanically resisted movements.
- More finely graded resistance than mechanical resistance.
- Resistance is adjusted throughout the ROM as the therapist responds to the patient's efforts or a painful arc.
- Muscle works maximally at all portions of the ROM.
- The range of joint movement can be carefully controlled by the therapist to protect healing tissues or to prevent movement into an unstable portion of the range.
- Useful for dynamic or static strengthening.
- Direct manual stabilization prevents substitute motions.
- Can be performed in a variety of patient positions.
- Placement of resistance is easily adjusted.
- Gives the therapist an opportunity for direct interaction with the patient to monitor the patient's performance continually.

### Disadvantages

- Exercise load (amount of resistance) is subjective; it cannot be measured or quantitatively documented for purposes of establishing a baseline and exercise-induced improvements in muscle performance.
- Amount of resistance is limited to the strength of the therapist; therefore, resistance imposed is not adequate to strengthen already strong muscle groups.
- Little value for strong muscle groups.
- Speed of movement is slow to moderate, which may not carry over to most functional activities.
- Cannot be performed independently by the patient to strengthen most muscle groups.
- Not useful in home program unless caregiver assistance is available.
- Labor- and time-intensive for the therapist.
- Impractical for improving muscular endurance; too time-consuming.

## Guidelines and Special Considerations

The general principles for the application of resistance exercises discussed in the preceding section of this chapter apply to manual resistance exercise. In addition, there are some special guidelines that are unique to manual resistance exercises that also should be followed when using this form of exercise. These guidelines apply to manual resistance applied in anatomical planes of motion, discussed in this section, and to manual resistance used in association with PNF, discussed in the following section.

### Body Mechanics of the Therapist

- Select a treatment table on which to position the patient that is a suitable height or adjust the height of the patient's bed, if possible, to enhance use of proper body mechanics.
- Assume a position close to the patient to avoid stresses on your low back and to maximize control of the patient's upper or lower extremity.
- Use a wide base of support to maintain a stable posture while manually applying resistance; shift your weight to move as the patient moves his or her limb.

### Application of Manual Resistance and Stabilization

- Review the principles and guidelines for placement and direction of resistance and stabilization (see Figs. 6.12 and 6.13). Stabilize the proximal attachment of the contracting muscle with one hand, when necessary, while applying resistance distally to the moving segment. Use appropriate hand placements (manual contacts) to provide tactile and proprioceptive cues to help the patient better understand in which direction to move.[269]
- Grade and vary the amount of resistance to equal the abilities of the muscle through all portions of the available ROM.

N O T E : It requires well developed skills on the part of the therapist to provide enough resistance to challenge but not overpower the patient's efforts, especially when the patient has significant weakness.

- Gradually apply and release the resistance so movements are smooth, not unexpected or uncontrolled.
- Hold the patient's extremity close to your body so some of the force applied is from the weight of your body not just the strength of your upper extremities. This allows you to apply a greater amount of resistance, particularly as the patient's strength increases.
- When applying manual resistance to alternating isometric contractions of agonist and antagonist muscles to develop joint stability, maintain manual contacts at all times as the isometric contractions are repeated. As a transition is made from one muscle contraction to another, no abrupt relaxation phase or joint movements should occur between the opposing contractions.

### Verbal Commands

- Coordinate the *timing* of the verbal commands with the application of resistance to maintain control when the patient initiates a movement.
- Use simple, direct verbal commands.
- Use different verbal commands to facilitate isometric, concentric, or eccentric contractions. To resist an *isometric* contraction, tell the patient to "Hold" or "Don't let me move you" or "Match my resistance." To resist a *concentric* contraction, tell the patient to "Push" or "Pull." To resist an *eccentric* contraction, tell the patient to "Slowly let go as I push or pull you."

### Number of Repetitions and Sets; Rest Intervals

- As with all forms of resistance exercise, the number of repetitions is dependent on the response of the patient.

- For manual resistance exercise, the number of repetitions of exercise is also contingent on the strength and endurance of the therapist.
- Build in adequate rest intervals for the patient *and* the therapist; after 8 to 12 repetitions, both the patient and the therapist begin to experience some degree of muscular fatigue.

## Techniques—General Background

The manual resistance exercise techniques described in this section are for the upper and lower extremities, performed concentrically in the anatomical planes of motion. The direction of limb movement would be the opposite if manual resistance were applied to an eccentric contraction. The exercises described are performed in non-weight-bearing positions and involve movements to isolate individual muscles or muscle groups.

Consistent with Chapter 3, most of the exercises described and illustrated in this section are performed with the patient in a *supine position.* Variations in the therapist's position and hand placements may be necessary, depending on the size and strength of the therapist and the patient. Alternate positions, such as prone or sitting, are described when appropriate or necessary. Ultimately, a therapist must be versatile and able to apply manual resistance with the patient in all positions to meet the needs of many patients with significant differences in abilities, limitations, and pathologies.

N O T E : In all illustrations in this section, the direction in which resistance (R) is applied is indicated with a solid arrow.

Opposite motions, such as flexion/extension and abduction/adduction, are often alternately resisted in an exercise program in which strength and balanced neuromuscular control in both agonists and antagonists are desired. Resistance to reciprocal movement patterns also enhances a patient's ability to reverse the direction of movement smoothly and quickly, a neuromuscular skill that is necessary in many functional activities. Reversal of direction requires muscular control of both prime movers and stabilizers and combines concentric and eccentric contractions to decrease momentum and make a controlled transition from one direction to the opposite direction of movement.

The use of manual resistance in diagonal patterns of motion associated with PNF are described and illustrated in the next section of this chapter. Additional exercises to increase strength, endurance, and neuromuscular control in the extremities can be found in Chapters 17 through 22. In these chapters many examples and illustrations of resisted eccentric exercises, exercises in weight-bearing (closed-chain) positions, and exercises in functional movement patterns are included. Resistance exercises for the cervical, thoracic, and lumbar spine are described and illustrated in Chapter 16.

## Upper Extremity

### Flexion of the Shoulder

**Hand Placement and Procedure**

- Apply resistance to the anterior aspect of the distal arm or to the distal portion of the forearm if the elbow is stable and pain-free (Fig. 6.14).
- Stabilization of the scapula and trunk is provided by the treatment table.

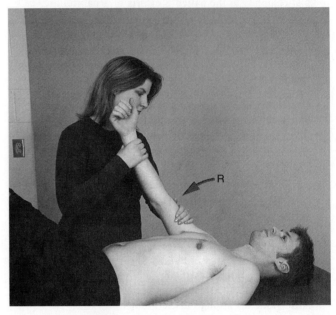

FIGURE 6.14 Resisted shoulder flexion.

### Extension of the Shoulder

**Hand Placement and Procedure**

- Apply resistance to the posterior aspect of the distal arm or the distal portion of the forearm.
- Stabilization of the scapula is provided by the table.

### Hyperextension of the Shoulder

The patient may be in the supine position, close to the edge of the table, side-lying, or prone so hyperextension can occur.

**Hand Placement and Procedure**

- Apply resistance in the same manner as for extension of the shoulder.
- Stabilize the anterior aspect of the shoulder if the patient is supine.
- If the patient is side-lying, adequate stabilization must be given to the trunk and scapula. This can usually be done if the therapist places the patient close to the edge of the table and stabilizes the patient with the lower trunk.
- If the patient is lying prone, manually stabilize the scapula.

## Abduction and Adduction of the Shoulder

### Hand Placement and Procedure

● Apply resistance to the distal portion of the arm with the patient's elbow flexed to 90°. To resist abduction (Fig. 6.15), apply resistance to the lateral aspect of the arm. To resist adduction, apply resistance to the medial aspect of the arm.
● Stabilization (although not pictured in Fig. 6.15) is applied to the superior aspect of the shoulder, if necessary, to prevent the patient from *initiating* abduction by shrugging the shoulder (elevation of the scapula).

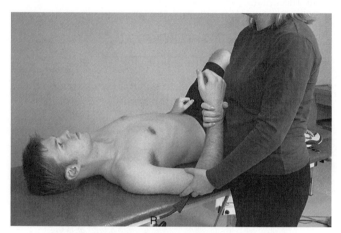

FIGURE 6.15 Resisted shoulder abduction.

PRECAUTION: Allow the glenohumoral joint to externally rotate when resisting abduction above 90° to prevent impingement.

### Elevation of the Arm in the Plane of the Scapula ("Scaption")

### Hand Placement and Procedure

● Same as previously described for shoulder flexion.
● Apply resistance as the patient elevates the arm in the plane of the scapula (30° to 40° anterior to the frontal plane of the body).[53,73,184]

NOTE: Although "scaption" is not a motion of the shoulder that occurs in one of the anatomical planes of the body, resistance in the scapular plane is thought to have its merits. The evidence is inconclusive[53,238,297] as to whether the torque-producing capabilities of the key muscle groups of the glenohumeral joint are greater when the arm elevates in the plane of the scapula versus the frontal or sagittal planes; however, the glenohumeral joint has been shown to be more stable, and there is less risk of impingement of soft tissues when strength training is performed in the scapular plane.[73] (See additional discussion in Chapter 17.)

## Internal and External Rotation of the Shoulder

### Hand Placement and Procedure

● Flex the elbow to 90° and position the shoulder in the plane of the scapula.
● Apply resistance to the distal portion of the forearm during internal rotation and external rotation (Fig. 6.16A).
● Stabilize at the level of the clavicle during internal rotation; the back and scapula are stabilized by the table during external rotation.

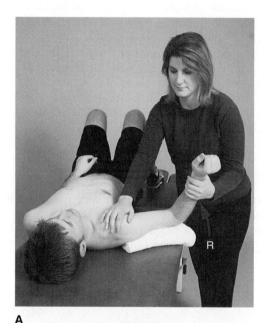

A

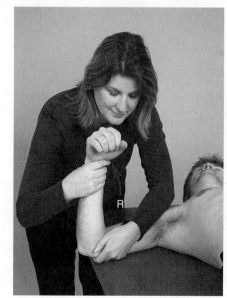

B

FIGURE 6.16 (A) Resisted external rotation of the shoulder with the shoulder positioned in flexion and abduction (approaching the plane of the scapula). (B) Resisted internal rotation of the shoulder with the shoulder in 90° of abduction.

### Alternate Procedure

Alternate alignment of the humerus (Fig. 6.16B). If the mobility and stability of the glenohumeral joint permit, the shoulder can be positioned in 90° of abduction during resisted rotation.

### Horizontal Abduction and Adduction of the Shoulder

#### Hand Placement and Procedure

- Flex the shoulder and elbow to 90° and place the shoulder in neutral rotation.
- Apply resistance to the distal portion of the arm just above the elbow during horizontal adduction and abduction.
- Stabilize the anterior aspect of the shoulder during horizontal adduction. The table stabilizes the scapula and trunk during horizontal abduction.
- To resist horizontal abduction from 0° to 45°, the patient must be close to the edge of the table while supine or be placed side-lying or prone.

### Elevation and Depression of the Scapula

#### Hand Placement and Procedure

- Have the patient assume a supine, side-lying, or sitting position.
- Apply resistance along the superior aspect of the shoulder girdle just above the clavicle during scapular elevation (Fig. 6.17).

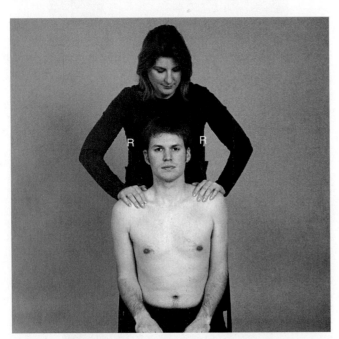

FIGURE 6.17 Elevation of the shoulders (scapulae), resisted bilaterally.

### Alternate Procedures: Scapular Depression

To resist unilateral scapular depression in the supine position, have the patient attempt to reach down toward the feet and push the hand into the therapist's hand. When the patient has adequate strength, the exercise can be performed to include weight bearing through the upper extremity by having the patient sit on the edge of a low table and lift the body weight with both hands.

### Protraction and Retraction of the Scapula

#### Hand Placement and Procedure

- Apply resistance to the anterior portion of the shoulder at the head of the humerus to resist protraction and to the posterior aspect of the shoulder to resist retraction.
- Resistance may also be applied directly to the scapula if the patient sits or lies on the side, facing the therapist.
- Stabilize the trunk to prevent trunk rotation.

### Flexion and Extension of the Elbow

#### Hand Placement and Procedure

- To strengthen the elbow flexors, apply resistance to the anterior aspect of the distal forearm (Fig. 6.18).

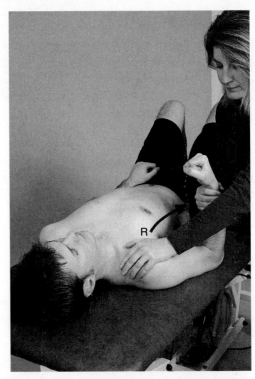

FIGURE 6.18 Resisted elbow flexion with proximal stabilization.

- The forearm may be positioned in supination, pronation, and neutral to resist individual flexor muscles of the elbow.
- To strengthen the elbow extensors, place the patient prone (Fig. 6.19) or supine and apply resistance to the distal aspect of the forearm.
- Stabilize the upper portion of the humerus during both motions.

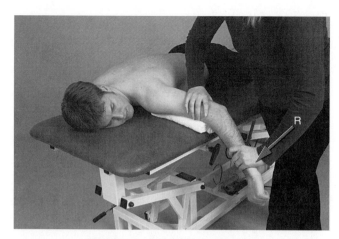

FIGURE 6.19 Resisted elbow extension.

## Pronation and Supination of the Forearm

### Hand Placement and Procedure

- Apply resistance to the radius of the distal forearm with the patient's elbow flexed to 90° (Fig. 6.20) to prevent rotation of the humerus.
- Do not apply resistance to the hand to avoid twisting forces at the wrist.

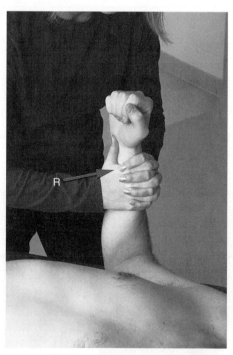

FIGURE 6.20 Resisted pronation of the forearm.

## Flexion and Extension of the Wrist

### Hand Placement and Procedure

- Apply resistance to the volar and dorsal aspects of the hand at the level of the metacarpals to resist flexion and extension, respectively (Fig. 6.21).
- Stabilize the volar or dorsal aspect of the distal forearm.

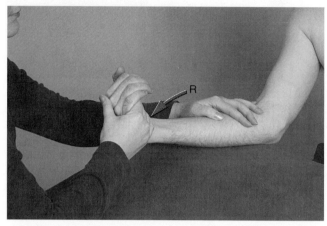

FIGURE 6.21 Resisted wrist flexion and stabilization of the forearm.

## Radial and Ulnar Deviation of the Wrist

### Hand Placement and Procedure

- Apply resistance to the second and fifth metacarpals alternately to resist radial and ulnar deviation.
- Stabilize the distal forearm.

## Motions of the Fingers and Thumb

### Hand Placement and Procedure

- Apply resistance just distal to the joint that is moving. Resistance is applied to one joint motion at a time (Figs. 6.22 and 6.23).
- Stabilize the joints proximal and distal to the moving joint.

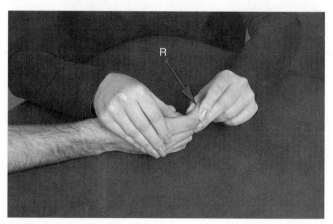

FIGURE 6.22 Resisted flexion of the proximal interphalangeal (PIP) joint of the index finger with stabilization of the metacarpophalangeal (MCP) and distal interphalangeal (DIP) joints.

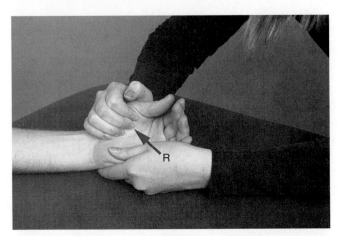

FIGURE 6.23 Resisted opposition of the thumb.

## Lower Extremity

### Flexion of the Hip with Knee Flexion

**Hand Placement and Procedure**

- Apply resistance to the anterior portion of the distal thigh (Fig. 6.24). Simultaneous resistance to knee flexion may be applied at the distal and posterior aspect of the lower leg, just above the ankle.
- Stabilization of the pelvis and lumbar spine is provided by adequate strength of the abdominal muscles.

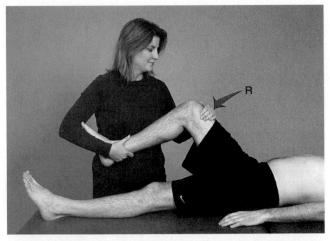

FIGURE 6.24 Resisted flexion of the hip with the knee flexed.

PRECAUTION: If, when the opposite hip is extended, the pelvis rotates anteriorly, and lordosis in the lumbar spine increases during resisted hip flexion, have the patient flex the opposite hip and knee and plant the foot on the table to stabilize the pelvis and protect the low back region.

### Extension of the Hip

**Hand Placement and Procedure**

- Apply resistance to the posterior aspect of the distal thigh with one hand and to the inferior and distal aspect of the heel with the other hand (Fig. 6.25).
- Stabilization of the pelvis and lumbar spine is provided by the table.

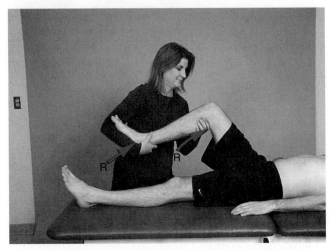

FIGURE 6.25 Resisted hip and knee extension with the hand placed at the popliteal space to prevent hyperextension of the knee.

### Hyperextension of the Hip
*Patient position*: prone.

**Hand Placement and Procedure**

- With patient in a prone position, apply resistance to the posterior aspect of the distal thigh (Fig. 6.26).
- Stabilize the posterior aspect of the pelvis to avoid motion of the lumbar spine.

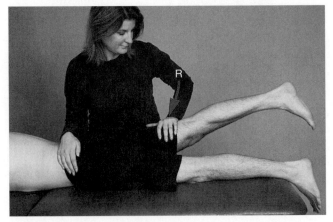

FIGURE 6.26 Resisted end-range hip extension with stabilization of the pelvis.

## Abduction and Adduction of the Hip

### Hand Placement and Procedure

● Apply resistance to the lateral and the medial aspects of the distal thigh to resist abduction (Fig. 6.27) and adduction, respectively, or to the lateral and medial aspects of the distal leg just above the malleoli if the knee is stable and pain-free.

● Stabilization is applied to the pelvis to avoid hip-hiking from substitute action of the quadratus lumborum and to keep the thigh in neutral position to prevent external rotation of the femur and subsequent substitution by the iliopsoas.

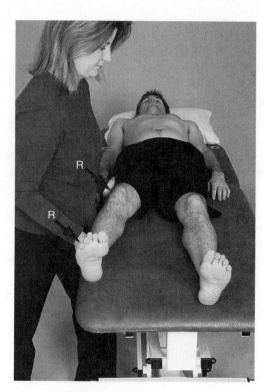

FIGURE 6.27 Resisted hip abduction.

## Internal and External Rotation of the Hip

*Patient position*: supine with the hip and knee extended.

### Hand Placement and Procedure

● Apply resistance to the lateral aspect of the distal thigh to resist external rotation and to the medial aspect of the thigh to resist internal rotation.

● Stabilize the pelvis.

*Patient position*: supine with the hip and knee flexed (Fig. 6.28).

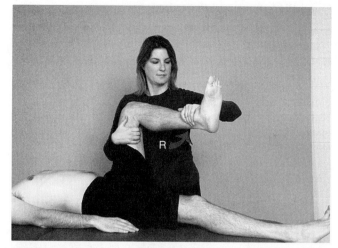

FIGURE 6.28 Resisted external rotation of the hip with the patient lying supine.

### Hand Placement and Procedure

● Apply resistance to the medial aspect of the lower leg just above the malleolus during external rotation and to the lateral aspect of the lower leg during internal rotation.

● Stabilize the anterior aspect of the pelvis as the thigh is supported to keep the hip in 90° of flexion.

*Patient position*: prone, with the hip extended and the knee flexed (Fig. 6.29).

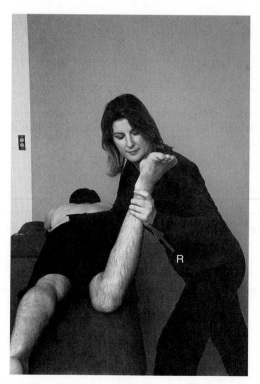

FIGURE 6.29 Resisted internal rotation of the hip with the patient lying prone.

## Hand Placement and Procedure

- Apply resistance to the medial and lateral aspects of the lower leg.
- Stabilize the pelvis by applying pressure across the buttocks.

### Flexion of the Knee

Resistance to knee flexion may be combined with resistance to hip flexion, as described earlier with the patient supine.

*Patient position*: prone with the hip extended (Fig. 6.30).

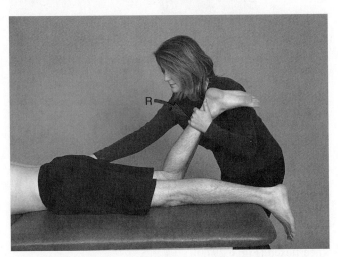

**FIGURE 6.30** Resisted knee flexion with stabilization of the hip.

### Hand Placement

- Apply resistance to the posterior aspect of the lower leg just above the heel.
- Stabilize the posterior pelvis across the buttocks.

The patient may also be sitting at the edge of a table with the hips and knees flexed and the trunk supported and stabilized.

### Extension of the Knee

### Alternate Patient Positions

- If the patient is lying supine on a table, the hip must be abducted and the knee flexed so the lower leg is over the side of the table. This position should not be used if the rectus femoris or iliopsoas is tight because it causes an anterior tilt of the pelvis and places stress on the low back.

- If the patient is prone, place a rolled towel under the anterior aspect of the distal thigh; this allows the patella to glide normally during knee extension.
- If the patient is sitting, place a rolled towel under the posterior aspect of the distal thigh (Fig. 6.31).

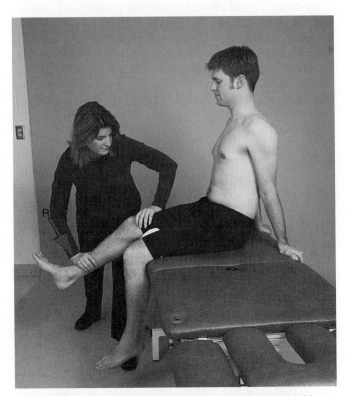

**FIGURE 6.31** Resisted knee extension with the patient sitting and stabilizing the trunk with the upper extremities and the therapist stabilizing the thigh.

### Hand Placement and Procedure

- Apply resistance to the anterior aspect of the lower leg.
- Stabilize the femur, pelvis, or trunk as necessary.

### Dorsiflexion and Plantarflexion of the Ankle

### Hand Placement and Procedure

- Apply resistance to the dorsum of the foot just above the toes to resist dorsiflexion (Fig. 6.32A) and to the plantar surface of the foot at the metatarsals to resist plantarflexion (Fig. 6.32B).
- Stabilize the lower leg.

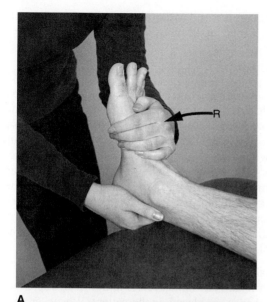

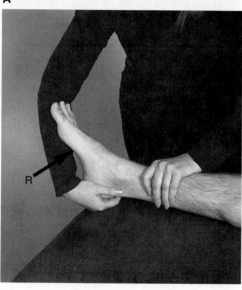

**FIGURE 6.32** (*A*) Resisted dorsiflexion. (*B*) Resisted plantarflexion of the ankle.

### Inversion and Eversion of the Ankle

#### Hand Placement and Procedure

● Apply resistance to the medial aspect of the first metatarsal to resist inversion and to the lateral aspect of the fifth metatarsal to resist eversion.

● Stabilize the lower leg.

### Flexion and Extension of the Toes

#### Hand Placement and Procedure

● Apply resistance to the plantar and dorsal surfaces of the toes as the patient flexes and extends the toes.

● Stabilize the joints above and below the joint that is moving.

## ● PROPRIOCEPTIVE NEUROMUSCULAR FACILITATION—PRINCIPLES AND TECHNIQUES

*Proprioceptive neuromuscular facilitation* (PNF) is an approach to therapeutic exercise that combines functionally based diagonal patterns of movement with techniques of neuromuscular facilitation to evoke motor responses and improve neuromuscular control and function. This widely used approach to exercise was developed during the 1940s and 1950s by the pioneering work of Kabat, Knott, and Voss.[165] Their work integrated the analysis of movement during functional activities with then-current theories of motor development, control, and learning and principles of neurophysiology as the foundations of their approach to exercise and rehabilitation. Long associated with neurorehabilitation, PNF techniques also have widespread application for rehabilitation of patients with musculoskeletal conditions that result in altered neuromuscular control of the extremities, neck, and trunk.[14,131,269,282]

PNF techniques can be used to develop muscular strength and endurance; facilitate stability, mobility, neuromuscular control, and coordinated movements; and lay a foundation for the restoration of function. PNF techniques are useful throughout the continuum of rehabilitation from the early phase of tissue healing when isometric techniques are appropriate to the final phase of rehabilitation when high-speed, diagonal movements can be performed against maximum resistance.

Hallmarks of this approach to therapeutic exercise are the use of diagonal patterns and the application of sensory cues—specifically proprioceptive, cutaneous, visual, and auditory stimuli—to elicit or augment motor responses. Embedded in this philosophy and approach to exercise is that the stronger muscle groups of a diagonal pattern facilitate the responsiveness of the weaker muscle groups. The focus of discussion of PNF in this chapter deals with the use of PNF patterns and techniques as an important form of resistance exercise for the development of strength, muscular endurance, and dynamic stability.

Although PNF patterns for the extremities can be performed unilaterally or bilaterally and in a variety of weight-bearing and non-weight-bearing positions, only unilateral patterns with the patient in a supine position are described and illustrated. In Chapter 4 of this text, the use of PNF stretching techniques—specifically contract–relax and hold–relax techniques or other variations—to increase flexibility are described. As noted in Chapter 3, diagonal patterns can also be used for passive and active ROM. Additional application of diagonal patterns for the extremities and trunk, some using resistance equipment, are described in the regional chapters later in this text.

## Diagonal Patterns

The patterns of movement associated with PNF are composed of *multijoint, multiplanar, diagonal,* and *rotational* movements of the extremities, trunk, and neck. Multiple muscle groups contract simultaneously. There are two pairs of diagonal patterns for the upper and lower extremities: diagonal 1 (D$_1$) and diagonal 2 (D$_2$). Each of these patterns can be performed in either flexion or extension. Hence, the terminology used is D$_1$Flexion or D$_1$Extension and D$_2$Flexion or D$_2$Extension of the upper or lower extremities. The patterns are identified by the motions that occur at proximal pivot points—the shoulder or the hip joints. In other words, a pattern is named by *the position of the shoulder or hip when the diagonal pattern has been completed.* Flexion or extension of the shoulder or hip is coupled with abduction or adduction as well as external or internal rotation. Motions of body segments distal to the shoulder or hip also occur simultaneously during each diagonal pattern. Table 6.9 summarizes the component motions of each of the diagonal patterns.

As mentioned, the diagonal patterns can be carried out unilaterally or bilaterally. Bilateral patterns can be done *symmetrically* (e.g., D$_1$Flexion of both extremities); *asymmetrically* (D$_1$Flexion of one extremity coupled with D$_2$Flexion of the other extremity); or *reciprocally* (D$_1$Flexion of one extremity and D$_1$ Extension of the opposite extremity). Furthermore, there are patterns specifically for the scapula or pelvis and techniques that integrate diagonal movements into functional activities, such as rolling, crawling, and walking. There are several in-depth resources that describe and illustrate the many variations and applications of PNF techniques.[268,269,287]

## Basic Procedures with PNF Patterns

A number of basic procedures that involve the application of multiple types of sensory cues are superimposed on the diagonal patterns to elicit the best possible neuromuscular responses.[268,269,287] Although the diagonal patterns can be used with various forms of mechanical resistance (e.g., free weights, simple weight-pulley systems, elastic resistance, or even an isokinetic unit), the interaction between the patient and therapist, a prominent feature of PNF, provides the greatest amount and variety of sensory input, particularly in the early phases of re-establishing neuromuscular control.

### Manual Contacts

The term *manual contact* refers to how and where the therapist's hands are placed on the patient. Whenever possible, manual contacts are placed over the agonist muscle groups or their tendinous insertions. These contacts allow the therapist to apply resistance to the appropriate muscle groups and cue the patient as to the desired direction of movement. For example, if wrist and finger extension is to be resisted, manual contact is on the dorsal surface of the hand and wrist. In the extremity patterns one manual contact is placed distally (where movement begins). The other manual contact can be placed more proximally, for example, at the shoulder or scapula. Placement of manual contacts is adjusted based on the patient's response and level of control.

| TABLE 6.9 | Component Motions of PNF Patterns: Upper and Lower Extremities | | | |
|---|---|---|---|---|
| Joints or Segments | Diagonal 1: Flexion (D$_1$Flx) | Diagonal 1: Extension (D$_1$Ext) | Diagonal 2: Flexion (D$_2$Flx) | Diagonal 2: Extension (D$_2$Ext) |
| | *UPPER EXTREMITY COMPONENT MOTIONS* | | | |
| *Shoulder* | *Flexion-adduction-external rotation* | *Extension-abduction-internal rotation* | *Flexion-abduction-external rotation* | *Extension-adduction-internal rotation* |
| Scapula | Elevation, abduction, upward rotation | Depression, adduction, downward rotation | Elevation, abduction, upward rotation | Depression, adduction downward rotation |
| Elbow | Flexion or extension | Flexion or extension | Flexion or extension | Flexion or extension |
| Forearm | Supination | Pronation | Supination | Pronation |
| Wrist | Flexion, radial deviation | Extension, ulnar deviation | Extension, radial deviation | Flexion, ulnar deviation |
| Fingers and thumb | Flexion, adduction | Extension, abduction | Extension, abduction | Flexion, adduction |
| | *LOWER EXTREMITY COMPONENT MOTIONS* | | | |
| *Hip* | *Flexion-adduction-external rotation* | *Extension-abduction-internal rotation* | *Flexion-abduction-internal rotation* | *Extension-adduction-external rotation* |
| Knee | Flexion or extension | Flexion or extension | Flexion or extension | Flexion or extension |
| Ankle | Dorsiflexion, inversion | Plantarflexion, eversion | Dorsiflexion, eversion | Plantarflexion, inversion |
| Toes | Extension | Flexion | Extension | Flexion |

## Maximal Resistance

The amount of resistance applied during dynamic concentric muscle contractions is the greatest amount possible that still allows the patient to move smoothly and without pain through the available range. Resistance should be adjusted throughout the pattern to accommodate to strong and weak components of the pattern.

## Position and Movement of the Therapist

The therapist remains positioned and aligned along the diagonal planes of movement with shoulders and trunk facing in the direction of the moving limb. Use of effective body mechanics is essential. Resistance should be applied through body weight, not only through the upper extremities. The therapist must use a wide base of support, move with the patient, and pivot over the base of support to allow rotation to occur in the diagonal pattern.

## Stretch

*Stretch stimulus.* The stretch stimulus is the placing of body segments in positions that lengthen the muscles that are to contract during the diagonal movement pattern. For example, prior to initiating $D_1$ Flexion of the lower extremity, the lower limb is placed in $D_1$ Extension.

Rotation is of utmost consideration because it is the rotational component that elongates the muscle fibers and spindles of the agonist muscles of a given pattern and increases the excitability and responsiveness of those muscles. The stretch stimulus is sometimes described as "winding up the part" or "taking up the slack."

*Stretch reflex.* The stretch reflex is facilitated by a rapid stretch (overpressure) just past the point of tension to an already elongated agonist muscle. The stretch reflex is usually directed to a distal muscle group to elicit a phasic muscle contraction to initiate a given diagonal movement pattern. The quick stretch is followed by sustained resistance to the agonist muscles to keep the contracting muscles under tension. For example, to initiate $D_1$ Flexion of the upper extremity, a quick stretch is applied to the already elongated wrist and finger flexors followed by application of resistance. A quick stretch can also be applied to any agonist muscle group at any point during the execution of a diagonal pattern to further stimulate an agonist muscle contraction or direct a patient's attention to a weak component of a pattern. (See additional discussion of the use of *repeated contractions* in the next section, which describes special PNF techniques.)

PRECAUTION: Use of a stretch reflex, even prior to resisted isometric muscle contractions, is not advisable during the early stages of soft tissue healing after injury or surgery. It is also inappropriate with acute or active arthritic conditions.

## Normal Timing

A *sequence* of distal to proximal, coordinated muscle contractions occurs during the diagonal movement patterns. The distal component motions of the pattern should be completed halfway through the pattern. Correct sequencing of movements promotes neuromuscular control and coordinated movement.

## Traction

Traction is the slight separation of joint surfaces theoretically to inhibit pain and facilitate movement during execution of the movement patterns.[268,269,287] Traction is most often applied during flexion (antigravity) patterns.

## Approximation

The gentle compression of joint surfaces by means of manual compression or weight bearing stimulates co-contraction of agonists and antagonists to enhance dynamic stability and postural control via joint and muscle mechanoreceptors.[268,269,287]

## Verbal Commands

Auditory cues are given to enhance motor output. The tone and volume of the verbal commands are varied to help maintain the patient's attention. A sharp verbal command is given simultaneously with the application of the stretch reflex to synchronize the phasic, reflexive motor response with a sustained volitional effort by the patient. Verbal cues then direct the patient throughout the movement patterns. As the patient learns the sequence of movements, verbal cues can be more succinct.

## Visual Cues

The patient is asked to follow the movement of a limb to further enhance control of movement throughout the ROM.

## Upper Extremity Diagonal Patterns

NOTE: All descriptions for hand placements are for the patient's right (R) upper extremity. During each pattern tell the patient to watch the moving hand. Be sure that rotation shifts *gradually* from internal to external rotation (or vice versa) throughout the range. By mid-range, the arm should be in neutral rotation. Manual contacts (hand placements) may be altered from the suggested placements as long as contact remains on the appropriate surfaces. Resist all patterns through the full, available ROM.

### $D_1$ Flexion

**Starting Position (Fig. 6.33A)**

Position the upper extremity in shoulder extension, abduction, and internal rotation; elbow extension; forearm pronation; and wrist and finger extension with the hand about 8 to 12 inches from the hip.

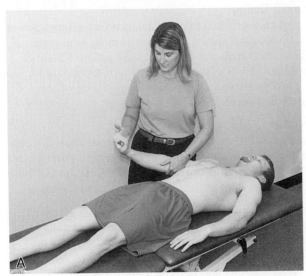

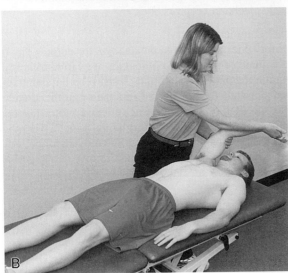

**FIGURE 6.33** (A) Starting position and (B) ending position for D$_1$ flexion of the upper extremity.

### Hand Placement
Place the index and middle fingers of your (R) hand in the palm of the patient's hand and your left (L) hand on the volar surface of the distal forearm or at the cubital fossa of the elbow.

### Verbal Commands
As you apply a quick stretch to the wrist and finger flexors, tell the patient "Squeeze my fingers, turn your palm up; pull your arm up and across your face," as you resist the pattern.

### Ending Position (Fig. 6.33B)
Complete the pattern with the arm across the face in shoulder flexion, adduction, external rotation; partial elbow flexion; forearm supination; and wrist and finger flexion.

## D$_1$ Extension

### Starting Position (Fig. 6.34A)
Begin as described for completion of D$_1$ Flexion.

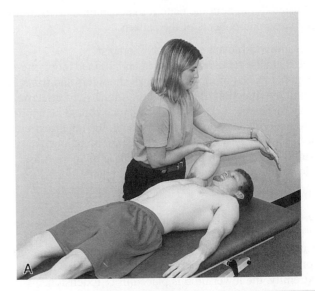

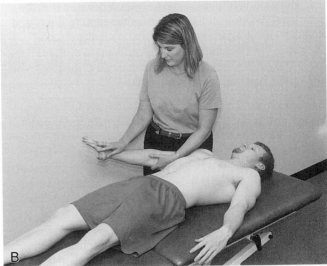

**FIGURE 6.34** (A) Starting position and (B) ending position for D$_1$ extension of the upper extremity.

### Hand Placements
Grasp the dorsal surface of the patient's hand and fingers with your (R) hand using a *lumbrical grip*. Place your (L) hand on the extensor surface of the arm just proximal to the elbow.

### Verbal Commands
As you apply a quick stretch to the wrist and finger extensors, tell the patient, "Open your hand" (or "Wrist and fingers up"); then "Push your arm down and out."

**Ending Position (Fig. 6.34B)**
Finish the pattern in shoulder extension, abduction, internal rotation; elbow extension; forearm pronation; and wrist and finger extension.

## D₂ Flexion

**Starting Position (Fig. 6.35A)**
Position the upper extremity in shoulder extension, adduction, and internal rotation; elbow extension; forearm pronation; and wrist and finger flexion. The forearm should lie across the umbilicus.

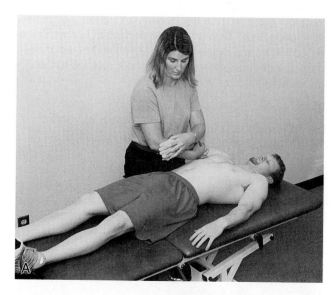

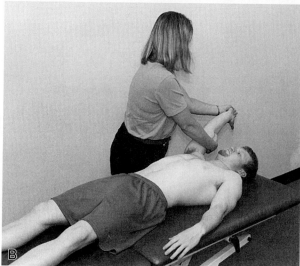

FIGURE 6.35 (*A*) Starting position and (*B*) ending position for D₂ flexion of the upper extremity.

**Hand Placement**
Grasp the dorsum of the patient's hand with your (L) hand using a lumbrical grip. Grasp the dorsal surface of the patient's forearm close to the elbow with your (R) hand.

**Verbal Commands**
As you apply a quick stretch to the wrist and finger extensors, tell the patient, "Open your hand and turn it to your face"; "Lift your arm up and out"; "Point your thumb out."

**Ending Position (Fig. 6.35B)**
Finish the pattern in shoulder flexion, abduction, and external rotation; elbow extension; forearm supination; and wrist and finger extension. The arm should be 8 to 10 inches from the ear; the thumb should be pointing to the floor.

## D₂ Extension

**Starting Position (Fig. 6.36A)**
Begin as described for completion of D₂ Flexion.

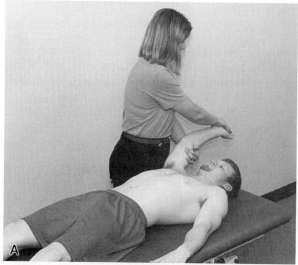

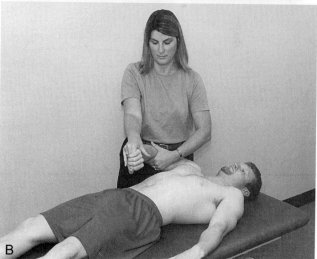

FIGURE 6.36 (*A*) Starting position and (*B*) ending position for D₂ extension of the upper extremity.

**Hand Placement**
Place the index and middle fingers of your (R) hand in the palm of the patient's hand and your (L) hand on the volar surface of the forearm or distal humerus.

**Verbal Commands**

As you apply a quick stretch to the wrist and finger flexors, tell the patient, "Squeeze my fingers and pull down and across your chest."

**Ending Position (Fig. 6.36B)**

Complete the pattern in shoulder extension, adduction, and internal rotation; elbow extension; forearm pronation; and wrist and finger flexion. The forearm should cross the umbilicus.

## Lower Extremity Diagonal Patterns

N O T E : Follow the same guidelines with regard to rotation and resistance as previously described for the upper extremity. All descriptions of hand placements are for the patient's (R) lower extremity.

### D₁ Flexion

**Starting Position (Fig. 6.37A)**

Position the lower extremity in hip extension, abduction, and internal rotation; knee extension; plantar flexion and eversion of the ankle; and toe flexion.

N O T E : This pattern may also be initiated with the knee flexed and the lower leg over the edge of the table.

**Hand Placement**

Place your (R) hand on the dorsal and medial surface of the foot and toes and your (L) hand on the anteromedial aspect of the thigh just proximal to the knee.

**Verbal Commands**

As you apply a quick stretch to the ankle dorsiflexors and invertors and toe extensors, tell the patient, "Foot and toes up and in; bend your knee; pull your leg over and across."

**Ending Position (Fig. 6.37B)**

Complete the pattern in hip flexion, adduction, and external rotation; knee flexion (or extension); ankle dorsiflexion and inversion; toe extension. The hip should be adducted across the midline, creating lower trunk rotation to the patient's (L) side.

### D₁ Extension

**Starting Position (Fig. 6.38A)**

Begin as described for completion of D₁ Flexion.

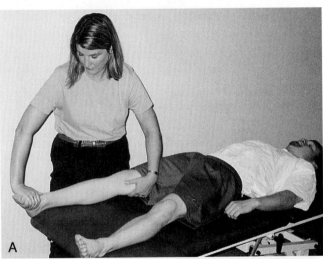

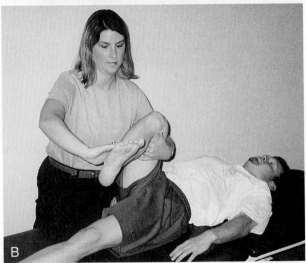

FIGURE 6.37 (A) Starting position and (B) ending position for D₁ flexion of the lower extremity.

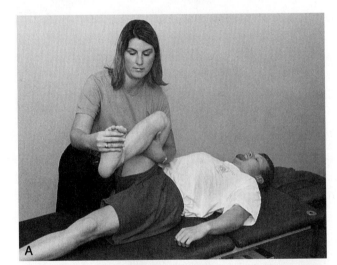

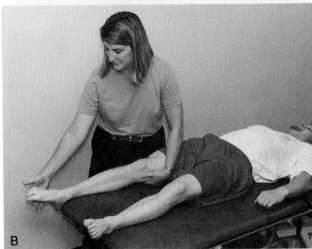

FIGURE 6.38 (A) Starting position and (B) ending position for D₁ extension of the lower extremity.

**Hand Placement**

Place your (R) hand on the plantar and lateral surface of the foot at the base of the toes. Place your (L) hand (palm up) at the posterior aspect of the knee at the popliteal fossa.

**Verbal Commands**

As you apply a quick stretch to the plantarflexors of the ankle and toes, tell the patient, "Curl (point) your toes; push down and out."

**Ending Position (Fig. 6.38B)**

Finish the pattern in hip extension, abduction, and internal rotation; knee extension or flexion; ankle plantarflexion and eversion; and toe flexion.

## D₂Flexion

**Starting Position (Fig. 6.39A)**

Place the lower extremity in hip extension, adduction, and external rotation; knee extension; ankle plantarflexion and inversion; and toe flexion.

**Hand Placement**

Place your (R) hand along the dorsal and lateral surfaces of the foot and your (L) hand on the anterolateral aspect of the thigh just proximal to the knee. The fingers of your (L) hand should point distally.

**Verbal Commands**

As you apply a quick stretch to the ankle dorsiflexors and evertors and toe extensors, tell the patient, "Foot and toes up and out; lift your leg up and out."

**Ending Position (Fig. 6.39B)**

Complete the pattern in hip flexion, abduction, and internal rotation; knee flexion (or extension); ankle dorsiflexion and eversion; and toe extension.

## D₂Extension

**Starting Position (Fig. 6.40A)**

Begin as described for the completion of D₂Flexion.

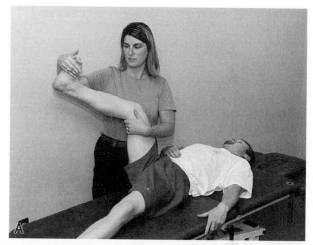

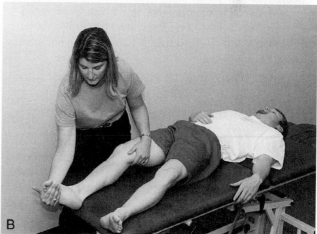

FIGURE 6.40 (A) Starting position and (B) ending position for D₂ extension of the lower extremity.

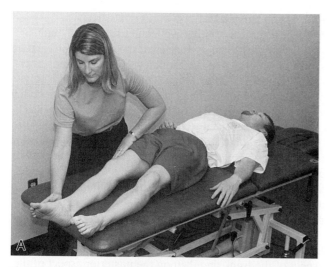

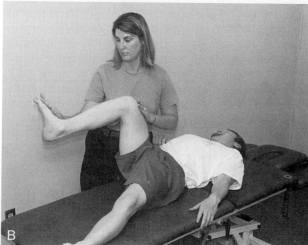

FIGURE 6.39 (A) Starting position and (B) ending position for D₂ flexion of the lower extremity.

### Hand Placement

Place your (R) hand on the plantar and medial surface of the foot at the base of the toes and your (L) hand at the posteromedial aspect of the thigh, just proximal to the knee.

### Verbal Commands

As you apply a quick stretch to the plantarflexors and invertors of the ankle and toe flexors, tell the patient, "Curl (point) your toes down and in; push your leg down and in."

### Ending Position (Fig. 6.40B)

Complete the pattern in hip extension, adduction, and external rotation; knee extension; ankle plantarflexion and inversion; and toe flexion.

## Specific Techniques with PNF

There are a number of specific techniques that may be used during the execution of a PNF pattern to stimulate weak muscles further and enhance movement or stability. These techniques are implemented selectively by the therapist to evoke the best possible response from the patient and to focus on specific treatment goals.

### Rhythmic Initiation

Rhythmic initiation is used to promote the ability to initiate a movement pattern. After the patient voluntarily relaxes, the therapist moves the patient's limb *passively* through the *available range* of the desired movement pattern several times so the patient becomes familiar with the sequence of movements within the pattern. It also helps the patient understand the *rate* at which movement is to occur. Practicing assisted or active movements (without resistance) also helps the patient learn a movement pattern.

### Repeated Contractions

Repeated, dynamic contractions, initiated with repeated quick stretches followed by resistance, are applied at any point in the ROM to strengthen a weak agonist component of a diagonal pattern.

### Reversal of Antagonists

Many functional activities involve quick reversals of the direction of movement. This is evident in diverse activities such as sawing or chopping wood, dancing, playing tennis, or grasping and releasing objects. The reversal of antagonists technique involves stimulation of a weak agonist pattern by first resisting static or dynamic contractions of the antagonist pattern. The reversals of a movement

pattern are instituted *just before* the previous pattern has been fully completed. The reversal of antagonists technique is based on Sherrington's law of *successive induction*.[247,260] There are two categories of reversal techniques available to strengthen weak muscle groups.

***Slow reversal.*** Slow reversal involves dynamic concentric contraction of a stronger agonist pattern immediately followed by dynamic concentric contraction of the weaker antagonist pattern. There is no voluntary relaxation between patterns. This promotes rapid, reciprocal action of agonists and antagonists.

***Slow reversal hold.*** Slow reversal hold adds an *isometric* contraction at the end of the range of a pattern to enhance end-range holding of a weakened muscle. With no period of relaxation, the direction of movement is then rapidly reversed by means of *dynamic* contraction of the agonist muscle groups quickly followed by isometric contraction of those same muscles. This is one of several techniques used to enhance dynamic stability, particularly in proximal muscle groups.

### Alternating Isometrics

Another technique to improve isometric strength and stability of the postural muscles of the trunk or proximal stabilizing muscles of the shoulder girdle and hip is alternating isometrics. Manual resistance is applied in a single plane on one side of a body segment and then on the other. The patient is instructed to "hold" his or her position as resistance is alternated from one direction to the opposite direction. No joint movement should occur. This procedure isometrically strengthens agonists and antagonists; and it can be applied to one extremity, to both extremities simultaneously, or to the trunk. Alternating isometrics can be applied with the extremities in open-chain or closed-chain positions.

For example, if a patient assumes a side-lying position, manual contacts are alternately placed on the anterior aspect of the trunk and then on the posterior aspect of the trunk. The patient is told to maintain (hold) the side-lying position as the therapist first attempts to push the trunk posteriorly and then anteriorly (Fig. 6.41A). Manual contacts are maintained on the patient as the therapist's hands are moved alternately from the anterior to posterior surfaces. Resistance is gradually applied and released. The same can be done unilaterally or bilaterally in the extremities (Fig. 6.41B).

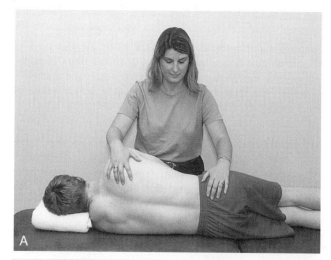

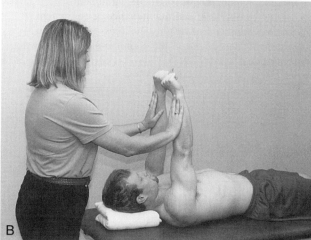

FIGURE 6.41  (A) Use of alternating isometrics to improve static strength of the proximal musculature by alternately placing both hands and applying resistance on the anterior aspect of the body and then on the posterior aspect of the body. (B) Use of alternating isometrics in the upper extremities.

### Rhythmic Stabilization

Rhythmic stabilization is used as a progression of alternating isometrics and is designed to promote stability through co-contraction of the proximal stabilizing musculature of the trunk as well as the shoulder and pelvic girdle regions of the body. Rhythmic stabilization is typically performed in weight-bearing positions to incorporate joint approximation into the procedure, hence further facilitating co-contraction. The therapist applies multidirectional, rather than unidirectional, resistance by placing manual contacts on opposite sides of the body and applying resistance *simultaneously* in opposite directions as the patient holds the selected position. Multiple muscle groups around joints must contract, most importantly the rotators, to hold the position.

For example, in the selected position, the patient is told to hold that position as one hand pushes against the posterior aspect of the body and the other hand simultaneously pushes against the anterior aspect of the body (Fig. 6.42). Manual contacts are then shifted to the opposite surfaces and isometric holding against resistance is repeated. There is no voluntary relaxation between contractions.

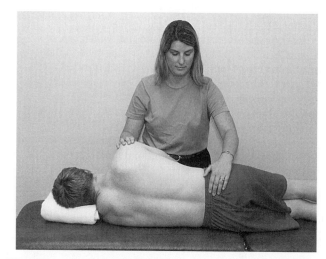

FIGURE 6.42  Use of rhythmic stabilization to improve stability of the trunk by simultaneously applying resistance in opposite directions to the anterior and posterior surfaces of the trunk, emphasizing isometric contractions of the trunk rotators.

Use of these special techniques, as well as others associated with PNF gives the therapist a significant variety of manual resistance exercise techniques to increase muscle strength and to promote dynamic stability and controlled mobility as the foundation of and in preparation for initiating task-specific skilled movements in a rehabilitation program.

## MECHANICAL RESISTANCE EXERCISE

*Mechanical resistance exercise* is any form of exercise in which resistance (the exercise load) is applied by means of some type of exercise equipment. Frequently used terms that denote the use of mechanical resistance are *resistance training*, *weight training*, and *strength training*.[6,8,9,14,16,118,236,314]

Mechanical resistance exercise is an integral component of rehabilitation and conditioning programs for individuals of all ages. However, use of mechanical resistance in an exercise program has some advantages and disadvantages (Box 6.14). The positive and negative qualities of specific types of exercise equipment are described in the last section of this chapter.

---

**BOX 6.14    Mechanical Resistance Exercise: Advantages and Disadvantages**

**Advantages**

- Establishes a quantitative baseline measurement of muscle performance against which improvement can be judged.
- Most appropriate during intermediate and advanced phases of rehabilitation when muscle strength is 4/5 or greater or when the strength of the patient exceeds the therapist's strength.
- Heavy exercise loads, far beyond that which can be applied manually by a therapist, can be used to induce a training effect for already strong muscle groups.
- Increases in level of resistance can be incrementally and quantitatively documented.
- Quantitative improvement is an effective source of motivation for the patient.
- Useful for improving dynamic or static muscular strength.
- Adds variety to a resistance training program.
- Practical for improving muscular endurance.
- Some equipment provides variable resistance through the ROM.
- High-velocity resistance training is possible and safe with some forms of mechanical resistance (hydraulic and pneumatic variable resistance machines, isokinetic units, elastic resistance). Potentially better carryover to functional activities than relatively slow-velocity manual resistance exercises.
- Appropriate for independent exercise in a home program after careful patient education and a period of supervision.

**Disadvantages**

- Not appropriate when muscles are very weak or soft tissues are in the very early stages of healing, with the exception of some equipment that provides assistance, support, or control against gravity.
- Equipment that provides constant external resistance maximally loads the muscle at only one point in the ROM.
- No accommodation for a painful arc (except with hydraulic, pneumatic, or isokinetic equipment).
- Expense for purchase and maintenance of equipment.
- With free weights and weight machines, gradation in resistance is dependent on the manufacturer's increments of resistance.

---

## Use in Rehabilitation

Mechanical resistance exercise is commonly implemented in rehabilitation programs to eliminate or reduce deficits in muscular strength, power, and endurance caused by an array of pathological conditions and to restore or improve functional abilities. Guidelines for integration of mechanical resistance exercises into an individualized rehabilitation program for patients with specific conditions are detailed in Chapters 16 through 22.

## Use in Conditioning Programs

There is a growing awareness through health promotion and disease prevention campaigns that training with weights or other forms of mechanical resistance is an important component of comprehensive conditioning programs to improve or maintain physical fitness and health throughout most of the life span. As in rehabilitation programs, resistance training complements aerobic training and flexibility exercises in conditioning programs. Guidelines for a balanced resistance training program for the healthy, but untrained adult (less than 50 to 60 years of age) recommended by the American College of Sports Medicine[8,9] and other resources[16,33,193] are summarized in Box 6.15.

## Special Considerations for Children and Older Adults

As noted previously, children and older adults often wish to, or may find it necessary to, engage in resistance training in a conditioning program to improve physical fitness, reduce health-related risk factors, or enhance physical

---

**BOX 6.15    Summary of Guidelines for Resistance Training in Conditioning Programs for Healthy Adults (< 50–60 years old)[8,9,16,32,193]**

- Prior to resistance training, perform warm-up activities followed by flexibility exercises.
- Perform dynamic exercises that target the major muscle groups of the body (approximately 8–10 muscle groups of the upper and lower extremities and trunk) for total body muscular fitness.
- Balance flexion-dominant (pulling) exercises with extension-dominant (pushing) exercises.
- Move through the full, available, and pain-free ROM.
- Include both concentric (lifting) and eccentric (lowering) muscle actions.
- Use *moderate*-intensity exercises: *at least* 8 to 12 repetitions per set.
- Perform 1 to 3 sets of each exercise for 8 to 12 repetitions per set.
- Use slow to moderate speeds of movement.
- Use rhythmic, controlled, nonballistic movements.
- Exercises should not interfere with normal breathing.
- Include rest intervals of 2 to 3 minutes between sets. While resting one muscle group, exercise a different muscle group.
- Frequency: two to three times per week.
- Increase intensity gradually (increments of approximately 5%) to progress the program as strength and muscular endurance improve.
- Whenever possible, train with a partner for feedback and assistance.
- Cool down after completion of exercises.
- After a layoff of more than 1 to 2 weeks, reduce the resistance and volume when reinitiating weight training.

performance. Resistance training can be safe and effective if exercise guidelines are modified to meet the unique needs of these two groups.

### Children and Resistance Training

Until the past decade or two, health professionals have been reluctant to support preadolescent youth participation in resistance training as a part of fitness programs because of concerns about possible adverse stress and injury to the immature musculoskeletal system, in particular, growth-plate injuries and avulsion fractures. Furthermore, a common assumption was that the benefits of resistance training were questionable in children.[26,90,91,93]

There is now a growing body of evidence that demonstrates that children do achieve health-related benefits from resistance training and can safely engage in closely supervised weight-training programs.[271,314] Use of body weight as a source of resistance and equipment specifically designed to fit a child contributes to program safety (Fig. 6.43). Training-induced strength gains in prepubescent children have been documented,[91,92,107,306] but sports related injury prevention remains of questionable benefit.[91,306] As with adults, information on the impact of strength training on the enhancement of functional motor skills is limited.

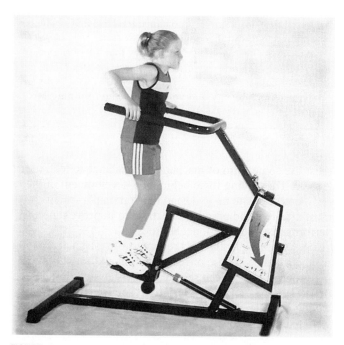

FIGURE 6.43 Us Youth resistance training on Kids-N-Motion® equipment (Triceps-Dip) specifically designed and sized for a child's use. *(Courtesy of Youth Fitness International, Moncks Corner, SC; www.youthfit.com/.)*

⦿ **Focus on Evidence**_____

Research has shown that, although some acute and chronic responses of children to exercise are similar to those of adults, other responses are quite different. For example,

children dissipate body heat less easily, fatigue more quickly, and may need more time to recover from exercise than young adults.[79,306,314] Such differences in response to resistance exercise must be addressed when designing and implementing strength training programs for children.

---

Accordingly, the American Academy of Pediatrics,[6] the American College of Sports Medicine,[8,314] and many health professionals support youth involvement in resistance training—but only if a number of special guidelines and precautions are consistently followed.[6,8,26,91,314] Although the risk of injury from resistance training is quite low,[32,93,271] exercise-induced soft tissue or growth-plate injuries have been noted if guidelines and precautions are not followed.[75] Special guidelines are summarized in Box 6.16.[6,8,32,91,107,271,314] Consistent with adult guidelines, a balanced program of dynamic exercise for major muscle groups includes warm-up and cool-down periods.

### Older Adults and Resistance Training

It is well known that muscle performance diminishes with age,[109,186,283,304] and deficits in muscle strength, power, and

---

**BOX 6.16** | **Resistance Training for Children: Special Guidelines and Special Considerations[6,8,9,32,91,314]**

- No formal resistance training for children less than 6 to 7 years of age.
- At age 6 to 7, introduce the concept of an exercise session initially using exercises without weights, then with light (only 1- or 2-pound) weights.
- Maintain *close* and *continuous supervision* by trained personnel or a parent who has received instruction.
- Focus on proper form, exercise technique, and safety (alignment, stabilization, controlled motion).
- Emphasize *low intensity* throughout childhood to avoid potential injury to a child's growing skeletal system and to joints and supportive soft tissues.
- Emphasize a variety of short-duration, play-oriented exercises to prevent boredom, overheating, and muscle fatigue.
- Perform warm-up activities for at least 5 to 10 minutes before initiating resistance exercises.
- Select low exercise loads that allow a *minimum* of 8 to 12[8,9,32] or 12 to 15[91] repetitions. Emphasize multijoint, combined movements.
- Perform only one to two sets of each exercise; rest at least 3 minutes between sets of exercises.
- Initially progress resistance training by increasing repetitions, not resistance, or by increasing the total number of exercises. Later, increase weight by no more than 5% at a time.[32,91]
- Limit the frequency to two sessions per week.
- Use properly fitting equipment that is designed or can be adapted for a child's size. Many weight machines cannot be adequately adjusted to fit a child's stature.

endurance are associated with a higher incidence of functional limitations and disability.[145,283] The extent to which decreasing muscle strength is caused by the normal aging process versus a sedentary lifestyle or an increasing incidence of age-related diseases, such as hypertension and osteoarthritis, is not clear.

A major goal of resistance training in older adults is to maintain or improve their levels of functional independence[8,35,47,210,267,283] and reduce the risk of age-related diseases.[47,210,283] As with young and middle-aged adults, older adults (less than age 60 to 65) benefit from regular exercise that includes aerobic activity, flexibility exercises, and resistance training. Even in previously sedentary older adults or frail elderly patients, a program of weight training has resulted in training-induced gains in muscle strength* and improvements in a number of parameters of physical function, such as balance, speed of walking, and the ability to rise from a chair.[36,97,145,210,226,267,294] It also has been suggested that strength training in the elderly population may minimize the incidence of falls.[32]

NOTE: The positive impact of resistance training on bone mineral density and slowing bone loss in older adults exercise is discussed in further detail in Chapter 11.

Although many of the guidelines for resistance training that apply to young and middle-aged adults (see Box 6.15) are applicable to healthy older adults, in general, resistance training for older adults should be more closely supervised and initially less rigorous than for younger populations of adults.[47,304] Accordingly, impaired balance, age-related postural changes, and poor vision that can compromise safety must be addressed if present. Also, because of age-related changes in connective tissue, there is a higher incidence of DOMS and greater muscle fiber damage in older versus young adults after heavy-resistance, high-volume strength training.[232]

Guidelines for safe but effective resistance training for older adults are listed in Box 6.17.[8,47,296] As with young adult and youth guidelines, proper warm-up and cool-down periods, a balanced program of dynamic exercises, controlled movements, and proper form and technique are equally important for older adults.

## SELECTED RESISTANCE TRAINING REGIMENS

For the past 50 to 60 years practitioners and researchers alike in rehabilitation and fitness settings have taken great interest in resistance exercise and functional training. As a result, many systems of exercise have been developed to improve muscle strength, power, and endurance. All of these systems are based on the overload principle, and

---

* See references 35, 36, 43, 120, 145, 179, 203, 213, 248, 267, 270, 304.

**BOX 6.17  Resistance Training for Older Adults (≥ 60–65 Years): Guidelines and Special Considerations[8,47,296]**

- Secure approval to initiate exercise from the participant's physician.
- Institute close supervision during the early phases of training to ensure safety.
- Monitor vital signs, particularly when the program is progressed.
- Perform at least 5 to 10 minutes of warm-up activities before each session of resistance exercises.
- Begin with low-resistance, low-repetition exercises, especially for eccentric exercises, to minimize loads on joints and to allow time for connective tissue as well as muscle to adapt.
- Emphasize low to moderate levels of resistance (at a level that permits 10–12 repetitions) for 6 to 8 weeks. Progress the program during this time by increasing repetitions. Later, increase resistance by small increments.
- Throughout the program avoid high-resistance exercises to avoid excessive stresses on joints.
- Perform resistance training two to three times weekly, allowing a 48-hour rest interval between sessions.
- Modify exercises for age-related postural changes, such as excessive kyphosis, that can alter the biomechanics of an exercise.
- Avoid flexion-dominant resistance training that could emphasize postural changes.
- When possible, use weight machines that allow the participant to perform exercises in a seated position to avoid loss of balance.
- Reduce the intensity and volume of weight training by 50% after a 1- to 2-week layoff.

most use some form of mechanical resistance to load the muscle. The driving force behind the development of these regimens seems to be to design the "optimal"—that is, the most effective and efficient—method to improve muscular performance and functional abilities.

Several frequently used regimens of resistance training for the advanced phase of rehabilitation and for conditioning programs have been selected for discussion in this section. They are progressive resistive exercise (PRE), circuit weight training, plyometric training (stretch-shortening drills), and isokinetic training regimens.

### Progressive Resistance Exercise

Progressive resistance exercise (PRE) is a system of dynamic resistance training in which a constant external load is applied to the contracting muscle by some mechanical means (usually a free weight or weight machine) and incrementally increased. The *repetition maximum* (RM) is used as the basis for determining and progressing the resistance.

### Focus on Evidence

The results of countless studies have demonstrated that PRE programs improve the force-generating capacity of muscle that may carry over to improvement in physical performance. It is important to note that the participants in many of these studies have been young, healthy adults, rather than patients with pathology and impairments.

However a systematic review of the literature[272] in 2005 indicated that PRE also was beneficial for patients with a variety of pathological conditions including musculoskeletal injuries, osteoarthritis, osteoporosis, hypertension, adult-onset (type II) diabetes, and chronic obstructive pulmonary disease. Specific findings of some of the studies identified in this systematic review are discussed in later chapters of this textbook

### Delorme and Oxford Regimens

The concept of PRE was introduced almost 60 years ago by DeLorme,[63-65] who originally used the term *heavy resistance training*[63] and later *load-resisting exercise*[64,65] to describe a new system of strength training. DeLorme proposed and studied the use of three sets of a 10 RM with *progressive loading* during each set. Other investigators[313] developed a regimen, the Oxford technique, with *regressive loading* in each set (Table 6.10).

The DeLorme technique builds a warm-up period into the protocol, whereas the Oxford technique diminishes the resistance as the muscle fatigues. Both regimens incorporate a rest interval between sets; both incrementally increase the resistance over time; and both have been shown to result in training-induced strength gains over time. In a randomized study comparing the DeLorme and Oxford regimens, no significant difference was found in adaptive strength gains in the quadriceps muscle group in older adults after a 9-week exercise program.[99]

Since the DeLormer and Oxford systems of training were first introduced, numerous variations of PRE protocols have been proposed and studied to determine an optimal intensity of resistance training, optimal number of repetitions and sets, optimal frequency, and optimal progression of loading. In reality, an ideal combination of these variables does not exist. Extensive research has shown that many combinations of exercise load, repetitions and sets, frequency, and rest intervals significantly improve strength.[16,103,169] In general, training-induced strength gains occur with two to three sets of 6 to 12 repetitions of a 6 to 12 RM.[8,9,16,32,103,118,169] This gives a therapist wide latitude when designing an effective weight-training program.

### DAPRE Regimen

Knowing when and by how much to increase the resistance in a PRE program to overload the muscle progressively is often imprecise and arbitrary. A common guideline is to increase the weight by 5% to 10% when all prescribed repetitions and sets can be completed easily without significant fatigue.[14,32] The Daily Adjustable Progressive Resistive Exercise (DAPRE) technique[163,164] is more systematic and takes into account the different rates at which individuals progress during rehabilitation or conditioning programs. The system is based on a 6 RM *working weight* (Table 6.11). The *adjusted working weight,* which is based on the maximum number of repetitions possible using the working weight in Set #3 of the regimen, determines the working weight for the next exercise session (Table 6.12).

N O T E : It should be pointed out that the recommended increases or decrease in the adjusted working weight are based on progressive loading of the quadriceps muscle group.

## Circuit Weight Training

Another system of training that employs mechanical resistance is *circuit weight training*.[30,118,169] A pre-established sequence (circuit) of continuous exercises[15] is performed in succession at individual exercise stations that target a variety of major muscle groups (usually 8 to 12) as an aspect of total body conditioning. An example of a circuit weight training sequence is shown in Box 6.18.

Each resistance exercise is performed at an exercise station for a specified number of repetitions and sets. Typically, repetitions are higher and intensity (resistance) is lower than in other forms of weight training. For example, two to three sets of 8 to 12 repetitions at 90% to 100% 10 RM or 10 to 20 repetitions at 40% to 50% 1 RM are per-

---

**TABLE 6.10    Comparison of Two PRE Regimens**

| DeLorme Regimen | Oxford Regimen |
| --- | --- |
| Determination of a 10 RM | Determination of a 10 RM |
| 10 reps @ 50% of the 10 RM | 10 reps @ 100% of the 10 RM |
| 10 reps @ 75% of the 10 RM | 10 reps @ 75% of the 10 RM |
| 10 reps @ 100% of the 10 RM | 10 reps @ 50% of the 10 RM |

---

**TABLE 6.11    DAPRE Technique**

| Sets | Repetitions | Amount of Resistance |
| --- | --- | --- |
| 1 | 10 | 50% 6 RM* |
| 2 | 6 | 75% 6 RM |
| 3 | Maximum possible | 100% 6 RM |
| 4 | Maximum possible | 100% adjusted working weight** |

*6 RM = working weight

**See Table 6.12 for calculation of the adjusted working weight.

| TABLE 6.12 | Calculation of the Adjusted Working Weight for the DAPRE Regimen | |
| --- | --- | --- |
| **Adjustment of Working Weight** | | |
| Repetitions in Set 3 | Set 4 | Next exercise session 3 |
| 0–2 | ↓ 5–10 lb | ↓ 5–10 lb |
| 3–4 | ↓ 0–5 lb | Same weight |
| 5–6 | Keep same weight | ↑ 5–10 lb |
| 7–10 | ↑ 5–10 lb | ↑ 5–15 lb |
| 11 or more | ↑ 10–15 lb | ↑ 10–20 lb |

formed,[19,193] with a minimum amount of rest (15 to 20 seconds) between sets and stations. The program is progressed by increasing the number of sets or repetitions, the resistance, the number of exercise stations, and the number of circuit revolutions.

*Exercise order* is an important consideration when setting up a weight training circuit.[16,30,166] Exercises with free weights or weight machines should alternate among upper extremity, lower extremity, and trunk musculature and between muscle groups involved in pushing or pulling actions. This enables one muscle group to rest and recover from exercise while exercising another group and, therefore, minimizes muscle fatigue. Ideally, larger muscle groups should be exercised before smaller muscle groups. Multijoint exercises that recruit multiple muscle groups should be performed before exercises that recruit an isolated muscle group to minimize the risk of injury from fatigue.

## Plyometric Training—Stretch–Shortening Drills

High-intensity, high-velocity exercises emphasize the development of muscular power and coordination. Reactive bursts of force in functional movement patterns are often necessary if a patient is to return to high-demand occupational, recreational, or sport-related activities. Plyometric

| BOX 6.18 | Example of a Resistance Training Circuit |
| --- | --- |
| Station #1: Bench press → #2: Leg press or squats → #3: Sit-ups → #4: Upright rowing → #5: Hamstring curls → #6: Prone trunk extension → #7: Shoulder press → #8: Heel raises → #9: Push-ups→ #10: Leg lifts or lowering | |

training is integrated into the advanced phase of rehabilitation as a mechanism to train the neuromuscular system to react quickly in order to prepare for activities that require rapid starting and stopping movements. This form of training is appropriate only for carefully selected patients.

### Definitions and Characteristics

*Plyometric training*,[37,193,284,286] also called *stretch-shortening drills*[302] or *stretch-strengthening drills*,[285] employs high-velocity eccentric to concentric muscle loading, reflexive reactions, and functional movement patterns. Plyometric training is defined as a system of high-velocity resistance training characterized by a rapid eccentric contraction during which the muscle elongates, immediately followed by a rapid reversal of movement with a resisted shortening contraction of the same muscle.[285,286,302] The rapid eccentric loading phase is the *stretch cycle*, and the concentric phase is the *shortening cycle*. The period of time between the stretch and shortening cycles is known as the *amortization phase*. It is important that the amortization phase is kept very brief by a rapid reversal of movements to capitalize on the increased tension in the muscle.

Body weight or an external form of loading, such as elastic bands or tubing or a weighted ball, are possible sources of resistance. An example of a stretch-shortening drill against the resistance of body weight is represented in Figure 6.44.

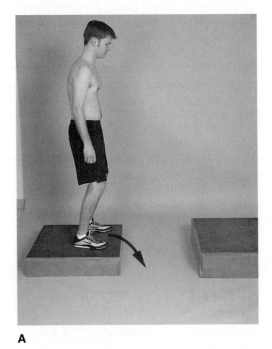

**A**

**FIGURE 6.44** Plyometric activity against the resistance of body weight. (*A*) Patient stands on a low platform;

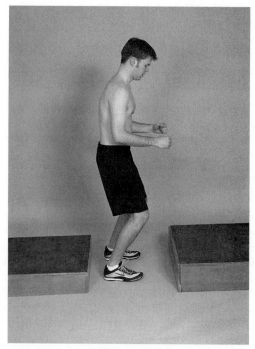

B

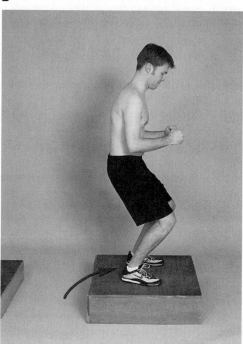

C

FIGURE 6.44 (continued) (*B*) jumps off the platform to the floor, controlling the impact with a loaded, lengthening contraction of the hip and knee extensors and plantarflexors—the stretch phase; and (*C*) then without delay jumps forward onto the next platform using a concentric contraction of the same muscle groups—the shortening phase.

| BOX 6.19 | Plyometric Activities for the Upper and Lower Extremities |

**Upper Extremities**
- Catching and throwing a weighted ball with a partner or against a wall: bilaterally then unilaterally
- Stretch-shortening drills with elastic tubing using anatomical and diagonal motions
- Dribbling a ball on the floor or against a wall
- Drop push-ups: from boxes to floor and back to boxes
- Clap push-ups

**Lower Extremities**
- Repetitive jumping on the floor: in place; forward/backward; side to side; diagonally to four corners; jump with rotation; zigzag jumping; later, jump on foam
- Vertical jumps and reaches
- Multiple jumps across a floor (bounding)
- Box jumping: initially off and freeze; then off and back on box increasing speed and height
- Side to side jumps (box to floor to box)
- Jumping over objects on the floor
- Hopping activities: in place; across a surface; over objects on the floor
- Depth jumps (advanced): jump from a box, squat to absorb shock, and then jump and reach as high as possible

Additional examples of plyometric training for the upper and lower extremities are noted in Box 6.19.

**Neurological and Biomechanical Influences**
Plyometric training is thought to utilize the series-elastic properties of soft tissues and the stretch reflex of the neuromuscular unit. The spring-like properties of the series-elastic components of muscle-tendon units create elastic energy during the initial phase (the stretch cycle) as the muscle contracts eccentrically and lengthens while loaded. This energy is briefly stored and then retrieved for use during the concentric contraction (shortening cycle) that follows. The storage and release of this elastic energy augments the force production of the concentric muscle contraction.[20,37,284]

Furthermore, the stretch-shortening cycle is thought to stimulate the proprioceptors of muscles, tendons, ligaments, and joints, increase the excitability of the neuromuscular receptors, and improve the reactivity of the neuromuscular system. The term *reactive neuromuscular training* has also been used to describe this approach to exercise. More specifically, the loaded, eccentric contraction (stretch cycle) is thought to prepare the contractile elements of the muscle for a concentric contraction (shortening cycle) by stimulation and activation of the monosynaptic stretch reflex.[37,78,284] Muscle spindles, the receptors that lie in parallel with muscle fibers, sense the length of a muscle and the velocity of stretch applied to a muscle and transmit this information to the CNS via afferent pathways. Impulses are then sent back to the muscle from the CNS, which reflexively facilitates activation of a shortening contraction of the stretched muscle (the shortening cycle).[184,193,250] Therefore, the more rapid the eccentric muscle contraction (the stretch), the more likely it is that the stretch reflex will be activated.

It has been suggested that the ability to use this stored elastic energy and neural facilitation is contingent on the velocity and magnitude of the stretch and the transition time between the stretch and shortening phases (the amortization phase).[37] During the amortization phase the muscle must reverse its action, switching from deceleration to acceleration of the load. A decrease in the amortization phase theoretically increases the force output during the shortening cycle.[20,37,284,286]

### Effects of Plyometric Training
The evidence to support the effectiveness of plyometric training to enhance physical performance is somewhat limited, with many resources citing opinion and anecdotal evidence. However, there is evidence indicating that plyometric training is associated with an increase in a muscle's ability to resist stretch, which may enhance the muscle's dynamic restraint capabilities.[20] There is also promising evidence to suggest that plyometric training is associated with a decreased incidence of lower extremity injury.[133,244,258]

 **Focus on Evidence**_____

In a prospective study by Hewett[133] two groups of high school-age female athletes were monitored during a season of participation in one of three sports (soccer, volleyball, and basketball). One group (n = 366) participated in a 6-week preseason training program, whereas the other group (n = 463) did not. The preseason training focused on jumping and landing techniques. At the end of the sport season there was a significantly higher incidence (3.6 times higher) of knee injury in the untrained group than in the trained group. The investigaators concluded that preseason plyometric training may reduce the risk of knee injury in female athletes possibly owing to increased dynamic knee stability.

---

### Application and Progression of Plyometric Training
Plyometric training is appropriate only in the later stage of rehabilitation of active individuals who must achieve a high level of physical performance in specific, high-demand activities.

***Contraindications.*** Plyometrics should not be used if inflammation, pain, or significant joint instability is present.

***Preparation for plyometrics.*** Prior to initiation of plyometric training, a patient should have an adequate base of muscle strength and endurance as well as flexibility of the muscles to be exercised. Criteria to begin plyometric training usually include an 80% to 85% level of strength and 90% to 95% ROM.[37]

***Specificity of training.*** A plyometric drill should be designed with specific functional activities in mind and should include movement patterns that replicate the desired activity.

***Progression.*** Parameters of plyometric training are progressed as follows.

- ***Speed of drills.*** Drills should be performed rapidly but safely. The rate of stretch of the contracting muscle is more important than the length of the stretch.[284] Emphasis should be placed on decreasing the reversal time from an eccentric to a concentric contraction (decreasing the amortization phase). This trains the muscle to generate tension in the shortest time possible. If a jumping activity is performed, for example, progression of the plyometric activity should center on reducing the time on the ground between each jump.
- ***Intensity.*** Increase the resistance applied but not enough to slow down the activity. Examples include use of a weighted vest, heavier Plyoballs (weighted balls), heavier grade elastic resistance, double-leg to single-leg jumping or hopping, or using higher height platforms. Intensity also involves progressing from simple to complex movements.
- ***Repetitions and frequency.*** Increase the number of repetitions of an activity *so long as proper form (technique) is maintained;* increase the number of plyometric exercises in a session; or increase the number of plyometric sessions in a week. A 48- to 72-hour recovery period is recommended.[37,284]

Box 6.20 summarizes sample activities for upper extremity plyometric training.[37,284,286,302] Programs, of course, must be individually designed and progressed to meet each patient's needs and goals. Note that prior to initiating plyometric activities a series of warm-up exercises must be performed.

PRECAUTIONS: As with other forms of high-intensity resistance training, special precautions must be followed to ensure patient safety.[37,284] These precautions are listed in Box 6.21.

## Isokinetic Regimens

It is well established that isokinetic training improves muscle performance. Its effectiveness in carryover to functional tasks is less clear. Studies support[86,202] and refute[127,229] that isokinetic training improves function. Ideally, when isokinetic training is implemented in a rehabilitation program, to have the most positive impact on function it should be

| BOX 6.20 | Sample Plyometric Sequence for the Upper Extremities |
| --- | --- |

- Warm-up activities
  - Trunk exercises holding lightweight ball: rotation, side-bending, wood-chopping
  - Upper extremity exercises in anatomical and diagonal planes of motion with light-grade elastic tubing
  - Prone push-ups
- Throwing motions with a weighted ball to and from a partner: bilateral chest press; bilateral overhead throw; bilateral side throw
- ER/IR against elastic tubing (90/90 position of shoulder and elbow)
- Diagonal patterns against elastic resistance
- Unilateral throwing motions with weighted ball: baseball throw; side throws
- Additional exercises
  - Trunk exercises holding weighted ball: abdominal curl-ups; back extension; sit-up and bilateral throw; long sitting throws
  - Clap push-ups
  - Prone push-ups from box to floor and back to box

| BOX 6.21 | Precautions for Plyometric Training |
| --- | --- |

- If high-stress, shock-absorbing activities are not permissible, do not incorporate plyometric training into a patient's rehabilitation program.
- If a decision is made to include plyometric activities in a rehabilitation program for children or elderly patients, select only beginning-level stretch-shortening drills against light resistance. Do not include high-impact, heavy-load activities—such as drop jumps or weighted jumps—that could place excessive stress on joints.
- Be sure the patient has adequate flexibility and strength before initiating plyometric exercises.
- Wear shoes that provide support for lower extremity plyometrics.
- *Always* warm-up prior to plyometric training with a series of active, dynamic trunk and extremity exercises.
- During jumping activities, emphasize learning techniques for a safe landing before progressing to rebounding.
- Progress repetitions of an exercise before increasing the level of resistance used or the height or length of jumps.
- For high-level athletes who progress to high-intensity plyometric drills, increase the rest intervals between sets and decrease the frequency of drills as the intensity of the drills increases.
- Allow adequate time for recovery with 48 to 72 hours between sessions of plyometric activities.
- Stop an exercise if a patient can no longer perform the plyometric activity with good form and landing technique because of fatigue.

performed at velocities that closely match or at least approach the expected velocities of movement of specific functional tasks. Because many functional movements occur at a variety of medium to fast speeds, isokinetic training is typically performed at medium and fast velocities.[5,55,60,84]

Current isokinetic technology makes it possible to approximate training speeds to velocities of movement during some lower extremity functions, such as walking.[55,308] In the upper extremities this is far less possible. Some functional movements in the upper extremities occur at exceedingly rapid velocities (e.g., more than 1000° per second for overhead throwing), which far exceed the capabilities of isokinetic dynamometers.[84]

It is also widely accepted that isokinetic training is relatively speed-specific, with only limited transfer of training (physiological overflow causing improvements in muscle performance at speeds other than the training speed).[149,278] Therefore, *speed-specific isokinetic training,* similar to the velocity of a specific functional task, is advocated.[5,57,84]

### Velocity Spectrum Rehabilitation
To deal with the problem of limited physiological overflow of training effects from one training velocity to another, a regimen called *velocity spectrum rehabilitation* (VSR) has been advocated.[55,84,103] With this system of training, exercises are performed across a range of velocities.[255]

N O T E : The guidelines for VSR that follow are for *concentric* isokinetic training. General guidelines for eccentric isokinetics are identified at the conclusion of this section.

***Selection of training velocities.*** Typically, medium (60° or 90° to 180°/sec) and fast (180° to 360°/sec) angular velocities are selected. Although isokinetic units are designed for testing and training at velocities faster than 360° per second, the fastest velocities usually are not used for training. This is because the limb must accelerate to the very fast, preset speed before encountering resistance from the torque arm of the dynamometer. Hence, the contracting muscles are resisted through only a small portion of the ROM.

It has been suggested that the effects of isokinetic training (improvements in muscle strength, power, or endurance) carry over only 15° per second from the training velocity.[55,149] Therefore, some VSR protocols use 30° per second increments for medium and fast velocity training. Of course, if a patient trains at medium and fast velocities (from 60° or 90° to 360°/sec) in one exercise session, this strategy necessitates nine different training velocities, giving rise to a time-consuming exercise session for one agonist/antagonist combination of muscle groups. A more common protocol is to use as few as three training velocities.[5,84,255]

***Repetitions, sets, and rest.*** A typical VSR protocol might have the patient perform one or two sets of 8 to 10 or as many as 20 repetitions of agonist/antagonist muscle groups (reciprocal training) at multiple velocities.[5,55,84] For example, at medium velocities (between 90° and 180°/sec) training could occur at 90°, 120°, 150°, and 180° per second. A second series would then be performed at decreasing velocities: 180°, 150°, 120°, and 90° per second. Because many combinations of repetitions, sets, and different training velocities lead to improvement in muscle performance, the therapist has many options when designing a VSR program. A 15- to 20-second rest between sets and a 60-second rest between exercise velocities has been recommended.[261] The recommended frequency for VSR is a maximum of three times per week.[5]

*Intensity.* Submaximal effort is used for a brief warm-up period on the dynamometer. This is not a replacement for a more general form of upper or lower body warm-up exercises, such as cycling or upper-extremity ergometry. When training to improve endurance, exercises are carried out at a submaximal intensity (effort) but at a maximal intensity to improve strength or power.

During the early stages of isokinetic training, it is useful to begin with submaximal isokinetic exercise at intermediate and slow velocities so the patient gets the "feel" of the isokinetic equipment and at the same time protects the muscle. As the program progresses, maximum effort can be exerted at intermediate speeds. Slow-speed training is eliminated when the patient begins to exert maximum effort. During the advanced stage of rehabilitation, maximum-effort, fast-velocity training is emphasized, so long as exercises are pain-free.[60] Additional aspects to a progression of isokinetic training regimens include short-arc to full-arc exercises (if necessary) and concentric to eccentric movements.[60]

PRECAUTION: Maximum-effort, slow-velocity training is rarely indicated because of the excessive shear forces produced across joint surfaces.[55,84]

### Eccentric Isokinetic Training: Special Considerations

As isokinetic technology evolved over several decades, eccentric isokinetic training became possible,[5,55,84,123] but few guidelines for eccentric isokinetic training and evidence of their efficacy are available. Guidelines developed to date are primarily based on clinical opinion or anecdotal evidence. Key differences in eccentric versus concentric isokinetic guidelines (intensity, repetitions, frequency, rest) are listed in Box 6.22. Several resources describe pathology-specific guidelines for eccentric isokinetic training based on clinical experience.[55,84,122,123]

PRECAUTIONS: Eccentric isokinetic training is appropriate only during the final phase of a rehabilitation program to continue to challenge individual muscle groups when isolated deficits in strength and power persist. Because of the robotic nature of eccentric isokinetic training, medium rather than fast training velocities are considered safer. A sudden, rapid, motor-driven movement of the dynamometer's torque arm against a limb could injure healing tissue.

---

**BOX 6.22   Key Differences in Eccentric Versus Concentric Isokinetic Training**

Eccentric isokinetic exercise is:

- Introduced only *after maximal* effort concentric isokinetic exercise can be performed without pain
- Implemented only after functional ROM has been restored
- Performed at slower velocities across a narrower velocity spectrum than concentric isokinetic exercise: usually between 60° and 120° per second for the general population and up to 180° per second for athletes
- Carried out at submaximal levels for a longer time frame to avoid extensive torque production and lessen the risk of DOMS
- Most commonly performed in a continuous concentric-eccentric pattern for a muscle group during training

---

 # EQUIPMENT FOR RESISTANCE TRAINING

There seems to be an almost limitless selection of exercise equipment on the market that is designed for resistance training. The equipment ranges from simple to complex, compact to space-consuming, and inexpensive to expensive. An assortment of simple but versatile handheld and cuff weights or elastic resistance products is useful in clinical and home settings, whereas multiple pieces of variable resistance equipment may be useful for advanced-level resistance training. Sources of information about new products on the market are the literature distributed by manufacturers, product demonstrations at professional meetings, and studies of these products reported in the research literature.

Although most equipment is *load resisting* (augments the resistance of gravity), a few pieces of equipment can be adapted to be *load assisting* (eliminates or diminishes the resistance of gravity) to improve the strength of weak muscles. Equipment can be used for static or dynamic, concentric or eccentric, and open-chain or closed-chain exercises to improve muscular strength, power, or endurance, neuromuscular stability or control, as well as cardiopulmonary fitness.

In the final analysis, the choice of equipment depends primarily on the individual needs, abilities, and goals of the person using the equipment. Other factors that influence the choice of equipment are the *availability*; the *cost* of purchase or maintenance by a facility or a patient; the *ease of use* (application or setup) of the equipment; the *versatility* of the equipment; and the *space requirements* of the equipment. Once the appropriate equipment has been selected, its safe and effective use is the highest priority. General principles for use of equipment are listed in Box 6.23.

| BOX 6.23 | General Principles for the Selection and Use of Equipment |
|---|---|

- Base the selection of equipment on a comprehensive examination and evaluation of the patient.
- Determine when in the exercise program the use of equipment should be introduced and when it should be altered or discontinued.
- Determine if the equipment could or should be set up and used independently by a patient.
- Teach appropriate exercise form before adding resistance with the equipment.
- Teach and supervise the application and use of the equipment before allowing a patient to use the equipment independently.
- Adhere to all safety precautions when applying and using the equipment.
  - Be sure all attachments, cuffs, collars, and straps are securely fastened and that the equipment is appropriately adjusted to the individual patient prior to the exercise.
  - Apply padding for comfort, if necessary, especially over bony prominences.
  - Stabilize or support appropriate structures to prevent unwanted movement and to prevent undue stress on body parts.
- If exercise machines are used independently, be certain that set-up and safety instructions are clearly illustrated and affixed directly to the equipment.
- If compatible with the selected equipment, use range-limiting attachments if ROM must be restricted to protect healing tissues or unstable structures.
- If the patient is using the equipment in a home program, give explicit instructions on how, when, and to what extent to change or adapt the equipment to provide a progressive overload.
- When making a transition from use of one type of resistance equipment to another, be certain that the newly selected equipment and method of set-up initially provides a similar level of torque production to the equipment previously employed to avoid insufficient or excessive loads.
- When the exercise has been completed:
  - Disengage the equipment and leave it in proper condition for future use.
  - Never leave broken or potentially hazardous equipment for future use.
- Set up a regular routine of maintenance, replacement, or safety checks for all equipment.

## Free Weights and Simple Weight–Pulley Systems

### Types of Free Weights
Free weights are graduated weights that are handheld or applied to the upper and lower extremities or trunk. They include commercially available dumbbells, barbells, weighted balls (Fig. 6.45), cuff weights, weighted vests, and even sandbags. Free weights can also be fashioned for a home exercise program from readily available materials and objects found around the home.

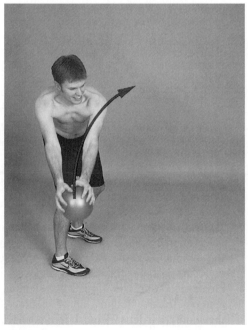
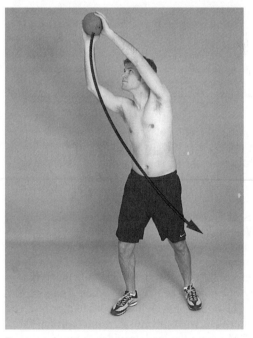

**A**            **B**

FIGURE 6.45 *(A, B)* Holding a weighted ball while performing combined patterns of movement provides resistance to upper extremity and trunk muscles and augments the resistance of body weight to lower extremity muscle groups during weight-bearing activities.

## Simple Weight–Pulley Systems

Free-standing or wall-mounted simple weight-pulley systems with weight-plates are commonly used for resisted upper and lower extremity or trunk exercises (Fig. 6.46). Permanent or interchangeable weights are available. Permanent weights are usually stacked with individual weight plates of 5- to 10-pound increments that can be easily adjusted by changing the placement of a single weight key.

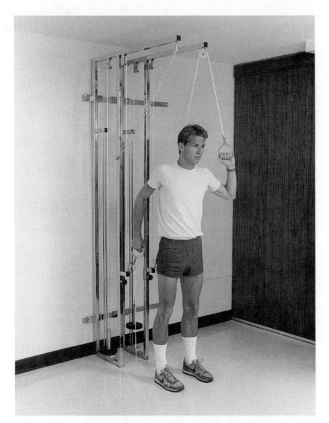

FIGURE 6.46 Multi Exercise Pulley Unit can be used to strengthen a variety of muscle groups. *(Courtesy of N–K Products Company, Inc., Soquel, CA.)*

N O T E : The simple weight-pulley systems described here are those that impose a relatively constant (fixed) load. Variable resistance weight machines, some of which incorporate pulleys into their designs, are discussed later in this section.

## Characteristics of Free Weights and Simple Weight–Pulley Systems

Free weights and weight-pulley systems are resistance equipment that impose a fixed (constant) load. The weight selected, therefore, maximally challenges the contacting muscle at only one portion of the ROM when a patient is in a particular position. The weight that is lifted or lowered can be no greater than what the muscle can control at the point in the ROM where the load provides the maximum

torque. In addition, there is no accommodation for a painful arc.

When using free weights, it is possible to vary the point in the ROM at which the maximum resistance load is experienced by changing the patient's position with respect to gravity or the direction of the resistance load. For example, shoulder flexion may be resisted with the patient standing or supine and holding a weight in the hand.

● *Patient position:* standing (Fig. 6.47): Maximum resistance is experienced and maximum torque is produced when the shoulder is at 90° of flexion. Zero torque is produced when the shoulder is at 0° of flexion. Torque again decreases as the patient lifts the weight from 90° to 180° of flexion. In addition, when the weight is at the side (in the 0° position of the shoulder), it causes traction force on the humerus; and when overhead, it causes compression force through the upper extremity.

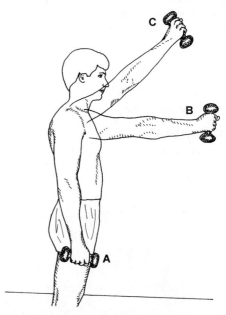

FIGURE 6.47 When the patient is standing and lifting a weight: (*A*) Zero torque is produced in the shoulder flexors when the shoulder is at 0° of flexion. (*B*) Maximum torque is produced when the shoulder is at 90° of flexion. (*C*) Torque again decreases as the arm moves from 90° to 180° of shoulder flexion.

● *Patient position:* supine (Fig. 6.48): Maximum resistance is experienced and maximum torque is produced when the shoulder is at 0° of flexion. Zero torque is produced at 90° of shoulder flexion. In this position the entire load creates a compression force. The shoulder flexors are not active between 90° and 180° of shoulder flexion. Instead, the shoulder extensors must contract eccentrically to control the descent of the arm and weight.

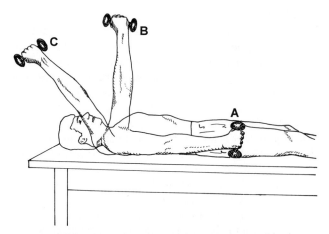

FIGURE 6.48 When the patient is supine and lifting a weight: (A) Maximum torque is produced at 0° of shoulder flexion. (B) Zero torque is produced at 90° of shoulder flexion. (C) The shoulder extensors are active and contract eccentrically against resistance from 90° to 180° of shoulder flexion.

The therapist must determine at which portion of the patient's ROM maximum strength is needed and must choose the optimum position in which the exercise should be performed to gain maximum benefit from the exercise.

Simple weight-pulley systems provide maximum resistance when the angle of the pulley is at right angles to the moving bone. As the angle of the pulley becomes more acute, the load creates more compression through the moving bones and joints and less effective resistance.

Unlike many weight machines, neither free weights nor pulleys provide external stabilization to guide the moving segment or restrict ROM. When a patient lifts or lowers a weight to an overhead position, muscles of the scapula and shoulder abductors, adductors, and rotators must synergistically contract to stabilize the arm and keep it aligned in the correct plane of motion. The need for concurrent contraction of adjacent stabilizing muscle groups can be viewed as an advantage or disadvantage. Because muscular stabilization is necessary to control the plane or pattern of movement, less resistance can be controlled with free weights than with a weight machine during the same movement pattern.

### Advantages and Disadvantages of Free Weights and Simple Weight-Pulley Systems

- Exercises can be set up in many positions, such as supine, side-lying, or prone in bed or on a cart, sitting in a chair or on a bench, or standing. Many muscle groups in the extremities and trunk can be strengthened by simply repositioning the patient.
- Free weights and simple weight-pulley systems typically are used for dynamic, non-weight-bearing exercises but also can be set up for isometric exercise and resisted weight-bearing activities.
- Stabilizing muscle groups are recruited; however, because there is no external source of stabilization and

movements must be controlled entirely by the patient, it may take more time for the patient to learn correct alignment and movement patterns.

- A variety of movement patterns is possible, incorporating single plane or multiplanar motions. An exercise can be highly specific to one muscle or generalized to several muscle groups. Movement patterns that replicate functional activities can be resisted.
- If a large enough assortment of graduated free weights is available, resistance can be increased by very small increments, as little as 1 pound at a time. The weight plates of pulley systems have larger increments of resistance, usually a minimum of 5 pounds per plate.
- Most exercises with free weights and weight-pulley systems must be performed slowly to minimize acceleration and momentum and prevent uncontrolled, end-range movements that could compromise patient safety. It is thought that the use of exclusively slow movements during strengthening activities has less carryover to many daily living activities than the incorporation of slow- and fast-velocity exercises into a rehabilitation program. However, a weighted ball can be used with catching and throwing exercises as part of plyometric training during the advanced phase of upper extremity rehabilitation.[302]
- Free weights with interchangeable disks, such as a barbell, are versatile and can be used for patients with many different levels of strength, but they require patient or personnel time for proper assembly.
- Bilateral lifting exercises with barbell weights often require the assistance of a spotter to ensure patient safety, thus increasing personnel time.

## Variable-Resistance Machines

Variable-resistance exercise equipment falls into two broad categories: specially designed weight-cable (weight-pulley) machines and hydraulic and pneumatic units. Both categories of equipment impose a variable load on the contracting muscles consistent with the changing torque-producing capabilities of the muscles throughout the available ROM.

### Variable Resistance Weight-Cable Systems

Variable-resistance weight-cable machines (Fig. 6.49) use a cam in their design. The cam (an elliptical or kidney-shaped disk) in the weight-cable system is designed to vary the load (torque) applied to the contracting muscle even though the weight selected remains the same. In theory, the cam is configured to replicate the length-tension relationship and resultant torque curve of the contracting muscle with the greatest amount of resistance applied in the mid-range. This system varies the external load imposed on the contracting muscle based on the physical dimensions of the "average" individual. How effectively this design provides truly accommodating resistance throughout the full ROM is debatable.

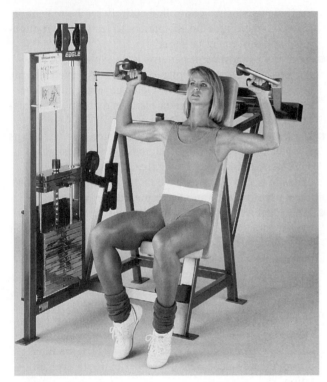

**FIGURE 6.49** Cybex/Eagle Fitness Systems shoulder press provides variable resistance throughout the range of motion. *(Courtesy of Cybex, Division of Lumex, Ronkonkoma, NY.)*

With each repetition of an exercise, the same muscle group contracts and is resisted concentrically and eccentrically. As with simple weight-pulley systems and free weights, exercises must be performed at relatively slow velocities, thus compromising carryover to many functional activities.

### Hydraulic and Pneumatic Variable–Resistance Units

Other variable-resistance machines employ hydraulic or pressurized pneumatic resistance to vary the resistance throughout the ROM. These units allow concentric, reciprocal muscle work to agonist and antagonist muscle groups but no eccentric work. Patients can safely exercise at fast velocities with these units. These units also allow a patient to accommodate for a pain-free arc.

### Advantages and Disadvantages of Variable-Resistance Machines

- The obvious advantage of these machines compared to constant load equipment is that the effective resistance is adjusted, at least to some extent, to a muscle's tension-generating capabilities throughout the ROM. The contracting muscle is loaded maximally at multiple points in the ROM, rather than just one small portion of the range.
- Most pieces of equipment are designed to isolate and exercise a specific muscle group. For example, resisted

squats are performed on one machine and hamstring curls on another. Some units, such as a leg press or shoulder press, strengthen multiple muscle groups simultaneously.

- Unlike functional movement, most machines allow only single-plane movements, although some newer units now offer a dual-axis design allowing multiplanar motions that strengthen multiple muscle groups and more closely resemble functional movement patterns.
- The equipment is adjustable to a certain extent to allow individuals of varying heights to perform each exercise in a well aligned position.
- Each unit provides substantial external stabilization to guide or limit movements. This makes it easier for the patient to learn how to perform the exercise correctly and safely and helps the patient maintain appropriate alignment without assistance or supervision.
- One of the main disadvantages of weight machines is the initial expense and ongoing maintenance costs. Multiple machines, usually 8 to 10 or more, must be purchased to target multiple major muscle groups. Multiple machines also require a large amount of space in a facility.

## Elastic Resistance Bands and Tubing

The use of elastic resistance products in therapeutic exercise programs has become widespread in rehabilitation and has been shown to be an effective method of providing resistance and improving muscle strength.[146] Despite the popularity of these products, not until the past 10 years has quantitative information been reported on the actual or relative resistance supplied by elastic products or the level of muscle activation during use.[135,136,147,152,221,223,245,275] These studies suggest that the effective use of elastic products for resistance training requires not only the application of biomechanical principles but also an understanding of the physical properties of elastic resistance material.

### Types of Elastic Resistance

Elastic resistance products, specifically designed for use during exercise, fall into two broad categories: elastic bands and elastic tubing. Elastic bands and tubing are produced by several manufacturers under different product names, the most familiar of which is Thera-Band® Elastic Resistance Bands and Tubing (Hygenic Corp., Akron, OH). Elastic bands are available in an assortment of grades or thicknesses. Tubing comes in graduated diameters and wall thickness that provide progressive levels of resistance. Color-coding denotes the thickness of the product and grades of resistance.

### Properties of Elastic Resistance— Implications for Exercise

A number of studies describing the physical characteristics of elastic resistance have provided quantitative information about its material properties. Knowledge of this information enables a therapist to use elastic resistance more effectively for therapeutic exercise programs.

***Effect of elongation of elastic material.*** Elastic resistance provides a form of variable resistance because the force generated changes as the material is elongated. Specifically, as it is stretched, the amount of resistance (force) produced by an elastic band or tubing increases depending on the *relative change* in the length of the material *(percentage of elongation/deformation)* from the start to the end of elongation. There is a relatively predictable and *linear* relationship between the percentage of elongation and the tensile force of the material.[136,147,152,223,245]

To determine the percentage of elongation, the stretched length must be compared to the resting length of the elastic material. The *resting length* of a band or tubing is its length when it is laid out flat and there is no stretch applied. The actual length of the material before it is stretched has no effect on the force imparted. Rather, it is the percentage of elongation that affects the tensile forces.[223]

The formula for calculating the percentage of elongation/deformation is[146,245]:

Percent of elongation = (stretched length − resting length) ÷ resting length × 100

Using this formula, if a 2-foot length of red tubing, for example, is stretched to 4 feet, the percentage of elongation is 100%. With this in mind, it is understandable why a 1-foot length of the same color tubing stretched to 2 feet (100% elongation) generates the same force as a 2-foot length stretched to 4 feet.[221,222]

Furthermore, the *rate* at which elastic material is stretched does not seem to have a significant effect on the amount of resistance encountered.[223] Consequently, when a patient is performing a particular exercise, so long as the percentage of elongation of the tubing is the same from one repetition to the next, the resistance encountered is the same regardless of whether the exercise is performed at slow or fast velocity.

***Determination and quantification of resistance.*** In order to make decisions based on evidence, rather than solely on clinical judgment, about the grade (color) of elastic material to select for a patient's exercise program, a number of studies have been done to quantify the resistance imparted by elastic bands or tubing.[136,147,152,223,245,275] These studies measured and compared the tensile forces generated by various grades of elastic bands or tubing in relation to the percentage of elongation of the material. The forces expected at specific percentages of elongation of each grade of tubing or bands can be calculated by means of linear regression equations. Detailed specifications about the material properties of one brand of elastic resistance products, Thera-Band,® are available at www.thera-bandacademy.com/.

During exercise, the percentage of deformation and resulting resistance (force) from the material is not the only factor that must be considered. The amount of torque (force × distance) imposed by the elastic on the bony lever is also an important consideration. Just because the tension produced by an elastic band or tubing increases as it is stretched, it does not mean that the imposed torque necessarily increases from the beginning to the end of an exercise. In addition to the resistance (force) imposed by the elastic material as it is stretched, the factor of the changing length of the moment arm as the angle of the elastic changes with respect to the moving limb affects the torque imparted by the elastic material.[147] Studies have indicated that bell-shaped torque curves occur, with the peak torque near mid-range during exercises with elastic material.[147,222] Careful scrutiny of these studies is necessary to determine if the elastic resistance is at a 90° angle to the moving limb at mid-range. As in all forms of dynamic resistance exercise, the length–tension relationship of the contracting muscle also affects its ability to respond to the changing load.

***Fatigue characteristics.*** It has been suggested that elastic resistance products tend to fatigue over time, which causes the material to lose some of its force-generating property.[146] That being said, the extent of *material fatigue* is dependent on the number of times the elastic band or tubing has been stretched (number of stretch cycles) and the percentage of deformation with each stretch.[245]

Studies have shown that the decrease in tensile force is significant but small, with much of the decrease occurring within the first 20[223] or 50[146] stretch cycles. However, in the former study, investigators found that after this small initial decrease in tensile force occurred there was no appreciable decrease in the force-generating potential of the tubing after more than 5000 cycles of stretch. In other words, a patient could perform 10 repetitions each of four different exercises, three times a day on a daily basis for 6 weeks with the same piece of tubing before needing to replace it.

Elastic materials also display a property called *viscoelastic creep*. If a constant load is placed on elastic material, in time it becomes brittle and eventually ruptures. Environmental conditions, such as heat and humidity, also affect the force-generating potential of elastic bands and tubing.[146]

### Application of Elastic Resistance

***Selecting the appropriate grade of material.*** The thickness (stiffness) of the material affects the level of resistance. A heavier grade of elastic generates greater tension when stretched and therefore imparts a greater level of resistance.[136,146,245] As already noted, corresponding levels of resistance have been published for the different grades of bands and tubing.

There is a question of whether similar colors of bands or tubing from different manufacturers may or may not provide similar levels of tension under the same conditions.

In a study[275] comparing similar colors and lengths of Thera-Band and Cando tubing (Cando Fabrication Enterprises, White Plains, NY), investigators measured (by means of a strain gauge) the forces generated under similar conditions. They found no appreciable differences between the two products except for the thinnest (yellow) and thickest (silver/gray) grades. In those two grades the Cando tubing produced approximately 30% to 35% higher levels of force than the Thera-Band product. Despite these small differences, it is prudent to use the same product with the same patient.

***Selecting the appropriate length.*** Elastic bands or tubing come in large rolls and can be cut in varying lengths depending on the specific exercise to be performed and the height of a patient or the length of the extremities. The length of the elastic material should be sufficient to attach it *securely* at both ends. It should be taut but not stretched (*resting length)* at the beginning position of an exercise.

Remember, the percentage of elongation of the material affects the tension produced. Accordingly, it is essential that the same length of elastic resistance is used each time a particular exercise is performed. Otherwise, the imposed load may be too little or too much from one exercise session to the next even though the same grade (thickness) of elastic is used.

***Securing bands or tubing.*** One end is often tied or attached to a fixed object (doorknob, table leg, or D-ring) or secured by having the patient stand on one end of the material. The other end is grasped or fastened to a nylon loop, which is then placed around a limb segment. The material can also be secured to a harness on a patient's trunk for resisted walking activities. The band or tubing can also be held in both hands or looped under both feet for bilateral exercise. Figure 6.50A–C depicts upper or lower extremity and trunk strengthening activities using elastic resistance.

***Setting up an exercise.*** With elastic resistance the muscle receives the maximum resistive force when the material is on a stretch and angled 90° to the lever arm (moving bone). The therapist should determine the limb position at which maximum resistance is desired and anchor the elastic material so it is at a right angle at that portion of the range. When the material is at an acute angle to the moving bone, there is less resistance but greater joint compressive force.

It is important to consistently set up the exercise in the same manner from one exercise session to the next. Each time a patient performs a specific exercise, in addition to using the same length of elastic material the patient should assume the same position. A resource by Page and Ellenbecker[221] described setups for numerous exercises using elastic resistance.

***Progressing exercises.*** Exercises can be progressed by increasing the number of repetitions of an exercise with the same grade of resistance or by using the next higher grade of elastic band or tubing.

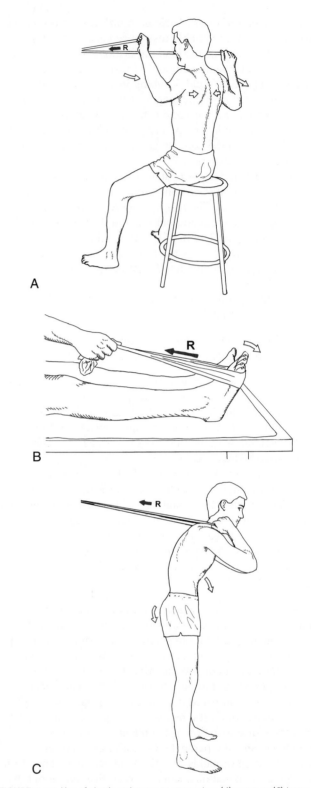

FIGURE 6.50 Use of elastic resistance to strengthen (*A*) upper or (*B*) lower extremity or (*C*) trunk musculature.

## Advantages and Disadvantages of Exercise with Elastic Resistance

### Advantages

- Elastic resistance products are *portable* and relatively *inexpensive*, making them an ideal choice for home exercise programs.
- Because elastic resistance is not significantly gravity-dependent, elastic bands and tubing are extremely *versatile*, allowing exercises to be performed in many combinations of movement patterns in the extremities and trunk and in many positions.[146,147,222]
- It is safe to exercise at moderate to fast velocities with elastic resistance because the patient does not have to overcome the inertia of a rapidly moving weight. As such, it is appropriate for plyometric training.

### Disadvantages

- One of the most significant drawbacks to the use of elastic resistance is the need to refer to a table of figures for quantitative information about the level of resistance for each color-coded grade of material. This makes it difficult to know which grade to select initially and to what extent changing the grade of the band or tubing changes the level of resistance.
- As with free weights, there is no source of stabilization or control of extraneous movements when an elastic band or tubing is used for resistance. The patient must use muscular stabilization to ensure that the correct movement pattern occurs.
- Although the effects of material fatigue are small with typical clinical use (up to 300% deformation in most exercises), elastic bands and tubing should be replaced on a routine basis to ensure patient safety.[146,245] If many individuals use the same precut lengths of bands or tubing, it may be difficult to determine how much use has occurred.
- Some elastic products contain latex, thus eliminating use by individuals with an allergy to latex. However, there are latex-free products on the market at a relatively comparable cost.

## Equipment for Closed-Chain Training

Many closed-chain exercises are performed in weight-bearing postures to develop strength, endurance, and stability across multiple joints. Typically, these exercises use partial or full body weight as the source of resistance. Examples in the lower extremities include squats, lunges, and step-ups or step-downs; and in the upper extremities they include push-ups or press-ups in various positions and pull-ups or chin-ups. These exercises can be progressed by simply adding resistance with handheld weights, a weighted belt or vest, or elastic resistance. Progressing from bilateral to unilateral weight bearing (when feasible) also increases the exercise load.

The following equipment is designed specifically for closed-chain training and has features to improve muscle performance across multiple joints.

### Body Weight Resistance— Multipurpose Exercise Systems

The Total Gym® system, for example, uses a glideboard, which can be set at 10 incline angles, that enables a patient to perform bilateral or unilateral closed-chain strengthening and endurance exercises in positions that range from partially reclining to standing (Fig. 6.51 A&B). The level of resistance on the Total Gym apparatus is increased or decreased by adjusting the angle of the glideboard on the incline.

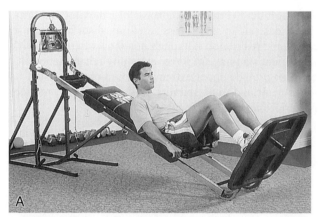

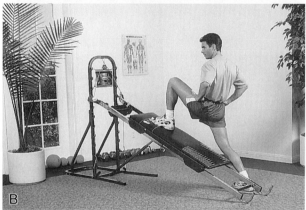

FIGURE 6.51 Closed-chain training: (*A*) in the semi-reclining position and (*B*) standing position using the Total Gym system. *(Courtesy of Total Gym, San Diego, CA.)*

Performance of bilateral and, later, unilateral squatting exercises in a semireclining position allows the patient to begin closed-chain training in a partially unloaded (partial weight-bearing) position early in the rehabilitation program. Later, the patient can progress to forward lunges (where the foot slides forward on the glideboard) while in a standing position.

N O T E : The Total Gym® system can also be set up for trunk exercises and open-chain exercises for the upper or lower extremities.

## Balance Boards

A balance board (wobble board) is used for proprioceptive training in the upper or lower extremities. One example is the BAPS (Biomechanical Ankle Platform) system. This system can be used in the standing position, the seated position (with the foot placed on the board) for ankle exercises, or in the quadriped position for upper extremity activities. Progressively increasing the size of the half spheres under the board or placing weights on the board makes the balance activity more challenging.

## Slide Boards

The ProFitter® (Fig. 6.52) consists of a moving platform that slides side to side across an elliptical surface against adjustable resistance. Although it is most often used with the patient standing for lower extremity rehabilitation, it can also provide upper extremity closed-chain resisted movements and trunk stability. Medial-lateral or anterior-posterior movements are possible.

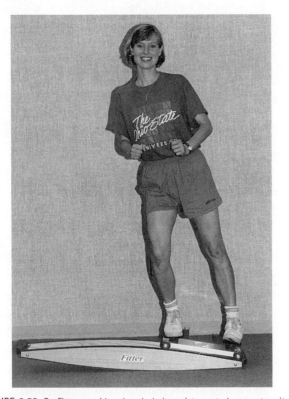

FIGURE 6.52 ProFitter provides closed-chain resistance to lower extremity musculature in preparation for functional activities.

## Mini-Trampolines (Rebounders)

Mini-trampolines enable the patient to begin gentle, bilateral or unilateral bouncing activities on a resilient surface to decrease the impact on joints. A patient can jog, jump, or hop in place. "Mini-tramps" that have a waist-height bar (attached to the frame) to hold onto provide additional safety.

## Reciprocal Exercise Equipment

Similar to other types of equipment that can be used for closed-chain training, reciprocal exercise devices strengthen multiple muscle groups across multiple joints. They also are appropriate for low-intensity, high-repetition resistance training to increase muscular endurance and reciprocal coordination of the upper or lower extremities and improve cardipulmonary fitness. They are often used for warm-up or cool-down exercises prior to and after more intense resistance training. Resistance is imparted by an adjustable friction device or by hydraulic or pneumatic resistance.

### Stationary Exercise Cycles

The stationary exercise cycle (upright or recumbent) is used to increase lower extremity strength and endurance. An upright cycle requires greater trunk control and balance than a recumbent cycle. A few exercise cycles provide resistance to the upper extremities as well. Resistance can be graded to challenge the patient progressively. Distance, speed, or duration of exercise can also be monitored.

The exercise cycle provides resistance to muscles during repetitive, nonimpact, and reciprocal movements of the extremities. Passive devices resist only concentric muscle activity as the patient performs pushing or pulling movements. Motor-driven exercise cycles can be adjusted to provide eccentric as well as concentric resistance. The placement of the seat can also be adjusted to alter the arc of motion that occurs in the lower extremities.

### Portable Resistive Reciprocal Exercise Units

A number of portable resistive exercisers are effective alternatives to an exercise cycle for repetitive, reciprocal exercise. One such product, the Chattanooga Group Exerciser® (Fig. 6.53), can be used for lower extremity exercise by placing the unit on the floor in front of a chair or wheelchair. This is particularly appropriate for a patient who is unable to get on and off an exercise cycle. In addition, it can be placed on a table for upper extremity exercise. Resistance can be adjusted to meet the abilities of individual patients.

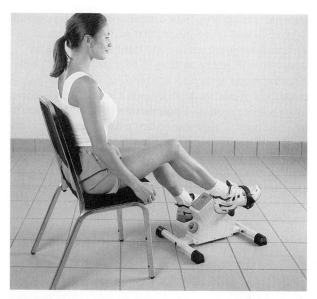

FIGURE 6.53 Resisted reciprocal exercise using the Chattanooga Exerciser. *(Courtesy of Chattanooga Group, Inc., Hixon, TN.)*

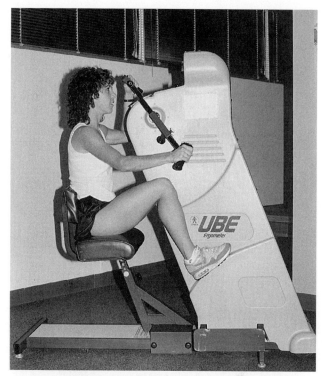

FIGURE 6.54 Upper Body Exerciser (UBE) is used for upper extremity strength and endurance training.

### Stair-Stepping Machines

The StairMaster® and the Climb Max 2000® are examples of a stepping machines that allow the patient to perform reciprocal pushing movements against adjustable resistance to make the weight-bearing activity more difficult. Stepping machines provide nonimpact, closed-chain strengthening as an alternative to walking or jogging on a treadmill. A patient can also kneel next to the unit and place both hands on the foot plates to use this equipment for upper extremity closed-chain exercises.

### Elliptical Trainers and Cross-Country Ski Machines

Elliptical trainers and cross-country ski machines also provide nonimpact, reciprocal resistance to the lower extremities in an upright, weight-bearing position. Variable incline adjustments of these units further supplement resistance options. Both types of equipment also incorporate sources of reciprocal resistance to the upper extremities into their designs.

### Upper Extremity Ergometers

Upper body ergometers (UBEs) provide resistance exclusively for the upper extremities (Fig. 6.54). Typically, the patient is seated, but the UBE can also be used with the patient in a standing position to lessen the extent of elevation of the arms necessary with each revolution. This is particularly helpful for patients with impingement syndromes of the shoulder.

## Equipment for Dynamic Stabilization Training

### Swiss Balls (Stability Balls)

Heavy-duty vinyl balls, usually 20 to 30 inches in diameter, are used for a variety of trunk and extremity stabilization exercises. A patient can also use elastic resistance or free weights while on the ball to increase the difficulty of exercises. Refer to Chapter 16 for descriptions of a number of dynamic stabilization exercises using stability balls.

### BodyBlade®

The BodyBlade® (Fig. 6.55) is a dynamic, reactive form of resistance equipment that uses the principle of inertia as the source of resistance to produce dynamic stability. While a patient drives the blade, rapidly, alternating contractions of agonist and antagonist muscle groups occur in an attempt to control the instability in three planes of motion dictated by movements of the blade. The greater the amplitude or flex of the blade, the greater the resistance. This provides progressive resistance that the patient controls.

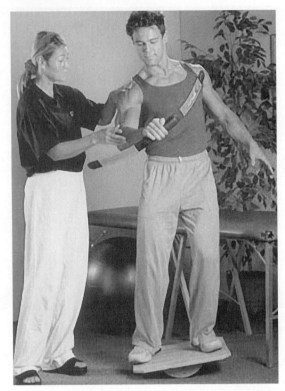

FIGURE 6.55 Dynamic stabilization exercises of the upper extremity and trunk using the BodyBlade. *(Courtesy of BodyBlade/Hymanson, Inc., Los Angeles, CA; 1-800-77BLADE, or 25233; www.bodyblade.com/.)*

Initially, the oscillating blade is maintained in various positions in space, particularly those positions in which dynamic stability is required for functional activities. The patient can progress the difficulty of the stabilization exercises by moving the upper extremity through various planes of motion (from sagittal to frontal and ultimately to transverse) as the blade oscillates. The goal is to develop proximal stability (a stable core) as a foundation of controlled mobility.

## Isokinetic Testing and Training Equipment

Isokinetic dynamometers (rate-limiting devices that control the velocity of motion) provide accommodating resistance during dynamic exercises of the extremities or trunk. The equipment supplies resistance proportional to the force generated by the person using the machine. The preset rate (degrees per second) cannot be exceeded no matter how vigorously the person pushes against the force arm. Therefore, the muscle contracts to its fullest capacity at all points in the ROM.

### Features of Isokinetic Dynamometers
New product lines of isokinetic equipment and improvements in existing equipment have been developed over the years. The Biodex isokinetic dynamometer (Fig. 6.56) is an example of a unit currently on the market. The specifications of the various manufacturers' dynamometers differ

somewhat. Features include computerized testing capabilities; passive and active modes that permit open-chain, concentric and eccentric testing and training; and velocity settings from 0° per second up to 500° per second for the concentric mode and up to 120° to 250° per second for the eccentric mode. Isokinetic units can be used for continuous passive motion. Computer programming allows limb movement within a specified range. Single-joint, uniplanar movements are most common, but some multiplanar movement patterns are possible. The Biodex dynamometer has attachments for multijoint, closed-chain exercises. Reciprocal training of agonist and antagonist and concentric/eccentric training of the same muscle group are both possible.

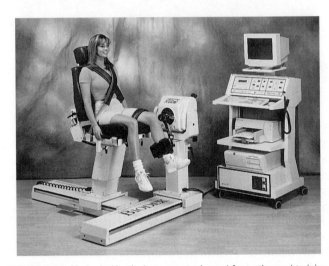

FIGURE 6.56 Biodex isokinetic dynamometer is used for testing and training. *(Courtesy of Biodex Medical Systems, Inc., Shirley, NY.)*

## Advantages and Disadvantages of Isokinetic Equipment

### Advantages

- Isokinetic equipment can provide maximum resistance at all points in the ROM as a muscle contracts.
- Both high- and low-velocity training can be done safely and effectively.
- The equipment accommodates for a painful arc of motion.
- As a patient fatigues, exercise can still continue.
- Isolated strengthening of muscle groups is possible to correct strength deficits in specific muscle groups.
- External stabilization keeps the patient and moving segment well aligned.
- Concentric and eccentric contractions of the same muscle group can be performed repeatedly, or reciprocal exercise of opposite muscle groups can be performed, allowing one muscle group to rest while its antagonist contracts; the latter method minimizes muscle ischemia.
- Computer-based visual or auditory cues provide feedback to the patient so submaximal to maximal work can be carried out more consistently.

## Disadvantages

- The equipment is large and expensive.
- Setup time and assistance from personnel are necessary if a patient is to exercise multiple muscle groups.
- The equipment cannot be incorporated into a home exercise program.
- Most units allow only open-chain (non-weight-bearing) movement patterns, which do not simulate most lower extremity functions and some upper extremity functions.
- Although functional movements typically occur in combined patterns and at many different velocities, most exercises are performed in a single plane and at a constant velocity.
- Although the range of concentric training velocities (up to 500°/sec) is comparable to some lower extremity limb speeds during functional activities, even the upper limits of this range cannot begin to approximate the rapid limb speeds that are necessary during many sports-related motions, such as throwing. In addition, the eccentric velocities available, at best, only begin to approach medium-range speeds, far slower than the velocity of movement associated with quick changes of direction and deceleration. Both of these limitations in the range of training velocities compromise carryover to functional goals.

## Equipment for Isometric Training

To complete the total picture of the importance of equipment for effective resistance training, isometric resistance exercises must also be addressed. One of the advantages of isometric training is that it is possible to perform a variety of exercises *without* equipment. For example, *multiple-angle isometrics* can be carried out by simply having the patient push against an immovable object, such as a door frame, a heavy table, a sofa, or a wall. Of course, manual resistance is also an effective means of strengthening muscles isometrically, particularly early in a rehabilitation program.

Many pieces of equipment designed for dynamic exercise can be adapted for isometric exercise. A weight-pulley system that provides resistance greater than the force-generating capacity of a muscle results in a static muscle contraction. Most isokinetic devices can be set up with the speed set at 0°/sec at multiple joint angles for isometric resistance at multiple points in the ROM. If elastic resistance or a pulley system is applied to the sound lower extremity, as the patient stands and bears full weight on the involved lower extremity, the muscles of the involved extremity must contract isometrically to hold the body in a stable, upright position as the sound extremity moves against the resistance.

## INDEPENDENT LEARNING ACTIVITIES

### Critical Thinking and Discussion

1. What physical findings from an examination and evaluation of a patient would lead you to determine that resistance exercises were an appropriate intervention?
2. What are the benefits and limitations of isometric, dynamic (constant or variable resistance), and isokinetic exercises?
3. What are the key changes that occur in muscle strength and endurance throughout the life span?
4. You have been asked to design a resistance exercise program as part of a total fitness program for a group of 7- to 9-year-old soccer players (boys and girls). Indicate the exercises you would include, the equipment you need, and the guidelines for intensity, volume, frequency, and rest.
5. Analyze five daily living tasks or recreational activities that you currently perform or would like to be able to perform effectively and efficiently. Identify what aspects of muscle performance (strength, power, endurance) and other parameters of function, such as mobility (flexibility), stability, balance, and coordinated movement, are involved in each of these tasks.
6. Develop an in-service instructional presentation that deals with the appropriate and effective use of elastic resistance products.
7. You have been asked to help design a circuit weight training sequence at a soon-to-open fitness facility at the outpatient treatment center where you work. Select equipment to meet the needs of beginning and advanced individuals. Establish general guidelines for intensity, repetitions and sets, order of exercise, rest intervals, and frequency.
8. Analyze the plyometric training activities listed in Box 6.19 and determine in which muscle groups training-induced gains in strength and power would occur and what functional tasks could each of the activities enhance.
9. Design a resistance-training program as part of a total fitness program for a group of older adults who participate in activities at a community-based senior citizen center. All participants are ambulatory and range in age from 65 to 85 years. Each has received clearance from his or her physician to participate in the program. What types of resistance equipment and levels of resistance would you recommend? Identify special precautions you would want to take.

### Laboratory Practice

1. Perform manual resistance exercise to all muscle groups of the upper and lower extremities in the following posi-

tions: supine, prone, side-lying, and sitting. What are the major limitations to effective, full-range strengthening in each of these positions?

2. Apply manual resistance exercises to each of the muscles of the wrist, fingers, and thumb.

3. Practice upper extremity and lower extremity $D_1$ and $D_2$ PNF exercises on your laboratory partner's right *and* left extremities.

4. Determine a 1 RM and 10 RM for the following muscle groups: shoulder flexors, shoulder abductors, shoulder external rotators, elbow flexors and extensors, hip abductors, hip flexors, knee flexors and extensors. Select one upper and one lower extremity muscle group. Determine a 1 RM or 10 RM with free weights in two positions. Determine where in the ROM maximum

resistance is encountered. Then determine a 1 RM or 10 RM with a pulley system. Compare your results.

5. Set up and safely apply exercises with elastic bands or tubing to strengthen the major muscle groups of the upper and lower extremities. Include a dynamic open-chain, a dynamic closed-chain, and an isometric exercise for each muscle group.

6. Demonstrate a series of simulated functional activities that could be used in the final stages of rehabilitation to continue to improve muscle performance as a transition into independent functional activities for a mail carrier, a nurse's aide who works in a skilled nursing facility, a ski instructor, a baseball player, and a daycare worker who cares for a group of active toddlers (each weighing approximately 25 pounds).

# REFERENCES

1. Abe, T, DeHoyos, DV, Pollock, ML, Garzarella, L: Time course for strength and muscle thickness changes following upper and lower body resistance training in men and women. Eur J Appl Physiol 81:174, 2000.
2. Abraham, WM: Factors in delayed muscle soreness. Med Sci Sports Exerc 9:11, 1977.
3. Ades, PA, et al: Weight training improves walking endurance in healthy elderly persons. Am J Internal Med 124:568, 1996.
4. Aitkens, S, et al: Moderate resistance exercise program. Its effects in slowly progressive neuromuscular disease. Arch Phys Med Rehabil 74:711, 1993.
5. Albert, MS, Wooden, MJ: Isokinetic evaluation and treatment. In Donatelli, RA (ed) Physical Therapy of the Shoulder, ed 3. Churchill Livingstone, New York, 1997, p 401.
6. American Academy of Pediatrics: Strength training by children and adolescents: policy statement. Pediatrics 107(6):1470–1472, 2001.
7. American Association of Cardiovascular and Pulmonary Rehabilitation: Guidelines for Cardiac Rehabilitation Programs, ed 3. Human Kinetics, Champaign, IL, 1999.
8. American College of Sports Medicine: ACSM's Guidelines for Exercise Testing and Prescription, ed 6, Lippincott Williams & Wilkins, Philadelphia, 2000.
9. American College of Sports Medicine: Position stand: progression models in resistance training for healthy adults. Med Sci Sports Exerc 34:364–380, 2002.
10. American Physical Therapy Association: Guide to Physical Therapist Practice, ed 2. Phys Ther 81:9–744, 2001.
11. Amiridis, IG, et al: Concentric and/or eccentric training-induced alterations in shoulder flexor and extensor strength. J Orthop Sports Phys Ther 25:26, 1997.
12. Antonio, J, Gonyea, WJ: Skeletal muscle fiber hyperplasia. Med Sci Sports Exerc 25:1333, 1993.
13. Armstrong, RB: Mechanisms of exercise-induced delayed onset muscular soreness: a brief review. Med Sci Sports Exerc 15:529–538, 1984.
14. Arnheim, DD, Prentice, WE: Principles of Athletic Training, ed 9. McGraw-Hill, Boston, 1997.
15. Augustsson, J, et al: Weight training of the thigh muscles using closed vs. open kinetic chain exercises: a comparison of performance enhancement. J Orthop Sports Phys Ther 27:3, 1998.
16. Baechle, TR, Earle, RW, Wathen, D: Resistance training. In Baechle, TR, Earle, RW (eds) Essentials of Strength Training and Conditioning, ed 2. Human Kinetics, Champaign, IL, 2000, p 395.
17. Baratta, R, et al: Muscular coactivation: the role of the antagonist musculature in maintaining knee stability. Am J Sports Med 16:113, 1988.
18. Barrett, DS: Proprioception and function after anterior cruciate ligament reconstruction. J Bone Joint Surg 73:83, 1991.
19. Beckham, SG, Earnest, CP: Metabolic cost of free weight circuit training. J Sports Med Physical Fitness 40(2):118–125, 2000.
20. Benn, C, et al: The effects of serial stretch loading on stretch work and stretch-shorten cycle performance in the knee musculature. J Orthop Sports Phys Ther 27:412, 1998.
21. Bennett, R, Knowlton, G: Overwork weakness in partially denervated skeletal muscle. Clin Orthop 12:22, 1958.
22. Bigland-Richie, B, Woods, J: Changes in muscle contractile properties and neural control during human muscle fatigue. Muscle Nerve 7:691, 1984.
23. Bishop, KN, et al: The effect of eccentric strength training at various speeds on concentric strength of the quadriceps and hamstring muscles. J Orthop Sports Phys Ther 13:226–229, 1991.
24. Blackard, DO, Jensen, RL, Ebben, WP: Use of EMG analysis in challenging kinetic chain terminology. Med Sci Sports Exerc 31:443, 1999.
25. Blackburn, JR, Morrissey, MC: The relationship between open and closed kinetic chain strength of the lower limb and jumping performance. J Orthop Sports Phys Ther 27:430, 1998.
26. Blimkie, C: Benefits and risks of resistance training in youth. In Cahill, B, Pearl, A (eds) Intensive Participation in Children's Sports. Human Kinetics, Champaign, IL, 1993, p 133.
27. Bonen, A, Belcastro, AN: Comparison of self-directed recovery methods on lactic acid removal rates. Med Sci Sports Exerc 8:176, 1976.
28. Bottomley, JM: Age-related bone health and pathophysiology of osteoporosis. Orthop Phys Ther Clin North Am 7:117, 1998.
29. Brask, B, Lueke, R, Sodeberg, G: Electromyographic analysis of selected muscles during the lateral step-up exercise. Phys Ther 64:324, 1984.
30. Brosky, JA, Wright, GA: Training for muscular strength, power and endurance and hypertrophy. In Nyland, J (ed) Clinical Decisions in Therapeutic Exercise: Planning and Implementation. Pearson Education, Upper Saddle River, NJ, 2006, pp 171–230.
31. Brunnstrom, S: Clinical Kinesiology. FA Davis, Philadelphia, 1962.
32. Bryant, CX, Peterson, JA, Graves, JE: Muscular strength and endurance. In Roitman, JL (ed) ACSM's Resource Manual for Exercise Testing and Prescription, ed 4. Lippincott Williams & Wilkins, Philadelphia, 2001, p 460.
33. Carron, AV, Bailey, DA: Strength development in boys from 10–16 years. Monogr Soc Res Child Dev 39:1, 1974.
34. Chandler, JM, Duncan, PW: Eccentric versus concentric force-velocity relationships of the quadriceps femoris muscle. Phys Ther 68:800, 1988.
35. Chandler, JM: Understanding the relationship between strength and mobility in frail older persons: a review of the literature. Top Geriatr Rehabil 11:20, 1996.
36. Chandler, JM, et al: Is lower extremity strength gain associated with improvement in physical performance and disability in frail, community-dwelling elders? Arch Phys Med Rehabil 79:24, 1998.
37. Chu, DA, Cordier, DJ: Plyometrics in rehabilitation. In Ellenbecker, TS (ed) Knee Ligament Rehabilitation. Churchill-Livingstone, New York, 2000, p 321.

38. Chung, F, Dean, E, Ross, J: Cardiopulmonary responses of middle-aged men without cardiopulmonary disease to steady-rate positive and negative work performed on a cycle ergometer. Phys Ther 79:476, 1999.

39. Clark, MA, Foster, D, Reuteman, P: Core (trunk) stabilization and its importance for closed kinetic chain performance. Orthop Phys Ther Clin North Am 9:119, 2000.

40. Clarkson, PM, Hubal, MJ: Exercise-induced muscle damage in humans. Am J Phys Med Rehabil 81(11 Suppl):S52–S69, 2002.

41. Clarkson, PM, Tremblay, I: Exercise induced muscle damage, repair and adaptation in humans. J Appl Physiol 65:1–6, 1988.

42. Connelly, DM, Vandervoort, AA: Effects of detraining on knee extensor strength and functional mobility in a group of elderly women. J Orthop Sports Phys Ther 26:340, 1997.

43. Connelly, DM, Vandervoort, AA: Improvement in knee extensor strength of institutionalized elderly women after exercise with ankle weights. Physiother Can 47:15, 1995.

44. Connolly, DA, Sayers, SP, McHugh, MP: Treatment and prevention of delayed onset muscle soreness. J Strength Cond Res 17:197–208, 2003.

45. Conroy, BP, Earle, RW: Bone, muscle and connective tissue adaptations to physical activity. In Beachle, TR (ed) Essentials of Strength Training and Conditioning. Human Kinetics, Champaign, IL, 1994, p 51.

46. Cook, TM, et al: EMG comparison of lateral step-up and stepping machine exercise. J Orthop Sports Phys Ther 16:108, 1992.

47. Corbin, DE: Exercise programming for older adults. In Roitman, JL (ed) ACSM's Resource Manual for Guidelines for Exercise Testing and Prescription, ed 4. Lippincott Williams & Wilkins, Philadelphia, 2001, p 529.

48. Corder, KP, et al: Effects of active and passive recovery conditions on blood lactate, rating of perceived exertion, and performance during resistance exercise. J Strength Conditioning Res 14:151, 2000.

49. Cress, ME, et al: Functional training: muscle structure, function and performance in older women. J Orthop Sports Phys Ther 24:4, 1996.

50. Cress, NM, Peters, KS, Chandler, JM: Eccentric and concentric force-velocity relationships of the quadriceps femoris muscle. J Orthop Sports Phys Ther 16:82–86, 1992.

51. Croarkin, E: Osteopenia: implications for physical therapists managing patients of all ages. PT Magazine Phys Ther 9:80, 2001.

52. Croarkin, E: Osteopenia in the patient with cancer. Phys Ther 79:196, 1999.

53. Cullan, E, Peat, M: Functional anatomy of the shoulder complex. J Orthop Sports Phys Ther 18:342, 1993.

54. Curtis, C, Weir, J: Overview of exercise responses in healthy and impaired states. Neurol Rep 20:13, 1996.

55. Davies, GJ: A Compendium of Isokinetics in Clinical Usage and Rehabilitation Techniques, ed 4. S & S Publishing, Onalaska, WI, 1992.

56. Davies, GJ: The need for critical thinking in rehabilitation. J Sports Rehabil 4:1, 1995.

57. Davies, GJ, Ellenbecker, TS: Application of isokinetics in testing and rehabilitation. In Andrews, JR, Harrelson, GL, Wilk, KE (eds) Physical Rehabilitation of the Injured Athlete, ed 2. WB Saunders, Philadelphia, 1998, p 219.

58. Davies, GJ, et al: The scientific and clinical rationale for the integrated approach to open and closed kinetic chain rehabilitation. Orthop Phys Ther Clin North Am 9:247, 2000.

59. Davies, GJ, Heiderscheit, BC, Clark, M: Open and closed kinetic chain rehabilitation. In Ellenbecker, TS (ed) Knee Ligament Rehabilitation. Churchill Livingstone, New York, 2000, p 219.

60. Davies, GJ, Zillmer, DA: Functional progression of a patient through a rehabilitation program. Orthop Phys Ther Clin North Am 9:103, 2000.

61. Davis, M, Fitts, R: Mechanisms of muscular fatigue. In Roitman, JL (ed) ACSM's Resource Manual for Guidelines for Exercise Testing and Prescription, ed 4. Lippincott Williams & Wilkins, Philadelphia, 2001, p 184.

62. Dean, E: Physiology and therapeutic implications of negative work: a review. Phys Ther 68:233, 1988.

63. DeLorme, TL: Heavy resistance exercise. Arch Phys Med Rehabil 27:607, 1946.

64. DeLorme, TL, Watkins, A: Progressive Resistance Exercise. Appleton-Century, New York, 1951.

65. DeLorme, T, Watkins, A: Technics of progressive resistance exercise. Arch Phys Med Rehabil 29:263, 1948.

66. Denegar, CR, et al: Influence of transcutaneous electrical nerve stimulation on pain, range of motion and serum cortisol concentration in females experiencing delayed onset muscle soreness. J Orthop Sports Phys Ther 11:100–103, 1989.

67. DeVine, K: EMG activity recorded from an unexercised muscle during maximum isometric exercise of contralateral agonists and antagonists. Phys Ther 61:898, 1981.

68. DeVries, HA: Electromyographic observations on the effects static stretching has on muscular distress. Res Q 32:468, 1961.

69. DeVries, HA: Quantitative electromyographic investigation of the spasm theory of muscle pain. Am J Phys Med Rehabil 45:119, 1966.

70. Dierking, JK, et al: Validity of diagnostic ultrasound as a measure of delayed onset muscle soreness. J Orthop Sports Phys Ther 30:116, 2000.

71. DiFabio, RP: Editorial: making jargon from kinetic and kinematic chains. J Orthop Sports Phys Ther 29:142, 1999.

72. Dillman CJ, Murray, TA, Hintermeister, RA: Biomechanical differences of open and closed-chain exercises with respect to the shoulder. J Sport Rehabil 3:228, 1994.

73. Donatelli, RA: Functional anatomy and mechanics. In Donatelli, RA (ed) Physical Therapy of the Shoulder, ed 4. Churchill Livingstone, St Louis, 2004, p 11.

74. Donnelly, AE, Clarkson, PM, Maughan, RJ: Exercise-induced damage: effects of light exercise on damaged muscle. Eur J Appl Physiol 64:350, 1992.

75. Doucette, SA, Child, DD: The effect of open and closed-chain exercise and knee joint position on patellar tracking in lateral patellar compression syndrome. J Orthop Sports Phys Ther 23:104, 1996.

76. Douris, PC: Cardiovascular response to velocity-specific isokinetic exercises. J Orthop Sports Phys Ther 13:28–32, 1991.

77. Draganich, LF, Jaeger, RJ, Kraji, AR: Coactivation of the hamstrings and quadriceps during extension of the knee. J Bone Joint Surg Am 71:1075, 1989.

78. Drury, DG: The role of eccentric exercise in strengthening muscle. Orthop Phys Ther Clin North Am 9:515, 2000.

79. Duarte, JA, et al: Exercise-induced signs of muscle overuse in children. Int J Sports Med 20:103, 1999.

80. Duncan, PW, et al: Mode and speed specificity of eccentric and concentric exercise training. J Orthop Sports Phys Ther 11:70–75, 1989.

81. Durstine, JL, Davis, PG: Specificity of exercise training and testing. In Roitman, JL (ed) ACSM's Resource Manual for Guidelines for Exercise Testing and Prescription, ed 4. Lippincott Williams & Wilkins, Philadelphia, 2001, p 484.

82. Dvir, Z: Isokinetics: Muscle Testing, Interpretations and Clinical Application. Churchill Livingstone, Edinburgh, 2004.

83. Edwards, BJ, Perry, HM: Age-related osteoporosis. Clin Geriatr Med 10:575, 1994.

84. Ellenbecker, TS: Isokinetics in rehabilitation. In Ellenbecker, TS (ed) Knee Ligament Rehabilitation. Churchill Livingstone, New York, 2000, p 277.

85. Ellenbecker, TS, Cappel, K: Clinical application of closed kinetic chain exercises in the upper extremities. Orthop Phys Ther Clin North Am 9:231, 2000.

86. Ellenbecker, TS, Davies, GJ, Rowinski, MJ: Concentric versus eccentric isokinetic strengthening of the rotator cuff. Am J Sports Med 16:64, 1988.

87. Ellenbecker, TS, Davies, GJ: Closed Kinetic Chain Exercise: A Comprehensive Guide to Multiple-Joint Exercises. Human Kinetics, Champaign, IL, 2001.

88. Escamilla, RF, et al: Biomechanics of the knee during closed kinetic chain and open kinetic chain exercises. Med Sci Sports Exerc 30:556, 1998.

89. Eston, R, Peters, D: Effects of cold water immersion symptoms of exercise-induced muscle damage. J Sports Sci 17:231, 1999.

90. Faigenbaum, A, et al: The effects of strength training and detraining on children. J Strength Conditioning Res 10:109, 1996.

91. Faigenbaum, AD, Bradley, DF: Strength training for the young athlete. Orthop Phys Ther Clin North Am 7:67, 1998.

92. Faigenbaum, AD, Westcott, WL, Loud, RL, Long, C: The effects of different resistance training protocols on muscular strength and endurance development in children. Pediatrics 104(1):e55, 1999.

93. Falk, B, Tenenbaum, G: The effectiveness of resistance training in children: a meta-analysis. Sports Med 22:176, 1996.

94. Fardy, P: Isometric exercise and the cardiovascular system. Phys Sportsmed 9:43, 1981.

95. Faust, MS: Somatic development of adolescent girls. Soc Res Child Dev 42:1, 1977.

96. Fees, M, Decker, T, Snyder-Mackler, L, Axe, MJ: Upper extremity weight training modifications for the injured athlete: a clinical perspective. Am J Sports Med 26:732–742, 1998.

97. Fiatarone, MA, et al: High-intensity strength training in nonagenarians. JAMA 263:3029, 1990.

98. Fillyaw, M, et al: The effects of long-term nonfatiguing resistance exercise in subjects with post-polio syndrome. Orthopedics 14:1252, 1991.

99. Fish, DE, Krabeck, DJ, Johnson-Greene, D, DeLeteur, BJ: Optimal resistance training: comparison of DeLorme with Oxford techniques. Am J Phys Med and Rehabil 92:903–909, 2003.

100. Fitzgerald, GK, et al: Exercise induced muscle soreness after concentric and eccentric isokinetic contractions. Phys Ther 7:505–513, 1991.

101. Fitzgerald, GK: Open versus closed kinetic chain exercise: issues in rehabilitation after anterior cruciate ligament surgery. Phys Ther 77:1747, 1997.

102. Fleck, SJ: Periodized strength training: a critical review. J Strength Condition Res 13:82, 1999.

103. Fleck, SJ, Kraemer, WJ: Designing Resistance Training Programs, ed 2. Human Kinetics, Champaign, IL, 1997.

104. Francis, KT: Delayed muscle soreness: a review. J Orthop Sports Phys Ther 5:10, 1983.

105. Francis, KT: Status of the year 2000 health goals for physical activity and fitness. Phys Ther 79:405, 1999.

106. Franklin, ME, et al: Effect of isokinetic soreness-inducing exercise on blood levels of creatine protein and creatine kinase. J Orthop Sports Phys Ther 16:208–214, 1992.

107. Freedson, PS, Ward, A, Rippe, JM: Resistance training for youth. In Grana, WA, et al (eds) Advances in Sports Medicine and Fitness, Vol 3. Year Book, Chicago, 1990, p 57.

108. Friden, J, Sjostrom, M, Ekblom, B: Myofibrillar damage following intense eccentric exercise in man. Int J Sports Med 4:170, 1983.

109. Frontera, WR, Larsson, L: Skeletal muscle function in older people. In Kauffman, TL (ed) Geriatric Rehabilitation Manual. Churchill Livingstone, New York, 1999, p 8.

110. Fry, AC: The role of training intensity in resistance exercise, overtraining and overreaching. In Kreider R, Fry, A, O'Toole M (eds) Overtraining in Sport. Human Kinetics, Champaign, IL, 1998, p 107.

111. Gajdosik, RL, Vander Linden, DW, Williams, AK: Concentric isokinetic torque characteristics of the calf muscles of active women aged 20 to 84 years. J Orthop Sports Phys Ther 29:181, 1999.

112. Gilligan, C, Checovich, MN, Smith, EL: Osteoporosis. In Skinner, JS (ed) Testing and Exercise Prescription in Special Cases, ed 2. Lea & Febiger, Philadelphia, 1993, p 127.

113. Gisolti, C, Robinson, S, Turrell, ES: Effects of aerobic work performed during recovery from exhausting work. J Appl Physiol 21:1767, 1966.

114. Gollnick, P, et al: Glycogen depletion patterns in human skeletal muscle fibers during prolonged work. J Appl Physiol 34:615, 1973.

115. Gollnick, PD, et al: Muscular enlargement and number of fibers in skeletal muscle of rats. J Appl Physiol 50:936, 1981.

116. Gonyea, WJ: Role of exercise in inducing increases in skeletal muscle fibre number. J Appl Physiol 48:424, 1980.

117. Gonyea, WJ, Ericson, GC, Bonde-Petersen, F: Skeletal muscle fiber splitting induced by weightlifting in cats. Acta Physiol Scand 99:105, 1977.

118. Graves, JE, Pollock, ML, Bryant, CX: Assessment of muscular strength and endurance. In: Roitman, JL (ed) ACSM's Resource Manual for Guidelines for Exercise Testing and Prescription, ed 4. Lippincott Williams & Wilkins, Philadelphia, 2001, p 376.

119. Greig, CA, Botella, J, Young, A: The quadriceps strength of healthy elderly people remeasured after 8 years. Muscle Nerve 16:6, 1993.

120. Grimby, G, et al: Training can improve muscle strength and endurance in 78–84 year old men. J Appl Physiol 73:2517, 1992.

121. Guyton, AC, Hall, JE: Textbook of Muscle Physiology, ed 10. WB Saunders, Philadelphia, 2000.

122. Hageman, PA, Gillaspie, D, Hall, LD: Effects of speed and limb dominance on eccentric and concentric isokinetic testing of the knee. J Orthop Sports Phys Ther 10:59, 1988.

123. Hageman, PA, Sorensen, TA: Eccentric isokinetics. In Albert, M (ed) Eccentric Muscle Training in Sports and Orthopedics, ed 2. Churchill Livingstone, New York, 1995, p 115.

124. Hagood, S, et al: The effect of joint velocity on the contribution of the antagonist musculature to knee stiffness and laxity. Am J Sports Med 18:182, 1990.

125. Harbst, KB, Wilder, PA: Neurophysiologic, motor control and motor learning basis of closed kinetic chain exercises. Orthop Phys Ther Clin North Am 9:137, 2000.

126. Hasson, S, et al: Therapeutic effect of high speed voluntary muscle contractions on muscle soreness and muscle performance. J Orthop Sports Phys Ther 10:499, 1989.

127. Heiderscheit, BC, McLean, KP, Davies, GJ: The effects of isokinetic vs. plyometric training on the shoulder internal rotators. J Orthop Sports Phys Ther 23:125, 1996.

128. Heiderscheit, BC, Rucinski, TJ: Biomechanical and physiologic basis of closed kinetic chain exercises in the upper extremities. Orthop Phys Ther Clin North Am 9:209, 2000.

129. Hellebrandt, FA, Houtz, SJ: Mechanisms of muscle training in man: experimental demonstration of the overload principle. Phys Ther Rev 36:371, 1956.

130. Herbison, GJ, Jaweed, MM, Ditunno, JF, et al: Effect of overwork during reinnervation of rat muscle. Exp Neurol 41:1, 1973.

131. Hertling, D, Kessler, RM: Management of Common Musculoskeletal Disorders: Physical Therapy Principles and Methods, ed 4. Lippincott Williams & Wilkins, Philadelphia, 2006.

132. Hettinger, T, Muller, EA: Muscle strength and muscle training. Arbeitsphysiol 15:111, 1953.

133. Hewett, TE: The effect of neuromuscular training on the incidence of knee injury in female athletes: a prospective study. Am J Sports Med 27(6):699–706, 1999.

134. Hill, DW, Richardson, JD: Effectiveness of 10% trolamine salicylate cream on muscular soreness induced by a reproducible program of weight training. J Orthop Sports Phys Ther 11:19–23, 1989.

135. Hintermeister, RA, et al: Electromyographic activity and applied load during shoulder rehabilitation exercises using elastic resistance. Am J Sports Med 26:210, 1998.

136. Hintermeister, RA, et al: Quantification of elastic resistance knee rehabilitation exercises. J Orthop Sports Phys Ther 28:40, 1998.

137. Hislop, HJ, Montgomery, J: Daniels and Worthingham's Muscle Testing: Techniques of Manual Examination, ed 7. WB Saunders, Philadelphia, 2002.

138. Hislop, HJ, Perrine, J: The isokinetic concept of exercise. Phys Ther 41:114, 1967.

139. Hislop, HJ: Quantitative changes in human muscular strength during isometric exercise. Phys Ther 43:21, 1963.

140. Ho, K, et al: Muscle fiber splitting with weight lifting exercise. Med Sci Sports Exerc 9:65, 1977.

141. Hopp, JF: Effects of age and resistance training on skeletal muscle: a review. Phys Ther 73:361, 1993.

142. Hought, T: Ergographic studies in muscular soreness. Am J Physiol 7:76, 1902.

143. Housh, D, Housh T: The effects of unilateral velocity-specific concentric strength training. J Orthop Sports Phys Ther 17:252–256, 1993.

144. Howell, JN, Chleboun, G, Conaster, R: Muscle stiffness, strength loss, swelling and soreness following exercise-induced injury in humans. J Physiol 464:183, 1993.

145. Hruda, KV, Hicks, AL, McCartney, N: Training for muscle power in older adults: effects on functional abilities. Can J Applied Phyiol 28(2):178–189, 2003.

146. Hughes, C, Maurice, D: Elastic exercise training. Orthop Phys Ther Clin North Am 9:581, 2000.

147. Hughes, CJ, et al: Resistance properties of Thera-Band® tubing during shoulder abduction exercise. J Orthop Sports Phys Ther 29:413, 1999.

148. Issacs, L, Pohlman, R, Craig, B: Effects of resistance training on strength development in prepubescent females. Med Sci Sports Exerc 265:210, 1994.

149. Jenkins, WL, Thackaberry, M, Killan, C: Speed-specific isokinetic training. J Orthop Sports Phys Ther 6:181, 1984.

150. Jenkins, WL, et al: A measurement of anterior tibial displacement in the closed and open kinetic chain. J Orthop Sports Phys Ther 25:49, 1997.

151. Jones, H: The Valsalva procedure: its clinical importance to the physical therapist. Phys Ther 45:570, 1965.

152. Jones, KW, et al: Predicting forces applied by Thera-Band® Tubing during resistive exercises [abstract]. J Orthop Sports Phys Ther 27:65, 1998.

153. Jonhagen, S, Ackermann, P, Eriksson, T, et al: Sports massage after eccentric exercise. Am J Sports Med 32(6):1499–1503, 2004.

154. Kadi, F, et al: Cellular adaptation of the trapezius muscle in strength-trained athletes. Histochem Cell Biol 111:189, 1999.

155. Kauffman, TL, Nashner, LM, Allison, LK: Balance is a critical parameter in orthopedic rehabilitation. Orthop Phys Ther Clin North Am 6:43, 1997.

156. Kelley, GA, Kelley, KS, Tran, ZV: Resistance training and bone mineral density in women: a meta-analysis of controlled trials. Am J Phys Med Rehabil 80:65–77, 2001.

157. Kelsey, DD, Tyson, E: A new method of training for the lower extremity using unloading. J Orthop Sports Phys Ther 19:218–223, 1994.

158. Kendall, FP, McCreary, EK, Provance, PG, et al: Muscles: Testing and Function with Posture and Pain, ed 5. Lippincott Williams & Wilkins, Philadelphia, 2005.

159. Kernozck, TW, McLean, KP, McLean, DP: Biomechanical and physiologic factors of kinetic chain exercise in the lower extremity. Orthop Phys Ther Clin North Am 9:151, 2000.

160. Kerr, D, Ackland, T, Maslen, B, et al: Resistance training over 2 years increases bone mass in calcium-replete postmenopausal women. J Bone Miner Res 16(1):175–181, 2001.

161. Kitai, TA, Sale, DG: Specificity of joint angle in isometric training. Eur J Appl Physiol 58:741, 1989.

162. Knapik, JJ, Mawadsley, RH, Ramos, MU: Angular specificity and test mode specificity of isometric and isokinetic strength training. J Orthop Sports Phys Ther 5:58, 1983.

163. Knight, KL: Knee rehabilitation by the daily adjustable progressive resistive exercise technique. Am J Sports Med 7:336, 1979.

164. Knight, KL: Quadriceps strengthening with DAPRE technique: case studies with neurological implications. Med Sci Sports Exerc 17:636, 1985.

165. Knott, M, Voss, DE: Proprioceptive Neuromuscular Facilitation, Patterns and Techniques, ed 2. Harper & Row, Philadelphia, 1968.

166. Kraemer, WJ, Bush, JA: Factors affecting the acute neuromuscular responses to resistance exercise. In Rotman, JL (ed) ACSM's Resource Manual for Guidelines for Exercise Testing and Prescription, ed 4. Lippincott Williams & Wilkins, Philadelphia, 2001, p 167.

167. Kraemer, WJ, Bush, JA, Wickham, RB, et al: Continuous compression as an effective therapeutic intervention in treating eccentric-exercise-induced muscle soreness. J Sport Rehabilitation 10:11–23, 2001.

168. Kraemer, WJ, Ratamess, NA: Physiology of resistance training: current issues. Orthop Phys Ther Clin North Am 9:467, 2000.

169. Kraemer, WJ, Duncan, ND, Volek, JS: Resistance training and elite athletes: adaptations and program considerations. J Orthop Sports Phys Ther 28:110, 1998.

170. Kraemer, WJ, et al: Influence of resistance training volume and periodization on physiological and performance adaptations in collegiate women tennis players. Am J Sports Med 28:626, 2000.

171. Kraemer, W, et al: Influence of compression therapy on symptoms following soft tissue injury from maximal eccentric exercise. J Orthop Sports Phys Ther 31:282, 2001.

172. Kraemer, WJ, Volek, JS, Fleck, SJ: Chronic musculoskeletal adaptations to resistance training. In Roitman, JL (ed) ACSM's Resource Manual for Guidelines for Exercise Testing and Prescription, ed 4. Lippincott Williams & Wilkins, Philadelphia, 2001, p 176.

173. Kuipers, H: Training and overtraining: an introduction. Med Sci Sports Exerc 30:1137, 1998.

174. Kvist, J, et al: Anterior tibial translation during different isokinetic quadriceps torque in anterior cruciate ligament deficient and nonimpaired individuals. J Orthop Sports Phys Ther 31:4, 2001.

175. Lane, JN, Riley, EH, Wirganowicz, PZ: Osteoporosis: diagnosis and treatment. J Bone Joint Surg Am 78:618, 1996.

176. LaStayo, PC, Woolf, JM, Lewek, MD, et al: Eccentric muscle contractions: their contributions to injury, prevention, rehabilitation, and sport. J Orthop Sports Phys Ther 33(10):557–571, 2003.

177. Lear, LJ, Gross, MT: An electromyographical analysis of the scapular stabilizing synergists during a push-up progression. J Orthop Sports Phys Ther 28:146, 1998.

178. Lefever, SL: Closed kinetic chain training. In Hall, CM, Brody, LT (eds) Therepeutic Exercise: Moving Toward Function, ed 2. Lippincott Williams & Wilkins, Philadelphia, 2005, pp 263–308.

179. Lemmer, JT, et al: Age and gender responses to strength training and detraining. Med Sci Sports Exerc 32:1505, 2000.

180. Lephart, SM, et al: Proprioception following ACL reconstruction. J Sports Rehabil 1:188, 1992.

181. Lephart, SM, et al: The effects of neuromuscular control exercises on functional stability in the unstable shoulder. J Athletic Training 33S:15, 1998.

182. Lephart SM, et al: The role of proprioception in rehabilitation of athletic injuries. Am J Sports Med 25:130, 1997.

183. Lephart, SM, Henry, TJ: The physiological basis for open and closed kinetic chain rehabilitation for the upper extremity. J Sport Rehabil 5:71, 1996.

184. Levangie, PK, Norkin, CC: Joint Structure and Function: A Comprehensive Analysis, ed 3. FA Davis, Philadelphia, 2001.

185. Liberson, WT: Brief isometric exercise. In Basmajian, JV (ed) Therapeutic Exercise, ed 3. Williams & Wilkins, Baltimore, 1978.

186. Lindle, RS, et al: Age and gender comparisons of muscle strength of 654 women and men aged 20–93 yr. J Appl Physiol 83:1581, 1997.

187. MacDougal, J, et al: Arterial pressure responses to heavy resistance exercise. J Appl Physiol 70:2498, 1991.

188. MacDougall, JD, Elder, GCB, Sale, DG, et al: Effect of training and immobilization on human muscle fibers. Eur J Appl Physiol 43:25–34, 1980.

189. MacDougall, JD: Hypertrophy or hyperplasia. In Komi, PV (ed) Strength and Power in Sport, ed 2. Blackwell Science, Oxford, 2003, pp 252–264.

190. MacKinnon, J: Osteoporosis: a review. Phys Ther 68:1533–1540, 1988.

191. Mair, SD, et al: The role of fatigue in susceptibility to acute muscle strain injury. Am J Sports Med 24:137, 1996.

192. Malina, R, Bouchard, C: Growth, maturation and physical activity. Human Kinetics, Champaign, IL, 1991.

193. McArdle, WD, Katch, FI, Katch, VL: Essentials of Exercise Physiology, ed 2. Lippincott Williams & Wilkins, Philadelphia, 2000.

194. McCarrick, MS, Kemp, JG: The effect of strength training and reduced training on rotator cuff musculature. Clin Biomech 15(1 Suppl):S42–S45, 2000.

195. McGee, C: Standard rehabilitation vs. standard plus closed kinetic chain rehabilitation for patients with shoulder pathologies: a rehabilitation outcomes study [abstract]. Phys Ther 79:S65, 1999.

196. McGill, SM, Cholewicki, J: Biomechanical basis of stability: an explanation to enhance clinical utility. J Orthop Sports Phys Ther 31:96–99, 2001.

197. Menkes, A, et al: Strength training increases regional bone mineral density and bone remodeling in middle-aged and older men. J Appl Physiol 74:2478, 1993.

198. Mikesky, AE, et al: Changes in muscle fiber size and composition in response to heavy resistance exercise. Med Sci Sports Exerc 23:1042, 1991.

199. Moffroid, M, et al: A study of isokinetic exercise. Phys Ther 49:735, 1969.

200. Moffroid, M, Whipple, R: Specificity of the speed of exercise. Phys Ther 50:1693, 1970.

201. Moffroid, MT, Kusick, ET: The power struggle: definition and evaluation of power of muscular performance. Phys Ther 55:1098, 1975.

202. Mont, MA, et al: Isokinetic concentric versus eccentric training of shoulder rotators with functional evaluation of performance enhancement in elite tennis players. Am J Sports Med 22:513, 1994.

203. Morganti, CM, et al: Strength improvements with 1 yr of progressive resistance training in older women. Med Sci Sport Exerc 27:906, 1995.

204. Moritani, T, deVries, HA: Neural factors vs. hypertrophy in the time course of muscle strength gain. Am J Phys Med Rehabil 58:115–130, 1979.

205. Morrissey, MC, Dreschler, WI, Morrissey, D, et al: Effects of distally fixated leg extensor resistance training on knee pain in the early period after anterior cruciate ligament reconstruction. Phys Ther 82:35–42, 2002.

206. Morrissey, MC, Harman, EA, Johnson, MJ: Resistance training modes: specificity and effectiveness. Med Sci Sport Exerc 27:648, 1995.
207. Mueller, MJ, Maluf, KS: Tissue adaptation to physical stress: a proposed "physical stress theory" to guide physical therapist practice, education and research. Phys Ther 82(4):383–403, 2002.
208. Mujika, I, Padilla, S: Muscular characteristics of detraining in humans. Med Sci Sports Exerc 33:1297–1303, 2001.
209. Muller, EA: Influence of training and inactivity on muscle strength. Arch Phys Med Rehabil 51:449, 1970.
210. Nelson, ME, et al: Effects of high-intensity strength training on multiple risk factors for osteoporotic fractures. JAMA 272:1909, 1994.
211. Newman, D: The consequences of eccentric contractions and their relationship to delayed onset muscle pain. Eur J Appl Physiol 57:353–359, 1988.
212. Newman, D, Jones, D, Clarkson, P: Repeated high force eccentric exercise effects on muscle pain and damage. J Appl Physiol 63:1381–1386, 1987.
213. Nichols, JF, et al: Efficacy of heavy-resistance training for active women over sixty: muscular strength, body composition and program adherence. J Am Geriatr Soc 41:205, 1993.
214. Nosaka, K, Clarkson, PM: Influence of previous concentric exercise on eccentric exercise-induced damage. J Sports Sci 15:477, 1997.
215. Nosaka, K, Clarkson, PM: Muscle damage following repeated bouts of high force eccentric exercise. Med Sci Sports Exerc 27:1263, 1995.
216. Oakley, CR, Gollnick, PD: Conversion of rat muscle fiber type: a time course study. Histochemistry 83:555, 1985.
217. Osternig, LR, et al: Influence of torque and limb speed on power production in isokinetic exercise. Am J Phys Med Rehabil 62:163–171, 1983.
218. O'Sullivan, SB: Strategies to improve motor control and motor learning. In O'Sullivan, SB, Schmitz, TJ (eds) Physical Rehabilitation: Assessment and Treatment. FA Davis, Philadelphia, 2001, p 363.
219. O'Sullivan, SB: Assessment of motor function. In O'Sullivan, SB, Schmitz, TJ (eds) Physical Rehabilitation: Assessment and Treatment, ed 4. FA Davis, Philadelphia, 2001, p 177.
220. Palmitier, RA, An, KN, Scott, CG, et al: Kinetic chain exercise in knee rehabilitation. Sports Med 11:402–413, 1991.
221. Page, P, Ellenbecker, TS (eds): The Science and Clinical Application of Elastic Resistance. Human Kinetics, Champaign, IL, 2003.
222. Page, P, McNeil, M, Labbe, A: Torque characteristics of two types of resistive exercise [abstract]. Phys Ther 80:S69, 2000.
223. Patterson, RM, Stegink Jansen, CW, Hogan, HA, Nassif, MD: Material properties of Thera-Band Tubing. Phys Ther 81(8): 1437–1445, 2001.
224. Petersen, SR, et al: The effects of concentric resistance training and eccentric peak torque and muscle cross-sectional area. J Orthop Sports Phys Ther 13:132–137, 1991.
225. Pomerantz, EM: Osteoporosis and the female patient. Orthop Phys Ther Clin North Am 3:71, 1996.
226. Porter, MM, Vandervoort, AA: High-intensity strength training for the older adult—a review. Top Geriatric Rehabil 10:61, 1995.
227. Pruitt, LA, et al: Weight-training effects on bone mineral density in early postmenopausal women. J Bone Miner Res 7:179, 1992.
228. Richardson, C, Hodges, P, Hides, J: Therapeutic Exercise for Lumbopelvic Stabilization, ed 2. Churchill Livingstone, Edinburgh, 2004.
229. Rivera, JE: Open versus closed kinetic rehabilitation of the lower extremity: a functional and biomechanical analysis. J Sports Rehabil 3:154, 1994.
230. Rockwell, JC, et al: Weight training decreases vertebral bone density in premenopausal women: a prospective study. J Clin Endocrinol Metab 71:988, 1990.
231. Rose, SJ, Rothstein, JM: Muscle mutability. Part 1. General concepts and adaptations to altered patterns of use. Phys Ther 62:1773–1787, 1982.
232. Roth, SM, et al: High-volume, heavy-resistance strength training and muscle damage in young and older women. J Appl Physiol 88:1112, 2000.
233. Rothstein, JM: Muscle biology: Clinical considerations. Phys Ther 62:1823, 1982.
234. Sale, DG: Neural adaptation to strength training. In Komi, PV (ed) Strength and Power in Sport ed 2. Blackwell Science, Oxford, 2003, pp 281–315.
235. Sale, DG: Neural adaptation to resistance training. Med Sci Sports Exerc 20:S135, 1988.
236. Sanders, MT: Weight training and conditioning. In Sanders, B (ed) Sports Physical Therapy. Appleton & Lange, Norwalk, CT, 1990.
237. Sapega, AA, Drillings, G: The definition and assessment of muscular power. J Orthop Sports Phys Ther 5:7, 1983.
238. Sapega, AA, Kelley, MJ: Strength testing about the shoulder. J Shoulder Elbow Surg 3:327, 1994.
239. Schueman, SE: The physical therapist's role in the management of osteoporosis. Orthop Phys Ther Clin North Am 7:199, 1998.
240. Scott, W, Stevens, J, Binder-Macleod, SA: Human skeletal muscle fiber type classifications. Phys Ther 81(11):1810–1816, 2001.
241. Seger, J, Arvidsson, B, Thortensson, A: Specific effects of eccentric and concentric training on muscle strength and morphology. Eur J Appl Physiol 79:49, 1998.
242. Servedio, FJ: Normal growth and development: physiologic factors associated with exercise and training in children. Orthop Phys Ther Clin North Am 6:417, 1997.
243. Shaw, JM, Witzke, KA, Winters, KM: Exercise for skeletal health and osteoporosis prevention. In Rotman, JL (ed) ACSM's Resource Manual for Guidelines for Exercise Testing and Prescription, ed 4. Lippincott Williams & Wilkins, Philadelphia, 2001, p 299.
244. Silvers, HJ, Mandelbaum, BR: Preseason conditioning to prevent soccer injuries in young women. Clin J Sports Med 11(3):206, 2001.
245. Simoneau, GG, et al: Biomechanics of elastic resistance in therapeutic exercise programs. J Orthop Sports Phys Ther 31:16–24, 2001.
246. Sinacore, DR, Bander, BL, Delitto, A: Recovery from a 1-minute bout of fatiguing exercise: characteristics, reliability and responsiveness. Phys Ther 74:234–241, 1994.
247. Sinaki, M, et al: Can strong back extensors prevent vertebral fractures in women with osteoporosis? Mayo Clin Proc 71:951, 1996.
248. Skelton, DA, et al: Effects of resistance training on strength, power and selected functional abilities of women aged 75 and older. J Am Geriatric Soc 43:1081, 1995.
249. Smith, CA: The warm up procedure: to stretch or not to stretch; a brief review. J Orthop Sports Phys Ther 19:12, 1994.
250. Smith, LK, Weiss, EL, Lehmkuhl, LD: Brunnstrom's Clinical Kinesiology, ed 5. FA Davis, Philadelphia, 1996.
251. Smith, MJ, Melton, P: Isokinetic vs. isotonic variable-resistance training. Am J Sports Med 9:275, 1981.
252. Snyder-Mackler, L, et al: Strength of the quadriceps femoris muscle and functional recovery after reconstruction of the anterior cruciate ligament. J Bone Joint Surg Am 77:1166, 1995.
253. Snyder-Mackler, L: Scientific rationale and physiological basis for the use of closed kinetic chain exercise in the lower extremity. J Sport Rehabil 5:2, 1996.
254. Soderberg, GL: Skeletal muscle function. In Currier, DP, Nelson, RM (eds) Dynamics of Human Biologic Tissues. FA Davis, Philadelphia, 1992, p 74.
255. Soderberg, GJ, Blaschak, MJ: Shoulder internal and external rotation peak torque through a velocity spectrum in differing positions. J Orthop Sports Phys Ther 8:518, 1987.
256. Solomonow, M, et al: The synergistic action of the anterior cruciate ligament and thigh muscles in maintaining joint stability. Am J Sports Med 15:207, 1987.
257. Stackhouse, SK, Reisman, DS, Binder-Macleod, SA: Challenging the role of pH skeletal muscle fatigue. Phys Ther 81(12):1897–1903, 2001.
258. Stanton, P, Purdam, C: Hamstring injuries in sprinting: the role of eccentric exercise. J Orthop Sports Phys Ther 10:343, 1989.
259. Staron, RS, et al: Skeletal muscle adaptations during the early phase of heavy-resistance training in men and women. J Appl Physiol 76:1247, 1994.
260. Steindler, A: Kinesiology of the Human Body under Normal and Pathological Conditions. Charles C Thomas, Springfield, IL, 1955.
261. Stiene, HA, et al: A comparison of closed kinetic chain and isokinetic joint isolation exercise in patients with patellofemoral dysfunction. J Orthop Sports Phys Ther 24:136, 1996.
262. Stone, MH, Karatzaferi, C: Connective tissue and bone responses to strength training. In Komi, PV (ed) Strength and Power in Sport, ed 2. Blackwell Science, Oxford, 2003, pp 343–360.
263. Stone, MH: Implications for connective tissue and bone alterations resulting from resistance exercise training. Med Sci Sports Exerc 20:S162, 1988.

264. Stone, WJ, Coulter, SP: Strength/endurance effects from three resistance training protocols with women. J Strength Conditioning Res 8:231, 1994.

265. Stout, JL: Physical fitness during childhood and adolescence. In Campbell, SK, Vander Linden, DW, Palisano, RJ (eds) Physical Therapy for Children, ed 2. WB Saunders, Philadelphia, 2000, p 141.

266. Straker, JS, Stuhr, PJ: Clinical application of closed kinetic chain exercises in the lower extremity. Orthop Phys Ther Clin North Am 9:185, 2000.

267. Sullivan, DH, Wall, PT, Bariola, JR, et al: Progressive resistance muscle strength training of hospitalized frail elderly. Am J Phys Med Rehabil 80:503–509, 2001

268. Sulivan, PE, Markos, PD, Minor, MAD: An Integrated Approach to Therapeutic Exercise, Reston, Reston, VA, 1982.

269. Sullivan, PE, Markos, PD: Clinical Decision Making in Therapeutic Exercise. Appleton & Lange, Norwalk, CT, 1995.

270. Taaffe, DR, et al: Once-weekly resistance exercise improves muscle strength and neuromuscular performance in older adults. J Am Geriatr Soc 47:1208, 1999.

271. Tanner, SM: Weighing the risks: strength training for children and adolescents. Phys Sports Med 21:105, 1993.

272. Taylor, NF, Dodd, KJ, Damiano, DL: Progressive resistance exercise in physical therapy: a summary of systemic reviews. Phys Ther 85:1208–1223, 2005.

273. Taylor, RA, et al: Knee position error detection in closed and open kinetic chain tasks during concurrent cognitive distraction. J Orthop Sports Phys Ther 28:81, 1998.

274. Tesch, PA, Thurstensson, A, Kaiser, P: Muscle capillary supply and fiber type characteristics in weight and power lifters. J Appl Physiol 56:35, 1984.

275. Thomas, M, Muller, T, Busse, MW: Comparison of tension in Thera-Band and Cando tubing. J Orthop Sports Phys Ther 32(11):576–578, 2002.

276. Thompson, LV: Skeletal muscle adaptations with age, inactivity and therapeutic exercise. J Orthop Sports Phys Ther 32(2):44–57, 2002.

277. Tiidus, PM: Manual massage and recovery of muscle function following exercise: a literature review. J Orthop Sports Phys Ther 25:107, 1997.

278. Timm, KE: Investigation of the physiological overflow effect from speed-specific isokinetic activity. J Orthop Sports Phys Ther 9:106, 1987.

279. Tippett, SR: Closed-chain exercise. Orthop Phys Ther Clin North Am 1:253–267, 1992.

280. Tomberlin, JP, et al: Comparative study of isokinetic eccentric and concentric quadriceps training. J Orthop Sports Phys Ther 14:31–36, 1991.

281. Tracy, BL, et al: Muscle quality. II. Effects of strength training in 65- to 75-year old men and women. J Appl Physiol 86:195, 1999.

282. Tyler, TF, Mullaney, M: Training for joint stability. In Nyland, J (ed) Clinical Decisions in Therapeutic Exercise: Planning and Implementation. Pearson Education, Upper Saddle River, NJ, 2006, pp 248–254.

283. Vandervoort, AA: Resistance exercise throughout life. Orthop Phys Ther Clin North Am 10(2):227–240, 2001.

284. Voight, M, Tippett, S: Plyometric exercise in rehabilitation. In Prentice, WE, Voight, ML (eds) Techniques in Musculoskeletal Rehabilitation. McGraw-Hill, New York, 2001, pp 167–178.

285. Voight, ML: Stretch strengthening: an introduction to plyometrics. Orthop Phys Ther Clin North Am 1:243–252, 1992.

286. Voight, ML, Draovitch, P: Plyometrics. In Albert, M (ed) Eccentric Muscle Training in Sports and Orthopedics, ed 2. Churchill Livingstone, New York, 1995, p 149.

287. Voss, DE, Ionta, MK, Myers, BJ: Proprioceptive Neuromuscular Facilitation, ed 3. Harper & Row, New York, 1985.

288. Waltrous, B, Armstrong, R, Schwane, J: The role of lactic acid in delayed onset muscular soreness. Med Sci Sports Exerc 1:380, 1981.

289. Warner, JJP, et al: Effect of joint compression on the inferior stability of the glenohumeral joint. J Shoulder Elbow Surg 8:31, 1999.

290. Weber, MD, Servedio, F, Woodall, WR: The effect of three modalities on delayed onset muscle soreness. J Orthop Sports Phys Ther 20:236–242, 1994.

291. Weir, JP, et al: The effect of unilateral concentric weight training and detraining on joint angle specificity, cross-training and the bilateral deficit. J Orthop Sports Phys Ther 25:264, 199.

292. Weir, JP, et al: The effect of unilateral eccentric weight training and detraining on joint angle specificity, cross-training and the bilateral deficit. J Orthop Sports Phys Ther 22:207, 1995.

293. Weir, JP, Housh, TJ, Wagner, LI: Electromyographic evaluation of joint angle specificity and cross-training following isometric training. J Appl Physiol 77:197, 1994.

294. Weiss, A, Suzuki, T, Bean, J, et al: High-intensity strength training improves strength and functional performance after stroke. Am J Phys Med Rehabil 79(4):369–376, 2000.

295. Weiss, LW, Coney, HD, Clark, FC: Gross measures of exercise-induced muscular hypertrophy. J Orthop Sports Phys Ther 30:141, 2000.

296. Wescott, WL: Strength Training Past 50. Human Kinetics, Champaign, IL, 1998.

297. Whitcomb, LJ, Kelley, MJ, Leiper, CI: A comparison of torque production during dynamic strength testing shoulder abduction in the coronal plane and the plane of the scapula. J Orthop Sports Phys Ther 21:227, 1995.

298. Wilder, PA: Muscle development and function. In Cech, D, Martin, S: Functional Movement Development Across the Life Span. WB Saunders, Philadelphia, 1995, p 13.

299. Wilk, K, Arrigo, C, Andrews, J: Closed and open kinetic chain exercise for the upper extremity. J Sports Rehabil 5:88, 1995.

300. Wilk, KE, et al: A comparison of tibiofemoral joint forces and electromyography during open and closed kinetic chain exercises. Am J Sports Med 24:518, 1996.

301. Wilk, KE, et al: Open and closed kinetic chain exercise for the lower extremity: theory and clinical application. Athletic Training Sports Health Perspect 1:336, 1995.

302. Wilk, KE, et al: Stretch-shortening drills for the upper extremities: theory and clinical application. J Orthop Sports Phys Ther 17:225–239, 1993.

303. Wilke, DV: The relationship between force and velocity in human muscle. J Physiol 110:249, 1950.

304. Williams, GN, Higgins, MJ, Lewek, MD: Aging skeletal muscle: physiologic changes and effects of training. Phys Ther 82(1):62–68, 2002.

305. Witvrouw, E, Danneels, L, Van Tiggelen, D, et al: Open versus closed kinetic chain exercises in patellofemoral pain: a 5-year prospective, randomized study. Am J Sports Med 32(5):1122–1130, 2004.

306. Woodall, WR, Weber, MD: Exercise response and thermoregulation. Orthop Phys Ther Clin North Am 7:1, 1998.

307. Wu, Y, et al: Relationship between isokinetic concentric and eccentric contraction modes in the knee flexor and extensor muscle groups. J Orthop Sports Phys Ther 26:143, 1997.

308. Wyatt, MP, Edwards, AM: Comparison of quadriceps and hamstrings torque values during isokinetic exercise. J Orthop Sports Phys Ther 3:348, 1981.

309. Yack, HJ, Colins, CE, Whieldon, T: Comparison of closed and open kinetic chain exercise in the anterior cruciate ligament deficient knee. Am J Sports Med 21:49, 1993.

310. Yack, HJ, Riley, LM, Whieldon, T: Anterior tibial translation during progressive loading the ACL-deficient knee during weight-bearing and nonweight-bearing isometric exercise. J Orthop Sports Phys Ther 20:247, 1994.

311. Yarasheski, KE, Lemon, PW, Gilloteaux, J: Effect of heavy resistance exercise training on muscle fiber composition in young rats. J Appl Physiol 69:434, 1990.

312. Zernicke, RF, Loitz-Ramage, B: Exercise-related adaptations in connective tissue. In Komi, PV (ed) Strength and Power in Sport, ed 2. Blackwell Science, Oxford, 2003, pp 96–113.

313. Zinowieff, AN: Heavy resistance exercise: the Oxford technique. Br J Phys Med 14:129, 1951.

314. Zwiren, LD, Manos, LM: Exercise testing and prescription considerations throughout childhood. In Roitman, JL (ed) ACSM's Resource Manual for Guidelines for Exercise Testing and Prescription, ed 4. Lippincott Williams & Wilkins, Philadelphia, 2001, p 520.

# Principles of Aerobic Exercise

Karen Holtgrefe, DHS, PT, OCS

Terri M. Glenn, PhD, PT

There are numerous sources from which to obtain information on training for endurance in athletes and healthy young people and for individuals with coronary heart disease. Information or emphasis on endurance training and the improvement of fitness in the individual who has other types of chronic disease or disability is beginning to emerge. Using the most recent research, the American College of Sports Medicine published basic guidelines for several of the more common chronic conditions.[2] This chapter uses information from well known sources to demonstrate that the physical therapist can use aerobic-type activity when working with either healthy individuals or patients with a variety of conditions. In addition, some fundamental information about cardiovascular and respiratory parameters in children and the elderly, as well as the young or middle-aged adult, is presented so the physical therapist can be prepared to treat individuals of all ages.

##  KEY TERMS AND CONCEPTS

### Fitness

Fitness is a general term used to describe the ability to perform physical work. Performing physical work requires cardiorespiratory functioning, muscular strength and endurance, and musculoskeletal flexibility. Optimum body composition is also included when describing fitness.

To become physically fit, individuals must participate regularly in some form of physical activity that uses large muscle groups and challenges the cardiorespiratory system. Individuals of all ages can improve their general fitness status by participating in activities that include walking, biking, running, swimming, stair climbing, cross-country skiing, and/or training with weights.

Fitness levels can be described on a continuum from poor to superior based on energy expenditure during a bout of physical work.[8,9,11] These ratings are often based on direct or indirect measurement of the body's maximum oxygen consumption ($\dot{V}O_{2\,max}$). Oxygen consumption is influenced by age, gender, heredity, inactivity, and disease.

### Maximum Oxygen Consumption

Maximum oxygen consumption ($\dot{V}O_{2\,max}$) is a measure of the body's capacity to use oxygen.[2,8,9,11] It is usually measured when performing an exercise that uses many large muscle groups such as swimming, walking, and running. It is the maximum amount of oxygen consumed per minute when the individual has reached maximum effort. It is usually expressed relative to body weight, as milliliters of oxygen per kilogram of body weight per minute (mL/kg per minute). It is dependent on the transport of oxygen, the oxygen-binding capacity of the blood, cardiac function, oxygen extraction capabilities, and muscular oxidative potential.

### Endurance

Endurance (a measure of fitness) is the ability to work for prolonged periods of time and the ability to resist fatigue.[8,9,11] It includes muscular endurance and cardiovascular endurance. Muscular endurance refers to the ability of an isolated muscle group to perform repeated contractions over a period of time, whereas cardiovascular endurance refers to the ability to perform large muscle dynamic exercise, such as walking, swimming, and/or biking for long periods of time.

### Aerobic Exercise Training (Conditioning)

Aerobic exercise training, or conditioning, is augmentation of the energy utilization of the muscle by means of an exercise program.[8,9,11] The improvement of the muscle's ability to use energy is a direct result of increased levels of oxidative enzymes in the muscles, increased mitochondrial density and size, and an increased muscle fiber capillary supply.

- Training is dependent on exercise of sufficient intensity, duration, and frequency.
- Training produces cardiovascular and/or muscular adaptation and is reflected in an individual's endurance.
- Training for a particular sport or event is dependent on the specificity principle[8,9,11]; that is, the individual improves in the exercise task used for training and may not improve in other tasks. For example, swimming may enhance one's performance in swimming events but may not improve one's performance in treadmill running.

### Adaptation

The cardiovascular system and the muscles used adapt to the training stimulus over time.[8,9,11] Significant changes can be measured in as little as 10 to 12 weeks.

Adaptation results in increased efficiency of the cardiovascular system and the active muscles. Adaptation represents a variety of neurological, physical, and biochemical changes in the cardiovascular and muscular systems. Performance improves in that the same amount of work can be performed after training but at a lower physiological cost.

Adaptation is dependent on the ability of the organism to change and the training stimulus threshold (the stimulus that elicits a training response). The person with a low level of fitness has more potential to improve than the one who has a high level of fitness.

Training stimulus thresholds are variable. The higher the initial level of fitness, the greater the intensity of exercise needed to elicit a significant change.

### Myocardial Oxygen Consumption

Myocardial oxygen consumption ($m\dot{V}O_2$) is a measure of the oxygen consumed by the myocardial muscle.[2,3,8,9,11] The need or demand for oxygen is determined by the heart rate (HR), systemic blood pressure, myocardial contractility, and afterload. Afterload is determined by the left ventricular wall tension and central aortic pressure. It is the ventricular force required to open the aortic valve at the beginning of systole. Left ventricular wall tension is primarily determined by ventricular size and wall thickness.

The ability to supply the myocardium with oxygen is dependent on the arterial oxygen content (blood substrate), hemoglobin oxygen dissociation, and coronary blood flow, which is determined by aortic diastolic pressure, duration of diastole, coronary artery resistance, and collateral circulation. In a healthy individual, a balance between myocardial oxygen supply and demand is maintained during maximum exercise. When the demand for oxygen is greater than the supply, myocardial ischemia results.

Persons who have coronary occlusion may not present with any type of chest pain (angina) until they need to exert themselves. This is because when the body works harder the heart rate increases, diastolic filling time decreases, and increased coronary blood flow is sacrificed by the reduced time for filling the coronary arteries. Without an adequate blood supply, the underlying cardiac tissue no longer receives the oxygen needed for metabolic activity, resulting in anginal pain.

Because the myocardial muscle extracts 70% to 75% of the oxygen from the blood during rest, its main source of supply during exercise is through an increase in coronary blood flow. The clinical relevance is described in Box 7.1.

## Deconditioning

Deconditioning occurs with prolonged bed rest, and its effects are frequently seen in the patient who has had an extended, acute illness or long-term chronic condition. Decreases in maximum oxygen consumption, cardiac output (stroke volume), and muscular strength occur rapidly. These effects are also seen, although possibly to a lesser degree, in the individual who has spent a period of time on bed rest without any accompanying disease process and in the individual who is sedentary because of lifestyle and increasing age. Deconditioning effects associated with bed rest are summarized in Box 7.2.

## Energy Systems, Energy Expenditure, and Efficiency

### Energy Systems

Energy systems are metabolic systems involving a series of biochemical reactions resulting in the formation of adenosine triphosphate (ATP), carbon dioxide, and water.[8,9,11] The cell uses the energy produced from the conversion of ATP to adenosine diphosphate (ADP) and phosphate (P) to perform metabolic activities. Muscle cells use this energy

BOX 7.2    Deconditioning Effects Associated With Bed Rest[3]

↓ Muscle mass
↓ Strength
↓ Cardiovascular function
↓ Total blood volume
↓ Plasma volume
↓ Heart volume
↓ Orthostatic tolerance
↓ Exercise tolerance
↓ Bone mineral density

for actin-myosin cross-bridge formation when contracting. There are three major energy systems. The intensity and duration of activity determine when and to what extent each metabolic system contributes.

### Phosphagen, or ATP-PC, System

The ATP-PC system (adenosine triphosphate–phosphocreatine) has the following characteristics.

● Phosphocreatine and ATP are stored in the muscle cell.
● Phosphocreatine is the chemical fuel source.
● No oxygen is required (anaerobic).
● When muscle is rested, the supply of ATP-PC is replenished.
● The maximum capacity of the system is small (0.7 mol ATP).
● The maximum power of the system is great (3.7 mol ATP/min).
● The system provides energy for short, quick bursts of activity.
● It is the major source of energy during the first 30 seconds of intense exercise.

### Anaerobic Glycolytic System

The anaerobic glycolytic system has the following characteristics.

● Glycogen (glucose) is the fuel source (glycolysis).
● No oxygen is required (anaerobic).
● ATP is resynthesized in the muscle cell.
● Lactic acid is produced (by-product of anaerobic glycolysis).
● The maximum capacity of the system is intermediate (1.2 mol ATP).
● The maximum power of the system is intermediate (1.6 mol ATP/min).
● The systems provide energy for activity of moderate intensity and short duration.
● It is the major source of energy from the 30th to 90th second of exercise.

### Aerobic System

The aerobic system has the following characteristics.

● Glycogen, fats, and proteins are fuel sources and are utilized relative to their availability and the intensity of the exercise.
● Oxygen is required (aerobic).
● ATP is resynthesized in the mitochondria of the muscle cell. The ability to metabolize oxygen and other substrates is related to the number and concentration of the mitochondria and cells.
● The maximum capacity of the system is great (90.0 mol ATP).
● The maximum power of the system is small (1.0 mol ATP/min).
● The system predominates over the other energy systems after the second minute of exercise.

### Recruitment of Motor Units

Recruitment of motor units is dependent on the rate of work. Fibers are recruited selectively during exercise.[8,9,11]

- Slow-twitch fibers (type I) are characterized by a slow contractile response, are rich in myoglobin and mitochondria, have a high oxidative capacity and a low anaerobic capacity, and are recruited for activities demanding endurance. These fibers are supplied by small neurons with a low threshold of activation and are used preferentially in low-intensity exercise.
- Fast-twitch fibers (type IIB) are characterized by a fast contractile response, have a low myoglobin content and few mitochondria, have a high glycolytic capacity, and are recruited for activities requiring power.
- Fast-twitch fibers (type IIA) have characteristics of both type I and type IIB fibers and are recruited for both anaerobic and aerobic activities.

## Functional Implications

- Bursts of intense activity (seconds) develop muscle strength and stronger tendons and ligaments. ATP is supplied by the phosphagen system.
- Intense activity (1 to 2 minutes) repeated after 4 minutes of rest or mild exercise enhances anaerobic power. ATP is supplied by the phosphagen and anaerobic glycolytic system.
- Activity with large muscles, which is less than maximum intensity for 3 to 5 minutes repeated after rest or mild exercise of similar duration, may develop aerobic power and endurance capabilities. ATP is supplied by the phosphagen, anaerobic glycolytic, and aerobic systems.
- Activity of submaximum intensity lasting 20 to 30 minutes or more taxes a high percentage of the aerobic system and develops endurance.

## Energy Expenditure

Energy is expended by individuals engaging in physical activity and is often expressed in kilocalories. Activities can be categorized as light, moderate or heavy by determining the energy cost. The energy cost of any activity is affected by mechanical efficiency and body mass. Factors that affect both walking and running are terrain, stride length, and air resistance.[8,9,11]

### Quantification of Energy Expenditure

Energy expended is computed from the amount of oxygen consumed. Units used to quantify energy expenditure are kilocalories and METs.

- A kilocalorie is a measure expressing the energy value of food. It is the amount of heat necessary to raise 1 kilogram (kg) of water 1°C. A kilocalorie (kcal) can be expressed in oxygen equivalents. Five kilocalories equal approximately 1 liter of oxygen consumed (5 kcal = 1 liter $O_2$).
- A MET is defined as the oxygen consumed (milliliters) per kilogram of body weight per minute (mL/kg). It is equal to approximately 3.5 mL/kg per minute.[2]

| BOX 7.3 | Daily Energy Expenditure |
| --- | --- |

The average individual engaged in normal daily tasks expends 1800 to 3000 kcal per day. Athletes engaged in intense training can use more than 10,000 kcal per day.

Data from Wilmore, JH, Costill, DL: Physiology of Sport and Exercise. Human Kinetics, Champaign, IL, 1994.

### Classification of Activities

Activities are classified as light, moderate, or heavy according to the energy expended or the oxygen consumed while accomplishing them.[8,9,11]

- Light work for the average male (65 kg) requires 2.0 to 4.9 kcal/min, or 6.1 to 15.2 mL $O_2$/kg per minute, or 1.6 to 3.9 METs. Strolling 1.6 km/hr, or 1.0 mph, is considered light work.
- Heavy work for the average male (65 kg) requires 7.5 to 9.9 kcal/min, or 23.0 to 30.6 mL $O_2$/kg per minute, or 6.0 to 7.9 METs. Jogging 8.0 km/hr, or 5.0 mph, is considered heavy work.
- Jogging 8.0 km/hr, or 5.0 mph, requires 25 to 28 mL $O_2$/kg per minute and is considered heavy work. The energy expended is equivalent to 8 to 10 kcal/min, or 7 to 8 METs.
- The energy expenditure necessary for most industrial jobs requires more than three times the energy expenditure at rest.
- Energy expenditure of certain physical activities can vary, depending on factors such as skill, pace, and fitness level (Box 7.3).

## Efficiency

Efficiency is usually expressed as a percentage[8,9,11] (Box 7.4).

Work output equals force times distance (W = F × D). It can be expressed in power units or work per unit of time (P = w/t). On a treadmill, work equals the weight of the subject times the vertical distance the subject is raised walking up the incline of the treadmill. On a bicycle ergometer, work equals the distance (which is the circumference of the flywheel times the number of revolutions) times the bicycle resistance.

Work input equals energy expenditure and is expressed as the net oxygen consumption per unit of time. With aerobic exercise, the resting volume of oxygen used per unit of time ($VO_2$ value) is subtracted from the oxygen consumed during 1 minute of the steady-state period.

| BOX 7.4 | Efficiency Expressed as a Percentage |
| --- | --- |

$$\text{Percent efficiency} = \frac{\text{useful work output}}{\text{energy expended or work input}} \times 100$$

- Steady state is reached within 3 to 4 minutes after exercise has started if the load or resistance is kept constant.
- In the steady-state period, $VO_2$ remains at a constant (steady) value.

Total net oxygen cost is multiplied by the total time in minutes the exercise is performed. The higher the net oxygen cost, the lower the efficiency in performing the activity. Efficiency of large muscle activities is usually 20% to 25%.

# PHYSIOLOGICAL RESPONSE TO AEROBIC EXERCISE

The rapid increase in energy requirements during exercise requires equally rapid circulatory adjustments to meet the increased need for oxygen and nutrients to remove the end-products of metabolism such as carbon dioxide and lactic acid and to dissipate excess heat. The shift in body metabolism occurs through a coordinated activity of all the systems of the body: neuromuscular, respiratory, cardiovascular, metabolic, and hormonal (Box 7.5). Oxygen transport and its utilization by the mitochondria of the contracting muscle are dependent on adequate blood flow in conjunction with cellular respiration.[8,9,11]

## Cardiovascular Response to Exercise

### Exercise Pressor Response
Stimulation of small myelinated and unmyelinated fibers in skeletal muscle involves a sympathetic nervous system (SNS) response. The central pathways are not known.[2,3,8,9,11]

- The SNS response includes generalized peripheral vasoconstriction in nonexercising muscles and increased myocardial contractility, an increased heart rate, and an increased systolic blood pressure. This results in a marked increase and redistribution of the cardiac output.
- The degree of the response equals the muscle mass involved and the intensity of the exercise.

---

**BOX 7.5  Factors Affecting the Response to Acute Exercise**

Ambient temperature, humidity, and altitude can affect the physiological responses to acute exercise. Diurnal fluctuations as well as changes associated with a female subject's menstrual cycle can affect these responses as well. Therefore, researchers control these factors as much as possible when evaluating the response to exercise.

---

### Cardiac Effects

- The frequency of sinoatrial node depolarization increases, as does the heart rate.
- There is a decrease in vagal stimuli as well as an increase in SNS stimulation.
- There is an increase in the force development of the cardiac myofibers. A direct inotropic response of the SNS increases myocardial contractility.

### Peripheral Effects

**Net Reduction in Total Peripheral Resistance**

- Generalized vasoconstriction occurs that allows blood to be shunted from the nonworking muscles, kidneys, liver, spleen, and splanchnic area to the working muscles.
- A locally mediated reduction in resistance in the working muscle arterial vascular bed, independent of the autonomic nervous system, is produced by metabolites such as $Mg^{2+}$, $Ca^{2+}$, ADP, and $P_{CO_2}$.
- The veins of the working and nonworking muscles remain constricted.

**Increased Cardiac Output**
The cardiac output increases because of the:

- Increase in myocardial contractility, with a resultant increase in stroke volume
- Increase in heart rate
- Increase in the blood flow through the working muscle
- Increase in the constriction of the capacitance vessels on the venous side of the circulation in both the working and nonworking muscles, raising the peripheral venous pressure

**Increase in Systolic Blood Pressure**
The increase in systolic blood pressure is the result of the augmented cardiac output.

## Respiratory Response to Exercise

- Respiratory changes occur rapidly, even before the initiation of exercise.[8,9,11] Gas exchange ($O_2$, $CO_2$) increases across the alveolar-capillary membrane by the first or second breath. Increased muscle metabolism during exercise results in more $O_2$ extracted from arterial blood resulting in an increase in venous $P_{CO_2}$ and $H^+$, an increase in body temperature, increased epinephrine, and increased stimulation of receptors of the joints and muscles. Any of these factors alone or in combination may stimulate the respiratory system. Baroreceptor reflexes, protective reflexes, pain, emotion, and voluntary control of respiration may also contribute to the increase in respiration.
- Minute ventilation increases as respiratory frequency and tidal volume increase.
- Alveolar ventilation, occurring with the diffusion of gases across the capillary-alveolar membrane, increases 10- to 20-fold during heavy exercise to supply the additional oxygen needed and excrete the excess $CO_2$ produced.

## Responses Providing Additional Oxygen to Muscle

### Increased Blood Flow

The increased blood flow to the working muscle previously discussed provides additional oxygen.

### Increased Oxygen Extraction

There is also extraction of more oxygen from each liter of blood. There are several changes that allow for this.

- A decrease of the local tissue $PO_2$ occurs because of the use of more oxygen by the working muscle. As the partial pressure of oxygen decreases, the unloading of oxygen from hemoglobin is facilitated.
- The production of more $CO_2$ causes the tissue to become acidotic (the hydrogen ion concentration increases) and the temperature of the tissue to increase. Both situations increase the amount of oxygen released from hemoglobin at any given partial pressure.
- The increase of red blood cell 2,3-diphosphoglycerate (DPG) produced by glycolysis during exercise also contributes to the enhanced release of oxygen.

### Oxygen Consumption

Factors determining how much of the oxygen is consumed are:

- Vascularity of the muscles.
- Fiber distribution.
- Number of mitochondria.
- Oxidative mitochondrial enzymes present in the fibers. The oxidative capacity of the muscle is reflected in the $a - \bar{v}O_2$ difference, which is the difference between the oxygen content of arterial and venous blood.

## TESTING AS A BASIS FOR EXERCISE PROGRAMS

Testing for physical fitness of healthy individuals should be distinct from graded exercise testing of convalescing patients, individuals with symptoms of coronary heart disease, or individuals who are 35 years or older but asymptomatic.[1,2] Regardless of the type of testing, the level of performance is based on the submaximum or maximum oxygen uptake ($\dot{V}O_{2\,max}$) or the symptom-limited oxygen uptake. The capacity of the individual to transport and utilize oxygen is reflected in the oxygen uptake. Readers are referred to publications by the American College of Sports Medicine[1,2] for additional information.

### Fitness Testing of Healthy Subjects

Field tests for determining cardiovascular fitness include the time to run 1.5 miles or the distance run in 12 minutes. These measures correlate well with $\dot{V}O_{2\,max}$, but their use is limited to young persons or middle-aged individuals who have been carefully screened and have been jogging or running for some time.[2,3]

Multistage testing can provide a direct measurement of $\dot{V}O_{2\,max}$ by analyzing samples of expired air.[1,2] Testing is usually completed in four to six treadmill stages, which progressively increase in speed and or grade. Each stage is 3 to 6 minutes long. Electrocardiographic (ECG) monitoring is performed during the testing. Maximum oxygen uptake can be determined when the oxygen utilization plateaus despite an increase in workload.

### Stress Testing for Convalescing Individuals and Individuals at Risk

Individuals undergoing stress testing should have a physical examination, be monitored by the ECG, and be closely observed at rest, during exercise, and during recovery (Fig. 7.1).

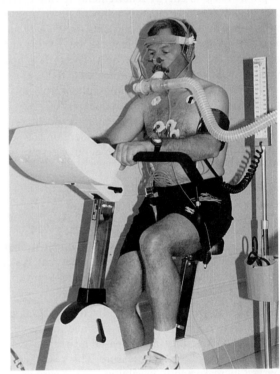

FIGURE 7.1 Placement of electrodes for the 12-lead exercise electrocardiogram used to determine heart rate and rhythm during the stress test.

### Principles of Stress Testing

The principles of stress testing include the following.[2,3]

- Changing the workload by increasing the speed and/or grade of the treadmill or the resistance on the bicycle ergometer.
- An initial workload that is low in terms of the individual's anticipated aerobic threshold.
- Maintaining each workload for 1 minute or longer.
- Terminating the test at the onset of symptoms or a definable abnormality of the ECG.
- When available, measuring the individual's maximum oxygen consumption.

## Purpose of Stress Testing

In addition to serving as a basis for determining exercise levels or the exercise prescription, the stress test:

- Helps establish a diagnosis of overt or latent heart disease.
- Evaluates cardiovascular functional capacity as a means of clearing individuals for strenuous work or exercise programs.
- Determines the physical work capacity in kilogram-meters per minute (kg-m/min) or the functional capacity in METs.
- Evaluates responses to exercise training and/or preventive programs.
- Assists in the selection and evaluation of appropriate modes of treatment for heart disease.
- Increases individual motivation for entering and adhering to exercise programs.
- Is used clinically to evaluate patients with chest sensations or a history of chest pain to establish the probability that such patients have coronary disease. It can also evaluate the functional capacity of patients with chronic disease.

## Preparation for Stress Testng

All individuals who are taking a stress test should:

- Have had a physical examination.
- Be monitored by ECG and closely observed at rest, during exercise, and during recovery.
- Sign a consent form.

PRECAUTIONS: Precautions to be taken are summarized in Box 7.6. They are applicable for both stress testing and the exercise program.[2,3]

---

| BOX 7.6 | Precautions for Stress Testing and Exercise Program |
|---|---|

Cardiopulmonary changes occur with stress testing and exercises; monitor and recognize the following.

- Monitor the pulse to assess abnormal increases in heart rate.
- Blood pressure increases with exercise approximately 7 to 10 millimeters (mm) of mercury (Hg) per MET of physical activity.
  - Systolic pressure should not exceed 220 to 240 mm Hg.
  - Diastolic pressure should not exceed 120 mm Hg.
- Rate and depth of respiration increase with exercise.
  - Respiration should not be labored.
  - The individual should have no perception of shortness of breath.
- The increase in blood flow while exercising, which regulates core temperature and meets the demands of the working muscles, results in changes in the skin of the cheeks, nose, and earlobes. They become pink, moist, and warm to the touch.

---

## Termination of Stress Testing

Endpoints requiring termination of the test period are[2]:

- Progressive angina.
- A significant drop in systolic pressure in response to an increasing workload.
- Lightheadedness, confusion, pallor, cyanosis, nausea, or peripheral circulatory insufficiency.
- Abnormal ECG responses including ST segment depression greater than 4 mm.
- Excessive rise in blood pressure.
- Subject wishes to stop.

## Multistage Testing

Each of the four to six stages lasts approximately 1 to 6 minutes. Differences in protocols involve the number of stages, magnitude of the exercise (intensity), equipment used (bicycle, treadmill), duration of stages, endpoints, position of body, muscle groups exercised, and types of effort (Box 7.7).[2,3]

Protocols have been developed for multistage testing. The most popular treadmill protocol is the Bruce protocol. Treadmill speed and grade are changed every 3 minutes. Speed increases from 1.7 mph up to 5.0 mph, and the initial grade of 10% increases up to 18% during the five stages.

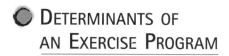

# DETERMINANTS OF AN EXERCISE PROGRAM

Just as testing for fitness should be distinct from stress testing for patients or individuals at high risk, training programs for healthy individuals are distinct from the exercise prescription for individuals with cardiopulmonary disease.

Effective endurance training for any population must produce a conditioning or cardiovascular response. Elicitation of the cardiovascular response is dependent on three critical elements of exercise: intensity, duration, and frequency.[2,3,8,9,11]

## Intensity

Determination of the appropriate intensity of exercise to use is based on the overload principle and the specificity principle.[2,3,8,9,11]

### Overload Principle

Overload is stress on an organism that is greater than that regularly encountered during everyday life. To improve cardiovascular and muscular endurance, an overload must be applied to these systems. The exercise load (overload) must be above the training stimulus threshold (the stimulus that elicits a training or conditioning response) for adaptation to occur.

Once adaptation to a given load has taken place, the training intensity (exercise load) must be increased for the

## BOX 7.7
### Case Example of an Exercise Stress Test

Mr. Smith is a 55-year-old sedentary man with a history of chest pain with exertion. He has undergone a stress test to assist in evaluating his angina. He is not taking any medications at the present time. He has been a smoker for 20 years.
• Resting electrocardiogram (ECG): normal

• Resting heart rate: 75 beats/min
• Age-predicted maximum heart rate: 165 beats/min
• Resting blood pressure: 128/86
• Resting respiration rate: 20 breaths/min
• Treadmill: Bruce protocol

| Stage | Heart Rate | Blood Pressure | Comments |
|---|---|---|---|
| 1 | 80 | | |
| | 84 | | |
| | 85 | 138/88 | No complaints |
| 2 | 88 | | |
| | 90 | | |
| | 92 | 142/90 | No complaints |
| 3 | 98 | | |
| | 100 | | |
| | 102 | 156/91 | Complaining of leg fatigue |
| 4 | 114 | | |
| | 116 | | |
| | 122 | 161/90 | Complaining of minimal chest pain |
| 5 | 133 | | |
| | 135 | | |
| | 137 | 174/89 | Complaining of severe chest pain; test terminated |

### Conclusion
The stress test was terminated because of complaints of severe chest pain accompanied by a drop in the ST segment of the ECG to 4 mm. The symptom-limited maximum heart rate was determined to be 137 beats/min. Maximum oxygen consumption was determined to be 32 mL/kg/min.

individual to achieve further improvement. Training stimulus thresholds are variable, depending on the individual's level of health, level of activity, age, and gender. The higher the initial level of fitness, the greater the intensity of exercise needed to elicit a change.

A conditioning response occurs generally at 60% to 90% maximum heart rate (50% to 85% $\dot{V}O_{2\,max}$) depending on the individual and the initial level of fitness.

• Seventy percent maximum heart rate is a minimal-level stimulus for eliciting a conditioning response in healthy young individuals.

• Sedentary or "deconditioned" individuals respond to a low exercise intensity, 40% to 50% of $\dot{V}O_{2\,max}$.
• The exercise does not have to be exhaustive to achieve a training response.
• Determining the maximum heart rate and the exercise heart rate for training programs provides the basis for the initial intensity of the exercise (Box 7.8).
• When the individual is young and healthy, the maximum heart rate can be determined directly from a maximum performance multistage test, extrapolated from a heart rate achieved on a predetermined submaximum test or, less accurately, calculated as 220 minus age.

## BOX 7.8
### Methods to Determine Maximum Heart Rate and Exercise Heart Rate

| Determine Maximum Heart Rate (HR) | Determine Exercise Heart Rate |
|---|---|
| • From multistage test (for young and healthy) | • Percentage of maximum heart rate (dependent on level of fitness) |
| • HR achieved in predetermined submaximum test | • Karvonen's formula (heart rate reserve) |
| • 220 minus age (less accurate) | Exercise heart rate = $HR_{rest}$ + 60–70% ($HR_{max}$ − $HR_{rest}$) |

- The exercise heart rate is determined in one of two ways: (1) as a percentage of the maximum heart rate (the percentage used is dependent on the level of fitness of the individual); and (2) using the heart rate reserve (Karvonen's formula). Karvonen's formula is based on the heart rate reserve (HRR), which is the difference between the resting heart rate ($HR_{rest}$) and the maximum heart rate ($HR_{max}$). The exercise heart rate is determined as a percentage (usually 60% to 70%) of the heart rate reserve plus the resting heart rate (see Box 7.8).
- When using Karvonen's formula, the exercise heart rate is higher than when using the maximum heart rate alone.

### Individuals at Risk

Maximum heart rate and exercise heart rate used for the exercise prescription for individuals at risk for coronary artery disease, individuals with coronary artery disease or other chronic disease, and individuals who are elderly are ideally identified based on their performance on the stress test. The maximum heart rate cannot be determined in the same manner as for the young and healthy.

- Assuming that an individual has an average maximum heart rate, using the formula 220 minus age produces substantial errors in prescribing the exercise intensity for these individuals.
- Maximum heart rate, which may be symptom-limited, is considered maximum. At no time should the exercise heart rate exceed the symptom-limited heart rate achieved on the exercise test.
- Individuals with cardiopulmonary disease may start exercise programs, depending on their diagnosis, as low as 40% to 60% of their maximum heart rate.

### Variables

Exercising at a high intensity for a shorter period of time appears to elicit a greater improvement in $\dot{V}O_{2\,max}$ than exercising at a moderate intensity for a longer period of time. However, as exercise approaches the maximum limit, there is an increase in the relative risk of cardiovascular complications and the risk of musculoskeletal injury.

- The higher the intensity and the longer the exercise intervals, the faster the training effect.
- Maximum oxygen consumption ($\dot{V}O_{2\,max}$) is the best measure of exercise intensity. Aerobic capacity and heart rate are linearly related; therefore, the maximum heart rate is a function of intensity.

### Specificity Principle

The specificity principle as related to the specificity of training refers to adaptations in metabolic and physiological systems depending on the demand imposed. There is no overlap when training for strength–power activities and training for endurance activities. Workload and work–rest periods are selected so training results in:

- Muscle strength without a significant increase in total oxygen consumption.
- Aerobic or endurance training without training the anaerobic systems.
- Anaerobic training without training the aerobic systems.
- Even when evaluating aerobic or endurance activities, there appears to be little overlap. When training for swimming events, the individual may not demonstrate an improvement in $\dot{V}O_{2\,max}$ when running.

## Duration

The optimal duration of exercise for cardiovascular conditioning is dependent on the total work performed, exercise intensity and frequency, and fitness level. Generally speaking, the greater the intensity of the exercise, the shorter the duration needed for adaptation; and the lower the intensity of exercise, the longer the duration needed.

A 20- to 30-minute session is generally optimal at 60% to 70% maximum heart rate. When the intensity is below the heart rate threshold, a 45-minute continuous exercise period may provide the appropriate overload. With high-intensity exercise, 10- to 15-minute exercise periods are adequate; three 5-minute daily periods are effective in some deconditioned patients.

## Frequency

Like duration, there is no clear-cut information provided on the most effective frequency of exercise for adaptation to occur. Frequency may be a less important factor than intensity or duration in exercise training. Frequency varies, dependent on the health and age of the individual. Optimal frequency of training is generally three to four times a week. If training is at low intensity, greater frequency may be beneficial. A frequency of two times a week does not generally evoke cardiovascular changes, although older individuals and convalescing patients may benefit from a program of that frequency.

***Recommendations.*** The American Heart Association Scientific Statement on physical activity and atherosclerotic heart disease as reported by Thompson et al.[12] recommends 30 minutes of moderate intensity aerobic exercise on most if not all days of the week. The Centers for Disease Control (CDC) supports these recommendations,[5] whereas the American College of Sports Medicine, as described by Pollock et al.,[10] recommends aerobic exercise 3 to 5 days/week at 65% to 90% maximum heart rate for 20 to 60 continuous or intermittent minutes. They further recommend that if the activity is lower intensity it should have a longer duration and that multiple bouts of exercise (no less than 10 minutes) may be accumulated throughout the day.

## Mode

- Many types of activity provide the stimulus for improving cardiorespiratory fitness. The important factor is that the exercise involves large muscle groups that are activated in a rhythmic, aerobic nature. However, the magnitude of the changes may be determined by the mode used.

- For specific aerobic activities such as cycling and running, the overload must use the muscles required by the activity and stress the cardiorespiratory system (specificity principle). If endurance of the upper extremities is needed to perform activities on the job, the upper extremity muscles must be targeted in the exercise program. The muscles trained develop a greater oxidative capacity with an increase in blood flow to the area. The increase in blood flow is due to increased microcirculation and more effective distribution of the cardiac output.
- Training benefits are optimized when programs are planned to meet the individual needs and capacities of the participants. The skill of the individual, variations among individuals in competitiveness and aggressiveness, and variation in environmental conditions must be considered.

## Reversibility Principle

The beneficial effects of exercise training are transient and reversible.

- Detraining occurs rapidly when a person stops exercising. After only 2 weeks of detraining, significant reductions in work capacity can be measured, and improvements can be lost within several months. A similar phenomenon occurs with individuals who are confined to bed with illness or disability: the individual becomes severely deconditioned, with loss of the ability to carry out normal daily activities as a result of inactivity.
- The frequency or duration of physical activity required to maintain a certain level of aerobic fitness is less than that required to improve it.

## ● EXERCISE PROGRAM

A carefully planned exercise program can result in higher levels of fitness for the healthy individual, slow the decrease in functional capacity of the elderly, and recondition those who have been ill or have chronic disease. There are three components of the exercise program: (1) a warm-up period, (2) the aerobic exercise period, and (3) a cool-down period.

## Warm-Up Period

Physiologically, a time lag exists between the onset of activity and the bodily adjustments needed to meet the physical requirements of the body. The purpose of the warm-up period is to enhance the numerous adjustments that must take place before physical activity.

### Physiological Responses
During this period there is:

- An increase in muscle temperature. The higher temperature increases the efficiency of muscular contraction by reducing muscle viscosity and increasing the rate of nerve conduction.
- An increased need for oxygen to meet the energy demands for the muscle. Extraction from hemoglobin is greater at higher muscle temperatures, facilitating the oxidative processes at work.
- Dilatation of the previously constricted capillaries with increases in the circulation, augmenting oxygen delivery to the active muscles and minimizing the oxygen deficit and the formation of lactic acid.
- Adaptation in sensitivity of the neural respiratory center to various exercise stimulants.
- An increase in venous return. This occurs as blood flow is shifted centrally from the periphery.

### Purposes
The warm-up also prevents or decreases:

- The susceptibility of the musculoskeletal system to injury.
- The occurrence of ischemic electrocardiographic (ECG) changes and arrhythmias.

### Guidelines
The warm-up should be gradual and sufficient to increase muscle and core temperature without causing fatigue or reducing energy stores. Characteristics of the period include:

- A 10-minute period of total body movement exercises, such as calisthenics, and walking slowly.
- Attaining a heart rate that is within 20 beats/min of the target heart rate.

## Aerobic Exercise Period

The aerobic exercise period is the conditioning part of the exercise program. Attention to the determinants of intensity, frequency, duration, and mode of the program, as previously discussed, has an impact on the effectiveness of the program. The main consideration when choosing a specific method of training is that the intensity be great enough to stimulate an increase in stroke volume and cardiac output and to enhance local circulation and aerobic metabolism in the appropriate muscle groups. The exercise period must be within the person's tolerance, above the threshold level for adaptation to occur, and below the level of exercise that evokes clinical symptoms.

In aerobic exercise, submaximum, rhythmic, repetitive, dynamic exercise of large muscle groups is emphasized.

There are four methods of training that challenge the aerobic system: continuous, interval (work relief), circuit, and circuit interval.

### Continuous Training

- A submaximum energy requirement, sustained throughout the training period, is imposed.
- Once the steady state is achieved, the muscle obtains energy by means of aerobic metabolism. Stress is placed primarily on the slow-twitch fibers.

The activity can be prolonged for 20 to 60 minutes without exhausting the oxygen transport system.

The work rate is increased progressively as training improvements are achieved. Overload can be accomplished by increasing the exercise duration.

In the healthy individual, continuous training is the most effective way to improve endurance.

### Interval Training

With this type of training, the work or exercise is followed by a properly prescribed relief or rest interval. Interval training is perceived to be less demanding than continuous training. In the healthy individual, interval training tends to improve strength and power more than endurance.

The relief interval is either a rest relief (passive recovery) or a work relief (active recovery); and its duration ranges from a few seconds to several minutes. Work recovery involves continuing the exercise but at a reduced level from the work period. During the relief period, a portion of the muscular stores of ATP and the oxygen associated with myoglobin that were depleted during the work period are replenished by the aerobic system; an increase in $\dot{V}O_{2\,max}$ occurs.

The longer the work interval, the more the aerobic system is stressed. With a short work interval, the duration of the rest interval is critical if the aerobic system is to be stressed (a work/recovery ratio of 1:1 to 1:5 is appropriate). A rest interval equal to one and a half times the work interval allows the succeeding exercise interval to begin before recovery is complete and stresses the aerobic system. With a longer work interval, the duration of the rest is not as important.

A significant amount of high-intensity work can be achieved with interval or intermittent work if there is appropriate spacing of the work–relief intervals. The total amount of work that can be completed with intermittent work is greater than the amount of work that can be completed with continuous training.

### Circuit Training

Circuit training employs a series of exercise activities. At the end of the last activity, the individual starts from the beginning and again moves through the series. The series of activities is repeated several times.

Several exercise modes can be used involving large and small muscle groups and a mix of static or dynamic effort.

Use of circuit training can improve strength and endurance by stressing both the aerobic and anaerobic systems.

### Circuit-Interval Training

Combining circuit and interval training is effective because of the interaction of aerobic and anaerobic production of ATP.

In addition to the aerobic and anaerobic systems being stressed by the various activities, with the relief interval there is a delay in the need for glycolysis and the production of lactic acid prior to the availability of oxygen supplying the ATP.

## Cool-Down Period

A cool-down period is necessary following the exercise period.

### Purpose

The purpose of the cool-down period is to:

Prevent pooling of the blood in the extremities by continuing to use the muscles to maintain venous return.

Prevent fainting by increasing the return of blood to the heart and brain as cardiac output and venous return decreases.

Enhance the recovery period with the oxidation of metabolic waste and replacement of the energy stores.

Prevent myocardial ischemia, arrhythmias, or other cardiovascular complications.

### Guidelines

Characteristics of the cool-down period are similar to those of the warm-up period.

Total-body exercises such as calisthenics and static stretching are appropriate.

The period should last 5 to 10 minutes.

## Application

Application of aerobic training is summarized in Box 7.9.

## PHYSIOLOGICAL CHANGES THAT OCCUR WITH TRAINING

Changes in the cardiovascular and respiratory systems as well as changes in muscle metabolism occur following endurance training. These changes are reflected both at rest and with exercise. It is important to note that all of the following training effects cannot result from one training program.

## Cardiovascular Changes

### Changes at Rest

A reduction in the resting pulse rate occurs in some individuals because of a decrease in sympathetic drive, with decreasing levels of norepinephrine and epinephrine; a decrease in atrial rate secondary to biochemical changes in the muscles and levels of acetylcholine, norepinephrine, and epinephrine in the atria; and an apparent increase in parasympathetic (vagal) tone secondary to decreased sympathetic tone

A decrease in blood pressure occurs in some individuals with a decrease in peripheral vascular resistance. The largest decrease is in systolic blood pressure and is most apparent in hypertensive individuals.

| BOX 7.9 | General Guidelines for an Aerobic Training Program |

- Establish the target heart rate and maximum heart rate.
- Warm up gradually for 5 to 10 minutes. Include stretching and repetitive motions at slow speeds, gradually increasing the effort.
- Increase the pace of the activity so the target heart rate can be maintained for 20 to 30 minutes. Examples include fast walking, running, bicycling, swimming, cross-country skiing, and aerobic dancing.
- Cool down for 5 to 10 minutes with slow, total body repetitive motions and stretching activities.
- The aerobic activity should be undertaken three to five times per week.
- To avoid injuries from stress, use appropriate equipment, such as correct footwear, for proper biomechanical support. Avoid running, jogging, or aerobic dancing on hard surfaces such as asphalt and concrete.
- To avoid overuse syndromes in structures of the musculoskeletal system, proper warm-up and stretching of muscles to be used should be performed. Progression of activities should be within the tolerance of the individual. Overuse commonly occurs when there is an increase in time or effort without adequate rest (recovery) time between sessions. Increase the repetitions or the time by no more than 10% per week. If pain begins while exercising or lasts longer than 4 hours after exercising, heed the warning and reduce the stress.
- Individualize the program of exercise. All people are not at the same fitness level and therefore cannot perform the same exercises. Any one exercise has the potential to be detrimental if attempted by someone not able to execute it properly. During recovery following an injury or surgery choose an exercise that does not stress the vulnerable tissue. Begin at a safe level for the individual and progress as the individual meets the desired goals.

- An increase in blood volume and hemoglobin may occur. This facilitates the oxygen delivery capacity of the system.

### Changes During Exercise

- A reduction in the pulse rate occurs in some individuals because of the mechanisms listed earlier in this section.
- Increased stroke volume may occur because of an increase in myocardial contractility and an increase in ventricular volume.
- Increased cardiac output may occur as a result of the increased stroke volume that occurs with maximum exercise but not with submaximum exercise. The magnitude of the change is directly related to the increase in stroke volume and the magnitude of the reduced heart rate.
- Increased extraction of oxygen by the working muscle occurs in some individuals because of enzymatic and biochemical changes in the muscle, as well as increased maximum oxygen uptake ($\dot{V}O_{2\,max}$). Greater $\dot{V}O_{2\,max}$ results in a greater work capacity. The increased cardiac output increases the delivery of oxygen to the working

muscles. The increased ability of the muscle to extract oxygen from the blood increases the utilization of the available oxygen.
- Decreased blood flow per kilogram of the working muscle may occur even though increasing amounts of blood are shunted to the exercising muscle. The increase in extraction of oxygen from the blood compensates for this change.
- Decreased myocardial oxygen consumption (pulse rate times systolic blood pressure) for any given intensity of exercise may occur as a result of a decreased pulse rate with or without a modest decrease in blood pressure. The product can be decreased significantly in the healthy subject without any loss of efficiency at a specific workload.

## Respiratory Changes

### Changes at Rest

- Larger lung volumes develop because of improved pulmonary function, with no change in tidal volume.
- Larger diffusion capacities develop because of larger lung volumes and greater alveolar-capillary surface area.

### Changes During Exercise

- Larger diffusion capacities occur for the same reasons as those listed previously; the maximum capacity of ventilation is unchanged.
- A smaller amount of air is ventilated at the same oxygen consumption occurs; maximum diffusion capacity is unchanged.
- The maximal minute ventilation is increased.
- Ventilatory efficiency is increased.

## Metabolic Changes

### Changes at Rest

- Muscle hypertrophy and increased capillary density occurs.
- The number and size of mitochondria are increased, increasing the capacity to generate ATP aerobically.
- The muscle myoglobin concentration increases, increasing the rate of oxygen transport and possibly the rate of oxygen diffusion to the mitochondria.

### Changes During Exercise

- A decreased rate of depletion of muscle glycogen at submaximum work levels may occur. Another term for this phenomenon is glycogen sparing. It is due to an increased capacity to mobilize and oxidize fat and increased fat-mobilizing and fat-metabolizing enzymes.
- Lower blood lactate levels at submaximum work may occur. The mechanism for this is unclear; it does not appear to be related to decreased hypoxia of the muscles.
- Less reliance on phosphocreatine (PC) and ATP in skeletal muscle and an increased capability to oxidize carbohydrate may result because of an increased oxidative potential of the mitochondria and an increased glycogen storage in the muscle.

N O T E : Ill health may influence metabolic adaptations to exercise.

## Other System Changes

Changes in other systems that occur with training include:

- Decrease in body fat
- Decrease in blood cholesterol and triglyceride levels
- Increased heat acclimatization
- Increase in the breaking strength of bones and ligaments and the tensile strength of tendons

## APPLICATION OF PRINCIPLES OF AN AEROBIC CONDITIONING PROGRAM FOR THE PATIENT WITH CORONARY DISEASE

Employing the principles of aerobic conditioning in physical therapy has been most dominant in program planning for the individual following a myocardial infarction (MI) or following coronary artery bypass surgery.[4,6,7]

During the past 20 to 25 years, there have been major changes in the medical management of these patients. The changes have included shortened hospital stays, more aggressive progression of activity for the patient following MI or cardiac surgery, and earlier initiation of an exercise program based on a low-level stress test prior to discharge from the hospital. An aerobic conditioning program, in addition to risk factor modification, is a dominant part of cardiac rehabilitation.

### Inpatient Phase (Phase I)

The inpatient phase of the program occurs in the hospital following stabilization of the patient's cardiovascular status after MI or coronary bypass surgery. Because the length of hospital care has decreased over the past few years, this time may be limited to 3 to 5 days. When hospital stays were longer, this phase often lasted 7 to 14 days and was referred to as phase 1 of the cardiac rehabilitation program.

#### Purpose
The purpose of the early portion of cardiac rehabilitation is to:

- Initiate risk factor education and address future modification of certain behaviors, such as eating habits and smoking.
- Initiate self-care activities and progress from sitting to standing to minimize deconditioning (1 to 3 days postevent).
- Provide an orthostatic challenge to the cardiovascular system (3 to 5 days postevent). This is usually accomplished by supervised ambulation. Ambulation is usually monitored electrocardiographically, as well as manually monitoring the heart rate, ventilation rate, and blood pressure.
- Prepare patients and family for continued rehabilitation and for life at home after a cardiac event.

---

> **BOX 7.10  Case Example of a Cardiac Rehabilitation Referral**
>
> Mr. Smith is referred and undergoes further evaluation to determine the cause of his chest pain. He is diagnosed with single vessel coronary artery disease. He is referred to cardiac rehabilitation.
>
> - Medications. Nitroglycerin as needed to relieve angina. Mr. Smith will attend cardiac rehabilitation three times per week for 8 to 12 weeks to improve his fitness level and attend smoking cessation classes. He will meet with a medical dietitian to discuss meal planning to lower his intake of fat and cholesterol.
> - Exercise prescription. Mr. Smith will exercise at an intensity lower than his anginal threshold. This intensity will be initially established at 60% to 65% of his maximum heart rate or 50% of his $\dot{V}o_{2\,max}$. He will exercise three times per week for 20 to 40 minutes, depending on his tolerance.

### Outpatient Phase (Phase II)

The outpatient phase of the program is initiated either upon discharge from the hospital or, depending on the severity of the diagnosis, 6 to 8 weeks later. This delay allows time for the myocardium to heal as well as time to monitor the patient's response to a new medical regimen. Participants are monitored via telemetry to determine heart rate and rhythm responses; blood pressure is recorded at rest and during exercise; and ventilation responses are noted. These programs usually last 6 to 8 weeks (Box 7.10).

#### Purpose
The purpose of the program is to:

- Increase the person's exercise capacity in a safe, progressive manner so adaptive cardiovascular and muscular changes occur. The early part of the program is referred to by some as "low-level" exercise training.
- Enhance cardiac functions and reduce the cardiac cost of work. This may help eliminate or delay symptoms such as angina and ST-segment changes in the patient with coronary heart disease.
- Produce favorable metabolic changes.
- Determine the effect of medications on increasing levels of activity.
- Relieve anxiety and depression.
- Progress the patient to an independent exercise program.

#### Guidelines
A symptom-limited exercise stress test is performed 6 to 12 weeks after hospital discharge (or as early as 2 to 4 weeks following discharge).

The exercise program is predominantly aerobic. Generally, for patients with functional capacities greater than 5 METs, the exercise prescription is based on the results of the symptom-limited test.

*Intensity.* The initial level of activity or training intensity may be as low as 40% to 60% of the maximum heart rate or 40% to 70% of the functional capacity defined in METs. The starting intensity is dictated by the severity of the diagnosis in concert with the individual's age and prior fitness level. The intensity is progressed as the individual responds to the training program.

*Duration.* The duration of the exercise session may be limited to 10 to 15 minutes at the start, progressing to 30 to 60 minutes as the patient's status improves. Each session usually includes 8- to 10-minute warm-up and cool-down periods.

*Frequency.* Participants often attend sessions offered three times per week.

*Mode.* The mode of exercise is usually continuous, using large muscle groups, such as stationary biking or walking. These activities allow ECG monitoring via telemetry.

*Method.* Circuit-interval exercise is a common method used with the patient during phase II. The patient can exercise on each modality at a defined workload, compared with exercising continuously on a bicycle or treadmill. As a result, the patient can:

- Perform more physical work.
- Exercise at a higher intensity—fitness may improve within a shorter period of time.
- Maintain lactic acid and the oxygen deficit at minimum levels.
- Exercise at a lower rate of perceived exertion.

*Weight training.* Low-level weight training may be initiated during the outpatient program, provided the individual has undergone a symptom-limited stress test. Resistive exercises should not produce ischemic symptoms associated with an increase in heart rate and systolic blood pressure. Therefore, heart rate and blood pressure should be monitored periodically throughout the exercise session. Starting weight may be calculated using 40% of a one repetition maximum (1-RM) effort.

*Progression.* Progression of the workload occurs when there have been three consecutive sessions (every-other-day sessions) during which the peak heart rate is below the target heart rate.

## Outpatient Program (Phase III)

The outpatient phase of cardiac rehabilitation includes a supervised exercise conditioning program, which is often continued in a hospital or community setting. Heart rate and rhythm are no longer monitored via telemetry. Participants are reminded to monitor their own pulse rate, and a supervisory person is available to monitor blood pressure.

### Purpose
The purpose of the program is to continue to improve or maintain fitness levels achieved during the phase II program.

### Guidelines

*Recreational activities.* Activities to maintain levels gained during phase II may include:

- Swimming, which incorporates both arms and legs. However, there is a decreased awareness of ischemic symptoms while swimming, especially when the skill level is poor.
- Outdoor hiking, which is excellent if on level terrain.

*Activities at 8 METs.*

- Jogging approximately 5 miles per hour
- Cycling approximately 12 miles per hour
- Vigorous down-hill skiing.

## Special Considerations

There are special considerations related to types of exercise and patient needs that must be recognized when developing conditioning programs for patients with coronary disease. Arm exercises elicit different responses than leg exercises.

- Mechanical efficiency based on the ratio between output of external work and caloric expenditure is lower than with leg exercises.
- Oxygen uptake at a given external workload is significantly higher for arm exercises than for leg exercises.
- Myocardial efficiency is lower with leg exercises than with arm exercises.
- Myocardial oxygen consumption (heart rate × systolic blood pressure) is higher with arm exercises than with leg exercises.

PRECAUTION: Patients with coronary disease complete 35% less work with arm exercises than with leg exercises before symptoms occur.

## Adaptive Changes

Adaptive changes following training of individuals with cardiac disease include:

- Increased myocardial aerobic work capacity.
- Increased maximum aerobic or functional capacity by predominantly widening the arteriovenous oxygen $(a - \bar{V}o_2)$ difference.
- Increased stroke volume following high-intensity training 6 to 12 months into the training program.
- Decreased myocardial demand for oxygen.
- Increased myocardial supply by the decreased heart rate and prolongation of diastole.
- Increased tolerance to a given physical workload before angina occurs.
- Significantly lower heart rate at each submaximum workload and therefore a greater heart rate reserve. When muscles are used that are not directly involved in the activity, the reduction in heart rate is not as great.
- Improved psychological orientation and, over time, an impact on depression scores, scores for hysteria, hypochondriasis, and psychoasthenia on the Minnesota Multiphasic Personality Inventory.

NOTE: Cardiovascular complications are prevented and/or reduced if the program includes appropriate selection of patients, continuous evaluation of each patient, medical supervision of the exercise throughout the training period, regular communication with the physician, specific instructions to patients about adverse symptoms, class size limitations to 30 or fewer patients, and maintenance of accurate records related to compliance to the program.

## ⬤ APPLICATIONS OF AEROBIC TRAINING FOR THE DECONDITIONED INDIVIDUAL AND THE PATIENT WITH CHRONIC ILLNESS

Deconditioned individuals, including those with chronic illness and the elderly may have major limitations in pulmonary and cardiovascular reserve that severely curtail their daily activities.

***Deconditioning.*** Implications of the changes due to deconditioning brought on by inactivity resulting from any illness or chronic disease are important to remember.

- There is decreased work capacity, which is a result of decreased maximum oxygen uptake and decreased ability to use oxygen and perform work. There is also decreased cardiac output, which is the major limiting factor.
- There is decreased circulating blood volume that can be as much as 700 to 800 mL. For some individuals, this results in tachycardia along with orthostatic hypotension, dizziness, and episodes of syncope when initially attempting to stand.
- There is a decrease in plasma and red blood cells, which increases the likelihood of life-threatening embothrombolic episodes and prolongation of the convalescent period.
- There is a decrease in lean body mass, which results in decreased muscle size and decreased muscle strength and ability to perform activities requiring large muscle groups. For example, the individual may have difficulty walking with crutches or climbing stairs.
- There is increased excretion of urinary calcium, which results from a decrease in the weight-bearing stimulus critical in maintaining bone integrity, in bone loss or osteoporosis, and in an increased likelihood of fractures upon falling because of osteoporosis.

***Reversal of deconditioning.*** Through an exercise program, the negative cardiovascular, neuromuscular, and metabolic functions can be reversed. This results in:

- A decrease in the resting heart rate, the heart rate with any given exercise load, and urinary excretion of calcium
- An increase in stroke volume at rest, stroke volume with exercise, cardiac output with exercise, total heart volume, lung volume (ventilatory volume), vital capacity, maximum oxygen uptake, circulating blood volume, plasma volume and red blood cells, and lean body mass
- A reversal of the negative nitrogen and protein balance
- An increase in levels of mitochondrial enzymes and energy stores
- Less use of the anaerobic systems during activity

## Adaptations for Disabilities, Functional Limitations, and Deconditioning

Individuals who have a physical disability or functional limitation should not be excluded from a conditioning program that can increase their fitness level. This includes individuals in wheelchairs or persons who have problems ambulating, such as those with paraplegia, hemiplegia, or amputation, and those with an orthopedic problem, such as arthrodesis.

- Adaptations must be made when testing the physically disabled using a wheelchair treadmill or more frequently using the upper extremity ergometer.
- Exercise protocols may emphasize upper extremities and manipulation of the wheelchair.
- It is important to remember that energy expenditure is increased when the gait is altered, and wheelchair use is less efficient than walking without impairment.

## Impairments, Goals, and Plan of Care

The goals of an aerobic exercise program are dependent on the initial level of fitness of the individual and on his or her specific clinical needs. The general goals are to decrease the deconditioning effects of disease and chronic illness and to improve the individual's cardiovascular and muscular fitness.

### Common Impairments

- Increased susceptibility to thromboembolic episodes, pneumonia, atelectasis, and the likelihood of fractures
- Tachycardia, dizziness, and orthostatic hypotension when moving from sitting to standing
- A decrease in general muscle strength, with difficulty and shortness of breath in climbing stairs
- A decrease in work capacity that limits distances walked and activities tolerated
- Increased heart rate and blood pressure responses (rate–pressure product) to various activities
- A decrease in the maximum rate–pressure product tolerated with angina or other ischemic symptoms appearing at low levels of exercise

### Goals

- Prevention of thromboembolic episodes, pneumonia, atelectasis, and fractures
- Decrease in the magnitude of the orthostatic hypotensive response
- Ability to climb stairs safely and without shortness of breath

> ### BOX 7.11  Guidelines for Initiating an Aerobic Exercise Program for the Deconditioned Individual and the Patient with Chronic Illness
>
> - Determine the exercise heart rate response that can be safely reached using the Karvonen formula as a guide, accounting for medical conditions, medications, and the individual's perceived exertion.
> - Initiate a program of activities for the patient that does not elicit a cardiovascular response over the exercise heart rate (e.g., walking, repetitive activities, easy calisthenics).
> - Provide patients with clearly written instructions about any activity they perform on their own.
> - Initiate an educational program that provides the patient with information about effort symptoms and exercise precautions, monitoring the heart rate, and modifications when indicated.

- Tolerance for walking longer measured distances and completing activities without fatigue or symptoms
- Decrease in the heart rate and blood pressure (rate–pressure product) at a given level of activity
- An increase in the maximum rate–pressure product tolerated without ischemic symptoms

### Outcomes

- Improved pulmonary, cardiovascular, and metabolic response to various levels of exercise
- Improved ability to complete selected activities with appropriate heart rate and blood responses to exercise

### Guidelines

Guidelines for establishing a safe program of intervention for the deconditioned individual and the convalescent patient with chronic illness are summarized in Boxes 7.11 and 7.12.

## ● AGE DIFFERENCES

Differences in endurance and physical work capacity among children, young adults, and middle-aged or elderly individuals are evident. Some comparisons are made between maximum oxygen uptake and the factors influencing it and among blood pressure, respiratory rate, vital capacity, and maximum voluntary ventilation in the different age categories. It is important when developing aerobic conditioning programs that these age-related differences are taken into consideration.

### Children

Between the ages of 5 and 15 there is a threefold increase in body weight, lung volume, heart volume, and maximum oxygen uptake.

> ### BOX 7.12  Guidelines for Progression of an Aerobic Training Program
>
> - Determine the maximum heart rate or symptom-limited heart rate by multistage testing with ECG monitoring.
> - Decide on the threshold stimulus (percentage of maximum or symptom-limited heart rate) that elicits a conditioning response for the individual tested and that can be used as the exercise heart rate.
> - Determine the intensity, duration, and frequency of exercise that results in attaining the exercise heart rate and a conditioning response.
> - Determine the mode of exercise to be used based on the individual's physical capabilities and interest.
> - Initiate an exercise program with the patient and provide clearly written instructions regarding the details of the program.
> - Educate the patient about:
>   - Effort symptoms and the need to cease or modify exercise when these symptoms appear and to communicate with the physical therapist and/or physician about these problems.
>   - Monitoring heart rate at rest as well as during and following exercise.
>   - The importance of exercising within the guidelines provided by the physical therapist.
>   - The importance of consistent long-term follow-up about the exercise program so it can be progressed within safe limits.
>   - The importance of modifying risk factors related to cardiac problems.

### Heart Rate

- Resting heart rate is on the average above 125 (126 in girls, 135 in boys) at infancy.
- Resting heart rate drops to adult levels at puberty.
- Maximum heart rate is age-related (220 minus age).

### Stroke Volume

- Stroke volume is closely related to size.
- Children 5 to 16 years of age have a stroke volume of 30 to 40 mL.

### Cardiac Output

- Cardiac output is related to size.
- Cardiac output increases with increasing stroke volume.
- The increase in cardiac output for a given increase in oxygen consumption is a constant throughout life: It is the same in the child as in the adult.

### Arteriovenous Oxygen Difference

- Children tolerate a larger $a - \bar{v}O_2$ difference than adults.
- The larger $a - \bar{v}O_2$ difference makes up for the smaller stroke volume.

## Maximum Oxygen Uptake ($\dot{V}O_{2\,max}$)

- The $\dot{V}O_{2\,max}$ increases with age up to 20 years (expressed as liters per minute).
- Before puberty, girls and boys show no significant difference in maximum aerobic capacity.
- Cardiac output in children is the same as in the adult for any given oxygen consumption.
- Endurance times increase with age until 17 to 18 years.

## Blood Pressure

- Systolic blood pressure increases from 40 mm Hg at birth to 80 mm Hg at age 1 month to 100 mm Hg several years before puberty. Adult levels are observed at puberty.
- Diastolic blood pressure increases from 55 to 70 mm Hg from 4 to 14 years of age, with little change during adolescence.

## Respiration

- Respiratory rate decreases from 30 breaths per minute at infancy to 16 breaths per minute at 17 to 18 years of age.
- Vital capacity and maximum voluntary ventilation are correlated with height, although the greater increase in boys than girls at puberty may be due to an increase in lung tissue.

## Muscle Mass and Strength

- Muscle mass increases through adolescence, primarily owing to muscle fiber hypertrophy and the development of sarcomeres. Sarcomeres are added at the musculotendinous junction to compensate for the required increase in length.
- Girls develop peak muscle mass between 16 and 20 years, whereas boys develop peak muscle mass between 18 and 25 years.
- Strength gains are associated with increased muscle mass in conjunction with neural maturation.

## Anaerobic Ability

- Children generally demonstrate a limited anaerobic capacity. This may be due to a limited amount of phosphofructokinase, a controlling enzyme in the glycolytic pathway.
- Children produce less lactic acid when performing anaerobically. This may be due to a limited glycolytic capacity.

# Young Adults

There are more data on the physiological parameters of fitness for the young and middle-aged adult than for children or the elderly.

## Heart Rate

- Resting heart rate reaches 60 to 65 beats per minute at 17 to 18 years of age (75 beats per minute in a sitting, sedentary young man).
- Maximum heart rate is age-related (190 beats per minute in the same sedentary young man).

## Stroke Volume

- The adult values for stroke volume are 60 to 80 mL (75 mL in a sitting, sedentary young man).
- With maximum exercise, stroke volume is 100 mL in that same sedentary young man.

## Cardiac Output for the Sedentary Young Man at Rest

- Cardiac output at rest is 75 beats per minute $\times$ 75 mL, or 5.6 liters per minute.
- With maximum exercise, cardiac output is 190 beats per minute $\times$ 100 mL, or 19 liters per minute.

## Arteriovenous Oxygen Difference (a − $vO_2$ Difference)

- Approximately 25% to 30% of the oxygen is extracted from blood as it runs through the muscles or other tissues at rest.
- In a normal, sedentary young man, it increases threefold (5.2 to 15.8 mL/dL blood) with exercise.

## Maximum Oxygen Uptake

- The difference in $\dot{V}O_{2\,max}$ between males and females is greatest in the adult.
- Differences in $\dot{V}O_{2\,max}$ between the sexes is minimal when $\dot{V}O_{2\,max}$ is expressed relative to lean body weight.
- In the sedentary young man, maximum oxygen uptake equals 3000 mL/min (oxygen uptake at rest equals 300 mL/min).

## Blood Pressure

- Systolic blood pressure is 120 mm Hg (average). At peak effort during exercise, values may range from as low as 190 mm Hg to as high as 240 mm Hg.
- Diastolic blood pressure is 80 mm Hg (average). Diastolic pressure does not change markedly with exercise.

## Respiration

- Respiratory rate is 12 to 15 breaths per minute.
- Vital capacity is 4800 mL in a man 20 to 30 years of age.
- Maximum voluntary ventilation varies considerably from laboratory to laboratory and is dependent on age and the surface area of the body.

## Muscle Mass and Strength

- Muscle mass increases with training as a result of hypertrophy. This hypertrophy can be the result of an increased number of myofibrils, increased actin and myosin, sarcoplasm, and/or connective tissue.
- Limited evidence suggests that the number of muscle fibers may increase, referred to as hyperplasia.
- As the nervous system matures, increased recruitment of motor units or decreased autogenic inhibition by Golgi tendon organs appears also to dictate strength gains.

## Anaerobic Ability

- Anaerobic training increases the activity of several controlling enzymes in the glycolytic pathway and enhances stored quantities of ATP and phosphocreatine.

● Anaerobic training increases the muscle's ability to buffer the hydrogen ions released when lactic acid is produced. Increased buffering allows the muscle to work anaerobically for longer periods of time.

## Older Adults

With increasing interest in the aged, data are appearing in the literature about this age group and their response to exercise.

### Heart Rate

● Resting heart rate is not influenced by age.
● Maximum heart rate is age-related and decreases with age (in very general terms, 220 minus age). The average maximum heart rate for men 20 to 29 years of age is 190 beats/min. For men 60 to 69 years of age, it is 164 beats/min.
● The amount that the heart rate increases in response to static and maximum dynamic exercise (hand grip) decreases in the elderly.

### Stroke Volume

Stroke volume decreases in the aged and results in decreased cardiac output.

### Cardiac Output

Cardiac output decreases on an average of 7.0 to 3.4 liters per minute from age 19 to 86 years.

### a − $\bar{v}o_2$ Difference

Arteriovenous oxygen difference decreases as a result of decreased lean body mass and low oxygen-carrying capacity.

### Maximum Oxygen Uptake

● According to cardiorespiratory fitness classification, if men 60 to 69 years of age of average fitness level are compared with men 20 to 29 years of age of the same fitness level, the maximum oxygen uptake for the older man is lower.
  • 20 to 29 years: 31 to 37 mL/kg per minute
  • 60 to 69 years: 18 to 23 mL/kg per minute

● Aerobic capacity decreases about 10% per decade when evaluating sedentary men. Maximum oxygen consumption decreases on an average from 47.7 mL/kg per minute at age 25 years to 25.5 mL/kg per minute at age 75 years. This decrease is not directly the result of age; athletes who continue exercising have significantly less decrease in $\dot{V}O_{2\,max}$ when evaluated over a 10-year period.

### Blood Pressure

Blood pressure increases because of increased peripheral vascular resistance.

● Systolic blood pressure of the aged is 150 mm Hg (average).
● Diastolic blood pressure is 90 mm Hg (average).
● If the definition of high blood pressure (stage II hypertension) is $\geq 160/100$, then 22% of men and 34% of women 65 to 74 years of age are hypertensive
● Using 150/95 mm Hg as a cutoff, 25% of individuals are hypertensive at age 50 years and 70% between the ages of 85 and 95 years.

### Respiration

● Respiratory rate increases with age.
● Vital capacity decreases with age. There is a 25% decrease in the vital capacity of the 50- to 60-year-old man compared with the 20- to 30-year-old man with the same surface area.
● Maximum voluntary ventilation decreases with age.

### Muscle Mass and Strength

● Generally, the strength decline with age is associated with a decrease in muscle mass and physical activity.
● The decrease in muscle mass is primarily due to a decrease in protein synthesis, in concert with a decline in the number of fast-twitch muscle fibers.
● Aging may also affect strength by slowing the nervous system's response time. This may alter the ability to recruit motor units effectively.
● Continued training as one ages appears to reduce the effects of aging on the muscular system.

# INDEPENDENT LEARNING ACTIVITIES

## ● Critical Thinking and Discussion

1. A 16-year-old cross-country runner is referred to the clinic where you are employed with the diagnosis of a right ankle sprain. You examine and evaluate him and develop a treatment plan for the ankle. You must also address his desire to return to competition when able.
  • Discuss the energy systems utilized with distance running.
  • Discuss the notion of sport specificity.
  • What aerobic exercises could the patient do to maintain his aerobic condition while his ankle heals but not stress the ankle?

2. You are an invited speaker at a senior citizen center for a lunchtime discussion of lifetime fitness and establishing an appropriate exercise program for individuals in this age category.
  • Discuss the definition of fitness.
  • Discuss the concept of the exercise prescription.
  • Describe the necessary precautions when dealing with the older population (both the older athlete and the untrained individual).

3. Explain the concepts of energy expenditure, oxygen consumption, and efficiency with regard to ambulating with an assistive device with each of these diagnoses:

rheumatoid arthritis, post-tibial fracture, and post-total-hip replacement.

4. Design an exercise program for the local fire fighters. Utilize the concepts of the aerobic energy systems, anaerobic energy system, and strength training.

5. You have been invited to speak to a group of elementary and preschool teachers about the importance of aerobic exercise for children. Explain the basic physiological differences between children and adults at rest with regard to heart rate, respiratory rate and metabolism, and their response to exercise.

# REFERENCES

1. American College of Sports Medicine: Exercise Management for Persons with Chronic Diseases and Disabilities, ed 2. Human Kinetics, Champaign, IL, 2003.
2. American College of Sports Medicine: ASCM's Guidelines for Exercise Testing and Prescription, ed 7. Lippincott Williams, & Wilkins, Philadelphia, 2005.
3. American College of Sports Medicine: Resource Manual for Guidelines for Exercise Testing and Prescription, ed 5. Lippincott Williams & Wilkins, Philadelphia, 2005.
4. Brannon, FJ, Foley, MW, Starr, JA, Saul, LM: Cardiopulmonary Rehabilitation: Basic Theory and Application, ed 3. FA Davis, Philadelphia, 1998.
5. Center for Disease Control and Prevention. Physical Activity for Everyone: Recommendations [website]. Available at: http://www.cdc.gov/nccdphp/dnpa/physical/recommendations/index.htm. Accessed March 2006.
6. Hillegass, S, Sadowsky, H: Essentials of Cardiopulmonary Physical Therapy, ed 2. WB Saunders, Philadelphia, 2001.
7. Irwin, S, Teckline, JS: Cardiopulmonary Physical Therapy, ed 4. CV Mosby, St. Louis, 2004.
8. McArdle, WD, Katch, FI, Katch VL: Essentials of Exercise Physiology, ed 3. Lippincott Williams & Wilkins, Philadelphia, 2005.
9. McArdle, WD, Katch, FI, Katch, VL: Exercise Physiology: Energy, Nutrition, and Human Performance, ed 5. Lippincott Williams & Wilkins, Philadelphia, 2001.
10. Pollock M, Gaesser G, Butcher J, et al. The recommended quantity and quality of exercise for developing and maintaining cardiorespiratory and muscular fitness, and flexibility in healthy adults. Med Sci Sports Exerc 30(6):975–991, 1998.
11. Powers, SK, Howley, ET: Exercise Physiology: Theory and Application, ed 4. McGraw-Hill, Boston, 2001.
12. Thompson P, Buchner D, Pina I, et al. Exercise and Physical Activity in the Prevention and Treatment of Atherosclerotic Cardiovascular Disease: AHA Scientific Statement. Circulation 107(24):3109–3116, 2003.

# Exercise for Impaired Balance

Anne D. Kloos, PT, PhD, NCS

Deborah Givens Heiss, PT, PhD, DPT, OCS

Loss of balance and falling are problems that affect individuals with a wide range of diagnoses. Physical therapists commonly evaluate balance and use balance training/exercises as either primary or secondary interventions for patients undergoing many types of rehabilitation programs. Because of the importance of balance assessment and treatment in clinical practice, The *Guide to Physical Therapist Practice* (2001)[4] has designated an entire preferred practice pattern (pattern 5A) to primary prevention/risk reduction for loss of balance and falling. The purpose of this chapter is to present an overview of key background terms and concepts related to balance, how balance control is normally achieved in humans for a variety of conditions, possible causes of balance impairments, and evidence-based assessments and interventions for enhancing all aspects of an individual's balance control.

##  BACKGROUND AND CONCEPTS

### Balance: Key Terms and Definitions

Balance, or postural stability, is a generic term used to describe the dynamic process by which the body's position is maintained in equilibrium. Equilibrium means that the body is either at rest (static equilibrium) or in steady-state motion (dynamic equilibrium). Balance is greatest when the body's center of mass (COM) or center of gravity (COG) is maintained over its base of support (BOS).

***Center of mass.*** The COM is a point that corresponds to the center of the total body mass and is the point where the body is in perfect equilibrium. It is determined by finding the weighted average of the COM of each body segment.[105]

***Center of gravity.*** The COG refers to the vertical projection of the center of mass to the ground. In the anatomical position, the COG of most adult humans is located slightly anterior to the second sacral vertebra[14] or approximately 55% of a person's height.[42]

***Momentum.*** Momentum is the product of mass times velocity. Linear momentum relates to the velocity of the body along a straight path, for example in the sagittal or transverse planes. Angular momentum relates to the rotational velocity of the body.

***Base of support.*** The BOS is defined as the perimeter of the contact area between the body and its support surface; foot placement alters the BOS and changes a person's postural stability.[81] A wide stance, such as is seen with many elderly individuals, increases stability, whereas a narrow BOS, such as tandem stance or walking, reduces it. So long as a person maintains the COG within the limits of the BOS, referred to as the *limits of stability*, he or she does not fall.

***Limits of stability.*** "Limits of stability" refers to the sway boundaries in which an individual can maintain equilibrium without changing his or her BOS (Fig. 8.1).[81] These

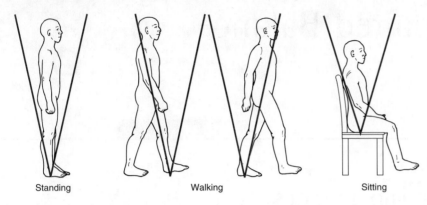

Standing    Walking    Sitting

FIGURE 8.1 Boundaries of the limits of stability while standing, walking, and sitting.

boundaries are constantly changing depending on the task, the individual's biomechanics, and aspects of the environment.[105] For example, the limits of stability for a person during quiet stance is the area encompassed by the outer edges of the feet in contact with the ground. Any deviations in the body's COM position relative to this boundary are corrected intermittently, producing a random swaying motion. For normal adults, the anteroposterior sway limit is approximately 12° from the most posterior to most anterior position.[82] Lateral stability varies with foot spacing and height; adults standing with 4 inches between the feet can sway approximately 16° from side to side.[80] However, a person sitting without trunk support has much greater limits of stability than when standing because the height of the COM above the BOS is less and the BOS is much larger (i.e., perimeter of the buttocks in contact with a surface).

***Ground reaction force and center of pressure.*** In accordance with Newton's law of reaction, the contact between our bodies and the ground due to gravity (action forces) is always accompanied by a reaction from it, the so-called ground reaction force.

The center of pressure (COP) is the location of the vertical projection of the ground reaction force.[124] It is equal and opposite to the weighted average of all the downward forces acting on the area in contact with the ground. If one foot is on the ground, the net COP lies within that foot. When both feet are on the ground, the net COP lies somewhere between the two feet, depending on how much weight is taken by each foot. When both feet are in contact, the COP under each foot can be measured separately. To maintain stability, a person produces muscular forces to continually control the position of the COG, which in turn changes the location of the COP. Thus the COP is a reflection of the body's neuromuscular responses to imbalances of the COG.[125] A force plate is traditionally used to measure ground reaction forces [in newtons (N)] and COP movements [in meters (m)].

## Balance Control

Balance is a complex motor control task involving the detection and integration of sensory information to assess the position and motion of the body in space and the execution of appropriate musculoskeletal responses to control body position within the context of the environment and task. Thus, balance control requires the interaction of the nervous and musculoskeletal systems and contextual effects (Fig. 8.2).

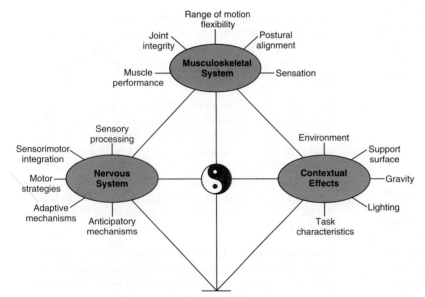

FIGURE 8.2 Interactions of the musculoskeletal and nervous systems and contextual effects for balance control.

- The *nervous system* provides the (1) sensory processing for perception of body orientation in space provided mainly by the visual, vestibular, and somatosensory systems; (2) sensorimotor integration essential for linking sensation to motor responses and for adaptive and anticipatory (i.e., centrally programmed postural adjustments that preceed voluntary movements) aspects of postural control; and (3) motor strategies for planning, programming, and executing balance responses.[44]
- *Musculoskeletal contributions* include postural alignment, musculoskeletal flexibility such as joint range of motion (ROM), joint integrity, muscle performance (i.e., muscle strength, power, and endurance), and sensation (touch, pressure, vibration, proprioception, and kinesthesia).
- *Contextual effects* that interact with the two systems are the environment whether it is closed (predictable with no distractions) or open (unpredictable and with distractions), the support surface (i.e., firm versus slippery, stable versus unstable, type of shoes), the amount of lighting, effects of gravity and inertial forces on the body, and task characteristics (i.e., well learned versus new, predictable versus unpredictable, single versus multiple tasks).

Even if all elements of the neurological and musculoskeletal systems are operating effectively, a person may fall if contextual effects force the balance control demands to be so high that the person's internal mechanisms are overwhelmed.

## Sensory Systems and Balance Control

Perception of one's body position and movement in space require a combination of information from peripheral receptors in multiple sensory systems including the visual, somatosensory (proprioceptive, joint, and cutaneous receptors), and vestibular systems.

### Visual System

The visual system provides information regarding (1) the position of the head relative to the environment; (2) the orientation of the head to maintain level gaze; and (3) the direction and speed of head movements because as your head moves, surrounding objects move in the opposite direction. Visual stimuli can be used to improve a person's stability when proprioceptive or vestibular inputs are unreliable by fixating the gaze on an object. Conversely, visual inputs sometimes provide inaccurate information for balance control, such as when a person is stationary and a large object such as a nearby bus starts moving, causing the person to have an illusion of movement.

### Somatosensory System

The somatosensory system provides information about the position and motion of the body and body parts relative to each other and the support surface. Information from muscle proprioceptors including muscle spindles and Golgi tendon organs (sensitive to muscle length and tension), joint receptors (sensitive to joint position, movement, and

stress), and skin mechanoreceptors (sensitive to vibration, light touch, deep pressure, skin stretch) are the dominant inputs for maintaining balance when the support surface is firm, flat, and fixed. However, when standing on a surface that is moving (e.g., on a boat) or on a surface that is not horizontal (e.g., on a ramp), inputs about body position with respect to the surface are not appropriate for maintaining balance; therefore, a person must rely on other sensory inputs for stability in these conditions.[105]

Information from joint receptors does not contribute greatly to conscious joint position sense. It has been demonstrated that local anesthetization of joint tissues and total joint replacement does not impair joint position awareness.[38,39] Muscle spindle receptors appear to be mostly responsible for providing joint position sense, whereas the primary role of joint receptors is to assist the gamma motor system in regulating muscle tone and stiffness to provide anticipatory postural adjustments and to counteract unexpected postural disturbances.[88]

### Vestibular System

The vestibular system provides information about the position and movement of the head with respect to gravity and inertial forces. Receptors in the semicircular canals (SCCs) detect angular acceleration of the head, whereas the receptors in the otoliths (utricle and saccule) detect linear acceleration and head position with respect to gravity. The SCCs are particularly sensitive to fast head movements, such as during walking or during episodes of imbalance (slips, trips, stumbles), whereas the otoliths respond to slow head movements, such as during postural sway.[43,105]

By itself, the vestibular system can give no information about the position of the body. For example, it cannot distinguish a simple head nod (head movement on a stable trunk) from a forward bend (head movement in conjunction with a moving trunk).[43] Consequently, additional information, particularly from mechanoreceptors in the neck, must be provided for the central nervous system (CNS) to have a true picture of the orientation of the head relative to the body.[88] The vestibular system uses motor pathways originating from the vestibular nuclei for postural control and coordination of eye and head movements. The vestibulospinal reflex brings about postural changes to compensate for tilts and movements of the body through vestibulospinal tract projections to antigravity muscles at all levels of the spinal cord. The vestibulo-ocular reflex stabilizes vision during head and body movements through projections from the vestibular nuclei to the nuclei that innervate extraocular muscles.

### Sensory Organization for Balance Control

Vestibular, visual, and somatosensory inputs are normally combined seamlessly to produce our sense of orientation and movement.[88] Incoming sensory information is integrated and processed in the cerebellum, basal ganglia, and supplementary motor area.[123] Somatosensory information has the fastest processing time for rapid responses, followed by visual and vestibular inputs.[123] When sensory inputs from one system are inaccurate owing to environmental conditions or injuries that decrease the information-processing rate, the CNS must suppress the inaccurate input and select and combine the appropriate sensory inputs from the other two systems. This adaptive process is called *sensory organization.* Most individuals can compensate well if one of the three systems is impaired; therefore, this concept is the basis for many treatment programs.

### Types of Balance Control

Functional tasks require different types of balance control, including (1) *static balance control* to maintain a stable antigravity position while at rest such as when standing and sitting; (2) *dynamic balance control* to stabilize the body when the support surface is moving or when the body is moving on a stable surface such as sit-to-stand transfers or walking; and (3) *automatic postural reactions* to maintain balance in response to unexpected external perturbations, such as standing on a bus that suddenly accelerates forward.

*Feedforward,* or *open loop motor control,* is utilized for movements that occur too fast to rely on sensory feedback (e.g., reactive responses) or for anticipatory aspects of postural control. *Anticipatory control* involves activation of postural muscles in advance of performing skilled movements, such as activation of posterior leg and back extensor muscles prior to a person pulling on a handle when standing[26] or planning how to navigate to avoid obstacles in the environment. *Closed loop control* is utilized for precision movements that require sensory feedback (e.g., maintaining balance while sitting on a ball or standing on a balance beam).

## Motor Strategies for Balance Control

To maintain balance, the body must continually adjust its position in space to keep the COM of an individual over

---

| BOX 8.1 | Factors Influencing Selection of Balance Strategies |
| --- | --- |

- Speed and intensity of the displacing forces
- Characteristics of the support surface
- Magnitude of the displacement of the center of mass
- Subject's awareness of the disturbance
- Subject's posture at the time of perturbation
- Subject's prior experiences

---

the BOS or to bring the COM back to that position after a perturbation. Horak and Nashner[45] described three primary movement strategies used by healthy adults to recover balance in response to sudden perturbations of the supporting surface (i.e., brief anterior or posterior platform displacements) called ankle, hip, and stepping strategies (Fig. 8.3). Factors that determine which strategy most effectively addresses a balance disturbance are identified in Box 8.1. Results of research examining the patterns of muscle activity underlying these movement strategies suggest that preprogrammed muscle synergies comprise the fundamental movement unit used to restore balance.[45,78,83] A synergy is a functional coupling of groups of muscles so they must act together as a unit; this organization greatly simplifies the control demands of the CNS.

The CNS uses three movement systems to regain balance after the body is perturbed: reflex, automatic, and voluntary systems. Table 8.1 summarizes the key characteristics of reflexes, automatic postural responses, and voluntary movements.[80] *"Stretch" reflexes* mediated by the spinal cord comprise the first response to external perturbations. They have the shortest latencies (< 70 ms), are independ-

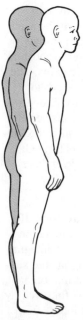
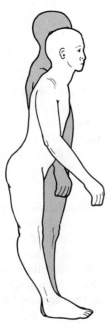
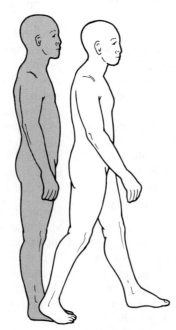

Ankle strategy          Hip strategy          Stepping strategy

FIGURE 8.3 Ankle, hip, and stepping strategies used by adults to control body sway.

| TABLE 8.1 | Characteristics of the Three Movement Systems for Balance Control Following Perturbations | | |
|---|---|---|---|
| Characteristic | Reflex | Automatic | Voluntary |
| Mediating pathway | Spinal cord | Brain stem/subcortical | Cortical |
| Mode of activation | External stimulus | External stimulus | External stimulus or self-stimulus |
| Comparative latency of response | Fastest | Intermediate | Slowest |
| Response | Localized to point of stimulus and highly stereotyped | Coordinated among leg and trunk muscles; stereotypical but adaptable | Coordinated and highly variable |
| Role in balance | Muscle force regulation | Resist disturbances | Generate purposeful movements |
| Factors modifying the response | Musculoskeletal or neurological abnormalities | Musculoskeletal or neurological abnormalities; configuration of support; prior experience | Musculoskeletal or neurological abnormalities; conscious effort; prior experience; task complexity |

Adapted from Nashner.[80]

ent of task demands, and produce stereotyped muscle contractions in response to sensory inputs. *Voluntary responses* have the longest latencies (> 150 ms), are dependent on task parameters, and produce highly variable motor outputs (e.g., reach for a nearby stable support surface or walk away from a destabilizing condition). *Automatic postural reactions* have intermediate latencies (80 to 120 ms) and are the first responses that effectively prevent falls. They produce quick, relatively invariant movements among individuals (similar to reflexes), but they require coordination of responses among body regions and are modifiable depending on the demands of the task (similar to voluntary responses). The reflex, automatic, and voluntary movement systems interact to ensure that the response matches the postural challenge.

### Ankle Strategy (Anteroposterior Plane)

In quiet stance and during small perturbations (i.e., slow-speed perturbations usually occurring on a large, firm surface), movements at the ankle act to restore a person's COM to a stable position. For small external perturbations that cause loss of balance in a forward direction (i.e., platform displacements in a backward direction), muscle activation usually proceeds in a distal to proximal sequence: gastrocnemius activity beginning about 90 to 100 ms after perturbation onset, followed by the hamstrings 20 to 30 ms later, and finally paraspinal muscle activation.[79,80] In response to backward instability, muscle activity begins in the anterior tibialis, followed by the quadriceps and abdominal muscles.

### Weight-Shift Strategy (Lateral Plane)

The movement strategy utilized to control mediolateral perturbations involves shifting the body weight laterally from one leg to the other. The hips are the key control

points of the weight-shift strategy. They move the COM in a lateral plane primarily through activation of hip abductor and adductor muscles, with some contribution from ankle invertors and evertors.[80]

### Suspension Strategy

The suspension strategy is observed during balance tasks when a person quickly lowers his or her body COM by flexing the knees, causing associated flexion of the ankles and hips.[81] The suspension strategy can be combined with the ankle or the weight-shift strategy to enhance the effectiveness of a balance movement.[81]

### Hip Strategy

For rapid and/or large external perturbations or for movements executed with the COG near the limits of stability, a hip strategy is employed.[80] The hip strategy uses rapid hip flexion or extension to move the COM within the BOS.[124] As the trunk rapidly rotates in one direction, horizontal (shear) forces are generated against the support surface in the opposite direction that move the COM in the opposite direction as the trunk.[81] The muscle activity associated with the hip strategy has been studied by having a person stand crosswise on a narrow balance beam while the support surface suddenly moves backward (i.e., person sways forward) or forward (i.e., person sways backward).[45] In response to a forward body sway, muscles are typically activated in a proximal to distal sequence: Abdominals beginning about 90 to 100 ms after perturbation onset followed by activation of the quadriceps. Backward body sway results in activation first of the paraspinals followed by the hamstrings. A person cannot use the hip strategy to restore balance while walking on slippery surfaces because the large horizontal forces generated cause the feet to slip.

## Stepping Strategy

If a large force displaces the COM beyond the limits of stability, a forward or backward step is used to enlarge the BOS and regain balance control. The uncoordinated step that follows a stumble on uneven ground is an example of a stepping strategy.

## Combined Strategies

Research has shown that movement response patterns to postural perturbations are more complex and variable than originally described by Nashner.[56] Most healthy individuals use combinations of strategies to maintain balance depending on the control demands. Balance control requirements vary depending on the task and the environment. For example, standing on a bus that is moving has higher control demands than standing on a fixed surface. Therefore, it is important during treatment of balance disorders to vary the task and environment so the person develops movement strategies for different situations.

# Balance Control Under Varying Conditions

## Balance During Stance

In quiet stance the body sways like an inverted pendulum about the ankle joint.[124] The balance goal is to keep the body's COM safely within the BOS. To accomplish this goal, an ankle strategy is utilized in which ankle muscles (i.e., ankle plantarflexors/dorsiflexors, invertors/evertors) are automatically and selectively activated to counteract body sway in different directions. Other muscles that are tonically active during quiet stance to maintain an erect posture are the gluteus medius and tensor fasciae latae, the iliopsoas to prevent hyperextension of the hip, and the thoracic paraspinals (with some intermittent abdominal activation).[9] Body alignment contributes to stability in quiet stance. Standing with the body in optimal body alignment allows the body to maintain balance with the least amount of muscle energy expenditure.[105]

## Balance with Perturbed Standing

Perturbations to balance in standing can be either internal (i.e., voluntary movement of the body) or external (i.e., forces applied to the body). Both types of perturbations involve activation of muscle synergies, but the response timing is proactive (i.e., anticipatory) for internally generated perturbations and reactive for externally generated perturbations.[124] Moving platform experiments have provided much information about the motor strategies (i.e., ankle, hip, and stepping strategies) and associated muscle activation patterns that result when a person is standing on a surface that unexpectedly translates or tilts.[57,77,79,80] With repetition of a platform perturbation, learning adaptation occurs that is characterized by a significant reduction in the reactive response.[70,77] For example, Nashner[77] found that upward rotation of a platform initially elicited reflex contractions of the gastrocnemius muscles of subjects, giving them the false impression that their bodies were falling forward; with repeated tilts the gastrocnemius response diminished, and by the fourth repetition it was completely absent.

Thus, prior experience and feedforward anticipatory control have an important influence on balance responses.

## Balance During Whole-Body Lifting

One of the most common ways that balance is challenged during everyday life is when lifting boxes or other large objects that are resting on the floor or at a level that is low relative to the person's COM (Fig. 8.4). Loss of balance during lifting may result in a fall, slip, or back injury.[6,94,103]

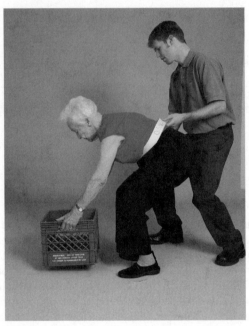

FIGURE 8.4 Balance during forward lifting with knees flexed.

During lifting the movement of the body toward the load disturbs the position of the COM. When a load is lifted in front of the body, the COM is shifted forward during flexion of the trunk and legs, which is an internal disturbance to balance. The COM is further displaced forward when the load is added to the hands, creating an external disturbance to balance. In this case, anticipatory postural adjustments are needed to match whole-body backward momentum (horizontal linear and angular) to the displacement of the body and magnitude of the expected load.[25,40,41] The CNS estimates the amount of momentum necessary for lifting the load based on previous experience with the load or other objects of similar physical properties (e.g., size, weight, and density).[41] The generation of backward horizontal linear momentum serves to keep the COM of the body within the base of support. The generation of angular momentum is essential for movement of the person with the load toward the upright posture.

The amount of whole-body momentum and the lifting force generated is scaled to the anticipated weight of the load.[41] When a heavy load is expected, sufficient levels of backward horizontal and angular momentum are needed to counteract the additional load, which tends to pull and rotate the body COM forward. Subtle differences in lifting

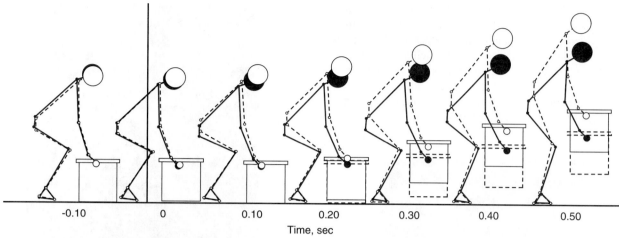

-0.10          0          0.10          0.20          0.30          0.40          0.50

Time, sec

FIGURE 8.5 Postural adjustments for lifting a heavy versus a light load. When subjects approach a load (indicated by the vertical bar at time 0), early in the lift subtle differences in the anticipatory postural adjustments are evident. When a heavy load is expected (dark circles) there is greater flexion of the trunk, hips, and knees compared to when a light load is expected (light circles). *(Adapted from Heiss et al.[41])*

posture, which reflect the underlying differences in momentum, occur when subjects lift a light load versus a heavy load (Fig. 8.5). Subjects tend to flex their hips and knees more and shift their weight back when lifting a heavy load (dark circles) than when lifting a light load (light circles).

Loss of balance during lifting can occur when subjects overestimate or underestimate the weight of the load.[40] When the load weight is overestimated, too much momentum is generated and the body tends to topple backward. Most subjects compensate for this loss of balance by taking a step backward. When the load weight is underestimated, too little momentum is generated and the body tends to topple forward, resulting in the load quickly coming back to the ground.

The lifting style does appear to affect the challenges to balance. Keeping the knees more extended during lifting (Fig. 8.6) reduces the risk of balance loss, especially when the quadriceps are weak. Research comparing lifting styles has found that loss of balance was more common when subjects used a style of lifting where the knees were more flexed compared to when the knees were straighter.[22,24,40,113]

Clinicians frequently instruct patients to use the leg lifting style, with the knees bent and the trunk erect, when lifting loads (Fig. 8.7).[73,108] This recommendation is based on the assumption that leg lifting imposes lower compression loads on the spine than other styles of lifting, such as the stoop lift, with the knees straight and the trunk flexed.[62] This assumption is likely true when the load to be lifted can be placed between the feet (Figs. 8.7 and 8.8). However, van Dieen and colleagues[116] found little evidence in the biomechanical literature to support that leg lifting generally results in lower loads on the spine than back lifting. Recent research, using sophisticated biomechanical models, indicates that leg lifting results in higher compression forces on the spine compared to back lifting when the load is not positioned between the legs.[19,28,58,92] Although researchers have consistently found that bending moments

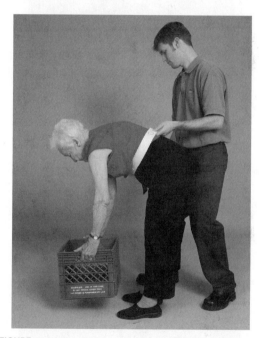

FIGURE 8.6 Balance during forward lifting with knees extended.

and fascial strain are substantially greater with the back lift compared to the squat lift,[5,28,29] the magnitude of the bending moments on the spine appear to be well below the threshold for injury.[1,28,115]

Based on the current literature, it appears that if the objective of training for lifting is to reduce the load on the lumbar spine, other factors that have a more substantial effect on reducing the load on the lumbar spine should be emphasized over the selection of a lifting style, especially when placing the load between the legs is not feasible. These factors include maintaining a neutral spine, slowing the lifting speed, optimizing the horizontal and vertical position of the load, avoiding asymmetrical lifts (because of the increased lateral and twisting moments on the spine) (Fig. 8.9), and reducing the load weight.[115] If maintaining balance is a concern, especially in the elderly, lifting styles in which the knees are more extended, such as with the semi-squat and stoop lift, are probably safer. In younger individuals with strong quadriceps, the straddle lift with one leg in front of the other to widen the base of support would reduce the risk of balance loss.

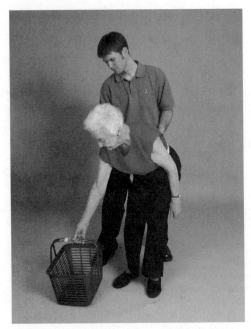

FIGURE 8.9 Side lift with the right trunk in lateral flexion and rotation results in high loads on the lumbar spine and should be avoided.

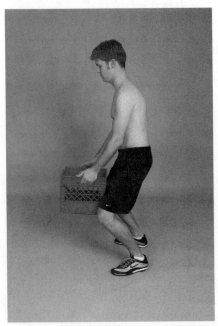

FIGURE 8.7 Squat lift with trunk erect and object placed between the feet.

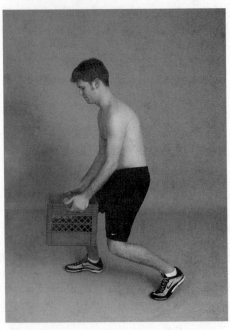

FIGURE 8.8 Straddle lift with trunk erect and object placed between the feet.

## Balance in Unperturbed Human Gait

During walking the COM is always outside the BOS except during the short double support period.[124] Therefore, the balance goal is to move the body outside the BOS by letting the body fall forward and yet prevent a fall. To accomplish this goal, a person must be able to maintain balance and posture of the upper body (i.e., head, arms, trunk) and vertical alignment of the body against gravity. Trunk and hip muscles (flexors/extensors in the sagittal plane; abductors/adductors in the frontal plane) keep the upper body balanced, and extensor muscles of the lower extremities prevent vertical collapse.[124,125] The ankle muscles control anterior/posterior or medial/lateral acceleration of the body's COG but are not able to prevent falls.[124] Fine motor control of the foot during the swing phase involving anticipatory activation of the ankle dorsiflexors ensures minimum toe clearance (0.55 cm) to prevent trips.[90]

# ⬤ IMPAIRED BALANCE

Impaired balance can be caused by injury or disease to any structures involved in the three stages of information processing (i.e., sensory input, sensorimotor integration, motor output generation).

## Sensory Input Impairments

Proprioceptive deficits have been implicated as contributing to balance impairments following lower extremity and trunk injuries or pathologies. Decreased joint position sense has been reported in individuals with recurrent ankle sprains,[13,33,34,37] knee ligamentous injuries,[7,89,100] degenerative joint disease,[8] and low back pain.[16,35,61] These same conditions have been associated with increased postural sway compared to that of controls.[2,18,27,33,34,61,74,122] It is unclear whether decreased joint position sense is due to changes in joint receptors or in muscle receptors.

Somatosensory, visual, or vestibular deficits may impair balance and mobility. Reduced somatosensation in the lower extremities caused by peripheral polyneuropathies in the aged and in individuals with diabetes are associated with balance deficits[95,97,106,114] and an increased risk for falls.[50,96] These individuals tend to rely more heavily on a hip strategy to maintain balance than do those without somatosensory deficits.[46] Visual loss or specific deficits in acuity, contrast sensitivity, peripheral field vision, and depth perception caused by disease, trauma, or aging can impair balance and lead to falls.[21,52] Individuals with damage to the vestibular system due to viral infections, traumatic brain injury (TBI), or aging may experience vertigo (a feeling of spinning) and postural instability. Black et al.[11] found that patients with severe bilateral loss of vestibular function are unable to use hip strategies even when standing crosswise on a narrow beam, although ankle strategies are unaffected.

## Sensorimotor Integration

Damage to the basal ganglia, cerebellum, or supplementary motor area impair processing of incoming sensory information, resulting in difficulty adapting sensory information in response to environmental changes and in disruption of anticipatory and reactive postural adjustments.[47,80,105] When stance is perturbed by platform translations, patients with Parkinson's disease tend to have a smaller than normal amplitude of movement due to co-activation of muscles on both sides of the body, while patients with cerebellar lesions typically demonstrate larger response amplitudes.[105]

Sensory organization problems that manifest as overreliance on one particular sense for balance control or a more generalized inability to select an appropriate sense for balance control when one or more senses give inaccurate information have been demonstrated in patients with a wide variety of neurological conditions.[105] Individuals who rely heavily on visual inputs (visually dependent) or somatosensory inputs (surface dependent) become unstable or fall under conditions where the preferred sense is either absent or inaccurate, whereas those with generalized adaptation problems are unstable in any condition in which a sensory input is not accurate.

## Biomechanical and Motor Output Deficits

Deficits in the motor components of balance control can be caused by musculoskeletal (i.e., poor posture, joint ROM limitations, decreased muscle performance) and/or neuromuscular system (i.e., impaired motor coordination, pain)

impairments. Postural malalignment, such as the typical thoracic kyphosis of the elderly, that shifts the COM away from the center of the BOS increases a person's chance of exceeding his or her limits of stability.[80] Because the legs operate as closed chains, impaired ROM or muscle strength at one joint can alter posture and balance movements throughout the entire limb. For example, restriction of ankle motion by contractures or wearing ankle-foot orthoses and/or ankle dorsiflexor weakness eliminates the use of an ankle strategy, resulting in increased use of hip and trunk muscles for balance control.[17,102] In individuals with neurological conditions (e.g., stroke, traumatic brain injury, Parkinson's disease), failure to generate adequate muscle forces due to abnormal tone, or impaired coordination of motor strategies may limit the person's ability to recruit muscles required for balance.[105] Pain can alter movements, reduce a person's normal stability limits, and if persistent produce secondary strength and mobility impairments.

## Deficits with Aging

Falls are common and are a major cause of morbidity, mortality, reduced functioning, and premature nursing home admissions in persons over age 65.[21,30,84,99,101] The most common risk factors associated with falls in the elderly are listed in Box 8.2. Most falls by the elderly are likely due to complex interactions between multiple risk factors. Clinicians are encouraged to follow published guidelines for the prevention of falls by older persons when prescribing fall prevention interventions.[3]

Declines in all sensory systems (somatosensory, vision, vestibular) and all three stages of information processing (i.e., sensory processing, sensorimotor integration, motor output) are found with aging.[64,105] In comparison to young adults, older adults have more difficulty maintaining balance when sensory inputs from more than one system are greatly reduced, particularly when they must rely solely on vestibular inputs for balance control.[110,127] Studies of

---

**BOX 8.2   Most Common Risk Factors for Falls Among the Elderly**

- Muscle weakness
- History of falls
- Gait deficit
- Balance deficit
- Use of assistive device
- Visual deficit
- Arthritis
- Impaired activities of daily living
- Depression
- Cognitive impairment
- Age > 80 years

From AGS Panel on Fall Prevention, 2001.[3]

response patterns to platform perturbations in older adults have demonstrated the following motor strategy changes compared to those of young adults.

- Slower-onset latencies[107,127]
- More frequent use of a hip strategy for balance control[48]
- Limitations in the ability to maintain balance when challenged with perturbations of increasing magnitude and velocity[65]

Impaired anticipatory postural adjustments prior to making voluntary movements have been demonstrated in older individuals and may explain the high incidence of falls during activities such as walking, lifting, and carrying objects.[32,51] Two reliable, valid, and sensitive tools for assessing fall risk in the elderly are the Tinetti Performance-Oriented Mobility Assessment (Tinetti Mobility Test [111]) and the Berg Balance Scale.[10]

Elderly individuals who have experienced one or more falls may develop fear of falling, which leads to a loss of confidence in a person's ability to perform routine tasks, restricted activity, social isolation, functional decline, depression, and decreased quality of life.[21,59] The fear of falling arises more often from a person's fear of institutionalization than a fear of injury.[49] Individuals with fear of falling demonstrate perceived stability limits that are reduced from their actual stability limits, and gait changes including decreased stride length, reduced speed, increased stride width, and increased double-support time.[20,69] It is important that clinicians screen patients for fear of falling with instruments such as the Activities Specific Balance Confidence (ABC) Scale[93] or the Falls Efficacy Scale[112] so evidence-based interventions that reduce fear of falling and promote physical, social, and functional activity are implemented.[15,109,120]

## Deficits from Medications

There is an increased risk of falling among older individuals who take four or more medications and among those taking certain medications (i.e., hypnotics, sedatives, tricyclic antidepressants, tranquilizers, antihypertensive drugs) due to dizziness or other side effects.[3,21] Individuals who have fallen should have their medications reviewed and altered or stopped as appropriate to prevent future falls.

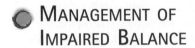

# MANAGEMENT OF IMPAIRED BALANCE

## Examination and Evaluation of Impaired Balance

The key elements of a comprehensive evaluation of individuals with balance problems include the following.

- A thorough history of falls (whether onset of falls is sudden versus gradual; the frequency and direction of falls; the environmental conditions, activities, and presence of dizziness, vertigo, or lightheadedness at time of the fall; current and past medications; presence of fear of falling)
- Assessments to identify sensory input (proprioceptive, visual, vestibular), sensory processing (sensorimotor integration, anticipatory and reactive balance control), and biomechanical and motor (postural alignment, muscle strength and endurance, joint ROM and flexibility, motor coordination, pain) impairments contributing to balance deficits
- Tests and observations to determine the impact of balance control system deficits on functional performance
- Environmental assessments to determine fall risk hazards in a person's home.[21]

Commonly used tests and measures for each of the three categories of balance assessments described in the *Guide to Physical Therapist Practice*[4] are presented in Table 8.2. Clinicians should carefully select a variety of tests and measures that assess all of the various types of balance control.

| TABLE 8.2 | Balance Assessments and Interventions | |
|---|---|---|
| **Category of Assessment** | **Clinical Tests/Measures** | **Interventions if Deficits Present** |
| **I. Balance*** | | |
| Static | Observations of patient maintaining different postures; Single-Leg Stance Test[119]; Romberg Test[85]; Stork Stand Test[53] | Vary postures<br>Vary support surface<br>Incorporate external loads |
| Dynamic | Observations of patient standing or sitting on unstable surface; Tinetti Performance-Oriented Mobility Assessment (POMA)[111]; Timed Up and Go Test (TUG)[91]; Berg Balance Scale[10]; Gait Abnormality Rating Scale (GARS)[118]; Dynamic Gait Index[105] | Moving support surfaces<br>Move head, trunk, arms, legs<br>Transitional and locomotor activities |

*(table continued on page 261)*

| Category of Assessment | Clinical Tests/Measures | Interventions if Deficits Present |
|---|---|---|
| Anticipatory (feedforward) | Observations of patient catching ball, opening doors, lifting objects of different weights; Functional Reach Test[31]; Multidirectional Reach Test[86] | Reaching<br>Catching<br>Kicking<br>Lifting<br>Obstacle course |
| Reactive (feedback) | Observation of patient's responses to pushes (small or large, slow or rapid, anticipated and unanticipated); Pull Test[76]; Backward Release[98]; Postural Stress Test[126] | Standing sway<br>Ankle strategy<br>Hip strategy<br>Stepping strategy<br>Perturbations |
| Sensory organization | Clinical Test of Sensory Integration on Balance Test (CTSIB) also called the "Foam and Dome" Test[104] | Reduce visual inputs<br>Reduce somatosensory cues |
| II. Balance during functional activities* | Physical Performance Test[117]; Barthel ADL Index[68]; Katz ADL Index[54]; Functional Independence Measure (FIM)[55]; Lawton Instrumental Activities of Daily Living Scale[60]; Progressive Mobility Skills Assessment Task[21] | Functional activities<br>Dual or multitask activities |
| III. Safety during gait, locomotion, or balance* | Observations; home assessments | Balance within stability limits; Environmental modifications; Assistive devices; External support |

* With or without the use of assistive, adaptive, orthotic, protective, supportive, or prosthetic devices or equipment.[4]

## Balance Training

There are many factors to consider when developing an intervention program for balance impairments. Most balance intervention programs require a multisystems approach. For example, an individual who has experienced prolonged bed rest or inactivity following an illness may require a program that includes stretching the lower extremities and trunk to improve postural alignment and mobility; strengthening exercises to improve motor performance; and dynamic, functional balance activities to improve the ability to perform daily activities safely. The following elaborates on the interventions suggested in Table 8.2, which are based on identified deficits in static, dynamic, anticipatory, and reactive control as well as problems involving sensory organization, function, and safety. For specific procedures to address musculoskeletal problems such as strength, joint mobility, flexibility, or posture refer to the chapters addressing these interventions or to chapters focused on specific regions of the body.

Because balance training often involves activities that challenge the patient's limits of stability, it is important that the therapist takes steps to ensure the patient's safety. Box 8.3 lists safety measures that should be considered and utilized to prevent falls and injuries during therapy.

### Static Balance Control
Activities to promote static balance control include having the patient maintain sitting, half-kneeling, tall kneeling,

and standing postures on a firm surface. More challenging activities include practice in the tandem and single-leg stance (Fig. 8.10), lunge, and squat positions. Progress these activities by working on soft surfaces (e.g., foam, sand, grass), narrowing the base of support, moving the arms, or closing the eyes. Provide resistance via handheld

---

**BOX 8.3  Safety During Balance Exercises**

1. Use a gait belt any time the patient practices exercises or activities that challenge or destabilize balance.
2. Stand slightly behind and to the side of the patient with one arm holding or near the gait belt and the other arm on or near the top of the shoulder (on the trunk, not the arm).
3. Perform exercises near a railing or in parallel bars to allow patient to grab when necessary.
4. Do not perform exercises near sharp edges of equipment or objects.
5. Have one person in front and one behind when working with patients at high risk of falling or during activities that pose a high risk of injury.
6. Check equipment to ensure that it is operating correctly.
7. Guard patient when getting on and off equipment (such as treadmills and stationary bikes).
8. Ensure that the floor is clean and free of debris.

weights or elastic resistance (Figs. 8.11 and 8.12). Add a secondary task (i.e., catching a ball or mental calculations) to further increase the level of difficulty (Fig. 8.13).

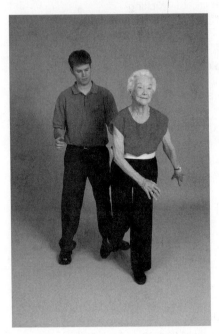

FIGURE 8.10 Balance during single leg stance.

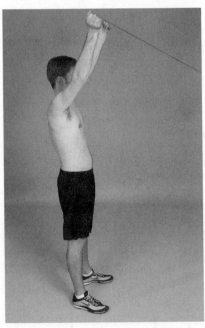

FIGURE 8.11 Balance while standing with resistance provided to the arms via elastic resistance.

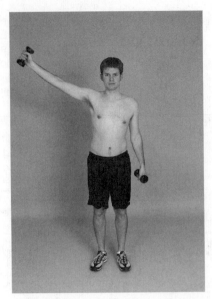

FIGURE 8.12 Balance while standing with arm abducting and holding a weight.

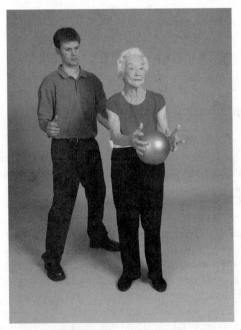

FIGURE 8.13 Balance while standing and catching a ball.

## Dynamic Balance Control

To promote dynamic balance control, interventions may involve the following.

- Have the patient maintain equal weight distribution and upright trunk postural alignment while on moving surfaces, such as sitting on a therapeutic ball, standing on wobble boards (Fig. 8.14), or bouncing on a mini-trampoline.

- Vary the position of the arms from out to the side to above the head (Fig. 8.16).

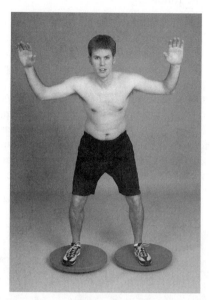

FIGURE 8.16  Balance while standing on wobble boards with arms above the head.

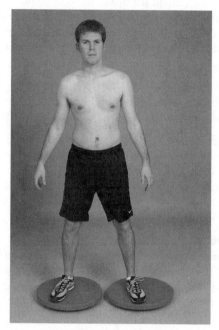

FIGURE 8.14  Balance while standing on wobble boards.

- Practice stepping exercises starting with small steps, then mini-lunges, to full lunges.
- Progress the exercise program to include hopping, skipping, rope jumping, and hopping down from small stool while maintaining balance.
- Have the patient perform arm and leg exercises while standing with normal stance, tandem stance, and single-leg stance (Fig. 8.17).

- Progress the activities by superimposing movements such as shifting the body weight, rotating the trunk, moving the head or arms (Fig. 8.15).

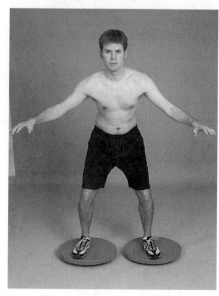

FIGURE 8.15  Balance while standing on wobble boards with arm movements.

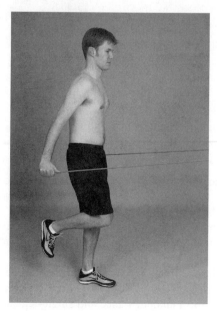

FIGURE 8.17  One-legged stance with resisted shoulder extension using elastic resistance.

## Anticipatory Balance Control

Have the patient practice anticipatory balance control by performing the following.

- Reach in all directions to touch or grasp objects, catching a ball, or kicking a ball.
- Use different postures for variation (e.g., sitting, standing, kneeling) and throwing or rolling the ball at different speeds and heights (Fig. 8.18).
- Use functional tasks that involve multiple parts of the body to increase the challenge to anticipatory postural control by having the patient lift objects of varying weight in different postures at varying speeds, open and close doors with different handles and heaviness, or maneuver through an obstacle course.

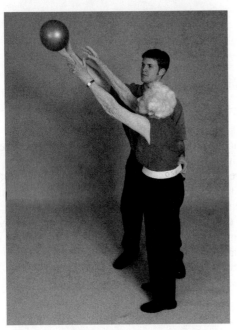

FIGURE 8.18 Balance when standing while reaching and catching the ball overhead.

## Reactive Balance Control

Have the patient train reactive balance control with the following activities.

- Have the patient work to gradually increase the amount of sway when standing in different directions while on a firm stable surface.
- To emphasize training of the *ankle strategy*, have the patient practice while standing on one leg with the trunk erect.
- To emphasize training of the *hip strategy*, have the patient walk on balance beams or lines drawn on the floor; perform tandem stance and single-leg stance with trunk bending; stand on a mini-trampoline, rocker balance, or sliding board.

- To emphasize the *stepping strategy*, have the patient practice stepping up onto a stool or stepping with legs crossed in front or behind other leg (e.g., weaving or braiding).
- To increase the challenge during these activities, add anticipated and unanticipated external forces. For example, have the patient lift boxes that are identical in appearance but of different weights; throw and catch balls of different weights and sizes; or while on a treadmill, suddenly stop/start the belt or increase/decrease the speed.

## Sensory Organization

Many of the activities previously described can be utilized while varying the reliance on specific sensory systems.

- To reduce or destabilize the *visual inputs*, have the patient close the eyes, wear prism glasses, or move the eyes and head together during the balance activity.
- To decrease reliance on *somatosensory cues*, patients can narrow the BOS, stand on foam, or stand on an incline board.

## Balance During Functional Activities

The therapist should focus on activities similar to the functional limitations identified in the evaluation. For example, if reaching is limited, the patient should work on activities such as reaching for a glass in a cupboard, reaching behind (as putting arm in a sleeve), or catching a ball off center. Having the patient perform two or more tasks simultaneously increases the level of task complexity. Practicing recreational activities the patient enjoys, such as golf, increases motivation for practice while challenging balance control (Fig. 8.19).

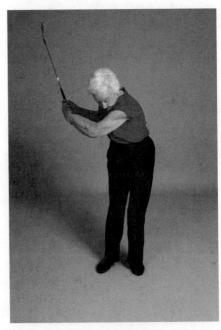

FIGURE 8.19 Functional balance during a golf swing.

## Safety During Gait, Locomotion, or Balance

To emphasize safety, the therapist should have the patient practice postural sway activities within the person's actual stability limits and progress dynamic activities with emphasis on promoting function. If balance deficits cannot be changed, environmental modifications, assistive devices, and increased family or external support may be required to ensure safety.

## Health and Environmental Factors

In addition to exercise and balance training activities, clinicians should address several other factors affecting balance to reduce the risk of falls.[67]

### Low Vision

To address low vision issues, encourage regular eye examinations with adjustments to lens prescriptions and cataract surgery, if necessary. Wearing a hat and sunglasses in bright sunlight, taking extra precautions when it is dark, and making sure lights are on when walking about the house at night are other recommendations. Advise patients to avoid using bifocal glasses when walking because single lens glasses are safest for improving depth perception and contrast sensitivity, especially on stairs.[66]

### Sensory Loss

For individuals with sensory loss in the legs, caution them to take extra care when walking on soft carpet or uneven ground and use a cane or other device if necessary. Recommend that they wear firm rubber shoes with low heels. Regular medical examinations should be encouraged to ensure that patients' blood glucose levels and other factors (i.e., cholesterol, lipids) are under control to minimize damage to sensory nerves from diseases such as diabetes and peripheral vascular disease. Advise patients to seek medical attention if they experience any symptoms of dizziness.

### Medications

Patients should be educated about the influence of certain medications, such as sedatives and antidepressants, on their risk of falling. For example, if such medications are used at night as a sleep aid, individuals should take extra precautions when getting up to use the bathroom.

## Evidence–Based Balance Exercise Programs

Mounting evidence from randomized clinical trials indicates that therapeutic exercise is an effective tool in the prevention of falls, especially if it is incorporated with a comprehensive strategy targeting health, environmental, and behavioral risk factors that contribute to falls.[36,72]

### Low Intensity Exercise Program for Elderly Who Have Low Physical Functioning

Morgan and colleagues[75] studied the effectiveness of a low intensity exercise program for elderly individuals who had recently experienced a brief period of bed rest due to ill-

---

### BOX 8.4 — Exercises for Elderly with Low Physical Functioning[75]

**Exercises While Sitting in a Chair**

**Set 1 (for the lower extremities)**
Extend leg up then back down
Raise up and down on toes then heels
March in place
Bring leg out to the side then back to the middle
Bring leg back toward the chair then forward again

**Set 2 (for the upper extremities)**
Bend arms towards shoulders then back down again
Push arms out away from chest then back again
Push arms up from shoulders then back down again
Raise shoulders up toward ears then back down again
Roll shoulders forward then backward
Raise arm to shoulder level and extend forearm upward toward ceiling then back down again
Bring elbows in then back out from chest

**Standing Exercises for Balance**
Bring leg in toward the middle then back out again
Rise up and down on heels and then toes
March in place
Keeping the trunk and hip straight, bend leg toward buttocks then back down
Squat down by bending at the knees and keeping back straight
Kick leg straight back behind body while not bending the knee
Kick leg in front of body while not bending the knee
Lunge leg out to the side then back toward the middle again
Lunge leg in back of the body then toward the front again
Practice standing on one leg, then the other, without holding onto the counter

---

ness. The program was found to be effective for reducing the risk of falls for up to 1 year after the intervention in individuals who scored less than 55 on the Physical Functioning component of the Short Form-36 (SF-36). The program did not reduce the fall risk in those who were more active (> 55 on the Physical Functioning scale). The participants attended exercise sessions in groups of five. The sessions lasted approximately 45 minutes, including rest and a cool-down period, and were attended three times per week for 8 weeks. The exercises were performed under the direction of a physical therapist with a physical therapist assistant. The program developed by Morgan and colleagues is provided in Box 8.4.

### Exercise Program for Elderly with Balance Deficits One Year After Stroke

Marigold and colleagues[71] investigated the effects of balance training on fall risk behavior in ambulatory, community-residing individuals who were at least 1 year

<br>

**BOX 8.5   Exercise Program for Elderly with Balance Deficits One Year After Stroke[71]**

Warm-up period consisting of 5 minutes of walking and light stretching

**Practice of Standing Postures**
Feet apart
Tandem
One-foot stance
Weight shifting

**Practice of Walking**
Variation in step length
Variation in speed
Tandem walking
Figure-of-eight walking
Stepping up and over low risers
Side stepping
Crossover stepping
Stepping over obstacles

**Perturbation Training**
Therapist pushes patient (reactions)
Patient pushes therapist (anticipatory)

**Other Exercises**
Sit-to-stand practice
Raising the knee rapidly while standing

**Level of challenge increased in above activities with**
Eyes closed
Foam surface under base of support

Cool-down period consisting of 5 minutes of walking and light stretching

---

poststroke. The 1-hour exercise sessions were performed in a group (ratio of instructor to participant was 1:3) at a community center three times per week for 10 weeks. The exercise program implemented by Marigold and colleagues,[71] provided in Box 8.5, led to improved postural reaction times and fewer falls in response to translations from a platform system.

### Program Incorporating Strengthening, Walking, and Functional Activities

Means and colleagues[72] investigated the effects of a program designed to improve balance in community-residing elders with or without a history of falls. The program incorporated activities such as stretching, strengthening, coordination exercises, body mechanics, balance training, survival training maneuvers, and walking for endurance. The participants attended 90-minute exercise sessions three times per week in groups of six to eight. The exercises were performed under the direction of a physical therapist. Initially, participants were encouraged to exercise at a "fairly light" level (equal to 11 on the 6- to 20-point Borg perceived exertion scale[12]). After the first week, participants were encouraged to exercise at a level of intensity

that was "somewhat hard" (equal to 13 on the Borg scale). Box 8.6 provides general guidelines for exercise repetitions, duration of endurance walking, and progression of the program.[72] The participants who attended this 6-week comprehensive exercise program showed a reduction in the time to complete an obstacle course (e.g., walking, climbing stairs, opening doors, getting up from a chair, stepping over objects) and in the number of fall and fall-related injuries for up to 6 months after participation.

### Multisystem Program Incorporating a Circuit of Activities to address Balance Impairments and Function

Nitz and Choy[87] investigated the efficacy of a balance training program that integrated individual and group exercises targeting strength, coordination, sensory systems (vision, perception, vestibular), cognition, reaction time, and static and dynamic stability. Community-residing elderly individuals with a recent history of falls were randomly assigned to two groups. One group participated in the balance training program that addressed multisystem activities. Table 8.3 provides the details of the balance exercise program, consisting of circuit training and group activities, from Nitz and Choy.[87] The control group participated in a more traditional group exercise program (e.g., see the program in Table 8.3). Participants in both groups received an education booklet on how to prevent falls in the home and attended a 1-hour exercise session once a week for 10 weeks. The exercises were led by a physical therapist assisted by one or two students when small group activities (six participants per group) were performed. After the intervention, both groups reported a reduction in the number of falls. The reduction in falls was greater in the group that performed the circuit training program; they also showed greater improvements in functional tests of the ability to perform activities of daily living. Although the circuit training program devised by Nitz and Choy[87] clearly incorporates many important activities to address multiple systems affecting balance, the results should be interpreted with caution because there was a small sample size and high proportion of dropouts throughout the study.

### Tai Chi for Balance Training

Tai Chi has become a popular form of exercise for balance training. Tai Chi is a traditional Chinese exercise program consisting of a sequence of whole-body movements that are performed in a slow, relaxed manner with an emphasis on awareness of posture alignment and synchronized breathing. Participants learn to control the displacement of the body COM while standing and increase their lower extremity strength and flexibility during the regimens of physical movement.[23] Some of the characteristics of Tai Chi exercise and the therapeutic rationale for why Tai Chi may affect posture and balance include the following.[121] The slow, continuous, even rhythm of the movements facilitates sensorimotor integration and awareness of the external environment (see Fig. 8.2). The emphasis on maintaining a vertical posture enhances postural alignment and perception

**BOX 8.6   Balance Exercise Program Incorporating Strengthening, Walking, and Functional Activities[72]**

**Week 1**
**Flexibility exercises** (5 repetitions, 15-second hold)
Hamstring stretch
Gluteus maximus and hip flexor stretch
Gastrocnemius and soleus stretch
Paraspinal stretch
**Strengthening exercises** (baseline determination of preferred elastic-band strengths for lower limb exercises—1 repetition maximum)
*Lower limb muscles* (elastic band: 1 set of 8–10 repetitions for each leg)
Quadriceps (sitting and straight-leg raises)
Hamstrings
Gluteus maximus
Gluteus medius
*Upper limb muscles* (5–10 repetitions)
Push-ups
*Abdominal muscles* (5 repetitions)
Curl-ups with arms behind head
**Instruction in body mechanics for**
Standing
Sitting
Lying
Lifting
Reaching
Carrying
Arising from floor
Ascending/descending stairs
**Baseline walking evaluation** (determine maximum comfortable distance)

**Week 2**
**Flexibility exercises** (as above)
**Strengthening exercises:** lower limb muscles (elastic band: 1 set of 10 repetitions, each leg), upper limb muscles (10 repetitions), abdominal muscles (5–10 repetitions)
**Postural exercises** (10 repetitions, 10-second hold)
Head and neck
Trunk

**Coordination exercises**
Reciprocal leg movements (10 repetitions, eyes closed)
Bridging (10 repetitions)
Sitting/standing (5 repetitions)
Braiding exercises (2 repetitions)
Reciprocal ankle motion (10 repetitions)
Rung ladder: forward stepping (2 repetitions)

**"Survival" maneuvers**
Floor recovery exercises—"how to get up if you should fall"

Ascending and descending stairs safely (individual practice)
**Endurance walking** (begin at 75–100% of baseline minutes walked; increase at comfortable pace)

**Week 3**
**Flexibility exercises** (5 repetitions, 20-second hold)
**Strengthening exercises:** lower limb (2 sets of 10 repetitions), upper limb (push-ups, 10–15 repetitions), abdominals (curl-ups, 10–15 repetitions)
**Postural exercises** (15 repetitions, 10-second hold)
**Coordination exercises** (repetitions increased)
**Survival maneuvers:** practice (floor recovery/stairs)
**Endurance walking** (0–6 minutes, comfortable pace)

**Week 4**
**Flexibility exercises** (5 repetitions, 25-second hold)
**Strengthening exercises:** lower limb (2–3 sets of 10 repetitions), upper limb (push-ups, 15 repetitions), abdominals (curl-ups, 15 repetitions)
**Postural exercises** (20 repetitions, 10-second hold)
**Coordination exercises** (repetitions increased)
Reciprocal legs (eyes closed)
Braiding (no holding, eyes open)
Rung ladder (forward, side, and backward stepping)
**Survival maneuvers:** practice (floor recovery/stairs)
**Endurance walking** (3–8 minutes, comfortable pace)

**Week 5**
**Flexibility exercises** (5 repetitions, 30-second hold)
**Strengthening exercises:** lower limb (3 sets of 10 repetitions), upper limb (push-ups, 15–20 repetitions), abdominals (curl-ups, 15–20 repetitions)
**Postural exercises** (25 repetitions, 10-second hold)
**Coordination exercises:** as above with increased repetitions, plus:
Braiding (no holding, eyes closed)
Reciprocal ankle dorsi/plantar flexion (25 repetitions)
**Survival maneuvers:** practice (floor recovery/stairs)
**Endurance walking** (6–10 minutes, comfortable pace)

**Week 6**
**Flexibility exercises** (5 repetitions, 30-second hold)
**Strengthening exercises:** lower limb (3 sets of 10 repetitions), upper limb (push-ups, 20 repetitions), abdominals (curl-ups, 15–20 repetitions)
**Postural exercises** (25 repetitions, 10-second hold)
**Coordination exercises** (as above with increased repetitions)
**Endurance walking** (8–12 minutes, comfortable pace)
**Survival maneuvers:** practice (floor recovery/stairs)

of orientation. The continuous weight shifting from one leg to the other facilitates anticipatory balance control, motor coordination, and lower-extremity strength. Finally, the large dynamic, flowing and circular movements of the extremities promote joint ROM and flexibility. These characteristics should be considered when recommending

Tai Chi classes to patients to ensure that instructors are following these principles and that patients are appropriate for these activities. Tai Chi performed while standing three times per week over a 6-month period reduced the number and risk of falls and improved balance in community-residing, but inactive, elderly individuals.[63]

| TABLE 8.3 | Circuit Training Program to Address Balance Impairments and Function[87] | |

| Activity | Responses targeted | Progression of Activity |
|---|---|---|
| Sit-to-stand-to-sit | Lower limb strength<br>Functional ability<br>Multiple tasks | Lower the height of the chair<br>Add/remove upper limb assistance<br>Hold an item in the hands, balance a cup with/without water on a saucer/tray<br>Add a cognitive task to the manual task |
| Stepping in all directions (forward, side, and back) | Choice step reaction time<br>Lower limb strength and coordination | Use a mirror to provide visual feedback<br>Increase speed of step<br>Perform stepping on a soft surface<br>Close eyes |
| Reaching to limits of stability | Challenging limits of stability<br>Vestibular stimulation and integration<br>Upper and lower limb strengthening | Stick objects on a wall in the front by reaching to limits in all directions up and down while keeping feet in one position<br>Lunge forward to pick up objects that are shifted to a high shelf to the side and behind, progress by reaching further and increasing the weight and size of objects |
| Step up and down | Lower limb strengthening and endurance<br>Step reaction time | Step up forward, backward, and sideways over blocks of various heights; increase height, repetitions, and speed of stepping |
| Ankle, hip, and upper limb balance strategy practice | Lower limb strengthening<br>Balance strategy training | Stand in front of a wall with toe touching a line 0.5 meter from the wall. Lean back toward the wall, keeping balance and dorsiflexing the feet and using arm movement to balance while lowering toward the wall |
| Sideways reach task | Mediolateral muscle strengthening in lower limbs<br>Vestibular stimulation and integration<br>Challenging limits of stability<br>Multiple tasks and confounded proprioceptive input | Stand between a high and a low table positioned on either side, pick up objects from one table and transfer to other table.<br>Move the tables farther apart and increase the weight and size of the objects to increase the challenge<br>Perform task while standing on an exercise mat on the floor |
| Ball games | Multiple tasks<br>Hand–eye coordination<br>Vestibular stimulation<br>Ballistic upper and lower limb activity | Use inflated beach balls and progress to smaller or harder balls or two or three balls at once<br>Add a cognitive task such as nominating an animal that starts with a G, while throwing and catching or kicking the ball |
| Card treasure hunt/sort into suits | Coping strategies with visual conflict<br>Vestibular stimulation and challenge of limits of stability | Prior to the session hide playing cards in the room such that to collect the cards the participants have to bend and look under furniture, reach up high, or detect the card from a visually confounding background. Red and black teams are possible and the team with the most cards returned to a collecting point inside 5 minutes is the winner.<br>Add the cognitive challenge of finding/sorting cards into order according to suit |

# INDEPENDENT LEARNING ACTIVITIES

## ● Critical Thinking and Discussion

1. A person is experiencing falls when arising from a chair. Using biomechanical principles of balance, what adjustments can the person immediately make to increase his or her stability and prevent falls?

2. Differentiate and describe several balance movements that rely primarily on feedforward or open-loop motor control versus those that utilize closed-loop control.

3. Review the ankle, hip, and stepping strategies and discuss how the strategies are elicited and what key muscles are activated to control balance.

4. Think about the times you have fallen in the past. What activity were you doing at the time that you fell? What musculoskeletal, neurological, and/or contextual factors contributed to the fall occurrence? What were the consequences of the fall? What differences would you expect between your falls and those experienced by an elderly person?

5. Differentiate and discuss treatment activities that you would use to train static, dynamic, anticipatory, reactive, and sensory organization aspects of balance control. Provide examples of how you would progress each of the activities.

6. For an elderly person with a history of falls, what aspects of the home environment might need to be modified to maximize the individual's safety and independence?

## ● Laboratory Practice

1. With a partner, mount a yardstick on the wall at the person's shoulder height. Measure the maximum amount of anterior and posterior sway by recording the maximum shoulder displacement during a 30-second period of quiet stance in each of the following conditions.
   - Standing on a firm surface with feet together, arms on hips, and eyes open.
   - Standing on a firm surface with feet together, arms on hips, and eyes closed.
   - Standing on a soft foam surface with feet together, arms on hips, and eyes open.
   - Standing on a soft foam surface with feet together, arms on hips, and eyes closed.
     For each of the conditions, what sensory inputs are available to the person for maintaining balance? How does the amount of sway vary with each condition and why?

2. With a partner, observe body movement during the following activities.

   - Standing with feet shoulder width apart, perform self-initiated forward and backward body sways progressing from small to large amplitudes.
   - Standing with feet apart, have your partner place his or her hand on your sternum and nudge you backward gently and then again with a larger force.
   - Standing with the feet placed heel to toe, have your partner gently nudge your backward.
   - Put on ankle-foot orthoses or ski boots that restrict ankle movements and have your partner gently nudge you backward.
     Which movement strategy is elicited with each activity and why?

3. Practice performing treatment activities that you would use to train static, dynamic, anticipatory, reactive, and sensory organization aspects of balance control as described in Table 8.2. Progress each of the activities to maximally challenge your balance.

## ● Case Studies

1. A 20-year-old male soccer player sustained a right mid-tibial fracture in a motor vehicle accident and was required to wear a long-leg rigid cast for 6 weeks. You are seeing the patient 1 week after cast removal for physical therapy. He would like to return to playing soccer but is currently unable to maintain balance on his right leg to kick a soccer ball. What underlying impairments might be causing this individual's balance problems, and how would you design an exercise program that would allow him to reach his goals?

2. A 75-year-old woman fell in her bathtub and sustained a right pelvic fracture, requiring bed rest for 2 weeks. You are seeing the patient in her home following her hospital discharge. She has generalized weakness, deconditioning, is unsteady on her feet, and is fearful of falling. Currently she is using a walker for ambulation. Prior to her fall, she was completely independent in all activities of daily living and enjoyed going on walks in her neighborhood in the evenings. Design a progressive balance program for this woman to restore her to her prior level of functioning.

3. A 70-year-old retiree has had bilateral knee replacement surgeries. He would like to resume his favorite hobby of boating but lacks confidence in his ability to balance under dynamic conditions. Design an exercise and balance training program that will help him return to his recreational pursuits. What suggestions do you have to increase his safety when boating? What if his hobby were golfing instead of boating? Compare and contrast the activities and exercises you would prescribe for these two different issues.

# REFERENCES

1. Adams MA, Hutton WC. Has the lumbar spine a margin of safety in forward bending? Clin Biomech 1:3–6, 1986.
2. Alexander KM, LaPier TL. Differences in static balance and weight distribution between normal subjects and subjects with chronic unilateral low back pain. J Orthop Sports Phys Ther 28:378–383, 1998.
3. American Geriatrics Society, British Geriatrics Society, American Academy of Orthopaedic Surgeons Panel on Fall Prevention. Guidelines for the prevention of falls in older persons. J Am Geriatr Soc 49:664–672, 2001.
4. American Physical Therapy Association: Guide to Physical Therapist Practice, ed 2. Phys Ther 81:9–746, 2001.
5. Anderson CK, Chaffin DB. A biomechanical evaluation of five lifting techniques. Appl Ergon 17:2–8, 1986.
6. Andersson G. Epidemiologic aspects of low back pain in industry. Spine 6:53–60, 1981.
7. Barrack JA, Skinner HB, Buckley S. Proprioception in the anterior cruciate deficient knee. Am J Sports Med 17:1–7, 1989.
8. Barrett DS, Cobb AG, Bentley G. Joint proprioception in normal, osteoarthritic and replaced knees. J Bone Joint Surg Br 73:53–56, 1991.
9. Basmajian JV, DeLuca CJ. Muscles Alive: Their Functions Revealed by Electromyography. 5th ed. Baltimore, Williams & Wilkins, 1985.
10. Berg KO, Wood-Dauphinee SL, Williams JI, Maki B. Measuring balance in the elderly: validation of an instrument. Can J Public Health 83(Suppl 2):S7–S11, 1992.
11. Black FO, Shupert CL, Horak FB, Nashner LM. Abnormal postural control associated with peripheral vestibular disorders. Prog Brain Res 76:263–275, 1988.
12. Borg G. Perceived exertion as an indicator of somatic stress. Scand J Rehabil Med 2:92–98, 1970.
13. Boyle J, Negus V. Joint position sense in the recurrently sprained ankle. Aust J Physiother 44:159–163, 1998.
14. Braune W, Fischer O. On the Centre of Gravity of the Human Body. Berlin, Springer-Verlag, 1984.
15. Brouwer BJ, Walker C, Rydahl SJ, Culham EG. Reducing fear of falling in seniors through education and activity programs: a randomized trial. J Am Geriatr Soc 51:829–834, 2003.
16. Brumagne S, Cordo P, Lysens R, Verschueren S, Swinnen S. The role of paraspinal muscle spindles in lumbosacral position sense in individuals with and without low back pain. Spine 25:989–994, 2000.
17. Burtner PA, Woollacott MH, Qualls C. Stance balance control with orthoses in a group of children with spastic cerebral palsy. Dev Med Child Neurol 41:748–757, 1999.
18. Byl NN, Sinnott PL. Variations in balance and body sway in middle-aged adults: subjects with healthy backs compared with subjects with low back dysfunction. Spine 16:325–330, 1991.
19. Chaffin DB, Page GB. Postural effects on biomechanical and psychophysical weight-lifting limits. Ergonomics 37:663–676, 1994.
20. Chamberlin ME, Fulwider BD, Sanders SL, Medeiros JM. Does fear of falling influence spatial and temporal gait parameters in elderly persons beyond changes associated with normal aging? J Gerontol A Biol Sci Med Sci 60:1163–1167, 2005.
21. Chandler JM, Duncan PW. Balance and falls in the elderly: issues in evaluation and treatment. In: Guccione AA, editor. Geriatric Physical Therapy. St. Louis, Mosby, 1993, pp. 237–251.
22. Chow DH, Cheng IY, Holmes AD, Evans JH. Postural perturbation and muscular response following sudden release during symmetric squat and stoop lifting. Ergonomics 48:591–607, 2005.
23. Christou EA, Yang Y, Rosengren KS. Taiji training improves knee extensor strength and force control in older adults. J Gerontol A Biol Sci Med Sci 58:763–766, 2003.
24. Commissaris D, Toussaint H. Load knowledge affects low-back loading and control of balance in lifting tasks. Ergonomics 40:559–575, 1997.
25. Commissaris D, Toussaint HM, Hirschfeld H. Anticipatory postural adjustments in a bimanual, whole-body lifting task seem not only aimed at minimising anterior-posterior centre of mass displacements. Gait Posture 14:44–55, 2001.
26. Cordo PJ, Nashner LM. Properties of postural adjustments associated with rapid arm movement. J Neurophysiol 47:187–302, 1982.
27. Cornwall MW, Murrell P. Postural sway following inversion sprain of the ankle. J Am Podiatr Med Assoc 81:243–247, 1991.
28. Dolan P, Earley M, Adams MA. Bending and compressive stresses acting on the lumbar spine during lifting activities. J Biomech 27:1237–1248, 1994.
29. Dolan P, Mannion AF, Adams MA. Passive tissues help the back muscles to generate extensor moments during lifting. J Biomech 27:1077–1085, 1994.
30. Donald IP, Bulpitt CJ. The prognosis of falls in elderly people living at home. Age Ageing 28:121–125, 1999.
31. Duncan PW, Weiner DK, Chandler J, Studenski S. Functional reach: a new clinical measure of balance. J Gerontol 45:M192–M197, 1990.
32. Frank JS, Patla AE, Brown JE. Characteristics of postural control accompanying voluntary arm movement in the elderly. Soc Neurosci Abstr 13:335, 1987.
33. Freeman MA, Dean MR, Hanham IW. The etiology and prevention of functional instability of the foot. J Bone Joint Surg Br 47:678–685, 1965.
34. Garn SN, Newton RA. Kinesthetic awareness in subjects with multiple ankle sprains. Phys Ther 68:1667–1671, 1988.
35. Gill KP, Callaghan MJ. The measurement of lumbar proprioception in individuals with and without low back pain. Spine 23:371–377, 1998.
36. Gillespie LD, Gillespie WJ, Robertson MC, Lamb SE, Cumming RG, Rowe BH. Interventions for preventing falls in elderly people. Cochrane Database Syst Rev CD000340, 2003.
37. Glencross D, Thornton E. Position sense following joint injury. J Sports Med Phys Fitness 21:23–27, 1981.
38. Grigg P. Articular neurophysiology. In: Zachazewski JE, McGee DJ, Quillen WS, editors. Athletic Injury Rehabilitation. Philadelphia, WB Saunders, 1996.
39. Grigg P, Finerman GA, Riley LH. Joint-position sense after total hip replacement. J Bone Joint Surg Am 55:1016–1025, 1973.
40. Heiss DG, Shields RK, Yack HJ. Balance loss when lifting a heavier-than-expected load: effects of lifting technique. Arch Phys Med Rehabil 83:48–59, 2002.
41. Heiss D, Shields R, Yack H. Anticipatory control of vertical lifting force and momentum during the squat lift with expected and unexpected loads. J Orthop Sports Phys Ther 31:708–729, 2001.
42. Hellebrandt FA, Tepper RH, Braun GL. Location of the cardinal anatomical orientation planes passing through the center of weight in young adult women. Am J Physiol 121:465, 1938.
43. Horak F, Shupert C. The role of the vestibular system in postural control. In: Herdman S, editor. Vestibular Rehabilitation. New York, FA Davis, 1994, p 22–46.
44. Horak FB. Postural orientation and equilibrium: what do we need to know about neural control of balance to prevent falls? Age Ageing 35(Suppl 2):ii7–ii11, 2006.
45. Horak FB, Nashner LM. Central programming of postural movements: adaption to altered support surface configurations. J Neurophysiol 55:1369–1381, 1986.
46. Horak FB, Nashner LM, Diener HC. Postural strategies associated with somatosensory and vestibular loss. Exp Brain Res 82:167–177, 1990.
47. Horak FB, Nutt JG, Nashner LM. Postural inflexibility in parkinsonian subjects. J Neurol Sci 111:46–58, 1992.
48. Horak FB, Shupert CL, Mirka A. Components of postural dyscontrol in the elderly: a review. Neurobiol Aging 10:727–738, 1989.
49. Howland J, Peterson EW, Levin WC, et al. Fear of falling among the community-dwelling elderly. J Aging Health 5:229–243, 1993.
50. Huang HC, Gau ML, Lin WC, George K. Assessing risk of falling in older adults. Public Health Nurs 20:399–411, 2003.
51. Inglin B, Woollacott M. Age-related changes in anticipatory postural adjustments associated with arm movements. J Gerontol 43:M105–M113, 1988.
52. Jack CI, Smith T, Neoh C, Lye M, McGalliard JN. Prevalence of low vision in elderly patients admitted to an acute geriatric unit in Liverpool: elderly people who fall are more likely to have low vision. Gerontology 41:280–285, 1995.
53. Johnson BL, Nelso JK. Practical Measurements for Evaluation in Physical Education, 4th ed. Minneapolis, Burgess, 1979.
54. Katz S, Downs TD, Cash HR, et al. Index of activities of daily living. Gerontologist 1:20–31, 1970.
55. Keith RA, Granger CV, Hamilton BB, Sherwin FS. The functional independence measure: a new tool for rehabilitation. Adv Clin Rehabil 1:6–18, 1987.

56. Keshner EA. Reflex, voluntary, and mechanical process in postural stabilization. In: Duncan PW, editor. Balance Proceedings of the APTA Forum. Alexandria, VA, American Physical Therapy Association, 1990.
57. Keshner EA, Woollacott M, Debu B. Neck and trunk muscle responses during postural perturbations in humans. Exp Brain Res 71:455–466, 1988.
58. Kingma I, Bosch T, Bruins L, van Dieen JH. Foot positioning instruction, initial vertical load position and lifting technique: effects on low back loading. Ergonomics 47:1365–1385, 2004.
59. Lachman ME, Howland J, Tennstedt S, et al. Fear of falling and activity restriction: the survey of activities and fear of falling in the elderly (SAFE). J Gerontol B Psychol Sci Soc Sci 53:43–50, 1998.
60. Lawton MP, Brody EM. Assessment of older people: self-maintaining and instrumental activities of daily living. Gerontologist 9:179–186, 1969.
61. Leinonen V, Kankaanpaa M, Luukkonen M, et al. Lumbar paraspinal muscle function, perception of lumbar position, and postural control in disc herniation-related back pain. Spine 28:842–848, 2003.
62. Leskinen TP, Stalhammar HR, Kuorinka IA, Troup J. A dynamic analysis of spinal compression with different lifting techniques. Ergonomics 26:595–604, 1983.
63. Li F, Harmer P, Fisher KJ, et al. Tai Chi and fall reductions in older adults: a randomized controlled trial. J Gerontol A Biol Sci Med Sci 60:187–194, 2005.
64. Light KE. Information processing for motor performance in aging adults. Phys Ther 70:820–826, 1990.
65. Lin SI, Woollacott MH, Jensen JL. Postural response in older adults with different levels of functional balance capacity. Aging Clin Exp Res 16:369–374, 2004.
66. Lord SR, Dayhew J, Howland A. Multifocal glasses impair edge-contrast sensitivity and depth perception and increase the risk of falls in older people. J Am Geriatr Soc 50:1760–1766, 2002.
67. Lord SR, Tiedemann A, Chapman K, et al. The effect of an individualized fall prevention program on fall risk and falls in older people: a randomized, controlled trial. J Am Geriatr Soc 53:1296–1304, 2005.
68. Mahoney FI, Barthel DW. Functional evaluation: the Barthel Index. Md State Med J 14:61–65, 1965.
69. Maki BE. Gait changes in older adults: predictors of falls or indicators of fear. J Am Geriatr Soc 45:313–320, 1997.
70. Maki BE, Whitelaw RS. Influence of expectation and arousal on center-of-pressure responses to transient postural perturbations. J Vestib Res 3:25–39, 1993.
71. Marigold DS, Eng JJ, Dawson AS, et al. Exercise leads to faster postural reflexes, improved balance and mobility, and fewer falls in older persons with chronic stroke. J Am Geriatr Soc 53:416–423, 2005.
72. Means KM, Rodell DE, O'Sullivan PS. Balance, mobility, and falls among community-dwelling elderly persons: effects of a rehabilitation exercise program. Am J Phys Med Rehabil 84:238–250, 2005.
73. Miller RL. When you lift, bend your knees. Occup Health Safety 45:46–47, 1976.
74. Mizuta H, Shiraishi M, Kubota K, et al. A stabilometric technique for evaluation of functional instability in the anterior cruciate ligament deficient knee. Clin J Sport Med 2:235–249, 1992.
75. Morgan RO, Virnig BA, Duque M, et al. Low-intensity exercise and reduction of the risk for falls among at-risk elders. J Gerontol A Biol Sci Med Sci 59:1062–1067, 2004.
76. Munhoz RP, Li JY, Kurtinecz M, et al. Evaluation of the pull test technique in assessing postural instability in Parkinson's disease. Neurology 62:125–127, 2004.
77. Nashner L. Adaptations of human movement to altered environments. Trends Neurosci 5:358–361, 1982.
78. Nashner L, Woollacott MH. The organization of rapid postural adjustments of standing humans: an experimental-conceptual model. In Talbott RE, Humphrey DR, editors. Posture and Movement. New York, Raven, 1979, p 243–257.
79. Nashner LM. Fixed patterns of rapid postural responses among leg muscles during stance. Exp Brain Res 30:13–24, 1977.
80. Nashner LM. Sensory, neuromuscular, and biomechanical contributions to human balance. In Duncan PW, editor. Balance Proceedings of the APTA Forum. Alexandria, VA, American Physical Therapy Association, 1990.
81. Nashner LM. The anatomic basis of balance in orthopaedics. In Wallman HW, editor. Orthopaedic Physical Therapy Clinics of North America: Balance. Philadelphia, WB Saunders, 2002.
82. Nashner LM, Shupert CL, Horak FB, Black FO. Organization of posture controls: an analysis of sensory and mechanical constraints. Prog Brain Res 80:411–418, 1989.
83. Nashner LM, Woollacott M, Tuma G. Organization of rapid responses to postural and locomotor-like perturbations of standing man. Exp Brain Res 36:463–476, 1979.
84. Nevitt MC. Falls in the elderly: risk factors and prevention. In Masdeu JC, Sudarsky L, Wolfson L, editors. Gait Disorders of Aging: Falls and Therapeutic Strategies. Philadelphia, Lippincott-Raven, 1997, p 13–36.
85. Newton RA. Review of tests of standing balance abilities. Br Injury 3:335–343, 1989.
86. Newton RA. Validity of the multi-directional reach test: a practical measure for limits of stability in older adults. J Gerontol A Biol Sci Med Sci 56:M248–M252, 2001.
87. Nitz JC, Choy NL. The efficacy of a specific balance-strategy training programme for preventing falls among older people: a pilot randomised controlled trial. Age Ageing 33:52–58, 2004.
88. Nolte J. The Human Brain: An Introduction to Its Functional Anatomy, 5th ed. St. Louis, Mosby, 2002.
89. Pap G, Machner A, Nebelung W, Awiszus F. Detailed analysis of proprioception in normal and ACL-deficient knees. J Bone Joint Surg Br 81:764–768, 1999.
90. Patla AE, Winter DA, Frank JS, Walt SE, Prasad S. Identification of age-related changes in the balance-control system. In Duncan PW, editor. Balance Proceedings of the APTA Forum. Alexandria, VA, American Physical Therapy Association, 1990.
91. Podsiadlo D, Richardson S. The timed "Up & Go": a test of basic functional mobility for frail elderly persons. J Am Geriatr Soc 39:142–148, 1991.
92. Potvin JR, McGill SM, Norman RW. Trunk muscle and lumbar ligament contributions to dynamic lifts with varying degrees of trunk flexion. Spine 16:1099–1107, 1991.
93. Powell LE, Myers AM. The Activities-specific Balance Confidence (ABC) scale. J Gerontol A Biol Sci Med Sci 50A:M28–M34, 1995.
94. Puniello MS, McGibbon CA, Krebs DE. Lifting characteristics of functionally limited elders. J Rehabil Res Dev 37:341–352, 2000.
95. Resnick HE, Vinik AI, Schwartz AV, et al. Independent effects of peripheral nerve dysfunction on lower-extremity physical function in old age: the Women's Health and Aging Study. Diabetes Care 23:1642–1647, 2000.
96. Richardson JK. Factors associated with falls in older patients with diffuse polyneuropathy. J Am Geriatr Soc 50:1767–1773, 2002.
97. Richardson JK, Ashton-Miller JA, Lee SG, Jacobs K. Moderate peripheral neuropathy impairs weight transfer and unipedal balance in the elderly. Arch Phys Med Rehabil 77:1152–1156, 1996.
98. Rose DJ. FallProof! A comprehensive balance and mobility program. Champaign, IL, Human Kinetics, 2003.
99. Rubenstein LZ, Josephson KR, Robbins AS. Falls in the nursing home. Ann Intern Med 121:442–451, 1994.
100. Safran MR, Allen AA, Lephart SM, et al. Proprioception in the posterior cruciate ligament deficient knee. Knee Surg Sports Traumatol Arthrosc 7:310–17, 1999.
101. Sattin RW. Falls among older persons: a public health perspective. Annu Rev Public Health 13:489–508, 1992.
102. Schenkman ML. Interrelationship of neurological and mechanical factors in balance ocntrol. In: Duncan PW, editor. Balance Proceedings of the APTA Forum. Alexandria, VA, American Physical Therapy Association, 1990.
103. Shu Y, Southard S, Shin G, Mirka GA. The effect of a repetitive, fatiguing lifting task on horizontal ground reaction forces. J Appl Biomech 21:260–270, 2005.
104. Shumway-Cook A, Horak F. Assessing the influence of sensory interaction of balance: suggestion from the field. Phys Ther 66:1548–1550, 1986.
105. Shumway-Cook A, Woollacott M. Motor Control: Theory and Practical Applications, 2nd ed. Lippincott Williams & Wilkins, 2001.
106. Simoneau GG, Ulbrecht JS, Derr JA, et al. Postural instability in patients with diabetic sensory neuropathy. Diabetes Care 17:1411–1421, 1994.

107. Studenski S, Duncan PW, Chandler J. Postural responses and effector factors in persons with unexplained falls: results and methodologic issues. J Am Geriatr Soc 39:229–234, 1991.

108. Sturdevant R. Prescription for workplace safety: bend and lift correctly to avoid back injuries. J Tennessee Med Assoc 86:457, 1993.

109. Taggart HM. Effects of Tai Chi exercise on balance, functional mobility, and fear of falling among older women. Appl Nurs Res 15:235–242, 2002.

110. Teasdale N, Stelmach GE, Breunig A. Postural sway characteristics of the elderly under normal and altered visual and support surface conditions. J Gerontol 46:B238–B244, 1991.

111. Tinetti ME. Performance-oriented assessment of mobility problems in elderly patients. J Am Geriatr Soc 34:119–126, 1986.

112. Tinetti M, Richman D, Powell L. Falls efficacy as a measure of fear of falling. J Gerontol 45:239–243, 1990.

113. Toussaint H, Commissaris DM, Beek P. Anticipatory postural adjustments in the back and leg lift. Med Sci Sports Exerc 29:1216–1224, 1997.

114. Uccioli L, Giacomini PG, Monticone G, et al. Body sway in diabetic neuropathy. Diabetes Care 18:339–344, 1995.

115. Van Dieen JH, van Dieen JH, Visser B, Visser B. Estimating net lumbar sagittal plane moments from EMG data: the validity of calibration procedures. J Electromyogr Kinesiol 9:309–315, 1999.

116. Van Dieen J, Hoozemans M, Toussaint H. Stoop or squat: a review of biomechanical studies on lifting techniques. Clin Biomech 14: 685–696, 1999.

117. VanSwearingen JM, Paschal KA, Bonino P, Chen TW. Assessing recurrent fall risk of community-dwelling, frail older veterans using specific tests of mobility and the physical performance test of function. J Gerontol A Biol Sci Med Sci 53:M457–M464, 1998.

118. VanSwearingen JM, Paschal KA, Bonino P, Yang JF. The modified Gait Abnormality Rating Scale for recognizing the risk of recurrent falls in community-dwelling elderly adults. Phys Ther 76:994–1002, 1996.

119. Vellas BJ, Wayne SJ, Romero L, et al. One-leg balance is an important predictor of injurious falls in older persons. J Am Geriatr Soc 45:735–738, 1997.

120. Walker JE, Howland J. Falls and fear of falling among elderly persons living in the community: occupational therapy interventions. Am J Occup Ther 45:119–122, 1991.

121. Wayne PM, Krebs DE, Wolf SL, et al. Can Tai Chi improve vestibulopathic postural control? Arch Phys Med Rehabil 85:142–152, 2004.

122. Wegener L, Kisner C, Nichols D. Static and dynamic balance responses in persons with bilateral knee osteoarthritis. J Orthop Sports Phys Ther 25:13–18, 1997.

123. Winstein CJ, Mitz AR. The motor system. II. Higher centers. In Cohen H, editor. Neuroscience for Rehabilitation. Philadelphia, JB Lippincott, 1993.

124. Winter DA. A.B.C. (Anatomy, Biomechanics and Control) of Balance During Standing and Walking. Waterloo, Ontario, Waterloo Biomechanics, 1995.

125. Winter DA, Patla AE, Frank JS, Walt SE. Biomechanical walking pattern changes in the fit and healthy elderly. Phys Ther 70:340–347, 1990.

126. Wolfson LI, Whipple R, Amerman P, Kleinberg A. Stressing the postural response: a quantitative method for testing balance. J Am Geriatr Soc 34:845–850, 1986.

127. Woollacott MH, Shumway-Cook A, Nashner LM. Aging and posture control: changes in sensory organization and muscular coordination. Int J Aging Hum Dev 23:97–114, 1986.

# Aquatic Exercise

## Robert Schrepfer, MS, PT

The use of water for healing purposes dates back several centuries. Near the end of the 19th century in Europe, and soon after in the United States, the use of an aquatic environment to facilitate exercise began to grow in popularity. In recent years, health care practitioners have increasingly utilized the aquatic medium to facilitate therapeutic exercises. The unique properties of the aquatic environment provide clinicians with treatment options that would otherwise be difficult or impossible to implement on land. Through the use of buoyant devices and varied depths of immersion the practitioner may position the patient supine, seated, kneeling, prone, side-lying, or vertically with any desired amount of weight bearing. Aquatic exercise has been successfully used for a wide variety of rehabilitation populations including pediatric, orthopedic, neurological, and cardiopulmonary patients.

## BACKGROUND AND PRINCIPLES FOR AQUATIC EXERCISE

## DEFINITION OF AQUATIC EXERCISE

*Aquatic exercise* refers to the use of multidepth immersion pools or tanks that facilitate the application of various established therapeutic interventions, including stretching, strengthening, joint mobilization, balance and gait training, and endurance training.

## GOALS AND INDICATIONS FOR AQUATIC EXERCISE

The specific purpose of aquatic exercise is to facilitate functional recovery by providing an environment that augments a patient's and/or practitioner's ability to perform various therapeutic interventions. The specific goals include:

- Facilitate range of motion (ROM) exercise*
- Initiate resistance training[6,18,28,36,38,40,52]
- Facilitate weight-bearing activities[38,39]
- Enhance delivery of manual techniques[4,5,54]
- Provide three-dimensional access to the patient[5,51,54]
- Facilitate cardiovascular exercise†
- Initiate functional activity replication‡
- Minimize risk of injury or reinjury during rehabilitation[4,18,60,61]
- Enhance patient relaxation[4,41,42]

## PRECAUTIONS AND CONTRAINDICATIONS TO AQUATIC EXERCISE

Although most patients easily tolerate aquatic exercise, the practitioner must consider several physiological and psychological aspects of immersion that affect selection of an aquatic environment.

### Precautions

#### Fear of Water
Fear of water can limit the effectiveness of any immersed activity. Fearful patients often experience increased symptoms during and after immersion because of muscle guarding, stress response, and improper form with exercise.[19,20] Often patients require an orientation period designed to provide instruction regarding the effects of immersion on balance, control of the immersed body, and proper use of flotation devices.[51]

#### Neurological Disorders
Ataxic patients may experience increased difficulty controlling purposeful movements.[51] Patients with heat-intolerant multiple sclerosis may fatigue with immersion in temperatures greater than 33°C.[51]

#### Seizures
Patients with controlled epilepsy require close monitoring during immersed treatment and must be compliant with medication prior to treatment.[51]

---

* See references 6, 18, 19, 28, 30, 32, 36, 38, 39, 40, 59.
† See references 3, 10, 12, 13, 15, 21, 23, 33, 45, 47, 48, 50–52, 58, 60.
‡ See references 6, 8, 19, 28, 30, 40, 51, 56, 59, 62, 63.

#### Cardiac Dysfunction
Patients with angina and abnormal blood pressure also require close monitoring. For patients with cardiac disease, low-intensity aquatic exercise may result in lower cardiac demand than similar land exercise.[35,44,47]

#### Small Open Wounds and Lines
Small, open wounds and tracheotomies may be covered by waterproof dressings. Patients with intravenous lines, Hickman lines, and other open lines require proper clamping and fixation.[51]

### Contraindications

- Incipient cardiac failure and unstable angina.
- Respiratory dysfunction; vital capacity of less than 1 liter.
- Severe peripheral vascular disease.
- Danger of bleeding or hemorrhage.
- Severe kidney disease: Patients are unable to adjust to fluid loss during immersion.
- Open wounds, colostomy, and skin infections such as tinea pedis and ringworm.
- Uncontrolled bowel or bladder: Bowel accidents require pool evacuation, chemical treatment, and possibly drainage.
- Water and airborne infections or diseases: Examples include influenza, gastrointestinal infections, typhoid, cholera, and poliomyelitis.
- Uncontrolled seizures: They create a safety issue for both clinician and patient if immediate removal from the pool is necessary.

## PROPERTIES OF WATER

The unique properties of water and immersion have profound physiological implications in the delivery of therapeutic exercise. To utilize aquatics efficiently, practitioners must have a basic understanding of the clinical significance of the static and dynamic properties of water as they affect human immersion and exercise.

### Physical Properties of Water

The properties provided by buoyancy,[4,8,19,37,51] hydrostatic pressure,[2,4,8,9,51] viscosity,[4,8,51] and surface tension[4,8,51] have a direct effect on the body in the aquatic environment.

#### Buoyancy (Fig. 9.1)

***Definition.*** Buoyancy is the upward force that works opposite to gravity.

***Properties.*** Archimedes' principle states that an immersed body experiences upward thrust equal to the volume of liquid displaced.

## Weight Bearing with Immersion

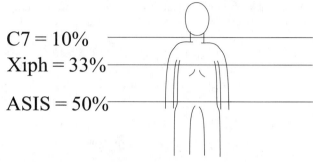

C7 = 10%
Xiph = 33%
ASIS = 50%

FIGURE 9.1 Percentage of weight bearing at various immersion depths.

### Clinical Significance

- Buoyancy provides the patient with relative weightlessness and joint unloading, allowing performance of active motion with increased ease.
- Buoyancy allows the practitioner three-dimensional access to the patient.

### Hydrostatic Pressure

**Definition.** Hydrostatic pressure is the pressure exerted on immersed objects.

#### Properties

- Pascal's law states that the pressure exerted by fluid on an immersed object is equal on all surfaces of the object.
- As the density of water and depth of immersion increase, so does hydrostatic pressure.

#### Clinical Significance

- Increased pressure reduces or limits effusion, assists venous return, induces bradycardia, and centralizes peripheral blood flow.
- The proportionality of depth and pressure allows patients to perform exercise more easily when closer to the surface.

### Viscosity

**Definition.** Viscosity is friction occurring between molecules of liquid resulting in resistance to flow.

**Properties.** Resistance from viscosity is proportional to the velocity of movement through liquid.

#### Clinical Significance

- Water's viscosity creates resistance with all active movements.

- Increasing the velocity of movement increases the resistance.
- Increasing the surface area moving through water increases resistance.

### Surface Tension

**Definition.** The surface of a fluid acts as a membrane under tension. Surface tension is measured as force per unit length.

#### Properties

- The attraction of surface molecules is parallel to the surface.
- The resistive force of surface tension changes proportionally to the size of the object moving through the fluid surface.

#### Clinical Significance

- An extremity that moves through the surface performs more work than if kept under water.
- Using equipment at the surface of the water increases the resistance.

### Hydromechanics

**Definition.** Hydromechanics comprise the physical properties and characteristics of fluid in motion.[4,8,51]

#### Components of Flow Motion

- *Laminar flow.* Movement where all molecules move parallel to each other, typically slow movement.
- *Turbulent flow.* Movement where molecules do not move parallel to each other, typically faster movements.
- *Drag.* The cumulative effects of turbulence and fluid viscosity acting on an object in motion.

#### Clinical Significance of Drag

- As the speed of movement through water increases, resistance to motion increases.
- Moving water past the patient requires the patient to work harder to maintain his/her position in pool.
- Application of equipment (glove/paddle/boot) increases drag and resistance as the patient moves the extremity through water.

### Thermodynamics

Water temperature has an effect on the body and, therefore, performance in an aquatic environment.[4,7,8,51]

### Specific Heat

**Definition.** Specific heat is the amount of heat (calories) required to raise the temperature of 1 gram of substance by 1°C.

***Properties.*** The rate of temperature change is dependent on the mass and the specific heat of the object.

### *Clinical Significance*

- Water retains heat 1000 times more than air.
- Differences in temperature between an immersed object and water equilibrate with minimal change in the temperature of the water.

### Temperature Transfer

- Water conducts temperature 25 times faster than air.
- Heat transfer increases with velocity. A patient moving through the water loses body temperature faster than an immersed patient at rest.

## Center of Buoyancy (Fig. 9.2)

Center of buoyancy, rather than center of gravity, affects the body in an aquatic environment.[4,8,51]

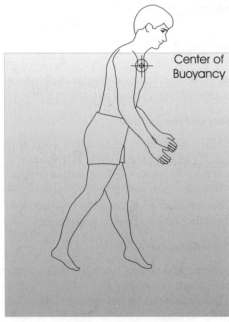

FIGURE 9.2 Center of buoyancy.

***Definition.*** The center of buoyancy is the reference point of an immersed object on which buoyant (vertical) forces of fluid predictably act.

***Properties.*** Vertical forces that do not intersect the center of buoyancy create rotational motion.

### *Clinical Significance*

- In the vertical position, the human center is located at the sternum.
- In the vertical position, posteriorly placed buoyancy devices cause the patient to lean forward; anterior buoyancy causes the patient to lean back.

- During unilateral manual resistance exercises the patient revolves around the practitioner in a circular motion.
- A patient with a unilateral lower extremity amputation leans toward the residual limb side when in a vertical position.
- Patients bearing weight on the floor of the pool (i.e., sitting, kneeling, standing) experience aspects of both the center of buoyancy and center of gravity.

## AQUATIC TEMPERATURE AND THERAPEUTIC EXERCISE

A patient's impairments and the intervention goals determine the water temperature selection. In general, utilize cooler temperatures for higher-intensity exercise and utilize warmer temperatures for mobility and flexibility exercise and for muscle relaxation.[4,7,14,51] The ambient air temperature should be 3°C higher than the water temperature for patient comfort. Incorrect water or ambient air temperature selection may adversely affect a patient's ability to tolerate or maintain immersed exercise.[*]

## Temperature Regulation

- Temperature regulation during immersed exercise differs from that during land exercise because of alterations in temperature conduction and the body's ability to dissipate heat.[4,8,19,37,51] With immersion there is less skin exposed to air, resulting in less opportunity to dissipate heat through normal sweating mechanisms.
- Water conducts temperature 25 times faster than air[11]—more if the patient is moving through the water and molecules are forced past the patient.
- Patients perceive small changes in water temperature more profoundly than small changes in air temperature.
- Over time, water temperature may penetrate to deeper tissues. Internal temperature changes are known to be inversely proportional to subcutaneous fat thickness.[11]
- Patients are unable to maintain adequate core warmth during immersed exercise at temperatures less than 25°C.[11]
- Conversely, exercise at temperatures greater than 37°C may be harmful if prolonged or maintained at high intensities. Hot water immersion may increase the cardiovascular demands at rest and with exercise.[53]
- In waist-deep water exercise at 37°C, the thermal stimulus to increase the heart rate overcomes the centralization of peripheral blood flow due to hydrostatic pressure.
- At temperatures greater than or equal to 37°C, cardiac output increases significantly at rest alone.[7,16]

## Mobility and Functional Control Exercise

- Aquatic exercises, including flexibility, strengthening, gait training, and relaxation, may be performed in temperatures between 26°C and 33°C.[4,8,51]

---

* See references 3, 11, 16, 19, 22, 27, 28, 37, 54, 56.

● Therapeutic exercise performed in warm water (33°C) may be beneficial for patients with acute painful musculoskeletal injuries because of the effects of relaxation, elevated pain threshold, and decreased muscle spasm.[4,8,51]

## Aerobic Conditioning

● Cardiovascular training and aerobic exercise should be performed in water temperatures between 26°C and 28°C. This range maximizes exercise efficiency, increases stroke volume, and decreases heart rate.[3,16,51,60]

● Intense aerobic training performed above 80% of a patient's maximum heart rate should take place in temperatures between 22°C and 26°C to minimize the risk of heat illness.[3,16,51,60]

# ● SPECIAL EQUIPMENT FOR AQUATIC EXERCISE

A large variety of equipment exists for use with aquatic exercise. Aquatic equipment is used to provide buoyant support to the body or an extremity, challenge or assist balance, and generate resistance to movement. By adding or removing equipment, the practitioner can progress exercise intensity.

## Collars, Rings, Belts, and Vests

Equipment designed to assist with patient positioning by providing buoyancy assistance can be applied to the neck, extremities, or trunk. Inflatable cervical collars are used for the supine patient to support the neck and maintain the head out of the water (Fig. 9.3). Flotation rings come in

various sizes and are used to support the extremities in any immersed position (Fig. 9.4). Often the rings are used at the wrists and ankles during manual techniques to assist with patient positioning and relaxation. Several types of belt exist that may be used to assist with buoyancy of an extremity or the entire body (Fig. 9.5). Belts and vests are used to position patients supine, prone, or vertically for shallow and deep water activities.

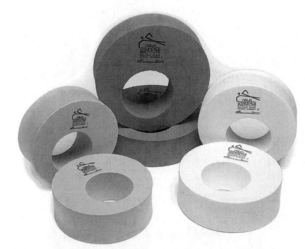

FIGURE 9.4 Flotation rings. *(Courtesy of Rothhammer International Inc., San Luis Obispo, CA.)*

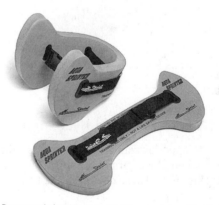

FIGURE 9.5 Buoyancy belts. *(Courtesy of Rothhammer International Inc., San Luis Obispo, CA.)*

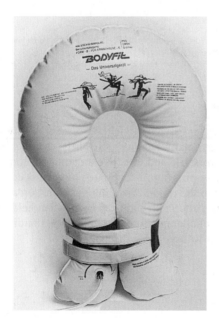

FIGURE 9.3 Cervical collar. *(Courtesy of Rothhammer International Inc., San Luis Obispo, CA.)*

## Swim Bars

Buoyant dumbbells (swim bars) are available in short and long lengths. They are useful for supporting the upper body or trunk in upright positions and the lower extremities in the supine or prone positions (Fig. 9.6). Patients can balance (seated or standing) on long swim bars in deep water to challenge balance, proprioception, and trunk strength.

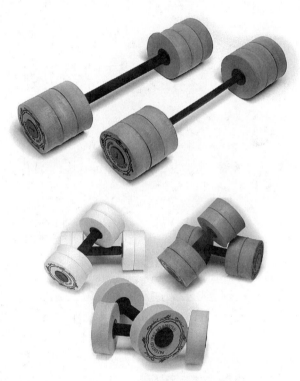

FIGURE 9.6  Swim bars. *(Courtesy of Rothhammer International Inc., San Luis Obispo, CA.)*

## Gloves, Hand Paddles, and Hydro-tone® Balls

Resistance to upper extremity movements is achieved by applying webbed gloves or progressively larger paddles to the hands (Fig. 9.7). These devices are not buoyant and,

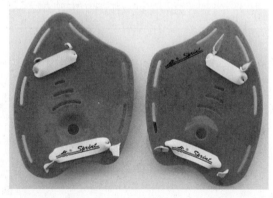

FIGURE 9.7  Hand paddles. *(Courtesy of Rothhammer International Inc., San Luis Obispo, CA.)*

therefore, only resist motion in the direction of movement. Hydro-tone® bells are large, slotted plastic devices that increase drag during upper extremity motions. The bells generate substantially more resistance than gloves or hand paddles.

## Fins and Hydro-tone® Boots

The application of fins or boots to the feet during lower extremity motions generates resistance by increasing the surface area moving through the water. Fins are especially useful for challenging hip, knee, and ankle strength. Hydro-tone® boots are most effective during deep water walking and running (Fig. 9.8).

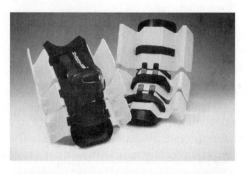

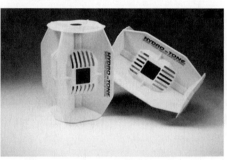

FIGURE 9.8  Hydro-tone boots and bells. *(Courtesy of Rothhammer International Inc., San Luis Obispo, CA.)*

## Kickboards

The shapes and styles of kickboards (Fig. 9.9) vary extensively among manufacturers. Nevertheless, kickboards remain a versatile and effective aquatic tool for augmenting any exercise program. Kickboards may be used to provide buoyancy in the prone or supine positions, create resistance to walking patterns in shallow water when held vertically, or used to challenge seated, kneeling, or standing balance in the deep water.

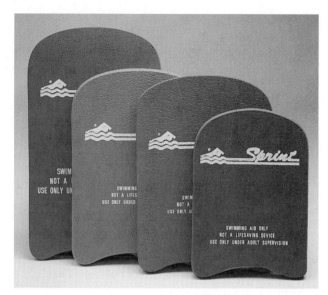

FIGURE 9.9 Kickboards. *(Courtesy of Rothhammer International Inc., San Luis Obispo, CA.)*

## EXERCISE INTERVENTIONS USING AN AQUATIC ENVIRONMENT

 STRETCHING EXERCISES

Patients may tolerate immersed stretching exercises better than land stretching because of the effects of relaxation, soft tissue warming, and ease of positioning. However, buoyancy creates an inherently less stable environment than the land. Therefore, careful consideration is warranted when recommending aquatic stretching.

### Manual Stretching Techniques

Manual stretching is typically performed with the patient supine in waist depth water with buoyancy devices at the neck, waist, and feet. Alternatively, the patient may be seated on steps. The buoyancy-supported supine position improves (versus land techniques) both access to the patient and control by the practitioner, as well as the position of the patient.

However, turbulence from wave activity can adversely affect both the patient and practitioner's ability to perform manual stretching. Difficulties may be experienced maintaining and perceiving the subtleties of end-range stretching and scapular stabilization in the supine buoyancy supported position. Anecdotal evidence indicates that careful consideration of all factors is warranted prior to initiating manual stretching in an aquatic environment.[5,54]

The manual stretching techniques described in this section are considered passive techniques but may be adapted to utilize muscle inhibition techniques. The principles of stretching are the same as those discussed in Chapter 4.

The following terms are used to describe the stretching techniques.

- *Practitioner position.* Describes the orientation of the practitioner to the patient.
- *Patient position.* Includes buoyancy-assisted (BA) seated or upright positioning and buoyancy-supported (BS) supine positioning.
- *Hand placement.* The fixed hand, which stabilizes the patient, is typically the same (ipsilateral) hand as the patient's affected extremity, and it is positioned proximally on the affected extremity. The movement hand, which guides the patient's extremity through the desired motion and applies the stretch force, is typically the opposite (contralateral) hand as the patient's affected extremity and is positioned distally.
- *Direction of movement.* Describes the motion of the movement hand.

### Cervical Spine: Flexion

**Practitioner Position**
Stand at the patient's head facing caudalward.

**Patient Position**
BS supine without cervical collar.

**Hand Placement**
Cup the patient's head with your hands, the forearms supinated and thumbs placed laterally. Alternatively, place your hands in a pronated position with the thumbs at the occiput. This results in a more neutral wrist position at end-range stretch.

**Direction of Movement**
As you flex the cervical spine, the patient has a tendency to drift away from you if care is not taken to perform the motion slowly.

### Cervical Spine: Lateral Flexion (Fig. 9.10)

**Practitioner Position**
Stand at the side facing the patient.

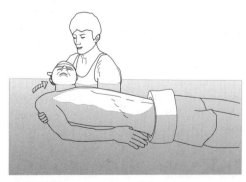

FIGURE 9.10 Hand placement and stabilization for stretching to increase cervical lateral flexion.

## Patient Position

BS supine without a cervical collar.

## Hand Placement

Reach the fixed hand dorsally under the patient and grasp the contralateral arm; support the head with the movement hand.

## Direction of Movement

Move the patient into lateral flexion and apply stretch force at desired intensity. This position prevents patient drift as the fixed hand stabilizes the patient against the practitioner.

### Thoracic and Lumbar Spine: Lateral Flexion/Side Bending (Fig. 9.11)

## Practitioner Position

Stand on the side opposite that to be stretched, facing cephalad with ipsilateral hips in contact (e.g., if stretching the left side of the trunk, the therapist's right hip is against patient's right hip).

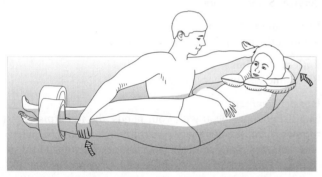

FIGURE 9.11 Hand placement and stabilization for stretching to increase lateral trunk flexion.

## Patient Position

BS supine, if tolerated. The patient's stretch side arm is abducted to end range to facilitate stretch.

## Hand Placement

Grasp the patient's abducted arm with the fixed hand; alternately, grasp at the deltoid if patient's arm is not abducted. The movement hand is at the lateral aspect of the lower extremity of the side to be stretched (more distal placement improves leverage with stretch).

## Direction of Movement

With the patient stabilized by your hip, pull the patient into lateral flexion. This technique allows variability in positioning and hand placement to isolate distinct segments of the spine.

### Shoulder Flexion (Fig. 9.12)

## Practitioner Position

Stand on the side to be stretched facing cephalad.

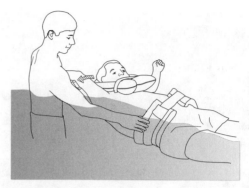

FIGURE 9.12 Hand placement and stabilization for stretching to increase shoulder flexion.

## Patient Position

BS supine with the affected shoulder positioned in slight abduction.

## Hand Placement

Grasp the buoyancy belt with the fixed hand; the movement hand is at the elbow of the affected extremity.

## Direction of Movement

After positioning the arm in the desired degree of abduction, direct the arm into flexion and apply the stretch force with the movement hand.

### Shoulder Abduction

## Practitioner Position

Stand on the affected side facing cephalad with your hip in contact with the patient's hip.

## Patient Position

BS supine.

## Hand Placement

Stabilize the scapula with the fixed hand; the movement hand grasps medially on the affected elbow joint.

## Direction of Movement

Guide the arm into abduction and apply the stretch force. The hip contact provides additional stabilization as the stretch force is applied.

### Shoulder External Rotation

## Practitioner Position

Stand lateral to the affected extremity facing cephalad.

## Patient Position

BS supine; position arm in desired degree of abduction with elbow flexed to 90°.

## Hand Placement

Grasp the medial side of the patient's elbow with the palmar aspect of the fixed hand while fingers hold laterally; grasp the midforearm with the movement hand.

**Direction of Movement**
Movement hand guides forearm dorsally to externally rotate the shoulder and apply stretch force.

### Shoulder Internal Rotation

**Practitioner Position**
Stand lateral to the patient's affected extremity facing caudalward.

**Patient Position**
BS supine; position arm in desired degree of abduction with elbow flexed to 90°.

**Hand Placement**
Stabilize the scapula with the dorsal aspect of the fixed hand entering from the axilla; the movement hand is at the distal forearm.

**Direction of Movement**
Direct the forearm palmarward and apply the stretch force. Use care to observe the glenohumeral joint to avoid a forward thrust and substitution.

### Hip Extension

**Practitioner Position**
Kneel on one knee at the patient's affected side.

**Patient Position**
BS supine with the hip extended and the knee slightly flexed.

**Hand Placement**
Stabilize the patient's affected extremity by hooking the top of the foot with your ipsilateral thigh. Grasp the buoyancy belt with the movement hand and guide the motion with the fixed hand on the knee.

**Direction of Movement**
Direct the patient caudally with the movement hand. To increase the stretch on the rectus femoris, lower the patient's knee in the water. Motion is performed slowly to limit spinal and pelvic substitution.

### Hip External Rotation

**Practitioner Position**
Face the lateral aspect of the patient's thigh with your ipsilateral arm under the patient's flexed knee.

**Patient Position**
BS supine; hip flexed 70° and knee flexed 90°.

**Hand Placement**
Grasp the buoyancy belt with the contralateral (fixed) hand while the ipsilateral (movement) hand grasps the thigh.

**Direction of Movement**
Externally rotate hip with the movement hand as the patient's body lags through water to create stretch force.

### Hip Internal Rotation

**Practitioner Position**
Face the lateral aspect of the involved thigh with the ipsilateral arm under the flexed knee.

**Patient Position**
BS supine, hip flexed 70° and knee flexed 90°.

**Hand Placement**
Stabilize the buoyancy belt with the contralateral (fixed) hand while grasping the thigh with the ipsilateral (movement) hand.

**Direction of Movement**
Internally rotate the hip as the patient's body lags through water to create the stretch force.

### Knee Extension with Patient on Steps

**Practitioner Position**
Half-kneel lateral to the affected knee with the ankle of the affected extremity resting on your thigh.

**Patient Position**
Semi-reclined on pool steps.

**Hand Placement**
Place one hand just proximal and one just distal to the knee joint.

**Direction of Movement**
Extend the patient's knee.

### Knee Flexion with Patient on Steps

**Practitioner Position**
Half-kneel lateral to the affected knee.

**Patient Position**
Semi-reclined on pool steps.

**Hand Placement**
Grasp the distal tibia with the ipsilateral hand; the contralateral hand stabilizes the lateral aspect of affected knee.

**Direction of Movement**
Apply the stretch force into flexion.

### Knee Flexion with Patient Supine (Fig. 9.13)

**Practitioner Position**
Half-kneel lateral to the affected knee with the dorsal aspect of the patient's foot hooked under the ipsilateral thigh.

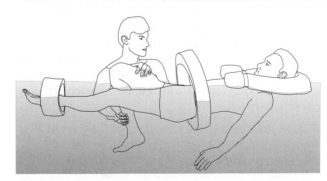

FIGURE 9.13 Hand placement and stabilization for stretching to increase knee flexion.

**Patient Position**
BS supine, affected knee flexed.

**Hand Placement**
Place the ipsilateral (fixed) hand on distal tibia and the contralateral (movement) hand on buoyancy belt to pull the body over the fixed foot.

**Direction of Movement**
Pull the patient's body over the fixed foot, creating the stretch to increase knee flexion. Lower the patient's knee into the water to extend the hip and increase the stretch on the rectus femoris. Perform the motion slowly to limit spinal and pelvic substitution.

### Hamstrings Stretch

**Practitioner Position**
Face the patient and rest the patient's affected extremity on your ipsilateral shoulder.

**Patient Position**
BS supine, knee extended.

**Hand Placement**
Place both hands at distal thigh.

**Direction of Movement**
Start in the squatting position and gradually stand to flex the hip and apply the stretch force. Maintain knee extension by pulling the patient closer and increasing the stretch.

## Self-Stretching with Aquatic Equipment

Often the intervention plan is to instruct the patient to perform independent stretching.* Self-stretching can be performed in either waist-depth or deep water. The patient frequently utilizes the edge of the pool for stabilization in both waist-depth and deep water.

Applying buoyancy devices may assist with stretching and increase the intensity of the aquatic stretch.[60] However, buoyancy devices are not required to achieve buoyancy-assisted stretching. That is, as buoyancy acts on any submersed extremity, correct patient positioning adequately produces a gentle stretch. The following guidelines describe the use of equipment for mechanical stretching; the descriptions apply similarly for use without buoyancy equipment. Providing verbal cueing and visual demonstration for patient positioning and form aids in achieving the desired stretching effects.

Positioning for self-stretching of every body part is not described in this section. Typically, positioning for immersed self-stretches reflects traditional land positioning.

The following terms are used to describe the self-stretching techniques.

- **Patient position**. Includes buoyancy-assisted (seated/upright), buoyancy-supported (supine), or vertical.
- **Buoyancy-assisted**. Using the natural buoyancy of water to "float" the extremity toward the surface.

---

* See references 6, 29, 43, 46, 48, 49, 51, 57, 63.

- **Equipment-assisted.** Includes use of buoyancy devices attached or held distally on an extremity.

The following are some examples of self-stretching.

### Shoulder Flexion and Abduction

**Patient Position**
Upright, neck level immersion.

**Equipment**
Small or large buoyant dumbbell or wrist strap.

**Direction of Movement**
Grasping the buoyant device with the affected extremity allows the extremity to float to the surface as the buoyancy device provides a gentle stretch.

### Hip Flexion (Fig. 9.14)

**Patient Position**
Upright, immersed to waist, or seated at edge of pool/on steps with hips immersed.

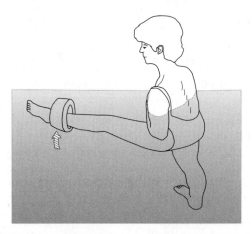

FIGURE 9.14 Self-stretching technique to increase hip flexion (stretch the hamstrings) using aquatic equipment.

**Equipment**
Small buoyant dumbbell or ankle strap. For hip flexion with knee flexion, place strap/dumbbell proximal to the knee. For hip flexion with knee extension (to stretch the hamstrings), place strap/dumbbell at the ankle.

**Direction of Movement**
Allow buoyancy device to float hip into flexion, applying stretch to hip extensors or hamstrings.

### Knee Extension

**Patient Position**
Seated on steps/edge of pool with knee in a position of comfort.

**Equipment**
Small dumbbell or ankle strap.

**Direction of Movement**
Allow buoyancy device to extend knee toward the surface applying stretch to increase knee extension.

### Knee Flexion

**Patient Position**
Stand immersed to waist with hip and knee in neutral position; increasing the amount of hip extension increases the stretch on the two joint knee extensors.

**Equipment**
Small dumbbell or ankle strap.

**Direction of Movement**
Allow buoyancy device to flex the knee toward the surface, applying stretch to knee extensors.

 STRENGTHENING EXERCISES

By reducing joint compression, providing three-dimensional resistance, and dampening perceived pain, immersed strengthening exercises may be safely initiated earlier in the rehabilitation program than traditional land strengthening exercises.[4] Both manual and mechanical immersed strengthening exercises typically are done in waist-depth water. However, some mechanical strengthening exercises may also be performed in deep water. Frequently, immersion alters the mechanics of active motion. For example, the vertical forces of buoyancy support the immersed upper extremity and alter the muscular demands on the shoulder girdle.[60] Furthermore, studies have demonstrated that lower extremity demand is inversely related to the level of immersion during closed-chain strengthening.[25]

## Manual Resistance Exercises

Application of aquatic manual resistance exercises for the extremities typically occurs in a concentric, closed-chain fashion.[5,54] Manual aquatic resistance exercises are designed to fixate the distal segment of the extremity as the patient contracts the designated muscle group(s). The practitioner's hands provide primary fixation and guidance during contraction. As the patient contracts his or her muscles, the body moves over or away from the fixed distal segment (generally over the fixed segment for the lower extremity and away from the fixed segment for the upper extremity). The patient's movement through the viscous water generates resistance; and the patient's body produces the drag forces. Verbal cueing by the practitioner is essential to direct the patient when to contract and when to relax, thereby synchronizing practitioner and patient.

Stabilization of the distal extremity segment is essential for maintaining proper form and isolating desired muscles. However, appropriate stabilization is not possible in the buoyancy-supported supine position for eccentric exercises or rhythmic stabilization of the extremities. The patient's body will have a tendency to tip and rotate in the water. In addition, the practitioner will have difficulty generating adequate resistance force, and the patient's body

will move easily across the surface of the water with minimal drag producing inadequate counterforce to the practitioner's resistance. When supine, some motions, including horizontal shoulder adduction and abduction, should be avoided because of the difficulty the patient may have isolating proper muscle groups. Nevertheless, for many motions, the aquatic environment allows closed-chain resistive training through virtually limitless planes of motion.

The following terms refer to manual resistance exercise in water.

- *Practitioner position.* Describes the orientation of the practitioner to the patient.
- *Patient position.* Buoyancy-supported (BS) in the supine position.
- *Hand placement.* The guide hand is generally the ipsilateral hand as the patient's affected extremity and typically is positioned more proximally. It directs the patient's body as muscles contract to move the body through the water. The resistance hand is generally the contralateral hand and typically is placed at the distal end of the contracting segment. More distal placement increases overall resistance.
- *Direction of movement.* Describes the motion of the patient.

### Shoulder Flexion/Extension (Fig. 9.15 A&B)

**Practitioner Position**
Face caudal, lateral to the patient's affected shoulder.

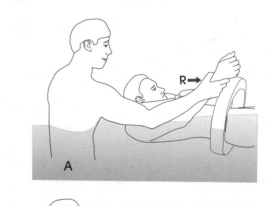

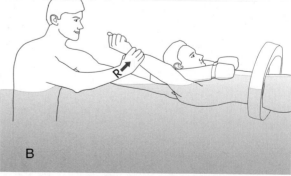

FIGURE 9.15 Manual resistance exercise for strengthening shoulder flexion, (A) start position, and (B) end position.

**Patient Position**
BS supine; affected extremity flexed to 30°.

**Hand Placement**
Place the palmar aspect of the guide hand at the patient's acromioclavicular joint. The resistance hand grasps the distal forearm. An alternative placement for the resistance hand may be the distal humerus; this placement alters muscle recruitment.

**Direction of Movement**
Active shoulder flexion against the resistance hand causes the body to move away from the practitioner. Active shoulder extension from a flexed position causes the body to glide toward the practitioner.

NOTE: The patient must be able to actively flex through 120° for proper resistance to be provided.

### Shoulder Abduction

**Practitioner Position**
Face medially, lateral to the patient's affected extremity.

**Patient Position**
BS supine; affected extremity in neutral.

**Hand Placement**
Place the palmar aspect of guide hand at the proximal humerus as the thumb wraps anteriorly and the fingers wrap posteriorly. Place the resistance hand at the lateral aspect of distal humerus.

**Direction of Movement**
The practitioner determines the amount of external rotation and elbow flexion. Active abduction against the resistance hand causes the body to glide away from the affected extremity and the practitioner.

### Shoulder Internal/External Rotation (Fig. 9.16 A&B)

**Practitioner Position**
Face medially on the lateral side of the patient's affected extremity.

**Patient Position**
BS supine; affected extremity's elbow flexed to 90° with the shoulder in the desired amount of abduction and initial rotation.

**Hand Placement**
Place the palmar aspect of the guide hand at the lateral aspect of the elbow. The resistance hand grasps the palmar aspect of the distal forearm. An alternative method requires the practitioner to "switch" hands. The practitioner's ipsilateral hand becomes the guide hand and grasps the buoyancy belt laterally. The practitioner's contralateral hand becomes the resistance hand, as described above. This approach allows improved stabilization; however, the practitioner loses contact with the patient's elbow and must cue the patient to maintain the desired degree of shoulder abduction during the exercise.

**Direction of Movement**
Active internal rotation by the patient against the resistance hand causes the body to glide toward the affected extremity; active external rotation causes the body to glide away from the affected extremity.

### Unilateral Diagonal Pattern $D_1$ Flexion/Extension of the Upper Extremity

**Practitioner Position**
Stand lateral to the patient's unaffected extremity and face medially and caudally.

**Patient Position**
BS supine; affected extremity internally rotated and pronated with slight forward flexion.

**Hand Placement**
Secure the medial and lateral epicondyles of the distal humerus with the guide hand. Place the resistance hand on the dorsal surface of the distal forearm.

**Direction of Movement**
Prior to contraction, cue the patient to execute the specific joint motions expected in the diagonal patterns. Active contraction through the $D_1$ flexion pattern causes the body to glide away from the practitioner. At the end position of $D_1$, secure the medial and lateral epicondyles of the distal humerus with the guide hand. The resistance hand will be on the palmar aspect of the distal forearm. From the flexed position, the practitioner cues the patient to contract through the $D_1$ extension pattern.

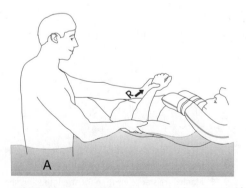
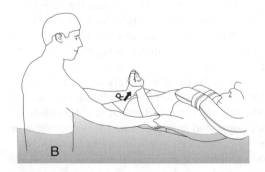

FIGURE 9.16 Manual resistance exercise for strengthening shoulder external rotation, (A) start position, and (B) end position.

## Unilateral Diagonal D₂ Flexion/Extension of the Upper Extremity (Fig. 9.17 A&B)

**Practitioner Position**
Stand lateral to the patient's affected shoulder, face medially and caudally.

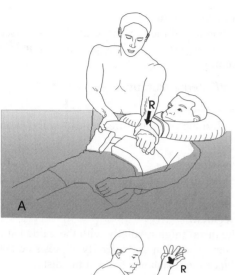

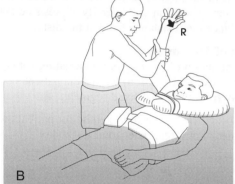

FIGURE 9.17 Manual resistance exercise for upper extremity unilateral diagonal D₂ flexion pattern, (A) start position, and (B) end position.

**Patient Position**
BS supine; affected extremity adducted and internally rotated.

**Hand Placement**
Secure the medial and lateral epicondyles of the distal humerus with the guide hand. Wrap the palmar aspect of the resistance hand on the dorsal wrist medial to the palmar surface.

**Direction of Movement**
Active movement through the D₂ flexion pattern causes the body to glide away from the practitioner. From the fully flexed position, cue the patient to then move into the D₂ extension pattern. This causes the body to glide toward the practitioner.

## Bilateral Diagonal D₂ Flexion/Extension of the Upper Extremities (Fig. 9.18 A&B)

**Practitioner Position**
Stand cephalad to patient, facing caudally.

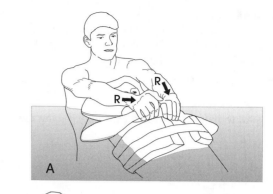

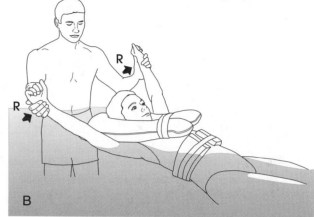

FIGURE 9.18 Manual resistance exercise for upper extremity bilateral diagonal D₂ pattern, (A) start position, and (B) end position.

**Patient Position**
BS supine; upper extremities adducted and internally rotated.

**Hand Placement**
Use both hands to provide resistance. Grasp the dorsal aspect of each of the patient's wrists, wrapping medially to the palmar surface.

**Direction of Motion**
Active contraction through the D₂ flexion pattern causes the body to glide away from the practitioner. From the fully flexed position, cue the patient to contract through D₂ extension, causing the patient to move toward the practitioner.

### Hip Adduction

**Practitioner Position**
Stand lateral to the patient's affected extremity and face medially.

**Patient Position**
BS supine; hip abducted.

**Hand Placement**
Place the guide hand on the buoyancy belt and the resistance hand on the patient's medial thigh.

### Direction of Movement

Active contraction of the hip adductors causes the affected leg to adduct as the contralateral leg and body glides toward the affected leg and the practitioner.

### Hip Abduction (Fig. 9.19)

**Practitioner Position**

Stand lateral to patient's affected extremity, facing medially.

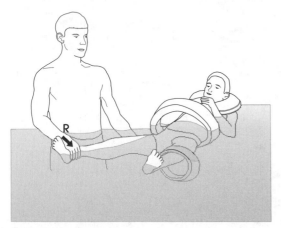

FIGURE 9.19 Manual resistance exercise for strengthening hip abduction with resistance applied to lateral aspect of the leg.

**Patient Position**

BS supine; hip adducted.

**Hand Placement**

Place the guide hand on the buoyancy belt or lateral thigh and the thumb and base of the resistance hand on the patient's lateral leg.

**Direction of Movement**

Active contraction of the hip abductors causes the affected leg to abduct as the contralateral leg and body glides away from the affected leg and the practitioner.

### Hip Flexion with Knee Flexion (Fig. 9.20)

**Practitioner Position**

Stand at the side of the patient's affected extremity, facing cephalad.

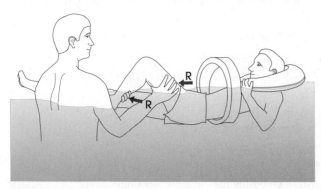

FIGURE 9.20 Manual resistance exercise for strengthening hip and knee flexion.

**Patient Position**

BS supine.

**Hand Placement**

Place the guide hand on the buoyancy belt or lateral hip. The resistance hand grasps proximal to the distal tibiofibular joint.

**Direction of Movement**

Active contraction of the hip and knee flexors causes the patient's body to glide toward the practitioner and fixed distal extremity.

### Hip Internal/External Rotation

**Practitioner Position**

Stand lateral to the patient's affected extremity, facing medially.

**Patient Position**

BS supine; hip in neutral at 0° extension with knee flexed to 90°.

**Hand Placement**

Contact the distal thigh medially with the guide hand for resisted internal rotation and laterally for resisted external rotation. Place the resistance hand at the distal leg.

**Direction of Movement**

Active contraction of hip rotators (alternating between internal and external rotation) causes the patient's body to glide away from the distal fixed segment.

P R E C A U T I O N : Avoid this exercise for patients with possible medial or lateral knee joint instability.

### Knee Extension

**Practitioner Position**

Stand at the patient's feet, facing cephalad.

**Patient Position**

BS supine.

**Hand Placement**

Place the guide hand at the patient's lateral thigh and the resistance hand on the dorsal aspect of the distal tibiofibular joint.

**Direction of Movement**

Active contraction of the quadriceps against the practitioner's resistance hand directs the body away from the practitioner as the knee extends.

### Ankle Motions

**Practitioner Position**

Stand lateral to the affected leg, facing caudally.

**Patient Position**

BS supine.

**Hand Placement**

The hand placement creates a short lever arm at the patient's ankle. As the patient moves through the resisted ankle motions, the patient's entire body moves through the water, producing a significant amount of drag and demand on the ankle complex.

PRECAUTION: For patients with ligamentous laxity and unstable ankles or compromised ankle musculature, the practitioner should cue the patient to avoid maximum effort during contraction to avoid potential injury.

### Ankle Dorsiflexion and Plantarflexion

**Hand Placement**

Place the guide hand on the lateral aspect of the leg and the resistance hand over the dorsal aspect of the foot to resist dorsiflexion and on the plantar aspect to resist plantarflexion.

**Direction of Movement**

The body moves toward the practitioner during dorsiflexion and away from the practitioner during plantarflexion.

### Ankle Inversion and Eversion

**Hand Placement**

Place the guide hand on the lateral aspect of the lower leg during inversion and on the medial aspect of tibia during eversion. To resist inversion grasp the dorsal medial aspect of the foot and to resist eversion grasp the lateral foot.

**Direction of Movement**

During inversion the body glides toward the practitioner, and during eversion the body glide aways from the practitioner.

### Dynamic Trunk Stabilization

By applying concepts utilized for spinal stabilization exercises on land (see Chapters 15 and 16), the practitioner can challenge the dynamic control and strength of the trunk muscles in the aquatic environment. The BS supine position creates a unique perceptual environment for the patient.

◉ *Dynamic trunk stabilization—frontal plane* (Fig. 9.21).

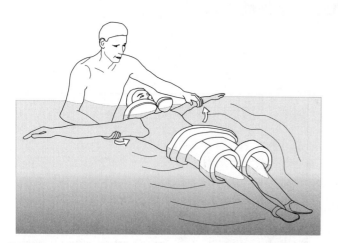

FIGURE 9.21 Isometric trunk stabilization exercise using side to side motions of the trunk.

**Practitioner Position**

Hold the patient at the shoulders or feet.

**Patient Position**

Typically, the patient is placed in a supine position with buoyancy devices at the neck, waist, and legs.

**Execution**

Have the patient identify his or her neutral spine position, perform a "drawing-in maneuver" (see Chapter 16), and maintain the spinal position (isometric abdominal contraction). Move the patient from side to side through the water; monitor and cue the patient to avoid lateral trunk flexion, an indication that the patient is no longer stabilizing the spine.

**Intensity**

Moving the patient through the water faster increases drag and exercise intensity. Holding the patient more distally increases exercise intensity.

◉ *Dynamic trunk stabilization—multidirectional.*

**Practitioner Position**

Stand at the shoulders or feet of the patient and grasp the patient's extremity to provide fixation as the patient contracts.

**Patient Position**

Typically, the patient is placed in a supine position with buoyancy devices at the neck, waist, and legs.

**Execution**

Instruct the patient to assume a neutral spine, perform the drawing-in maneuver, and "hold" the spine stable. Instruct the patient to perform either unilateral or bilateral resisted extremity patterns while maintaining a neutral spine and abdominal control. Monitor and cue the patient to avoid motion at the trunk, an indication that the patient is no longer stabilizing with the deep abdominal and spinal muscles. Upper extremity motions include shoulder flexion, abduction, and diagonal patterns. Lower extremity motions include hip and knee flexion and hip abduction and adduction.

**Intensity**

Unilateral patterns are more demanding than bilateral patterns. Increasing speed or duration increases exercise intensity.

## Independent Strengthening Exercises

Often patients perform immersed strengthening exercises independently. Because the resistance created during movement through water is speed-dependent, patients are able to control the amount of work performed and thedemands imposed on contractile elements.[4,24,51] Typically, positioning and performance of equipment-assisted strengthening activities in water reflect that of traditional land exercise. However, the aquatic environment allows patients to assume many positions (supine, prone, side-lying, seated, vertical). Attention to specific patient positioning allows the practitioner to utilize the buoyant properties of water and/or the buoyant and resistive properties of equipment that can either assist or resist patient movement.[31,34] Before initiating immersed strengthening activities, patients should be oriented to the effects of speed and surface area on resistance. Specific exercises for mechanical strengthening of every body part are not described. Only selected exercises are discussed and illustrated to reinforce major concepts and principles of application.

The following terms are used for equipment-assisted exercise.

- **Buoyancy assisted (BA):** Vertical movement directed parallel to vertical forces of buoyancy that assist motion (patient may use buoyant equipment to assist with motion).

- **Buoyancy supported (BS):** Horizontal movement with vertical forces of buoyancy eliminating or minimizing the need to support an extremity against gravity (patient may use buoyant equipment to assist with motion).
- **Buoyancy resisted (BR):** Movement directed against or perpendicular to vertical forces of buoyancy, creating drag (performed without equipment).
- **Buoyancy superresisted (BSR):** Use of equipment generates resistance by increasing the total surface area moving through water by creating greater drag. Increasing the speed of motion through water generates further drag.

### Extremity Strengthening Exercises (Fig. 9.22 A–E)

The most common aquatic upper and lower extremity strengthening exercises are outlined in Box 9.1.[1,31,34] Typically, patients are positioned standing immersed to shoulder level for upper extremity strengthening and to mid-trunk level for lower extremity strengthening. How-

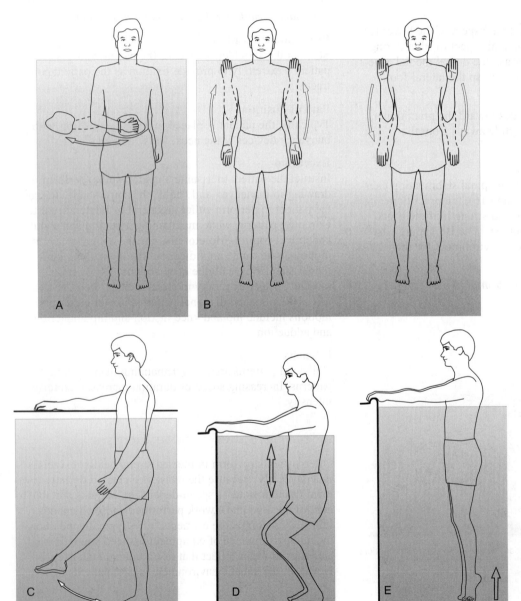

FIGURE 9.22 Mechanical resistance for strengthening (A) shoulder internal and external rotation, (B) elbow flexion and extension, (C) hip flexion and extension, (D) functional squatting, and (E) ankle plantarflexion. *(Adapted from Bates and Hanson.[6])*

| BOX 9.1 | Summary of Motions Used for Upper and Lower Strengthening Exercises |
|---|---|
| **Shoulder** | Flexion/extension |
| | Abduction/adduction |
| | Horizontal abduction/adduction |
| | Internal/external rotation |
| | Unilateral diagonals |
| | Bilateral diagonals |
| **Elbow** | Flexion/extension |
| | Diagonals |
| | Push/pull |
| **Hip** | Flexion/extension |
| | Abduction/adduction |
| | Internal/external rotation |
| | Unilateral diagonals |
| | Bilateral diagonals |
| **Knee** | Flexion/extension |
| | Diagonals |

| BOX 9.2 | Summary of Lumbar Spine-Strengthening Exercises |
|---|---|
| **Standing** | Walking patterns: forward, backward, lateral, lunge walk, high stepping |
| | Unilateral/bilateral stance with upper extremity motions |
| **Semi-reclined** | Bicycling |
| | Hip abduction/adduction |
| | Flutter kick |
| | Bilateral lower extremity PNF patterns |
| | Unilateral/bilateral hip and knee flexion/extension |
| **Supine** | Bridging with long dumbbell placed at knees |
| | Swimming kicks |
| **Prone** | Swimming kicks |
| **Deep water** | Vertical stabilization exercises; abdominal bracing with arm and leg motions in the pike and iron-cross positions |
| | Seated on dumbbell; abdominal bracing and balance while performing unilateral or bilateral arm motions |
| | Standing on a kickboard or dumbbell; abdominal bracing and balance while performing bicycling motions and/or arm motions |

ever, many exercises may be performed with the patient positioned vertically in deep water. The prone or supine position is useful when practitioners wish to progress patients or when patients require position-specific or sports-specific strengthening. Some exercises, most notably bilateral lower extremity diagonals, require the patient to be positioned supine, prone, or vertical in deep water.

## Lumbar Spine Strengthening

Spinal stabilization may be performed in shallow, mid-depth, or deep water levels. Typically, patients are instructed to maintain a neutral spine with the drawing-in maneuver (see Chapter 16) while performing functional activities or moving the extremities. The patient's ability to stabilize the spine can be challenged by increasing the duration of the activity, the speed or surface area moving through water, and by the addition of buoyant devices in the deep water. The exercises are summarized in Box 9.2.

## Trunk-Strengthening Exercises: Standing

● **Walking patterns.** Holding a kickboard vertically in the water increases resistance.
● **Unilateral and bilateral stance during upper extremity motions.** The buoyant and turbulent forces of the water require co-contraction of the trunk muscles to stabilize the immersed body; using equipment (Hydro-tone bells, paddles, resistive tubing) to increase resistance increases the need for co-contraction of the trunk muscles.

## Trunk-Strengthening Exercises: Semi-Reclined

Patients may use noodles, dumbbells, or kickboards for support. The practitioner can further challenge the patient by having him or her hold buoyant equipment, such as paddles, and then stabilize the trunk against the movement. A variety of lower extremity movements are suggested in Box 9.2.

## Trunk-Strengthening Exercises: Supine

Various swimming kicks are used in the supine position. Instruct the patient to concentrate on the drawing-in maneuver and on maintaining the neutral spine position while moving the legs. Bridging while maintaining a neutral spine can be done with a long dumbbell placed at the knees.

## Trunk-Strengthening Exercises: Prone

In the prone position, various swimming kicks, such as the flutter kick, are used while the patient performs the drawing-in maneuver and maintains a neutral spine.

## Trunk-Strengthening Exercises in Deep Water

Stabilization exercises performed in deep water with the patient positioned vertically typically require the patient to brace with the abdominal muscles. Emphasize identifying the neutral spine, activating the drawing-in maneuver, and holding the spine in the stable position while performing the various activities. Utilize any combination of unilateral or bilateral upper and/or lower extremity motions to further challenge the stabilization effort. Add equipment devices to the hands or legs for additional resistance and increased challenge when the patient can maintain good stabilization control. Variations include:

● Altering trunk positions such as the pike position or the iron-cross position.
● Sitting on a dumbbell and bicycling forward or backward or moving the upper extremities through any combination of motions.

◉ Standing on a kickboard or dumbbell and moving the upper extremities through various combinations of motions, first without then with equipment. Such standing activities typically induce obligatory abdominal bracing and challenges to balance.

# ◯ AEROBIC CONDITIONING

Aquatic exercise that emphasizes aerobic/cardiovascular conditioning can be an integral component of many rehabilitation programs. Aerobic/cardiovascular exercise typically takes place with the patient suspended vertically in deep water pools without the feet touching the pool bottom. Alternative activities that may be performed in mid-level water, 4 to 6 feet in depth, include jogging, swimming strokes, immersed cycling, and immersed treadmill. Understanding the various treatment options, physiological responses, monitoring methods, proper form, and equipment selection allows the clinician to use this form of exercise effectively and safely in a rehabilitation program.

## Treatment Interventions

*Deep-water walking/running (Fig. 9.23).* Deep water walking and running are the most common vertical deep-water cardiovascular endurance exercises. Alternatives include cross-country motions and high-knee marching. Deep-water cardiovascular training, which may be used as a precursor to mid-water or land-based cardiovascular training, eliminates the effects of impact on the lower extremities and spine.

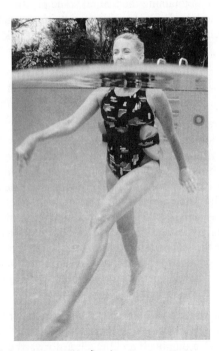

FIGURE 9.23 Deep water walking/jogging. *(Courtesy of Rothhammer International Inc. San Luis Obispo, CA.)*

The patient can be tethered to the edge of the pool to perform deep-water running in those pools with limited space. Some small tanks provide resistance jets for the patient to move against.

*Mid-water jogging/running (immersed treadmill running).* Mid-water aerobic exercise, which may be used as a precursor to land training, lessens the effects of impact on the spine and lower extremities. As a patient's tolerance to impact improves, mid-water jogging may be performed in progressively shallower depths to provide increased weight bearing and functional replication. In pools with limited space, tethering with resistive tubing can provide resistance.

*Immersed equipment.* Immersed equipment includes an immersed cycle, treadmill, or upper body ergometer.

*Swimming strokes.* For patients able to tolerate the positions necessary to perform various swim strokes (neck and shoulder ROM and prone, supine, or side-lying positions), swimming can be an excellent tool to train and improve cardiovascular fitness. Swimming may elicit significantly higher elevations of heart rate, blood pressure, and $\dot{V}O_{2max}$ than other aquatic activities. Swimming contributes the added benefit of hip and trunk strengthening for some patients with spinal conditions.

PRECAUTION: Recommending swimming for poorly skilled swimmers with cardiac compromise may adversely challenge the patient's cardiovascular system.

## Physiological Response to Deep–Water Walking/Running

Various physiological responses to deep-water walking and running have been reported.[*]

### Cardiovascular Response
Patients without cardiovascular compromise may experience dampened elevation of heart rate, ventilation, and $\dot{V}O_{2max}$ compared to similar land-based exercise. During low-intensity exercise, cardiac patients may experience lower cardiovascular stresses.[22,23] As exercise intensity increases, cardiovascular stresses approach those of related exercise on land.[23,35]

### Training Effect
Patients experience carryover gains in $\dot{V}O_{2max}$ from aquatic to land conditions.[45] Additionally, aquatic cardiovascular training maintains leg strength and maximum oxygen consumption in healthy runners.[33,45,58,60]

## Proper Form for Deep–Water Running

### Instruction for Beginners
Proper instruction is important to ensure correct form because many beginners experience a significant learning curve.[8] Once immersed, the patient should maintain a neu-

---

[*] See references 3, 10, 12, 13, 15, 21, 27, 33, 55, 58.

tral cervical spine and slightly forward flexed trunk with the arms at the sides. During running the hips should alternately flex to approximately 80° with the knee extended and then extend to neutral as the knee flexes.

### Accommodating Specific Patient Populations

For patients with positional pain associated with spinal conditions, a posterior buoyancy belt helps maintain a slightly forward flexed position, and a flotation vest helps maintain more erect posture and a relatively extended spine. Patients with unilateral lower extremity amputations may have difficulty maintaining a vertical position. Placing the buoyancy belt laterally (on the contralateral side of the amputation) allows the patient to remain vertical more easily.

## Exercise Monitoring

### Monitoring Intensity of Exercise

- *Rate of perceived exertion.* Because skill may affect technique, subjective numerical scales depicting perceived effort may inadequately identify the level of intensity for novice deep-water runners. However, at both submaximal and maximal levels of exertion, subjective numerical rating of effort appears to correlate adequately with the heart rate during immersed exercise.[10,13,26,33]

- *Heart rate.* Because of the physiological changes that occur with neck level immersion, various adjustments have been suggested in the literature to lower the immersed maximum heart rate during near-maximum cardiovascular exercise.[12,13,17,50,60] The suggested decreases range from 7 to 20 beats per minute.[17,50,60] The immersed heart rate can be reliably monitored manually or with water-resistant electronic monitoring devices.

### Monitoring Beginners

Care should be taken to monitor regularly the cardiovascular response of novice deep-water runners or patients with known cardiac, pulmonary, or peripheral vascular disease. Novice deep-water runners may experience higher levels of perceived exertion and $\dot{V}O_{2max}$ than they would during similar land exercise.[26]

## Equipment Selection

### Deep Water Equipment

Selection of buoyancy devices should reflect the desired patient posture, comfort, and projected intensity level. The most common buoyant device for deep-water running is the flotation belt positioned posteriorly (see Fig. 9.5). Patients presenting with injuries or sensitivity of the trunk may require an alternative buoyant device, such as vests, flotation dumbbells, or noodles. Providing the patient with smaller buoyant equipment (i.e., smaller belts, fewer noodles) requires the patient to work harder to maintain adequate buoyancy, thereby increasing the intensity of the activity. Fins and specially designed boots can be applied to the legs and feet to add resistance. Also, bells or buoyant dumbbells can be held in the hands to increase resistance (see Fig. 9.8).

### Midwater Equipment

Specially designed socks can help eliminate the potential problem of skin breakdown on the feet during impact activities, such as running. Patients can run against a forced current or tethered with elastic tubing for resistance. Using noodles around the waist or running while holding a kickboard increases the amount of drag and resistance against which the patient must move.

## INDEPENDENT LEARNING ACTIVITIES

### ● Case Studies

POSTOPERATIVE ARTHROSCOPIC KNEE MENISCECTOMY
Mike is a 54-year-old man who tore his right medial meniscus playing basketball. He is 2 weeks status post-arthroscopic débridement of the torn piece of cartilage. Mike has returned to his desk job as a computer programmer but has a strong desire to return to his active workout schedule and weekend sports leagues. The surgeon has told Mike that he has no limitations except pain.
**Past Medical History:** Mike is healthy with no prior medical problems. He has never had an injury that made him miss more than a few days of sports participation.
**Functional Status:** Mike is ambulating without assistive devices, but he limps slightly because of a stiff knee. He is able to go up and down stairs but only one step at a time and has to lead with his left leg.
**Musculoskeletal Status:** Mike has only minimal swelling of the right knee. He rates his pain as a 1 out of 10 at rest and a 3 out of 10 with activity. His active knee ROM is 5°

to 100°. He has normal ROM in the remaining joints of the right leg. Mike is able to perform a straight leg raise and has good quadriceps contraction. Manual muscle testing reveals 4/5 quadriceps strength, 4/5 hamstring and gastrocsoleus strength. He has good patellofemoral joint mobility.
**Physician Referral:** The prescription Mike's physician gave him states "Evaluate and treat right knee, S/P arthroscopic meniscal débridement; may utilize land and aquatic exercise for ROM and strength."

- Formalize a program to utilize the shallow water (4-ft depth) to start Mike with independent exercises for strength and flexibility.
- Describe what manual techniques you might be able to perform with Mike for strength or flexibility.
- As Mike progresses to full ROM and near-normal strength, how could you use aquatics to replicate the demands of basketball?
- What can Mike do in the pool to maintain his cardiovascular fitness while his knee heals?

## CALF TEAR

Cecily is a 30-year-old weather anchor who happens to be an elite marathon runner. Four days ago she was running up a hill and felt a "pulling" in her left calf just distal to the knee. She decided to run in a 10K marathon the next day but had to quit after about 5K because of a sharp pain in her calf. The doctor has told her to use crutches and remain 25% weight bearing for the next 3 days. After that she can gradually begin to increase the weight she puts through the leg over the next week. The doctor has told Cecily that she should be full weight bearing in 1 week and able to run in 3 weeks. Cecily is anxious to return to her intensive training schedule.

**Past Medical History:** Cecily is healthy with no prior medical problems. She has worn orthotic inserts in her shoes for "flat feet" for as long as she can remember. She says she has pulled her left calf several times during a running career that goes back to high school.

**Functional Status:** Cecily enters the facility ambulating with crutches. She is putting about 25% of her weight through her left foot. She is able to perform stairs without difficulty using the crutches and/or a railing.

**Musculoskeletal Status:** Cecily has a visible bruise at the medial head of the left gastrocnemius muscle belly. She is very tender to palpation there and has some swelling. She rates her pain at rest as 1 on a 10-point scale and her pain with activity as 2. Her ankle ROM is normal for all motions actively and passively with the exception of dorsiflexion. She dorsiflexes actively 5° and passively 8°. You grade her ankle strength as 5/5 except for plantarflexion, which you grade as a 4–/5; this may be limited due to pain. You also notice that her left hip flexors, quadriceps, and hamstrings are all tight.

**Physician Referral:** The prescription that Cecily's doctor gives her states "Aquatic therapy; evaluate and treat for left calf strain: gait training, ROM, strength. Progress to land as tolerated."

- Write up a program to address Cecily's dysfunctions and impairments utilizing the aquatic environment.
- At what depth of mid-water does Cecily need to be to gait train in the water and still maintain 25% weight bearing?
- Write up a program for the deep water to help Cecily maintain her high level of cardiovascular fitness.
- What equipment might be useful to assist her with independent stretching in the deep water and for cardiovascular training in the deep water?

## CHRONIC LOW BACK PAIN

Develop an aquatic program for a patient who has chronic low back pain and needs a comprehensive flexibility and strengthening program for the legs and trunk. The patient has only one visit approved by the insurance company. However, the patient has a pool in his or her back yard that gradually goes from 3 feet to 7 feet in depth. The 7-foot deep area is only 10 feet long and 5 feet wide. The patient has no other medical problems that would limit his or her performance of the aquatic program.

# REFERENCES

1. Abidin, MR, et al: Hydrofitness devices for strengthening upper extremity muscles. J Burn Care Rehabil 9:199, 1988.
2. Arborelius, M, Balldin, UI, et al: Hemodynamic changes in man during immersion with the head above water. Aerospace Med 43:592, 1972.
3. Avellini, BA, Shapiro, Y, Pandolf, KB: Cardio-respiratory physical training in water and on land. Eur J Appl Physiol 50:255, 1983.
4. Babb, R, Muntzer, E: Hydrotherapy: whirlpools to aquatic pools. In: Michlovitz SL (ed) Thermal Agents In Rehabilitation. FA Davis, Philadelphia, 1990.
5. Babb, R, Simelson-Warr, A: Manual techniques of the lower extremities in aquatic physical therapy. J Aquatic Phys Ther 4(2):7, 1996.
6. Bates, A, Hanson, N: Aquatic Exercise Therapy: A Comprehensive Approach to Use of Aquatic Exercise in Treatment of Orthopedic Injuries. Swystun & Swystun, British Columbia, Canada, 1992.
7. Bazett, HC, Maxfield, ME, Blithe, MD: Effect of baths at different temperature on oxygen exchange and on the circulation. Am J Physiol 119:93, 1938.
8. Becker, BE, Cole, AJ (eds): Comprehensive Aquatic Therapy. Butterworth-Heinemann, London, 1997.
9. Begin, R, Epstein, M, Sackner, MA, et al: Effects of water immersion to the neck on pulmonary circulation and tissue volume in man. J Appl Physiol 60:293, 1976.
10. Brennan, DK, Michaud, TJ, et al: Gains in aquarunning peak oxygen consumption after eight weeks of aqua run training (abstract). Med Sci Sports Exerc 24:S23, 1992.
11. Bullard, RW, Rapp, GM: Problems of body heat loss in water immersion. Aerospace Med 41:1269, 1970.
12. Butts, NK, Tucker, M, Greening, C: Physiologic responses to maximal treadmill and deep water running in men and women. Am J Sports Med 19:612, 1991.
13. Butts, NK, Tucker, M, Smith, R: Maximal responses to treadmill and deep water running in high school female cross country runners. Res Q Exerc Sport 62:236, 1991.
14. Campion, M: Hydrotherapy: Principles and Management. Butterworth-Heinemann, London, 1997.
15. Cassady, SL, Neilsen, DH: Cardiorespiratory responses to calisthenics performed with upper and lower extremities on land and in water at given cadences. Phys Ther 72:532, 1992.
16. Choukroun, ML, Varene, P: Adjustments in oxygen transport during head-out immersion in water at different temperatures. J Appl Physiol 68:1475, 1990.
17. Christie, JL, et al: Cardiovascular regulation during head-out immersion exercise. J Appl Physiol 69:657, 1990.
18. Croce, P, Gregg, JR: Keeping fit when injured. Clin Sports Med 10:181, 1991.
19. Duffield, MH, Skinner, AT, Thompson, AM: Duffield's Exercise In Water. Bailliere Tindall, London, 1983.
20. Egan, S: Reduction of anxiety in aquaphobics. Can J Appl Sports Sci 6:68, 1981.
21. Evans, FW, Cureton, KJ, Purvis, JW: Metabolic and circulatory responses to walking and jogging in water. Res Q Exerc Sport 49:442, 1987.
22. Fernhall, B, Congdon, K, Manfredi, T: ECG response to water and land based exercise in patients with cardiovascular disease. J Cardiopulm Rehabil 10:5, 1990.
23. Fernhall, B, Manfredi, TG, Congdon, K: Prescribing water-based exercise from treadmill and arm ergometry in cardiac patients. Med Sci Sports Exerc 24:139, 1992.
24. Frey Law, LA, Smidt, GL: Underwater forces produced by the Hydro-Tone bell. J Orthop Sports Phys Ther 23:267, 1996.
25. Fuller, RA, Dye, KK, Cook, NR, Awbrey, BJ. The activity levels of the vastus medialis oblique muscle during a single leg squat on the land and at varied water depths. J Aquatic Phys Ther 7(1):13, 1999.

26. Gehring, M, Keller, B, Brehm, B: Physiological responses to deep water running in competitive and non-competitive runners (abstract). Med Sci Sports Exerc 24:S23, 1992.
27. Gleim, GW, Nicholas, JA: Metabolic costs and heart rate responses to treadmill walking in water at different depths and temperatures. Am J Sports Med 17:248, 1989.
28. Golland, A: Basic hydrotherapy. Physiotherapy 67(9):258, 1981.
29. Green, J, et al: Home exercises are as effective as outpatient hydrotherapy for osteoarthritis of the hip. Br J Rheumatol 32:812, 1993.
30. Hall, J, Skevington, SM, et al: A randomized and controlled trial of hydrotherapy in rheumatoid arthritis. Arthritis Care Res 9(3):206, 1996.
31. Harrison, RA: A quantitative approach to strengthening exercises in the hydrotherapy pool. Physiotherapy 65:60, 1980.
32. Harrison, RA: Tolerance of pool therapy by ankylosing spondylitis patients with low vital capacities. Physiotherapy 67:296, 1981.
33. Hertler, L, Provost-Craig, M, Sestili, D, et al: Water running and the maintenance of maximal oxygen consumption and leg strength in runners (abstract). Med Sci Sports Exerc 24:S23, 1992.
34. Hillman, MR, Matthews, L, Pope, JM: The resistance to motion through water created with hydrotherapy table-tennis bats. Physiotherapy 73:570, 1987.
35. Johnson, BK, Adamcyk, J, Stromme, SG, Tennoe, KO: Comparison of oxygen uptake and heart rate during exercises on land and in water. Phys Ther 57:3, 1977.
36. Kelsey, DD, Tyson, E: A new method of training for the lower extremity using unloading. J Orthop Sports Phys Ther 19(4):218, 1994.
37. Kolb, ME: Principles of underwater exercise. Phys Ther Rev 37:361, 1957.
38. Lawson, GE: An overview of aquatic rehabilitation therapy. Top Clin Chiro 3(9):82, 1996.
39. Langridge, JC, Phillips, D: Group hydrotherapy exercises for chronic low back pain sufferers. Physiotherapy 74:269, 1988.
40. LeFort, SM, Hannah, TE: Return to work following an aquafitness and muscle strengthening program for the low back injured. Arch Phys Med Rehabil 75:1247, 1994.
41. Levine, BA: Use of hydrotherapy in reduction of anxiety. Psychol Rep 55:226, 1984.
42. Mano, T, Iwase, S, Yamazaki, Y, Saito, M: Sympathetic nervous adjustments in man to simulated weightlessness induced by water immersion. Sngyo Ika Daigaku Zasshi 7(Suppl):215, 1985.
43. McGrath, AM, Johnson, AS, Moeller, JM: The effects of hamstring stretching on land versus water (abstract). Phys Ther 73(6):S30, 1993.
44. McMurray, RG, Fieselman, CC, et al: Exercise hemodynamics in water and on land in patients with coronary artery disease. J Cardiopulm Rehabil 8:69, 1988.

45. Michaud, TL, Brennan, DK, et al: Aquarun training and changes in treadmill running maximal oxygen consumption (abstract). Med Sci Sports Exerc 24:S23, 1992.
46. Norton, CO, Shaha, S, Stewart, L: Aquatic versus traditional therapy: contrasting effectiveness for acquisition rates (abstract). Phys Ther 73(6):S10, 1993.
47. Perk, J, Perk, L, Boden, C: Cardiopulmonary adaptation of COPD patient to physical training on land and in water. Eur Respir J 9:248, 1996.
48. Prins, J, Cutner, D: Aquatic therapies in the rehabilitation of athletic injuries. Clin Sports Med 18(2):447, 1999.
49. Revay, S, Dahlstrom, M, Dalen, N: Water exercise versus instruction for self-training following a shoulder fracture. Int J Rehabil Res 15, 1992.
50. Ritchie, SE, Hopkins, WG: The intensity of exercise in deep-water running. Int J Sports Med 12:27, 1991.
51. Ruoti, RG, Morris, DM, Cole, AJ: Aquatic Rehabilitation. Lippincott, Philadelphia, 1997.
52. Ruoti, RG, Troup, JT, Berger, RA: The effects of nonswimming water exercise on older adults. J Orthop Sports Phys Ther 19(3):140, 1994.
53. Sagawas, S, et al: Water temperature and intensity of exercise in maintenance of thermal equilibrium. J Appl Physiol 65:2413, 1988.
54. Schrepfer, R, Babb, R: Manual techniques of the shoulder in aquatic physical therapy. J Aquatic Phys Ther 6(1):11, 1998.
55. Sheldahl, LM, Clifford, PS, et al: Effects of head-out water immersion on response to exercise training. J Appl Physiol 60:1878, 1986.
56. Simmons, V, Hansen, PD: Effectiveness of water exercise on postural mobility in the well elderly: an experimental study on balance enhancement. J Gerontol 51A:M233, 1996.
57. Speer, KP, Cavanaugh, JT, et al: A role for hydrotherapy in shoulder rehabilitation. Am J Sports Med 21(6):850,1993.
58. Svendenhag, J, Seger, J: Running on land and in water: comparative exercise physiology. Med Sci Sports Exerc 24:1155, 1992.
59. Templeton, MS, Booth, DL, O'Kelly, WD: Effects of aquatic therapy on joint flexibility and functional ability in subjects with rheumatic disease. J Orthop Sports Phys Ther 6:376, 1996.
60. Thein, JM, Brody, LT: Aquatic-based rehabilitation and training for the elite athlete. J Orthop Sports Phys Ther 27(1):32, 1998.
61. Tovin, BJ, Wolf, SL, et al: Comparison of the effects of exercise in water and on land on the rehabilitation of patients with intra-articular anterior cruciate ligament reconstructions. Phys Ther 74:710, 1994.
62. Whitlach, S, Adema, R: Functional benefits of a structured hot water group exercise program. Activities Adaptation Aging 20(3):75, 1996.
63. Woods, DA: Rehabilitation aquatics for low back injury: functional gains or pain reduction. Clin Kinesth 43:96, 1989.

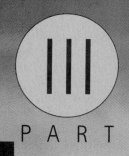

# Principles of Intervention

## III
### PART

# 10

**CHAPTER**

# Soft Tissue Injury, Repair, and Management

The proper use of therapeutic exercise in the management of musculoskeletal disorders depends on determining the impairments, functional limitations, or disabilities. In many cases it is possible to identify the musculoskeletal structure involved and its stage of inflammation or recovery. Examination of the involved region is an important prerequisite for identifying the anatomical structure or structures that are causing the impairments and limiting function and also for determining whether the tissue is in the acute, subacute, or chronic stage of recovery. This chapter and subsequent chapters in this book have been written with the assumption that the reader has a background in examination, evaluation, and program planning to be able to assess impairments and develop functional goals. Utilizing the principles presented in this chapter, the reader should be able to design therapeutic exercise programs that meet the goals and choose techniques for intervention that are at an appropriate intensity for the stage of healing of connective tissue disorders. Subsequent chapters in this section deal with specific joint, soft tissue, bony, and nerve lesions as well as common surgical interventions.

## ◉ SOFT TISSUE LESIONS

### Examples of Soft Tissue Lesions– Musculoskeletal Disorders

◉ **Strain:** Overstretching, overexertion, overuse of soft tissue. Tends to be less severe than a sprain. Occurs from slight trauma or unaccustomed repeated trauma of a minor degree.[6] This term is frequently used to refer specifically to some degree of disruption of the musculotendinous unit.[13]

- **Sprain:** Severe stress, stretch, or tear of soft tissues, such as joint capsule, ligament, tendon, or muscle. This term is frequently used to refer specifically to injury of a ligament and is graded as first- (mild), second- (moderate), or third- (severe) degree sprain.[13]
- **Dislocation:** Displacement of a part, usually the bony partners in a joint resulting in loss of the anatomical relationship and leading to soft tissue damage, inflammation, pain, and muscle spasm.
- **Subluxation:** An incomplete or partial dislocation of the bony partners in a joint that often involves secondary trauma to surrounding soft tissue.
- **Muscle/tendon rupture or tear:** If a rupture or tear is partial, pain is experienced in the region of the breach when the muscle is stretched or when it contracts against resistance. If a rupture or tear is complete, the muscle does not pull against the injury, so stretching or contraction of the muscle does not cause pain.[8]
- **Tendinous lesions/tendinopathy:** *Tenosynovitis* is inflammation of the synovial membrane covering a tendon. *Tendinitis* is inflammation of a tendon; there may be resulting scarring or calcium deposits. *Tenovaginitis* is inflammation with thickening of a tendon sheath. *Tendinosis* is degeneration of the tendon due to repetitive microtrauma.
- **Synovitis:** Inflammation of a synovial membrane; an excess of normal synovial fluid in a joint or tendon sheath caused by trauma or disease.
- **Hemarthrosis:** Bleeding into a joint, usually due to severe trauma.
- **Ganglion:** Ballooning of the wall of a joint capsule or tendon sheath. Ganglia may arise after trauma, and they sometimes occur with rheumatoid arthritis.
- **Bursitis:** Inflammation of a bursa.
- **Contusion:** Bruising from a direct blow, resulting in capillary rupture, bleeding, edema, and an inflammatory response.
- **Overuse syndromes, cumulative trauma disorders, repetitive strain injury:** Repeated, submaximal overload and/or frictional wear to a muscle or tendon resulting in inflammation and pain.

## Clinical Conditions Resulting from Trauma or Pathology

In many conditions involving soft tissue, the primary pathology is difficult to define or the tissue has healed with limitations, resulting in secondary loss of function. The following are examples of clinical manifestations resulting from a variety of causes, including those listed under the previous section.

- **Dysfunction:** Loss of normal function of a tissue or region. The dysfunction may be caused by adaptive shortening of the soft tissues, adhesions, muscle weakness, or any condition resulting in loss of normal mobility.
- **Joint dysfunction:** Mechanical loss of normal joint play in synovial joints; commonly causes loss of function and

pain. Precipitating factors may be trauma, immobilization, disuse, aging, or a serious pathological condition.[24]
- **Contractures:** Adaptive shortening of skin, fascia, muscle, or a joint capsule that prevents normal mobility or flexibility of that structure.
- **Adhesions:** Abnormal adherence of collagen fibers to surrounding structures during immobilization, after trauma, or as a complication of surgery, which restricts normal elasticity and gliding of the structures involved.
- **Reflex muscle guarding:** Prolonged contraction of a muscle in response to a painful stimulus. The primary pain-causing lesion may be in nearby or underlying tissue, or it may be a referred pain source. When not referred, the contracting muscle functionally splints the injured tissue against movement. Guarding ceases when the painful stimulus is relieved.
- **Intrinsic muscle spasm:** Prolonged contraction of a muscle in response to the local circulatory and metabolic changes that occur when a muscle is in a continued state of contraction. Pain is a result of the altered circulatory and metabolic environment, so the muscle contraction becomes self-perpetuating regardless of whether the primary lesion that caused the initial guarding is still irritable (Fig. 10.1). Spasm may also be a response of muscle to viral infection, cold, prolonged periods of immobilization, emotional tension, or direct trauma to muscle.[24]
- **Muscle weakness:** A decrease in the strength of muscle contraction. Muscle weakness may be the result of a systemic, chemical, or local lesion of a nerve of the central or peripheral nervous system or the myoneural junction. It may also be the result of a direct insult to the muscle or simply due to inactivity.
- **Myofascial compartment syndromes:** Increased interstitial pressure in a closed, nonexpanding, myofascial compartment that compromises the function of the blood vessels, muscles, and nerves. It results in ischemia and irreversible muscle loss if there is no intervention.[4] Causes include, but are not limited to, fractures, repetitive trauma, crush injuries, skeletal traction, and restrictive clothing, wraps, or casts.

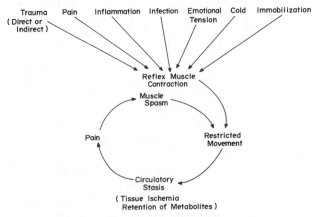

FIGURE 10.1 Self-perpetuating cycle of muscle spasm.

| TABLE 10.1 | Characteristics and Clinical Signs of the Stages of Inflammation, Repair, and Maturation of Tissue | | |
|---|---|---|---|
| **Acute Stage: Inflammatory Reaction** | | **Subacute Stage: Repair and Healing** | **Chronic Stage: Maturation and Remodeling** |

**Characteristics**

| Acute Stage | Subacute Stage | Chronic Stage |
|---|---|---|
| Vascular changes | Removal of noxious stimuli | Maturation of connective tissue |
| Exudation of cells and chemicals | Growth of capillary beds into area | Contracture of scar tissue |
| Clot formation | Collagen formation | Remodeling of scar |
| Phagocytosis, neutralization of irritants | Granulation tissue | Collagen aligns to stress |
| Early fibroblastic activity | Very fragile, easily injured tissue | |

**Clinical signs**

| Acute Stage | Subacute Stage | Chronic Stage |
|---|---|---|
| Inflammation | Decreasing inflammation | Absence of inflammation |
| Pain before tissue resistance | Pain synchronous with tissue resistance | Pain after tissue resistance |

**Physical therapy intervention**

| PROTECTION PHASE | CONTROLLED-MOTION PHASE | RETURN-TO-FUNCTION PHASE |
|---|---|---|
| Control effects of inflammation Modalities | Promote healing; develop mobile scar | Increase strength and alignment of scar; develop functional independence |
| Selective rest/immobilization | Nondestructive active, resistive, open- and closed-chain stabilization, and muscular endurance exercises, carefully progressed in intensity and range | Progressive stretching, strengthening, endurance training, functional exercises, and specificity drills |
| Promote early healing and prevent deleterious effects of rest | | |
| Passive movement, massage, and muscle setting with caution | | |

## Severity of Tissue Injury

● *Grade 1 (first-degree)*. Mild pain at the time of injury or within the first 24 hours. Mild swelling, local tenderness, and pain occur when the tissue is stressed.[13,14]

● *Grade 2 (second-degree)*. Moderate pain that requires stopping the activity. Stress and palpation of the tissue greatly increase the pain. When the injury is to ligaments, some of the fibers are torn, resulting in some increased joint mobility.[13,14]

● *Grade 3 (third-degree)*. Near-complete or complete tear or avulsion of the tissue (tendon or ligament) with severe pain. Stress to the tissue is usually painless; palpation may reveal the defect. A torn ligament results in instability of the joint.[13,14]

## Irritability of Tissue: Stages of Inflammation and Repair

After any insult to connective tissue, whether it is from mechanical injury (including surgery) or chemical irritant, the vascular and cellular response is similar (Table 10.1).[5] Tissue irritability, or sensitivity, is the result of these responses and is usually divided into three stages of inflammation and repair with the following clinical signs and symptoms.

### Acute Stage (Inflammatory Reaction)

During the acute stage, the signs of inflammation are present; they are swelling, redness, heat, pain at rest, and loss of function. When testing the range of motion (ROM),

movement is painful, and the patient usually guards against the motion before completion of the range is possible (Fig. 10.2A). The pain and impaired movement are from the altered chemical state that irritates the nerve endings, increased tissue tension due to edema or joint effusion, and muscle guarding, which is the body's way of immobilizing a painful area. This stage usually lasts 4 to 6 days unless the insult is perpetuated.

### Subacute Stage (Repair and Healing)

During the subacute stage, the signs of inflammation progressively decrease and eventually are absent. When testing ROM, the patient may experience pain synchronous with encountering tissue resistance at the end of the available ROM (Fig. 10.2B). Pain occurs only when the newly developing tissue is stressed beyond its tolerance or when tight tissue is stressed. Muscles may test weak, and function is limited as a result of the weakened tissue. This stage usually lasts 10 to 17 days (14 to 21 days after the onset of injury) but may last up to 6 weeks in some tissues with limited circulation, such as tendons.[9]

### Chronic Stage (Maturation and Remodeling)

There are no signs of inflammation during the chronic stage. There may be contractures or adhesions that limit range, and there may be muscle weakness limiting normal function. Connective tissue continues to strengthen and remodel during this stage. A stretch pain may be felt when testing tight structures at the end of their available range (Fig. 10.2C). Function may be limited by muscle weakness, poor endurance, or poor neuromuscular control.

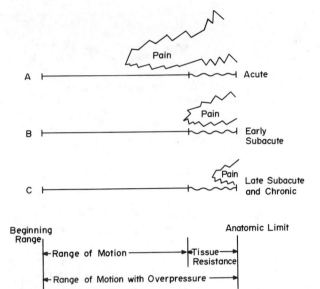

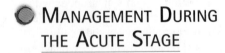

FIGURE 10.2 Pain experienced with ROM when involved tissue is in the (A) acute stage, (B) early subacute stage, and (C) late subacute or chronic stage.

This stage may last 6 months to 1 year depending on the tissue involved and amount of tissue damage.

### Chronic Inflammation (Overuse Syndrome)

An overuse syndrome is a state of prolonged inflammation. There are symptoms of increased pain, swelling, and muscle guarding that last more than several hours after activity. There are also increased feelings of stiffness after rest, loss of ROM 24 hours after activity, and progressively greater stiffness of the tissue as long as the irritation persists.

### Chronic Pain Syndrome

Chronic pain syndrome is a state that persists longer than 6 months. It includes pain that cannot be linked to a source of irritation or inflammation and functional limitations and disability that include physical, emotional, and psychosocial parameters.

## ● MANAGEMENT DURING THE ACUTE STAGE

### Tissue Response—Inflammation

The inflammation stage involves cellular, vascular, and chemical responses in the tissue. During the first 48 hours after insult to soft tissue, vascular changes predominate. Exudation of cells and solutes from the blood vessels takes place, and clot formation occurs. During this period, neutralization of the chemical irritants or noxious stimuli, phagocytosis (cleaning up of dead tissue), early fibroblastic activity, and formation of new capillary beds begin. These physiological processes serve as a protective mechanism as well as a stimulus for subsequent healing and repair.[5] Usually this stage lasts 4 to 6 days unless the insult is perpetuated.

## Management Guidelines—Protection Phase

The therapist's role during the protection phase of intervention is to control the effects of the inflammation, facilitate wound healing, and maintain normal function in unaffected tissues and body regions. The information provided here is summarized in Box 10.1.

### Patient Education

Inform the patient about the expected duration of symptoms (4 to 6 days), what he or she can do during this stage, any precautions or contraindications, and what to expect when the symptoms lessen. Patients need reassurance that the acute symptoms are usually short-lived, and they need to learn what is safe to do during this stage of healing.

### Protection of the Injured Tissue

To minimize musculoskeletal pain and promote healing, protection of the part affected by the inflammatory process is necessary during the first 24 to 48 hours. This is usually provided by rest (splint, tape, cast), cold (ice), compression, and elevation. Depending on the type and severity of the injury, manual methods of pain and edema control, such as massage and gentle (grade I) joint oscillations, may be beneficial. Depending on the part involved, protection with assistive devices for ambulation may be required.

### Prevention of Adverse Effects of Immobility

Complete or continuous immobilization should be avoided whenever possible as it can lead to adherence of the developing fibrils to surrounding tissue, weakening of connective tissue, and changes in articular cartilage.[8,20,21,24]

The *long-term goal of treatment* is the formation of a strong, mobile scar at the site of the lesion so there is complete and painless restoration of function. Initially, the network of fibril formation is random. It acquires an organized arrangement depending on the mechanical forces acting on the tissue. To influence the development of an organized scar, begin treatment during the acute stage, when tolerated, with carefully controlled *passive movements*.

*Tissue-specific movement.* Tissue-specific movements should be directed to the structure involved to prevent abnormal adherence of the developing fibrils to surrounding tissue and thus avoid future disruption of the scar. Tissue-specific techniques are described below.

*Intensity.* The intensity (dosage) of movement should be gentle enough so the fibrils are not detached from the site of healing. Too much movement too soon is painful and reinjures the tissue. The dosage of passive movement depends on the severity of the lesion. Some patients tolerate no movement during the first 24 to 48 hours; others tolerate only a few degrees of gentle passive movement. Continuous passive movement (CPM) (see Chapter 3) has been useful immediately after various types of surgery to joints; intra-articular, metaphyseal, and diaphyseal fractures; surgical release of extra-articular contractures and adhesions; and other selected conditions.[20,21] Any movement tolerated at this stage is beneficial, but it must *not*

## BOX 10.1
## MANAGEMENT GUIDELINES—Acute Stage/Protection Phase

**Impairments:**
Inflammation, pain, edema, muscle spasm
Impaired movement
Joint effusion (if the joint is injured or if there is arthritis)
Decreased use of associated areas

| Plan of Care | Intervention (up to 1 week postinjury) |
|---|---|
| 1. Educate the patient. | 1. Inform patient of anticipated recovery time and how to protect the part while maintaining appropriate functional activities. |
| 2. Control pain, edema, spasm. | 2. Cold, compression, elevation, massage (48 hours).<br>Immobilize the part (rest, splint, tape, cast).<br>Avoid positions of stress to the part.<br>Gentle (grade I) joint oscillations with joint in pain-free position. |
| 3. Maintain soft tissue and joint integrity and mobility. | 3. Appropriate dosage of passive movements within limit of pain, specific to structure involved.<br>Appropriate dosage of intermittent muscle setting or electrical stimulation. |
| 4. Reduce joint swelling if symptoms are present. | 4. May require medical intervention if swelling is rapid (blood).<br>Provide protection (splint, cast). |
| 5. Maintain integrity and function of associated arease. | 5. Active-assistive, free, resistive, and/or modified aerobic exercises, depending on proximity to associated areas and effect on the primary lesion.<br>Adaptive or assistive devices as needed to protect the part during functional activities. |

**Precautions:** The proper dosage of rest and movement must be used during the inflammatory stage. Signs of too much movement are increased pain or increased inflammation.

**Contraindications:** Stretching and resistance exercises should not be performed at the site of the inflamed tissue.

increase the inflammation or pain. Active movement is usually *contraindicated* at the site of an active pathological process unless it is a chronic disease, such as rheumatoid arthritis.

***General movement.*** Active movement is appropriate in neighboring regions to maintain integrity in uninjured tissue and to aid in circulation and lymphatic flow.

### Specific Interventions and Dosages

PRECAUTION: If the movement increases pain or inflammation, it is either of too great a dosage or it should not be done. Extreme care must be used with movement at this stage.

***Passive range of motion.*** Passive range of motion (PROM) within the limit of pain is valuable for maintaining mobility in joints, ligaments, tendons, and muscles as well as improving fluid dynamics and maintaining nutrition in the joints.[20,21] Initially, the range is probably very small.[25] Stretching at this stage is contraindicated. Any motion gained from the PROM techniques is because of decreased pain, swelling, and muscle guarding.

***Low-dosage joint mobilization techniques.*** Grade I or II distraction and glide techniques have the benefit of improving fluid dynamics in the joint to maintain cartilage health. These techniques may also reflexively inhibit or gate the perception of pain. Low-dosage joint mobilizations are beneficial with joint pathologies and any other

connective tissue injury that affects joint motion during the acute stage.

***Muscle setting.*** Gentle isometric muscle contractions performed intermittently and at a very low intensity so as not to cause pain or joint compression have several purposes. The pumping action of the contracting muscle assists the circulation and, therefore, fluid dynamics. If there is muscle damage or injury, the setting techniques are done with the muscle in the shortened position to help maintain mobility of the actin-myosin filaments without stressing the breached tissue. If there is joint injury, the position during the setting techniques is dictated by pain; usually the resting position for the joint is most comfortable. If tolerated, the intermittent setting techniques are performed in several positions.

***Massage.*** Massage serves the purpose of moving fluid; and if it is applied cautiously and gently to injured tissue, it may assist in preventing adhesions. Tendinous lesions are treated with a gentle dosage applied transverse to the fibers to smooth roughened surfaces or to maintain mobility of the tendon in its sheath. When applied, the tendon is kept taut. When treating muscle lesions, the muscle is usually kept in its shortened position so as not to separate the healing breach.[8]

### Interventions for Associated Areas
During the protection phase, maintain as normal a physiological state as possible in related areas of the body. Include techniques to maintain or improve the following.

*Range of motion.* These techniques may be done actively or passively, depending on the proximity to and the effect on the injured tissue.

*Muscle performance.* Resistance may be applied at an appropriate dosage to muscles not directly related to the injured tissue to prepare the patient for use of assistive devices, such as crutches or a walker, and to improve functional activities.

*Functional activities.* Supportive or adaptive devices may be necessary depending on area of injury and expected functional activities.

*Circulation.* The circulation is helped by performing functional activities and by using supportive elastic wraps, by elevating the part, and by using appropriate massage and muscle-setting techniques.

# MANAGEMENT DURING THE SUBACUTE STAGE

## Tissue Response—Repair and Healing

During the second to fourth days after tissue injury, the inflammation begins to decrease, the clot starts resolving, and repair of the injured site begins. This usually lasts an additional 10 to 17 days (14 to 21 days after the onset of injury) but may last up to 6 weeks.

The synthesis and deposition of collagen characterize this stage. Noxious stimuli are removed, and capillary beds begin to grow into the area. Fibroblastic activity, collagen formation, and granulation tissue development increase. Fibroblasts are present in tremendous numbers by the fourth day after injury and continue in large number until about day 21.[22] The fibroblasts produce new collagen, and this immature collagen replaces the exudate that originally formed the clot. In addition, myofibroblastic activity begins about day 5, causing scar shrinkage (contraction).[22] Wound closure usually takes 5 to 8 days in muscle and skin and 3 to 6 weeks in tendons and ligaments.[9]

During this stage, the immature connective tissue that is produced is thin and unorganized. It is extremely fragile and easily injured if overstressed, yet proper growth and alignment can be stimulated by appropriate tensile loading in the line of normal stresses for that tissue. At the same time, adherence to surrounding tissues can be minimized.[7]

## Management Guidelines— Controlled Motion Phase

The therapist's role during this stage is critical. The patient feels much better because the pain is no longer constant, and active movement can begin. It is easy to begin too much movement too soon or be tempted to approach intervention cautiously and not progress rapidly enough. Understanding the healing process and tissue response to stresses underlies the critical decisions that are made throughout this phase of intervention. The key is to initiate and progress *nondestructive* exercises and activities (i.e., exercises and activities that are within the tolerance of the healing tissues, which can then respond without reinjury or inflammation). The information that follows is summarized in Box 10.2.

### Patient Education

Inform the patient about what to expect at this stage, the time frame for healing, and what signs and symptoms indicate that he or she is pushing beyond tissue tolerance. Encourage the patient to return to normal activities that do not exacerbate symptoms, but caution against returning to recreational, sports, or work-related activities that would be detrimental to the healing process. Teach the patient a home exercise program and help him or her adapt work and recreational activities that are consistent with intervention strategies so the patient becomes an active participant in the recovery process.

### Management of Pain and Inflammation

Pain and inflammation decrease as healing progresses. Criteria for initiating active exercises and stretching during the early subacute stage include decreased swelling, pain that is no longer constant, and pain that is not exacerbated by motion in the available range.

*Monitor activities and exercises.* As new exercises are introduced or as the intensity of exercises is progressed, monitor the patient's response, so if symptoms warrant the intensity of exercise can be modified.

**PRECAUTION:** The new tissue being developed is fragile and easily interrupted. The patient often feels good and returns to normal activity too soon, causing exacerbation of symptoms. Exercises progressed too vigorously or functional activities begun too early can be injurious to the fragile, newly developing tissue and therefore may delay recovery by perpetuating the inflammatory response.[22,26] However, if movement is not progressed, the new tissue adheres to surrounding structures and eventually becomes a source of pain and limited tissue mobility.

### Initiation of Active Exercises

Because of the restricted use of the injured region, there is muscle weakness even in the absence of muscle pathology. The subacute phase is a transition period during which *active* exercises within the pain-free range of the injured tissue can begin and be progressed to muscular endurance and strengthening exercises with care, keeping within the tolerance of the healing tissues (nondestructive motion). If activity is kept within a safe intensity and frequency, symptoms of pain and swelling progressively decrease each day. Patient response is the best guide to how quickly or vigorously to progress. Clinically, if signs of inflammation increase or the ROM progressively decreases, the intensity of the exercise and activity must decrease because chronic inflammation has developed and a retracting scar will become more limiting.[2,3,15]

**BOX 10.2**

MANAGEMENT GUIDELINES—Subacute Stage/Controlled Motion Phase

**Impairments:**
Pain when end of available ROM is reached
Decreasing soft tissue edema
Decreasing joint effusion (if joints are involved)
Developing soft tissue, muscle, and/or joint contractures
Developing muscle weakness from reduced usage
Decreased functional use of the part and associated areas

| Plan of Care | Intervention (up to 3 weeks postinjury) |
|---|---|
| 1. Educate the patient. | 1. Inform patient of anticipated healing time and importance of following guidelines. Teach home exercises and encourage functional activities consistent with plan; monitor and modify as patient progresses. |
| 2. Promote healing of injured tissues. | 2. Monitor response of tissue to exercise progression; decrease intensity if inflammation increases. Protect healing tissue with assistive devices, splints, tape, or wrap; progressively increase amount of time the joint is free to move each day and decrease use of assistive device as strength in supporting muscles increases. |
| 3. Restore soft tissue, muscle, and/or joint mobility. | 3. Progress from passive to active-assistive to active ROM within limits of pain. Gradually increase mobility of scar, specific to structure involved. Progressively increase mobility of related structures if they are tight; use techniques specific to tight structure. |
| 4. Develop neuromuscular control, muscle endurance, and strength in involved and related muscles. | 4. Initially, progress multiple-angle isometric exercises within patient's tolerance; begin cautiously with mild resistance. Initiate AROM and protected weight bearing and stabilization exercises. As ROM, joint play, and healing improve, progress isotonic exercises with increased repetitions. Emphasize control and proper mechanics. Progress resistance later in this stage. |
| 5. Maintain integrity and function of associated areas. | 5. Apply progressive strengthening and stabilizing exercises, monitoring effect on the primary lesion. Resume low-intensity functional activities involving the healing tissue that do not exacerbate the symptoms. |

**Precautions:** The signs of inflammation or joint swelling normally decrease early in this stage. Some discomfort will occur as the activity level is progressed, but it should not last longer than a couple of hours. Signs of too much motion or activity are resting pain, fatigue, increased weakness, and spasm.

***Multiple-angle, submaximal isometric exercises.*** Submaximal isometric exercises are used during the early subacute stage to initiate control and strengthening of the muscles in the involved region in a nonstressful manner. They may also help the patient become aware of using the correct muscles. The intensity and angles for resistance are determined by the absence of pain.

● To initiate isometric exercise in an injured, healing muscle, place it in the shortened or relaxed position so the new scar is not pulled from the breached site.[7,22]

● To initiate isometric exercises when there is joint pathology, the resting position for the joint may be the most comfortable position. The intensity of contraction should be kept below the perception of pain.

***Active range of motion exercises.*** Active range of motion (AROM) activities in pain-free ranges are used to develop control of the motion. Initially, isolated, single plane motions are used. Emphasize control of the motion using light-resistive, concentric exercises of involved muscle and muscles needed for proper joint mechanics. Use of combined motions or diagonal patterns may facilitate contraction of the desired muscles, but care must be taken not to use patterns of motion dominated by stronger muscles, with the weaker muscles not effectively participating at this early stage. Do not stress beyond the ability of the involved or weakened muscles to participate in the motion.

***Muscular endurance.*** Exercises for muscle endurance are emphasized during the subacute phase because slow-twitch muscle fibers are the first to atrophy when there is joint swelling, trauma, or immobilization. Initially, only active ROM is used, with emphasis on control. Later during the healing phase, low-intensity, high-repetition exercise using light resistance is used rather than high-intensity resistance. The therapist must be certain that the patient is using correct motor patterns without substitution and is informed of the importance of stopping the exercise or activity when the involved muscle fatigues or involved tissue develops symptoms. For example, if the patient is doing shoulder flexion or abduction activities, substitution with scapular elevation should be avoided; or if the patient is doing leg-lift exercises, proper stabilization of the pelvis and the spine is important to ensure safety and correct motor learning.

*Protected weight-bearing exercises.* Partial weight bearing within the tolerance of the healing tissues may be used early to load the region in a controlled manner and stimulate stabilizing co-contractions in the muscles. Reinforcement from the therapist helps develop awareness of appropriate muscle contractions and helps develop control while the patient shifts his or her weight in a side-to-side or anterior-to-posterior motion. As tolerated by the patient, progress by increasing the amplitude of movement or by decreasing the amount of support or protection. Resistance is added to progress strength in the stabilizing muscles.

PRECAUTION: Eccentric and heavy-resistance exercises (such as PRE) may cause added trauma to muscle and are not used in the early subacute stage after muscle injury when the weak tensile quality of the healing tissue could be jeopardized.[16] For nonmuscular injuries, eccentric exercises may not reinjure the part, but the resistance should be limited to a low intensity at this stage to avoid delayed-onset muscle soreness. (This is in contrast to using eccentric exercises to facilitate and strengthen weak muscles when there has been no injury to take advantage of greater tension development with less energy in eccentric contractions, which is described in Chapter 6.)

### Initiation and Progression of Stretching

Restricted motion during the acute stage and adherence of the developing scar usually cause decreased flexibility in the healing tissue and related structures in the region. To increase mobility and stimulate proper alignment of the developing scar, initiate stretching techniques that are specific to the tissues involved. More than one technique may have to be used to regain the ROM.

*Warm the tissues.* Use modalities or active ROM to increase the tissue temperature and relax the muscles for ease in stretching.

*Inhibition techniques.* Muscles that are not relaxed interfere with joint mobilization and passive stretching of inert tissue. If necessary, utilize hold–relax techniques first to be able to take the tissues to the end of their available range.

*Joint mobilization.* If there is decreased joint play restricting range, it is important to begin stretching with joint mobilization techniques. Use grade III sustained or grade III and IV oscillation techniques to restore some of the joint slide prior to physiological stretching so as to mini-

mize excessive compression of vulnerable cartilage. Joint distraction and gliding techniques are applied to stretch restricting capsular tissue (see Chapter 5 for the principles and techniques of joint mobilization).

*Stretching techniques.* Use of passive stretching techniques, self-stretching, and prolonged mechanical stretching are used to increase the extensibility of inert connective tissue, which permeates every structure in the body. These techniques are interspersed with neuromuscular inhibition techniques to relax and elongate the muscles crossing the joints (see Chapter 4 for the principles and techniques of stretching).

*Massage.* Various types of massage can be used for their soft tissue mobilizing effects. For example, cross-fiber friction massage is used to mobilize ligaments and incision sites so they move freely across the joint. Cross-fiber massage is also used at the site of muscle scar tissue or tendon adhesions to gain mobility of the scar tissue. The intensity and duration of the technique is progressively increased as the tissue responds.

*Use of the new range.* The patient must use the new range to maintain any extensibility gained with the stretching maneuvers and to develop control of the new range. Teach home exercises that include light resistance using the agonist in the new range as well as self-stretching techniques. Also help the patient incorporate the new range into his or her daily activities.

### Correction of Contributing Factors

Continue to maintain or develop as normal a physiological and functional state as possible in related areas of the body. Correct postural stability problems or muscle length and strength imbalances that could have contributed to the problem. Resume low-intensity functional activities as the patient tolerates without exacerbating symptoms. Continue to reassess the patient's progress and understanding of the controlled activities.

## ⬤ MANAGEMENT DURING THE CHRONIC STAGE

### Tissue Response—Maturation and Remodeling

Scar retraction from activity of the myofibroblasts is usually complete by the 21st day and the scar stops increasing in size, so from day 21 to day 60 there is a predominance of fibroblasts that are easily remodeled.[22] The process of maturation begins during the late subacute stage and continues for several months. The maturation and remodeling of the scar tissue occurs as collagen fibers become thicker and reorient in response to stresses placed on the connective tissue. Remodeling time is influenced by factors that affect the density and activity level of the fibroblasts, including the amount of time immobilized, stress placed on the tissue, location of the lesion, and vascular supply.

## Maturation of Tissue

The primary differences in the state of the healing tissue between the late subacute and chronic stages are the improvement in quality (orientation and tensile strength) of the collagen and the reduction of the wound size during the chronic stages. The quantity of collagen stabilizes; and there is a balance between synthesis and degradation. Depending on the size of the structure or degree of injury or pathology, healing, with progressively increasing tensile quality in the injured tissue, may continue for 12 to 18 months.[9,17,22]

## Remodeling of Tissue

Because of the way immature collagen molecules are held together (hydrogen bonding) and adhere to surrounding tissue, they can be easily remodeled with gentle and persistent treatment. This is possible for up to 10 weeks. If not properly stressed, the fibers adhere to surrounding tissue and form a restricting scar. As the structure of collagen changes to covalent bonding and thickens, it becomes stronger and resistant to remodeling. At 14 weeks, the scar tissue is unresponsive to remodeling. Consequently, an old scar has a poor response to stretch.[7] Treatment under these conditions requires either adaptive lengthening in the tissue surrounding the scar or surgical release.

# Management Guidelines— Return to Function Phase

The therapist's role during this phase is to design a progression of exercises that safely stress the maturing connective tissue in terms of both flexibility and strength so the patient can return to his or her functional and work-related activities. Individuals returning to high-intensity activities require more intense exercises to prepare the tissues to withstand the stresses and train the neuromuscular system to respond to the demands of the activity.

Because remodeling of the maturing collagen occurs in response to the stresses placed on it, it is important to use controlled forces that duplicate normal stresses on the tissue. Maximum strength of the collagen develops in the direction of the imposed forces. Pain that the patient now experiences arises only when stress is placed on restrictive contractures or adhesions or when there is soreness due to increased stress of resistive exercise. To avoid chronic or recurring pain, the contractures must be stretched or the adhesions broken up and mobilized. Excessive or abnormal stresses leads to reinjury and chronic inflammation, which can be detrimental to the return of function. The information that follows is summarized in Box 10.4.

## Patient Education

Unless there is restrictive scar tissue requiring manual techniques for intervention, the patient becomes more responsible for carrying out the exercises in the plan of treatment. Instruct the patient in biomechanically safe progressions of resistance and self-stretching and how to self-monitor for detrimental effects and signs of excessive stress (Box 10.3). Establish guidelines for what must be

attained to return safely to recreational, sport, or work-related activities. Re-examine and evaluate the patient's progress and modify the exercises as progress is noted or if problems develop. Recommend modifications in living, work, or sport activities if they are contributing to the patient's impairments and preventing return to desired activities.

## Considerations for Progression of Exercises

Free joint play within a useful (or functional) ROM is necessary to avoid joint trauma. If joint play is restricted, joint-mobilizing techniques should be used. These stretching techniques can be vigorous so long as no signs of increased irritation result.

Joint motion without adequate muscle support causes trauma to that joint, or faulty neuromuscular patterns will be used as functional activities are attempted. Zohn and Mennell[26] recommended that the criterion for strength should be a muscle test grade of 4 on a 5-point scale in lower extremity musculature before discontinuing use of supportive or assistive devices for ambulation. Although this advice was given during the 1970s, it emphasizes the importance of muscle support in the protection of joints.

- To increase strength when there is a loss of joint play, use multiple-angle isometric exercises.
- Once joint play within the available ROM is restored, use resistive dynamic exercises within the available range. This does not imply that normal ROM needs to be present before initiating dynamic exercises but that joint play within the available range should be present (see Chapter 5 for information on joint play).

In summary, joint dynamics and muscle strength and flexibility should be balanced as the injured part is progressed to functional exercises.

## Progression of Stretching

Stretching of any restricting contractures or adhesions should be specific to the tissue involved using manual tech-

**BOX 10.4**

## MANAGEMENT GUIDELINES—Chronic Stage/Return to Function Phase

**Impairments:**
Soft tissue and/or joint contractures and adhesions that limit normal ROM or joint play
Decreased muscle performance: weakness, poor endurance, poor neuromuscular control
Decreased functional usage of the involved part
Inability to function normally in an expected activity

| Plan of Care | Interventions (>3 weeks postinjury) |
|---|---|
| 1. Educate the patient. | 1. Instruct patient in safe progressions of exercises and stretching. Monitor understanding and compliance. Teach ways to avoid reinjuring the part. Teach safe body mechanics. Provide ergonomic counseling. |
| 2. Increase soft tissue, muscle and/or joint mobility. | 2. Stretching techniques specific to tight tissue: <br>• Joint and selected ligaments (joint mobilization). <br>• Ligaments, tendons and soft tissue adhesions (cross-fiber massage). <br>• Muscles (neuromuscular inhibition, passive stretch, massage, and flexibility exercises). |
| 3. Improve neuromuscular *control,* strength, muscle endurance. | 3. Progress exercises: <br>• Submaximal to maximal resistance. <br>• Specificity of exercise using resisted concentric and eccentric, weight bearing and non-weight-bearing. <br>• Single plane to multiplane motions. <br>• Simple to complex motions, emphasizing movements that simulate functional activities. <br>• Controlled proximal stability, superimpose distal motion. <br>• Safe biomechanics. <br>• Increase time at slow speed; progress complexity and time; progress speed and time. |
| 4. Improve cardiovascular endurance. | 4. Progress aerobic exercises using safe activities. |
| 5. Progress functional activities. | 5. Continue using supportive and/or assistive devices until the ROM is functional with joint play, and strength in supporting muscles is adequate. Progress functional training with simulated activities from protected and controlled to unprotected and variable. Continue progressive strengthening exercises and advanced training activities until the muscles are strong enough and able to respond to the required functional demands. |

**Precautions:** There should be no signs of inflammation. Some discomfort will occur as the activity level is progressed, but it should not last longer than a couple of hours. Signs that activities are progressing too quickly or with too great a dosage are joint swelling, pain that lasts longer than 4 hours or that requires medication for relief, a decrease in strength, or fatiguing more easily.

niques such as joint mobilization, myofascial massage, neuromuscular inhibition techniques, and passive stretching in addition to instruction in self-stretching (see Chapters 4 and 5 and the self-stretching exercises described in Chapters 16 to 22). At this stage, progress the intensity and duration of the stretching maneuvers so long as no signs of increased irritation persist beyond 24 hours.

### Progression of Exercises for Muscle Performance: Developing Neuromuscular Control, Strength, and Endurance

As the patient's tissues heal, not only does treatment progress to stimulate proper maturation and remodeling in the healing tissue, but emphasis is also placed on con-

trolled progressive exercises designed to prepare the patient to meet the functional outcomes.

● If the patient is not using some of the muscles because of inhibition, weakness, or dominance of substitute patterns, isolate the desired muscle action or use unidirectional motions to develop awareness of muscle activity and control of the movement.

● Progress exercises from isolated, unidirectional, simple movements to complex patterns and multidirectional movements requiring coordination with all muscles functioning for the desired activity.[23]

● Progress strengthening exercises to simulate specific demands including both weight-bearing and non-weight-bearing (closed and open chain) and both eccentric and concentric contractions.

- Progress trunk stabilization, postural control, and balance exercises as well as coordinate with extremity motions for effective total body movement patterns.[23]
- Teach safe body mechanics and have the patient practice activities that replicate his or her work environment.
- Often overlooked but of importance in preventing injury associated with fatigue is developing muscular endurance in the prime mover muscles and stabilizing muscles as well as cardiovascular endurance.

### Return to High-Demand Activities

Patients who must return to activities with greater-than-normal demand, such as is required in sports participation and heavy work settings, are progressed further to more intense exercises including plyometrics, agility training, and skill development. Develop exercise drills that simulate the work[12] or sport[2,23] activities using a controlled environment with specific, progressive resistance and plyometric drills. As the patient demonstrates capabilities, increase the repetitions and speed of the movement. Progress by changing the environment and introducing surprise and uncontrolled events into the activity.[1,23]

The importance of proper education to teach a safe progression of exercises and how to avoid damaging stresses cannot be overemphasized. To return to the activity that caused the injury prior to regaining functional pain-free motion, strength, endurance, and skill to match the demands of the task would probably result in recurring injury and pain.

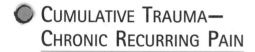

# CUMULATIVE TRAUMA— CHRONIC RECURRING PAIN

## Tissue Response—Chronic Inflammation

When connective tissue is injured, it goes through a healing process of repair, which was described in the preceding sections. However, in connective tissue that is repetitively stressed beyond the ability to repair itself, the inflammatory process is perpetuated. Proliferation of fibroblasts with increased collagen production and degradation of mature collagen leads to a predominance of new, immature collagen. This has an overall weakening effect on the tissue. In addition, myofibroblastic activity continues, which may lead to progressive limitation of motion.[22] Efforts to stretch the inflamed tissue perpetuate irritation and progressive limitation.

## Etiology of Chronic Inflammation Leading to Prolonged or Recurring Pain

***Overuse, cumulative trauma, repetitive strain.*** These are terms descriptive of the repetitive nature of the precipitating event.[10] Repetitive microtrauma or repeated strain over-

load over time results in structural weakening, or fatigue breakdown, of connective tissue, with collagen fiber cross-link breakdown and inflammation. Initially, the inflammatory response from the microtrauma is subthreshold but eventually builds to the point of perceived pain and resulting dysfunction.

***Trauma.*** Trauma that is followed by superimposed repetitive trauma results in a condition that never completely heals. This may be the result of too early return to high-demand functional activities before the original injury has properly healed. The continued reinjury leads to the symptoms of chronic inflammation and dysfunction.

***Reinjury of an "old scar."*** Scar tissue is not as compliant as surrounding, undamaged tissue. If the scar adheres to the surrounding tissues or is not properly aligned to the stresses imposed on the tissue, there is an alteration in the force transmission and energy absorption. This region becomes more susceptible to injury with stresses that normal, healthy tissue could sustain.

***Contractures or poor mobility.*** Faulty postural habits or prolonged immobility may lead to connective tissue contractures that became stressed with repeated or vigorous activity.

## Contributing Factors

By the nature of the condition, there is usually some factor that perpetuates the problem. Not only should the tissue at fault and its stage of pathology be identified, but the *mechanical cause* of the repetitive trauma needs to be defined. Evaluate for faulty mechanics or faulty habits that may be sustaining the irritation. Possibilities include:

- *Imbalance between the length and strength of the muscles* around the joint, leading to faulty mechanics of joint motion or abnormal forces through the muscles.
- *Rapid or excessive repeated eccentric demand* placed on muscles not prepared to withstand the load, leading to tissue failure, particularly in the musculotendinous region.[16]
- *Muscle weakness* or an inability to respond to excessive strength demands that results in muscle fatigue with decreased contractility and shock-absorbing capabilities and increased stress to supporting tissues.[16]
- *Bone malalignment or weak structural support* that causes faulty joint mechanics of force transmission through the joints (poor joint stability as in a flat foot).[18]
- *Change in the usual intensity or demands* of an activity such as an increase or change in an exercise or a training routine or change in job demands.[16]
- *Returning to an activity too soon after an injury* when the muscle-tendon unit is weakened and not ready for the stress of the activity.[11]
- *Sustained awkward postures or motions*, placing parts of the body at a mechanical disadvantage, leading to postural fatigue or injury.

● *Environmental factors* such as a work station not ergonomically designed for the individual, excessive cold, continued vibration, or inappropriate weight-bearing surface (for standing, walking, or running), which may contribute to any of the previous factors.

● *Age-related factors* such that a person attempts activities that could be done when younger but his or her tissues are no longer in condition to withstand the sustained stress.[19]

● *Training errors,* such as using improper methods, intensity, amount, equipment, or condition of the participant, which lead to abnormal stresses.[18]

● *A combination of several contributing factors* are frequently seen that cause the symptoms.

## Management Guidelines— Chronic Inflammation

When the patient has symptoms and signs of chronic inflammation, it is imperative that treatment begins by controlling the inflammation—in other words, treat it as an acute condition. Once the inflammation is under control, treatment progresses to dealing with the impairments and functional limitations. Management guidelines are summarized in Box 10.5.

---

### BOX 10.5
### MANAGEMENT GUIDELINES—Chronic Inflammation/Cumulative Trauma Syndromes

**Impairments:**

Pain in the involved tissue of varying degrees:
- Only after doing repetitive activities
- When doing repetitive activities as well as after
- When attempting to do activities; completion of demands prevented
- Continued and unremitting

Soft tissue, muscle, and/or joint contractures or adhesions that limit normal ROM or joint play
Muscle weakness and poor muscular endurance in postural or stabilizing muscles as well as primary muscle at fault
Imbalance in length and strength between antagonistic muscles; biomechanical dysfunction
Decreased functional use of the region
Faulty position or movement pattern perpetuating the problem

| Plan of Care | Interventions During Chronic Inflammation |
|---|---|
| 1. Educate the patient. | 1. Counsel as to cause of chronic irritation and need to avoid stressing the part while inflamed. Adapt the environment to decrease tissue stress. Home exercise program to reinforce therapeutic interventions. |
| 2. Promote healing; decrease pain and inflammation. | 2. Cold, compression, massage. Rest to the part (stop mechanical stress, splint, tape, cast). |
| 3. Maintain integrity and mobility of involved tissue. | 3. Nonstressful passive movement, massage, and muscle setting within limits of pain. |
| 4. Develop support in related regions. | 4. Posture training. Stabilization exercises. |

| Plan of Care | Interventions—Controlled Motion and Return to Function Phases |
|---|---|
| 1. Educate the patient. | 1. Ergonomic counseling in ways to prevent recurrence. Home instruction in safe progression of stretching and strengthening exercises. Instruction on signs of too much stress (see Box 10.3). |
| 2. Develop strong, mobile scar. | 2. Friction massage. Soft tissue mobilization. |
| 3. Develop a balance in length and strength of the muscles. | 3. Correct cause of faulty muscle and joint mechanics with appropriately graded stretching and strengthening exercises. |
| 4. Progress functional independence. | 4. Train muscles to function according to demand; provide alternatives or support if it cannot. Train coordination and timing. Develop endurance. |
| 5. Analyze job/activity. | 5. Adapt home, work, sport environment/tools. |

**Precaution:** If there is progressive loss of range of motion as the result of stretching, do not continue to stretch. Reevaluate the condition and determine if there is still a chronic inflammation with contracting scar or if there is protective muscle guarding. Emphasize stabilizing the part and training in safe adaptive patterns of motion.

## Chronic Inflammation—Acute Stage

When the inflammatory response is perpetuated because of continued tissue irritation, the inflammation must be controlled to avoid the negative effects of continued tissue breakdown and excessive scar formation.

● In addition to the use of modalities and resting the part, it is imperative to identify and modify the mechanism of chronic irritation with appropriate biomechanical counseling. This requires cooperation from the patient. Describe to the patient how the tissue reacts and breaks down under continued inflammation and explain the strategy of intervention. Using illustrations—such as what happens when a person repeatedly hits a thumbnail with a hammer or repeatedly scrapes a skin area before it heals—helps the patient visualize the repeated trauma occurring in the musculoskeletal problem and understand the need to quit "hitting the sore."

● Initially, allow only nonstressful activities.

● Initiate exercises at *nonstressful* intensities in the involved tissues, as with any acute lesion, and at appropriate corrective intensities in related regions without stressing the involved tissues.

## Subacute and Chronic Stages of Healing Following Chronic Inflammation

Once the constant pain from the chronic inflammation has decreased, progress the patient through an exercise program with controlled stresses until the connective tissue in the involved region has developed the ability to withstand the stresses imposed by the functional activities.

● Locally, if there is a chronic, contracted scar that limits range or continually becomes irritated with microrup-

tures, mobilize the scar in the tissue using friction massage, soft tissue manipulation, or stretching techniques. If inflammation results from the stretching maneuvers, treat it as an acute injury. Because chronic inflammation can lead to proliferation of scar tissue and contraction of the scar, progressive loss of range is a warning sign that the intensity of stretching is too vigorous.

● Muscle guarding could be a sign that the body is attempting to protect the part from excessive motion. In this case, the emphasis is on developing stabilization of the part and training in safe adaptive patterns of motion.

● Identify the cause of the faulty muscle and joint mechanics. Strengthening and stabilization exercises, in conjunction with working or recreational adaptations, are necessary to minimize the irritating patterns of motion.

● Because chronic irritation problems frequently result from an inability to sustain repetitive activities, muscle endurance is an appropriate component of the muscle re-education program. Consider endurance in the postural stabilizers as well as in the prime movers of the desired functional activity.

● As when treating patients in the chronic stage of healing, progress exercises to develop functional independence. The exercises become specific to the demand and include timing, coordination, and skill.

● Work-conditioning and work-hardening programs may be used to prepare the person for return to work; training in sports-specific exercises is important for returning an individual to sports.

**N O T E :** Specific overuse syndromes are covered in detail in the respective chapters associated with the involved region.

## INDEPENDENT LEARNING ACTIVITIES

● **Critical Thinking and Discussion**

1. Your patient has experienced an injury to a muscle; describe the symptoms that he or she will experience during each stage of inflammation and repair and describe the principles of the exercise intervention that should be used during each stage. Once you have identified the principles, choose a commonly injured muscle, such as the hamstrings, and describe the symptoms, test

results, goals treatment plan, and actual interventions that you would use for each stage of intervention.

2. Do the same activity as in #1 except use a ligamentous injury, such as strain of the humeroulnar ligament or anterior talofibular ligament.

3. Describe the mechanism of injury for common overuse syndromes, such as lateral epicondylitis or shin splints, and explain the differences between such an injury and an acute traumatic injury.

## REFERENCES

1. Arnheim, DD, Prentice, WE: Principles of Athletic Training, ed 3. McGraw-Hill, Boston, 1997.
2. Bandy, WD: Functional rehabilitation of the athlete. Orthop Phys Ther Clin North Am 1:269, 1992.
3. Barrick, EF: Orthopedic trauma. In Kauffman, TL (ed) Geriatric Rehabilitation Manual. Churchill Livingstone, New York, 1999.
4. Boissonnault, WG, Goodman, CC: Bone, joint and muscle disorders. In Goodman, CC, Guller KS, Boissonnault, WG (eds) Pathology: Implications for the Physical Therapist, ed 2. Saunders, Philadelphia, 2003, p 929

5. Boissonnault, WG, Goodman, CC: Introduction to pathology of the musculoskeletal system. In Goodman, CC, Guller KS, Boissonnault, WG (eds) Pathology: Implications for the Physical Therapist, ed 2. Saunders, Philadelphia, 2003, p 821.
6. Cailliet, R: Soft tissue pain and disability, ed 3. Davis, Philadelphia, 1996.
7. Cummings, GS, Tillman, LJ: Remodeling of dense connective tissue in normal adult tissues. In Currier, DP, Nelson, RM (eds) Dynamics of Human Biologic Tissues. Davis, Philadelphia, 1992, p 45.
8. Cyriax, J: Textbook of Orthopaedic Medicine, Vol 1. Diagnosis of Soft Tissue Lesions, ed 8. Bailliere & Tindall, London, 1982.

9. Enwemeka, CS: Connective tissue plasticity: ultrastructural, biomechanical, and morphometric effects of physical factors on intact and regenerating tendons. J Orthop Sports Phys Ther 14(5):198, 1991.

10. Guidotti, TL: Occupational repetitive strain injury. Am Fam Physician 45:585, 1992.

11. Hawley, DJ: Health status assessment. In Wegener, ST (ed): Clinical Care in the Rheumatic Diseases. American College of Rheumatology, Atlanta, 1996.

12. Isernhagen, SJ: Exercise technologies for work rehabilitation programs. Orthop Phys Ther Clin North Am 1:361, 1992.

13. Keene, J, Malone, TR: Ligament and muscle-tendon unit injuries. In Malone, TR, McPoil, TG, Nitz, AJ (eds) Orthopaedic and Sports Physical Therapy, ed 3. CV Mosby, St Louis, 1997, p 135.

14. Kellet, J: Acute soft tissue injuries: a review of the literature. Med Sci Sports Exerc 18:489, 1986.

15. McGinty, JB (ed): Operative Arthroscopy. Lippincott-Raven, Philadelphia, 1996.

16. Noonan, TJ, Garrett, WE: Injuries at the myotendinous junction. Clin Sports Med 11:783, 1992.

17. Noyes, FR, Keller, CS, et al: Advances in understanding of knee ligament injury, repair and rehabilitation Med Sci Sports Exerc 16:427, 1984.

18. Pease, BJ: Biomechanical assessment of the lower extremity. J Orthop Phys Ther Clin North Am 3:291, 1994.

19. Puffer, JC, Zachazewski, JE: Management of overuse injuries. Am Fam Physician 38:225, 1988.

20. Salter, RB: Continuous Passive Motion, A Biological Concept. Williams & Wilkins, Baltimore, 1993.

21. Salter, RB: Textbook of Disorders and Injuries of the Musculoskeletal System, ed 3. Williams & Wilkins, Baltimore, 1999.

22. Tillman, LJ, Cummings, GS: Biologic mechanisms of connective tissue mutability. In Currier, DP, Nelson, RM (eds) Dynamics of Human Biologic Tissues. Davis, Philadelphia, 1992, p 1.

23. Wilk, KE, Arrigo, C: An integrated approach to upper extremity exercises. J Orthop Phys Ther Clin North Am 1:337, 1992.

24. Woolf, CJ: Generation of acute pain: Central mechanisms. Br Med Bull 47:523, 1991.

25. Wynn Parry, CB, Stanley, JK: Synovectomy of the hand. Br J Rheumatol 32:1089, 1993.

26. Zohn, D, Mennell, J: Musculoskeletal Pain: Principles of Physical Diagnosis and Physical Treatment. Little, Brown, Boston, 1976.

# Joint, Connective Tissue, and Bone Disorders and Management

General guidelines and principles for developing exercise interventions for patients with soft tissue lesions were presented in the previous chapter. The purpose of this chapter is to present principles of management of selected pathologies that affect joints, connective tissue, and bone. Characteristics of arthritis, fibromyalgia, myofascial pain syndrome, osteoporosis, and fractures are described in conjunction with the effects of therapeutic exercise on impairments associated with these pathological conditions.

## ● ARTHRITIS—ARTHROSIS

*Arthritis* is inflammation of a joint. There are many types of arthritis, both inflammatory and noninflammatory, that affect joints and other connective tissues in the body. The most common types treated by therapists are rheumatoid arthritis and osteoarthritis. *Arthrosis* is limitation of a joint without inflammation. Unless the cause of the joint problems is known, such as recent trauma or immobility, medical intervention is necessary to diagnose and medically manage the pathology. Traumatic arthritis may require aspiration if there is bloody effusion. The therapist manages the physical impairments and functional restrictions that are the results of the underlying pathology.

## Clinical Signs and Symptoms

Signs and symptoms common to all types of arthritic conditions generally include the following.

### Impaired Mobility

The patient usually presents with signs typical of joint involvement that include a characteristic pattern of limitation (called a capsular pattern), usually a firm end-feel (unless acute; then the end-feel may be guarded), decreased and possibly painful joint play, and joint swelling (effusion).[28] Additional signs and symptoms may be present depending on the specific disease process. Table 11.1 summarizes the characteristic signs and symptoms of osteoarthritis and rheumatoid arthritis.

Arthrosis may be present if the individual is recovering from a fracture or other problem requiring immobilization. There is limited joint play along with other connective tissue and muscular contractures limiting ROM.

### Impaired Muscle Performance

Examination of the patient by the therapist should include identifying any mechanical imbalances in flexibility and strength in supporting muscles. This is important because poor muscle support allows the joint to be more susceptible to trauma; conversely, good muscle support helps protect an arthritic joint. Any asymmetry of muscle pull may be a deforming force; and if it cannot be corrected with exercises, splinting or bracing may be necessary to prevent progressive deformity. Stabilizing muscles are often inhibited when there are swollen or restricted joints. Strength returns with decreased swelling and increased joint mobility, so it is important to protect the joints when they are swollen and the muscles are weak.

## TABLE 11.1  Comparison of Osteoarthritis and Rheumatoid Arthritis[4,11,25,57,69,70]

| Characteristics | Osteoarthritis | Rheumatoid Arthritis |
| --- | --- | --- |
| Age of onset | Usually after age of 40 | Usually begins between age 15 and 50 |
| Progression | Usually develops slowly over many years in response to mechanical stress | May develop suddenly, within weeks or months |
| Manifestations | Cartilage degradation, altered joint architecture, osteophyte formation | Inflammatory synovitis and irreversible structural damage to cartilage and bone |
| Joint involvement | Affects a few joints (usually asymmetrical) typically<br>—DIP, PIP, 1st CMC of hands<br>—Cervical and lumbar spine<br>—Hips, knees, 1st MTP of feet | Usually affects many joints, usually bilateral; typically<br>—MCP and PIP of hands, wrists, elbows, shoulders<br>—Cervical spine<br>—MTP, talonavicular and ankle |
| Joint signs and symptoms | Morning stiffness (usually less than 30 min), increased joint pain with weight-bearing and strenuous activity; crepitus and loss of ROM | Redness, warmth, swelling, and prolonged morning stiffness; increased joint pain with activity |
| Systemic signs and symptoms | None | General feeling of sickness and fatigue, weight loss and fever; may develop rheumatoid nodules, may have ocular, respiratory, hematological, and cardiac symptoms |

## Impaired Balance

Patients may develop balance deficits because of altered or decreased sensory input from joint mechanoreceptors and muscle spindle. This is particularly a problem with weight-bearing joints.[74]

## Functional Limitations

The ability to carry out home, community, work-related, or social activities may be minimally to significantly restricted. Adaptive and assistive devices may be used by the patient to improve function or help prevent possible deforming forces. A variety of classification systems and functional instruments have been developed for use in clinical studies as well as routine practice to measure patient function and outcomes in response to interventions.[24]

## Rheumatoid Arthritis

Rheumatoid arthritis (RA) is an autoimmune, chronic, inflammatory, systemic disease primarily affecting the synovial lining of joints as well as other connective tissue. It is characterized by a fluctuating course, with periods of active disease and remission. The onset and progression vary from mild joint symptoms with aching and stiffness to abrupt swelling, stiffness, and progressive deformity.[4,8,32,50] The criteria for classification of RA are summarized in Box 11.1.

## Characteristics of RA

● There are usually periods of exacerbation (flare) and remission.[4,8,32] Joints are characteristically involved with early inflammatory changes in the synovial membrane, peripheral portions of the articular cartilage, and sub-

chondral marrow spaces. In response, granulation tissue (pannus) forms, covers, and erodes the articular cartilage, bone, and ligaments in the joint capsule. Adhesions may form, restricting joint mobility. With progression of the disease, cancellous bone becomes exposed. Fibrosis, ossific ankylosis, or subluxation may eventually cause deformity and disability (Figs. 11.1, 11.2, 11.3).[4,50]

● Inflammatory changes also occur in tendon sheaths (tenosynovitis); and if subjected to recurring friction, the tendons may fray or rupture.

### BOX 11.1  Criteria for Diagnosis of Rheumatoid Arthritis[5]

1. Morning stiffness in and around the joints, lasting at least 1 hour before maximal improvement
2. At least three joint areas simultaneously have soft tissue swelling or fluid observed by a physician
3. Swelling in the wrist, metacarpophalangeal (MCP), or proximal interphalangeal (PIP) joints
4. Symmetrical arthritis—bilateral involvement of PIP, MCP, or metatarsophalangeal (MTP) joints may occur without absolute symmetry
5. Rheumatoid nodules
6. Serum rheumatoid factor
7. Radiographic changes including erosions or periarticular osteopenia in hand and/or wrist joints

NOTE: RA is defined by the presence of at least four of these seven criteria. Nos. 1–4 must have been present for at least 6 weeks.

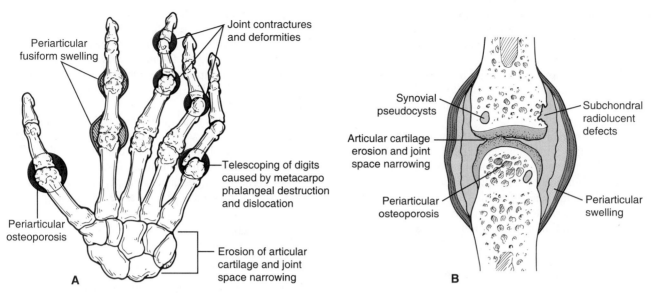

FIGURE 11.1  (*A*) Radiographic hallmarks and typical joint deformities with rheumatoid arthritis in small joints of the wrist and hand. (*B*) Radiographic hallmarks of rheumatoid arthritis in large joints.

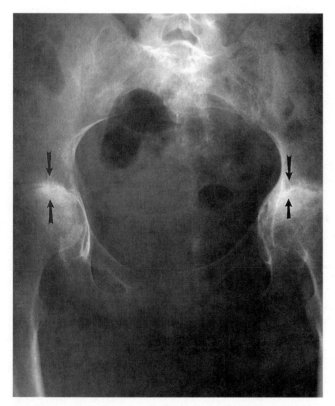

FIGURE 11.2  Advanced rheumatoid arthritis of the hip joints. Note that the destruction caused by rheumatoid arthritis involves the entire joint space and the bony regions on either side of the joint space. *(From McKinnis,[36] p 56, with permission.)*

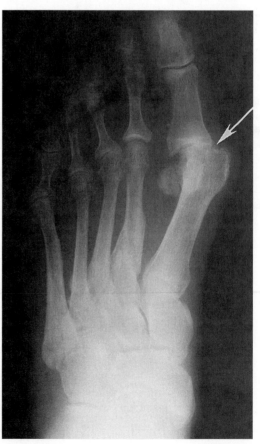

FIGURE 11.3  Rheumatoid arthritis of the foot. First metatarsophalangeal joint shows severe *erosion* of the joint surface with *subluxation* of the metatarsal (arrow). *(From McKinnis,[36] p 60, with permission.)*

● Extra-articular pathological changes sometimes occur; they include rheumatoid nodules, atrophy and fibrosis of muscles with associated muscular weakness, fatigue, and mild cardiac changes.

● Progressive deterioration and decline in the functional level of the individual attributed to the muscular changes and progressive muscle weakness is often seen.[13]

● The degree of involvement varies. Some individuals experience mild symptoms that require minor lifestyle changes and mild anti-inflammatory medications. Others experience significant pathological changes in the joints that require major adaptations in lifestyle. Loss of joint function is irreversible, and often surgery is needed to decrease pain and improve function. Early recognition is essential during the initial stages, with referral to a rheumatologist for diagnosis and medical management to control the inflammation and minimize joint damage.[11]

### Signs and Symptoms—Periods of Active Disease

● With synovial inflammation there is effusion and swelling of the joints, which cause aching and limited motion. Joint stiffness is prominent in the morning. Usually there is pain on motion; and a slight increase in skin temperature can be detected over the joints. Pain and stiffness worsen after strenuous activity.

● Onset is usually in the smaller joints of the hands and feet, most commonly in the proximal interphalangeal joints. Usually symptoms are bilateral.

● With progression, the joints become deformed and may ankylose or subluxate.

● Pain is often felt in adjoining muscles; and eventually muscle atrophy and weakness occur. Asymmetry in muscle strength and alterations in the line of pull of muscles and tendons add to the deforming forces.

● The person often experiences nonspecific symptoms such as low-grade fever, loss of appetite and weight, malaise, and fatigue.

### Principles of Management—Active Inflammatory Period of RA

Management guidelines are summarized in Box 11.2.

● *Joint protection.* Because periods of active disease may last several months to more than a year, education in the overall treatment plan, safe activity, and joint protection (Box 11.3) begins as soon as possible.[34] It is imperative to involve the patient in the management so he or she learns how to conserve energy and avoid potential deforming stresses during activities and when exercising.

---

**BOX 11.2**

## MANAGEMENT GUIDELINES—Rheumatoid Arthritis/Active Disease Period

**Impairments:**
Tenderness and warmth over the involved joints with joint swelling
Muscle guarding and pain on motion
Joint stiffness and limited motion
Muscle weakness and atrophy
Potential deformity and ankylosis from the degenerative process and asymmetric muscle pull
Fatigue, malaise, sleep disorders
Restricted ADLs and IADLs

| Plan of Care | Interventions |
|---|---|
| 1. Educate the patient. | 1. Inform the patient on importance of rest, joint protection, energy conservation, and performance of ROM. Teach home exercise program and activity modifications that conserve energy and minimize stress to vulnerable joints. |
| 2. Relieve pain and muscle guarding and promote relaxation. | 2. Modalities. Gentle massage. Immobilize in splint. Relaxation techniques. |
| 3. Minimize joint stiffness and maintain available motion. | 3. Passive or active-assistive ROM within limits of pain, gradual progression as tolerated. Gentle joint techniques using grade I or II oscillations. |
| 4. Minimize muscle atrophy. | 4. Gentle isometrics in pain-free positions, progression to ROM when tolerated. |
| 5. Prevent deformity and protect the joint structures. | 5. Use of supportive and assistive equipment for all pathologically active joints. Good bed positioning while resting. Avoidance of activities that stress the joints. |

**Precautions:** Respect fatigue and increased pain; do not overstress osteoporotic bone or lax ligaments.
**Contraindications:** Do not stretch swollen joints or apply heavy resistance exercise that cause joint stress.

## BOX 11.3 Principles of Joint Protection[30,49]

- Monitor activities and stop when discomfort or fatigue begins to develop.
- Use frequent but short episodes of exercise (three to five sessions per day) rather than one long session.
- Alternate activities to avoid fatigue.
- Decrease level of activities or omit provoking activities if joint pain develops and persists for more than 1 hour after activity.
- Maintain a functional level of joint ROM and muscular strength and endurance.
- Balance work and rest to avoid muscular and total body fatigue.
- Increase rest during flares of the disease.
- Avoid deforming positions.
- Avoid prolonged static positioning; change positions during the day every 20 to 30 minutes.
- Use stronger and larger muscles and joints during activities whenever possible.
- Use appropriate adaptive equipment.

● *Energy conservation.* It is important that the patient learns to respect fatigue and, when tired, rests to minimize undue stress to all the body systems. Because inflamed joints are easily damaged and rest is encouraged to protect the joints, the patient is taught how to rest the joints in nondeforming positions and to intersperse rest with ROM.

● *Joint mobility.* Gentle grade I and II distraction and oscillation techniques are used to inhibit pain and minimize fluid stasis. Stretching techniques are not performed when joints are swollen.

● *Exercise.* The type and intensity of exercise varies depending on the symptoms. The patient is encouraged to do active exercises through as much range of motion (ROM) as possible (not stretching). If active exercises are not tolerated owing to pain and swelling, passive ROM is used. Once symptoms of pain and signs of swelling are controlled with medication, exercises can progress as if subacute.

NOTE: Therapeutic exercises cannot positively alter the pathological process of RA; but if administered carefully, they can help prevent, retard, or correct the mechanical limitations and deforming forces that occur, especially during the early stages of the disease, and therefore help maintain function.

● *Functional training.* Activities of daily living (ADL) may need to be modified in order to protect the joints. If necessary, splints and assistive devices should be used to provide protection.

PRECAUTIONS: Secondary effects of steroidal medications may include osteoporosis and ligamentous laxity, so exercises should not cause excessive stress to bones or joints.

CONTRAINDICATIONS: Stretching techniques should not be performed across swollen joints. When there is effusion, limited motion is the result of excessive fluid in the joint space. Forcing motion on the distended capsule overstretches it, leading to subsequent hypermobility (or subluxation) when the swelling abates. It may also increase the irritability of the joint and prolong the joint reaction.

### Principles of Management—Subacute and Chronic Stages of RA

As the intensity of pain, joint swelling, morning stiffness, and systemic effects diminish, the disease is considered subacute. Often medications can decrease the acute symptoms so the patient can function as if in the subacute stage. The chronic stage occurs between exacerbations. This may be very short in duration, or it may last many years.

The treatment approach is the same as with any subacute and chronic musculoskeletal disorder, except appropriate precautions must be taken because the pathological changes from the disease process make the parts more susceptible to damage.

● To improve function, exercise should be aimed at improving flexibility, muscle performance, and cardiopulmonary endurance.[13]
● Nonimpact or low-impact conditioning exercises such as swimming and bicycling, performed within the tolerance of the individual with RA, improve aerobic capacity and physical activity and decrease depression and anxiety.[6,39,77] Group activities such as water aerobics also provide social support in conjunction with the activity.

PRECAUTIONS: The joint capsule, ligaments, and tendons may be structurally weakened by the rheumatic process (also as a result of using steroids), so the dosage of stretching and joint mobilization techniques used to counter any contractures or adhesions must be carefully graded.

CONTRAINDICATIONS: Vigorous stretching or manipulative techniques.

 **Focus on Evidence** _____

The results of a study[73] of patients with active but medically controlled RA demonstrated that subjects who participated in a carefully supervised intensive exercise program showed greater improvement in function and muscle strength, a greater decrease in the number of clinically active joints, and a faster rate of diminished disease activity compared to the control group of patients who participated in a program of ROM and isometric exercise. The intensive exercises included isokinetic resistance to the knees at 70% maximum voluntary contraction and angular velocity at 60°/sec, isometric exercises at 70% maximum voluntary contraction, bicycling at 60% of the age-predicted maximum for 15 minutes, and ROM exercises. All exercises were adjusted to the pain tolerance of the individual when needed. The primary conclusion of this study was that there is no evidence that patients with active disease should be prevented from vigorous exercise so long as fatigue and pain are respected. The study did not look at joint erosion or cartilage damage.

In a systematic outcomes review, investigators found that moderate or high-intensity exercise in patients with RA has a minimal effect on disease activity and radiological evidence of damage in the hands and feet, but that there is insufficient radiological evidence to determine the effect in large joints. The reviewers also reported that long-term moderate- or high-intensity exercises (individualized to protect radiologically damaged joints) improve aerobic capacity, muscle strength, functional ability, and psychological well-being in patients with RA.[17]

## Osteoarthritis—Degenerative Joint Disease

Osteoarthritis (OA) is a chronic degenerative disorder primarily affecting the articular cartilage of synovial joints, with eventual bony remodeling and overgrowth at the margins of the joints (spurs and lipping) (Fig. 11.4). There is also progression of synovial and capsular thickening and joint effusion.

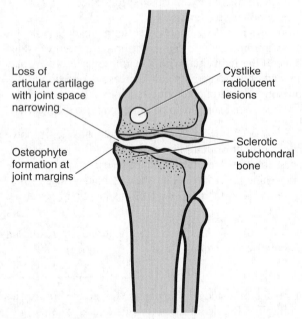

FIGURE 11.4 Radiographic hallmarks of osteoarthritis. *(From McKinnis,[36] p 63, with permission.)*

### Characteristics of OA

● With degeneration, there may be capsular laxity as a result of bone remodeling and capsule distention, leading to hypermobility or instability in some ranges of joint motion. With pain and decreased willingness to move, contractures eventually develop in portions of the capsule and overlying muscle, so as the disease progresses motion becomes more limited.[18,25,71]

● Although the etiology of OA is not known, mechanical injury to the joint due to a major stress or repeated minor stresses and poor movement of synovial fluid when the joint is immobilized are possible causes. Rapid destruc-

tion of articular cartilage occurs with immobilization because the cartilage is not being bathed by moving synovial fluid and is thus deprived of its nutritional supply.[8]

● OA is also genetically related, especially in the hands and hips and to some degree in the knees.[18] Other risk factors that show a direct relationship to OA are obesity, weakness of the quadriceps muscles, joint impact, or sports with repetitive impact and twisting (e.g., soccer, baseball pitching, football), and occupational activities such as jobs that require kneeling and squatting with heavy lifting.[17]

● The cartilage splits and thins out, losing its ability to withstand stress. As a result, crepitation or loose bodies may occur in the joint. Eventually, subchondral bone becomes exposed. There is increased density of the bone along the joint line, with cystic bone loss and osteoporosis in the adjacent metaphysis. During the early stages, the joint is usually asymptomatic because the cartilage is avascular and aneural, but pain becomes constant in later stages.

● Affected joints may become enlarged. Heberden's nodes (enlargement of the distal interphalangeal joint of the fingers) and Bouchard's nodes (enlargement of the proximal interphalangeal joints) are common.

● Most commonly involved are weight-bearing joints (hips and knees), the cervical and lumbar spine, and the distal interphalangeal joints of the fingers and carpometacarpal joint of the thumb (Figs. 11.5 and 11.6).

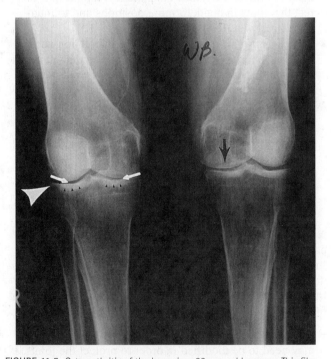

FIGURE 11.5 Osteoarthritis of the knees in a 66-year-old woman. This film was taken under weight-bearing conditions. At the patient's right knee, osteoarthritis is evidenced by narrowed joint space (white arrows), osteophyte formation at the joint margins (large white arrowhead), and sclerotic subchondral bone (small black arrowheads) of both the medial and lateral tibial plateaus. At the patient's left knee, it is interesting to note that in the area of minimal weight-bearing stress the subchondral bone has lost density, and rarefaction is present on the medial aspect of the joint. *(From McKinnis,[36] p 64, with permission.)*

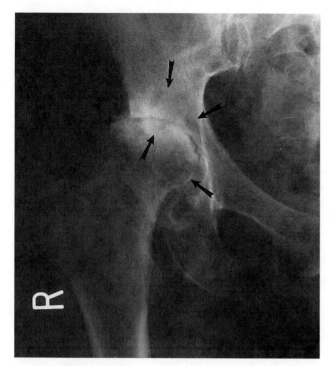

FIGURE 11.6 Severe osteoarthritis of the hip with pseudocysts. The radiolucent cyst-like areas (*arrows*) are caused by intrusion of synovial fluid into areas of subchondral bone that have become weakened by microfractures. *(From McKinnis,[36] p 64, with permission.)*

## Principles of Management—Osteoarthritis

Pain, joint stiffness, decreased muscle performance, and decreased aerobic capacity affect the quality of life and increase the risk for disability for the individual with OA.[19] Therapeutic exercise and manual therapy interventions are important in the comprehensive management of OA. Management guidelines are summarized in Box 11.4.

- *Patient instruction.* Education includes teaching the patient about the disease of OA, how to protect the joints while remaining active, and how to manage the symptoms. The patient is instructed in a home program of safe exercises to improve muscle performance, ROM, and endurance.
- *Pain management—early stages.* Pain and feelings of "stiffness" are common complaints during the early stages. Pain usually occurs because of excessive activity and stress on the involved joint and is relieved with rest. Brief periods of stiffness occur in the morning or after periods of inactivity. This is due to gelling of the involved joints after periods of inactivity.[2] Movement relieves the stasis and feelings of stiffness. It is important to find a balance between activity and rest and to correct biomechanical stresses in order to prevent, retard, or correct the mechanical limitations.
- *Pain management—late stages.* During the late stages of the disease, pain is often present at rest. The pain is probably from secondary involvement of subchondral

## BOX 11.4
## MANAGEMENT GUIDELINES—Osteoarthritis

**Impairments:**
Pain with mechanical stress or excessive activity
Pain at rest in the advanced stages
Stiffness after inactivity
Limitation of motion
Muscle weakness
Decreased proprioception and balance
Functional limitations in ADLs and IADLs

| Plan of Care | Intervention |
|---|---|
| 1. Educate the patient. | 1. Teach about deforming forces and prevention. Teach home exercise program to reinforce interventions and minimize symptoms. |
| 2. Decrease effects of stiffness. | 2. Active ROM Joint-play mobilization techniques. |
| 3. Decrease pain from mechanical stress and prevent deforming forces. | 3. Splinting and/or assistive equipment to minimize stress or to correct faulty biomechanics, strengthen supporting muscles. Alternate activity with periods of rest. |
| 4. Increase ROM. | 4. Stretch muscle, joint, or soft tissue restrictions with specific techniques. |
| 5. Improve neuromuscular control, strength, and muscle endurance. | 5. Low-intensity resistance exercises and muscle repetitions. |
| 6. Improve balance. | 6. Balance training activities. |
| 7. Improve physical conditioning. | 7. Nonimpact or low-impact aerobic exercise. |

**Precautions:** When strengthening supporting muscles, increased pain in the joint during or following resistive exercises probably means that too great a weight is being used or stress is being placed at an inappropriate part of the ROM. Analyze the joint mechanics and at what point during the range the greatest compressive forces are occurring. Maximum resistance exercise should not be performed through that ROM.

bone, synovium, and the joint capsule. In the spine, if bony growth encroaches on the nerve root, there may be radicular pain. Pain that cannot be managed with activity modification and analgesics is usually an indication for surgical intervention.

- *Assistive and supportive devices and activity.* With progression of the disease, the bony remodeling, swelling, and contractures alter the transmission of forces through the joint, which further perpetuates the deforming forces and creates joint deformity. Functional activities become more difficult; and adaptive or assistive devices, such as a raised toilet seat, cane, or walker, may be needed to decrease painful stresses and maintain function. Shock-absorbing footwear may decrease the stresses in OA of the knees.[18] Aquatic therapy and group-based exercise in water decreases pain and improves physical function in patients with lower extremity OA.[14]
- *Resistance exercise.* Progressive weakening in the muscle occurs either from inactivity or from inhibition of the neuronal pools. Weak muscles may add to the joint dysfunction.[1] Strong muscles protect the joint. Resistance exercises, within the tolerance of the joint, should be part of the patient's exercise program. When performing resistive exercises, it is important to avoid deforming forces and heavy weights that the patient cannot control or that cause joint pain. Adaptations include the use of multiple-angle isometrics in pain-free positions, applying resistance only through arcs of motion that are not painful, and use of a pool to decrease weight-bearing stresses and improve functional performance.[21]
- *Stretching and joint mobilization.* Stretching and joint mobilization techniques are used to increase mobility. The patient should be taught self-stretching/flexibility exercises and the importance of movement to counteract the developing restrictions.

###  Focus on Evidence

In a single-blind, randomized clinical trial of 109 patiends with OA of the hip, specific manipulations and mobilizations of the hip joint were reported to have a greater success rate than active exercise for improving muscle function and joint motion. Outcomes measured were perceived improvement after treatment (81% vs. 50%), pain, stiffness, hip function, and ROM.[26]

- *Balance activities.* Joint position sense may be impaired.[74] Balance exercises are described in Chapter 8. Nontraditional forms of exercise such as Tai Chi have been found to be effective for improving balance in patients with OA.[66]
- *Aerobic conditioning.* The patient should be instructed in low-, moderate-, or high-intensity exercises designed to improve cardiopulmonary function.[10] The choice of exercise should have low impact on the joints, such as walking, biking, and swimming. Jogging, jumping, and activities that cause repetitive intensive loading should be avoided.

###  Focus on Evidence

Two systematic reviews of studies designed to examine evidence of the effects of exercise in the management of hip and knee OA describe support for aerobic exercise and strengthening exercises to reduce pain and disability.[51,52] The consensus of expert opinion cited by Roddy[51] is that there are few contraindications and that exercise is relatively safe in patients with OA, but that exercise should be individualized and patient-centered with consideration for age, co-morbidity, and general mobility.

In another study that followed 285 patients with knee OA for 3 years, investigators found that factors that protected the individuals from poor functional outcomes included strength and activity level, as well as factors such as mental health, self-efficacy, and social support.[55]

##  FIBROMYALGIA AND MYOFASCIAL PAIN SYNDROME

Fibromyalgia (FM) and myofascial pain syndrome (MPS) are chronic pain syndromes that are often confused and interchanged. Each has a distinct proposed etiology. Individuals with FM process nociceptive signals differently from individuals without FM,[48] and individuals with MPS have localized changes in the muscle.[59] Although there are some similarities, the differences are significant and determine the method of treatment. They are summarized in Table 11.2.

### Fibromyalgia

Fibromyalgia, as defined by the American College of Rheumatology,[75] is a chronic condition characterized by

| TABLE 11.2 | Similarities and Differences between Fibromyalgia and Myofascial Pain Syndrome |
| --- | --- |
| **Fibromyalgia** | **Myofascial Pain Syndrome** |
| **Similarities** | |
| Pain in muscles | |
| Decreased range of motion | |
| Postural stresses | |
| **Differences** | |
| Tender points | Trigger points in muscle |
| Poor sleep | Referred patterns of pain |
| No referred patterns of pain | Tight band of muscle |
| Fatigue | |

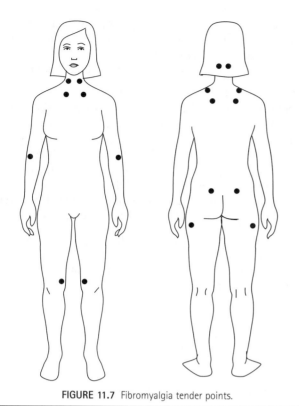

FIGURE 11.7 Fibromyalgia tender points.

widespread pain that covers half the body (right or left half, upper or lower half) and has lasted for more than 3 months. Additional symptoms include 11 of 18 tender points at specific sites throughout the body (Fig. 11.7), nonrestorative sleep, and morning stiffness. A final common problem is fatigue with subsequent diminished exercise tolerance.[75,76]

### Characteristics of FM
The characteristics of FM include the following.[1,29,67]

- The first symptoms of FM can occur at any age but usually appear during early to middle adulthood.
- For more than 30% of those diagnosed, the symptoms develop after physical trauma such as a motor vehicle accident or a viral infection.
- Although the symptoms vary from individual to individual, there are several hallmark complaints. Pain is usually described as muscular in origin and is predominantly reported to be in the scapula, head, neck, chest, and low back.
- Another common report is a significant fluctuation in symptoms. Some days an individual may be pain-free, whereas other days the pain is markedly increased. Most individuals report that when they are in a cycle where the symptoms are diminished they try to do as much as possible. This is usually followed by several days of worsening symptoms and an inability to carry out their normal daily activities. This is often the response to exercise.

- Individuals with FM have a higher incidence of tendonitis, headaches, irritable bowel, temporal mandibular joint dysfunction, restless leg syndrome, mitral valve prolapse, anxiety, depression, and memory problems.

### Contributing Factors to a Flare
Although FM is a noninflammatory, nondegenerative, nonprogressive disorder, several factors may affect the severity of symptoms. These factors include environmental stresses, physical stresses, and emotional stresses. FM is not caused by these various stresses, but it is aggravated by them.

- Environmental stresses include weather changes, especially significant changes in barometric pressure, cold, dampness, fog, and rain. An additional environmental stress is fluorescent lights.
- Physical stresses include repetitive activities, such as typing, playing piano, vacuuming; prolonged periods of sitting and/or standing; and working rotating shifts.
- Emotional stresses are any normal life stresses.

### Management—Fibromyalgia
Research supports the use of exercise,[33,47,53] particularly aerobic exercise, to reduce the most common symptoms associated with FM.

 **Focus on Evidence** _____

An evidence report from the Cochrane Collaborative[12] summarized the findings of 16 randomized trials related to FM and exercise. The reviewers concluded that aerobic exercise was beneficial in reducing FM symptoms and improving exercise capacity, and resistance exercises might be beneficial in reducing symptoms. Flexibility exercises, however, could not be recommended because the exercise was inadequately described in the studies.

One limitation of the research in this area is the description of the intensity and progression of the activity. Although all of the trials reviewed for the Cochrane report followed the American College of Sports Medicine (ACSM) guidelines[3] for aerobic activity and resistance training, only one recent study[37] investigated the intensity of the exercise prescription. The researchers reported that individuals with FM who exercised (walking) at a very low intensity (25% to 60% target heart rate) had better outcomes than those who exercised according to the ACSM recommendations.

_____

In addition to exercise, interventions include:

- Prescription medication
- Over-the-counter medication
- Instruction in pacing activities, in an attempt to avoid fluctuations in symptoms
- Avoidance of stress factors
- Decreasing alcohol and caffeine consumption
- Diet modification.

## Myofascial Pain Syndrome

Myofascial pain syndrome is defined as a chronic, regional pain syndrome.[38] The hallmark classification of MPS comprises the myofascial trigger points (MTrPs) in a muscle which have a specific referred pattern of pain (Fig. 11.8).[58,59] The *trigger point* is defined as a hyperirritable area in a tight band of muscle. The pain from these points is described as dull, aching, and deep. Additional impairments from the trigger points include decreased ROM when the muscle is being stretched, decreased strength in the muscle, and increased pain with muscle stretching. The trigger points may be active (producing a classic pain pattern) or latent (asymptomatic unless palpated).

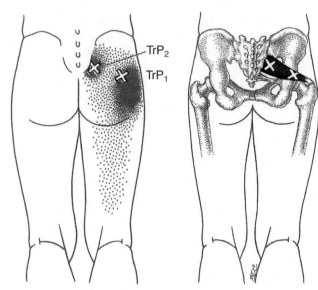

FIGURE 11.8 Composite pattern of pain (dark red) referred from trigger points (TrPs) (Xs) in the right piriformis muscle (medium red). The lateral X (TrP$_1$) indicates the most common TrP location. The red stippling locates the spillover part of the pattern that may be felt as less intense pain than that of the essential pattern (solid red). The spillover pain may be absent. *(From Travell, JG, Simmons, DG: Myofascial Pain and Dysfunction: The Trigger Point Manual: The Lower Extremities, Vol 2. Williams & Wilkins, Baltimore, 1992, p 188, with permission.)*

### Possible Causes of Trigger Points

Although the etiology of trigger points is not completely understood, some potential causes are[58-60]:

- Chronic overload of the muscle that occurs with repetitive activities or that maintain the muscle in a shortened position.
- Acute overload of muscle, such as slipping and catching oneself, picking up an object that has an unexpected weight, or following trauma such as in a motor vehicle accident.
- Poorly conditioned muscles compared to muscles that are exercised on a regular basis.
- Postural stresses such as sitting for prolonged periods of time, especially if the workstation is not ergonomically correct, and leg length differences.
- Poor body mechanics with lifting and other activities.

### Management—Myofascial Pain Syndrome

Treatment consists of three main components: eliminating the trigger point, correcting the contributing factors, and strengthening the muscle.[31,58,59] If the cause of the trigger point is a chronic overload of the muscle, the contributing factor should be eliminated prior to addressing the trigger point. When ROM is restored and the trigger point has been addressed, muscle strengthening is initiated. Several techniques are used to eliminate trigger points.

- Contract–relax–passive stretch done repeatedly until the muscle lengthens
- Contract–relax–active stretch also done in repetition
- Trigger point release
- Spray and stretch
- Dry needling or injection

## OSTEOPOROSIS

*Osteoporosis* is a disease of the bone that leads to decreased mineral content and weakening of the bone. This weakening may lead to fractures, especially of the spine, hip, and wrist. Approximately 10 million Americans have osteoporosis, 80% of them women.[43] The diagnosis of osteoporosis is determined by the T score of a bone mineral density (BMD) scan. The *T score* is the number of standard deviations (SD) above or below a reference value (young, healthy Caucasian women). The World Health Organization (WHO) has established the following criteria.[41]

- Normal: −1.0 or higher
- Osteopenia: −1.1 to −2.4
- Osteoporosis: −2.5 or less

### Risk Factors

***Primary osteoporosis.*** Risk factors for developing primary osteoporosis include being postmenopausal, Caucasian or Asian descent, family history, low body weight, little or no physical activity, and smoking.[43] Additional risk factors include prolonged bed rest and advanced age.

***Secondary osteoporosis.*** Secondary osteoporosis develops owing to other medical conditions (i.e., gastrointestinal diseases, hyperthyroidism, chronic renal failure, excessive alcohol consumption) and the use of certain medications such as glucocorticoids.[41] Regardless of etiology, osteoporosis is detected radiographically by cortical thinning, osteopenia (increased bone radiolucency), trabecular changes, and fractures (Figs. 11.9 and 11.10).[36]

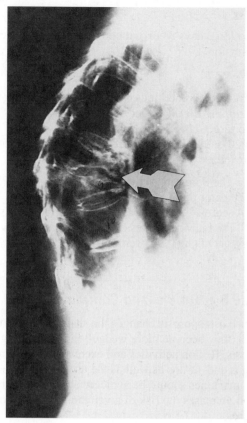

FIGURE 11.9 Osteoporosis of the spine with multiple compression fractures. The arrow points to the T8-T9 disc space, which is deformed by the collapse of these two vertebrae from multiple compression fractures. This 94-year-old woman has severe kyphosis of the thoracic spine (also known as a gibbous deformity) accentuated by vertebral collapse at multiple levels. *(From McKinnis,[36] p 66, with permission.)*

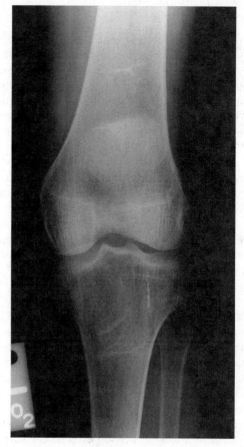

FIGURE 11.10 Osteoporosis is evident in this knee by the accentuation of the remaining trabeculae. The trabeculae have diminished in number and thickness, and the remaining vertically oriented trabeculae stand out as thin, delicate line images. *(From McKinnis,[36] p 66, with permission.)*

## Prevention of Osteoporosis

The National Osteoporosis Foundation (NOF) recommends four ways to prevent osteoporosis.[43]

- Diet rich in calcium and vitamin D
- Weight-bearing exercise
- Healthy lifestyle with moderate alcohol consumption and no smoking
- Testing bone for its density and medication if needed

Bone is living tissue, continually replacing itself in response to the daily demands placed on it. Normally this continual replacement keeps our bone at its optimum strength. Cells in bone called osteoclasts resorb bone, especially if calcium is needed for particular body functions and not enough is obtained in the diet. Another type of cell, the osteoblast, builds bone. This cycle is usually kept in balance with bone resorption equaling bone replacement until the third decade of life. At this point, peak bone mass should be reached. With increasing age there is shift to greater resorption. For women, resorption is accelerated during menopause owing to the decrease in estrogen.[44]

### Physical Activity

Physical activity has been shown to have a positive affect on bone remodeling. In children and adolescents, this activity may increase the peak bone mass. In adults, it has been shown to maintain or increase bone density; and in the elderly, it has been shown to reduce the effects of age-related or disuse-related bone loss.[42] Maintenance of, or an increase in, bone density is important for preventing fractures associated with osteoporosis. Weak bones due to osteoporosis have been attributed to causing more than 1.5 million fractures per year at a cost of $17 billion dollars. Many of these individuals never return to their previous functional level.[43]

### Effects of Exercise

Muscle contraction (e.g., strengthening exercises, resistance training) and mechanical loading (weight bearing) deform bone. This deformation stimulates osteoblastic activity and improves BMD.[61]

### ● Focus on Evidence _____

Dalsky et al.[16] compared postmenopausal women (55 to 70 years old) who did weight-bearing exercise (walking, jogging, stair climbing) with a sedentary control group. The BMD of the exercising group increased significantly during short-term exercise (9 months) and long-term exercise (22 months) compared to the control group. Interestingly, the effects of the exercise were reversed when the subjects discontinued the exercise program (most of the women returned to within 1.1% of their original BMD), indicating that exercise must be continued to have a lasting effect.

Similar results were reported by Nelson et al.[45,46] in two different research projects. The first study examined the effect of a 1-year walking program and increased dietary calcium on the BMD of the lumbar spine and femoral neck. The second study compared a high-intensity strength-training program with untreated controls and the effect on BMD of the lumbar spine and femoral neck. In both studies the subjects were postmenopausal women approximately 50 to 70 years old. In the 1-year walking program, the lumbar spine BMD increased significantly but not the femoral neck BMD. In the high-intensity strength training program, the lumbar spine and femoral neck BMD increased significantly.

Bloomfield et al.[7] compared healthy postmenopausal women doing non-weight- bearing exercise (bicycle ergometry) with sedentary control subjects and assessed the changes in BMD of the lumbar spine and femoral neck. The exercise group rode a bicycle ergometer 3 days/week for 8 months. The tension was set at 60% to 80% of each subject's maximum heart rate as determined by initial $\dot{V}O_{2max}$ testing. The workload was increased over time. Results showed a significant increase in BMD of the lumbar spine in the exercisers.

---

## Recommendations for Exercise

The NOF recommends weight-bearing exercise in the prevention of osteoporosis but does not specify what type of exercise or how often it should be done. Based on current research, the following recommendations are made.[7,16,20,22,23,27,40,45,46,56,61-65,68,72]

### Mode

- Weight-bearing exercise, such as walking, jogging, climbing stairs
- Non-weight-bearing exercise, such as with a bicycle ergometer
- Resistance (strength) training

### Frequency

- Two to three days/week with one day of rest between each session

### Intensity

- At 80% of one repetition maximum (1 RM) with resistance training for the upper extremities
- One to three sets of 8 to 12 repetitions
- At 16/20 on the Borg scale of perceived exertion for trunk exercise

N O T E : The Borg rate of perceived exertion scale (RPE) is a good indicator of how difficult an exercise is for an individual.[9] A score of 16/20 is based on a 15-grade RPE scale (6 to 20). The individual rates how hard he or she is working (7 = very, very light; 13 = somewhat hard; 19 = very, very hard).

## Exercise Precautions and Contraindications

- Because osteoporosis changes the shape of the vertebral bodies (they become more wedge-shaped), leading to kyphosis, flexion activities and exercise such as supine curl-ups and sit-ups as well as the use of sitting abdominal machines should be avoided. Stress into spinal flexion increases the risk of a vertebral compression fracture.
- Avoid combining flexion and rotation of the trunk to reduce stress on the vertebrae and the vertebral discs.
- When performing resistance exercise, it is important to increase the intensity progressively but within the structural capacity of the bone.

N O T E : Refer to Chapter 6 for a discussion of pathological fractures and precautions that should be taken during exercise, identified in Box 6.12

##  FRACTURES—POST-TRAUMATIC IMMOBILIZATION

A fracture is a structural break in the continuity of a bone, an epiphyseal plate, or a cartilaginous joint surface.[54] When there is a fracture, some degree of injury also occurs to the soft tissues surrounding the bone. Depending on the site of the fracture, the related soft tissue injury could be serious if a major artery or peripheral nerve is also involved. If the fracture is more central, the brain, spinal cord, or viscera could be involved. Causes and types of fractures are summarized in Table 11.3 and are illustrated in Figures 11.11, 11.12, and 11.13.

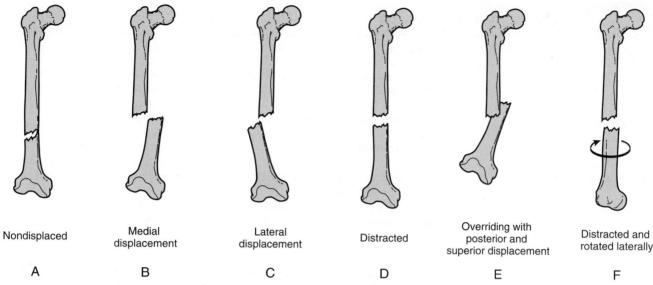

**FIGURE 11.11** *(A–F)* The *position* of fracture fragments may be described by how the *distal* fragment displaces in relationship to the *proximal* fragment. *(From McKinnis,[36] p 86, with permission.)*

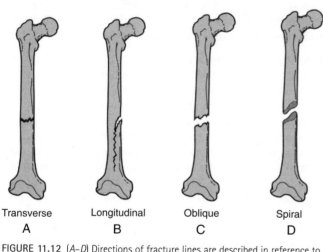

**FIGURE 11.12** *(A–D)* Directions of fracture lines are described in reference to the longitudinal axis of the bone. *(From McKinnis,[36] p 87, with permission.)*

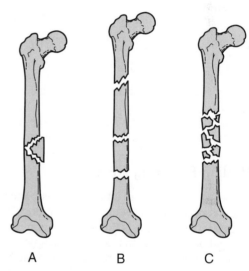

**FIGURE 11.13** *Comminuted* fractures are fractures with more than two fragments. Some frequently occurring comminuted fracture patterns are *(A)* the wedge-shaped or butterfly pattern and *(B)* a two- or three-segmented level fracture. *(C)* Other fractures with multiple fragments, be it several or several hundred, are still described as comminuted. *(From McKinnis,[36] p 87, with permission.)*

A fracture is identified by[54]:

- **Site:** diaphyseal, metaphyseal, epiphyseal, intra-articular
- **Extent:** complete, incomplete
- **Configuration:** transverse, oblique or spiral, comminuted (two or more fragments)
- **Relationship of the fragments:** undisplaced, displaced
- **Relationship to the environment:** closed (skin in tact), open (fracture or object penetrated the skin)
- **Complications:** local or systemic; related to the injury or to the treatment

The diagnosis, reduction, alignment, and immobilization for healing of a fracture are medical procedures and are not discussed in this text. There are times, though, when the therapist provides the initial screening following a traumatic event or examines a patient following repetitive microtrauma; moreover, a patient may sustain an injury

| TABLE 11.3 | Causes and Types of Fractures[54] | |
|---|---|---|
| **Force** | **Effect on Bone** | **Type of Fracture** |
| Bending (angulatory) | Long bone bends causing failure on convex side of bend | Transverse or oblique fracture Greenstick fracture in children |
| Twisting (torsional) | Spiral tension failure in long bone | Spiral fracture |
| Straight pulling (traction) | Tension failure from pull of ligament or muscle | Avulsion fracture |
| Crushing (compression) | Usually in cancellous bone | Compression fracture Torus (buckle) fracture in children |
| Repetitive microtrauma | Small crack in bone unaccustomed to the repetitive/rhythmic stress | Fatigue fracture or stress fracture |
| Normal force on abnormal bone | Such as with osteoporosis, bony tumor, or other diseased bone | Pathological fracture |

while at a therapy session. Hence, the therapist must be aware of symptoms and signs of a potential fracture. If a fracture is suspected, refer the patient for radiographic examination, medical diagnosis, and management. Box 11.5 summarizes the typical symptoms and signs of a possible fracture.

## Risk Factors

Risk factors for fracture include[8]:

- Sudden impact (e.g., accidents, abuse, assult)
- Osteoporosis (women > men)
- History of falls (expecially with increased age, low body mass index, and low levels of physical activity

## Bone Healing Following a Fracture

Fracture healing has (1) an inflammatory phase where there is hematoma formation and cellular proliferation; (2) a reparative phase where there is callous formation uniting the breach and ossification; and (3) a remodeling phase where there is consolidation and remodeling of the bone.[8,54]

### Cortical Bone

When the dense cortical bone of the shaft of a long bone is fractured, the tiny blood vessels are torn at the site, result-

ing in internal bleeding followed by normal clotting. The amount of bleeding depends on the degree of fracture displacement and amount of soft tissue injury in the region. The early stages of healing take place in the hematoma. Osteogenic cells proliferate from the periosteum and endosteum to form a thick callus, which envelopes the fracture site. At this stage the callus does not contain bone and is therefore radiolucent.

- As the callus starts to mature, the osteogenic cells differentiate into osteoblasts and chondroblasts. Initially, the chondroblasts form cartilage near the fracture site, and the osteoblasts form primary woven bone.
- *Stage of clinical union.* When the fracture site is firm enough that it no longer moves, it is clinically united. This occurs when the temporary callus consisting of the primary woven bone and cartilage surrounds the fracture site. The callus gradually hardens as the cartilage ossifies (endochondral ossification). On radiographic examination, the fracture line is still apparent, but there is evidence of bone in the callus. Usually at this stage, immobilization is no longer required. Movement of the related joints is allowed with the caution of avoiding deforming forces at the site of the healing fracture. When assessing the site, no movement of the fracture site or pain should be felt by the patient or therapist.
- *Stage of radiological union.* The bone is considered radiographically healed, or consolidated, when the temporary callus has been replaced by mature lamellar bone. The callus is resorbed, and the bone returns to normal.
- *Rigid internal fixation.* Sometimes it is necessary to apply an internal fixation device, such as a rod or a plate with screws, surgically to protect a healing bone. This allows the bone to be kept stable as it heals, but disuse osteoporosis of the bone under the device occurs because normal stresses are transmitted through the device and bypass the bone. Therefore, the fixation device is removed once the fracture is united in order to reverse the osteoporosis. Following removal of the rod or plate, the bone must be protected from excessive stress for several months until the osteoporosis is reversed.

| BOX 11.5 | Symptoms and Signs of a Possible Fracture |
|---|---|

The following should alert the therapist to a possible fracture.
- History of a fall, direct blow, twisting injury, accident
- Localized pain aggravated by movement
- Muscle guarding with passive movement
- Decreased function of the part
- Swelling, deformity, abnormal movement (may or may not be obvious)
- Sharp, localized tenderness at the site

---

**BOX 11.6  Types of Abnormal Healing of Fractures**

*Malunion*: The fracture heals in an unsatisfactory position resulting in a bony deformity.
*Delayed union*: The fracture takes longer than normal to heal.
*Nonunion*: The fracture fails to unite with a bony union. There may be a *fibrous union* or a *pseudoarthrosis*.

---

**BOX 11.7  Complications of Fractures[8]**

- *Swelling* that is contained within a compartment (fascial compartment or tight cast) leading to nerve and circulatory compromise.
- *Fat embolism* (may occur with fracture in bones with the most marrow, such as long bones and the pelvis) that migrates to the lungs and blocks pulmonary vessels. This is potentially life-threatening.
- *Problems with fixation devices* such as displacement of screws and breakage of wires.
- *Infection* that occurs locally or systemically.
- *Refracture*.
- *Delayed or malunion*.

---

- **Time for healing.** Healing time varies with age of the patient, the location and type of fracture, whether it was displaced, and the blood supply to the fragments. Healing is assessed by the physician using radiological and clinical examinations. Generally, children heal within 4 to 6 weeks, adolescents within 6 to 8 weeks, and adults within 10 to 18 weeks.[8]
- **Abnormal healing.** Abnormal healing is summarized in Box 11.6.

### Cancellous Bone

When the sponge-like lattice of the trabeculae of cancellous bone (in the metaphysis of long bones and bodies of short bones and flat bones) fractures, healing occurs primarily through formation of an intenal callus (endosteal) callus. There is a rich blood supply and a large area of bony contact, so union is more rapid than in dense cortical bone. Cancellous bone is more susceptible to compression forces, resulting in crush or compression fractures. If the surfaces of the fracture are pulled apart, which may occur during reduction of the fracture, healing is delayed.

### Epiphyseal Plate

If a fracture involves the epiphyseal plate, there may be growth disturbances and bony deformity as the skeleton continues to mature. The prognosis for growth disturbances depends on the type of injury, age of the child, blood supply to the epiphysis, method of reduction, and whether it is a closed or open injury.

## Principles of Management— Period of Immobilization

### Local Tissue Response

With immobilization, there is connective tissue weakening, articular cartilage degeneration, muscle atrophy, and contracture development as well as sluggish circulation.[8,15,35] In addition, there is soft tissue injury with bleeding and scar formation.[53,54] Because immobilization is necessary for bone healing, the soft tissue scar cannot become organized along lines of stress as it develops. Early, nondestructive motion within the tolerance of the fracture site is ideal but usually not feasible unless there is some type of internal fixation to stabilize the fracture site. It is important to keep structures in the related area in a state as near normal as possible by using appropriate exercises without jeopardizing alignment of the fracture site while it is healing. The

therapist must be alert to complications that can occur following a fracture (summarized in Box 11.7).

### Immobilization in Bed

If bed rest or immobilization in bed is required, as with skeletal traction, secondary physiological changes occur systematically throughout the body. General exercises for the uninvolved portions of the body are initiated to minimize these problems.

### Functional Adaptations

If there is a lower extremity fracture, alternate modes of ambulation, such as use of crutches or a walker, are taught to the patient who is allowed out of bed. The choice of device and gait pattern depends on the fracture site, the type of immobilization, and the functional capabilities of the patient. The patient's physician should be consulted to determine the amount of weight bearing allowed. Management guidelines are summarized in Box 11.8.

## Postimmobilization Period

### Signs and Symptoms

- There is decreased ROM, joint play, and muscle flexibility. Muscle atrophy with weakness and poor muscle endurance occur, as well as pain in the structures that have been immobilized.
- Initially, the patient experiences pain as movement begins, but it should progressively decrease as joint movement, muscle strength, and ROM improve.
- If there was soft tissue damage at the time of the fracture, an inelastic scar restricts tissue mobility in the region of the scar.

### Principles of Management—Postimmobilization

Management guidelines are summarized in Box 11.9

Consultation with the referring physician is necessary to determine if there is clinical or radiological healing. Until the fracture site is radiologically healed, care should be used any time stress is placed across the fracture site, such as when applying resistance or a stretch force or during weight-bearing activities. Once radiologically healed,

## BOX 11.8
## MANAGEMENT GUIDELINES—Postfracture/Period of Immobilization

**Impairments:**
Initially, inflammation and swelling
In the immobilized area, progressive muscle atrophy, contracture formation, cartilage degeneration, and decreased circulation
Potential overall body weakening if confined to bed
Functional limitations imposed by the fracture site and method of immobilization used

| Plan of Care | Intervention |
|---|---|
| 1. Educate the patient. | 1. Teach functional adaptations.<br>Teach safe ambulation, bed mobility. |
| 2. Decrease effects of inflammation during acute period. | 2. Ice, elevation. |
| 3. Decrease effects of immobilization. | 3. Intermittent muscle setting.<br>Active ROM to joints above and below immobilized region. |
| 4. If patient is confined to bed, maintain strength and ROM in major muscle groups. | 4. Resistive exercises to major muscle groups not immobilized, especially in preparation for future ambulation. |

the bone has normal structural integrity and can withstand normal stress.

The patient is examined to identify impairments and determine the current functional status, activity level, and desired outcome. ROM, joint mobility, and muscle performance as well as any other impairments are measured and documented. Usually all of the joint and periarticular tissues are affected in the region that was immobilized.

Typical interventions include:

● *Joint mobilization.* Joint mobilization techniques are effective for regaining lost joint play without traumatizing the articular cartilage or stressing the fracture site.[28] Intervention begins with gentle stretches (grades III and IV) and progresses in intensity as joint reaction becomes predictable.

## BOX 11.9
## MANAGEMENT GUIDELINES—Postfracture/Postimmobilization

**Impairments:**
Pain with movement, which progressively decreases
Decreased ROM
Decreased joint play
Scar tissue adhesions
Decreased strength and endurance

| Plan of Care | Interventions |
|---|---|
| 1. Educate the patient. | 1. Inform patient of limitations until fracture site is radiologically healed.<br>Teach home exercises that reinforce interventions. |
| 2. Provide protection until radiologically healed. | 2. Use partial weight bearing in lower extremity and nonstressful activities in the upper extremity. |
| 3. Initiate active exercises. | 3. Active ROM, gentle multiangle isometrics. |
| 4. Increase joint and soft tissue mobility. | 4. Initiate joint play stretching techniques (using grades III and IV) with the force applied proximal to the healing fracture site.<br>For muscle stretching, apply the force proximal to the healing fracture site until radiologically healed. |
| 5. Increase strength and muscle endurance. | 5. As the ROM increases and the bone heals, initiate resistive and repetitive exercises. |
| 6. Improve cardiorespiratory fitness. | 6. Initiate safe aerobic exercises that do not stress the fracture site until it is healed. |

**Precautions:** No stretch or resistive forces distal to the fracture site until the bone is radiologically healed. No excessive joint compression or shear for several weeks after the period of immobilization. Use protected weight bearing until the site is radiologically healed.

● *Stretching and muscle inhibition.* Hold–relax and agonist-contraction techniques are used during the post-immobilization period because the intensity can be controlled by the patient's tolerance. It is important to monitor the intensity of contraction and to not apply the resistive or stretch force beyond the fracture site until there is radiological healing of the bone in order to avoid a bending force across the fracture site. Once the bone is radiologically healed, the stretch force can be applied beyond the fracture site.

● *Functional activities.* The patient can resume normal activities with caution. During the early postimmobilization period it is important to not traumatize the weakened muscle, cartilage, bone, and connective tissue. Partial weight bearing must be continued for several weeks after a lower extremity fracture until the fracture site is completely healed and able to tolerate full weight bearing.

● *Muscle performance: strengthening and muscle endurance.* For 2 to 3 weeks following immobilization, because neither the bone nor cartilage can tolerate excessive compressive or bending forces, exercises are initiated with light isometrics. As joint play and ROM improve, progression is made to light resistance through the available range. The resistive force should be applied proximal to the fracture site until the bone is radiologically healed.

● *Scar tissue mobilization.* If there is restricting scar tissue, manual techniques to the mobilize the scar are used. The choice of technique depends on the tissue involved.

## INDEPENDENT LEARNING ACTIVITIES

### ● Critical Thinking and Discussion

1. Your patient sustained a traumatic knee joint injury in an automobile accident. There is joint effusion, limited ROM, and decreased joint play 2 days after the accident. The patient guards against motion as you approach the end of the available range. Identify the principles of treatment, the goals, and plan of care for this patient. Describe and practice specific therapeutic techniques that you would use for intervention and describe how you would progress the techniques through the stages of healing.

2. Develop a program of interventions for a patient with osteoarthritis in the knees who has pain when ascending and descending steps and has difficulty standing up from a chair. What examination procedures do you want to do? What functional tests do you want to document? How would the program differ for an individual with symptoms of rheumatoid arthritis during a period of active disease (the acute phase)? During a period of remission (the chronic phase)?

3. Describe your plan of care and list specific interventions for a 55-year-old woman who is postmenopausal and has early signs of osteoporosis. What patient instructions would be important to include?

4. An individual sustained a fracture 6 weeks ago, and the limb was just removed from the cast. How does treatment differ from that of other traumatic conditions 6 weeks postinjury? Describe what precautions you will follow and why they are important.

5. Your patient was involved in a motor vehicle accident 6 months ago. You saw her 3 months ago, but now she has returned with a diagnosis of fibromyalgia (FM). Her physician recommends exercise. Describe your treatment program, taking into consideration the characteristics of FM and the benefits and problems of exercise in this population.

6. Your new patient is a secretary who presents with upper back and neck pain. She describes a gradual onset. She reports sitting at a computer for 6 to 8 hours each day and having to take phone calls on a regular basis as well. You examine the patient and find several active myofascial trigger points. Describe your course of treatment for this patient. How will you address the effect her work has on her problem?

## REFERENCES

1. American College of Rheumatology: Fibromyalgia Fact Sheet [Website]. Accessed on January 12, 2006. Available at: http://www.rheuma tology.org/public/factsheets/fibromya_new.asp?/.

2. American College of Rheumatology Subcommittee on Osteoarthritis Guidelines: Recommendations for the medical management of osteoarthritis of the hip and knee: 2000 update. Arthritis Rheum 43(9):1905, 2000.

3. American College of Sports Medicine's Guidelines for Exercise Testing and Prescription, ed 6. Lippincott Williams & Wilkins, Philadelphia, 2000.

4. Anderson, RJ: Rheumatoid arthritis: clinical and laboratory features. In Klippel, JH (ed) Primer on the Rheumatic Diseases, ed 12. Arthritis Foundation, Atlanta, 2001, p 218.

5. Arnett, FC, Edworthy, SM, Bloch, DA, et al: The American Rheumatism Association 1987 revised criteria for the classification of rheumatoid arthritis. Arthritis Rheum 31:315, 1988.

6. Bilberg, A, Ahlmen, M, Mannerkorpi, K: Moderately intensive exercise in a temperate pool for patients with rheumatoid arthritis: a randomized controlled study. Rheumatology (Oxford) 44(4):502–508, 2005.

7. Bloomfield S, Williams N, et al: Non-weightbearing exercise may increase lumbar spine bone mineral density in healthy postmenopausal women. Am J Phys Med Rehabil 72(4):204–209, 1993.

8. Boissonnault, WG, Goodman, CC: Bone, joint, and soft tissue disorders. In Goodman, CC, Fuller, KS, Boissonnault, WG (eds) Pathology: Implications for the Physical Therapist, ed 2. WB Saunders, Philadelphia, 2003, p 929.

9. Borg, G, Hassmen, P, Lagerstrom, M: Perceived exertion related to heart rate and blood lactate during arm and leg exercise. Eur J Appl Physiol 65:679–685, 1987.

10. Brosseau, L, MacLeay, L, et al: Intensity of exercise for the treatment of osteoarthritis. Cochrane Database Syst Rev CD004259(2), 2003.

11. Bruce, ML, Peck, B: New rheumatoid arthritis treatments. Holistic Nurs Pract 19(5):197, 2005.

12. Busch A, Schachter CL, et al: Exercise for treating fibromyalgia syndrome. Cochrane Review. In: The Cochrane Library, Issue 3, 2004. John Wiley, Chichester, UK.

13. Clark, SR, Burckhardt, CS, Bennett, RM: The use of exercise to treat rheumatic disease. In Goldberg, L, Elliot, DL (eds) Exercise for Prevention and Treatment of Illness. FA Davis, Philadelphia, 1994, p 83.

14. Cochrane, T, Davey, RC, Matthes Edwards, SM: Randomised controlled trial of the cost-effectiveness of water-based therapy for lower limb osteoarthritis. Health Technol Assess 9(31):1–114, 2005.

15. Cummings, GS, Tillman, LJ: Remodeling of dense connective tissue in normal adult tissues. In Currier, DP, Nelson, RM (eds) Dynamics of Human Biologic Tissues. FA Davis, Philadelphia, 1992, p 45.

16. Dalsky G, Stocke K, Ehsani A, et al: Weight-bearing exericse training and lumbar bone mineral content in postmenopausal women. Ann Intern Med 108:824–828, 1988.

17. De Jong, Z, Vlieland, TP: Safety of exercise in patients with rheumatoid arthritis. Curr Opin Rheumatol 17(2):177–182, 2005.

18. Felson, DT, Lawrence, RC, Dieppe, PA, et al: Osteoarthritis: new insights. Part 1. The disease and its risk factors. Ann Intern Med 133(8):635, 2000.

19. Felson, DT, Lawrence, RC, Hockberg, MC, et al: Osteoarthritis: new insights. Part 2. Treatment approaches. Ann Intern Med 133(9):726, 2000.

20. Fiatorone M, O'Neill E, Ryan N, et al. Exercise training and nutritional supplementation for physical fraily in very elderly people. N Engl J Med 30(25):1769–1775, 1994.

21. Foley, A, Halbert, J, et al: Does hydrotherapy improve strength and physical function in patients with osteoarthritis—a randomized controlled trial comparing a gym based and a hydrotherapy based strengthening programme. Ann Rheum Dis 62(12):1162–1167, 2003.

22. Frontera W, Meredith C, O'Reilly K, et al: Strength conditioning in older men: skeletal muscle hypertrophy and improved function. J Appl Physiol 64(3):1038–1044, 1988.

23. Halle J, Smidt G, et al: Relationship between trunk muscle torque and bone mineral content of the lumbar spine and hip in healthy postmenopausal women. Phys Ther 70(11):690–699, 1990.

24. Hawley, DJ: Health status assessment. In Wegener, ST (ed) Clinical Care in the Rheumatic Diseases. American College of Rheumatology, Atlanta, 1996.

25. Hockberg, MC: Osteoarthritis: clinical features and treatment. In Klippel, JH (ed) Primer on the Rheumatic Diseases, ed 11. Arthritis Foundation, Atlanta, 1997, p 218.

26. Hoeksma, HL, Dekker, J, Ronday, HK, et al: Comparison of manual therapy and exercise therapy in osteoarthritis of the hip: a randomized clinical trial. Arthritis Rheum 51(5):722–729, 2004.

27. Kaelin ME, Swank AM, Adams KJ, et al: Cardiopulmonary responses, muscle soreness, and injury during the one repetition maximum assessment in pulmonary rehabilitation patients. J Cardiopulm Rehabil 19(6):366–372, 1999.

28. Kaltenborn, F: Manual Mobilization of the Extremity Joints: The Kaltenborn Method of Joint Examination and Treatment. Vol I. The Extremities, ed 5. Olaf Norlis Bokhandel, Oslo, 1999.

29. Krsnich-Shriwise S: Fibromyalgia syndrome: an overview. Phys Ther. 77:68–75, 1997.

30. Leonard, JB: Joint protection for inflammatory disorders. In Lichtman, DM, Alexander, AH (eds) The Wrist and Its Disorders, ed 2. WB Saunders, Philadelphia, 1997, p 1377.

31. Lewit K, Simons D: Myofascial pain: relief by post-isometric relaxation. Arch Phys Med Rehabil 65:452–456, 1984.

32. Margolis, S, Flynn, JA: Arthritis: The Johns Hopkins White Papers. The Johns Hopkins Medical Institutions, Baltimore, 2000.

33. Martin L, Nutting A, Macintosh B, et al: An exercise program in the treatment of fibromyalgia. J Rheumatol 23:1050–1053, 1996.

34. Matteson, EL: Rheumatoid arthritis: treatment. In Klippel, JH (ed) Primer on the Rheumatic Diseases, ed 12. Arthritis Foundation, Atlanta, 2001, p 225.

35. McDonough, A: Effect of immobilization and exercise on articular cartilage: a review of literature. J Orthop Sports Phys Ther 3:2, 1981.

36. McKinnis, LN: Fundamentals of Musculoskeletal Imaging, ed 2. FA Davis, Philadelphia, 1999.

37. Meyer BB, Lemley KJ: Utilizing exercise to affect the symptomology of fibromyalgia: a pilot study. Med Sci Sports Exerc 32(10):1691–1697, 2000.

38. Meyer, H: Myofascial pain syndrome and its suggested role in the pathogenesis and treatment of fibromyalgia syndrome. Curr Pain Headache Rep 6:274–283, 2002.

39. Minor, MA, et al: Efficacy of physical conditioning exercise in patients with rheumatoid arthritis and osteoarthritis. Arthritis Rheum 32:1396, 1989.

40. Morganti C, Nelson M, Fiatarone M, et al: Strength improvements with 1 yr of progressive resistance training in older women. Med Sci Sports Exerc 27(6):906–912, 1995.

41. National Institutes of Health Consensus Development Panel. Osteoporosis prevention, diagnosis, and therapy. JAMA 285:785–795, 2001.

42. National Institutes of Health Osteoporosis and Related Bone Diseases: Peak Bone Mass in Women [website]. Available at: http://www.osteo.org.

43. National Osteporosis Foundation: Disease Statistics [website]. Available at: http://www.nof.org/osteoporosis/stats.htm/. Accessed February 2003.

44. Nelson M: Strong Women, Strong Bones. Berkley Publishing Group. New York, 2000.

45. Nelson M, Fisher E, Dilmanian FA, et al: A 1-y walking program and increased dietary calcium in postmenopausal women: effects on bone. Am J Clin Nutr 53:1304–1311, 1991.

46. Nelson M, Fiatarone M, Morganti C, et al: Effects of high-intensity strength training on multiple risk factors for osteoporotic fractures: a randomized controlled trial. JAMA 272(24):1909–1914, 1994.

47. Nichols D, Glenn T: Effects of aerobic exercise on pain perception, affect, and level of disability in individuals with fibromyalgia. Phys Ther 74(4):327–332, 1994.

48. Pellemer, SR, Bradley, LA, Crofford, LJ, et al: The neuroscience and endocrinology of fibromyalgia. Arthritis Rheum 40(11):1928–1939, 1997.

49. Phillips, CA: Therapist's management of patients with RA. In Lichtman, DM, Alexander, AH (eds) The Wrist and Its Disorders, ed 2. WB Saunders, Philadelphia, 1997, p 1345.

50. Pincus, T: Rheumatoid arthritis. In Wegener, ST (ed) Clinical Care in the Rheumatic Diseases. American College of Rheumatology, Atlanta, 1996, p 147.

51. Roddy, E, Zhang, W, Doherty, M, et al: Evidence-based recommendations for the role of exercise in the management of osteoarthritis of the hip or knee—the MOVE consensus. Rheumatology 44(1):67–73, 2005.

52. Roddy, E, Zhang, W, Doherty, M: Aerobic walking or strengthening exercise for osteoarthritis of the knee? A systematic review. Ann Rheum Dis 64(4):544–548, 2005.

53. Rooks D, Silverman C, Kantrowitz F: The effects of progressive strength training and aerobic exercise on muscle strength and cardiovascular fitness in women with fibromyalgia: a pilot study. Arthritis Care Res 47:22–28, 2002.

54. Salter, RB: Textbook of Disorders and Injuries of the Musculoskeletal System, ed 3. Williams & Wilkins, Baltimore, 1999.

55. Sharma, L, Cahue, S, Song, J, et al: Physical functioning over three years in knee osteoarthritis: role of psychosocial, local mechanical, and neuromuscular factors. Arthritis Rheum 48(12):3359–3370, 2003.

56. Shaw C, McCully K, Posner J.: Injuries during the one repetition maximum assessment in the elderly. J Cardiopulm Rehabil 15(4):283–287, 1995.

57. Simon, LS: Arthritis: new agents herald more effective symptom management. Geriatrics 54(6):37, 1999.

58. Simons D, Travell J, Simons L: Myofascial Pain and Dysfunction: The Trigger Point Manual, Vol 1, ed 2. Williams & Wilkins, Baltimore, 1999.

59. Simons D: Review of enigmatic MTrPs as a common cause of enigmatic musculoskeletal pain and dysfunction. J Electromyogr Kinesiol 14:95–107, 2004.

60. Simons D: Clinical and etiological update of myofascial pain from trigger points. J Musculoskel Pain 4:93–121, 1996.

61. Sinaki M: Effect of physical activity on bone mass. Curr Opin Rheumatol 1996;8:376–383.

62. Sinaki M, Wahner H, et al: Efficacy of nonloading exercises in prevention of vertebral bone loss in postmenopausal women: a controlled trial. Mayo Clin Proc 64:762–769, 1989.

63. Sinaki M, Wollan P, et al: Can strong back extensors prevent vertebral fractures in women with osteoporosis? Mayo Clin Proc 71:951–956, 1996.

64. Smith E, Smith P, et al: Bone evolution decrease in exercising middle-aged women. Calcif Tissue Int 36:S129–S138, 1984.

65. Snow-Harter C, Bouxsein M, Lewis B, et al: Effects of resistance and endurance exercise on bone mineral status of young women: a randomized exercise intervention trial. J Bone Miner Res 7(7):761–769, 1992.

66. Song, R, Lee EO, et al: Effect of Tai Chi exercise on pain, balance, muscle strength, and perceived difficulties in physical functioning in older women with osteoarthritis: a randomized clinical trial. J Rheumatol 30(9):2039–2044, 2003.

67. Starlanyl D, Copeland M: Fibromyalgia and Chronic Myofascial Pain Syndrome. New Harbinger Publications, Oakland, 1996.

68. Suleiman S, Nelson M, Li F, et al: Effect of calcium intake and physical activity level on bone mass and turnover in healthy, white, postmenopausal women. Am J Clin Nutr 66:937–943, 1997.

69. The Arthritis Foundation's Guide to Good Living with Osteoarthritis. Arthritis Foundation, Atlanta, 2000.

70. The Arthritis Foundation's Guide to Good Living with Rheumatoid Arthritis. Arthritis Foundation, Atlanta, 2000.

71. Threlkeld, JA, Currier, DP: Osteoarthritis: effects on synovial joint tissues. Phys Ther 68:346, 1988.

72. Tsuzuku S, Shimokata H, Ikegami Y, et al: Effects of high versus low-intensity resistance training on bone mineral density in young males. Calcif Tissue Int 68:342–347, 2001.

73. Van den Ende, CH, Breedveld, FC, le Cessie, S, et al: Effect of intensive exercise on patients with active rheumatoid arthritis: a randomised clinical trial. Ann Rheum Dis 59(8):615, 2000.

74. Wegener, L, Kisner, C, Nichols, D: Static and dynamic balance responses in persons with bilateral knee osteoarthritis. J Orthop Sports Phys Ther 25:13, 1997.

75. Wolfe F, Smythe HA, Yunus MB: The American College of Rheumatology 1990 criteria for the classification of fibromyalgia: report of the Multicenter Criteria Committee. Arthritis Rheum 33:160–172, 1990.

76. Wolfe W: Diagnosis of fibromyalgia. J Musculoskel Med 7(7):53–69, 1990.

77. Ytterberg, SR, Mahowald, ML, Krug, HE: Exercise for arthritis. Baillieres Clin Rheumatol 8(1):161–189, 1994.

# Surgical Interventions and Postoperative Management

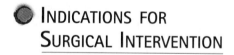

## 12

CHAPTER

An array of injuries, diseases, and disorders of the musculoskeletal system that affect muscles, tendons, ligaments, cartilage, fascia, joint capsules, or bones can cause impairment of the upper or lower extremities or the spine, resulting in functional limitation and disability to such an extent that surgical intervention is required. Ideally, surgery is preceded by a comprehensive examination and evaluation of a patient's impairments and functional status coupled with preoperative patient education and followed by a planned course of postoperative rehabilitation.

This chapter provides an overview of indications for surgical intervention for musculoskeletal pathology, considerations for preoperative management, factors that influence the outcomes of surgery, general guidelines for management during progressive phases of postoperative rehabilitation, and potential complications that can interfere with the achievement of optimal functional outcomes after surgery. The chapter concludes with an overview of the many types of orthopedic surgery that may be undertaken for the management of musculoskeletal conditions of the upper and lower extremities.

Descriptions of selected surgical procedures for common injuries or disorders of each region of the extremities are described in Chapters 17 through 22. In these chapters, guidelines and progressions for postoperative management of specific surgeries are presented that are based on the principles of tissue healing and exercise prescription addressed in Chapter 10 rather than adherence to specific protocols. These principles can be applied by the therapist when designing exercise interventions for patients under-

going current surgical procedures and can also be applied as a basis of rehabilitation in the future as surgical interventions change and evolve.

## ○ INDICATIONS FOR SURGICAL INTERVENTION

Many acute, recurring, or chronic musculoskeletal conditions can be successfully managed with conservative (nonoperative) measures, including rest, protection with splinting or use of assistive devices, medication, therapeutic exercise, manual therapy, and functional training, as well as the use of physical agents or electrotherapy. However, if a conservative program has not been successful and one or more impairments continue to significantly compromise a patient's ability to function or if the severity of a patient's condition is such that nonoperative management is not an appropriate option, surgical intervention becomes the treatment of choice. Indications for a variety of musculoskeletal surgeries are identified in Box 12.1.[11,13,47,56,58]

## ○ GUIDELINES FOR PREOPERATIVE AND POSTOPERATIVE MANAGEMENT

Although surgical intervention can correct or reduce adverse effects and impairments (e.g., pain, deformity, instability) associated with musculoskeletal pathology, a carefully planned and progressed rehabilitation program is essential for a patient to achieve optimal functional outcomes after surgery. In an ideal situation, rehabilitation begins with patient education before surgery and continues after surgery with direct intervention from a therapist followed by long-term self-management by the patient.

## Considerations for Preoperative Management

Contact with a patient prior to preplanned, elective surgery is advisable whether it occurs on a one-to-one basis between therapist and patient or in a group setting. In the health care environment of the past two to three decades, authorization for a preoperative visit with an individual patient has become increasingly difficult. However, preoperative contact with a group of patients scheduled for similar surgeries may be possible. The benefits of preoperative contact with a patient are noted in Box 12.2.

There are two main aspects of preoperative management: a comprehensive examination and evaluation of a patient's preoperative status and patient education.

### Preoperative Examination and Evaluation

If a preoperative visit is approved for an individual patient, it enables a therapist to perform a comprehensive, systematic examination to document the patient's impairments

and functional status prior to surgery.[46,57] By evaluating the findings of the examination, a therapist can identify the patient's needs, anticipated goals, and expected functional outcomes as a result of the surgery.

Testing and measurement of the following areas are of particular importance for determining realistic goals and functionally relevant outcomes of surgery and postoperative rehabilitation.[57]

- *Pain.* Quantitatively measure the patient's level of pain with a visual analog scale or a scale that identifies the degree of pain with specific functional activities.
- *Range of motion and joint integrity.* Measure both active and passive range of motion (ROM) of the involved joint or extremity and compare it to the ROM of the uninvolved areas. Check the stability and mobility of joints.
- *Integrity of the skin.* Note the presence of scars from previous injuries or surgeries, particularly those that are adherent and restrict mobility of skin.
- *Muscle performance (strength and endurance).* Evaluate muscle strength of the affcted areas, recognizing that pain adversely affects strength. Assess the functional strength of unaffected body segments in anticipation of postoperative ambulation with assistive devices, transfers, and activities of daily living (ADL).
- *Posture.* Identify the patient's preferred positions for comfort and any postural abnormalities that may affect ROM and function.
- *Gait analysis.* Analyze the gait characteristics, type of supportive or protective devices currently used, and degree of weight bearing tolerated during ambulation. Note any inequality in leg lengths.
- *Functional status.* Identify the patient's preoperative functional limitations and abilities and his or her perception of disability using a quantitative, self-report measurement tool.

N O T E : These areas of the examination are also components of the initial and subsequent postoperative evaluations during rehabilitation.

### Preoperative Patient Education—Methods and Rationale

Patient education can be initiated preoperatively, either during an individual instruction session with a patient or in a group setting with patients planning to undergo similar surgeries. Some large, acute-care facilities, for example, have reported descriptions of programs for patients scheduled for joint replacement surgery that focus on preoperative group instruction by team members from several disciplines, incuding nursing, physical therapy, and occupational therapy.[26,35,39] The group program may also include a tour of the operating and recovery rooms. It is believed that programs such as these help a patient understand what to expect the day of surgery and during the early postoperative days and may alleviate some of a patient's anxiety about the surgery and hospital experience.

Preoperative instruction gives a patient an opportunity to become familiar with wound care, any special precautions that must be followed after surgery, and the use of assistive or supportive equipment such as crutches, a splint, or a sling.[46,57] Of equal importance, it enables a patient to practice and learn early postoperative exercises without being hampered by postoperative pain or the side effects of pain medication, such as disorientation and drowsiness.[46,57] If surgery is scheduled on an outpatient basis, which is a growing trend, preoperative instruction enables a patient to be safe at home during the early postoperative days and to begin postoperative exercises at home the day of or after surgery before follow-up by a therapist at a later time.

### Components of Preoperative Patient Education

- *Overview of the plan of care.* Explain the general plan of care the patient can expect during the postoperative period.
- *Postoperative precautions.* Advise the patient of any precautions or contraindications to positioning, movement, or weight bearing that must be followed postoperatively.
- *Bed mobility and transfers.* Teach the patient how to move in bed or perform wheelchair transfers safely, incorporating necessary postoperative precautions.
- *Initial postoperative exercises.* Teach the patient any exercises that will be started during the very early postoperative period. These often include:
  - Deep-breathing and coughing exercises.
  - Active ankle exercises (pumping exercises), if possible, to prevent venous stasis and decrease the risk of deep vein thrombosis.
  - Gentle muscle-setting exercises of immobilized joints.
- *Gait training.* Teach the use of any supportive devices, such as crutches or a walker, that may be needed for protected weight bearing during ambulation after surgery.
- *Wound care.* Explain or reinforce postoperative care of the incision for optimal wound healing.

## Considerations for Postoperative Management

A well planned rehabilitation program, composed of a carefully progressed sequence of therapeutic exercise and functional training and ongoing patient education, is fundamental to the patient's postoperative care. Appropriate rehabilitative management takes many factors into consideration, any of which may affect the components and progression of a patient's postoperative program. These factors are noted in Box 12.3. Each of the factors also influences the postoperative functional outcomes for a patient and the ultimate success of the surgical procedure.

To design a safe, effective, efficient rehabilitation program for a patient, a therapist must understand the indications and rationale for a particular surgical procedure, must become familiar with the procedure itself, must be aware of special precautions related to the surgery, and must communicate effectively with the patient and surgeon.

### Postoperative Examination and Evlauation

Every individually designed postoperative rehabilitation program must be based on initial and ongoing examinations of a patient. In addition to the components of a preoperative examination noted previously in this section, an assessment of integumentary integrity is important after

---

**BOX 12.3 Factors That Influence the Components, Progression, and Outcomes of a Postoperative Rehabilitation Program**

- Extent of tissue pathology or damage
  - Size or severity of the lesion
- Type and unique characteristics of the surgical procedure
- Patient-related factors
  - Age, extent of preoperative impairments, and functional limitations
  - Health history, particularly use of medications and diabetes
  - Lifestyle history, including use of tobacco
  - Needs, goals, expectations, and social support
  - Level of motivation and ability to adhere to an exercise program
- Stage of healing of involved tissues
- Characteristics of types of tissues involved
  - Response to immobilization and remobilization
- Integrity of structures adjacent to involved tissues
- Philosophy of the surgeon

---

surgery. The incision should be inspected before and after each exercise session to identify any evidence of wound infection or delayed healing. Inspection of the surgical site includes the items noted in Box 12.4.

### Phases of Postoperative Rehabilitation

Postoperative rehabilitation is typically divided into phases, containing goals and suggested interventions for each phase. Phases are identified in several ways: by the overlapping phases of tissue healing (acute/inflammation, subacute/proliferative, chronic remodeling), by the level of difficulty of activities (initial, intermediate, advanced), by the degree of protection of healing tissues (maximum, moderate, minimum protection), or simply by sequential numbering (e.g., I, II, III).

As with nonoperative management of musculoskeletal pathology, these phases reflect the stages of healing of involved soft tissue and bone. In addition, phases of postoperative rehabilitation must take into account the characteristics of the surgical procedure, such as the type of surgical approach or tissue fixation.

---

**BOX 12.4 Inspection of the Surgical Incision**

- Check for signs of redness or tissue necrosis along the incision(s) and around sutures.
- Palpate along the incision and note signs of tenderness and edema.
- Palpate to determine evidence of increased heat.
- Check for signs of drainage; note color and amount of drainage on the dressing.
- Note the integrity of an incision across a joint *during and after* exercise.
- As the incision heals, check the mobility of the scar.

During each phase of postoperative rehabilitation, the goals and the plan of care, including therapeutic exercise interventions, change. For example, early after surgery, the emphasis of management focuses on minimizing pain, preventing postoperative complications, and retaining a safe level of functional mobility while protecting the surgical site. Later, as tissues heal and the patient recovers from surgery, interventions are directed toward restoring or improving ROM, strength, neuromuscular control, stability, balance, and muscular and cardiopulmonary endurance as well as the patient's ability to perform all necessary and desired functional activities.

Phases of postoperative rehabilitation do not take into account the individual qualities, needs, and abilities of each patient. Therefore, they are not prescriptive but, rather, are intended as general guidelines for management. To develop an individualized rehabilitation program for a patient, suggested guidelines for each phase should be modified based on the results of ongoing postoperative examination of the patient.

Without disregarding the differences among various surgical procedures and the fact that each patient's recovery after surgery is unique, guidelines for postoperative rehabilitation in this section are divided into three broad, overlapping phases based on the degree of protection of operated structures. The characteristics of these three phases are as follows.

● *Maximum protection phase.* This is the initial postoperative period when protection of operated tissues is paramount in the presence of tissue inflammation and pain. After some surgeries immobilization of the operated area is necessary during this phase. After other surgeries it is advisable to place low-level stresses on operated tissues soon after surgery, making early passive or assisted ROM within a protected range or within a patient's toler-ance permissable. In both situations, muscle-setting exercises to prevent muscle atrophy also are indicated. The time frame for maximum protection ranges from a few days or a week to a month or 6 weeks depending on the type of surgery and type of tissues involved.

● *Moderate protection phase.* This is the intermediate phase of rehabilitation when inflammation has subsided, pain and tenderness are minimal, and tissues are able to withstand gradually increasing levels of stress. Criteria for progression to this phase often include the absence of pain at rest and the availaability of at least limited pain-free movement of the operated extremity. Restoring ROM and normal arthrokinematics while tissues continue to heal and remodel, improving neuromuscular control and stability, and gradually increasing strength are emphasized during this phase. Depending on the healing characteristics of the operated tissues, this phase typically begins around 4 to 6 weeks postoperatively and continues for an additional 4 to 6 weeks.

● *Minimum protection/return to function phase.* During this advanced phase, little to no protection of operated tissues is required. To progress to this phase, full or almost full, pain-free active ROM should be available, and the joint capsule (if involved) should be clinically stable. Strength necessary to begin this phase varies widely after different procedures. Rehabilitation focuses on restoring functional strength and participating in gradually progressed functional activities. This phase begins anywhere from 6 to 12 weeks postoperatively and may continue until 6 months postoperatively or beyond.

Box 12.5 summarizes management guidelines for postoperative rehabilitation, including common impairments that must be addressed and a plan of care with suggested goals and interventions for each phase of rehabilitation.

---

**BOX 12.5**

MANAGEMENT GUIDELINES—Postoperative Rehabilitation

**Impairments:**
Postoperative pain because of disruption of soft tissue
Postoperative swelling
Potential circulatory and pulmonary complications
Joint stiffness or limitation of motion because of injury to soft tissue and necessary postoperative immobilization
Muscle atrophy because of immobilization
Loss of strength for functional activities
Limitation of weight bearing
Potential loss of strength and mobility in unoperated joints

**Maximum Protection Phase**

| Plan of Care | Interventions |
|---|---|
| 1. Educate the patient in preparation for self-management. | 1. Instruction in safe positioning and limb movements and special postoperative precautions or contraindications. |
| 2. Decrease postoperative pain, muscle guarding, or spasm. | 2. Relaxation exercises. Use of modalities such as transcutaneous nerve stimulation (TNS), cold, or heat. Continuous passive motion (CPM) during the early postoperative period. |

| Plan of Care | Interventions |
|---|---|
| 3. Prevent wound infection. | 3. Instruction or review of proper cleaning and dressing the incision. |
| 4. Minimize postoperative swelling. | 4. Elevation of the operated extremity.<br>Active muscle pumping exercises at the distal joints.<br>Use of compression garment.<br>Gentle distal-to-proximal massage.[69] |
| 5. Prevent circulatory and pulmonary complications such as deep vein thrombosis, pulmonary embolus, or pneumonia. | 5. Active exercises to distal musculature.<br>Deep-breathing and coughing exercises. |
| 6. Prevent unnecessary, residual joint stiffness, or soft tissue contractures. | 6. CPM or passive or active-assistive ROM initiated in the immediate postoperative period. |
| 7. Minimize muscle atrophy across immobilized joints. | 7. Muscle-setting exercises. |
| 8. Maintain motion and strength in areas above and below the operative site. | 8. Active and resistive ROM exercises to unoperated areas. |
| 9. Maintain functional mobility while protecting the operative site. | 9. Adaptive equipment and assistive devices. |

## Moderate Protection/Controlled Motion Phase

| Plan of Care | Interventions |
|---|---|
| 1. Educate the patient. | 1. Teach the patient to monitor the effects of the exercise program and make adjustments if swelling or pain increases. |
| 2. Gradually restore soft-tissue and joint mobility. | 2. Active-assistive or active ROM within limits of pain.<br>Joint mobilization procedures. |
| 3. Establish a mobile scar. | 3. Gentle massage across and around the maturing scar. |
| 4. Strengthen involved muscles and improve joint stability. | 4. Multiple-angle isometrics against increasing resistance.<br>Alternating isometrics and rhythmic stabilization procedures.<br>Dynamic exercise against light resistance in open- and closed-chain positions.<br>Light functional activities with operated limb. |

## Minimum Protection/Return to Function Phase

| Plan of Care | Interventions |
|---|---|
| 1. Continue patient education. | 1. Emphasize gradual but progressive incorporation of improved muscle performance, mobility, and balance into functional activities. |
| 2. Prevent reinjury or postoperative complications. | 2. Reinforce self-monitoring and review the signs and symptoms of excessive use; identify unsafe activities. |
| 3. Restore full joint and soft-tissue mobility, if possible. | 3. Joint stretching (mobilization) and self-stretching techniques. |
| 4. Maximize muscle performance, dynamic stability, and neuromuscular control. | 4. Progressive strengthening exercises using higher loads and speeds and combined movement patterns.<br>Integrate movements and positions into exercises that simulate functional activities. |
| 5. Restore balance and coordinated movement. | 5. Progressive balance and coordination training. |
| 6. Acquire or relearn specific motor skills. | 6. Apply principles of motor learning (appropriate practice and feedback during task-specific training). |

**Precautions:** In addition to the precautions already addressed that relate to the stages of tissue repair and healing, there are several additional precautions that are of particular importance to the postsurgical patient.

- Avoid positions, movements, or weight bearing that could compromise the integrity of the surgical repair.

- Keep the wound clean to avoid postoperative infection. Monitor for wound drainage and signs of systemic or local infection, such as elevated temperature.

- Avoid vigorous/high-intensity stretching or resistance exercises with soft tissues, such as muscles, tendons, or joint capsules that have been repaired or reattached for at least 6 weeks to ensure adequate healing and stability.

- Modify level and selection of physical activities, if necessary, to prevent premature wear and tear of repaired or reconstructed soft tissues and joints.

N O T E : The descriptions of each phase noted in Box 12.4 are general and inclusive of rehabilitation after a variety of surgical interventions. Guidelines that include goals and suggested interventions for each of the phases of postoperative rehabilitation are described for specific surgeries at each region of the extremities in Chapters 17 to 22.

### Time-Based and Criterion-Based Progression

Time frames for each phase of rehabilitation vary dramatically from one procedure to another. For example, immediately after an arthroscopic meniscectomy, the maximum protection phase during which movement of the operated joint is limited to passive or assisted motion within a protected range may extend for only 1 day postoperatively. However, after a complex tendon repair in the hand, maximum protection may be required for several weeks.

Although published descriptions of postoperative rehabilitation typically include estimated time frames for each phase of a program, these time periods must be viewed only as general guidelines. Determining a patient's readiness to advance from one phase of postoperative rehabilitation to the next should not be based solely on time but also on the patient's attainment of predetermined criteria, such as the absence of pain or restoration of a particular amount of ROM or level of strength. However, at this time most published guidelines and protocols are time-based and provide little or no information for making criterion-based decisions.

### Putting Postoperative Rehabilitaion into Perspective

Postoperative rehabilitation is often a lengthy process. Given the limited number of justifiable therapy sessions available for postoperative management, it is highly unlikely for a therapist to have direct, ongoing contact with a patient through all phases of a rehabilitation program. Consequently, the key to successful postoperative outcomes is effective self-management that includes therapist-directed perioperative patient education followed by a home program of selected interventions—in particular, a progression of exercises that have been carefully taught and are periodically monitored and modified by the therapist during each phase of rehabilitation.

## Potential Postoperative Complications

There are a number of serious complications that may be encountered after surgery, any one of which can adversely affect the outcomes of surgery and postoperative rehabilitation. Complications are sometimes classified as early (within 6 months after surgery) and late. Potential complications are noted in Box 12.6.[3,13,34,58,60,62]

### Reducing Risks of Postoperative Complications

Aspects of preoperative patient education and interventions in a postoperative rehabilitation program are directed toward reducing the risks for a number of these complications.

---

### BOX 12.6   Potential Postoperative Complications

- Increased risk of pulmonary complications, including pneumonia or atelectasis
- Local or systemic infection
- Deep vein thrombosis or pulmonary embolism
- Delayed wound healing
- Muscle function deficits secondary to tourniquet compression and resulting ischemia or nerve compression
- Failure, loosening, or displacement of internal fixation devices
- Delayed union of bone after fracture, osteotomy, or joint fusion
- Rupture of incompletely healed soft tissue after repair or reconstruction
- Subluxation or dislocation of joint surfaces or implants
- Nerve entrapment from scar tissue resulting in pain or sensory changes
- Adhesions and scarring leading to contractures of soft tissues and joint hypomobility
- Loosening of joint implants secondary to periprosthetic osteolysis

---

***Pulmonary complications.*** The risk of pulmonary complications is highest during the early postoperative period. General anesthesia and use of pain medication increase the risk of this complication as does extended confinement to bed. Deep breathing exercises initiated on the day of surgery and early standing and ambulation may reduce the risk of pneumonia or atelectasis.

***Deep vein thrombosis.*** Although there is an increased risk of development of a deep vein thrombosis (DVT) in all patients who have undergone surgery, this risk is particularly increased after total joint replacement arthroplasty of the hip and knee.[19,67] In addition to medical/pharmacological management with administration of perioperative anticoagulant drugs,[19,67] 1 minute of active ankle pumping exercises performed at regular intervals during the day has been shown to increase venous blood flow (for up to 30 minutes after exercise) and decrease venous stasis in the calf after total hip replacement surgery.[45] Therefore, ankle pumping exercises are thought to decrease the risk of developing a DVT. Early ambulation (before day 2) after surgery also promotes circulation and reduces the risk of a DVT.[67]

***Subluxation or dislocation after joint surgery.*** If a joint capsule has been incised during surgery, as is the case for total joint replacement or a repaired labrum for a history of joint dislocation, there is an increased risk of postoperative dislocation. This risk can be reduced through patient education and exercise instruction. For example, a pre- or postoperative program typically includes teaching a patient proper use of a removable immobilization device, such as a splint or sling, and what positions to avoid during exercises and ADL.

***Restricted motion from adhesions and scar tissue formation.*** Movement of the operated area as early as possible after surgery with ROM exercises or continuous passive motion (CPM) within a safe range is directed at maintaining the extensibility of soft tissues as they heal and preventing postoperative contractures.

***Failure, displacement, or loosening of internal fixation.*** Excessive or premature weight bearing prior to bony healing after open reduction and internal fixation of a fracture can cause loss of bone-to-bone apposition of the fracture site. Heavy lifting after a soft tissue repair in the upper extremity can cause rupture of sutured, but incompletely healed, tissues. Proper use of supportive devices, such as crutches or a walker, to control weight bearing during ambulation and appropriate progression of exercises and functional activities can reduce the risk of these postoperative complications.

## OVERVIEW OF COMMON ORTHOPEDIC SURGERIES AND POSTOPERATIVE MANAGEMENT

Surgical management of musculoskeletal conditions encompasses many operative procedures and combinations of procedures involving a variety of tissues and structures, including muscles, tendons, joint capsules, cartilage, ligaments, fascia, nerves, and bones. Orthopedic surgery procedures can be divided into several broad categories including repair, reattachment, reconstruction, stabilization, replacement, realignment, transfer, release, resection (excision), fixation, and fusion.[17,41,47,58] Examples of specific procedures in these categories are identified in Table 12.1.

The purpose of this final section of the chapter is to provide brief descriptions of some surgical procedures in these categories and a broad overview of the place of therapeutic exercise in postoperative rehabilitation. Chapters 17 through 22 contain more extensive background and descriptions of selected surgical procedures and progres-

sions of postoperative management for each region of the upper and lower extremities. For more detailed descriptions of specific surgeries and operative techniques for musculoskeletal conditions from the orthopedic surgeon's perspective, many textbooks and journals are available for reference.[17,30,44,50,61] In addition, to design and implement safe and effective postoperative exercise programs for individual patients, a therapist needs a clear understanding of the unique aspects of each patient's surgery. This information is available in the operative report in a patient's medical record and further obtained through close communication with the surgeon.

**NOTE:** In the general descriptions of various orthopedic procedures found in this chapter, the duration of immobilization, and the initiation, progression, and intensity of exercise vary according to differences in surgical technique, the philosophy of the surgeon, and the nature of each patient's responses during postoperative rehabilitation.

### Surgical Approaches—Open, Arthroscopic, and Arthroscopically Assisted Procedures

#### Open Procedure
An open surgical procedure involves an incision of adequate length and depth through superficial and deep layers of skin, fascia, muscles, and joint capsule so the operative field can be fully visualized by the surgeon during the procedure.[43,58] The term *arthrotomy* is used to describe an open procedure in which the joint capsule is incised and joint structures are exposed. Open approaches are necessary for surgeries, such as joint replacement, arthrodesis, internal fixation of fractures, and for some soft tissue repairs and reconstruction, such as tendon or ligament tears. There is extensive disturbance of soft tissues during an open procedure that requires a lengthy period of rehabilitation while soft tissues heal.

#### Arthroscopic Procedure
*Arthroscopy* is used as a diagnostic tool and as a means of treating a variety of intra-articular disorders.[2,44,55,63] Arthro-

| TABLE 12.1 | General Methods and Examples of Musculoskeletal Surgeries |
|---|---|
| **Surgical Methods** | **Examples of Procedures** |
| Repair | Tenorrhaphy, tendon repair; meniscus or ligament repair; articular cartilage repair |
| Release or decompression | Myotomy, tenotomy, fasciotomy; capsulotomy; tenolysis; muscle-tendon lengthening; retinacular release; arthroscopic subacromial decompression |
| Resection or removal | Synovectomy, meniscectomy, capsulectomy; débridement and lavage; laminectomy; excision of soft tissue or bony neoplasms |
| Realignment or stabilization | Tendon transfer, tenodesis; extensor mechanism realignment; capsulorrhaphy, capsular shift; osteotomy |
| Reconstruction or replacement | Tenoplasty; capsulolabral reconstruction; ligamentous reconstruction; chondroplasty; arthroplasty |
| Fusion or fixation for bony union | Arthrodesis; open reduction with internal fixation |

scopic procedures are typically performed on an outpatient basis and often under local anesthesia.

Arthroscopy involves several very small incisions (portals) in the skin, muscle, and joint capsule for insertion of an endoscope to visualize the interior of the joint by means of a camera. Miniature, motorized surgical tools are inserted through the portals and are used to repair tissues in or around the joint, remove loose bodies, or débride the joint surfaces. Arthroscopic techniques are most often used for surgical procedures at the shoulder and knee.[2,43,44,55,63]

Procedures include ligament, tendon, and capsule repairs or reconstruction, débridement of joints, meniscectomy, articular cartilage repair, and synovectomy. Because the incisions for the portals are so small, there is minimal disturbance of soft tissues during arthroscopic procedures. Therefore, rehabilitation *usually* but not always can proceed more quickly than after an open procedure.

### Arthroscopically Assisted Procedure

An arthroscopically assisted procedure uses arthroscopy for a portion of the procedure but also requires an open surgical field for selected aspects of the operative procedure.[2,43,44] This sometimes is referred to as a "mini-open" procedure.[28]

## Use of Tissue Grafts

In a number of orthopedic procedures to repair damaged structures, tissue grafts are implanted during the repair process. For example, soft tissue grafts are routinely used to reconstruct ligaments of the knee or ankle. Grafts are also used in articular cartilage repair procedures and many bony procedures.

### Types of Graft

Tissue grafts can be placed into several categories: autografts, allografts, and synthetic grafts.[38]

*Autograft.* An autograft, also referred to as an *autogenous* or *autologous graft*, uses a patient's own tissue harvested from a donor site in the body. Patellar tendon grafts, for example, have been used for more than two decades for intra-articular anterior or posterior cruciate ligament reconstruction.[53] More recently, autografts have been used for osteochondral implantation for repair of small, localized articular defects of the femoral condyles.[18]

*Allograft.* An allograft uses fresh or cryopreserved tissue that comes from a source other than the patient, typically from a cadaveric donor. This type of graft is used when an autograft in a previous surgery has failed or when an appropriate autograft is not available.

*Synthetic grafts.* Materials such as Gore-Tex and Dacron offer an alternative to human tissue and have been used on a limited basis for ligament reconstruction in the knee. However, synthetic ligaments, to date, have had a high rate of failure and have not held up well over time.[18] Implantation of synthetic ligaments has also been associated with chronic synovitis of the knee.

---

**BOX 12.7    Risks with Use of Autografts and Allografts**

**Autografts**

- Necessitates two surgical procedures for the patient
- Damage to or weakening of otherwise healthy tissue at the donor site

**Allografts**

- Potential disease transmission from the donor
- Decreased graft strength as the result of sterilization
- Greater risk of graft failure due to immunological rejection
- Insufficient availability of cadaveric tissues due to limited resources
- Not an option for articular cartilage implantation because cryopreservation destroys articular chondrocytes

---

The risks and drawbacks associated with autografts and allografts are summarized in Box 12.7.

## Repair, Reattachment, Reconstruction, Stabilization, or Transfer of Soft Tissues

Surgical repair, reattachment, or reconstruction of soft tissues may be necessary after severe injury of a muscle, tendon, or ligament.[1,36,47] Surgical reconstruction and stabilization of a joint capsule may be indicated to reduce excessive capsular laxity contributing to instability of the joint.[42,68] Transfer of a muscle-tendon unit may be required to improve stability of an unstable joint or to enhance neuromuscular control and function.

Although there are numerous surgeries that fall into this category, in all instances a therapist must always consider the effects of immobilization and remobilization and the characteristics of healing of the types of soft tissue involved when designing a postoperative exercise program.

### Muscle Repair

A complete tear or rupture of a muscle is unusual, but it may occur if a muscle that is already in a state of contraction takes a direct blow or is forcibly stretched.[1,16]

**Procedure**

Immediate surgical repair of a severe tear or even complete rupture of a muscle is uncommon because inflammation affects the texture of muscle tissue, making it difficult to hold sutures in place. A patient can achieve a more satisfactory outcome with a late repair (approximately 48 to 72 hours after injury) after acute symptoms have decreased. The muscle is reopposed, sutured, and immobilized so it is initially held in a *shortened* position as it begins to heal.[1,47,58]

**Postoperative Management**

- Muscle-setting exercise of the sutured muscle may be initiated immediately after surgery.

- When the immobilization is removed, active ROM, emphasizing controlled motion within a protected range, may be started to regain joint mobility and prevent contractures.
- Weight bearing is partially restricted until the patient achieves a functional level of strength and flexibility in the repaired muscle.
- Low-load, high-repetition resistance exercises are progressed very gradually to protect the healing muscle and should not elicit pain.
- Vigorous stretching or return to a full level of activity are contraindicated until soft tissue healing is complete—as long as 6 to 8 weeks postoperatively.

## Tendon Repair

When a tendon tears or rupturess in a young person, it is usually the result of severe trauma.[1,52] In an elderly person with a history of chronic impingement, it is usually the result of progressive deterioration of a tendon coupled with a sudden, unusual motion.[6] Tendons usually rupture at musculotendinous or tendo-osseous junctions.[52] Common sites of acute tear or rupture are the bicipital tendon at the shoulder or the Achilles tendon.[1]

In patients with chronic tenosynovitis of the hand and wrist, the extensor tendons can erode over time and may eventually rupture along the dorsum of the hand.[7,13] The superficial tendons of the hand and foot are also vulnerable to injuries, particularly lacerations, that may require surgical repair. The flexor tendons of the fingers, for example, are commonly severed as the result of a deep laceration to the palm of the hand.

Aside from the acute pain that occurs at the time of injury to a tendon, a complete tear, rupture, or laceration causes loss of the ability to generate tension in the muscle-tendon unit and results in weakness but little pain. With a partial tear there is significant pain during an active muscle contraction or stretch of the muscle-tendon unit.[1]

### Procedure

A complete tear or laceration of a tendon should be reaired immediately or within a few days after injury. Otherwise, the tendon begins to retract, making reattachment difficult. After the tendon is sutured, the repaired muscle-tendon unit is maintained in a shortened position, as with complete tear of a muscle. A longer immobilization period may be required for a repaired tendon than for a repaired muscle because the vascular supply to tendons is poor.[24,27] However, remobilization involving a limited degree of tensile forces on the repaired tendon, is initiated as early as possible to prevent or minize adhesions that can hinder tendon gliding.

### Postoperative Management

- Muscle setting is begun immediately after surgery to prevent adhesions of the tendon to the sheath or surrounding tissues and to promote alignment of healing tissue. If it is possible to remove the immobilization for brief periods of exercise, *passive* motion or active contraction of a muscle group that is an antagonist of the repaired muscle tendon within a protected range also may be permissible within a few days after surgery.[7,15]
- Controlled antigravity motions are initiated after the repaired tendon has had several weeks to heal.
- Weight bearing may be restricted after an upper or lower extremity tendon repair, and heavy lifting activities are often contraindicated for as long as 6 to 8 weeks after an upper extremity repair.
- Because the muscle-tendon unit must be held in a shortened position for several weeks, regaining full range may be difficult. However, vigorous stretching and high-intensity resistance exercise should not be initiated until at least 8 weeks, when healing of the tendon has occurred.[15]

N O T E : For detailed information on postoperative rehabilitation after repair of tendons in the shoulder, fingers, or ankle, refer to Chapters 17, 19, and 22, respectively.

## Ligament Repair or Reconstruction

After a large or complete tear of a ligament or when a ligament cannot be approximated for healing through closed reduction, surgical intervention through repair or reconstruction is warranted. Repair involves approximating and suturing the torn ligameant, whereas reconstruction is accomplished with a tissue graft taken from a donor site. The knee, ankle, and elbow joints are the more common sites of injury and surgical intervention.[36]

### Procedures

There are many surgical procedures that involve ligamentous repair or reconstruction. What is common to these surgeries is that postoperatively the joint is held in a position that places a safe level of tension on the sutured or reconstructed ligament during the healing process.[37,41,54] The duration of immobilization varies with the site and severity of injury and the type of repair or reconstruction that was done.[2,11,16,58]

### Postoperative Management

Rehabilitation after ligament surgery emphasizes early but protected motion and progressive strengthening and weight-bearing activities to load the healing tissues consistently but safely.[37,53,54] How quickly the rehabilitation program is progressed depends on many factors, such as the type of repair or reconstruction that was done. For example, rehabilitation after anterior cruciate ligament (ACL) reconstruction utilizing a patellar tendon graft and bone-to-bone fixation can be progressed more rapidly than after a soft tissue stabilization procedure involving transfer of the iliotibial band or hamstrings to stabilize the knee.[16,25,41] The rate of advancement also depends on the site of the repair or reconstruction. For example, support should be worn and weight bearing restricted for an extended period of time if the repair is at a potentially unstable joint and until muscle power can adequately protect the joint.

Generally, postoperative rehabilitation after ligamentous surgery is a lengthy process. For patients wishing to return to high-demand work or sports activities after knee ligament surgery, for example, it may take at least 6 months or as long as a year of rehabilitation.[25,41]

NOTE: Rehabilitation after reconstruction of ligaments of the knee and ankle is addressed in Chapters 21 and 22.

## Capsule Stabilization and Reconstruction

A joint capsule with excessive laxity cannot act as a source of restraint to maintain appropriate stability of the joint. In turn, hyperlaxity of the capsule can be an underlying cause of symptomatic instability of a joint, ranging from subluxation to gross instability and recurrent dislocation. Joints particularly vulnerable to instability are those with little inherent stability, most notably the glenohumeral joint.

In some instances an individual is predisposed to joint instability because capsular laxity and joint hypermobility are congenital, affecting many joints in the body. More often, joint instability is caused by an acute capsular injury as the result of traumatic dislocation or by progressive joint laxity as the result of repetitive stresses applied to the capsule when the joint is in extreme positions.[42] The latter is seen most often in athletes participating in sports, such as baseball and tennis, that involve repetitive, end-range shoulder motions.[65]

Surgical stabilization or reconstruction of a joint capsule is indicated for a patient with traumatic dislocation with associated capsular or labral avulsion or fracture, recurrent dislocation or symptomatic subluxation despite a course of nonoperative treatment, or an irreducible (fixed) dislocation.[42,55,65,71]

### Procedures

Surgical procedures designed to reduce capsular laxity and joint volume and restore or improve joint stability fall into several categories and are performed using an open or a arthroscopic approach. An open procedure, necessitating arthrotomy, is used if an open reduction of the joint is required or if there is extensive damage to the labrum, avulsion of the capsule, or a fracture. An arthroscopic approach typically is used to reduce capsular laxity and for some reconstructive procedures.[42,71]

Examples of stabilization and reconstruction procedures at the glenohumeral joint used for anterior, posterior, inferior, or multidirectional instabilities include the following.

*Capsulorrhaphy (capsular shift).* For capsulorrhaphy, using an arthroscopic or an open approach, a specific portion of the capsule is incised and tightened by overlapping and then suturing the redudant tissue.

*Capsulolabral reconstruction.* Capsulolabral reconstruction involves arthroscopic or open repair of a capsular lesion and labral tear (e.g., a Bankart lesion as the result of a traumatic anterior dislocation) by reattaching the labrum to the rim of the glenoid combined with stabilization of the capsule.

NOTE: With these procedures, a tendon transfer and bony procedure may also be performed to augment joint stability.

*Electrothermally assisted capsulorrhaphy.* For electrothermally assisted capsulorrhaphy, using an arthroscopic approach, thermal energy (laser or radiofrequency) is delivered to the capsule to shrink selective portions.[68]

### Postoperative Management

After any joint stabilization or reconstruction procedure, the goal of postoperative management is to restore a balance of joint stability and functional motion while protecting the joint capsule and other repaired tissues during healing. The duration of the immobilization period and the selection and progression of postoperative exercises and functional activities depend, in part, on the preoperative direction of the instability, the surgical approach, the type of stabilization or reconstruction procedure and tissue fixation, and the quality of the patient's tissue.

Postoperative exercise focuses on the following.

- To restore ROM, initially active motions are emphasized within a protected range during early rehabilitation. Movements that place stress on the portion of the capsule that was tightened or repaired are progressed cautiously.
- When strengthening exercises are permissible in the program, emphasis is placed on strengthening the dynamic stabilizers of the joint.

NOTE: Detailed progressions of postoperative exercises after surgical stabilization of the shoulder are presented in Chapter 17.

## Tendon Transfer or Realignment

The transfer or realignment of a muscle-tendon unit alters the line of pull of a muscle. This may be indicated, for example, to improve the stability of an unstable shoulder joint or to stabilize a chronically dislocating patella. Although a realignment procedure slightly alters the line of pull, it does not change the *action* of the muscle-tendon unit. For instance, after an extensor mechanism realignment, the quadriceps remains an extensor of the knee.

A tendon transfer from one bony surface to another is sometimes indicated for a patient with a significant neurological deficit to prevent deformity and improve functional control. With this type of procedure, not only is the line of pull of the muscle-tendon unit altered, the *action* of the muscle is also changed. For example, transfer of the distal attachment of the flexor carpi ulnaris to the dorsal surface of the wrist changes the action of the muscle-tendon unit from a flexor to an extensor of the wrist. This procedure may be indicated for a child with cerebral palsy to prevent wrist flexion contracture and improve active wrist extension for functional grasp.[58]

### Procedures

During a tendon transfer or realignment procedure, usually the distal attachment of the muscle-tendon unit is removed from its bony insertion and reattached to a different bone, to a different location on the same bone, or to adjacent soft tissues.[47,58] The muscle-tendon unit is then immobilized in a shortened position for a period of time.

## Postoperative Management

◉ As with a tendon repair, early muscle setting and protected motion are important to maintain tendon gliding. Resisted movements are progressed cautiously and gradually to protect the reattached tendon.

◉ If the purpose of the transfer was to change the function of the muscle, biofeedback and electrical muscle stimulation are often used to help a patient learn to control the new action of the transferred muscle-tendon unit.[58]

N O T E : Rehabilitation after tendon transfer for rheumatoid arthritis of the hand and wrist is described in Chapter 19. Chapter 21 contains information on rehabilitation after realignment of the patellar tendon for chronic patellofemoral dysfunction.

## Release, Lengthening, or Decompression of Soft Tissues

Soft tissues may be incised or sectioned to improve ROM, prevent or minimize progressive deformity, or relieve pain. Procedures include *myotomy*, *tenotomy*, or *fasciotomy*.[11,47,58]

Surgical release of soft tissues may be indicated for a young patient with severe arthritis and resulting contractures in whom joint replacement is not advisable or as a preliminary procedure in adults prior to joint replacement.[13] Releases are also performed in patients with myopathic and neuropathic diseases, such as muscular dystrophy and cerebral palsy, to improve functional mobility.[58] Release of soft tissues to achieve decompression of tissues and relieve pain may be indicated for a patient with an impingement or compartmental syndrome, such as shoulder impingement or carpal tunnel syndrome.[11,47]

### Procedures

During release or lengthening of a shortened muscle group, a portion of the muscle-tendon unit is surgically sectioned and fibrotic tissues are incised. A tendon can also be partially incised, as in a Z-lengthening to allow greater extensibility. The incised structures are then immobilized in a *lengthened* position except during exercise.[47,58] Some form of splinting or bracing in the corrected position in conjunction with exercise is always used postoperatively to maintain the gained ROM.

During decompression procedures, fasciae that are causing pressure on muscles, tendons, or nerves may be released or removed. Some decompression procedures, for example at the shoulder, also involve removal of osteophytes or alteration of bony structures that are creating excessive pressure on soft tissues.

### Postoperative Management

◉ CPM and/or active-assistive ROM is typically initiated within a day or two after surgery. As soft tissue healing progresses, this is followed by active ROM through the gained ranges.[11,58]

◉ Strengthening of the antagonists of the lengthened muscle and use of the gained ROM during functional activities also are started early to maintain active control of movement within the newly gained range.

## Joint Procedures

Orthopedic surgery involving the joints of the upper and lower extremeites is performed most frequently for management of pain and dysfunction associated with arthritis or acute injury, such as a labral tear in the hip or shoulder joint. Surgical interventions for arthritis range from arthroscopic débridement of a joint or removal of proliferated synovium to total joint replacement arthroplasty or joint fusion. An overview of stabilization and reconstruction procedures for the joint capsule was discussed earlier in this section of the chapter.

### Synovectomy

Synovectomy involves removal of the synovium (lining of the joint) in the presence of chronic joint inflammation. It is typically done in patients who have rheumatoid arthritis with chronic proliferative synovitis but minimal articular changes.[13,32,46,70] It is indicated if medical management has failed to alleviate joint inflammation for 4 to 6 months.

### Procedure

Synovectomy of a joint is usually performed using an arthroscopic approach and is most commonly performed on the knee, elbow, wrist, and metacarpophalangeal (MCP) joints.[7,13,32,46,70] When synovium proliferates in the synovial sheaths of tendons, it is referred to as *tenosynovitis*. Removal of excessive synovium from tendon sheaths is known as a *tenosynovectomy*. This procedure is most often done for chronic synovitis of the wrist to clear synovium from the extensor tendons of the hand and, as such, is also called a *dorsal clearance* procedure.[13,46,70]

Although synovium tends to regenerate, resection of the inflamed synovium temporarily relieves pain and swelling and is thought to protect articular cartilage or tendons from enzymatic damage.[13,32]

### Postoperative Management

◉ If an arthroscopic approach is used, passive or assisted ROM exercises (or CPM) and muscle-setting exercises are begun immediately or within 24 to 48 hours after surgery. Exercises quickly progress to active ROM. After synovectomy of the knee, for example, partial weight bearing as tolerated during ambulation progresses to full weight bearing by 10 to 14 days. After wrist or elbow synovectomy, lifting heavy objects is restricted for several weeks.

◉ After open synovectomy, progression of exercises and ADL proceeds more slowly.

◉ Progression of the rehabilitation program is based on the patient's response to exercise as well as the overall response to medication for the primary inflammatory disease. Every effort should be made to avoid excessive exercise or activity that could increase joint pain or swelling.[7,46,70]

N O T E : Rehabilitation after synovectomy of the knee is presented in detail in Chapter 21.

## Articular Cartilage Procedures

Surgical intervention for repair of articular cartilage defects (osteochondral lesions) has proven to be particularly challenging because of the limited capacity of this type of connective tissue to heal.[18] However, several procedures for the symptomatic knee or ankle have been developed for this purpose. Selection criteria for one procedure over another are based on the size of the chondral lesion and patient-related factors such as age and the ability to participate in the rehabilitation process.

### Procedures

***Arthroscopic débridement.*** Débridement of a joint involves arthroscopic removal of fibrillated cartilage, unstable chondral flaps, and loose bodies (fragments of cartilage or bone) in a joint.[13] Osteophytes also may be resected. This procedure is most often indicated to relieve joint pain and biomechanical "catching" during joint movement.

***Abrasion arthroplasty, subchondral drilling, and microfracture.*** Several arthroscopic procedures are used to promote healing of small chondral defects in symptomatic joints through stimulation of a marrow-based repair response leading to local ingrowth of cartilagenous repair tissue (fibrocartilage).[18,33,63] Lesions of the medial femoral condyle and the posterior aspect of the patella are most often treated with one of these procedures.

Abrasion arthroplasty, also known as *abrasion chondroplasty,* and subchondral drilling involve abrasion or drilling of an articular surface to the superficial layer of subchondral bone with a motorized, arthroscopic burr or drill. The positive effects of these procedures have been questionable, at best, and possibly no more effective for symptom relief than arthroscopic débridement alone.[18]

N O T E : Although rehabilitation after these procedures is quite protracted, the benefits appear to be short-lived because the fibrocartilage replacement tissue lacks the qualities of hyaline cartilage and therefore tends to deteriorate readily after ingrowth.[11,18]

A newer technique, microfracture of articular cartilage, is designed for repair of very small osteochondral defects ($<1.5$ cm$^2$). This procedure involves the use of a nonmotorized arthroscopic awl to penetrate the subchondral bone systematically and expose the bone marrow. Initial studies of this procedure suggest that microfracture relieves symptoms more effectively than abrasion arthroplasty or subchondral drilling, possibly because use of a nonmotorized instrument reduces the potential for tissue damage due to thermal necrosis.[18]

***Chondrocyte transplantation.*** Chondrocyte transplantation, also known as *autologous chondrocyte implantation,*[29] is designed to stimulate growth of hyaline cartilage for repair of focal defects of articular cartilage and prevention of progressive deterioration of joint cartilage leading to osteoarthritis.[12,18,29,33,48] It was introduced as an alternative to abrasion arthroplasty during the mid-1990s for full-thickness, symptomatic focal chondral and osteochondral defects (2.5 to 4.0 cm$^2$) of the knee, specifically lesions of the femoral condyles or patella.[12]

Chondrocyte transplantation occurs in two stages. First, healthy articular cartilage is harvested arthroscopically from the patient. Chondrocytes are extracted from the articular cartilage, cultured for several weeks, and processed in a laboratory to increase the volume of healthy tissue. The second phase is the implantation phase, which currently requires arthrotomy (open procedure). After the chondral defect sites are débrided and covered with a periosteal patch, millions of autologous chondrocytes are injected under the patch and into the articular defect.[18]

***Osteochondral autografts and allografts.*** Unlike transplantation of chondrocytes, ostechondral grafts involve transplantation of *intact* articular cartilage along with some underlying bone, resulting in a bone-to-bone graft. Several procedures fall within this category. An *autogenous osteochondral graft* (an autograft) procedure harvests a patient's own articular cartilage from a donor site.[18] As noted previously (see Box 12.7), a drawback to this type of articular graft is damage to the donor site, specifically the creation of an osteochondral defect at the donor site. To lessen concerns about damage to a patient's articular donor site, *osteochondral mosaicplasty* was developed.[9] During this procedure, small-diameter osteochondral plugs are retrieved from a donor site and press-fit into the chondral defect.

In contrast, an *osteochondral allograft* procedure transplants intact articular cartilage from a cadaveric donor. However, only fresh, intact grafts, which are in limited supply and can be stored for only a few days, can be used. This is because freezing the graft material prior to storage for later use kills the articular chondrocytes, thus causing graft failure.

### Postoperative Management

Rehabilitation after all of the articular cartilage procedures described in this section, with the exception of arthroscopic débridement, is a slow and arduous process.[12,18,29,33,48] Exercise is an important aspect of postoperative management at each stage of rehabilitation. Early passive motion, sometimes with CPM, and protected weight bearing are essential to promote the maturation and maintain the health of implanted chondrocytes or an osteochondral graft. Full weight bearing is allowable by 8 to 9 weeks. A well controlled program of progressive exercises continues for 6 months to a year to achieve optimal functional outcomes.[29]

N O T E : More detailed information on rehabilitation after procedures to repair articular cartilage and osteochondral lesions is presented in Chapter 21.

### Arthroplasty

Any reconstructive joint procedure, with or without joint implant, designed to relieve pain and improve funtion is referred to broadly as arthroplasty. This definition encompasses several categories of arthroplasty.

## Procedures

***Excision arthroplasty.*** Excision arthroplasty, also known as *resection arthroplasty*, involves removing periarticular bone from one or both articular surfaces. A space is left where fibrotic (scar) tissue is laid down during the healing process.[13,46,56] Excision arthroplasty has been performed in a variety of joints, including the hip, elbow, wrist, and foot, to alleviate pain. Although an old procedure and less frequently used now than in the past, this type of arthroplasty is still considered appropriate in selected cases. Resection of the head of the radius for late-stage arthritis of the radiohumeral joint[20] or a severe comminuted fracture of the radial head[49] and resection of the distal ulna (Darrach procedure) for late-stage arthritis of the distal radioulnar joint[22] are still used as primary procedures to reduce pain. However, excision arthroplasty of the hip (Girdlestone procedure) now is used as a salvage procedure, for example, after a failed total hip replacement where revision arthroplasty is not feasible.[13]

Despite the usefulness of excision arthroplasty, there are also a number of disadvantages.

- Possible joint instability
- In the hip, significant leg length discrepancy and poor cosmetic result because of shortening of the operated extremity
- Persistent muscular imbalance and weakness

N O T E : Rehabilitation after excision arthroplasty of the radial head is discussed in Chapter 18.

***Excision arthroplasty with implant.*** For excision arthroplasty with implant, after removing the articular surface, an artificial implant is fixed in place to help in the remodeling of a new joint. This is sometimes called *implant resection arthroplasty.*[20,46,62] The implant usually is made of a flexible silicone material and becomes encapsulated by fibrous tissue as the joint reforms.

***Interposition arthroplasty.*** Interposition arthroplasty essentially is biological resurfacing of a joint to provide a new articulating surface. After the involved joint surface is débrided, a foreign material is placed (interposed) between the two joint surfaces.[5,46] A variety of materials may be used to cover the joint surface, including fascia, Silastic material, or metal.[56]

This type of arthroplasty is used most often in young patients with incapacitating pain and loss of function resulting from severe deterioration of an articular surface in whom joint replacement arthroplasty is not appropriate. Some examples of interpositional arthroplasty are resurfacing of the glenoid fossa with fascia[5] and tendon interposition arthroplasty of the carpometacarpal (CMC) joint of the thumb.[21]

***Joint replacement arthroplasty.*** Joint replacement arthroplasty includes *total joint replacement arthroplasty* and *hemireplacement arthroplasty.* Total joint replacement is a common reconstructive procedure to relieve pain and improve function in patients with severe joint

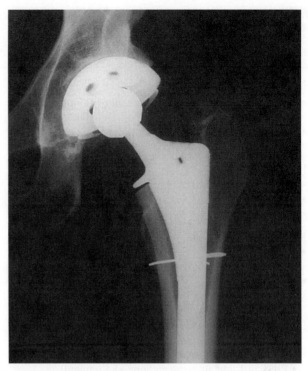

FIGURE 12.1 Total hip replacement arthroplasty. Both the acetabular and femoral portions of the joint have been replaced with prosthetic components. *(From McKinnis, LN: Fundamentals of Musculoskeletal Imaging, ed 2. FA Davis, Philadelphia, 2005, p 312, with permission.)*

degeneration associated with late-stage arthritis (Fig. 12.1).[13,14,43,46,50,56,62]

Total joint replacement procedures involve resecting both affected articulating surfaces of a joint and replacing them with artificial components, whereas hemireplacement arthroplasty involves resection and replacement of just one of the articulating surfaces of a joint.[13,46,50] In addition to use for late-stage arthritis when only one articulating surface of a joint has deteriorated, hemireplacement is also an option after femoral neck and proximal humeral fractures.[13]

- *Materials, designs, and methods of fixation.* Prosthetic replacements have been developed and refined for almost every joint of the extremities but have been used more frequently and successfully at the hip and knee than in the smaller joints of the foot and hand.[13,46,50,56] The materials, designs, and methods of fixation used for joint replacement arthroplasty are summarized in Box 12.8. Prosthetic implants are made of inert materials, specifically metal alloys, high-density polyethylene (plastic) material, and sometimes ceramic material. Because the biomechanical features of each joint are unique, there are a multitude of prosthetic designs. Component designs range from unconstrained (resurfacing) with no inherent stability to semiconstrained and fully constrained (articulated) designs that provide stability to an unstable joint. In almost all designs, one articular surface is metal and the other is plastic. The choice of fixation is

---

**BOX 12.8** Materials, Designs, and Methods of Fixation for Joint Replacement Arthroplasty

**Implant Materials**
- Rigid: inert metal (cobalt-chrome alloy, titanium alloy, or ceramic)
- Semirigid: plastic (high-density polymers such as polyethylene)

**Implant Designs**
- Unconstrained (resurfacing): no inherent stability
- Semiconstrained
- Fully constrained (articulated): inherent stability

**Methods of Fixation**
- Cemented
  - Acrylic cement (polymethylmethacrylate)
- Noncemented
  - Biological fixation (microscopic ingrowth of bone into a porous-coated prosthetic surface)
  - Macrointerlock between a nonporous component and bone with a bioactive compound applied to the component to improve osseous integration
  - Press fit (tight fit between bone and implant)
  - Screws, bolts, or nails
- Hybrid
  - Noncemented component for one joint surface and cemented component for opposing joint surface

---

based, in part, on the anticipated loads that will be placed on the prosthetic implants over time. Cemented fixation, using an acrylic-based cement (polymethylmethacrylate) eventually tends to break down at the bone–cement interface, resulting in mechanical loosening of the implant and pain.[13,50,60] Therefore, cemented fixation is used primarily for older or sedentary patients who are unlikely to place high stresses on the implants. Bio-ingrowth fixation, a form of cementless fixation, is achieved by growth of bone into the porous-coated exterior surface of an implant. It is thought that this form of fixation, which is advocated for younger, more active patients, is less likely to loosen over time.[13,50,60] Most recently, a nonporous, cementless prosthetic implant has been developed that is used with a bioactive compound that stimulates bone growth. Fixation is achieved by a macrointerlock between the implant and adjacent bone.[50]

N O T E : Descriptions of implants are reviewed, joint by joint, in Chapters 17 through 22.

◉ *Minimally invasive versus traditional arthroplasty.*
A recent advance in joint replacement arthroplasty that may have a significant impact on postoperative rehabilitation and outcomes is the development of minimally invasive surgical techniques that involve less disturbance of soft tissues than traditional arthroplasty. Currently, minimally invasive procedures are being used for total

hip and total knee replacement.[4,10,66] Although traditional hip and knee replacement procedures have provided excellent reults for several decades,[13,14,51,60] they impose substantial trauma to skin, muscles, and the joint capsule, leading to significant postoperative pain, which in turn affects the length of time required for postoperative recovery. Compared to surgical techniques used for traditional hip and knee replacement arthroplasty, minimally invasive procedures use smaller skin incisions, less muscle splitting to expose the joint, and less disruption to the capsule in preparation for insertion of prosthetic implants. For example, in a minimally invasive hip replacement, one or two small incisions ($<10$ cm in length) are used rather than a single incision (15 to 30 cm long involving extensive muscle splitting) that is typically used in a traditional hip replacement.[10] A 2-year follow-up indicates that patients who underwent minimally invasive total knee replacement had less pain, better early motion, and a shorter hospital stay than patients who had standard knee replacement surgery.[66] Research is ongoing to determine if the long-term results of minimally invasive procedures are equal to the long-term outcomes of traditional arthroplasty while enabling a patient to recover more rapidly after surgery, participate in accelerated rehabilitation, and return to full activity in less time.

◉ *Contraindications to joint replacement arthroplasty.*
Despite the positive functional outcomes after joint replacement arthroplasty, not every patient with advanced joint disease is a candidate for these procedures. Contraindications are noted in Box 12.9.[13,46,56] Although opinions vary as to which of these contraindications are absolute versus relative, there is general agreement that infection is of the utmost concern.

### Postoperative Management
Postoperative management, including therapeutic exercise interventions, after selected types of joint replacement arthroplasty of major joints of the extremities is described in detail in Chapters 17 through 22.

### Arthrodesis
Arthrodesis is surgical fusion of the surfaces of a joint. It is indicated as a primary surgical intervention in cases of severe joint pain associated with late-stage arthritis and

---

**BOX 12.9** Contraindications to Total Joint Arthroplasty

- Active infection in the joint
- Chronic osteomyelitis
- Systemic infection
- Substantial loss of bone or malignant tumors that prohibit adequate implant fixation
- Significant paralysis of muscles surrounding the joint
- Neuropathic joint
- Inadequate patient motivation

| TABLE 12.2 | Optimal Positions for Arthrodesis |
|---|---|
| **Joint** | **Position** |
| Shoulder | At 15°–30° of abduction and flexion and 45° of internal rotation: a position so the hand can reach the mouth |
| Elbow | Dominant upper extremity: 70°–90° of flexion and midposition of the forearm; nondominant limb: more extension for assisting during tasks |
| Wrist | Slight extension |
| MCP of the thumb | At 20° of flexion |
| Hip | At 10°–15° of flexion to allow ambulation and comfortable sitting |
| Ankle | |
| Tibiotalar joint | Neutral (90°) or slight equinus for women who wear low heels |
| Subtalar joint | Neutral to valgus |
| Spine | Neutral so normal lordosis or kyphosis is maintained |

joint instability in which mobility of the joint is a lesser concern.[8,13,59,62,64] Arthrodesis of the extremity joints is also reserved for patients with significant weakness of muscles surrounding a joint as the result of neurological abnormalities, such as a peripheral neuropathy of the ankle or a severe brachial plexus injury.[47,58] In addition, it may be the only salvage procedure available for a patient with a failed total joint arthroplasty who is not a candidate for revision arthroplasty.[40]

Arthrodesis is most frequently used in the cervical or lumbar spine, wrist, thumb, and ankle but has also been used in selected instances in the shoulder and hip. For example, arthodesis of one or more joints of the ankle and foot (Fig. 12.2) is the procedure most often used to relieve pain associated with severe arthritis.[59,64]

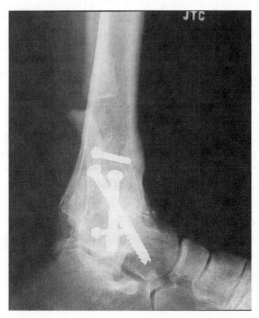

**FIGURE 12.2** Arthrodesis (surgical fusion with internal fixation of the ankle). *(From Logerstedt, DS, Smith, HL. Postoperative Management of the Foot and Ankle. Independent Study Course 15.2. Postoperative Management of Orthopedic Surgeries. Orthopedic Section, APTA, Inc., La Crosse, WI, 2005, with permission.)*

Optimal positions for arthrodesis are listed in Table 12.2. The optimal position is somewhat dependent on the functional needs or goals of each patient and may vary slightly in some joints, such as the elbow and ankle. For example, the optimal position for elbow fusion in the dominant upper extremity is usually between 70° and 90°. However, in the nondominant limb, the elbow must be in more extension for assistive activities.[8] For a woman, the optimal position for arthrodesis of the ankle might be in slightly greater plantarflexion than for a man to allow a woman to wear shoes with a slightly higher heel height.[58]

Although arthrodesis eliminates pain and creates stability in an involved joint, it is not without its disadvantages. Because loads are transferred to joints above and below the fused joint, there is the potential of developing excessive stresses leading to pain and hypermobility at those joints over time.

### Procedure

Fusion of joint surfaces in the position of maximum function is achieved with internal fixation (i.e., pins, nails, screws, plates, bone grafts). The joint is initially immobilized in a cast above and below the site of arthrodesis for 6 to 12 weeks postoperatively. Later, an orthotic device is used until complete bony healing and ankylosis has occurred.[59]

### Postoperative Management

- Because no movement is possible in the fused joint, ROM and strength must be maintained above and below the operated joint.
- Weight bearing is restricted until there is evidence of bony healing.

## Extra-articular Bony Procedures

Two of the more common reasons for surgical intervention involving bony structures outside a joint are fractures that require open reduction combined with internal fixation and deformity or malalignment of bone, sometimes associated with arthritis.

## Open Reduction and Internal Fixation of Fractures

Fractures are managed with either closed or open reduction. The process of bone healing and fracture management, addressed in Chapter 11, apply regardless of the method of reduction. In most instances in which open reduction is required, some type of internal fixation device is used to stabilize and maintain the alignment of the fracture site as it heals.

### Procedures

During surgery after the fracture site is exposed, any number of internal fixation devices, such as pins, nails, screws, plates, or rods, may be used to align and stabilize the bone fragments.[17,58] Intertrochanteric fracture of the femur, for example, is commonly stabilized with a compression plate and screws, as shown in Figure 12.3. After a fracture has healed, a second surgery may be necessary to remove some or all of the internal fixation devices, which tend to migrate over time.

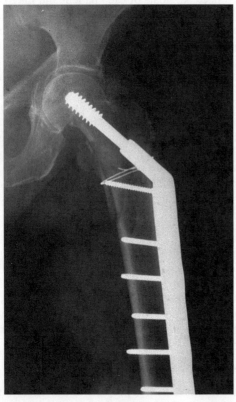

FIGURE 12.3 Intertrochanteric fracture of the left femur, fixed with compression plate and screws. *(From McKinnis, LN: Fundamentals of Musculoskeletal Imaging, ed 2. FA Davis, Philadelphia, 2005, p 67, with permission.)*

### Postoperative Management

Maintaining stability of the fracture site so bony healing can occur and getting the patient up and out of bed as early as possible are the main priorities postoperatively. The progression of rehabilitation after surgical stabilization of a fracture is dependent not only on factors such as the type and severity of fracture and the patient's age

and health status but also on the method(s) of internal fixation used.

Some fixation methods eliminate the need for external immobilization of the fracture site (e.g., with a cast), thereby enabling a patient to begin assisted or active movement of the involved limb and protected weight bearing shortly after surgery. However, with other fractures external immobilization and restricted weight bearing are necessary even with the use of internal fixation.[17,58]

During postoperative management not only must the fracture site be protected as it heals, soft tissues injured at the time the fracture occurred and further damaged when exposing the field during surgery must also be managed appropriately as they heal.

N O T E : Surgical interventions and postoperative management after hip fracture are discussed in Chapter 20.

### Osteotomy

Osteotomy—the surgical cutting and realignment of bone—is an extra-articular procedure indicated for the management of impairments associated with a number of musculoskeletal disorders. It is most often performed at the knee or hip.[13,14] Osteotomy is used, for example, to reduce pain and correct deformity in selected patients, such as a young adult with moderate, focal articular degeneration in the medial compartment and a varus deformity of the knee as the result of osteoarthritis[31,46] or a child with severe hip joint deterioration and pain secondary to congenital dysplasia or Legg-Calvé-Perthes disease (avascular necrosis of the head of the femur).[46,47]

In both of these examples, cutting and realigning bone near the involved joint shifts weight bearing loads to intact joint surfaces, thus reducing joint pain and reducing further deterioration of the involved articular cartilage.[13,14,58] It is also thought that redistributing loads on joint surfaces may stimulate the growth of fibrocartilage in the unloaded compartment of the joint.[14,23] A successful osteotomy delays the need for total joint replacement in patients who will most likely require revision arthroplasty sooner than the average patient with degenerative arthritis.

Osteotomy is also used to correct angular or rotational deformities of bone occurring in congenital or developmental disorders, such congenital dislocation of the hip, acquired hip dislocation in cerebral palsy, or congenital foot deformities.[58] Osteotomy is also necessary for surgically shortening or lengthening a bone to correct a severe leg length discrepancy.[17,58]

### Procedures

Numerous procedures are classified as osteotomies. Several examples are:

- *High tibial, lateral wedge osteotomy* followed by screw-plate fixation to correct a varus deformity, change the mechanical axis of the knee, and shift the the load to the lateral joint surface in a patient with degenerative arthritis of the medial compartment of the knee[31]
- *Medial wedge osteotomy* of the distal femur to correct a valgus deformity of the knee and shift weight-bearing

loads away from the deteriorated cartilage in the lateral compartment of the knee[46]

- *Intertrochanteric osteotomy* of the proximal femur, which repositions the femoral head to change the area where weight bearing occurs for a patient with arthitis or avascular necrosis of the hip[46]
- *Periacetabular osteotomy*, which repositions the acetabulum, to improve coverage of the head of the femur for a patient with congenital dysplasia of the hip and recurrent dislocation that could not be manged efffectively by nonoperative methods, such as splinting

During an osteotomy, muscles and other soft tissues may have to be reflected to expose the operative field and then reattached or repositioned. As with any type soft tissue repair, muscle-tendon units disturbed during surgery must be protected from excessive stress postoperatively.

### Postoperative Management

The primary concern of postoperative management is maintaining bone-to-bone apposition for healing of the osteotomy. Some procedures allow early joint motion and protected weight bearing because internal fixation maintains apposition of the osteotomy fragments. Others require additional external (cast) immobilization of the joints above and below the osteotomy site until bony union occurs, which may take as long as 8 to 12 weeks.[23,46,56] Full functional recovery after osteotomy may take about up to 6 months.

Postoperative exercises, when permissible, include the following.

- If immobilization in a cast is necessary, the patient can begin active ROM of the joints above and below the site of the osteotomy to prevent joint stiffness and undue muscle weakness.
- When motion and weight bearing are allowed, either immmediately after surgery or when the cast is removed, active-assistive and active exercise progressing to light resistive exercise are performed to restore joint ROM and strength (see discussion of management of fractures after immobilization in Chapter 11).
- Weight bearing typically is protected for 4 to 6 weeks or more.

## INDEPENDENT LEARNING ACTIVITIES

### Critical Thinking and Discussion

1. You have been asked to develop a preoperative patient education program for a group of individuals who are scheduled to undergo either total hip or knee replacement arthroplasty. What topics should be covered in your presentation, and why are they important for prospective patients to understand?

2. You are seeing an elderly patient for the first time who yesterday underwent an open reduction with internal fixation of a fracture of the hip (proximal femur). What would be the priorities of your initial examination of this patient? What is the general emphasis of postoperative management, including goals and interventions, during the maximum, moderate,

and minimum protection phases of postoperative rehabilitation?

3. Briefly describe the various surgical interventions for repair of articular cartilage.

4. Differentiate among the following types of soft tissue or bony surgeries primarily used in the management of arthritis: arthrodesis, arthroplasty, articular cartilage repair, débridement, osteotomy, and synovectomy. Briefly describe each surgery and compare and contrast postoperative management with respect to the use of therapeutic exercise.

5. Discuss the similarities and differences of postoperative management of the following soft tissue surgeries: muscle repair, tendon repair, tendon transfer, ligament reconstruction, repair of a joint capsule, tenotomy or myotomy, and decompression procedures.

## REFERENCES

1. Anderson, MK, Hall, SJ: Fundamentals of Sports Injury Management. Williams & Wilkins, Baltimore, 1997.
2. Andrews, JR, Timmerman, LA (eds) Diagnostic and operative arthroscopy. WB Saunders, Philadelphia, 1997.
3. Armstrong, AD, Galatz, LM: Complications of total elbow arthroplasty. In Williams, GR, Yamaguchi, K, Tamsey, ML, Galatz, LM (eds) Shoulder and Elbow Arthroplasty. Lippincott Williams & Wilkins, Philadelphia, 2005, 459–473.
4. Baerga-Varela, L, Malanga, GA: Rehabilitation and minimally invasive surgery. In Hozack, M, et al (eds) Minimally Invasive Total Joint Arthroplasty. Springer Verlag, Heidelberg, 2004, pp 2–5
5. Ball, CM, Yamaguchi, K: Interpositional arthroplasty. In Williams, GR, Yamaguchi, K, Tamsey, ML, Galatz, LM (eds) Shoulder and

Elbow Arthroplasty. Lippincott Williams & Wilkins, Philadelphia, 2005, pp 49–56.
6. Barrick, EF: Orthopedic trauma. In Kauffman, TL (ed) Geriatric Rehabilitation Manual. Churchill Livingstone, New York, 1999.
7. Batts Shanku, CD: Rheumatoid arthritis. In Hansen, RA, Atchison, B (eds) Conditions in Occupational Therapy, ed 2. Lippincott Williams & Wilkins, Philadelphia, 2000.
8. Beckenbaugh, RD: Arthrodesis. In Morrey, BF (ed) The Elbow and Its Disorders. WB Saunders, Philadelphia, 2000, p 751.
9. Berlet, GC, Mascia, A, Miniaci, A: Treatment of unstable osteochondritis dessicans lesions of the knee using autogenous osteochondral grafts (mosaicplasty). Arthroscopy 15:312–316, 1999.
10. Berry, DJ, Berger, RA, Callaghan, JJ, et al: Minimally invasive total hip arthroplasty: development, early results, and critical analysis. J Bone Joint Surg Am 85:2235–2246, 2003.

11. Brinker, M, Miller, M: Fundamentals of Orthopedics. WB Saunders, Philadelphia, 1999.

12. Brittberg, M, et al: Treatment of deep cartilage defects in the knee with autologous chondrocyte transplantation. N Engl J Med 331:889, 1994.

13. Buckwalter, JA, Ballard, WT: Operative treatment of arthritis. In Klippel, JH, (ed) Primer on the Rheumatic Diseases (ed 12). Arthritis Foundation, Atlanta, 2001, pp 613–623.

14. Buckwalter, JA, Lohmander, S: Operative treatment of osteoarthritis. J Bone Joint Surg Am 76:1405, 1994.

15. Burks, R, Burke, W, Stevanovic, M: Rehabilitation following repair of a torn latissimus dorsi tendon. Phys Ther 86(3):411–423, 2006.

16. Canavan, PK: Rehabilitation in Sports Medicine: A Comprehensive Guide. Appleton & Lange, Stamford, CT, 1998.

17. Chapman, M: Chapman's Orthopaedic Surgery ed 3 (Vols 1–4) Lippincott Williams & Wilkins, Philadelphia, 2004.

18. Chu, CR: Cartilage therapies: chondrocyte transplantation, osteochondral allografts, and autografts. In Pedowitz, RA, O'Connor, JJ, Akeson, WH (eds) Daniel's Knee Injuries: Ligament and Cartilage Structure, Function, Injury and Repair, ed 2. Lippincott Williams & Wilkins, Philadelphia, 2003, pp 227–237.

19. Comp, PC, Spiro, TE, Friedman, RJ, et al: Prolonged noxaparin therapy to prevent venous thromboembolism after primary hip or knee replacement. J Bone Joint Surg Am 83:336–343, 2001.

20. Cooney, WP: Elbow arthroplasty: historical perspective and current concepts. In Morrey, BF (ed) The Elbow and Its Disorders, ed 3. WB Saunders, Philadelphia, 2000, p 581.

21. Cooney III, WP: Arthroplasty of the thumb axis. In Morrey, BF (ed) Joint Replacement Arthroplasty, ed 3. Churchill Livingstone, Philadelphia, 2003, pp 204–225.

22. Cooney III, WP, Berger, RA: The distal radioulnar joint. In Morrey, BF (ed): Joint Replacement Arthroplasty, ed 3. Churchill Livingstone, Philadelphia, 2003, pp 226–243.

23. Coventry, MB, Ilstrup, DM, Wallrichs, SL: Proximal tibial osteotomy: a critical long-term study of eighty-seven cases. J Bone Joint Surg Am 75:196, 1993.

24. Cummings, GS, Tillman, LJ: Remodeling of dense connective tissue in normal adult tissues. In Currier, DP, Nelson, RM (eds) Dynamics of Human Biologic Tissues. FA Davis, Philadelphia, 1992, p 45.

25. D'Amato, M, Bach, BR: Knee injuries. In: Brotzman, SB, Wilk, KE (eds) Clinical Orthopedic Rehabilitation, ed 2. Mosby, Philadelphia, 2003, pp 251–370.

26. D'Lima, DD, et al: The effect of preoperative exercise on total knee replacement outcomes. Clin Orthop 326:174, 1996.

27. Enwemeka, CS: Connective tissue plasticity: ultrastructural, biomechanical, and morphometric effects of physical factors on intact and regenerating tendons. J Orthop Sports Phys Ther 14(5):198, 1991.

28. Fealey, S, Kingham, TP, Altchek, DW: Mini-open rotator cuff repair using a two-row fixation technique: outcomes analysis in patients with small, moderate, and large rotator cuff tears. Arthroscopy 18(6):665–670, 2002.

29. Gillogly, SD, Voight, M, Blackburn, T: Treatment of articular cartilage defects of the knee with autologous chondrocyte implantation. J Orthop Sports Phys Ther 28(4):241, 1998.

30. Green, DP, Hotchkiss, RN, Pederson, WC, Wolfe, SW (eds) Green's Operative Hand Surgery, ed 5. Churchill Livingstone, Philadelphia, 2005.

31. Hart, JA, Sekel, R: Osteotomy of the knee: is there a seat at the table? J Arthoplasty 4(Suppl 1):45–49, 2002.

32. Hatrup, SJ: Synovectomy. In Morrey, BF (ed) Reconstructive Surgery of the Joints, ed 2. Churchill Livingstone, New York, 1996, p 1599.

33. Irrgang, JJ, Pezzullo, D: Rehabilitation following surgical procedures to address articular cartilage lesions in the knee. J Orthop Sports Phys Ther 28(4):232, 1998.

34. Jacobson, MD, et al: Muscle function deficits after tourniquet ischemia. Am J Sports Med 22(3):372, 1994.

35. Jones, RE, Blackburn, WD: Joint replacement surgery preoperative management. Bull Rheum Dis 47(4):5, 1998.

36. Keene, J, Malone, TR: Ligament and muscle-tendon unit injuries. In Malone, TR, McPoil T, Nitz, AJ (eds) Orthopaedic and Sports Physical Therapy, ed 3. CV Mosby, St. Louis, 1997, p 135.

37. Khatod, M, Akerson, WH: Ligament injury and repair. In Pedowitz, RA, O'Connor, JJ, Akeson, WH (eds) Daniel's Knee Injuries: Liga-

ment and Cartilage Structure, Function, Injury and Repair, ed 2. Lippincott Williams & Wilkins, Philadelphia, 2003, pp 185–201.

38. Kim, CW, Pedowitz, RA: Principles of surgery. Part A. Graft choice and the biology of graft healing. In Pedowitz, RA, O'Connor, JJ, Akeson, WH (eds) Daniel's Knee Injuries: Ligament and Cartilage Structure, Function, Injury and Repair, ed 2. Lippincott Williams & Wilkins, Philadelphia, 2003, pp 435–455.

39. King, L: Case study: physical therapy management of hip osteoarthritis prior to total hip arthroplasty. J Orthop Sports Phys Ther 26(1):35, 1997.

40. Kitaoka, HB: Complications of replacement arthroplasty of the ankle. In Morrey, BF (ed) Joint Replacement Arthroplasty, ed 3. Churchill Livingstone, Philadelphia, 2003, pp 1151–1171.

41. Laimins, PD, Powell, SE: Principles of surgery. Part C. Anterior cruciate ligament reconstruction: techniques past and present. In Pedowitz, RA, O'Connor, JJ, Akeson, WH (eds) Daniel's Knee Injuries: Ligament and Cartilage Structure, Function, Injury and Repair, ed 2. Lippincott Williams & Wilkins, Philadelphia, 2003, pp 227–223

42. Matsen, FA, et al: Glenohumeral instability. In Rockwood, Jr, CA, Matsen III, FA, Wirth, MA, Lippitt, SB (eds) The Shoulder, Vol 2, ed 3. Saunders, Philadelphia, 2004, p 655.

43. Matsen, FA, et al: Glenohumeral arthritis and its management. In Rockwood, Jr, CA, Matsen III, FA, Wirth, MA, Lippit, SB (eds) The Shoulder, Vol 2, ed 3. Saunders, Philadelphia, 2004, p 879.

44. McGinty, JB: Operative Arthroscopy, ed 3. Lippincott Williams & Wilkins, Philadelphia, 2003.

45. McNally, MA, Mollan, RAB: The effect of active movement of the foot on venous blood flow after total hip replacement. J Bone Joint Surg Am 79:1198–1201, 1997.

46. Melvin, JL, Gall, V (eds): Rheumatologic Rehabilitation Series, Vol 5: Surgical Rehabilitation. American Occupational Therapy Association, Bethesda, 1999.

47. Mercier, LR: Practical Orthopedics, ed 4. Mosby, St. Louis, 1995.

48. Minas, T, Nehrer, S: Current concepts in the treatment of articular cartilage defects. Orthopedics 20:525, 1997.

49. Morrey, BF: Radial head fracture. In Morrey, BF (ed) The Elbow and Its Disorders, ed 3. WB Saunders, Philadelphia, 2000, p 341.

50. Morrey, BF (ed): Joint Replacement Arthroplasty, ed 3. Churchill Livingstone, Philadelphia, 2003.

51. NIH Consensus Development Panel on Total Hip Replacement. JAMA 273:1950, 1995.

52. Noonan, TJ, Garrett, WE: Injuries at the myotendinous junction. Clin Sports Med 11:783, 1992.

53. Noyes, FR, Butler, DL, Grood, ES, et al: Biomechanical analysis of human ligament grafts used in knee ligament repairs and reconstructions. J Bone Joint Surg Am 66:334, 1984.

54. Noyes, FR, Keller, CS, et al: Advances in understanding of knee ligament injury, repair and rehabilitation Med Sci Sports Exerc 16:427, 1984.

55. Peterson, CA, Alteck, DW, Warren, RE: Shoulder arthroscopy. In Rockwood, CA, Matsen, FA (eds) The Shoulder, Vol 2, ed 2. WB Saunders, Philadelphia, 1998, p 290.

56. Richterman, I, Keenan, MA: Surgical Interventions. In Walker, JM, Helewa, A: Physical Therapy in Arthritis. WB Saunders, Philadelphia, 1996.

57. Roach, JA, Tremblay, LM, Bowers, DL: A preoperative assessment and education program: implementation and outcomes. Patient Educ Couns 25:83, 1995.

58. Salter, RB: Textbook of Disorders and Injuries of the Musculoskeletal System, ed 3. Williams & Wilkins, Baltimore, 1999.

59. Saltzman, CL, Johnson, KA: Surgery of the ankle and foot. In Sledge, CB, et al (eds) Arthritis Surgery. WB Saunders, Philadelphia, 1994, p 818.

60. Scott, RD: Total Knee Arthroplasty. Saunders, Philadelphia, 2006.

61. Scott, WN (ed) Insall & Scott's Surgery of the Knee, ed 4. Churchill Livingstone, Philadelphia, 2006.

62. Sledge, CB: Introduction to surgical management. In Sledge, CB, et al (eds) Arthritis Surgery. WB Saunders, Philadelphia, 1994.

63. Tasto, JP, Tradonsky, S, Cohen, BS, Hunt, TJ: Surgical decisions and treatment alternatives—meniscal tears, malalignment, chondral injury and chronic arthrosis. In Pedowitz, RA, O'Connor, JJ, Akeson, WH (eds) Daniel's Knee Injuries: Ligament and Cartilage Structure, Func-

tion, Injury and Repair, ed 2. Lippincott Williams & Wilkins, Philadelphia, 2003, pp 567–586.

64. Thomas, RH, Daniels, TR: Ankle arthritis. J Bone Joint Surg Am 85:923–936, 2003.

65. Tibone, JE, McMahon, PJ: Biomechanics and pathologic lesions in the overhead athlete. In Innotti, JP, Williams, GR (eds) Disorders of the Shoulder: Diagnosis and Management. Lippincott Williams & Wilkins, Philadelphia, 1999, p 233.

66. Tria, Jr, AJ: Advances in minimally invasive total knee arthroplasty. Orthopedics 26(8 Suppl):859–863, 2003.

67. White, RH, Geltner, S, Newman, JM, et al: Predictors of rehospitalization for symptomatic venous thromboembolism after total hip arthroplasty. N Engl J Med 343:1758–1764, 2000.

68. Wilk, KE, Andrews, JR: Rehabilitation following thermal assisted capsular shrinkage of the glenohumeral joint: current concepts. J Orthop Sports Phys Ther 32(6):268–287, 2002.

69. Woolf, CJ: Generation of acute pain: central mechanisms. Br Med Bull 47:523, 1991.

70. Wynn Parry, CB, Stanley, JK: Synovectomy of the hand. Br J Rheumatol 32:1089, 1993.

71. Zazzali, MS, Wad, VB, Harrera, J, et al: Shoulder instability. In Donatelli, RA (ed) Physical Therapy of the Shoulder, ed 4. Churchill Livingstone, St. Louis, 2004, pp 483–505.

# Peripheral Nerve Disorders and Management

13
CHAPTER

Therapeutic exercise and related manual therapy techniques would not be possible without the nervous system and all its components activating, controlling, and modifying the motor system responses as well as receiving and interpreting feedback from the variety of sensory receptors throughout the body. Because of their intimate proximity to all the structures in the trunk and extremities, nerves may become stressed or injured with various musculoskeletal conditions, postures, and repetitive microtraumas resulting in symptoms, impairments, and functional limitations. Highlights of the anatomy and results of injury to the peripheral nervous system are reviewed in the first section of this chapter for the purpose of laying the foundation for management guidelines, including therapeutic exercise and manual therapy interventions, that are described in the remainder of the chapter. In the treatment of patients with musculoskeletal impairments, often the therapist does not think of the components of the central nervous system. Even though this chapter primarily deals with the peripheral nervous system, acknowledgment that the central nervous system plays a key role in the initiation and control of movement is a must. The reader is referred to Chapter 8 for consideration of motor control in the total rehabilitation of the individual.

349

The development of a plan of care and intervention techniques differs for patients with impairments due to nerve involvement. Nerve injuries may result in significant functional limitations due to paralysis and deformity. Utilizing the principles presented in this chapter, along with the knowledge and skills of examination and evaluation of the neural, muscular, and skeletal systems, the reader should be able to design therapeutic exercise programs that meet the goals and choose techniques for intervention that are appropriate for patients who have limitations due to injury or mobility restrictions of the peripheral nervous system. Also included in this chapter is a section on the complex regional pain syndrome and autonomic nervous system involvement that results in reflex sympathetic dystrophy.

## REVIEW OF PERIPHERAL NERVE STRUCTURE

### Nerve Structure

Peripheral components of the neuromuscular system include the alpha and gamma motor neurons, their axons, and the skeletal muscles they innervate; the sensory neurons and their receptors located in the connective tissues, joints, and blood vessels; and the neurons of the autonomic nervous system. Connective tissue surrounds each axon (endoneurium) as well as fascicles (perineurium) and entire nerve fibers (epineurium).[41,62] The axolemma is the surface membrane of axon. Schwann cells lie between the axolemma and endoneurium; they form myelin, which functions to insulate the axon as well as speed the conduction of action potentials along the nerve fiber. The exceptions are very small fibers that are unmyelinated. A peripheral nerve may consist of a single fascicle or consist of several fascicles.[41] The structure of a peripheral nerve with its connective tissue and vascular layers is illustrated in Figure 13.1, and the location of their cell bodies is summarized in Box 13.1.

### Nervous System Mobility Characteristics

Butler[7] described the peripheral and central nervous systems as a continuous tissue tract; simply stated, it is like an H on its side. Structurally and functionally, there is continuity of the connective tissues, of the impulse transmission between the neurons, and with the chemical flow

---

| BOX 13.1 | Content of Peripheral Nerves |

Peripheral nerves contain a mix of motor, sensory, and sympathetic neurons.

- *Alpha motor neuron (somatic efferent fibers)*: cell bodies located in anterior column of spinal cord; innervates skeletal muscles
- *Gamma motor neurons (efferent fibers)*: cell bodies located in lateral columns of spinal cord; innervates intrafusal muscle fibers of the muscle spindle
- *Sensory neurons (somatic afferent fibers)*: cell bodies located in the dorsal root ganglia; innervates sensory receptors
- *Sympathetic neurons (visceral afferent fibers)*: cell bodies located in sympathetic ganglia; innervates sweat glands, blood vessels, viscera, and glands

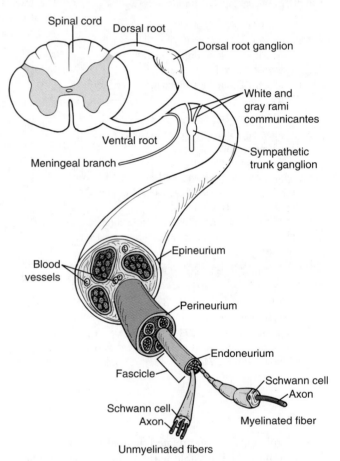

FIGURE 13.1 Peripheral nerve and its connective tissue coverings.

of neurotransmitters. The system is designed to be mobile and deform while at the same time to be able to conduct impulses.

When a joint moves and tension is placed on a nerve bed, nerve gliding is toward the moving joint (convergence); and when tension is relieved, nerve gliding is away from the moving joint (divergence). Initially, excursion of the nerve occurs adjacent to the moving joint, but excursion of the nerve progresses more distant from the moving joint as limb movement continues.[62]

Substantial mobility in the nervous system is needed for an individual to move during functional activities. With movement of an extremity, before there is increased tension in the nerve itself the whole peripheral nerve moves and there is movement between connective tissues and neural tissues. The mobility is allowed without undue stress on the nerve tissue because:

● The arrangement of the spinal cord, nerve roots, and plexes allows mobility. If any part of the H is placed under tension, the force can be dissipated throughout the system.
● The nerves themselves are wavy and can straighten when tension is applied.
● The connective tissue around the individual nerves and bundles of nerves (epineurium, perineurium, endoneurium) absorb tensile forces before the nerve itself stretches.

Cadaveric and in vivo ultrasound studies of median nerve mobility and strain have shown nerve movement of 5 to 10 mm depending on the position and motion of each of the joints in the upper extremity and neck, as well as a wavy appearance when on a slack (unloaded) and a straightening of the nerve when under tension.[17] Strain calculated in the stretch position (see upper limb tension test for the median nerve described in the section on Neural Tension Impairments) was 2.5% to 3.0%.[17]

## Common Sites of Injury to Peripheral Nerves

Injury to the nerves of the peripheral nervous system can occur anywhere along the pathway from the nerve roots to their termination in the tissues of the trunk and extremities. As each nerve courses from the intervertebral foramina to its peripheral destination, there are sites that increase its susceptibility to either tension or compression. Symptoms and signs of nerve impairments are sensory changes or loss and motor weakness in the distribution of the involved nerve fibers. Because nerves are composed of innervated connective tissue and blood vessels surround the axons, ischemic pain or tension pain may also occur when these tissues are stressed. Also, because peripheral nerves include sympathetic fibers, autonomic responses might occur. Whenever neurological symptoms and signs are present, the entire nerve should be tested for mobility and signs of compression at key points along its pathway.

In this section, primary sites of compression, tension, or injury are identified for the peripheral nerves in the upper and lower quarter regions including their origins at the nerve roots and pathways through each of the plexuses.

### Nerve Roots

Nerve roots emerge from the spinal canal and traverse the foramina of the spine where they can become impinged as a result of various pathologies of the spine that reduce the space in the foramina, such as degenerative disc disease (DDD), degenerative joint disease (DJD), disc lesions, and spondylolisthesis. With reduced spinal canal or foraminal space (stenosis), extension, side bending, or rotation to the side of the stenosis further decreases the space where the nerve root courses and may cause or perpetuate symptoms. If adhesions place tension on a nerve root, nerve mobility tests (described later in this chapter) can reproduce symptoms when the spine is side-bent (laterally flexed) away from the side causing the symptoms. When involved, symptoms and signs include sensory changes and/or loss of motor function in the respective dermatome and myotome patterns (Fig. 13.2 and Box 13.2). Nerve roots of the upper quarter include C5 through T1 and those of the lower quarter L1 through S3. Management guidelines for individuals with nerve root symptoms are described in Chapter 15.

| BOX 13.2 | Key Muscles for Testing Upper and Lower Quarter Myotomes[38] |
|---|---|

**Upper Quarter**

| | |
|---|---|
| C1-2 | Cervical flexion |
| C3 | Cervical side flexion |
| C4 | Scapular elevation |
| C5 | Shoulder abduction |
| C6 | Elbow flexion and wrist extension |
| C7 | Elbow extension and wrist flexion |
| C8 | Thumb extension |
| T1 | Finger abduction |

**Lower Quarter**

| | |
|---|---|
| L1-2 | Hip flexion |
| L3 | Knee extension |
| L4 | Ankle dorsiflexion |
| L5 | Big toe extension |
| S1 | Ankle eversion and plantar flexion, hip extension |
| S2 | Knee flexion |
| S3 | No specific test action; intrinsic foot muscles (except abductor hallucis) |

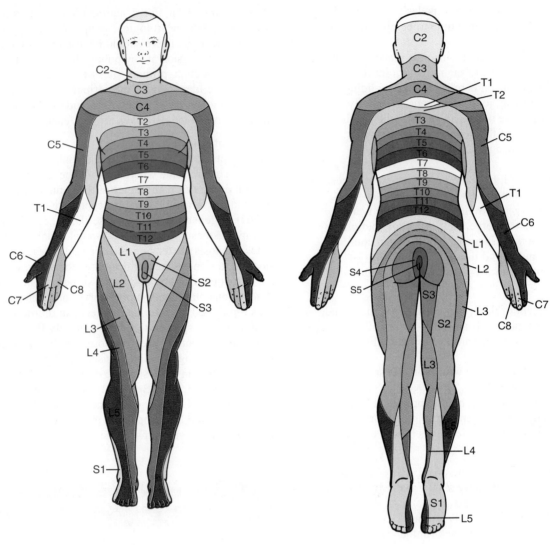

**FIGURE 13.2** Dermatomes—anterior and posterior views.

## Brachial Plexus

After emerging from the foramina, the nerve fibers divide into anterior and posterior primary rami. Vasomotor fibers from the sympathetic trunk join the anterior primary rami to course within the brachial plexus and peripheral nerves to the extremities. The brachial plexus is formed by the anterior primary divisions of the C5-T1 nerve roots (Fig. 13.3). The plexus functions as the distribution center for organizing the contents of each peripheral nerve. In addi-

tion, Butler[8] suggested that the weave pattern in the brachial plexus contributes to the mobility of the nerves such that when tension is placed on any one peripheral nerve the tension is transmitted to several cervical nerve roots rather than just one nerve root.

The brachial plexus courses through the region known as the thoracic outlet. There are three primary sites for compression or entrapment of the neurovascular structures in this region.

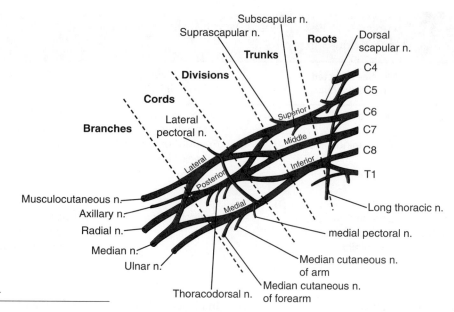

FIGURE 13.3 Brachial plexus.

- Interscalene triangle, bordered by the scalenus anterior and medius muscles and first rib
- Costoclavicular space between the clavicle superiorly and the first rib inferiorly
- Axillary interval between the anterior deltopectoral fascia, the pectoralis minor, and the coracoid process
- Structural anomalies such as a cervical rib or malunion of a clavicular fracture may compress or entrap a portion of the plexus

When vascular and/or neurological symptoms are caused by impairments in the thoracic outlet, it is commonly referred to as thoracic outlet syndrome. Characteristics of this syndrome and management guidelines are described later in the chapter.

Other injuries to the brachial plexus include:

- **Upper plexus injuries (C5,6):** The most common injury to the plexus involves compression or tearing of the upper trunk. The mechanism involves shoulder depression and lateral flexion of the neck to the opposite side. There is loss of abduction and lateral rotation of the shoulder and weakness in elbow flexion and forearm supination (waiter's tip position). Erb's palsy occurs with birth injuries when the shoulder is stretched downward, although Benjamin[5] cautioned that there are maternal and infant factors that could contribute this

injury in addition to the applied forces during delivery. A "stinger" occurs with injuries as might occur when playing football and the individual lands on the upper torso and shoulder with the head/neck laterally flexed in the opposite direction.
- **Middle plexus injuries (C7):** Rarely seen alone.
- **Lower plexus injuries (C8,T1):** Usually due to compression by a cervical rib or stretching the arm overhead. Klumpke's paralysis (paralysis of the intrinsics of the hand) occurs in birth injuries when the baby presents with its arm overhead.[5]
- **Complete or total injury of the plexus:** Complete paralysis from a total brachial plexus injury may occur as a complication of birth; it is known as Erb-Klumpke's paralysis and is associated with Horner's syndrome in one-third of those severely affected.[5]

### Peripheral Nerves in the Upper Quarter

The brachial plexus terminates in five primary peripheral nerves that are responsible for innervating the tissues of the upper extremity: musculocutaneous, axillary, median, ulnar, and radial nerves. Patterns of impairments from muscle weaknesses for each of these nerves are summarized in Table 13.1. Common sites for compression or tension injuries for each of the nerves are described in this section.

**TABLE 13.1    Patterns of Muscle Weakness and Functional Loss with Peripheral Nerve Injuries in the Upper Extremity**

| Nerve | Muscles Affected With Nerve Injury | Common Causes of Nerve Injury | Deformity | Primary Functional Loss |
|---|---|---|---|---|
| Axillary (C5,6) | Deltoid<br><br>Teres minor | Dislocation of shoulder<br>Fracture of surgical neck of humerus | "Square shoulder" from deltoid muscle atrophy | Weakness in shoulder abduction and lateral rotation; see shoulder shrugging and lateral bending of trunk to abduct/flex arm |
| Musculo-cutaneous (C5-7) | Coracobrachialis<br>Biceps brachii<br>Brachialis | Projectile wounds | Atrophy (flatness) along flexor surface of upper arm | Weakness in elbow flexion especially with forearm supinated; may have slight subluxation of head of humerus |
| Median (C6-8, T1) | Forearm<br>• Pronator teres<br>• Palmaris longus<br>• Flexor digitorum profundus (radial portion)<br>• Flexor carpi radialis<br>• Flexor digitorum superficialis<br>• Flexor pollicis longus<br>• Pronator quadratus<br>Wrist and hand<br>• Opponens pollicis<br>• Abductor pollicis brevis<br>• Flexor pollicis brevis (superficial head)<br>• Lumbricales I and II | Impingement in hypertrophied pronator teres<br><br><br>Compression in carpal tunnel | Ape hand with atrophy in the thenar eminence | Absent forearm pronation, weak grip; no thumb abduction and opposition therefore unable to do tip-to-tip, tip-to-pad, and pad-to-pad prehension. |
| Ulnar (C8, T1) | Forearm<br>• Flexor carpi ulnaris<br>• Flexor digitorum profundus (ulnar portion)<br>Wrist and hand<br>• Abductor, opponens, and flexor digiti minimi<br>• Lumbricales III and IV<br>• Interossei<br>• Adductor pollicis<br>• Flexor pollicis brevis (deep head) | Cubital tunnel<br>Impingement between heads of flexor carpi ulnaris<br><br>Compression in tunnel of Guyon at the wrist | Partial claw with atrophy between the metacarpals, with atrophy of hypothenar eminence and ulnar drifting of little finger | Use of 4th and 5th digits for spherical and cylindrical power grips, thumb for adduction, and finger abduction and adduction are lost |
| Radial (C5-8, T1) | Triceps brachii and anconeus<br>Brachialis<br>Brachioradialis<br>Extensor carpi radialis longus and brevis and ulnaris<br>Extensor digitorum communis and digiti quinti<br>Supinator<br>Abductor pollicis longus<br>Extensor pollicis longus and brevis | Axilla<br>Musculospiral groove<br>Radial neck | Wrist drop | With high lesions affecting the triceps cannot push; weak supination; unable to make fist or grip objects unless wrist is stabilized in extension |

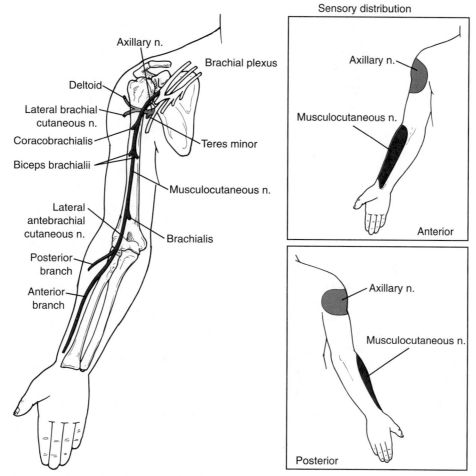

Sensory distribution

FIGURE 13.4 Sensory and motor innervations of the axillary (C5,6) and musculocutaneous (C5,6) nerves.

## Axillary Nerve: C5,6

The axillary nerve (Fig. 13.4) emerges from the posterior cord of the brachial plexus; it passes laterally through the axilla, sends a branch to the teres minor muscle, courses behind the surgical neck of the humerus, and innervates the deltoid muscle and overlying skin. The axillary nerve is vulnerable to injury with dislocation of the shoulder and fractures of the surgical neck of the humerus. If the upper trunk of the brachial plexus is stretched or injured, it affects the function of the axillary nerve. Shoulder abduction and lateral rotation are impaired when this nerve is affected.

## Musculocutaneous Nerve: C5,6

The musculocutaneous nerve (Fig. 13.4) emerges from the lateral cord of the brachial plexus and crosses the axilla with the median nerve; it pierces and innervates the coracobrachialis and then travels distally to innervate the biceps and brachialis muscles. It continues between these muscles to the flexor surface of the elbow; after emerging from the deep fascia at the elbow, is becomes the lateral cutaneous nerve of the forearm. Isolated impingement of this nerve is not common; injury to the lateral cord or the

upper trunk of the brachial plexus affects the musculocutaneous nerve. When affected, the patient is unable to flex the elbow with the forearm supinated and may have some instability in the shoulder.

## Median Nerve: C6-8

Bundles from the medial and lateral cords of the brachial plexus unite in the uppermost part of the arm to form the median nerve (Fig. 13.5). It courses the medial aspect of the humerus to the elbow, where it is deep in the cubital fossa under the bicipital aponeurosis, medial to the tendon of the biceps and brachial artery; it then moves into the forearm between the two heads of the pronator teres muscle. Hypertrophy of this muscle can compress the median nerve, producing symptoms that mimic carpal tunnel syndrome except that the forearm muscles (pronator teres, wrist flexors, extrinsic finger flexors) are involved in addition to the intrinsic muscles.

To enter the hand, the median nerve passes through the carpal tunnel at the wrist with the flexor tendons. The carpal tunnel is covered by the thick, relatively inelastic transverse carpal ligament. Entrapment of the median nerve in the tunnel, called carpal tunnel syndrome,

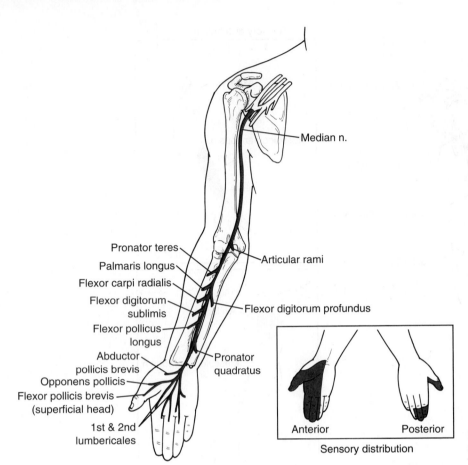

Median n.

Pronator teres

Palmaris longus

Flexor carpi radialis

Flexor digitorum sublimis

Flexor pollicus longus

Abductor pollicis brevis

Opponens pollicis

Flexor pollicis brevis (superficial head)

1st & 2nd lumbericales

Articular rami

Flexor digitorum profundus

Pronator quadratus

Anterior          Posterior

Sensory distribution

FIGURE 13.5 Sensory and motor innervations of the median nerve (C6-8, T1).

causes sensory changes and progressive weakness in the muscles innervated distal to the wrist resulting in ape-hand deformity (thenar atrophy and thumb in the plane of the hand). Characteristics of this syndrome and management guidelines are described later in the chapter. The branch innervating the opponens muscle hooks over the carpal ligament two-thirds of the way up the thenar eminence and can be entrapped separately.[29]

## Ulnar Nerve: C8, T1

The ulnar nerve (Fig. 13.6) emerges from the medial cord of the brachial plexus at the lower border of the pectoralis minor and descends the arm along the medial side of the humerus. It passes posterior to the elbow joint in the groove between the medial epicondyle of the humerus and the olecranon of the ulna. The groove is covered by a fibrous sheath, which forms the cubital tunnel. The nerve possesses considerable mobility to stretch around the elbow as it flexes, although the nerve can be easily irritated at this site owing to its superficial location. It then passes between the humeral and ulnar heads of the flexor carpi ulnaris muscle, another site where impingement could occur. The only extrinsic muscles innervated by the ulnar nerve are the flexor carpi ulnaris and ulnar half of the flexor digitorum profundus.

The ulnar nerve enters the hand through a trough formed by the pisiform bone and hook of the hamate bone and is covered by the volar carpal ligament and palmaris brevis muscle, forming the tunnel of Guyon. Trauma or entrapment in this region causes sensory changes and progressive weakness of muscles innervated distal to the site,

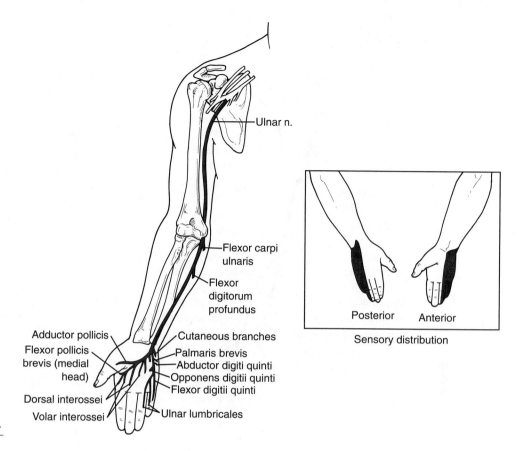

Posterior   Anterior

Sensory distribution

FIGURE 13.6 Sensory and motor innervations of the ulnar nerve (C8, T1).

resulting in partial claw-hand deformity. Injury to the nerve after it bifurcates leads to partial involvement, depending on the site of injury.[29] Characteristics of ulnar nerve impingement in the tunnel and management guidelines are described later in the chapter.

### Radial Nerve: C6-8, T1

The radial nerve (Fig. 13.7) emerges directly from the posterior cord of the brachial plexus at the lower border of the pectoralis minor. As it descends in the arm it winds around the posterior aspect of the humerus in the musculospiral groove and continues to the radial aspect of the elbow. In the arm it innervates the triceps, anconeus, and upper portion of the extensor and supinator group of the forearm. Injury to this nerve may occur with shoulder dislocations and mid-humeral fractures. Also known to all therapists is "crutch palsy," a condition of nerve compression caused by leaning on axillary crutches. "Saturday night palsy" occurs when sleeping with the person's head on the arm that is slung over the back of a chair or open car window. The triceps is involved only if the compression or injury to the nerve occurs close to the axilla.

At the elbow the radial nerve pierces the lateral muscular septum anterior to the lateral epicondyle and passes under the origin of the extensor carpi radialis brevis; it then divides into a superficial and a deep branch. The deep branch may become entrapped as it passes under the edge of the extensor carpi radialis brevis and the fibrous slit in the supinator, causing progressive weakness in the wrist and finger extensor and supinator muscles (except the extensor carpi radialis longus, which is innervated proximal to the bifurcation). Impingement may occur here and may be erroneously called tennis elbow (lateral epicondylitis—see Chapter 18). The deep branch passes around the

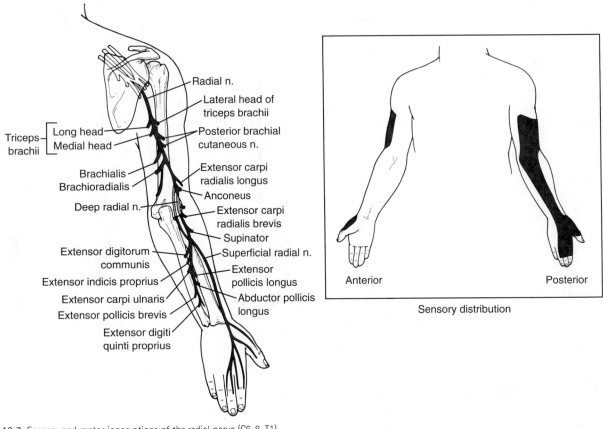

**FIGURE 13.7** Sensory and motor innervations of the radial nerve (C6-8, T1).

neck of the radius and may be injured with a radial head fracture. The superficial radial nerve may undergo direct trauma that causes sensory changes in the distribution of the nerve.

The radial nerve enters the hand on the dorsal surface as the superficial radial nerve, which is sensory only; therefore, injury to it in the wrist or hand does not cause any motor weakness. The influence of the radial nerve on hand musculature is entirely proximal to the wrist. Injury proximal to the elbow results in wrist drop and inability to actively extend the wrist and fingers. This affects the length–tension relationship of the extrinsic finger flexors, resulting in an ineffective grip unless the wrist is splinted in partial extension. Injury of the mid-forearm affect onlys the supinator muscle and extrinsic abductor and extensor pollicis muscles.

### Lumbosacral Plexus

The lumbar plexus is formed by the anterior primary divisions of the nerve roots L1, L2, L3, and part of L4 (Fig. 13.8A); the sacral plexus is formed from L4, L5, S1, and parts of S2 and S3 (Fig. 13.8B). As with the brachial plexus, the branches and divisions of the LS plexus organize the content of each of the peripheral nerves coursing into the lower extremity. In addition, the anterior primary rami of the plexus receive postganglionic sympathetic fibers from the sympathetic chain that innervate blood vessels, sweat glands, and piloerector muscles in the lower extremity. Isolated injuries to the lumbar plexus or sacral plexus are not common; symptoms more commonly arise from disc lesions or spondylitic deformities that affect one or more nerve roots or from tension or compression of specific peripheral nerves.

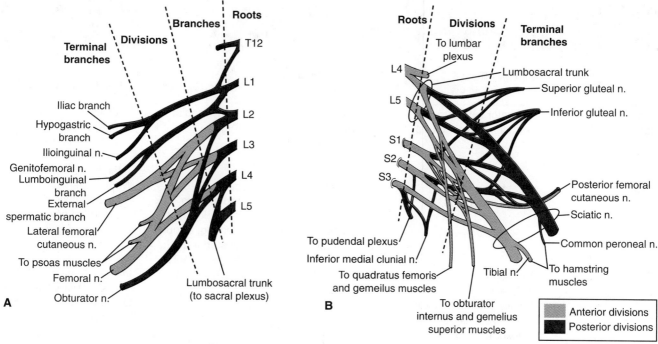

FIGURE 13.8 Lumbar plexus (*A*) and sacral plexus (*B*).

## Peripheral Nerves in the Lower Quarter

The lumbosacral plexus terminates in three primary peripheral nerves, which are responsible for innervating the tissues of the lower extremity. They are the femoral and obturator nerves from the lumbar plexus and the sciatic nerve from the sacral plexus. Patterns of impairments from muscle weakness for each of these nerves are summarized in Table 13.2. Common sites for compression or tension injuries are described in this section.

### Femoral Nerve: L2-4

The femoral nerve (Fig. 13.9) arises from the three posterior divisions of the lumbar plexus. It emerges from the lateral border of the psoas muscle superior to the inguinal ligament and descends underneath the

| TABLE 13.2 | Patterns of Muscle Weakness and Functional Loss With Peripheral Nerve Injuries in the Lower Extremity | | | |
|---|---|---|---|---|
| **Nerve** | **Muscles Affected With Nerve Injury** | **Common Sites of Nerve Compression/Tension or Causes of Nerve Injury** | **Deformity/Symptoms** | **Primary Functional Loss** |
| Femoral (L2-4) | Illiacus Sartorius Pectineus Quadriceps group | Pelvic or upper femur fractures, during reduction of congenital dislocation of the hip, or from pressure during a forceps labor and delivery | Atrophy in anterior thigh | Weakness or inability to flex thigh and extend knee. Gait and weight-bearing disturbances: unable to control knee flexion during loading response or hip flexion to initiate swing |

(table continued on page 360)

**TABLE 13.2** Patterns of Muscle Weakness and Functional Loss With Peripheral Nerve Injuries in the Lower Extremity (continued)

| Nerve | Muscles Affected With Nerve Injury | Common Sites of Nerve Compression/Tension or Causes of Nerve Injury | Deformity/Symptoms | Primary Functional Loss |
|---|---|---|---|---|
| Obturator (L2-4) | Obturator externus Adductor muscle group | Similar to femoral nerve. Pressure from gravid uterus and difficult labor | Atrophy medial thigh | Difficulty crossing the legs. Impaired adduction and external rotation of thigh |
| Sciatic | Hamstring group Adductor magnus | Compression from tight piriformis muscle; hip dislocation; fracture of the femur | "Sciatica"—pain radiating in posterior thigh and leg; atrophy posterior thigh, leg, and foot | Weak knee flexion and loss of ankle and foot control affecting all phases of gait |
| Tibial (L4 – S3) | Plantar flexors Popliteus Tibialis posterior, flexor digitorum longus and flexor hallucis longus | | Atrophy in calf | Inability to plantar flex ankle or flex the toes. Gait impairment in terminal stance |
| *Distal to ankle* • Medial and lateral plantar nerves | *Distal to ankle* • Abductor hallucis, flexor hallucis brevis, lumbricales, interossei, and quadratus plantae | *Ankle and foot* • Compromise in tarsal tunnel Irritation from pes planus or pes cavus | Foot deformities such as pes cavus and claw toes; foot strain, painful heel | |
| Common peroneal (L4-S2) • Deep peroneal nerve | Ankle dorsiflexors Toe extensors Peroneus tertius | Compression from crossing legs; injury from fracture at head/neck of fibula | *Deep peroneal nerve* • Foot drop • May develop pes valgus | Gait impairment during the loading response with foot slap and during swing phase with excessive hip flexion (steppage gait) to clear the toes |
| • Superficial peroneal nerve | Peroneus longus and brevis | | *Superficial peroneal nerve* • May develop equinovarus | |

ligament to the femoral triangle, lateral to the femoral artery, to innervate the sartorius and quadriceps muscle group. The iliopsoas is supplied superior to the ligament. Injuries to the nerve may occur with trauma, such as fractures of the upper femur or pelvis, during reduction of congenital dislocation of the hip, or from pressure during a forceps labor and delivery—resulting in weakness of hip flexion and loss of knee extension. Symptoms may occur from neuritis in diabetes mellitus.

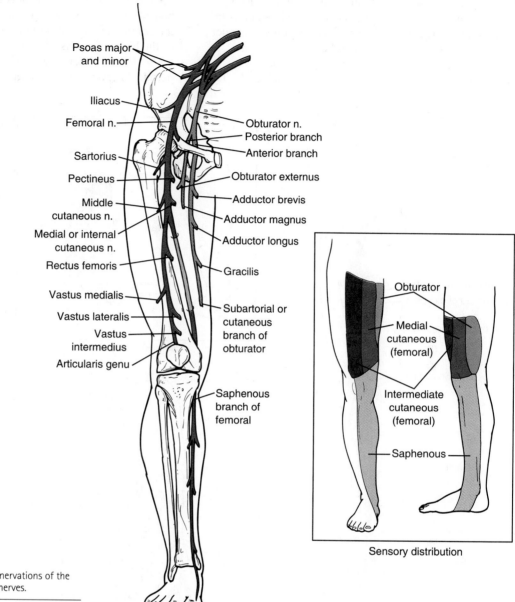

FIGURE 13.9 Sensory and motor innervations of the femoral (L2-4) and obturator (L2-4) nerves.

## Obturator Nerve: L2-4

The obturator nerve (Fig. 13.9) arises from the three anterior divisions of the lumbar plexus. It descends through the obturator canal in the medial obturator foramen to the medial side of the thigh to innervate the adductor muscle group and obturator externus. Isolated injury to this nerve is rare, although uterine pressure and damage during labor may cause the injury. If damaged, adduction and external rotation of the thigh are impaired, with the individual having difficulty crossing his or her legs.

## Sciatic Nerve: L4,5, S1–3

The sciatic nerve (Fig. 13.10) emerges from the sacral plexus as the largest nerve in the body; its component parts, the tibial and common peroneal nerves, can be differentiated in the common sheath. Muscles in the buttock region (external rotators and gluteal muscles) are innervated by small nerves from the sacral plexus, which emerge proximal to formation of the sciatic nerve. The sciatic nerve exits the pelvis through the greater sciatic foramen and typically courses below, although sometimes through, the piriformis muscle. Piriformis syndrome may occur from a shortened muscle, causing compression and irritation of the nerve at this site. The nerve is protected under the gluteus maximus as it courses between the ischial tuberosity and greater trochanter, although injury may occur in this region with hip dislocation or reduction. The tibial portion of the sciatic nerve innervates the biarticular hamstring muscles and a portion of the adductor magnus; the common peroneal portion innervates the short head of the biceps femoris. Proximal to the popliteal fossa, the sciatic nerve terminates when the tibial and common peroneal nerves emerge as separate structures.

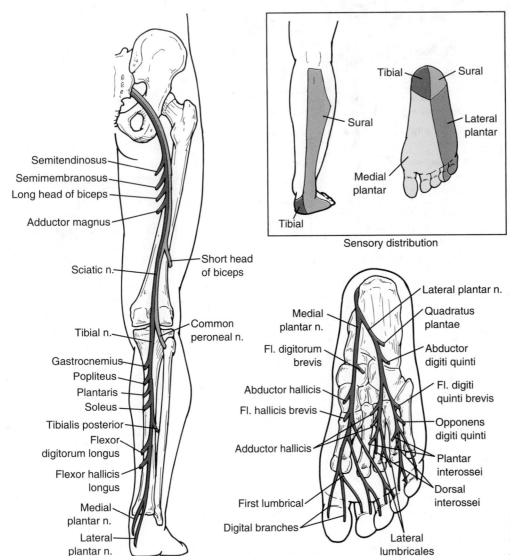

FIGURE 13.10 Sensory and motor innervations of the sciatic nerve (L4,5, S1-3) and tibial nerve (L4,5, S1-3).

## Tibial/Posterior Tibial Nerve: L4,5, S1–3

The tibial nerve (Fig. 13.10) forms from the anterior primary rami of the sacral plexus, courses with the common peroneal nerve as the sciatic nerve, and then emerges as a separate nerve proximal to the popliteal fossa. After coursing through the popliteal fossa, it sends a branch that joins a branch from the common peroneal nerve to form the sural nerve and continues on as the posterior tibial nerve. In the leg, it innervates the muscles of the posterior compartment, including the plantar flexors, popliteus, tibialis posterior, and extrinsic toe flexors.

In its approach to the foot, the nerve occupies a groove behind the medial malleolus along with the tendons of the tibialis posterior, flexor hallucis longus, and flexor digitorum longus; the groove is covered by a ligament, forming a tunnel. Entrapment usually from a space-occupying lesion is known as tarsal tunnel syndrome. The nerve then divides into the medial and lateral plantar and calcaneal nerves.

*Plantar and calcaneal nerves.* The plantar and calcaneal nerves may become entrapped as they turn under the medial aspect of the foot and pass through openings in the abductor hallucis muscle, especially with overpronation of the foot, which stresses the nerves against the fibrous-edged openings in the muscle.[29] Symptoms elicited are similar to acute foot strain (tenderness at the posteromedial plantar aspect of the foot), painful heel (inflamed calcaneal nerve), and pain in a pes cavus foot.[29] The medial and lateral plantar nerves innervate all the intrinsic muscles of the foot except the extensor digitorum brevis. The innervation pattern of the lateral plantar nerve in the foot corresponds to the ulnar nerve in the hand, and the medial plantar nerve corresponds to the median nerve. Weakness and postural changes in the foot such as pes cavus and clawing of the toes may occur with nerve compression or injury.

## Common Peroneal Nerve: L4,5, S1,2

After it bifurcates from the sciatic nerve in the knee region, the common peroneal nerve (Fig. 13.11) passes between the biceps femoris tendon and lateral head of the gastrocnemius muscle, sends a branch to join the tibial nerve and form the sural nerve, and then comes laterally around the fibular neck and passes through an opening in the peroneus longus muscle. Pressure or force against the nerve in this region can cause neuropathy, including sensory changes and weakness in the muscles of the anterior and lateral compartments of the leg. Injury also occurs subsequent to fracture of the head of the fibula, from rupture of the lateral collateral ligament of the knee, or from a tightly applied cast. Also, most people have experienced their "foot falling asleep" from sustained pressure when crossing their legs. The common peroneal nerve bifurcates just below the neck of the fibula into the superficial and deep peroneal nerves.

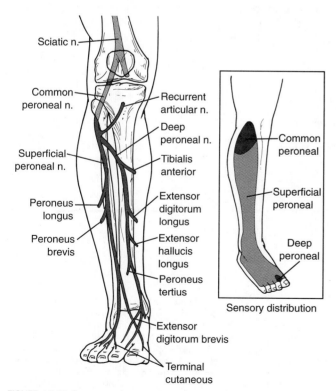

FIGURE 13.11 Sensory and motor innervations of the peroneal nerve (L4,5, S1,2).

***Superficial peroneal nerve.*** The superficial peroneal nerve descends along the anterior part of the fibula, innervating the peroneus longus and brevis muscles and continues on with cutaneous innervations. Injury to just this nerve primarily affects eversion. Over time, equinovarus may develop from unopposed inversion.

***Deep peroneal nerve.*** The deep peroneal nerve descends the leg along the interosseous membrane and distal tibia, innervating the ankle dorsiflexors, toe extensors, and peroneus tertius. In the foot it innervates the extensor digitorum brevis. Injury to the deep peroneal nerve results in foot drop and unopposed eversion during gait. Over time, pes valgus may develop.

## IMPAIRED NERVE FUNCTION

## ● NERVE INJURY AND RECOVERY

Peripheral nerve injury may result in motor, sensory, and/or sympathetic impairments. In addition, pain may be a symptom of nerve tension or compression because the connective tissue and vascular structures surrounding and in the peripheral nerves are innervated and the peripheral nerve function is sensitive to hypoxic states. Knowing the mechanism of injury and the clinical signs and symptoms help the clinician determine the potential outcome for the patient and develop a plan of care.[55]

### Mechanisms of Nerve Injury

Nerves are mobile and capable of considerable torsion and lengthening owing to their arrangement. Yet they are susceptible to various types of injury including[6,55]:

● Compression (sustained pressure applied externally such as tourniquet or internally such as from bone, tumor, or soft tissue impingement resulting in mechanical or ischemic injury)
● Laceration (knife, gunshot, surgical complication, injection injury)
● Stretch (excessive tension, tearing from traction forces)
● Radiation
● Electricity (lightening strike, electrical malfunction)

Injury may be complete or partial and produces symptoms based on the location of the insult.

Biomechanical injuries to the peripheral nervous system result most commonly from friction, compression, and stretch.[6,7] Secondary injury can be from blood or edema. Compressive forces can affect the microcirculation of the nerve, causing venous congestion and reduction of axoplasmic transport,[40] thus blocking nerve impulses; if sustained, it can cause nerve damage. The endoneurium helps maintain fluid pressure and may provide cushioning for nerves, especially when close to the surface and subject to greater pressure.

The insult can be acute from trauma or chronic from repetitive trauma or entrapment. Sites where a peripheral nerve is more vulnerable to compression, friction, or tension include tunnels (soft tissue, bony, fibro-osseous), branches of the nervous system (especially if the nerve has an abrupt angle), points where a nerve is relatively fixed when passing close to rigid structures (across a bony prominence), and at specific tension points.

Response to injury can be pathophysiological or pathomechanical, leading to symptoms derived from adverse tension on the nervous system. Results may be intraneural and/or extraneural.[7]

- *Intraneural.* Pathology that affects the conducting tissues (e.g., hypoxia or demyelination) or connective tissues of the nerve (e.g., scarring of epineurium or irritation of dura mater) may restrict the elasticity of the nervous system itself.
- *Extraneural.* Pathology that affects the nerve bed (e.g., blood), adhesions of epineurium to another tissue (e.g., a ligament), and swelling of tissue adjacent to a nerve (e.g., foraminal stenosis) may restrict the gross movement of the nervous system in relation to surrounding tissues.

## Classification of Nerve Injuries

Nerve injuries are classified using either the Seddon or Sunderland classification systems; both are based on structural and functional changes that occur in the nerve with various degrees of damage.[6,55,57] These systems describe the degree of injury to nerve substructures and the effect on prognosis. Seddon's system describes three levels of pathology: neuropraxia, axonotmesis, and neurotmesis. Sunderland's classification details five levels of injury and

potential for recovery. The characteristics of Seddon's classification of nerve injuries are summarized in Box 13.3 and are compared with Sunderland's classification in Fig. 13.12.

---

**BOX 13.3    Seddon's Classification and Characteristics of Nerve Injury[55,57]**

**Neuropraxia**
- Segmental demyelination
- Action potential slowed or blocked at point of demyelination; normal above and below point of compression
- Muscle does not atrophy; temporary sensory symptoms
- *Cause:* mild ischemia from nerve compression or traction
- Recovery is usually complete

**Axonotmesis**
- Loss of axonal continuity but connective tissue coverings remain intact
- Wallerian degeneration distal to lesion
- Muscle fiber atrophy and sensory loss
- *Cause:* prolonged compression or stretch causing infarction and necrosis
- Recovery is incomplete—surgical intervention may be required

**Neurotmesis**
- Complete severance of nerve fiber with disruption of connective tissue coverings
- Wallerian degeneration distal to lesion
- Muscle fiber atrophy and sensory loss
- *Cause:* gunshot or stab wounds, avulsion, rupture
- No recovery without surgery—recovery depends on surgical intervention and correct regrowth of individual nerve fibers in endoneural tubes

---

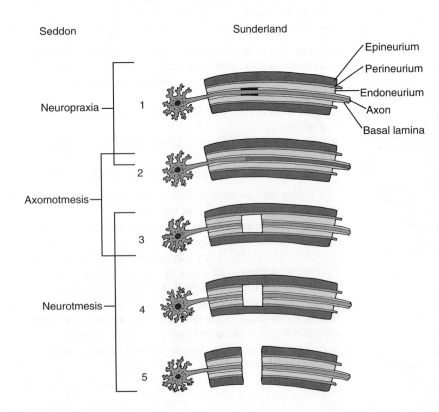

FIGURE 13.12 Comparison of Sunderland's and Seddon's classifications of nerve injuries. (1) First degree injury (neuropraxia): minimal structural disruption—complete recovery; (2) second degree (axonotmesis): complete axonal disruption with wallerian degeneration—usually complete recovery; (3) third degree (may be either axonotmesis or neurotmesis)—disruption of axon, and endoneurium—poor prognosis without surgery; (4) fourth degree (neurotmesis): disruption of axon, endoneurium, and perineurium—poor prognosis without surgery; (5) fifth degree (neurotmesis) complete structural disruption—poor prognosis without microsurgery.[55]

## Recovery of Nerve Injuries

Nerve tissue that has become irritated from tension, compression, or hypoxia may not have permanent damage and shows signs of recovery when the irritating factors are eliminated.[8] When the nerve has been injured, recovery is dependent on several factors including the extent of injury to the axon and its surrounding connective tissue sheath, the nature and level of the injury, the timing and technique of the repair (if necessary), and the age and motivation of the person.[6,18,20,54,64]

- *Nature and level of injury.* The more damage to the nerve and tissues, the more tissue reaction and scarring occur. Also, the proximal aspect of a nerve has greater combinations of motor, sensory and sympathetic fibers, so disruption there results in a greater chance of mismatching the fibers, thus affecting regeneration. Regeneration is often said to occur at a rate of 1 inch per day,[18] but rates from 0.5 to 9.0 mm per day have been reported based on the nature and severity of the injury, duration of denervation, condition of the tissues, and whether surgery is required.[6]
- *Timing and technique of repair.* Laceration or crush injuries that disrupt the integrity of the entire nerve require surgical repair. Timing of the repair is critical, as is the skill of the surgeon and technique used to align the segments accurately and avoid tension at the suture line for optimal nerve regeneration. Different regenerative potential outcomes following nerve repair have also been reported based on groupings of specific nerves.[50]
  - Excellent regenerative potential: radial, musculocutaneous, and femoral nerves
  - Moderate regenerative potential: median, ulnar, and tibial nerves
  - Poor regenerative potential: peroneal nerve
- *Age and motivation of the patient.* The nervous system must adapt and relearn use of the pathways once regeneration occurs. Motivation and age play a role in this, especially in the very young and the elderly.[50]

Smith[54] described five possible outcomes of nerve regeneration.

- Exact reinnervation of its native target organ with return of function
- Exact reinnervation of its native target organ but no return of function due to degeneration of the end organ
- Wrong receptor reinnervated in the proper territory, improper input
- Receptor reinnervation in wrong territory causing false localization of input
- No connection with an end organ

## Management Guidelines— Recovery from Nerve Injury

In general, recovery from nerve injury can be viewed as occurring in three phases.

- **Acute phase:** This is early after injury or after surgery, when the emphasis is on healing and prevention of complications.
- **Recovery phase:** This is when reinnervation occurs. Emphasis is on retraining and re-education.
- **Chronic phase:** This occurs when the potential for reinnervation has peaked and there are significant residual deficits. The emphasis is training compensatory function.

Management needs to consider not only nerve healing but tissue healing in general (see Chapter 10).[15] Management guidelines for the three phases of recovery from peripheral nerve injury are summarized in Box 13.4.

### Acute Phase

Following injury or immediately after surgery (e.g., following decompression and release or following repair of a lacerated nerve), there may be a brief period of immobilization to protect the nerve, minimize inflammation, and minimize tension at the injured/repaired site. As soon as allowed:

- *Movement.* Begin range of motion (ROM) to minimize joint and connective contractures and adhesions. This is dictated by the surgeon and type of surgery.
- *Splinting or bracing.* Splinting or bracing may be necessary to prevent deformities due to strength imbalances (use of a radial nerve splint to prevent wrist drop, a median nerve splint to position the thumb in opposition, a plantarflexion splint to prevent foot drop) and to prevent undue stress on the healing nerve tissue.

---

**BOX 13.4**
MANAGEMENT GUIDELINES—Recovery from Peripheral Nerve Injury

*Acute phase:* immediately after injury or surgery

- *Immobilization:* time dictated by surgeon
- *Movement:* amount and intensity dictated by type of injury and surgical repair
- *Splinting or bracing:* may be necessary to prevent deformities
- *Patient education:* protection of the part (see Box 13.5)

*Recovery phase:* signs of reinnervation (muscle contraction, increased sensitivity)

- *Motor retraining:* muscle "hold" in the shortened position
- *Desensitization:* multiple textures for sensory stimulation; vibration
- *Discriminative sensory reeducation:* identification of objects with, then without, visual cues

*Chronic phase:* reinnervation potential peaked with minimal or no signs of neurological recovery

- *Compensatory function:* compensatory function is minimized during the recovery phase but is emphasized when full neurological recovery does not occur
- *Preventive care:* emphasis on lifelong care to involved region (see Box 13.5)

◎ *Patient education.* The patient must learn to protect the extremity to avoid injury due to loss of sensation.

## Recovery Phase

The recovery phase begins with signs of reinnervation (volutional muscle contraction and hypersensitivity). With nerve regeneration and recovery, begin:

◎ *Motor retraining.* When signs of volutional muscle contraction occur, the muscle is positioned in its shortened position; the patient is asked to hold. Electrical stimulation may be used to reinforce this active effort. When the muscles demonstrate control of some range, begin gravity-eliminated, active-assistive ROM. Continue to protect the weak muscles with a splint or brace.

◎ *Desensitization.* As nerves regenerate, the person experiences increased sensitivity (hypersensitivity) in the area that had previously been without sensation. Use a graded series of modalities and procedures to decrease the irritability and increase awareness.[54]

- Use multiple types of textures or contact for sensory stimulation (cotton, rough material, sandpaper of various grades, Velcro). The textures can be wrapped around dowel rods for finger manipulation or stroking along skin. Contact particles such as cotton balls, beans, macaroni, sand, or other material with various degrees of roughness can be placed in tubs or cans where the patient can run the hand or foot through the material. Have the patient begin manipulating or placing the extremity in the least irritating texture for 10 minutes. As tolerance improves, progress to the next texture of slightly more irritating but tolerable stimulus. Maximum progress occurs when the most irritating texture is tolerated.
- Vibration can also be used. Pattern of recovery after nerve injury is pain (hypersensitivity), perception of slow vibration (30 cps), moving touch, constant touch, rapid vibration (256 cps), and awareness from proximal to distal.[55]

◎ *Discriminative sensory re-education.* This is the process of retraining the brain to recognize a stimulus once the hypersensitivity diminishes. Begin by using a moving touch stimulus, such as the eraser end of a pencil, and stroke over the area. The patient first watches, then closes his or her eyes and tries to identify where touch occurred. Progress from stroking to using constant touch. When the patient is able to localize constant touch, progress to identification of familiar objects of various sizes, shapes, and textures. For the hand, use familiar household and personal care objects, such as keys, eating utensils, blocks, toothbrush, and safety pins. For the feet, have the patient walk on various surfaces, such as grass, sand, wood, pebbles, and uneven surfaces.

◎ *Patient education.* Instruct the patient to resume use of the extremity gradually while monitoring pain, swelling, or any discoloration; if necessary, modify

---

> | **BOX 13.5** | **Patient Instructions for Preventive Care After Nerve Injury** |
>
> *While the nerve is regenerating, or if nerve recovery is incomplete*
>
> - Inspect skin regularly; provide prompt treatment of wounds or blisters
> - Compensate for dryness with massage creams or oils
>
> *In the upper extremity*
>
> - Avoid handling hot, cold, sharp, or abrasive objects
> - Avoid sustained grasps; change use of tools frequently
> - Redistribute hand pressure by building up the size of the handles
> - Wear protective gloves
>
> *In the lower extremity*
>
> - Wear protective shoes that fit properly
> - Inspect feet regularly for pressure points (reddened area) and modify shoes or provide protection if they occur
> - Do not walk barefoot, especially in the dark or on rough surfaces
> - Shift weight frequently when standing for long periods

or temporarily avoid any aggravating activities. While the nerve is recovering or if nerve recovery is incomplete, teach the patient preventive care to avoid injury (see Box 13.5).

## Chronic Phase

When the potential for reinnervation has peaked and there are minimal or no signs of reinnervation, emphasize training for compensatory function. The person will probably have to continue to wear the supportive splint or brace, and preventive care must continue indefinitely.

## ◉ NEURAL TENSION DISORDERS

Normally, the nervous system has considerable mobility to adapt to the wide range of movements imposed on it by daily activities. Still, there are sites where nerves are vulnerable to increased pressure or tension, especially when excessive or repetitive stresses or strains are imposed on the tissues surrounding the nerves or on the nerves themselves. If a nerve is compressed as it passes near a bony structure or through a confined space, undue tension may be placed on it as movement occurs proximal or distal to that site. This may be magnified if there is adhesive scar tissue or swelling that restricts mobility. When examining a patient, the therapist needs to be alert to symptoms described by the patient and be able to understand and interpret positive signs that are detected with testing maneuvers. This section summarizes the tests of provocation and describes the techniques that have been reported to mobilize components of the nervous system in order to improve the patient's outcome.[7]

## Symptoms and Signs of Nerve Mobility Impairment

### History

Vascular and mechanical factors can lead to nerve pathology. Pain is the most common symptom. Sensory responses, reported as stretch pain or paresthesia, occur when tissues are in the neural stretch position.[11] Clinical reasoning is used to understand the possible mechanism of injury, such as pathological insult to the nervous tissue or surrounding tissues or symptoms from movement patterns that place tension on the neural tissues and reproduce symptoms.

### Tests of Provocation

Neurodynamic test maneuvers are performed to detect tension signs in the neural tissue. The upper limb tension test (ULTT), upper limb neurodynamic test (ULNT), straight leg raise (SLR), and slump test are familiar terms that describe various tests and procedures. The reader is referred to textbooks by Butler for greater details and variations of these tests.[7,8] Points regarding the tests:

- Because the test positions place stress across multiple joints, every joint in the chain must be tested separately for range, mobility, and symptom provocation prior to nerve tension testing so any restriction that occurs during the test is not the result of joint or periarticular tissue limitations. Coppieters et al.[11] demonstrated that the stretch position altered the available ROM and sensory responses in 35 normal male subjects during neurodynamic testing and reiterated the importance of looking at other influences prior to neural-tension testing.
- Additional tests include nerve palpation, sensation testing, reflex testing, and muscle testing.[39]
- The test positions and maneuvers used to detect nerve tension and mobility are the same as the treatment positions and maneuvers.
- Tension signs are stretch pain or paresthesias that occur when the neurological system is stretched across multiple joints and is relieved when one of the joints in the chain is moved out of the stretch position. Therefore, the examiner carefully elongates the nerve across each joint in succession until there is symptom provocation (this is described in detail in the techniques section). When symptoms occur, the final position is noted. It is important to recognize that in highly irritable or restrictive conditions full range is not possible. Once symptoms are provoked, the examiner moves one of the joints in the chain out of the stretch position to see if the symptoms are relieved. This may then be repeated with each of the joints in the chain until the examiner understands the mobility pattern of the nerve.

## Causes of Symptoms

Butler[7] proposed that symptoms are the result of tension being placed on some component of the nervous system. If compression is preventing normal mobility, tension signs occur when the nerve is stressed either proximal or distal to the site of compression. Restriction of movement can be from inflammation and scarring between the nerve and the tissue through which it runs or from actual changes in the nerve itself.[7]

NOTE: Cadavaric and in vivo ultrasound imaging studies[17,24,27] have demonstrated that movement and tension placed on nerve tissue occurs with various neck, shoulder girdle, and upper extremity postures and movements. However DiFabio[16] cautioned that there is lack of evidence that neural tension tests are "sensitive and specific indicators of impairments caused by abnormal neural mobility" or that neural tissue can be mobilized independently of other structures. As with many manual testing techniques, the sensitivity and validity of the tests have yet to be determined. The efficacy of interventions based on these maneuvers has been presented in the literature,[26] although evidence is lacking to support or refute this approach to intervention with patients who demonstrate positive signs.

## Principles of Management

The principles of treatment are similar to those of any mobilization technique.[7]

- The intensity of the maneuver should be related to irritability of the tissue, patient response, and change in symptoms. The greater the irritability, the more gentle the technique.
- If the restriction is primarily tension, the stretch force is applied into the tissue resistance, held for 15 to 20 seconds, released, and then repeated several times.
- Neurological symptoms of tingling or increased numbness should not last when the stretch is released.
- Application of the techniques requires positioning the individual at the point of tension (symptoms just begin), then either passively or having the patient actively move one joint in the pattern in such a way as to stretch and then release the tension. Moving different joints in the pattern while maintaining the elongated position on the other joints changes the forces on the nerves.
- After several treatments and the tissue response is known, the patient is taught self-stretching.

## Neural Testing and Mobilization Techniques for the Upper Quadrant

### Median Nerve (Fig. 13.13)

*Patient position and procedure:* Begin with the patient supine; sequentially apply shoulder girdle depression, then slightly abduct the shoulder, extend the elbow, laterally rotate the arm, and supinate the forearm. Wrist, finger, and

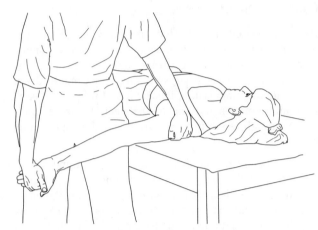

FIGURE 13.13 Position of maximum stretch on the median nerve includes shoulder girdle depression; shoulder abduction; elbow extension; shoulder external rotation and supination of the forearm; wrist, finger, and thumb extension; and finally contralateral cervical side flexion.

thumb extensions are then added; finally, the shoulder is taken into greater abduction. The full stretch position includes contralateral cervical side flexion. While maintaining the stretch position, move one joint at a time a few degrees in and out of the stretch position, such as wrist extension and flexion or elbow flexion and extension.

This maneuver is beneficial when examining and treating symptoms related to median nerve distribution, problems with shoulder girdle depression (e.g., thoracic outlet syndrome), and carpal tunnel syndrome.[7]

### Radial Nerve (Fig. 13.14)

*Patient position and procedure:* Begin with the patient supine; sequentially apply shoulder girdle depression, then slightly abduct the shoulder, extend the elbow, then medially rotate the arm and pronate the forearm. Keep the elbow

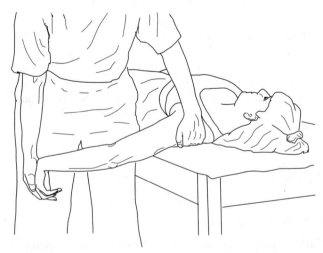

FIGURE 13.14 Position of maximum stretch on the radial nerve includes shoulder girdle depression; shoulder abduction; elbow extension; shoulder medial rotation and forearm pronation; wrist, finger, and thumb flexion; wrist ulnar deviation; and finally contralateral cervical side flexion.

in extension and add wrist, finger, and thumb flexion, and finally ulnar deviation of the wrist. The full stretch position includes contralateral side flexion of the cervical spine. While maintaining the stretch position, move one joint at a time a few degrees in and out of the stretch position, such as wrist extension and flexion.

This maneuver is important when examining and treating symptoms that are related to shoulder girdle depression, radial nerve distribution, and disorders such as tennis elbow and deQuervain's syndrome.[7]

### Ulnar Nerve (Fig. 13.15)

*Patient position and procedure:* Begin with the patient supine. Sequentially apply wrist extension and forearm supination followed by elbow flexion (full range); then add shoulder girdle depression. Maintain this position and add shoulder lateral rotation and abduction. In the final position the patient's hand is near his or her ear with fingers pointing posteriorly. In the full stretch position, contralateral side flexion of the cervical spine is added. While maintaining the overall stretch position, move one joint at a time a few degrees in and out of the stretch position, such as elbow extension and flexion.

This maneuver is important when symptoms are related to the C-8 and T-1 nerve roots, lower brachial plexus, ulnar nerve, and disorders such as medial epicondylitis.[7]

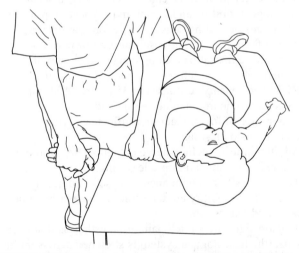

FIGURE 13.15 Position of maximum stretch on the ulnar nerve includes shoulder girdle depression; shoulder external rotation and abduction; elbow flexion; forearm supination and wrist extension; and finally contralateral cervical side flexion.

## Neural Testing and Mobilization Techniques for the Lower Quadrant

### Sciatic Nerve: Straight-Leg Raising with Ankle Dorsiflexion (Fig. 13.16)

*Patient position and procedure:* The patient is supine. Lift the lower extremity in the straight-leg raise (SLR) position and add ankle dorsiflexion. Several variations may be

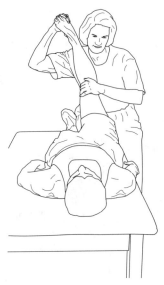

FIGURE 13.16 Position of stretch on the sciatic nerve includes straight-leg raising with adduction and internal rotation of the hip and dorsiflexion of the ankle.

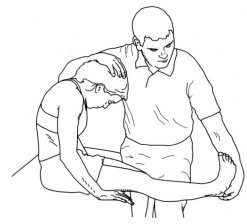

FIGURE 13.17 Slump-sitting with neck, thorax, and low back flexed, knee extended, and ankle dorsiflexed just to the point of tissue resistance and symptom reproduction.

done; ankle dorsiflexion, ankle plantar flexion with inversion, hip adduction, hip medial rotation, and passive neck flexion.[7] The maneuver may also be performed long-sitting (slump-sitting position—see below) and side-lying. These various positions of the lower extremity and neck are used to differentiate tight or strained hamstrings from possible sites of restriction or nerve mobility in the lumbosacral plexus and sciatic nerve.[21,63]

Once the position that places tension on the involved neurological tissue is found, maintain the stretch position and then move one of the joints a few degrees in and out of the stretch position, such as ankle plantarflexion and dorsiflexion or knee flexion and extension.

● Ankle dorsiflexion with eversion places more tension on the tibial tract.
● Ankle dorsiflexion with inversion places tension on the sural nerve.
● Ankle plantarflexion with inversion places tension on the common peroneal tract.
● Adduction of the hip while doing SLR places further tension on the nervous system because the sciatic nerve is lateral to the ischial tuberosity; medial rotation of the hip while doing SLR also increases tension on the sciatic nerve (see Fig. 13.16).
● Passive neck flexion while doing SLR pulls the spinal cord cranially and places the entire nervous system on a stretch.

### Slump-Sitting (Fig. 13.17)

*Patient position and procedur:* Begin with the patient sitting upright. Have the patient slump by flexing the neck, thorax, and low back. Apply overpressure to cervical spine. Dorsiflex the ankle and then extend the knee as much as possible to the point of tissue resistance and symptom reproduction. Release the overpressure on the spine and

have the patient actively extend the neck to see if symptoms decrease. Increase and release the stretch force by moving one joint in the chain a few degrees, such as knee flexion and extension or ankle dorsiflexion and plantar flexion.

### Femoral Nerve: Prone Knee Bend (Fig. 13.18)

*Patient position and procedure:* Prone with the spine neutral (not extended) and the hips extended to 0°. Flex the knee to the point of resistance and symptom reproduction. Pain in the low back or neurological signs (change in sensation in the anterior thigh) are considered positive for upper lumbar nerve roots and femoral nerve tension. Thigh pain could be rectus femoris tightness. It is important not to hyperextend the spine to avoid confusion with nerve root pressure from decreased foraminal space or facet pain from spinal movement. Flex and extend the knee a few degrees to apply and release tension.

Alternate position and procedure: Side-lying with the involved leg uppermost. Stabilize the pelvis and extend the hip with the knee flexed until symptoms are reproduced. Maintain knee flexion, release, and apply tension across the hip by moving it a few degrees at a time.

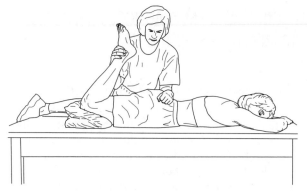

FIGURE 13.18 Position of stretch on the femoral nerve; prone lying with the spine neutral, hip extended to zero degrees, and knee flexed. It is important to maintain the spine in neutral and not allow it to extend.

## Prevention

These maneuvers may be used to prevent restrictive adhesions from developing if done early during treatment after an acute injury or surgery.

### Precautions and Contraindications to Neural Tension Testing and Treatment

There is incomplete scientific understanding of the pathology and mechanisms occurring when mobilizing the nervous system.[7] Use caution with the stretch force; neurological symptoms of tingling or increased numbness should not last when the stretch is released. The clinician should always use caution and perform a thorough systems review and screening examination to rule out "red flag" conditions prior to neural tension testing and treatment.[8]

### PRECAUTIONS

- Know what other tissues are affected by the positions and maneuvers.
- Recognize the irritability of the tissues involved and do not aggravate the symptoms with excessive stress or repeated movements.
- Identify whether the condition is worsening and the rate of worsening. A rapidly worsening condition requires greater care than a slowly progressing condition.
- Use care if there is an active disease or pathology affecting the nervous system.
- Watch for signs of vascular compromise. The vascular system is in close proximity to the nervous system and at no time should show signs of compromise when mobilizing the nervous system.

### CONTRAINDICATIONS

- Acute or unstable neurological signs
- Cauda equina symptoms related to the spine including changes in bowel or bladder control and perineal sensation
  - Spinal cord injury or symptoms
  - Neoplasm and infection

## MUSCULOSKELETAL DIAGNOSES INVOLVING IMPAIRED NERVE FUNCTION

##  THORACIC OUTLET SYNDROME

The thoracic outlet is the region along the pathway of the brachial plexus from just distal to the nerve roots exiting the intervertebral foramen to the lower border of the axilla (Fig. 13.19). The outlet is bordered medially by the scalenus anterior, medius, and posterior and the first rib; posteriorly by the upper trapezius and scapula; anteriorly by the clavicle, coracoid, pectoralis minor, and deltopectoral fascia; and laterally by the axilla. The plexus enters

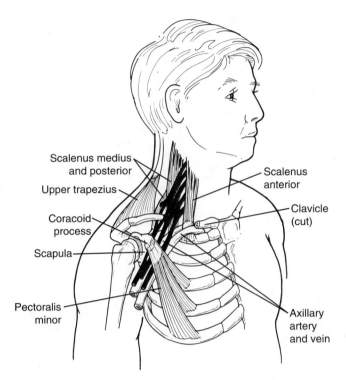

**FIGURE 13.19** Region of the thoracic outlet bordered medially by the scalene muscle and first rib; posteriorly by the upper trapezius and scapula; anteriorly by the clavicle, coracoid, pectoralis minor, and deltopectoral fascia; and laterally by the axilla.

the outlet between the scalenus anterior and medius; the subclavian artery runs posterior to the scalenus anterior; and the subclavian vein runs anterior to the scalenus anterior. The blood vessels join the brachial plexus and course together under the clavicle, over the first rib, and under the coracoid process posterior to the pectoralis minor. Vascular and/or upper extremity neurological symptoms that are not consistent with nerve root or peripheral nerve dermatome and myotome patterns should lead the therapist to suspect thoracic outlet problems.[34]

## Related Diagnoses

Thoracic outlet syndrome (TOS) encompasses a variety of clinical problems in the shoulder girdle region. The diagnosis itself is controversial because of the clinical complexity and variability in presentation that involve upper extremity neurological and vascular symptoms, including pain, paresthesia, numbness, weakness, discoloration, swelling, loss of pulse, ulceration, gangrene, and in some cases Raynaud's phenomenon. Patients also complain of headaches, which may be related to posture, tension, or vascular compromise. Diagnoses that have been used to describe TOS include cervical rib, scalenus anticus syndrome, costoclavicular syndrome, subcoracoid-pectoralis minor syndrome, droopy shoulder syndrome, and hyperabduction syndrome.[14,19,46,56,59,60,67] Commonly accepted medical diagnoses include:

- Neurogenic TOS—true TOS. This condition is rare. The patient presents with some anatomical abnormality such as cervical rib or elongated C7 transverse process. The patient describes paresthesias and pain along the medial border of the arm and experiences muscle weakness; there is atrophy in the intrinsic muscles of the hand. There are also positive electromyographic (EMG) findings. The condition is often misdiagnosed as carpal tunnel syndrome.
- Nonspecific "symptomatic" neurogenic TOS. This condition is similar to true TOS, but there are no anatomical abnormalities detected by radiography, no muscle atrophy, and no EMG findings. Often there is a postural component. Most TOS complaints fall into this category.
- Vascular syndromes—arterial. In some cases there is a small incidence of arterial compression. This condition is rare and is usually the result of structural abnormalities such as cervical rib. There is compression of the artery with arm motion, especially overhead usage. If the arm fatigues with overhead usage, the person may have to adapt work habits that avoid risk from repetitive trauma to the artery.
- Vascular syndromes—venous. Compression of the subclavian vein does not typically occur in TOS; venous symptoms would be from some other cause, such as thrombosis. Acute thrombosis (sudden, painful swelling with bluish discoloration of the arm) is usually dealt with medically, but the therapist should always be suspicious of unexplained swelling of the arm. Effort thrombosis could occur from sudden maximal arm use, or there could be insidious onset of swelling with prolonged use. If these occur, the patient's physician should be contacted.

## Etiology of Symptoms

Walsh[67] has identified three causative factors for TOS that could be interrelated or exist separately: compressive neuropathy, faulty posture, and entrapment.

- ***Compressive neuropathy.*** Compression of the neurovascular structures can occur if there is a decrease in the size of the area through which the brachial plexus and subclavian vessels pass. Compression can result from muscle hypertrophy in the scalenes or pectoralis minor, anatomical anomalies such as cervical rib or fractured clavicle, adaptive shortening of fascia, or a space-occupying lesion.
- ***Faulty posture.*** Changes in posture, particularly forward head with increased thoracic kyphosis, protracted scapulae, and forward shoulders narrow the spaces through which the neurovascular structures pass. Specifically, adaptive shortening of the scaleni and pectoralis minor muscles can potentially compress the neurovascular tissues or can cause repetitive trauma and adhesions with overuse.[42] If the angle of the clavicle falls below the level of the sternoclavicular joint, the shoulder girdle causes traction on the plexus.[59] In addition, the clavicle

can compress the neurovascular structures against the first rib.

Other contributing factors to postural stresses include hypertrophy of breast tissue leading to postural fatigue or pressure from undergarment support straps, and carrying a heavy briefcase, suitcase, or shoulder purse that causes pressure across the shoulder girdle, fatigue in the scapular stabilizers, or traction across the shoulder girdle tissues.

NOTE: A study reported by Pascarelli and Hsu[47] of 485 patients with work-related upper quarter pain and symptoms indicated that 70% of patients displayed posture-elated neurogentic TOS as a key factor in a series of cascading events, including 78% with protracted shoulders, 71% with forward head posture, 50% with hyperlaxity of fingers and elbows, 20% with sympathetic dysfunction, 64% with cubital tunnel, 60% with medial epicondylitis, 70% with peripheral muscle weakness, and other miscellaneous conditions such as carpal tunnel syndrome. Wood and Biondi[72] pointed out that among 165 patients with TOS 44% also had compression of a nerve distally, most commonly in the carpal tunnel (41 cases).

A surgical study reported findings that pathological adhesions of the brachial plexus to the scalenus muscle led to nerve fiber distraction as the mechanism behind the symptoms and suggested that the restrictive adhesions were directly related to long-standing postural deviations and myofascial pain syndrome.[12]

- ***Entrapment of the neural tissue from scar tissue or pressure.*** Entrapment affects the ability of nerve tissue of the brachial plexus to tolerate tension as it courses through the various tissues in the thoracic outlet. A possible explanation was offered in a review article by Carotti[13] wherein the pain–immobility–fibrosis loop that occurs after trauma (e.g., following an acceleration-extension motor vehicle injury) leads to the development of adhesions, which cause or perpetuate TOS symptoms. The Halstead test[39] and the upper limb tension test for the median nerve[7] (see Fig. 13.14) place the brachial plexus and median nerve on a stretch and with symptoms may indicate restricted nerve gliding. The Halstead test also may obliterate the radial pulse indicating vascular entrapment. Wilson et al.[72] described a cadaver study that demonstrated tension placed on the subclavian artery with either ipsilateral or contralateral side-bending of the cervical spine during the TOS testing maneuvers. They suggested that this could be the source of pain or tension symptoms even prior to signs of vascular pathology (decreased pulse, pallor, skin temperature).[72]

Contributing factors in the development of TOS are summarized in Box 13.6.

## Location of Compression or Entrapment and Tests of Provocation

There are three primary sites for compression or entrapment of the neurovascular structures that lead to tension or compression signs.[67]

**BOX 13.6    Summary of Contributing Factors to Thoracic Outlet Syndrome**

There is wide latitude of motion in the various joints of the shoulder complex that may result in compression or impingement of the nerves or vessels in TOS.

- *Postural variations*, such as a forward head or round shoulders, lead to associated muscle shortening in the scalene, levator, subscapularis, and pectoralis minor muscles and a depressed clavicle.
- *Postural stress*, such as carrying a heavy suitcase, brief case, or purse can place stress across the shoulder girdle, creating pressure in the thoracic outlet or traction on the brachial plexus.
- *Respiratory patterns* that continually use the action of the scalene muscles to elevate the upper ribs lead to hypertrophy of these muscles. Also, the elevated upper ribs decrease the space under the clavicle.
- *Congenital factors* such as an accessory rib, a long transverse process of the C-7 vertebra, or other anomalies in the region can reduce the space for the vessels. A traumatic or arteriosclerotic insult can also lead to TOS symptoms.
- *Traumatic injuries*, such as clavicular fracture or subacromial dislocations of the humeral head, can injure the plexus and vessels, leading to TOS symptoms.
- *Hypertrophy or scarring* in the pectoralis minor muscles can lead to TOS symptoms.
- *Injuries* that result in inflammation, scar tissue formation, and adhesions can restrict nerve tissue mobility when tension is placed on the nerve. This may occur anywhere from the intervertebral foramina at the spine to the distal-most portion of the peripheral nerve. There are nerve tension signs from restricted mobility.

- **Interscalene triangle:** bordered by the scalenus anterior and medius muscles and the first rib. If these muscles are hypertrophied, tight, or have anatomical variations, they may compress the proximal portion of the brachial plexus normal mobility of the neural tissues with head and arm movements.

  Symptoms from dysfunction in this area are reproduced with Adson's maneuver, which stretches the scalene muscles and places tension on the nerves. If the artery is compressed, there is also a decreased pulse.[38] Palpation of the scalene muscles may also provoke symptoms.
- **Costoclavicular space:** between the clavicle superiorly and the first rib inferiorly. Compression of the neurovascular bundle can occur between the clavicle and first rib, especially if the clavicle is depressed for periods of time, as occurs when carrying a heavy suitcase or shoulder bag or with a faulty, slouched posture. A fractured clavicle or anomalies in the region can also lead to symp-

toms. An elevated first rib, which can occur with first rib subluxation or upper thoracic breathing (as with asthma or chronic emphysema), also narrows the costoclavicular space.

Symptoms caused by a depressed clavicle are reproduced when the shoulders are retracted and depressed as with the Military Brace Test.[38] If, when in this posture, a patient is asked to take in a breath and symptoms are reproduced, the rib elevation is causing the symptoms. The mobility of the clavicle and first rib should also be tested.
- **Axillary interval:** between the anterior deltopectoral fascia, the pectoralis minor, and the coracoid process. Compression or restricted movement of the neurovascular structures may occur in this region if the pectoralis minor is tight owing to faulty posture with the scapula tipped forward or to repetitive overuse.

Holding the arms in an elevated position places a stretch on the lower branches of the brachial plexus and blood vessels. If there is poor neurovascular mobility and tension is placed on the brachial plexus, a patient experiences reproduction of symptoms when the arm is abducted. In addition, if the person does repetitive opening and closing of the hand and there is increased ischemic pain (Roos test),[38] there is vascular compromise. Palpation pressure against the pectoralis minor reproduces the neurological symptoms if the muscle is tight.

## Common Impairments in TOS

- Intermittent brachial plexus and vascular symptoms of pain, paresthesia, numbness, weakness, discoloration, and swelling
- Muscle length–strength imbalance in the shoulder girdle with tightness in anterior and medial structures and weakness in posterior and lateral structures
- Faulty postural awareness in the upper quarter
- Poor endurance in the postural muscles
- Shallow respiratory pattern characterized by upper thoracic breathing
- Poor clavicular and anterior rib mobility
- Nerve tension symptoms when the brachial plexus is placed on a stretch

## Common Functional Limitations/Disabilities

- Sleep disturbances that could be from excessive pillow thickness or arm posture
- Inability to carry briefcase, suitcase, purse with shoulder strap, or other weighted objects on the involved side
- Inability to maintain prolonged overhead reaching position
- Inability to do sustained computer or desk work, cradling a telephone receiver between head and involved shoulder, or prolonged periods driving a car

## Nonoperative Management of TOS

If the symptoms demonstrate that there is inflammation, treatment is first directed at eliminating the provoking mechanism and controlling the inflammation. Conservative interventions usually precede surgery. The primary emphasis of management is to decrease the mechanical pressure by increasing the mobility of tissues in the thoracic outlet region, preventing recurrence of the compression loads by correcting the postural alignment, and developing endurance to maintain correct posture.[2,33,67]

A program with interventions that specifically address the presenting impairments should be developed by the clinician (Box 13.7). Secondary or associated complaints such as myofascial trigger points, glenohumeral joint pathology, cervical pathology, or distal peripheral neuropathies should be identified and appropriate interventions incorporated into the program.[67] The following should be considered.

- *Patient education.* Teach the patient how to modify or eliminate provoking postures and activities and provide a home exercise program that includes flexibility, muscle performance, and postural exercises (see Chapter 14). Emphasize the importance of compliance to reduce the stresses on the nerve and vascular structures.
- *Nerve tissue mobility.* Use nerve mobilization maneuvers if nerve tension tests are positive.[71] These are described earlier in this chapter.
- *Joint, muscle, and connective tissue mobility.* Use manual and self-stretching techniques to address any mobility impairments. Restricted joint mobility might be present in the glenohumeral, sternoclavicular, or first costotransverse articulations. Common muscle restrictions with an impaired postural component include but are not limited to the scalene, levator scapulae, pectoralis minor, pectoralis major, anterior portion of the intercostals, and short suboccipital muscles. Identification of exercises to increase mobility are listed in Chapter 14 (section on posture exercises).
- *Muscle performance.* Develop a program to improve control and endurance in the postural muscles. Common weaknesses include but are not limited to scapular adductors and upward rotators, shoulder lateral rotators, deep anterior throat cervical flexor muscles, and thoracic extensors. Identification of postural exercises to improve muscle performance are listed in Chapter 14 (section on posture exercises).
- *Respiratory patterns and elevated upper ribs.* Teach abdominodiaphragmatic or bi-basilar breathing patterns and relaxation of the upper thorax (see Chapter 25) if the patient tends to use apical breathing patterns and has increased tension in the scalene muscles.
- *Functional independence.* Increase patient awareness and ability to manage symptoms through education. Have patients actively involved in all aspects of their program and interventions.

---

**BOX 13.7  Summary of Guidelines for Management of Thoracic Outlet Syndrome**

*Educate the patient*

- Teach posture correction
- Teach how to modify provoking stresses
- Teach safe exercises for home exercise program

*Correct impaired posture*

- See Chapter 14

*Mobilize restricted neurological tissue*

- Nerve mobilization techniques if testing is positive for restricted mobility

*Mobilize restricted joints, connective tissue, and muscle*

- Tissue-specific manual techniques to restricted structures if testing is positive for restricted mobility
- Self-stretching exercises for restricted muscle flexibility

*Improve muscle performance*

- Develop control and endurance in postural muscles
- Progress strengthening exercises

*Correct faulty breathing patterns*

- Relax upper thorax
- Teach abdominodiaphragmatic or bi-basilar breathing patterns

*Progress functional independence*

- Involve patient in all aspects of program

---

PRECAUTIONS: Shoulder girdle exercises cause worsening of symptoms in some patients; or they may be progressing favorably, then symptoms worsen. Worsening of neurological or vascular symptoms may indicate axonal disruption or vascular compromise. Refer the patient to his or her physician; surgical decompression may be indicated.

##  CARPAL TUNNEL SYNDROME

The carpal tunnel is a confined space between the carpal bones dorsally and the transverse carpal ligament (flexor retinaculum) volarly (Fig. 13.20). In this region the median nerve is susceptible to pressure as it courses through the tunnel with the extrinsic finger flexor tendons on their way into the hand. Carpal tunnel syndrome (CTS) is characterized by the sensory loss and motor weakness that occur when the median nerve is compromised in the carpal tunnel. Anything that decreases the space in the carpal tunnel or causes the contents of the tunnel to enlarge could compress or restrict the mobility of the median nerve, causing a compression or traction injury and neurological symptoms distal to the wrist.[23,40]

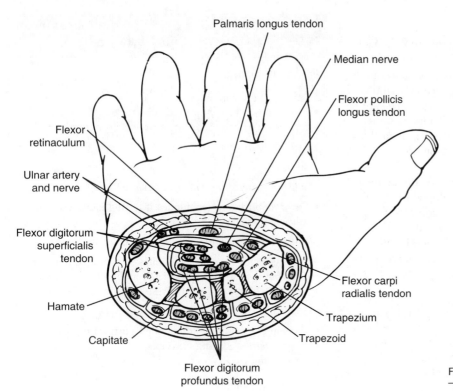

**FIGURE 13.20** Boundaries of the carpal tunnel.

## Etiology of Symptoms

Etiologic factors include synovial thickness and scarring in the tendon sheaths (tendinosis) or irritation, inflammation, and swelling (tendinitis) as a result of repetitive or sustained wrist flexion, extension, or gripping activities or sustained pressure. Because of this CTS is frequently classified as a cumulative trauma or overuse syndrome. Swelling of the wrist joint due to trauma to the carpals (e.g., a fall or blow to the wrist), a fracture of the carpals, pregnancy (hormonal changes and water retention), rheumatoid arthritis, or osteoarthritis could decrease the carpal tunnel space. Awkward wrist postures (flexion or extension), compressive forces from sustained equipment usage, and vibration against the carpal tunnel could also lead to median nerve compression and trauma.[4]

## Tests of Provocation

In a recent review on the sensitivity and specificity of the various tests used when screening for CTS, MacDermid and Doherty,[36] summarized the key signs and symptoms that increase the probability of diagnosing CTS.

*History.* Sensory changes in the median nerve distribution of the hand (excluding the palm, which is innervated by the palmar cutaneous branch of the median nerve arising proximal to the carpal tunnel); nocturnal numbness and pain relieved by flicking the wrists.

*Observation and provocation tests.* Thenar atrophy and/or weakness, positive Phalen's test (sustained wrist flexion), loss of two-point discrimination, and positive Tinel's sign (tapping the median nerve).[38]

Because there can be other causes of median nerve symptoms, such as tension, compression, or restricted mobility of the nerve roots in the cervical intervertebral foramen, of the brachial plexus in the thoracic outlet, or of the median nerve as it courses through tissues in the forearm region (pronator syndrome and anterior interosseous nerve syndrome),[32] each of these sites must be examined to rule them out or determine if any is the cause of the median nerve symptoms[24,32] (see Fig. 13.5).

With nerve irritability it is possible to develop what is known as a double crush injury[7,35,37,42] so the nerve develops symptoms at other areas along its course as well as at the primary site. Wood and Biondi[73] reported that 41 of 165 patients with TOS also had carpal tunnel syndrome, which they attributed to the lessened ability of the nerves to withstand distal compression when irritated proximally. In contrast, Seror[52,53] reported a lack of evidence supporting a relationship between unambiguous CTS in true neurogenic TOS (< 1/100), although disputed neurogenic TOS was frequently found (mild to moderate clinical symptoms and signs) even when there was no significant findings on electrodiagnostic tests.[52]

## Common Impairments

- Increasing pain in the hand with repetitive use
- Progressive weakness or atrophy in the thenar muscles and first two lumbricales (ape hand deformity)
- Tightness in the adductor pollicis and extrinsic extensors of the thumb and digits 2 and 3
- Irritability or sensory loss in the median nerve distribution (see Fig. 13.5)

● Possible decreased joint mobility in the wrist and meta-carpophalangeal joints of the thumb and digits 2 and 3
● May develop sympathetic changes

## Common Functional Limitations/Disabilities

● Decreased prehension in tip-to-tip, tip-to-pad, and pad-to-pad activities requiring fine neuromuscular control of thumb opposition
● May not use the area of the hand where there is decreased sensation
● Inability to perform provoking sustained or repetitive wrist motion, such as cashier checkout scanning, assembly line work, fine tool manipulation, typing, or manipulation of a computer mouse

## Nonoperative Management of CTS

In patients with mild to moderate symptoms, conservative intervention is directed toward minimizing or eliminating the causative factor[36,44] (Box 13.8). Considerations include:

● *Nerve protection.* Initially, the wrist may have to be splinted to provide rest from the provoking activity. Splint the wrist in the neutral position so there is minimal pressure in the tunnel.[40]
● *Activity modification and patient education.* Identify faulty wrist or upper extremity postures and activities. Modify activities to keep the wrist in neutral and to reduce forceful prehension. Teach the patient about the mechanisms of compression and their effect on the circulation and nerve pressure as well as how to modify or eliminate provoking postures and activities. Teach the patient safe exercises for a home exercise program. Emphasize the importance of compliance to reduce stresses on the nerve and tendinous structures. Also, instruct the patient to observe areas with decreased sensitivity to avoid tissue injury (see Box 13.5)
● *Mobility*
  • *Joint mobilization.* If there is restricted joint mobility, mobilize the carpals for increased carpal tunnel space. See Figure 5.39 and its description in Chapter 5.
  • *Tendon-gliding exercises.* Teach the patient tendon-gliding exercises for mobility in the extrinsic tendons; they should be performed gently to prevent increased swelling. See Figure 19.17 and the description in the exercise section of Chapter 19.
  • *Median nerve mobilization.*[7,51] The six positions for median nerve mobilization in the wrist and hand are illustrated in Figure 13.21. Begin with position A and progress to each succeeding position until the median nerve symptoms just begin to be provoked (tingling). That is the maximum position to use. Sustain that position for 5 to 30 seconds without making the symptoms worse. Then alternate between that position and the preceding position. When the patient can be moved into that position without symptoms, progress to the next stretch position and repeat the mobilizing routine. The mobilization exercise should be done three or four times per day so long as symptoms are not exacerbated.

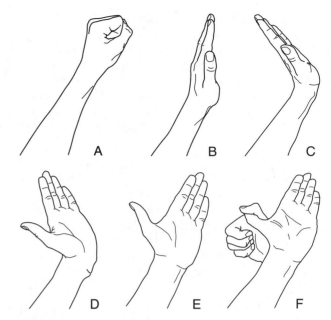

**FIGURE 13.21** Positions for median nerve glides and mobilization in the hand: (*A*) wrist neutral with fingers and thumb flexed; (*B*) wrist neutral with fingers and thumb extended; (*C*) wrist and fingers extended, thumb neutral; (*D*) wrist, fingers, and thumb extended; (*E*) wrist, fingers, and thumb extended and forearm supinated; (*F*) wrist, fingers, and thumb extended, forearm supinated, and thumb stretched into extension.

Additional median nerve mobilization techniques, including the entire upper extremity and neck, can be added if symptoms warrant (See Figure 13.14 and the description of principles earlier in this chapter under upper limb tension.)

 **Focus on Evidence** _____

A recent study documented a significant improvement in symptoms in patients treated conservatively with tendon-gliding and median nerve-gliding exercises. Only 43% of patients in the experimental group who performed the nerve mobilization exercises underwent subsequent surgical release of the carpal tunnel compared to 71% in the control group.[51]

● *Muscle performance*
  • *Gentle multiple-angle muscle-setting exercises.* Initially, gentle muscle-setting exercises are the only resistance exercises done. It is important that they do not provoke symptoms.
  • *Strengthening and endurance exercises.* Add dynamic strengthening and endurance exercises when symptoms are not increased with isometric exercises and there is full tendon- and nerve-gliding without symptoms or edema. Utilize exercises that prepare the patient for a return to functional activities.
  • *Speed, coordination, endurance, and fine finger dexterity.* Emphasize these activities when the symptoms are no longer provoked. Utilize activities that develop tip-to-tip and tip-to-pad prehension in order to improve use

of the thenar muscles as well as areas of the skin that may have decreased sensation.

 *Functional independence.* Teach the patient how to monitor his or her hand for recurrence of symptoms and the provoking factors and how to modify activities to decrease nerve injury. Usually, sustained wrist flexion, ulnar deviation, and repetitive wrist flexion and extension combined with gripping and pinching are the most aggravating motions.

### ◉ Focus on Evidence

In a Cochrane review of 21 trials involving 884 people, a hand brace significantly alleviated symptoms of CTS after 4 weeks; and in one trial involving 21 people, symptoms were significantly diminished after 3 weeks with carpal bone mobilization (compared to no intervention). Other evidence supported the use of oral steroids, ultrasound, and yoga.[44]

## Surgical Intervention and Postoperative Management

If conservative measures do not relieve the nerve symptoms or the neurological symptoms are severe (persistent, numbness, weakness, pain, decreased functional use of the hand),[36] surgical decompression involving transaction of the transverse carpal ligament is performed to increase the volume of the carpal tunnel and relieve the compressive forces on the median nerve. Also, any scar tissue is excised. Surgery may be an open carpal tunnel release or endoscopically assisted carpal tunnel release.[40] Therapy may be initiated after surgery if there are restrictions or muscle weakness. Use exercise and mobilization techniques that deal with the impairments and functional loss.

Pain in the thenar and hypothenar eminences may result from the release and flattening of the palmar arch (pillar pain). Immediately after surgery there is loss of the wrist pulley in the long finger flexor system due to release of the flexor retinaculum. Therefore, time must be allowed for healing to prevent bowstringing of the flexor tendons at the wrist. The wrist may be immobilized 7 to 10 days postoperatively in slight extension with the fingers free to move.

### ◉ Focus on Evidence

A study by Cook et al.[10] looked at the value of splinting the wrist after surgery versus initiating range of motion (ROM) exercises on the first postoperative day with 50 consecutive patients and concluded that splinting the wrist following open release was detrimental. The primary concern is preventing bowstringing of the extrinsic flexor tendons, and therefore the authors recommended exercising the fingers and wrist separately.[10]

### Maximum Protection Phase

Usually a bulky dressing or splint is used following surgery. When allowed, remove the protective splinting during therapy.

PRECAUTION: Avoid active wrist flexion past neutral as well as active finger flexion with the wrist flexed during the first 10 days after surgery. Use extreme caution for up to 3 weeks postoperatively to prevent bowstringing of the flexor tendons through the flexor retinaculum.

 *Patient education.* Educate the patient on expectations for recovery. The impairments of decreased strength in grip and pinch as well as pillar pain should resolve within 3 to 6 months.[40] This is related to the changed length–tension relationship of the thenar muscles due to cutting the transverse carpal ligament. Neurological symptoms should resolve with time, with light touch returning first.[40]

◉ *Wound management, control of edema and pain.*

◉ *Active tendon-gliding and nerve-gliding exercises.* Tendon-gliding (see Fig. 19.17) and nerve-gliding (see Fig. 13.21) exercises are important to prevent adhesion formation from restricting motion in the carpal tunnel. Include forearm supination and elbow extension as nerve symptoms allow.[4,49]

---

| BOX 13.8 | Summary of Guidelines for Nonoperative Management of Carpal Tunnel Syndrome |
|---|---|

*Protect the nerve*

- Splint wrist in neutral
- Protect areas in decreased sensitivity

*Modify activity and educate the patient*

- Teach patient about provoking activities and how to modify them
- Teach safe exercises for home exercise program
- Teach patient how to protect areas of decreased sensitivity in the hand (see Box 13.5)

*Mobilize restricted joints, connective tissue, and muscle/tendon*

- Mobilize carpals if restricted
- Tendon gliding exercises
- Median nerve mobilization exercises

*Improve muscle performance*

- Gentle multi-angle muscle setting
- Progress to resistance and endurance
- Fine-finger dexterity

*Progress functional independence*

- Involve patient in all aspects of program
- Self monitoring of symptoms

### Exercises

- Active finger and thumb flexion/extension, abduction/adduction, and thumb opposition with the wrist stabilized in moderate wrist extension
- Active wrist extension; this may be combined with passive wrist flexion with the splint removed.
- Active radial and ulnar deviation of the wrist (with the splint removed and the wrist supported in slight extension), pronation and supination of the forearm, and all shoulder and elbow motions.

## Moderate and Minimum Protection Phases

The sutures are usually removed around the 10th to 12th postoperative day, and more active treatment is allowed.[49] The patient should be able to return to full activity by 6 to 12 weeks. Impairments may include residual weakness and sensory deficits, persistent edema, limited motion, hypersensitivity, and pain.

Suggested interventions include:

- **Scar tissue mobilization.** Use soft tissue mobilization to the palmar fascia and scar.
- **Progressive stretching and joint mobilization of restricted tissue.** If restricted, lengthen the abductor pollicis brevis and opponens pollicis. Mobilize restricted tendons or nerve tissue (same techniques as described previously except with a stretch force).
- **Muscle performance.** Begin strengthening exercises 4 weeks after surgery with isometric exercises. Progress to grip and pinch exercises by 6 weeks. Emphasize strength, coordination, and endurance toward functional goals. Wrist and hand exercises are described and illustrated in detail in Chapter 19.
- **Dexterity exercises.** Begin as soon as signs of motor recovery occur. Suggestions include picking up small objects using pad-to-pad, tip-to-tip, and tip-to pad prehension patterns, turning over cards, stacking checkers, writing, and holding the perimeter of a jar lid and having the thumb move around the edge in a circumduction motion.
- **Sensory stimulation and discriminative sensory reeducation.** Desensitization of hypersensitive skin is a priority. As the nerve recovers, help desensitize and reprogram awareness.[54] These techniques were described earlier in the chapter. Educate the patient about the progression of nerve recovery such that an area that had absence of sensation will have increased sensitivity and pain as it recovers. Symptoms usually subside within 1 to 6 months.

### ◉ Focus on Evidence

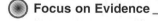

A recent Cochrane database systems review analyzed surgical versus nonsurgical treatment for CTS and, based on the evidence, concluded that surgical treatment relieves symptoms significantly better than splinting, and that the long-term outcomes favored surgical intervention.[65] They did not study patients with mild symptoms.

# COMPRESSION IN TUNNEL OF GUYON

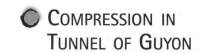

## Etiology of Symptoms

Injury or irritation of the ulnar nerve in the tunnel between the hook of the hamate and pisiform results from sustained pressure, such as prolonged handwriting or leaning forward onto extended wrists while biking; from repetitive use of the gripping action of the fourth and fifth fingers, as with knitting, tying knots, or using pliers and staplers; or from trauma, such as falling on the ulnar border of the wrist.

## Tests of Provocation

There can be other causes of ulnar nerve symptoms, such as tension, compression, or restricted mobility of the nerve roots in the cervical intervertebral foramen, the brachial plexus in the thoracic outlet, or the ulnar nerve as it courses through the bicipital groove; or there could be impingement between the heads of the flexor carpi ulnaris muscle. Therefore, each of these sites must be examined to rule out or determine if any is the cause of the symptoms[42] (see Fig. 13.6). In addition, with nerve irritability it is possible to develop what is known as a double crush injury[7] so the nerve develops symptoms at other areas along its course as well as at the primary site.

**History.** Description of symptoms in the little finger and ulnar side of the ring finger; history of provoking activity.

**Observation and tests.** May have atrophy in the hypothenar eminence and present with partial claw (see Table 13.1); positive Tinel's sign (tapping ulnar nerve) over the tunnel of Guyon.

## Common Impairments

- Pain and paresthesia along the ulnar side of the palm of the hand and digits in the distribution of the ulnar nerve (see Fig. 13.6)
- Progressive weakness or atrophy in the intrinsic muscles innervated by the ulnar nerve
- Restricted mobility in the extrinsic finger flexor and extensor muscles
- Possible restricted mobility of the pisiform

## Common Functional Limitations/Disabilities

- Decreased grip strength
- Unable to use fourth and fifth digits for spherical or cylindrical power grips
- Decreased ability to perform provoking activity

## Nonoperative Management

- Follow the same guidelines as for CTS. Modify the provoking activity, avoid pressure to the base of the palm of the hand, and provide rest with a cock-up splint.
- Ulnar nerve mobilization: Move the wrist into extension and radial deviation, then apply overpressure stretch into extension against the ring and little finger. Include forearm pronation and elbow flexion to move the nerve in a proximal direction. To test and mobilize the entire ulnar nerve, see Figure 13.15.

## Surgical Release and Postoperative Management

After release of the ulnar tunnel, the wrist is immobilized 3 to 5 days; then treatment begins with gentle ROM. Follow the same guidelines as with carpal tunnel surgery but with ulnar nerve mobilization techniques.

# COMPLEX REGIONAL PAIN SYNDROME: REFLEX SYMPATHETIC DYSTROPHY AND CAUSALGIA

Reflex sympathetic dystrophy (RDS) and causalgia are former diagnoses that are now classified as complex regional pain syndromes I and II, respectively (CPRS type I and CPRS type II) (Box 13.9). This revised taxonomic system was developed by a consensus conference in 1993 to

---

**BOX 13.9  Classification and Clinical Features of Complex Regional Pain Syndromes[58]**

CRPS type I (reflex sympathetic dystrophy)
- Develops after an initiating noxious event
- Spontaneous pain or allodynia/hyperalgesia
- Edema, vascular abnormalities
- Abnormal sudomotor activity
- Non-nerve origin

CRPS type II (causalgia)
- Develops after nerve injury
- Not limited to territory of injured nerve
- Edema; skin blood flow abnormality
- Abnormal sudomotor activity

Clinical Features of CRPS (in addition to the differences listed above)
- Symptoms more marked distally in an extremity
- Symptoms progress in intensity and spread proximally
- Symptoms vary with time
- Disproportion of symptoms in relation to the causing event
- A specific diagnosis, such as diabetes or fibromyalgia, has been excluded

---

clarify confusion about the meaning and interpretation of the previous diagnoses.[28,58,66] Basically, this is a grouping of complex painful disorders that develop as a consequence of trauma affecting the extremities with or without an obvious nerve lesion.[3]

## Related Diagnoses and Symptoms

Common synonyms used in the past for RSD include shoulder-hand syndrome, Sudeck's atrophy, reflex neurovascular dystrophy, traumatic angiospasm or vasospasm, and sympathetically maintained pain (SMP).[1,9,28,58,66] SMP is frequently a component of CPRS but is not a distinct diagnosis in itself. Pain is a key feature; other symptoms and signs may include sensory abnormalities (spontaneous burning pain and allodynia), autonomic dysfunction, trophic changes, impairment of motor function, and emotional/psychological responses.[3,66] The difference between CRPS types I and II is whether a nerve injury was involved (see Box 13.9).

## Etiology and Symptoms

The underlying mechanism that stimulates the onset of these syndromes is unclear.[1] They usually develop in association with a persistent, painful lesion, such as a painful shoulder; after a cardiovascular accident or myocardial infarction; with cervical osteoarthritis; after trauma such as a fracture or sprain; with burns or immobilization; or after surgery or cardiac catheterization.[1] There may or may not be an obvious nerve lesion.

The sympathetic nervous system is usually involved in CPRS type I (RSD); it is described as unstable owing to its continuous activity and leads to progressive ischemia, pain, abnormal pseudomotor activity, and trophic changes that are characteristically produced by dysfunction in the autonomic nervous system. Wasner et al.[69] demonstrated the origin of the autonomic dysfunction in one patient and two normal subjects to be in the central nervous system. Some individuals may have similar symptoms of intense burning pain and sensitivity suggestive of sympathetically maintained pain, yet are unresponsive to sympathetic blocks. The term "sympathetically independent pain" (SIP) is used to describe this sensory abnormality.[3,48] CPRS may be the result of various organic or psychiatric disorders that involve the nervous system.[43]

## Three Stages of CRPS Type I (RSD)[1,30]

- **Stage I:** acute/reversible stage. This stage of vasodilation lasts 3 weeks to 6 months. Pain, the predominant feature, is usually out of proportion to the severity of the injury. There is hyperhidrosis, warmth, erythema, rapid nail growth, and edema in the distal extremity (Fig. 13.22).

N O T E : It is important to recognize the early symptoms because early intervention may prevent progression.

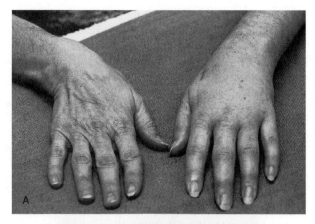

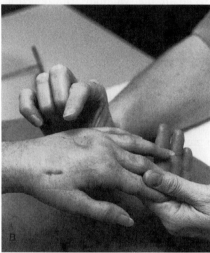

FIGURE 13.22 (A) In the early stages of reflex sympathetic dystrophy, generalized edema is present. This edema is often localized over the dorsum of the hand in the metacarpal and proximal interphalangeal joint areas. (B) The edema is usually of a pitting nature, as indicated by the indentation that remains once the pressure is removed.

- **Stage II:** dystrophic or vasoconstriction (ischemic) stage. This stage lasts 3 to 6 months. It is characterized by sympathetic hyperactivity, burning pain, and hyperesthesia exacerbated by cold weather. There is mottling and coldness, brittle nails, and osteoporosis.
- **Stage III:** atrophic stage. This stage is characterized by pain either decreasing or becoming worse and by severe osteoporosis. Muscle wasting and contractures may occur. The condition can last for months or years, but spontaneous recovery often occurs within 18 to 24 months.

## Common Impairments

- Pain or hyperesthesia at the shoulder, wrist, or hand out of proportion to the injury.
- Limitation of motion develops. Typically, the shoulder develops limitation in a capsular pattern with most restriction in lateral rotation and abduction. In the wrist and hand, the most common restrictions are limited wrist

extension and metacarpophalangeal and proximal interphalangeal flexion.
- Edema of the hand and wrist secondary to circulatory impairment of the venous and lymphatic systems, which in turn precipitates stiffness in the hand.
- Vasomotor instability.
- Trophic changes in the skin.

As the condition progresses, the pain subsides but limitation of motion persists. The skin becomes cyanotic and shiny, the intrinsic muscles of the hand atrophy, subcutaneous tissue in the fingers and palmar fascia thicken, nail changes occur, and osteoporosis develops.

## Management

### Early Intervention (Box 13.10)

It is a progressive disorder unless vigorous intervention is used during the acute stage.[68] The best intervention is prevention when it is recognized that development of CRPS type I (RSD) is a possibility, such as when there has been trauma to the extremity or when the extremity is immobilized. It requires that the therapist motivate the patient to move the entire extremity safely, minimize edema and vascular stasis with elevation and activity of the distal segments (squeeze and open hand with upper extremity lesions, or ankle pumping and toe curls with lower extremity lesions), and be alert to the development of adverse symptomatology.

| BOX 13.10 | Summary of Guidelines for Management of Complex Regional Pain Syndrome Type I (RSD) |
|---|---|

**Stage I (early intervention)**

*Relieve pain and control edema*
- Modalities
- Retrograde massage
- Elevate, elastic compression

*Increase mobility (specific to involved tissues)*
- Tendon gliding in the hand
- Nerve mobilization

*Improve muscle performance*
- Stress loading in quadruped position
- Distraction

*Improve total body circulation*
- Low impact aerobic exercise

*Desensitize the area*
- Desensitization techniques for brief periods 5×/day

*Educate the patient*
- Teach interventions that deal with variable vasomotor responses; when to use heat, cold, gentle exercises

Medical intervention is a necessity to manage this syndrome. The physician may choose to utilize analgesics, sympatholytic drugs, local anesthetic blocks, stellate ganglion blocks, spinal cord stimulation, or upper thoracic sympathectomy or may use oral steroids or intramuscular medication.[30] Because there is often an emotional or psychological component, medical intervention includes therapies to manage this area (antidepressants). This is done in conjunction with active exercise (including exercise in warm water) to manage physical impairments and functional limitations.

◉ *Pain and edema control.* Use modalities such as ultrasound, vibration, transcutaneous electrical nerve stimulation (TENS), or ice. Utilize retrograde massage. Elevate and use elastic compression when not undergoing pneumatic compression treatment.
◉ *Mobility.* In the early stages, use gentle, active exercises to manage the increasing stiffness.[31] Have the patient actively contract the musculature while the part is held near the end of the pain-free range. It is important to avoid increasing painful reactions that would decrease mobility. Support and have the patient actively move each joint for a short period of time. They should follow this program of brief motion frequently throughout the day.
  • In the hand, include tendon glide exercises (see Chapter 19, Fig. 19.17)
  • Butler[7] suggested that there may be adverse tension in the sympathetic trunk influencing sympathetic activity and therefore suggested mobilization of the nervous system, as described earlier in this chapter
◉ *Muscle performance.* Facilitate active muscle contractions. Include joints proximal to the symptoms (shoulder/hip); they often develop restrictions due to pain or lack of use. Use both dynamic and isometric exercise and alternating controlled stress loading (compressive loading) with distraction activities for neuromuscular control as well as afferent fiber stimulation. The objective is to provide tissue stress with minimal joint motion. Suggested exercises include[68,70]:
  • Stress load the upper extremity by scrubbing with a brush in the quadruped position, beginning at 3 minutes and incrementally increasing to 10 minutes three times a day. For the lower extremity, utilize progressive weight-bearing activities.
  • Distraction by carrying 1 to 5 pounds up to 10 minutes at a time frequently throughout the day
◉ *Total body circulation and cardiac output.* Initiate a program of low-impact aerobic exercises.
◉ *Desensitization.* Utilize desensitization techniques for brief periods five times per day, such as having the patient work with various textures and tap or vibrate over the sensitive area. The patient is instructed to wear a protective glove during activities of daily living (described earlier in the chapter).

◉ *Patient education.* Emphasize the importance of following the program of increased activity. Teach the patient interventions that deal with the variable vasomotor responses with the use of gentle heat when at home, gentle exercises for short periods throughout the day, and use of associated parts of the extremity.

PRECAUTION: It is important to not exacerbate the patient's pain and underlying pathology. If there is increased sensitivity, use caution when touching sensitive areas. Maintain continuous contact to avoid the irritation of "make-and-break" contact over the sensitive area especially if utilizing massage for edema control.[68] When the patient presents with hypersensitivity, painful stretching or manipulations exacerbate the symptoms. Utilize gentle active exercises and light massage, for short periods, throughout the day.[31]

### Intervention—Stages II and III

◉ *Pain management.* Modalities are often used as palliative interventions prior to or in conjunction with exercise to minimize pain.[68]
◉ *Desensitization.* Progress the desensitization techniques to increase the patient's tolerance to various textures.
◉ *Mobility.* Use joint mobilization, neuromobilization, and stretching techniques to address tissues limiting mobility. Because of the pain and significant limitations, little progress is sometimes seen with the stretching maneuvers, so surgical intervention may be required to gain motion.[61]
◉ *Muscle performance.* Develop an exercise program to improve strength, endurance, and overall functional performance that meets the specific needs of the patient.

PRECAUTION: Use caution with stretching and resistive exercises due to osteoporosis. Pain continues to be a variable, and therefore the initiation of any therapeutic exercise or manual therapy techniques should be carefully monitored to minimize exacerbation of symptoms.

 **Focus on Evidence** _____

Evidence supports effective use of physical therapy with early intervention (acute stage), but there is contradictory evidence for its effectiveness during the later stages.[22,25] In one study, the primary predictors for success and satisfaction with patients during the chronic phase after 6 months of therapy (evaluated at 12 months) was with the patient group that began therapy at a higher baseline of function, higher baseline ROM and strength, and less baseline pain.[25] Because of the variability in presenting symptoms and signs, therapeutic interventions should be adapted to the patient at each visit.[68]

# INDEPENDENT LEARNING ACTIVITIES

## ● Critical Thinking and Discussion

1. Your patient describes intermittent sensory changes in the index and middle finger. What are the possible causes? What tests would you use to examine this patient? What results would lead you to determine nerve mobility restrictions?

2. You have a new client who describes intermittent tingling and sensations of heaviness in his hands whenever working with his hands in an overhead position. He is an auto mechanic and frequently has to work this way. Identify possible causes of these symptoms. What is usually the source of "tingling" sensations? What may be the source of the "heaviness" feelings? Why would the overhead position cause both vascular and neurological symptoms? Identify possible sites that could cause these symptoms. What tests would you use to confirm or rule out your hypotheses?

3. A 19-year-old patient presents with the medical diagnosis of complex regional pain syndrome type I (RSD) and the following history.[45]

   • Three-month history of midfoot pain that increases with standing more than 5 minutes or running. Symptoms have increased over the past 3 weeks.

   • Stress fracture to the navicular was detected on radiography, so patient was placed in a BK non-weight-bearing cast.

   • Foot discomfort increased and became more diffuse, radiating into the lateral forefoot and digits even after pain medications were prescribed.

   • Symptoms increased with burning or stinging pain, edema, and discoloration of the digits.

   • Examination 3 weeks after cast applied: digits cool, edematous, hyperesthetic, and hyperhidrotic. Passive and active motions of ankle and toes were moderately painful. Radiographs showed diffuse osteoporosis.

What would be your goals for this patient? Develop a program of interventions.

4. Identify and describe everyday activities and/or positions that mimic the nerve tension test positions. These activities/positions may be patient complaints that indicate further nerve tension testing. For example, getting into a car by straightening the leg and ducking the head mimics the "slump" position.

## ● Laboratory Practice

1. With your laboratory partner, practice each of the nerve tension positions. Demonstrate how you would mobilize restrictions for each of the nerves.

2. Practice each of the thoracic outlet tests and describe the mechanics of each test. Identify and practice techniques you could use to increase mobility or reduce compression on the brachial plexus at each of the sites where compression or tension might occur. Design an exercise program and progression for managing impairments that could cause TOS symptoms.

3. Practice sensory stimulation and reintegration techniques by doing each of the following.

   • Gather 10 pieces of material of various textures. Place them in order of least irritating to most irritating. Practice sensory stimulation techniques by gently rubbing each material across your fingers.

   • Use five plastic tubs or buckets. Place each of the following in a container: dry peas or beans, spiral macaroni, sand, fine gravel, seeds. Practice sensory stimulation by moving your hand (or foot) through each of the textures.

   • Have your laboratory partner place several familiar household items in a bag (e.g., key, dime, penny, can opener). Without looking, attempt to identify each one.

## REFERENCES

1. Aprile, AE: Complex regional pain syndrome. AANA J 65(6):577–560, 1997.

2. Baker, CL, Liu, SH: Neurovascular injuries to the shoulder. J Orthop Sports Phys Ther 18:361, 1993.

3. Baron, R, Maier, C: Reflex sympathetic dystrophy: skin blood flow, sympathetic vasoconstrictor reflexes and pain before and after surgical sympathectomy. Pain 67:317–326, 1996.

4. Baxter-Petralia, P, Penney, V: Cumulative trauma. In Stanley, BG, Tribuzi, SM (eds) Concepts in Hand Rehabilitation. FA Davis, Philadelphia, 1992, p 419.

5. Benjamin, K: Injuries to the brachial plexus: mechanisms of injury and identification of risk factors. Adv Neonatal Care 5(4):181–189, 2005.

6. Burnett, MG, Zager, EL: Pathophysiology of peripheral nerve injury: a brief review. Neurosurg Focus 16(5):1–7, 2004.

7. Butler, DS: Mobilization of the Nervous System. Churchill Livingstone, New York, 1991.

8. Butler, DS: The Sensitive Nervous System. Noigroup Publications, Adelaide, Australia, 2000.

9. Cailliet, R: Shoulder Pain, ed 3. FA Davis, Philadelphia, 1991.

10. Cook AD, Szabo RM, et al: Early mobilization following carpal tunnel release: a prospective randomized study. J Hand Surg [Br] 20(2):228–230, 1995.

11. Coppieters, MW, Stappaerts, KH, et al: Addition of test components during neurodynamic testing: effect on range of motion and sensory responses. J Orthop Sports Phys Ther 31(5):226, 2001.

12. Crotti, FM, Carai, A, Carai, M, et al: TOS pathophysiology and clinical features. Acta Neurochir Suppl 92:7–12, 2005.

13. Crotti, FM, Carai, A, Carai, M, et al: Post-traumatic thoracic outlet syndrome (TOS). Acta Neurochir Suppl 92:13–15, 2005.

14. Cuetter, AC, Bartoszek, DM: The thoracic outlet syndrome: controversies, overdiagnosis, overtreatment, and recommendations for management. Muscle Nerve 12:410, 1989.

15. Dagum, AB: Peripheral nerve regeneration, repair, and grafting. J Hand Ther 11(2):111–117, 1998.

16. DiFabio, RP: Neural mobilization: the impossible [editorial]. J Orthop Sports Phys Ther 31(5):224–225, 2001.
17. Dilley, A, Lynn, B, et al: Quantitative in vivo studies of median nerve sliding in response to wrist, elbow, shoulder and neck movements. Clin Biomech 18:899–907, 2003.
18. Ehni, BL: Treatment of traumatic peripheral nerve injury. Am Fam Physician 43(3):897–905, 1991.
19. Fahey, VA: Thoracic outlet syndrome. J Cardiovasc Nurs 1:12, 1987.
20. Flores AJ, Lavernia, CJ, Owens, PW: Anatomy and physiology of peripheral nerve injury and repair. Am J Orthop 29(3):167–173, 2000.
21. George, SZ: Differential diagnosis and treatment for a patient with lower extremity symptoms. J Orthop Sports Phys Ther 30(8):468, 2000.
22. Guisel, A, Gill, JM, Witherell, P: Complex regional pain syndrome: which treatments show promise? J Fam Pract 54(7):599–603, 2005.
23. Hunter, JM, Davlin, LB, Defus, LM: Major neuropathies of the upper extremity: the median nerve. In Hunter, JM, Mackin, EJ, Callahan, AD (eds) Rehabilitation of the Hand: Surgery and Therapy, Vol II, ed 4. CV Mosby, St. Louis, 1995, p 905.
24. Julius, A, Lees, R, et al: Shoulder posture and median nerve sliding. BMC Musculoskel Disord 5:23, 2004.
25. Kemler, MA, Rijks, CP, de Vet, HC: Which patients with chronic reflex sympathetic dystrophy are most likely to benefit from physical therapy? J Manipulative Phys Ther 24(4):272–278, 2001.
26. Kietrys, DM: Neural mobilization: an appraisal of the evidence regarding validity and efficacy. Orthop Pract 15(4):18–20, 2003.
27. Kleinrensink GJ, Stoeckart, R, et al: Upper limb tension tests as tools in the diagnosis of nerve and plexus lesions: anatomical and biomechanical aspects. Clin Biomech 15(1):9–14, 2000.
28. Koman, LA, Smith, BP, Smith TL: Reflex sympathetic dystrophy (complex regional pain syndromes—types 1 and 2). In Mackin, EJ, Callahan, AD, et al (eds) Rehabilitation of the Hand and Upper Extremities, ed 5. Mosby, St. Louis, 2002, p 1695.
29. Kopell, H, Thompson, W: Peripheral Entrapment Neuropathies, ed 2. Robert Krieger, Huntington, NY, 1976.
30. Kurvers, HA: Reflex sympathetic dystrophy: facts and hypotheses. Vasc Med 3(3):207–214, 1998.
31. Lankford, LL: Reflex sympathetic dystrophy. In Hunter, JM, Mackin, EJ, Callahan, AD (eds) Rehabilitation of the Hand: Surgery and Therapy, ed 4. CV Mosby, St. Louis, 1995, p 779.
32. Lee, MJ, LaStayo, PC: Pronator syndrome and other nerve compressions that mimic carpal tunnel syndrome. J Orthop Sprots Phys Ther 34(10):601–609, 2004.
33. Lindgren, KA: Conservative treatment of thoracic outlet syndrome: a 2-year follow-up. Arch Phys Med Rehabil 78:373–378, 1007.
34. Lord, J, Rosati, JM: Thoracic Outlet Syndromes, Vol 23. Ciba. Summit, NJ, 1971.
35. Lundborg, G, Dahlin, LB: Anatomy, function, and pathophysiology of peripheral nerves and nerve compression. Hand Clin 12(2):185–192, 1996.
36. MacDermid, JC, Doherty, T: Clinical and electrodiagnostic testing of carpal tunnel syndrome: a narrative review. J Orthop Sports Phys Ther 34(10):565–588, 2004.
37. Mackinnon, SE: Pathophysiology of nerve compression. Hand Clin 18:231–241, 2002.
38. Magee, DJ: Orthopedic Physical Assessment, ed 4. WB Saunders, Philadelphia, 2002.
39. Matheson, JW: Neural mobilization: the need for more answers [letter to the editor]. J Orthop Sports Phys Ther 31(9):518, 2001.
40. Michlovitz, SL: Conservative Interventions for carpal tunnel syndrome. J Orthop Sports Phys Ther 34(10):589–600, 2004.
41. Nitz, AJ: Effects of acute pressure on peripheral nerve structure and function. In Currier, D, Nelson, R (eds) Dynamics of Human Biologic Tissues. FA Davis, Philadelphia, 1992.
42. Novak, CB: Upper extremity work-related musculoskeletal disorders: a treatment perspective. J Orthop Sports Phys Ther 34(10):628–637, 2004.
43. Ochoa, J: Reflex sympathetic dystrophy: fact and fiction [editorial]. Am Family Phys 56(9):2182, 1997.
44. O'Connor, D, Marshall, S, Massy-Westropp, N: Non-surgical treatment (other than steroid injection) for carpal tunnel syndrome. Cochrane Database Syst Rev CD003219:(1), 2003.
45. Osher, L, Young, G, et al: Reflex sympathetic dystrophy syndrome. J Am Podiatric Med Assoc 83(5):276–283, 1993.
46. Pang, D, Wessel, HB: Thoracic outlet syndrome. Neurosurgery 22:105, 1988.
47. Pascarelli, EF, Hsu, YP: Understanding work-related upper extremity disorders: clinical findings in 485 computer users, musicians, and others. J Occup Rehabil 11(1):1–21, 2001.
48. Price, DD, Bennett, GJ, Rafii, A: Psychophysical observations on patients with neuropathic pain relieved by a sympathetic block. Pain 36:273–288, 1989.
49. Provinciali, L, Giattini, A, et al: Usefulness of hand rehabilitation after carpal tunnel surgery. Muscle Nerve 23:211, 2000.
50. Roganovic, Z: Factors influencing the outcome of nerve repair. Voj Pregl 55(2):119–131, 1998.
51. Rozmaryn, LM, Dovelle, S, et al: Nerve and tendon gliding exercises and the conservative management of carpal tunnel syndrome. J Hand Ther 11:171, 1998.
52. Seror, P: Frequency of neurogenic thoracic outlet syndrome in patients with definite carpal tunnel syndrome: an electrophysiological evaluation in 100 women. Clin Neurophysiol 116(2):259–263, 2005.
53. Seror, P: Symptoms of thoracic outlet syndrome in women with carpal tunnel syndrome. Clin Neurophysiol 116(10):2324–2329, 2005.
54. Skirven, T: Nerve Injuries. In Stanley, BG, Tribuzi, SM (eds) Concepts in Hand Rehabilitation. FA Davis, Philadelphia, 1992, p 322.
55. Smith, KL: Nerve Response to Injury and Repair. In Mackin, EJ, Callahan, AD, et al (eds): Rehabilitation of the Hand and Upper Extremities, ed 5. CV Mosby, St. Louis, 2002, pp 583–598.
56. Smith, K: The thoracic outlet syndrome: a protocol of treatment. J Orthop Sports Phys Ther 1:89, 1979.
57. Smith, MB: The peripheral nervous system. In Goodman, CC, Fuller, KS, Boissonnault, WG: Pathology: Implications for the Physical Therapist. Saunders, Philadelphia, 2003, pp 1140–1173.
58. Stanton-Hicks, M, et al: Reflex sympathetic dystrophy: changing concepts and taxonomy. Pain 63:127, 1995.
59. Sucher, BM: Thoracic outlet syndrome: a myofascial variant. Part 1. Pathology and diagnosis. J Am Osteopath Assoc 90:686, 1990.
60. Sucher, BM: Thoracic outlet syndrome: a myofascial variant. Part 2. Treatment. J Am Osteopath Assoc 90:810, 1990.
61. Taylor Mullins, PA: Reflex sympathetic dystrophy. In Stanley, BG, Tribuzi, SM (eds) Concepts in Hand Rehabilitation, FA Davis, Philadelphia, 1992, p 446.
62. Topp, KS, Boyd, BS: Structure and biomechanics of peripheral nerves: nerve responses to physical stresses and implications for physical therapist practice. Phys Ther 86(1):92–109, 2006.
63. Turl, SE, George, KP: Adverse neural tension: a factor in repetitive hamstring strain. J Orthop Sports Phys Ther 27:16, 1998.
64. Varitimidis, SE, Sotereanos, DV: Partial nerve injuries in the upper extremity. Hand Clin 16(1):141–149, 2000.
65. Verdugo, RJ, Salinas RS, et al: Surgical versus non-surgical treatment for carpal tunnel syndrome. Cochrane Database Syst Rev CD001552 (3):2002.
66. Walker, SM, Cousins, MJ: Complex regional pain syndromes: including "reflex sympathetic dystrophy" and "causalgia." Anaesth Intensive Care 25:113, 1997.
67. Walsh, MT: Therapist management of thoracic outlet syndrome. J Hand Ther April-June:131, 1994.
68. Walsh, MT, Muntzer, E: Therapist's management of complex regional pain syndrome (reflex sympathetic dystrophy) In Mackin, EF, Callahan AD, et al (eds) Rehabilitation of the Hand and Upper Extremities, ed 5. CV Mosby, St. Louis, 2002, p 1707.
69. Wasner, G, Heckmann, K et al: Vascular abnormalities in acute reflex sympathetic dystrophy (CRPS I): complete inhibition of sympathetic nerve activity with recovery. Arch Neurol 56(5):613–620, 1999.
70. Watson, HK, Carlson, L: Treatment of reflex sympathetic dystrophy of the hand with an active "stress loading" program. J Hand Surg 12(5):779–785, 1987.
71. Wehbe, MA, Schlegel, JM: Nerve gliding exercises for thoracic outlet syndrome. Hand Clin 20(1):51–55, 2004.
72. Wilson, S, Selvaratnam, P, Briggs, D: Strain at the subclavian artery during the upper limb tension test. Aust Physiother 40(4):243, 1994.
73. Wood, VE, Biondi, J: Double-crush nerve compression in thoracic-outlet syndrome. J Bone Joint Surg Am 72(1):85–87, 1990.

# Exercise Interventions by Body Region

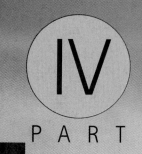

## 14
CHAPTER

## The Spine and Posture: Structure, Function, Postural Impairments, and Management Guidelines

*Posture* is a "position or attitude of the body, the relative arrangement of body parts for a specific activity, or a characteristic manner of bearing one's body."[68] It is alignment of the body parts whether upright, sitting, or recumbent. It is described by the positions of the joints and body segments and also in terms of the balance between the muscles crossing the joints. Impairments in the joints, muscles, or connective tissues may lead to faulty postures; or, conversely, faulty postures may lead to impairments

in the joints, muscles, and connective tissues as well as symptoms of discomfort and pain. Many musculoskeletal complaints can be attributed to stresses that occur from repetitive or sustained activities when in a habitually faulty postural alignment. This chapter reviews the structural relationships of the spine and extremities to normal and abnormal posture and describes the mechanisms that control posture. Common postural impairments and general guidelines for their management are described. Specific exercises for the various body regions are highlighted in this chapter and are described in detail in the succeeding chapters in this section of the text (see Chapters 15 to 22).

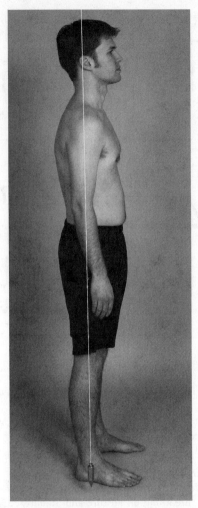

FIGURE 14.1 Lateral view of standard postural alignment. A plumb line is typically used for reference and represents the relationship of the body parts with the line of gravity. Surface landmarks are slightly anterior to the lateral malleolus, slightly anterior to the axis of the knee joint, through the greater trochanter (slightly posterior to the axis of the hip joint), through the bodies of the lumbar and cervical vertebrae, through the shoulder joint and through the lobe of the ear.

## POSTURE AND BIOMECHANICAL INFLUENCES

## ⬤ ALIGNMENT

### Curves of the Spine

The adult spine is divided into four curves: two *primary*, or posterior, curves, so named because they are present in the infant and the convexity is posterior; and two *compensatory*, or anterior, curves, so named because they develop as the infant learns to lift the head and eventually stand, and the convexity is anterior.

- Anterior curves are in the cervical and lumbar regions. *Lordosis* is a term also used to denote an anterior curve, although some sources reserve the term lordosis to denote abnormal conditions such as those that occur with a sway back.[42]
- Posterior curves are in the thoracic and sacral regions. *Kyphosis* is a term used to denote a posterior curve. Kyphotic posture refers to an excessive posterior curvature of the thoracic spine.[42]
- The curves and flexibility in the spinal column are important for withstanding the effects of gravity and other external forces.[52]
- The structure of the bones, joints, muscles, and inert tissues of the lower extremities are designed for weight bearing; they support and balance the trunk in the upright posture. Lower extremity alignment and function are described in greater detail in each of the extremity chapters (see Chapters 20 to 22).

### Postural Alignment

It is critical to understand the influence of gravity on the structures of the trunk and lower extremities when looking at posture and function. Gravity places stress on the structures responsible for maintaining the body upright and therefore provides a continual challenge to stability and efficient movement. For a weight-bearing joint to be stable, or in equilibrium, the gravity line of the mass must fall exactly through the axis of rotation, or there must be a force to counteract the moment caused by gravity. In the body, the counterforce is provided by either muscle or inert structures.[44,68] In addition, the standing posture usually involves a slight anterior/posterior swaying of the body of about 4 centimeters (cm), so muscles are necessary to control the sway and maintain equilibrium.

In the upright posture, the line of gravity transects the spinal curves, which are balanced anteriorly and posteriorly, and it is close to the axis of rotation in the lower extremity joints. The following describes the standard of a balanced upright posture (Fig. 14.1).

*Ankle.* For the ankle, the gravity line is anterior to the joint so it tends to rotate the tibia forward about the ankle. Stability is provided by the plantarflexor muscles, primarily the soleus muscle.

*Knee.* The normal gravity line is anterior to the knee joint, which tends to keep the knee in extension. Stability is provided by the anterior cruciate ligament, posterior capsule (locking mechanism of the knee), and tension in the muscles posterior to the knee (the gastrocnemius and hamstring muscles). The soleus provides active stability by pulling posteriorly on the tibia. With the knees fully extended, no muscle support is required at that joint to maintain an upright posture; but if the knees flex slightly, the gravity line shifts posterior to the joint, and the quadriceps femoris muscle must contract to prevent the knee from buckling.

***Hip.*** The gravity line at the hip varies with the swaying of the body. When the line passes through the hip joint, there is equilibrium, and no external support is necessary. When the gravitational line shifts posterior to the joint, some posterior rotation of the pelvis occurs, which is controlled by tension in the hip flexor muscles (primarily the iliopsoas). During relaxed standing, the iliofemoral ligament provides passive stability to the joint, and no muscle tension is necessary. When the gravitational line shifts anteriorly, stability is provided by active support of the hip extensor muscles.

***Trunk.*** Normally, the gravity line in the trunk goes through the bodies of the lumbar and cervical vertebrae, and the curves are balanced. Some activity in the muscles of the trunk and pelvis helps maintain the balance (this is described in greater detail in the following sections). As the trunk shifts, contralateral muscles contract and function as guy wires. Extreme or sustained deviations are supported by inert structures.

***Head.*** The center of gravity of the head falls anterior to the atlanto-occipital joints. The posterior cervical muscles contract to keep the head balanced. In postures in which the head is forward, greater demand is placed on these muscles. At the extreme of flexion, tension in the ligamentum nuchae prevents further motion.

## 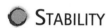 STABILITY

So long as the line of gravity from the center of mass falls within the base of support, a structure is stable. Stability is improved by lowering the center of gravity or increasing the base of support. In the upright position, the body is relatively unstable because it is a tall structure with a small base of support. When the center of gravity falls outside the base of support, the structure either falls or some force must act to keep the structure upright. Both inert and dynamic structures support the body against gravitational and other external forces. The inert osseous and ligamentous structures provide passive tension when a joint reaches the end of its range of motion (ROM). Muscles act as dynamic guy wires, responding to perturbations by providing counterforces to the torque of gravity as well as stability within the ROM so stresses are not placed on the inert tissues.

### Postural Stability in the Spine

Spinal stability is described in terms of three subsystems: passive (inert structures/bones and ligaments), active (muscles), and neural control.[18,60] The three subsystems are interrelated and can be thought of as a three-legged stool; if any one of the legs is not providing support, it affects the stability of the whole.[62] Instability of a spinal segment is often a combination of tissue damage, insufficient muscular strength or endurance, and poor neuromuscular control.[3]

### Inert Structures: Influence on Stability

Penjabi[59,60] described the ROM of any one segment as being divided into an *elastic zone* and a *neutral zone*. When spinal segments are in the neutral zone (midrange/neutral range) the inert joint capsules and ligaments provide minimal passive resistance to motion and therefore minimal stability. As a segment moves into the elastic zone, the inert structures provide restraint as passive resistance to the motion occurs. When a structure limits movement in a specific direction, it provides stability in that direction.[9,28] In addition to the inert tissues providing passive stability when limiting motion, the sensory receptors in the joint capsules and ligaments sense position and changes in position. Stimulation of these receptors provides feedback to the central nervous system, thus influencing the neural control system.[28] Table 14.1 summarizes the stabilizing features of the osteoligamentous tissues in the spine.

### Muscles: Influence on Stability

#### Role of Global and Core Muscle Activity

The muscles of the neck and trunk not only act as prime movers or as antagonists to movement caused by gravity during dynamic activity, they are important stabilizers of the spine.[7,8,10,21-23,32,49,50,71] Without the dynamic stabilizing activity from the trunk muscles, the spine would collapse in the upright position.[12] Both superficial (global) and deep (core) muscles function to maintain the upright posture. The global muscles, being multisegmental, are the large guy wires that respond to external loads imposed on the trunk that shift the center of mass (Fig. 14.2A). Their reaction is direction-specific to control spinal orientation.[3,32] The global muscles are unable to stabilize individual spinal segments except through compressive loading because they have little or no direct attachment to the vertebrae. If an individual segment is unstable, compressive loading from the global guy wires may lead to or perpetuate a painful situation as stress is placed on the inert tissues at the end of the range of that segment (Fig. 14.2B).

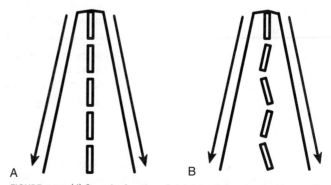

FIGURE 14.2 (*A*) Guy wire function of global trunk muscles provide overall stability against perturbations. (*B*) Instability in the multisegmental spine cannot be controlled by the global trunk muscle guy wires. Compressive loading from the long guy wires leads to stress on the inert tissues at the end ranges of the unstable segment.

**TABLE 14.1    Stabilizing Features of Inert Tissues in the Spine**

| Structure | Feature | Limits |
|---|---|---|
| *Facet joint orientation*<br>Cervical spine facets oriented in frontal plane with oblique angulation toward transverse plane | Allows free forward bending (flexion) and backward bending (extension) | Capsule taut at end of flexion; joint surfaces approximate at end of extension |
| Thoracic spine facets: upper spine similar to cervical, mid to lower facets more in sagittal plane | Rotation, side bending, and forward bending are allowed to various degrees by the facets | Facets are not as restricting as ribs and spinous processes |
| Lumbar spine facets in sagittal plane with some curvature in frontal plane[8] | Forward and backward bending allowed | Restricts rotation; frontal plane orientation provides stability at end of range in flexion[71] |
| *Ribs* | Ribs approximate on side of spinal concavity with any motion | Restricts forward bending, side bending, and rotation in the thoracic region |
| *Spinous processes* | Spinous processes approximate with extension; the longer the process the greater the restriction | Restricts extension, especially in the thoracic region; may approximate in lumbar region with flexible individual |
| *Intervertebral disks* | Greater the ratio of disk thickness to vertebral height the greater the mobility | Cervical spine (ratio 2:5) most mobile<br>Lumbar spine (ratio 1:3)<br>Thoracic spine (ratio 1:5) least mobile |
| Annulus fibrosus | Organized concentric rings behave similar to ligaments[8] | Some fibers are taut whichever direction the spinal segment rotates or sheers[43] |
| *Ligaments* | Slack midrange, taut at end of range | Forward bending limited by the interspinous and supraspinous ligaments, capsular ligaments, ligamentum flavum, and posterior longitudinal ligament.[61]<br>Backward bending limited by the anterior longitudinal ligament<br>Side bending limited by the contra-lateral intertransverse ligaments, ligamentum flavum, and capsular ligaments<br>Rotation limited by the capsular ligaments |
| *Thoracolumbar (lumbodorsal) fascia* | Extensive fascial system consists of several layers surrounding erector spinae and quadratus lumborum; has static and dynamic function | Limits end-range of forward bending of the lumbar spine[8]<br>(See also dynamic stabilizing function) |
| *Muscles* | Muscles with normal elasticity do not cause limitations of spinal movement; normally provide dynamic stability and control | When muscles develop contractures, they restrict movement opposite to their direction of contraction |

The deeper, core muscles, which have segmental attachments, respond regardless of direction of motion.[32] They provide dynamic support to individual segments in the spine and help maintain each segment in a stable position so the inert tissues are not stressed at the limits of motion (Fig. 14.3). Both the global and core musculature play critical roles in providing stability to the multisegmental spine. Table 14.2 summarizes the stabilizing characteristics of the global and core musculature.

## TABLE 14.2 Stabilizing Features of Muscles Controlling the Spine

| Global Muscles | Core Muscles |
|---|---|
| *Characteristics*<br>• Superficial: farther from axis of motion<br>• Cross multiple vertebral segments<br>• Produce motion and provide large guy wire function<br>• Compressive loading with strong contractions | • Deep: closer to axis of motion<br>• Attach to each vertebral segment<br>• Control segmental motion; segmental guy wire function<br>• Greater percentage of type I muscle fibers for muscular endurance |
| *Lumbar region*<br>• Rectus abdominis<br>• External and internal obliques<br>• Quadratus lumborum (lateral portion)<br>• Erector spinae<br>• Iliopsoas | • Transversus abdominis<br>• Multifidus<br>• Quadratus lumborum (deep portion)<br>• Deep rotators |
| *Cervical region*<br>• Sternocleidomastoid<br>• Scalene<br>• Levator scapulae<br>• Upper trapezius<br>• Erector spinae | • Rectus capitis anterior and lateralis<br>• Longus colli |

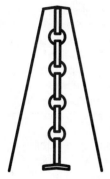

**FIGURE 14.3** Deep core muscles attached to each spinal segment provide segmental stability.

### Role of Muscle Endurance
Strength is critical for controlling large loads or responding to large and unpredictable loads (such as during heavy labor, sports, or falls); but only about 10% of maximum contraction is needed to provide stability in usual situations.[3] Slightly more might be needed in a segment damaged by disk disease or ligamentous laxity when muscles are called on to compensate for the deficit in the passive support.[3] Greater percentages of type I fibers than type II fibers are found in all back muscles, which is reflective of their postural and stabilization function.[54] Inactivity has been shown to change muscle fiber composition and may be one reason for decreased function in patients with low back pain.[54]

 **Focus on Evidence**

In a study that looked at 17 mechanical factors and the occurrence of low back pain in 600 subjects (ages 20 through 65), poor muscular endurance in the back extensors muscles had the greatest association with low back pain.[56]

### Muscle Control in the Lumbar Spine
The focus of recent research has been on the role of the transversus abdominis (TrA) and multifidus muscles and their function as core stabilizers. These deep muscles have segmental attachments in the lumbar spine and are therefore able to provide segmental control and stiffness. Studies have shown that the deep fibers of the multifidi and TrA are the first muscles to become active when there is postural disturbance from rapid extremity movements.[32,][35-37,51] Other deep muscles that theoretically play a role in segmental stability but to this point in time have been difficult to assess because of their depth include the intersegmental muscles (rotators and intertransversarii muscles) and deep fibers of the quadratus lumborum. General muscle function and stabilizing actions of the muscles of the spine are summarized in Table 14.3.

***Abdominal muscles (Fig. 14.4).*** The rectus abdominis (RA), external oblique (EO), and internal oblique (IO) muscles are large, multisegmental global muscles and are important guy wires for stabilizing the spine against postural perturbations. The transversus abdominis (TrA) is

## TABLE 14.3    Muscles of the Spine and Their Stabilizing Function

| Muscles | Prime Action | Stabilizing Function |
|---|---|---|
| *Lumbar spine* <br> Rectus abdominis (RA) | Trunk flexion (sit-up and curl-up exercises)[49] | • Stabilizes pelvis against anterior rotation forces[65] <br> • Provides long guy wire stability with backward bending (extension) loads on the spine |
| Internal obliques (IO) and external obliques (EO) | Bilateral contraction causes trunk flexion; EO on one side with IO on contralateral side together cause diagonal trunk rotation with flexion; EO and IO on same side cause side bending of trunk | • Controls against external loads that would cause backward bending or side bending of the spine <br> • Stabilizes pelvis (along with rectus abdominis) against anterior rotation forces <br> • Contracts in bracing maneuver to stiffen spine; increases compressive load <br> • Contracts with transverses abdominis to increase intra-abdominal pressure[11] and place tension on thoracolumbar fascia to unload spine[33] |
| Transversus abdominis (TrA) | Contributes to rotation[11] | • Creates tension via thoracolumbar fascia and increases intra-abdominal pressure to provide segmental stability <br> • Activates with "drawing-in" maneuver for core spinal stability[64,72] |
| Quadratus lumborum (QL) | Pelvic hiking and side bending of the spine | • Provides frontal and sagittal plane stability[49] <br> • Stabilizes ribs against pull of the diaphragm during inspiration[4] <br> • Deep fibers provide segmental stability to lumbar vertebrae |
| Multifidus | Spinal extension and contralateral rotation | • Stabilizes spine against flexion and rotation moments and contralateral side flexion moments. <br> • Provides core stability and segmental stiffness (deep fibers) <br> • Activated with the "drawing in" and bracing maneuvers for spinal stabilization[64] |
| Intersegmental rotators and intertransversarii | These muscles are rich in muscle spindles and may function to sense vertebral position and motion more so than to produce torque for movement | • Theoretically, these muscles are in position to make small segmental adjustments to stabilize against perturbations to posture |
| Superficial erector spinae (ES) muscles (iliocostalis, longissimus, spinalis) | Primary trunk extensors; extend thorax on pelvis causing spinal backward bending; also side bending and posterior translation of the vertebrae | • Antagonist to gravity—control movement of trunk during forward bending activities <br> • Long guy wires that provide global stability to the trunk by responding to external loads and preventing the trunk from falling over |
| Iliopsoas (iliacus and psoas major) | Primary hip flexors and indirectly lumbar extensors; Iliopsoas creates an anterior shear on the lumbar vertebrae | • This muscle complex does not function as a spinal stabilizer in normal standing.[2,49] <br> • Iliacus stabilizes the pelvis and hip joints and thus indirectly influences spinal posture <br> • Psoas assists in stabilizing the lumbar spine in the frontal plane, especially when a heavy load is applied to the contralateral side[2] |

| Muscles | Prime Action | Stabilizing Function |
|---|---|---|
| *Cervical spine* | | |
| Sternocleidomastoid and scalene group | Bilateral contraction causes cervical flexion; unilateral contraction causes side bending with contralateral rotation and flexion When the neck is stabilized, the scalenes elevate the upper ribs during inspiration, and the sternocleidomastoids (SCM) elevate the clavicles and sternum, which assists in inspiration | • Balance the head on the thorax against the forces of gravity when the center of mass is posterior |
| Upper trapezius and cervical erector spinae | Bilateral contraction causes cervical and capital extension; unilateral contraction causes side bending | • Balance the head on the thorax against the forces of gravity when the center of mass is anterior |
| Levator scapulae | The levator scapulae works with the upper trapezius to elevate the scapulae | • Supports the posture of the scapulae |
| Longus colli; rectus capitis anterior and lateralis | Craniocervical flexors; longus colli is the prime mover for cervical retraction (axial extension) | • Provides core (segmental) stability to cervical spine |

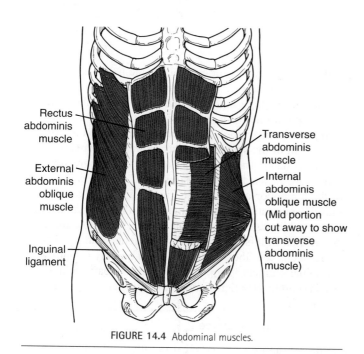

Rectus abdominis muscle

External abdominis oblique muscle

Inguinal ligament

Transverse abdominis muscle

Internal abdominis oblique muscle (Mid portion cut away to show transverse abdominis muscle)

FIGURE 14.4 Abdominal muscles.

around the abdomen and lumbar vertebrae. Only the TrA is active with both isometric trunk flexion and extension, whereas the other abdominal muscles have decreased activity with resisted extension. This is attributed to the stabilization function of the TrA.[11]

Early electromyographic research studies of the activity of the deeper abdominal muscles in their stabilization function was done with surface electrodes and did not discriminate activity between the TrA and IO. By using ultrasound imaging techniques, insertion of fine-needle electrodes into the various muscles has produced evidence

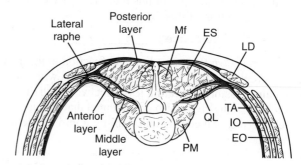

Lateral raphe

Posterior layer

Mf ES

LD

Anterior layer

Middle layer

PM

QL

TA

IO

EO

FIGURE 14.5 Transverse section in the lumbar region shows the relationships of the three layers of the thoracolumbar fascia to the muscles in the region and their attachments to the spine. ES, erector spinae; Mf, multifidus; TA, transversus abdominis; IO, internal obliques; EO, external obliques; LD, latissimus dorsi; PM, psoas major; QL, quadratus lumborum muscles.

the deepest of the abdominal muscles and responds uniquely to postural perturbations. It attaches posteriorly to the lumbar vertebrae via the posterior and middle layers of the thoracolumbar fascia (Figs. 14.5 and 14.6) and through its action develops tension that acts like a girdle of support

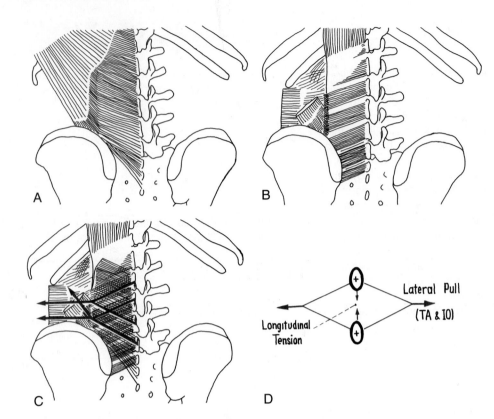

FIGURE 14.6 Orientation and attachments of the posterior layer of the thoracolumbar fascia. From the lateral raphe, (A) the fibers of the superficial lamina are angled inferiorly and medially, and (B) the fibers of the deep lamina are angled superiorly and medially. (C) Tension in the angled fibers of the posterior layer of the fascia is transmitted to the spinous processes in opposing directions, resisting separation of the spinous processes. (D) Diagrammatic representation of a lateral pull at the lateral raphe, resulting in tension between the lumbar spinous processes that oppose separation, thus providing stability to the spine. (A–C. Adapted from Bogduck and MacIntosh,[7] pp. 166–167, 169, with permission. D. Adapted from Gracovetsky et al.,[21] p. 319, with permission.)

of differing functions between these two muscles with perturbations to balance in healthy individuals as well as those who have low back pathology.[30] The TrA responds with anticipitatory activity, with rapid arm and leg movements, no matter in which direction the limb movement occurs, and coordinates with respiration during these stabilizing activities.[32,36,37] The TrA also has a coordinated link with the perineum and pelvic floor muscle function (see Chapter 23).[6,13,53,66,67] The "drawing-in" maneuver is used to activate the TrA voluntarily and, with training, produces the most independent activity of this muscle.[64,72] (See Chapter 16 for a description of this maneuver.)

### ● Focus on Evidence

It has been shown that activation and function in the TrA changes (delayed and more phasic) in patients with low back pain, possibly indicating less effective stabilizing action.[29,32] Studies have also documented that training this muscle for postural control and stability improves the long-term outcome.[25]

*Multifidus and erector spinae muscles (Fig. 14.7).* The erector spinae muscles are the long, multisegmental extensors that begin as a large musculotendinous mass over the sacral and lower lumbar vertebrae. They are impor-

tant global guy wires for controlling the trunk against postural perturbations. The multifasciculed multifidi muscle group has a high distribution of type I fibers and large capillary network, emphasizing its role as a tonic stabilizer. Its segmental attachments are able to control movement of the spinal segments as well as increase spinal stiffness. The multifidus, along with the erector spinae are encased by the posterior and middle layers of the lumbodorsal fascia (see Fig. 14.5), so bulk and muscle contraction increases tension on the fascia, adding to the stabilizing function of the fascia (see below for a description of this mechanism). In patients with low back impairment, the fibers of the multifidi quickly atrophy at the spinal segment[26]; and a moth-eaten appearance has been reported in patients undergoing surgery for lumbar disk disease.[63]

### ● Focus on Evidence

Evidence supports the idea that training with specific exercises increases the function of the multifidi as well as the erector spinae in general.[14,25,27]

*Thoracolumbar (lumbodorsal) fascia.* The thoracolumbar fascia is an extensive fascial system in the back that consists of several layers.[7,8,21-23,50] It surrounds the erector

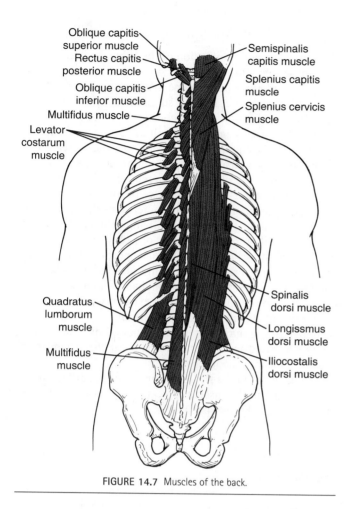

FIGURE 14.7 Muscles of the back.

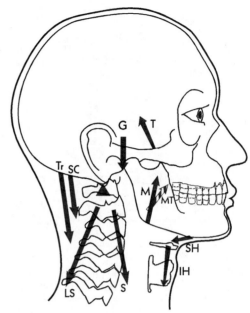

FIGURE 14.8 Head balance on the cervical spine. The posterior cervical muscles (trapezius and semispinalis capitis) counter the weight of the head. The mandibular elevating muscles (masseter, temporalis, medial pterygoid) maintain jaw elevation opposing the mandibular depression force of gravity and tension in the anterior throat muscles (suprahyoid and infrahyoid groups). The scalene and levator muscles stabilize against the posterior and anterior translatory forces on the cervical vertebrae. Tr, trapezius; SC, semispinalis capitis; M, masseter; T, temporalis; MT, medial pterygoid; SH, suprahyoid; IH, infrahyoid; S, scalene; LS, levator scapulae; G, center of gravity; ▲, axis of motion.

spinae, multifidi, and quadratus lumborum, thus providing support to these muscles when they contract[22] (see Fig. 14.5). Increased bulk in these muscles increases tension in the fascia, perhaps contributing the stabilizing function of these muscles.

The aponeurosis of the latissimus dorsi and fibers from the serratus posterior inferior, internal oblique, and transverse abdominis muscles blend together at the lateral raphe of the thoracolumbar fascia, so contraction in these muscles increases tension through the angled fascia, providing stabilizing forces for the lumbar spine[22] (see Fig. 14.6).

### Muscle Control in the Cervical Spine
The fulcrum of the head on the spine is through the occipital/atlas joints. The center of gravity of the head is anterior to the joint axis and therefore has a flexion moment. The weight of the head is counterbalanced by the cervical extensor muscles (upper trapezius and cervical erector spinae). Tension and fatigue in these muscles, as well as in the levator scapulae (which supports the posture of the scapulae), is experienced by most people who experience postural stress to the head and neck (Fig. 14.8). The posi-

tion of the mandible and the tension in the muscles of mastication are influenced by the postural relationship between the cervical spine and head.

***Mandible.*** The mandible is movable structure that is maintained in its resting position with the jaw partially closed through action of the mandibular elevators (masseter, temporalis, and internal pterygoid muscles).

***Suprahyoid and infrahyoid group.*** The anterior throat muscles assist with swallowing and balancing the jaw against the muscles of mastication. These muscles also function to flex the neck when rising from the supine position. With a forward head posture, they, along with the longus colli, tend to be stretched and weak so the person lifts the head with the sternocleidomastoid (SCM) muscles.

***Rectus capitis anterior and lateralis, longus colli, and longus capitis (Fig. 14.9).*** The deep craniocervical flexor muscles have segmental attachments and provide dynamic support to the cervical spine and head.[24] The longus colli is important in the action of axial extension (retraction) and works with the SCM for cervical flexion. Without the seg-

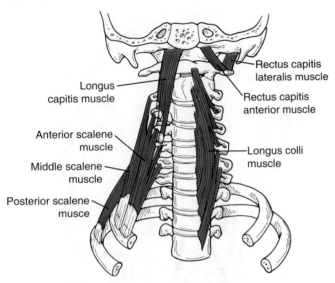

Longus capitis muscle

Anterior scalene muscle

Middle scalene muscle

Posterior scalene musce

Rectus capitis lateralis muscle

Rectus capitis anterior muscle

Longus colli muscle

FIGURE 14.9 Deep core musculature in the cervical spine: rectus capitis anterior and lateralis, longus colli, longus capitis, and scalene muscles.

mental influence of the longus colli, the SCM would cause increased cervical lordosis when attempting flexion.[5]

**Multifidus.** With its segmental attachments, the multifidus is thought to have a core stabilizing function in the cervical spine similar to its function in the lumbar region (see Fig. 14.7).[24]

### Neurological Control: Influence on Stability

The muscles of the neck and trunk are activated and controlled by the nervous system, which is influenced by peripheral and central mechanisms in response to fluctuating forces and activities. Basically, the nervous system coordinates the response of muscles to expected and unexpected forces at the right time and by the right amount by modulating stiffness and movement to match the various imposed forces.[3,15,32]

**Feedforward control and spinal stability.** The central nervous system activates the trunk muscles in anticipation of the load imposed by limb movement to maintain stability in the spine.[37] Research has demonstrated that there are feedforward mechanisms that activate postural responses of all trunk muscles preceding activity in muscles that move the extremities[32,35,37] and that anticipatory activation of the transversus abdominis and deep fibers of the multifidus is independent of the direction or speed of the postural disturbance.[30,31,36,51] The more superficial trunk muscles vary in response depending on the direction of arm and leg movement, reflective of their postural guy wire function, which controls displacement of the center of mass when the body changes configuration.[32,37] There are reported differences in patterns of muscle recruitment in patients with low back pain with delayed recruitment of the transversus abdominis in all movement directions and delayed recruitment of the rectus abdominis, erector spinae, and oblique abdominal muscles specific to the direction of movement compared to healthy subjects.[33]

## Effects of Limb Motion on Spinal Stability

Without adequate stabilization of the spine, contraction of the limb-girdle musculature transmits forces proximally and causes motions of the spine that place excessive stresses on spinal structures and the supporting soft tissue. For example, stabilization of the pelvis and lumbar spine by the abdominal muscles against the pull of the iliopsoas muscle is necessary during active hip flexion to avoid increased lumbar lordosis and anterior shearing of the vertebrae. Stabilization of the ribs by the intercostal and abdominal muscles is necessary for an effective pushing force from the pectoralis major and serratus anterior muscles.

Localized fatigue in the stabilizing spinal musculature may occur with repetitive activity or heavy exertion. There is a greater chance of injury in the supporting structures of the spine when the stabilizing muscles fatigue. Marras and Granata[47] reported significant changes in motion patterns between the spine and lower extremity joints as well as significant changes in muscle recruitment patterns with repetitive lifting during an extended period of time, resulting in decreased spinal compression but increased anterior/posterior shear in the lumbar spine.

Imbalances in the flexibility and strength of the hip, shoulder, and neck musculature cause asymmetrical forces on the spine and affect posture.

## Effects of Breathing on Posture and Stability

Inspiration and thoracic spine extension elevate the rib cage and align the spine. The intercostal muscles function as postural muscles to stabilize and move the ribs; and they act as a dynamic membrane between the ribs to prevent sucking in and blowing out of the soft tissue with the pressure changes during respiration.[4] The stabilizing function of the TrA also works in conjunction with the diaphragm in a feedforward response to rapid arm motions. Contraction of the diaphragm and increased intra-abdominal pressure occur prior to rapid arm movement, irrespective of the phase of respiration or the direction of the arm motion.[32,34] The tonic activities of the TrA and diaphragm are modulated to meet respiratory demands during both inspiration and expiration and provide stability to the spine when there are repetitive limb movements.[28,29]

### Intra-abdominal Pressure and the Valsalva Maneuver

During the Valsalva maneuver, contraction of the TrA, IO, and EO muscles increase intra-abdominal pressure.[11] Contraction of the TrA alone pushes the abdominal contents up against the diaphragm; therefore, to complete the enclosed chamber, the diaphragm and pelvic floor muscles contract in synchrony with the TrA.[53] This mechanism has several effects that improve spinal stability: The increased pressure in the enclosed chamber unloads the compressive forces on the spine (Fig. 14.10). It also increases the stabilizing effect by pushing out against the abdominal muscles, increasing their length–tension relationship and tension on the thoracolumbar fascia (Fig. 14.11).[23]

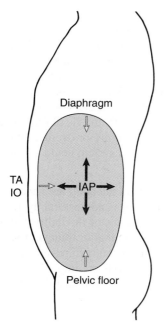

FIGURE 14.10 Coordinated contraction of the transversus abdominis, diaphragm, and pelvic floor musculature increases intra-abdominal pressure, which unloads the spine as well as provides stability.

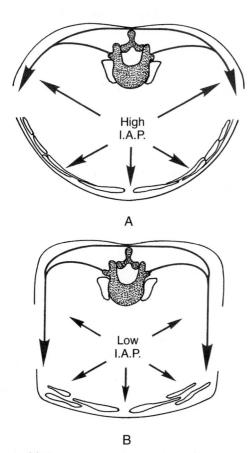

FIGURE 14.11 (A) Increased intra-abdominal pressure (IAP) pushes outward against the transversus abdominis and internal obliques, creating increased tension on the thoracolumbar fascia, resulting in improved spinal stability. (B) Reduced pressure decreases the stabilizing effect. *(Adapted from Gracovetsky,[23] p. 114, with permission.)*

The Valsalva maneuver is a technique frequently used by individuals lifting heavy loads and potentially has cardiovascular risks (see Chapter 6), so it is recommended that individuals be taught to exhale while maintaining the abdominal contractions to decrease the risks. In addition, Hodges et al.[34] found that if a static expulsive effort is maintained (holding the breath while contracting the abdominal muscles), activation of the transverse abdominis is delayed. Because activation of the transversus abdominis is necessary for segmental spinal stability, expiration during exertion reinforces this stabilizing function.

## IMPAIRED POSTURE

Impaired posture is classified in *The Guide to Physical Therapist Practice*, second edition, under the Musculoskeletal Diagnostic Classification Pattern B: Impaired Posture.[1]

## ● ETIOLOGY OF PAIN

### Effect of Mechanical Stress

The ligaments, facet capsules, periosteum of the vertebrae, muscles, anterior dura mater, dural sleeves, epidural areolar adipose tissue, and walls of blood vessels are innervated and responsive to nociceptive stimuli.[44] Mechanical stress to pain-sensitive structures, such as sustained stretch to ligaments or joint capsules or compression of blood vessels, causes distention or compression of the nerve endings, which leads to the experience of pain. This type of stimulus occurs in the absence of an inflammatory reaction. It is not a pathological problem but a mechanical one because signs of acute inflammation with constant pain are not present. Relieving the stress to the pain-sensitive structure relieves the pain stimulus, and the person no longer experiences pain. If the mechanical stresses exceed the supporting capabilities of the tissues, breakdown ensues. If it occurs without adequate healing, musculoskeletal disorders or overuse syndromes with inflammation and pain affect function without an apparent injury (see Chapter 10). Relieving the mechanical stress (i.e., correcting the posture) along with decreasing the inflammation is important.

### Effect of Impaired Postural Support from Trunk Muscles

Little muscle activity is required to maintain upright posture; but with total relaxation of muscles, the spinal curves become exaggerated, and passive structural support is called on to maintain the posture. When there is continued end-range loading, strain occurs with creep and fluid redistribution in the supporting tissues, making them vulnerable to injury.[70]

Continual exaggeration of the curves leads to postural impairment and muscle strength and flexibility imbalances as well as other soft tissue restrictions or hypermobility. Muscles that are habitually kept in a stretched position tend to test weaker because of a shift in the length-tension curve; this is known as *stretch weakness*.[42] Muscles kept in a habitually shortened position tend to lose their elasticity. These muscles test strong only in the shortened position but become weak as they are lengthened.[20] This is known as *tight weakness*.[20]

## Effect of Impaired Muscle Endurance

Endurance in muscles is necessary to maintain postural control. Sustained postures require continual, small adaptations in the stabilizing muscles to support the trunk against fluctuating forces. Large repetitive motions also require muscles to respond so as to control the activity. In either case, as the muscles fatigue, the mechanics of performance change and the load is shifted to the inert tissues supporting the spine at the end ranges.[69] As described above, with poor muscular support and a sustained load on the inert supporting tissues, creep and distention occur, causing mechanical stress. In addition, injuries occur more frequently after a lot of repetitive activity or long periods of work and play when there is muscle fatigue.

## Pain Syndromes Related to Impaired Posture

### Postural Fault and the Postural Pain Syndrome

A *postural fault* is a posture that deviates from normal alignment but has no structural limitations. *Postural pain syndrome* refers to the pain that results from mechanical stress when a person maintains a faulty posture for a prolonged period; the pain is usually relieved with activity. There are no abnormalities in muscle strength or flexibility; but if the faulty posture continues, strength and flexibility imbalances eventually develop.

### Postural Dysfunction

*Postural dysfunction* differs from the postural pain syndrome in that adaptive shortening of soft tissues and muscle weakness are involved. The cause may be prolonged poor postural habits, or it may be a result of contractures and adhesions formed during the healing of tissues after trauma or surgery. Stress to the shortened structures causes pain. In addition, strength and flexibility imbalances may predispose the area to injury or overuse syndromes that a normal musculoskeletal system could sustain.

### Postural Habits

Good postural habits in the adult are necessary to avoid postural pain syndromes and postural dysfunction. Also, careful follow-up in terms of flexibility and posture training exercises is important after trauma or surgery to prevent impairments from contractures and adhesions. In the child, good postural habits are important to avoid abnormal stresses on growing bones and adaptive changes in muscle and soft tissue.

## ● COMMON FAULTY POSTURES: CHARACTERISTICS AND IMPAIRMENTS

The head, neck, thorax, lumbar spine, and pelvis are all interrelated; and deviations in one region affect the other areas. In this section, the lumbopelvic and cervicothoracic regions and typical muscle length–strength impairments for each region are described separately for clarity of presentation.

### Pelvic and Lumbar Region

#### Lordotic Posture

Lordotic posture (Fig. 14.12A) is characterized by an increase in the lumbosacral angle (the angle that the superior

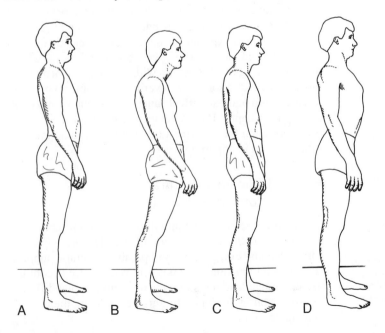

A   B   C   D

FIGURE 14.12  (*A*) Lordotic posture characterized by an increase in the lumbosacral angle, increased lumbar lordosis, increased anterior tilting of the pelvis, and hip flexion. (*B*) Relaxed or slouched posture characterized by excessive shifting of the pelvic segment anteriorly, resulting in hip extension, and shifting of the thoracic segment posteriorly, resulting in flexion of the thorax on the upper lumbar spine. A compensatory increased thoracic kyphosis and forward head placement are also seen. (*C*) Flat low-back posture characterized by a decreased lumbosacral angle, decreased lumbar lordosis, and posterior tilting of the pelvis. (*D*) Flat upper back and cervical spine characterized by a decrease in the thoracic curve, depressed scapulae, depressed clavicle, and an exaggeration of axial extension (flexion of the occiput on the atlas and flattening of the cervical lordosis).

border of the first sacral vertebral body makes with the horizontal, which optimally is 30°), an increase in lumbar lordosis, and an increase in the anterior pelvic tilt and hip flexion.[9] It is often seen with increased thoracic kyphosis and forward head and is called *kypholordotic posture.*[42]

**Potential Muscle Impairments**

● Mobility impairment in the hip flexor muscles (iliopsoas, tensor fasciae latae, rectus femoris) and lumbar extensor muscles (erector spinae)
● Impaired muscle performance due to stretched and weak abdominal muscles (rectus abdominis, internal and external obliques, and transversus abdominis)

**Potential Sources of Symptoms**

● Stress to the anterior longitudinal ligament.
● Narrowing of the posterior disk space and narrowing of the intervertebral foramen. This may compress the dura and blood vessels of the related nerve root or the nerve root itself, especially if there are degenerative changes in the vertebra or disk.[9]
● Approximation of the articular facets. The facets may become weight bearing, which may cause synovial irritation and joint inflammation.

**Common Causes**
Sustained faulty posture, pregnancy, obesity, and weak abdominal muscles are common causes.

## Relaxed or Slouched Posture
The relaxed or slouched posture (Fig. 14.12B) is also called *swayback.*[42] The amount of pelvic tilting is variable, but usually there is a shifting of the entire pelvic segment anteriorly, resulting in hip extension, and shifting of the thoracic segment posteriorly, resulting in flexion of the thorax on the upper lumbar spine. This results in increased lordosis in the lower lumbar region, increased kyphosis in the thoracic region, and usually a forward head. The position of the mid and upper lumbar spine depends on the amount of displacement of the thorax. When standing for prolonged periods, the person usually assumes an asymmetrical stance in which most of the weight is borne on one lower extremity with pelvic drop (lateral tilt) and hip abduction on the unweighted side. This affects frontal plane symmetry.

**Potential Muscle Impairments**

● Mobility impairment in the upper abdominal muscles (upper segments of the rectus abdominis and obliques), internal intercostal, hip extensor, and lower lumbar extensor muscles and related fascia
● Impaired muscle performance due to stretched and weak lower abdominal muscles (lower segments of the rectus abdominis and obliques), extensor muscles of the lower thoracic region, and hip flexor muscles

**Potential Sources of Symptoms**

● Stress to the iliofemoral ligaments, the anterior longitudinal ligament of the lower lumbar spine, and the

posterior longitudinal ligament of the upper lumbar and thoracic spine. With asymmetrical postures, there is also stress to the iliotibial band on the side of the elevated hip. Other frontal plane asymmetries may also be present and are described in the following section.
● Narrowing of the intervertebral foramen in the lower lumbar spine that may compress the blood vessels, dura, and nerve roots, especially with arthritic conditions.
● Approximation of articular facets in the lower lumbar spine.

**Common Causes**
As the name implies, this is a relaxed posture in which the muscles are not used to provide support. The person yields fully to the effects of gravity, and only the passive structures at the end of each joint range (e.g., ligaments, joint capsules, bony approximation) provide stability. Causes may be attitudinal (the person feels comfortable when slouching), fatigue (seen when required to stand for extended periods), or muscle weakness (the weakness may be the cause or the effect of the posture). A poorly designed exercise program—one that emphasizes thoracic flexion without balancing strength with other appropriate exercises and postural training—may perpetuate these impairments.

## Flat Low-Back Posture
Flat low-back posture (Fig. 14.12C) is characterized by a decreased lumbosacral angle, decreased lumbar lordosis, hip extension, and posterior tilting of the pelvis.

**Potential Muscle Impairments**

● Mobility impairment in the trunk flexor (rectus abdominis, intercostals) and hip extensor muscles
● Impaired muscle performance due to stretched and weak lumbar extensor and possibly hip flexor muscles

**Potential Sources of Symptoms**

● Lack of the normal physiological lumbar curve, which reduces the shock-absorbing effect of the lumbar region and predisposes the person to injury
● Stress to the posterior longitudinal ligament
● Increase of the posterior disk space, which allows the nucleus pulposus to imbibe extra fluid and, under certain circumstances, may protrude posteriorly when the person attempts extension

**Common Causes**
Continued slouching or flexing in sitting or standing postures; overemphasis on flexion exercises in general exercise programs

## Cervical and Thoracic Region

### Round Back (Increased Kyphosis) with Forward Head
The round back with forward head posture (see Fig. 14.12B) is characterized by an increased thoracic curve, protracted scapulae (round shoulders), and forward (protracted) head. A *forward head* involves increased flexion of the lower cervical and the upper thoracic regions, increased

extension of the upper cervical vertebra, and extension of the occiput on C1. There also may be temporomandibular joint dysfunction with retrusion of the mandible.

### Potential Muscle Impairments

◉ Mobility impairment in the muscles of the anterior thorax (intercostal muscles), muscles of the upper extremity originating on the thorax (pectoralis major and minor, latissimus dorsi, serratus anterior), muscles of the cervical spine and head that attached to the scapula and upper thorax (levator scapulae, sternocleidomastoid, scalene, upper trapezius), and muscles of the suboccipital region (rectus capitis posterior major and minor, obliquus capitis inferior and superior).

◉ Impaired muscle performance due to stretched and weak lower cervical and upper thoracic erector spinae and scapular retractor muscles (rhomboids, middle trapezius), anterior throat muscles (suprahyoid and infrahyoid muscles), and capital flexors (rectus capitis anterior and lateralis, superior oblique longus colli, longus capitis).

◉ With temporomandibular joint symptoms, the muscles of mastication may have increased tension (pterygoid, masseter, temporalis muscles).

### Potential Sources of Symptoms

◉ Stress to the anterior longitudinal ligament in the upper cervical spine and posterior longitudinal ligament in the lower cervical and thoracic spine

◉ Fatigue of the thoracic erector spinae and scapular retractor muscles

◉ Irritation of facet joints in the upper cervical spine

◉ Narrowing of the intervertebral foramina in the upper cervical region, which may impinge on the blood vessels and nerve roots, especially if there are degenerative changes

◉ Impingement on the neurovascular bundle from anterior scalene or pectoralis minor muscle tightness (see Thoracic Outlet Syndrome in Chapter 13)

◉ Strain on the neurovascular structures of the thoracic outlet from scapular protraction[38]

◉ Impingement of the cervical plexus from levator scapulae muscle tightness

◉ Impingement on the greater occipital nerves from a tight or tense upper trapezius muscle, leading to tension headaches

◉ Temporomandibular joint pain from faulty head, neck, and mandibular alignment and associated facial muscle tension

◉ Lower cervical disk lesions from the faulty flexed posture

### Common Causes

The effects of gravity, slouching, and poor ergonomic alignment in the work or home environment. Occupational or functional postures requiring leaning forward or tipping the head backward for extended periods, faulty sitting postures such as working at an improperly placed computer keyboard or screen, relaxed postures, or the end result of a faulty pelvic and lumbar spine posture are common causes of forward head posture. Causes are similar to the relaxed lumbar posture or the flat low-back posture, where there is continued slouching, and overemphasis on flexion exercises in general exercise programs.

### Flat Upper Back and Neck Posture

The flat upper back and neck posture (Fig. 14.12D) is characterized by a decrease in the thoracic curve, depressed scapulae, depressed clavicles, and decreased cervical lordosis with increased flexion of the occiput on atlas. It is associated with an exaggerated military posture but is not a common postural deviation. There may be temporomandibular joint dysfunction with protraction of the mandible.

### Potential Muscle Impairments

◉ Mobility impairment in the anterior neck muscles, thoracic erector spinae and scapular retractors, and potentially restricted scapular movement, which decreases the freedom of shoulder elevation

◉ Impaired muscle performance in the scapular protractor and intercostal muscles of the anterior thorax

### Potential Sources of Symptoms

◉ Fatigue of muscles required to maintain the posture

◉ Compression of the neurovascular bundle in the thoracic outlet between the clavicle and ribs

◉ Temporomandibular joint pain and occlusive changes.

◉ Decrease in the shock-absorbing function of the kypholordotic curvature, which may predispose the neck to injury.

### Common Cause

As noted above, this is not a common postural deviation and occurs primarily with exaggeration of the military posture.

### Scoliosis

Scoliosis usually involves the thoracic and lumbar regions. Typically, in right-handed individuals, there is a mild right thoracic, left lumbar S-curve, or a mild left thoracolumbar C-curve. There may be asymmetry in the hips, pelvis, and lower extremities.

*Structural scoliosis* involves an irreversible lateral curvature with fixed rotation of the vertebrae (Fig. 14.13A). Rotation of the vertebral bodies is toward the convexity of the curve. In the thoracic spine, the ribs rotate with the vertebrae so there is prominence of the ribs posteriorly on the side of the spinal convexity and prominence anteriorly on the side of the concavity. A posterior rib hump is detected on forward bending in structural scoliosis (Fig. 14.13B).[45]

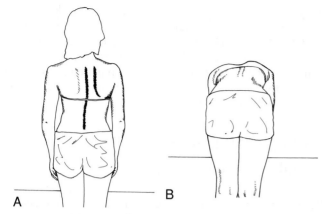

FIGURE 14.13 (A) Mild right thoracic left lumbar structural scoliosis with prominence of the right scapula. (B) Forward bending produces a slight posterior rib hump, indicating fixed rotation of the vertebrae and rib cage.

*Nonstructural scoliosis* is reversible and can be changed with forward or side bending and with positional changes such as lying supine, realignment of the pelvis by correction of a leg-length discrepancy, or with muscle contractions. It is also called *functional* or *postural scoliosis*.

**Potential Muscle Impairments**

- Mobility impairment in structures on the concave side of the curves.
- Impaired muscle performance due to stretch and weakness in the musculature on the convex side of the curves.
- If one hip is adducted, the adductor muscles on that side have decreased flexibility and the abductor muscles are stretched and weak. The opposite occurs on the contralateral extremity.[42]
- With advanced structural scoliosis, cardiopulmonary impairment may restrict function.

**Potential Sources of Symptoms**

- Muscle fatigue and ligamentous strain on the side of the convexity
- Nerve root irritation on the side on the concavity

**Common Causes: Structural Scoliosis**
Neuromuscular diseases or disorders (e.g., cerebral palsy, spinal cord injury, progressive neurological or muscular diseases), osteopathic disorders (e.g., hemivertebra, osteomalacia, rickets, fracture), and idiopathic disorders in which the cause is unknown are common causes of structural scoliosis.

**Common Causes: Nonstructural Scoliosis**
Leg-length discrepancy (structural or functional), muscle guarding or spasm from a painful stimuli in the back or neck, and habitual or asymmetrical postures are common causes of nonstructural scoliosis.

## Frontal Plane Deviations from Lower Extremity Asymmetries

Any lower extremity inequality has an effect on the pelvis that, in turn, affects the spinal column and structures supporting it.[17] When dealing with spinal posture, it is imperative to assess lower extremity alignment, symmetry, foot posture, ROM, muscle flexibility, and strength. See Chapters 20 through 22 for principles, procedures, and techniques for treating the hip, knee, ankle, and foot. Frontal plane deviations may also be seen with faulty postural habits such as perpetually standing with a pelvic drop on one side as frequently seen with slouched postures. This may result in muscle imbalances in the hip and spine and an apparent leg-length discrepancy.

**Characteristic Deviations when Standing with Weight Equally Distributed to Both Lower Extremities (Fig.14.14)**
An elevated ilium on the long leg (LL) side and lowered on the short leg (SL) side is the characteristic deviation.

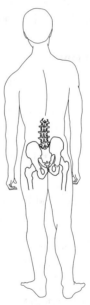

FIGURE 14.14 Frontal plane asymmetries. Pictured is an individual with a long leg and elevated ilium on the right side. Typically, hip adduction, vertical sacroiliac (SI) joint, side bending toward and rotation opposite that of the lumbar spine, and compensations in thoracic and cervical spine are seen on the long-leg side.

- This puts the LL side in hip adduction with greater shear stress and the SL side in hip abduction with greater compression stress.
- The sacroiliac (SI) joint on the LL side is more vertical with greater shear stress; on the SL side it is more horizontal with greater compression stress.
- Side bending of the lumbar spine toward the LL side coupled with rotation in the opposite direction.

● This compresses the intervertebral disk on the LL side and distracts the disk on the SL side; it also causes torsional stress.
● There is extension and compression of the lumbar facets on the LL side (concave portion of the curve) and flexion and distraction of the lumbar facets on the SL side (convex portion of the curve).
● There is narrowing of the intervertebral foramina on the LL side.
● The thoracic and cervical spine has compensatory scoliosis in the opposite direction.

**Potential Muscle Impairments**

● Mobility impairment from decreased flexibility in the hip adductors on the LL side and abductors on the SL side. There may also be asymmetrical differences in the iliopsoas, quadratus lumborum, piriformis, erector spinae, and multifidus muscles, with those on the concave side of the curve or the LL side having decreased flexibility.
● Impaired muscle performance from stretched and weakened muscles that typically includes hip adductors on the SL side, abductors on the LL side, and in general muscles on the convex side of the curve.

**Potential Sources of Symptoms**

● Greater shear forces occur in the hip and SI joints on the LL side, which increases stress in the supporting ligaments and decreases the load-bearing surface in the joint. Degenerative changes occur more frequently in hips on the LL side.[16]
● Stenosis in the lumbar intervertebral foramina on the LL side may cause vascular congestion or nerve root irritation.
● Lumbar facet compression and irritation on the LL side.
● Disk breakdown from torsional and asymmetrical forces.
● Muscle tension, fatigue, or spasm in response to asymmetrical loading and response.
● Lower extremity overuse syndromes.

**Common Causes**
Asymmetry in the lower extremities may result from structural or functional deviations at the hip, knee, ankle, or foot. Common functional problems include unilateral flat foot and imbalances in the flexibility of muscles. The resulting asymmetrical ground reaction forces transmitted to the pelvis and back may lead to tissue breakdown and overuse, particularly as a person ages, becomes overweight, or is generally deconditioned from inactivity.[62]

## MANAGEMENT OF IMPAIRED POSTURE

Faulty posture underlies many spinal and extremity disorders. Often by simply correcting the underlying postural stresses the primary symptoms can be minimized or even alleviated. Because of this the following guidelines may become a part of many of the interventions. Headaches are often a symptom of faulty posture; and management guidelines for tension or cervical headaches are described at the end of this section. Exercises for use with postural impairments and headaches related to impaired posture are referred to in this section and are described in detail in the respective chapters that follow.

## ● GENERAL MANAGEMENT GUIDELINES

Before developing a plan of care and selecting interventions for management, evaluate the findings from the examination of the patient, including the history, review of systems, and specific tests and measures, and document the findings.

● Postural alignment (sitting and standing), balance, and gait
● ROM, joint mobility, and flexibility
● Muscular strength and endurance for repetitions and holding
● Ergonomic assessment if indicated
● Body mechanics
● Cardiopulmonary endurance/aerobic capacity, breathing pattern

Common impairments and a summary of the information that follows on management of patients with impaired posture are summarized in Box 14.1.

### Postural Alignment: Proprioception and Control

Initially, good alignment may be prevented because of restricted mobility of muscle or connective tissue or malalignment of a vertebral segment, but developing patient awareness of balanced posture and its effects should begin as soon as possible in the treatment program in conjunction with stretching and muscle-training maneuvers.

#### Active Control of Spinal Movement
Isolate each body segment and train the patient how to move that segment. If one region is out of alignment, it is likely that there are compensatory deviations in the alignment throughout the spine. Therefore, total posture correction, including lower extremity alignment, should be emphasized. Direct the patient's attention to the feel of proper movement and muscle contraction and relaxation. It may be useful to have the patient assume an extreme corrected posture, then ease away from the extreme toward midposition, and finally hold the corrected posture. Use reinforcement techniques such as:

● *Verbal reinforcement.* As you interact with the patient, frequently interpret the sensations of muscle contraction and spinal positions that he or she should be feeling.

## BOX 14.1
## MANAGEMENT GUIDELINES—Impaired Posture

### Impairments
- Pain (including headaches) from mechanical stress to sensitive structures and from muscle tension
- Mobility impairment from muscle, joint, or fascial restrictions
- Impaired muscle performance associated with an imbalance in muscle length and strength between antagonistic muscle groups
- Impaired muscle performance associated with poor muscular endurance
- Insufficient postural control of stabilizing muscles
- Decreased cardiopulmonary endurance
- Altered kinesthetic sense of posture associated with poor neuromuscular control and prolonged faulty postural habits
- Lack of knowledge of healthy spinal control and mechanics

| Plan of Care | Intervention |
|---|---|
| 1. Develop awareness and control of spinal alignment in a variety of positions | 1. Teach procedures to develop active control of spinal and extremity movement |
| 2. Learn awareness between posture and pain | 2. Demonstrate relationship of symptoms with sustained or repetitive postures |
| 3. Increase mobility in restricting muscles, joints, fascia | 3. Manual stretching and joint mobilization; teach self-stretching |
| 4. Develop neuromuscular control, strength, and endurance in postural and extremity muscles | 4. Stabilization exercises; progress repetitions and challenge; progress to dynamic strengthening exercises |
| 5. Learn safe body mechanics | 5. Functional exercises to prepare for safe mechanics |
| 6. Learn to correct stress provoking postures/activities | 6. Adapt work, home, recreational environment |
| 7. Learn stress management/relaxation | 7. Relaxation exercises and postural stress relief |
| 8. Improve aerobic capacity | 8. Implement and progress an aerobic exercise program |
| 9. Develop healthy exercise habits for self-maintenance | 9. Integration of a fitness program, regular exercise and safe body mechanics into daily life |

- *Visual reinforcement.* Use mirrors so the patient can see how he or she looks, what it takes to assume correct alignment, and then how it feels when properly aligned. Verbally reinforce what the patient sees.
- *Tactile reinforcement.* Help the patient position the head and trunk in correct alignment and touch the muscles that need to contract to move and hold the parts in place.

### Axial Extension (Cervical Retraction) to Decrease a Forward Head Posture

*Patient position and procedure:* Sitting or standing, with arms relaxed at the side. Lightly touch above the lip under the nose and ask the patient to lift the head up and away (Fig. 14.15A). Verbally reinforce the correct movement of tucking the chin in and straightening the spine, and draw attention to the way it feels. Have the patient move to the extreme of the correct posture and then return to midline.

### Scapular Retraction

*Patient position and procedure:* Sitting or standing. For tactile and proprioceptive cues, gently resist movement of the inferior angle of the scapulae and ask the patient to pinch them together (retraction). Suggest that the patient imagine "holding a quarter between the shoulder blades." The patient should not extend the shoulders or elevate the scapulae (Fig. 14.15B).

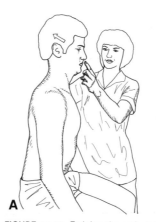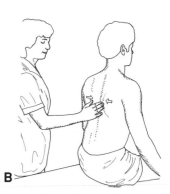

FIGURE 14.15 Training the patient to correct (*A*) forward-head posture and (*B*) protracted scapulae.

### Pelvic Tilt and Neutral Spine

*Patient position and procedure:* Sitting, then standing with the back against a wall. Teach the patient to roll the pelvis forward and backward to isolate an anterior and posterior pelvic tilt. After the patient has learned to isolate the movement, instruct him or her to practice control of the pelvis and lumbar spine by moving from extreme lordosis to extreme flat back and then assume mild lordosis. Identify the mid position as the "neutral spine" so the patient becomes familiar with the term. Show that the hand should be able to easily slip between the back and the wall and that he or she can then feel the back with one side of the hand and the wall with the other side. If the patient has difficulty tilting the pelvis, suggest that he or she imagine that the pelvis is a bushel basket with a rounded bottom and the waist is the rim of the basket. Have the patient then imagine and practice tipping the basket forward and backward and then finding the neutral spine position.

### Thoracic Spine

*Patient position and procedure:* Standing. The position of the thorax affects the posture of the lumbar spine and pelvis; consequently, the feel of thoracic movement is incorporated in posture training for the lumbar spine. As the patient assumes a mildly lordotic posture, have him or her breathe in and lift the rib cage (extension). Guide him or her to a balanced posture, not an extremely extended posture. Standing with the back against a wall (as in the pelvic tilt training above) encourages thoracic extension.

### Total Spinal Movement and Control

*Patient position and procedure:* Sitting. Instruct the patient to curl the entire spine by first flexing the neck, then the thorax, and then the lumbar spine. Give cues for unrolling by first touching the lumbar spine as the patient extends it, then the thoracic spine as he or she extends it and takes in a breath to elevate the rib cage. Then direct attention to adducting the scapulae while you gently resist the motion and then lifting the head in axial extension while you give slight pressure against the upper lip (see Fig. 14.15). Verbally and visually reinforce the correct posture when it is obtained.

## Relationship of Impaired Posture and Pain

Have the patient assume the faulty posture and wait. When he or she begins to feel discomfort, point out the posture and then instruct how to correct it and notice the feeling of relief. Many patients do not accept such a simple relationship between stress and pain, so draw their attention to noticing what posture they are in (including when at work, home, driving/riding in a car, or in bed) when their symptoms develop and how they can control the discomfort with the techniques they have been taught.

### Reinforcement

It is not possible for a person always to maintain good posture. Therefore, to reinforce proper performance, teach the patient to use cues throughout the day to check posture. For example, instruct the patient to check the posture every time he or she walks past a mirror, waits at a red traffic light while driving a car, sits down for a meal, enters a room, or begins talking with someone. Find out what daily routines the patient has that could be used for reinforcement or reminders; instruct the patient to practice and report the results. Provide positive feedback as the patient becomes actively involved in the relearning process.

### Postural Support

If necessary, provide external support with a postural splint or tape to prevent the extreme posture of round shoulders and protracted scapulae. These supports help train correct muscle functioning by acting as a reminder for the patient to assume correct posture when he or she slouches. Also, by preventing the position of stretch from occurring, stretch weakness can be corrected. These devices should be used only on a temporary basis for training so the patient does not become dependent on them.

## Joint, Muscle, and Connective Tissue Mobility Impairments

Common muscle imbalances in length and strength were described in the previous section on impaired postures. Stretching procedures and joint mobilization techniques are described in Chapters 4 and 5, respectively; and selected manual stretching and mobilization with movement techniques are described in the chapters for each region of the body (see Chapters 16 through 22). Although any structure could be involved, particularly following an injury or pathological condition, most typically seen are the muscle flexibility impairments identified in Box 14.2. Included are references for self-stretching/flexibility exercises for each muscle group. Specific instructions and precautions are

---

> **BOX 14.2   Stretching Techniques for Common Mobility Impairments**
>
> - *Suboccipital region:* self-stretch with capital nodding (see Fig. 16.4 in Chapter 16)
> - *Levator scapulae:* self-stretch with scapular depression and cervical flexion and rotation to the opposite side (see Fig. 17.35 in Chapter 17)
> - *Scalenes:* self-stretch with axial extension, side bend neck opposite and then rotate neck toward side of restriction (see position Fig. 16.3 in Chapter 16)
> - *Pectoralis major and anterior thorax:* self-stretch with corner stretches (see Fig. 17.31 in Chapter 17) or lying supine on a foam roll placed longitudinally under the spine (see Fig. 16.1B in Chapter 16)
> - *Latissimus dorsi:* self-stretch lying supine on a foam roll, reach arms overhead (see Fig. 16.1A in Chapter 16)
> - *Lumbar and hip extensors:* self-stretch lying supine, bring knees to chest; or quadruped position, move buttocks back over the feet (see Figs. 16.7 and 16.8 in Chapter 16)
> - *Lumbar and hip flexors:* self-stretch with prone press-ups or standing back bends (see Fig. 16.9 in Chapter 16)
> - *Tensor fascia lata:* self-stretch either side-lying or standing. Extend, laterally rotate, then adduct the hip (see Figs. 20.16 and 20.17 in Chapter 20)
> - *Hamstring:* self-stretch with a straight-leg maneuver either lying supine or long-sitting (see Figs. 20.14 and 20.15 in Chapter 20)
> - *Gastrocsoleus (heel cords):* self-stretch in a forward stride position with the heel of the back leg maintained on the floor, or stand on an incline board or edge of a step (see Fig. 22.8 in Chapter 22)

| BOX 14.3 | Training and Strengthening Techniques for Common Muscle Impairments |
|---|---|

- Activate and learn control of the longus colli and deep capital flexors (see Figs. 16.18B and 16.38 in Chapter 16)
- Lower cervical extension (see Fig. 16.19 in Chapter 16)
- Scapular retraction and shoulder lateral rotation (see Fig. 16.24 in Chapter 16 and Figs. 17.45 and 17.46 in Chapter 17)
- Lumbar spinal stabilization (see Figs. 16.26 through 16.36 plus accompanying text in Chapter 16)
- Hip abduction; posterior gluteus medius (see Fig. 20.17 in Chapter 20 for position; lift leg for resistance)

described in the text accompanying the pictures in the respective chapters.

## Impaired Muscle Performance

Typically impaired posture muscles that support the body in sustained postures succumb to the effects of gravity, become less active,[58] and develop stretch weakness.[42] Strengthening alone does not correct this problem, so any exercises must be done in conjunction with posture training for control, as described earlier in this section. In addition, exercises for muscular endurance are necessary to prepare the muscles to function over an extended period of time. Finally, environmental adaptations must be made to minimize the stresses of sustained and repetitive postures. Muscles that typically demonstrate stretch weakness or poor postural endurance are identified in Box 14.3. In-depth descriptions of the exercises are in the chapters identified.

## Body Mechanics

Muscle strengthening for safe body mechanics includes not only strengthening specific muscles but also functional activities that prepare the body for specific stresses that it is required to do for a particular function, as identified in Box 14.4. Instruction in body mechanics is described in detail in Chapter 16 in the section Functional Training.

| BOX 14.4 | Functional Exercises in Preparation for Safe Body Mechanics |
|---|---|

- Upper extremity pulling and pushing (see Fig. 17.56 in Chapter 17)
- Wall slides—progress to squatting and squatting with lifting (see Fig. 20.24 in Chapter 20)
- Lunges—progress to lunges with lifting and with pushing and pulling (see Fig. 20.23 in Chapter 20)

## Stress Provoking Postures and Activities: Relief and Prevention

It is critical to help the patient adapt postures and activities that are performed on a sustained or repetitive basis at work, at home, recreationally, or socially if they are contributing to the postural stresses and musculoskeletal disorders.[57] It may be necessary to use a lumbar pillow for support or to modify the work environment (workstation) to relieve sustained stressful postures. There are many resources, such as the Occupational Safety and Health Administration (OSHA) web site and others (http://www.osha.gov/SLTC/ergonomics/index.html or http://ergo.human.cornell.edu/) with links that provide information on ergonomic assessment and adaptation to work environments to relieve postural stress and musculoskeletal disorders.

⬤ **Focus on Evidence**_____

*Supporting evidence*: There is strong evidence, documented in a 3-year prospective study of 632 newly hired computer users, that a computer workstation may be the source of symptoms if the chair, desk, keyboard, mouse, and monitor are improperly positioned for the individual.[19,46] There is also mixed evidence, summarized in a systematic study of the literature on the relationship of posture and repetitive stresses in the work environment, regarding the development of low back pain.[73]

## Stress Management/Relaxation

A component of the educational process is to teach the individual how to relax tense muscles and relieve postural stress. Muscle relaxation techniques can be incorporated throughout the day to relieve postural stress, and conscious relaxation training increases patient awareness and control over tension in the muscles.

N O T E : These techniques are not appropriate for managing acute pain due to inflammation, joint swelling, or disk derangements.

### Muscle Relaxation Techniques

Whenever discomfort develops from maintaining a constant posture or from sustaining muscle contractions for a period of time, active ROM in the opposite direction aids in taking stress off supporting structures, promoting circulation, and maintaining flexibility. All motions are performed slowly, through the full range, with the patient paying particular attention to the feel of the muscles. Repeat each motion several times.

### Cervical and Upper Thoracic Region

*Patient position and procedure:* Sitting with the arms resting comfortably on the lap, or standing. Instruct the patient to:

- Bend the neck forward and backward. (Backward bending is contraindicated with symptoms of nerve root compression.)

- Side bend the head in each direction; then rotate the head in each direction.
- Roll the shoulders; protract, elevate, retract, and then relax the scapulae (in a position of good posture).
- Circle the arms (shoulder circumduction). This is accomplished with the elbows flexed or extended, using either small or large circular motions with the arms pointing either forward or out to the side. Both clockwise and counterclockwise motions should be performed, but conclude the circumduction by going forward, up, around, and then back, so the scapulae end up in a retracted position. This has the benefit of helping retrain proper posture.

**Lower Thoracic and Lumbar Region**

*Patient position and procedure:* Sitting or standing. If standing, the feet should be shoulder-width apart with the knees slightly bent. Have the patient place the hands at the waist with the fingers pointing backward. Instruct the patient to:

- Extend the lumbar spine by leaning the trunk backward (see Fig. 16.9*B*). This is particularly beneficial when the person must sit or stand in a forward-bent position for prolonged periods.
- Flex the lumbar spine by contracting the abdominal muscles, causing a posterior pelvic tilt; or if there are no signs of a disk problem, the patient can bend the trunk forward while sitting, dangling the arms toward the floor. This motion is beneficial when the person stands in a lordotic or swayback posture for prolonged periods. "Toe-touching" exercises are not advocated for individuals with low-back impairments because of the stress placed on the low back structures.
- Side bend in each direction.
- Rotate the trunk by turning in each direction while keeping the pelvis facing forward.
- Stand up and walk around at frequent intervals when sitting for extended periods.

**Conscious Relaxation Training for the Cervical Region**
Specific techniques for the cervical region develop the patient's kinesthetic awareness of a tensed or relaxed muscle and how consciously to reduce tension in the muscle. In addition, if done with posture training techniques in mind, as described earlier in the chapter, the patient can be helped to recognize decreased muscular tension when the head is properly balanced and the cervical spine is aligned in midposition.

*Patient position and procedure:* Sitting comfortably with arms relaxed, such as resting on a pillow placed on the lap; the eyes are closed. Position yourself next to the patient to use tactile cues on the muscles and help position the head as necessary. Have the patient perform the following activities in sequence.

- Use diaphragmatic breathing and breathe in slowly and deeply through the nose, allowing the abdomen to relax and expand; then relax and allow the air to be expired through the relaxed open mouth. This breathing is reinforced after each of the following activities.
- Next, relax the jaw. The tongue rests gently on the hard palate behind the front teeth with the jaw slightly open. If the patient has trouble relaxing the jaw, have him or her click the tongue and allow the jaw to drop. Practice until the patient feels the jaw relax and the tongue rests behind the front teeth. Follow with relaxed breathing.
- Slowly flex the neck. As the patient does so, direct the attention to the posterior cervical muscles and the sensation of how the muscles feel. Use verbal cues such as, "Notice the feeling of increased tension in your muscles as your head drops forward."
- Then slowly raise the head to neutral, inhale slowly, and relax. Help the patient position the head properly and suggest that he or she note how the muscles contract to lift the head, then relax once the head is balanced.
- Repeat the motion; again direct the patient's attention to the feeling of contraction and relaxation in the muscles as he or she moves. Imagery can be used with the breathing such as "fill your head with air and feel it lift off your shoulders as you breathe in and relax."
- Then go through only part of the range, noting how the muscles feel.
- Next, just think of letting the head drop forward and then tightening the muscles (setting); then think of bringing the head back and relaxing. Reinforce to the patient the ability to influence the feeling of contraction and relaxation in the muscles.
- Finally, just think of tensing the muscles and relaxing, letting the tension go out of the muscles even more. Point out that he or she feels even greater relaxation. Once the patient learns to perceive tension in muscles, he or she can then consciously think of relaxing the muscles. Emphasize the fact that the position of the head also influences muscle tension. Have the patient assume various head postures and then correct them until the feeling is reinforced.

**Modalities and Massage**
Once acute symptoms are under control, the use of modalities and massage are minimized or decreased so the patient learns self-management through exercises, relaxation, and posture retraining and does not become dependent on external applications of interventions for comfort.

## Healthy Exercise Habits

It is important to integrate a progression of postural control into all stabilization exercises, aerobic conditioning, and functional activities (see Chapter 16). The patient is carefully observed as greater challenges to activities are performed; and, if necessary, reminders are provided to find the neutral spinal position and to initiate contraction of the stabilizing muscles prior to the activity. For example, when reaching overhead, the patient learns to contract the abdominal muscles to maintain a neutral spine position and not allow the spine to extend into a painful or unstable range. This is incorporated into body mechanics, such as when going from picking up and lifting to placing an object on a high shelf, or into sport activities when reaching up to block or throw a ball. Once developed under your guidance, encourage the patient to continue with a healthy lifestyle, fitness level, and body mechanics.

# ⬤ TENSION HEADACHE/ CERVICAL HEADACHE

Headaches are a common complaint with impaired posture. About 15% to 20% of chronic and recurrent headaches are diagnosed as cervical headaches and are related to musculoskeletal impairments.[41] Often there is associated tension in the posterior cervical muscles, pain at the attachment of the cervical extensors, and/or pain radiating across the top and side of the scalp.

## Causes

There are many factors that may cause a cervical headache.[48] Headaches may follow soft tissue injury or may be caused by faulty or sustained postures, nerve irritation or impingement (the greater occipital nerve emerges through the neck extensor muscles where they attach at the base of the skull), or sustained muscle contraction (from faulty posture or emotional tension) leading to ischemia. With cervical headaches, the joints and ligaments of the upper cervical spine are often inflamed or in dysfunction. Headaches may be related to temporomandibular joint dysfunction (see Chapter 15) or other conditions such as allergies or sinusitis, or there may be vascular or autonomic involvement as with migraine or cluster headaches.[55] Whatever the cause, there usually is a cycle of pain, muscle contraction, decreased circulation, and more pain, which leads to decreased function and potential soft tissue and joint impairments.

## Presenting Signs and Symptoms

Differentiating cervical headaches and related impairments in the musculoskeletal system from other kinds of headaches, such as cluster or migraine headaches, is important for developing a plan of care that effectively manages the headaches. Although there is overlap in symptomatology, the following are usually associated with cervical headaches.[41]

*History and symptoms include*:

- Unilateral headaches or bilateral headaches with one side predominant
- Pain in the neck or suboccipital region that spreads into the head
- Intensity can fluctuate between mild, moderate, or severe
- Precipitated by sustained neck postures or movements
- May be precipitated by stress (also common with other types of headache)
- May be related to trauma, degenerative joint disease, or a sedentary lifestyle and postural stresses
- More prevalent in females but no familial tendency

*Musculoskeletal impairments include*:

- Joint impairment in the upper cervical spine (pain and motion restrictions)
- Impaired muscle performance (impaired tonic postural control and endurance in upper and deep cervical flexors and possibly multifidus and small posterior suboccipital muscles)[41]
- Impaired shoulder girdle/scapular posture with related muscle imbalances
- Impaired lumbar posture with related muscle imbalances[48]
- Impaired neural tissue from pressure or inflammation in the upper cervical/suboccipital region
- Impaired neuromotor control

## General Management Guidelines

Management is directed toward reversing the physical impairments, including posture correction, stress management, and prevention of future episodes.[41]

### Pain Management
Modalities, massage, and muscle-setting exercises are used to break into the cycle of pain and muscle tension.

### Mobility Impairments and Impaired Muscle Performance
Examine the flexibility and strength of the muscles in the cervical, upper thoracic, shoulder girdle, and lumbar spine and design an exercise program to regain a balance in flexibility and neuromuscular control in conjunction with posture correction and training as described in the previous section (see Boxes 14.2 and 14.3). Interventions that have been reported to decrease the intensity and incidence of cervical headaches include the following.[41,48]

- Increase joint mobility in the cervical spine and flexibility in the suboccipital muscles to relieve tension in that region as well as be able to activate and train the deep cervical flexors for control of capital flexion and cervical retraction. Control and support from the deep/core muscles is the foundation of management.
- Utilize cervical stabilization exercises as described in detail in Chapter 16, emphasizing tonic holding of the core muscles in isolation from the global muscles.[41]
- Train the lower trapezius, rhomboids, and serratus anterior muscles in tonic holding postures (described in Chapter 17) to improve control of scapulothoracic posture.

### Stress Management
If the person is in tension-producing situations, relaxation techniques, ROM and muscle-setting techniques, and proper spinal mechanics are taught.

 **Focus on Evidence**_____

A multicenter, randomized, controlled study of 200 individuals with cervicogenic headache looked at the effectiveness of manipulative therapy and a low-load exercise program alone and in combination compared to a control group. It found that both interventions reduced headache frequency and intensity and reduced neck pain compared to that in the control group, and that the effects were maintained at the 12-month follow-up.[39] The exercise intervention primarily consisted of training postural control of the longus colli and other deep neck flexors (see Chapter 16 for a description of the cervical stabilization exercises) as well as the serratus anterior and lower trapezius muscles (see Chapter 17 for a description of the scapular stabilizing exercises) and increasing muscular endurance. Postural correction exercises were also performed throughout the day and progressed to isometric resistance and flexibility exercises.

## Prevention

Underlying the prevention of future episodes of cervical headaches is education of the patient to correct postural stresses, to maintain a healthy balance in the length and strength of the postural muscles, and to adapt the home, work, or recreational environment to minimize sustained or repetitive faulty postural alignment.

# INDEPENDENT LEARNING ACTIVITIES

## ● Critical Thinking and Discussion

1. What are the functional differences between the way the cervical spine and lumbar spine are used in daily activities?
2. Explain how faulty posture can cause painful symptoms.
3. Explain why a "one-size-fits-all" exercise program for posture correction cannot benefit everyone, or how it may be detrimental to some individuals. Discuss this in relation to each of the faulty postures described in this chapter.

## ● Laboratory Practice

1. Practice identifying the effects various postures have on the various regions of the spine; that is, what happens to the cervical and lumbar spine when in supine, prone, side-lying, sitting, and standing postures. Does the spine tend to move into flexion or extension. Determine what is needed to change the position; that is, if flexion is emphasized in a particular posture, what is needed to move the spine into a more neutral (mid-range) position?
2. Identify and feel what happens to the various portions of the spine when moving from one position to another (i.e., rolling supine to prone and return, moving from supine to sit, sit to stand and reverse). What happens to the lumbar spine and pelvis when walking; how is this affected if the person has a hip flexion contracture, or a contracture in the external rotators of the hip?
3. Examine the standing posture of a classmate; then examine the joint ROM, muscle flexibility, and muscle strength. Identify any muscle imbalances in length and strength; then design an intervention program to influence change in the impairments. Use the guidelines presented in this chapter and summarized in Box 14.1 as well as Chapters 16 through 22 for suggested exercises and their safe application.
4. Identify and compare the similarities and differences in flexibility and muscle weakness between a person with excessive lumbar lordosis and an anterior pelvic tilt and a person with a slouched posture who stands with the pelvis shifted forward and the thorax flexed. What effect does each pelvic posture have on the hip position, and what muscles would develop restricted mobility? Usually in the slouched posture the thorax and upper lumbar spine are flexed; would the curl-up exercise be beneficial, or would it contribute to this problem? Develop an exercise program that addresses the common flexibility and strength impairments without reinforcing the faulty posture.

## ● Case Studies

CASE 1
Your patient is a 35-year-old computer programmer who is referred to you because of pain symptoms in the right cervical, posterior shoulder, and arm regions as well as discomfort from frequent tension headaches. The symptoms get progressively worse when at work; usually the pain begins within 1 hour, and it is 6/10 by lunchtime. The same cycle occurs in the afternoon. There is occasional "tingling" in the thumb and index finger. The symptoms have progressively worsened over the last 3 months, ever since being placed in a priority job. Recreational activities include tennis and reading; the tennis does not cause symptoms, but reading makes the headaches worse.

Examination reveals forward head and round shoulder posture. Capital flexion 50% range, cervical rotation and side bending are each 80% range, shoulder external rotation is 75°. There is restricted flexibility in the pectoralis major, pectoralis minor, levator scapulae, and scalene muscles. Cervical quadrant test reproduces the tingling in the right hand; all other neurological tests are negative. Strength of the suprahyoid and infrahyoid muscles, scapular retractors, and shoulder lateral rotators is 4/5.

- What is provoking the patient's symptoms and signs? What are the functional limitations? What is the prognosis?
- Identify impairment and functional outcome goals.
- Establish a program of intervention. How can you progress this person to functional independence?

## CASE 2

A 51-year-old auto mechanic is referred to physical therapy because of pain symptoms in the left buttock and posterior thigh. The symptoms are worse when standing and reaching overhead for more than 15 minutes, which is what he does when working on a car that is up on the racks. Carrying heavy objects (> 50 lb), standing, and walking for more than a half-hour increase the symptoms. There is no precipitating incident, but the symptoms have been recurrent over the past year. Symptoms also increase with the recreational activity of backpacking. Symptoms ease when in the rocker recliner, lying on a couch with knees bent, or when hugging knees to chest.

Examination reveals swayback posture when standing; decreased flexibility in the low back, gluteus max-

imus, hamstrings (straight leg raising to 60°), and upper abdominals; and increased pain with backward bending. Strength of the lower abdominals is 3/5. He is able to do repetitive lunges and partial squats for a maximum of 20 seconds.

- What is provoking the patient's symptoms and signs? What are the functional limitations? What is the prognosis?
- Identify impairment and functional outcome goals.
- Establish a program of intervention. Use the taxonomy of motor tasks discussed in Chapter 1 (see Figs. 1.6 and 1.7 and accompanying text) to develop a progression of exercises and tasks to progress this person to functional independence.

## REFERENCES

1. American Physical Therapy Association: Guide to Physical Therapist Practice, ed 2. Phys Ther 81:139, 2001.
2. Andersson E, et al: The role of the psoas and iliacus muscles for stability and movement of the lumbar spine, pelvis and hip. Scand J Med Sci Sports 5:10, 1995.
3. Barr, KP, Griggs, M, Cadby, T: Lumbar stabilization: core concepts and current literature. Part 1. Am J Phys Med Rehabil 84:473–480, 2005.
4. Basmajian, JV: Muscles Alive, ed 4. Williams & Wilkins, Baltimore, 1979.
5. Beazell, JR: Dysfunction of the longus colli and its relationship to cervical pain and dysfunction: a clinical case presentation. J Manual Manipulative Ther 6(1):12–16, 1998.
6. Bo, K, Sherburn, M, Allen, T: Transabdominal ultrasound measurement of pelvic floor muscle activity when activated directly or via a transverse abdominis muscle contraction. Neurourol Urodyn 22: 582–588, 2003.
7. Bogduk, N, MacIntosh, JE: The applied anatomy of the thoracolumbar fascia. Spine 9:164, 1984.
8. Bogduk, N, Twomey, LT: Clinical Anatomy of the Lumbar Spine. Churchill-Livingstone, New York, 1987.
9. Cailliet, R: Low Back Pain Syndrome, ed 4. FA Davis, Philadelphia, 1988.
10. Cholewicki J, Panjabi MM, Khachatryan A: Stabilizing function of trunk flexor-extensor muscle around a neutral spine posture. Spine 22(19):2207–2212, 1997.
11. Cresswell, AG, Grundstrom, H, Thorstensson, A: Observations on intra-abdominal pressure and patterns of abdominal intra-muscular activity in man. Acta Physiol Scand 144:409, 1992.
12. Crisco, J: Stability of the human ligamentous lumbar spine. Clin Biomech 7:19–32, 1992.
13. Critchley, D: Instructing pelvic floor contraction facilitates transversus abdominis thickness increase during low-abdominal hollowing. Physiother Res Int 7(2):65–75, 2002.
14. Danneels, L, Cools, A, Vanderstraeten G, et al: The effects of three different training modalities on the cross-sectional area of the paravertebral muscles. Scand J Med Sci Sports 11:335–351, 2001.
15. Ebenbichler, GR, Oddsson, L, et al: Sensory-motor control of the lower back: implications for rehabilitation. Med Sci Sports Exerc 33(11):1889–1898, 2001.
16. Farfan, HF, et al: The effects of torsion on the lumbar intervertebral joints: the role of torsion in the production of disc degeneration. J Bone Joint Surg Am 52(3):468, 1970.
17. Friber, O: Clinical symptoms and biomechanics of lumbar spine and hip joint in leg length inequality. Spine 8:643, 1983.
18. Fritz, JM, Erhard, RD, Hagen, BF: Segmental instability of the lumbar spine. Phys Ther 78(8):889, 1998.
19. Gerr, F, Marcus, M, et al: A prospective study of computer users. I. Study design and incidence of musculoskeletal symptoms and disorders. Am J Ind Med 41:221–235, 2002.
20. Gossman, M, Sahrmann, S, Rose, S: Review of length-associated changes in muscle. Phys Ther 62:1977, 1982.
21. Gracovetsky, S, Farfan, H, Helleur, C: The abdominal mechanism. Spine 10:317, 1985.
22. Gracovetsky, S, Farfan, H: The optimum spine. Spine 11:543, 1986.
23. Gracovetsky, S: The Spinal Engine. Springer-Verlag Wein, New York, 1988.
24. Grant, R, Jull, G, Spencer, T: Active stabilization training for screen based keyboard operators—a single case study. Aust Physiother 43(4):235–232, 1997.
25. Hides, JA, Jull GA, Richardson, CA: Long-term effects of specific stabilizing exercises for first-episode low back pain. Spine 26:243, 2001.
26. Hides, JA, Stokes, MJ, et al: Evidence of lumbar multifidus muscle wasting ipsilateral to symptoms in patients with acute/subacute low back pain. Spine 19(2):165–172, 1994.
27. Hides, JA, Richardson, CA, Jull, GA: Multifidus muscle recovery is not automatic after resolution of acute, first-episode low back pain. Spine 21:2763–2769, 1996.
28. Hodges, P, Gandevia, SC: Changes in intra-abdominal pressure during postural and respiratory activation of the human diaphragm. J Appl Physiol 89:967–976, 2000.
29. Hodges, P, Gandevia, SC: Activation of the human diaphragm during a repetitive postural task. J Physiol 522:165–175, 2000.
30. Hodges, PW, Richardson, CA: Altered trunk muscle recruitment in people with low back pain with upper limb movement at different speeds. Arch Phys Med Rehabil 80(9):1005, 1999.
31. Hodges, PW, Richardson, CA: Transversus abdominis and the superficial abdominal muscles are controlled independently in a postural task. Neurosci Lett 265(2):91, 1999.
32. Hodges, P, Cresswell, A, Thorstensson, A: Preparatory trunk motion accompanies rapid upper limb movement. Exp Brain Res 134:69–79, 1999.
33. Hodges, PW, Richardson, CA: Delayed postural contraction of transversus abdominis in low back pain associated with movement of the lower limb. J Spinal Disord 11(1):46, 1998.
34. Hodges, PW, Gandevia, SC, Richardson, CA: Contractions of specific abdominal muscles in postural tasks are affected by respiratory maneuvers. J Appl Physiol 83(3):753, 1997.
35. Hodges, PW, Richardson, CA: Relationship between limb movement speed and associated contraction of the trunk muscles. Ergonomics 40(11):1220, 1997.
36. Hodges, PW, Richardson, CA: Feedforward contraction of transversus abdominis is not influenced by direction of arm movement. Exp Brain Res 114(2):362, 1997.
37. Hodges, PW, and Richardson, CA: Contraction of the abdominal muscles associated with movement of the lower limb. Phys Ther 77(2): 132, 1997.
38. Julius, A, Lees, R, et al: Shoulder posture and median nerve sliding. BMC Musculoskel Disord 5:23, 2004.
39. Jull, G, Trott, P, Potter, H, et al: A randomized controlled trial of exercise and manipulative therapy for cervicogenic headache. Spine 27(17):1835–1834, 2002

40. Jull, G, Barrett, C, et al: Further clinical clarification of the muscle dysfunction in cervical headache. Cephalalgia 19:179–185, 1999.

41. Jull, G: Management of cervical headache. Manual Ther 2(4):182–190, 1997.

42. Kendall, FP, McCreary, EK, Provance, PG: Muscle Testing and Function, ed 4. Williams & Wilkins, Baltimore, 1993.

43. Klein, JA, Hukins, DWL: Collagen fiber orientation in the annulus fibrosus of intervertebral disc during bending and torsion measured by x-ray defraction. Biochim Biophys Acta 719:98, 1982.

44. Levangie, P, Norkin, C: Joint Structure and Function: A Comprehensive Analysis, ed 3. FA Davis, Philadelphia, 2001.

45. Lovell, WWQ, Winter, RB (eds): Pediatric Orthopedics, ed 2. Lippincott, Philadelphia, 1986.

46. Marcus, M, Gerr, F, et al: A prospective study of computer users. II. Postural risk factors for musculoskeletal symptoms and disorders. Am J Ind Med 41:236–249, 2002.

47. Marras, WS, Granata, KP: Changes in trunk dynamics and spine loading during repeated trunk exertions. Spine 22(21):2564, 1997.

48. McDonnell, MK, Sahrmann, SA, Van Dillen, L: A specific exercise program and modification of postural alignment for treatment of cervicogenic headache: a case report. J Orthop Sports Phys Ther 35(1):3–15, 2005.

49. McGill, SM: Low back exercises: evidence for improving exercise regimens. Phys Ther 78(7):754, 1998.

50. McGill, SM, Norman, RW: Low back biomechanics in industry: the prevention of injury through safer lifting. In Grabiner, M (ed) Current Issues in Biomechanics. Human Kinetics, Champaign, IL, 1993.

51. Moseley, GL, Hodges, PW, Gandevia, SC: Deep and superficial fibers of the lumbar multifidus muscle are differently active during voluntary arm movements. Spine 27:E29036, 1996.

52. Neumann, DA: Kinesiology of the Musculoskeletal System; Foundations for Physical Rehabilitation. Mosby, St. Louis, 2002.

53. Neumann, P, Gill, V: Pelvic floor and abdominal muscle interaction: EMG activity and intra-abdominal pressure. Int Urogynecol J 13: 125–132, 2002.

54. Ng, JK-F, et al: Relationship between muscle fiber composition and functional capacity of back muscles in healthy subjects and patients with back pain. J Orthop Sports Phys Ther 27(6):389, 1998.

55. Nicholson, GG, Gaston, J: Cervical headache. J Orthop Sports Phys Ther 31(4):184, 2001.

56. Nourbakhsh, MR, Arab, AM: Relationship between mechanical factors and incidence of low back pain. J Orthop Sports Phys Ther 32(9):447–460, 2002.

57. Novak, CB: Upper extremity work-related musculoskeletal disorders: a treatment perspective. J Orthop Sprots Phys Ther 34(10):628–637, 2004.

58. O'Sullivan, PB, Grahamslaw, KM, et al: The effect of different standing and sitting postures on trunk muscle activity in a pain-free population. Spine 27(11):1238–1244, 2002.

59. Penjabi, MM: The stabilizing system of the spine. Part I. Function, dysfunction, adaptation, and enhancement. J Spinal Disord 5:383–389, 1992.

60. Penjabi, MM: The stabilizing system of the spine. Part II. Neutral zone and instability hypothesis. J Spinal Disord 5:390–397, 1992.

61. Panjabi, MM, Geol, VK, Takata, K: Physiologic strains in the lumbar spinal ligaments. Spine 7:192, 1982.

62. Porterfield, JA: Dynamic stabilization of the trunk. J Orthop Sports Phys Ther 6:271, 1985.

63. Richardson, C, Hodges, P, Hides, J: Therapeutic Exercise for Lumbopelvic Stabilization: A Motor Control Approach for the Treatment and Prevention of Low Back Pain, ed 2. Churchill Livingstone, Edinburgh, 2004.

64. Richardson, CA, et al: Techniques for active lumbar stabilisation for spinal protection: a pilot study. Aust J Physiother 38:105, 1992.

65. Richardson, CA, Toppenberg, R, Jull, G: An initial evaluation of eight abdominal exercises for their ability to provide stabilisation for the lumbar spine. Aust J Physiother 36:6, 1990.

66. Sapsford, RR, Hodges, PW, Richardson, CA, et al: Co-activation of the abdominal and pelvic floor muscles during voluntary exercises. Neurol Urodynam 20:31–42, 2001.

67. Sapsford, RR, Hodges, PW: Contraction of the pelvic floor muscles during abdominal maneuvers. Arch Phys Med Rehabil 82:1081–1088, 2001.

68. Smith, LK, Weiss, EL, Lehmhuhl, LD: Brunnstrom's Clinical Kinesiology, ed 5. FA Davis, Philadelphia, 1996.

69. Sparto, PJ, Parnianpour, M, et al: The effect of fatigue on multijoint kinematics, coordination, and postural stability during a repetitive lifting test. J Orthop Sports Phys Ther 25(1):3–11, 1997.

70. Twomey, LT: A rationale for the treatment of back pain and joint pain by manual therapy. Phys Ther 72:885, 1992.

71. Twomey, T, Taylor, JR: Sagittal movements of the human lumbar vertebral column: a quantitative study of the role of the posterior vertebral elements. Arch Phys Med Rehabil 64:322, 1983.

72. Urquhart, DM, Hodges, PW, et al: Abdominal muscle recruitment during a range of voluntary exercises. Manual Ther 10(2):144–153, 2005.

73. Waddell, G, Burton, AK: Occupational health guidelines for the management of low back pain at work: evidence review. Occup Med 51(2):124–135, 2001.

# The Spine: Impairments, Diagnoses, and Management Guidelines

15

In theory, treating impairments and functional limitations related to the tissues of the spinal column and trunk is the same as treating tissues of the extremities. The major complicating factor in the spine is the close proximity of key structures to the spinal cord and nerve roots. The challenge for the therapist is to recognize the complex functional relationships of the facet joints, the intervertebral joints, the muscles, the fascia, and the nervous system and know how to examine and evaluate the individual who presents with pain and functional limitations. Activity, rather than prolonged bed rest, is accepted as important in the management of patients with spinal and postural pain,[2,72,100] but defining what are beneficial and safe activities during the process of healing and rehabilitation is the task of the therapist.

The medical model of diagnosis does not lend itself to direct therapeutic exercise intervention strategies, particularly because patients' complaints of back or neck pain often do not relate to specific pathologies. Efforts are being made to determine the most effective way to categorize patients with symptoms affecting spine and trunk function in order to be more accurate with outcome research.[22,23,27,64,65,85,92] In addition, results from research studies are beginning to provide the criteria for predicting outcomes in subgroups of patients with back pain so therapists can better identify the interventions that are more likely to result in positive outcomes.[5,8,17,35,58] The approach described in this text supports the importance of treatment based on presenting impairments and movement disorders while respecting the pathomechanics, pathophysiology, and precautions of specific medical diagnoses.

The content of this chapter has three major emphases. The first section summarizes the highlights of the anatomy and function of the spine. The second section reviews the pathology and pathomechanics of spinal structures. The focus of the third section is on principles and guidelines for managing patients with impaired function in the spine. This section includes principles of interventions for the broad categories of acute, subacute, and chronic spinal conditions as well as for the subcategories of specific impairments. Techniques geared toward treating unique impairments are described in these sections. Because the function of the temporomandibular joint (TMJ) is closely related to the cervical spine, management guidelines for impairments related to the TMJ are also described. General therapeutic exercise techniques of intervention for all spinal and postural impairments are described in Chapter 16. Chapters 14, 15, and 16 are written with the assumption that the reader has completed or is concurrently taking a course in examination and evaluation of posture and the spine.

## ⬡ REVIEW OF THE STRUCTURE AND FUNCTION OF THE SPINE

Postural alignment and spinal stability are described in detail in Chapter 14.

## Functional Components of the Spine

Functionally, the spinal column is divided into anterior and posterior pillars (Fig. 15.1).[16,56]

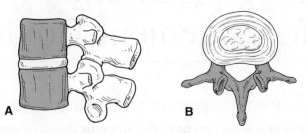

FIGURE 15.1 Spinal segment showing (A) the anterior weight-bearing, shock-absorbing portion, and (B) the posterior gliding mechanism and lever system for muscle attachments.

- The *anterior pillar* is made up of the vertebral bodies and intervertebral disks and is the hydraulic, weight-bearing, shock-absorbing portion of the spinal column.
- The *posterior pillar*, or vertebral arch, is made up of the articular processes and facet joints, which provide the gliding mechanism for movement. Also part of the posterior unit are the bony levers, the two transverse processes and spinous process, to which the muscles attach and function to cause and control motions and provide spinal stability.

## Motions of the Spinal Column

Motion of the spinal column is described both globally and at the functional unit or motion segment. The *functional unit* is comprised of two vertebrae and the joints in between (typically, two zygapophyseal facet joints and one intervertebral disk). Generally, the axis of motion for each unit is in the nucleus pulposus of the intervertebral disk. Because the spine can move from top down or bottom up, motion at a functional unit is defined by what is occurring with the anterior portion of the body of the superior vertebra (Fig. 15.2).

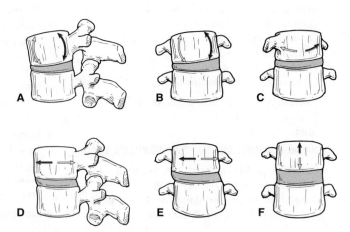

FIGURE 15.2 Motions of the spinal column. (A) Flexion/extension (forward/backward bending). (B) Lateral flexion (side bending). (C) Rotation. (D) Anterior/posterior shear. (E) Lateral shear. (F) Distraction/compression.

***Sagittal plane motion.*** Motion in the sagittal plane results in flexion (forward bending) or extension (backward bending). With flexion, the anterior portion of the bodies approximate and the spinous processes separate; with extension, the anterior portion of the bodies separate and the spinous processes approximate.

***Frontal plane motion.*** Motion in the frontal plane results in lateral flexion (side bending) to the left or right. With side bending the lateral edges of the vertebral bodies approximate on the side toward which the spine is bending and separate the opposite side.

***Transverse plane motion.*** Motion in the transverse plane results in rotation. Rotation to the right results in relative movement of the body of the superior vertebrae to the right and its spinous process to the left; the opposite occurs with rotation to the left. If movement occurs from the pelvis upward, the motion is still defined by the relative motion of the top vertebra.

***Anterior/posterior shear.*** Shear occurs when the body of the superior vertebra translates forward or backward on the vertebra below.

***Lateral shear.*** Lateral shear occurs when the body of the superior vertebra translates sideways on the vertebra below.

***Distraction/compression.*** Separation or approximation occurs with a longitudinal force, either away from or toward the vertebral bodies.

## Structure and Function of Intervertebral Disks

The intervertebral disk, consisting of the annulus fibrosus and nucleus pulposus, is one component of a three-joint complex between two adjacent vertebrae. The structure of the disk dictates its function (Fig. 15.3).[16,45,56,59]

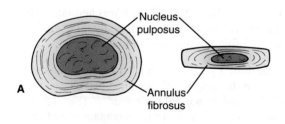

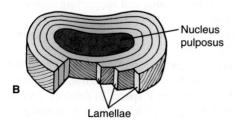

FIGURE 15.3 Intervertebral disk. (*A*) The annular rings enclose the nucleus pulposus, providing a mechanism for dissipating compressive forces. (*B*) Orientation of the layers of the annulus provide tensile strength to the disk with motions in various directions.

***Annulus fibrosus.*** The outer portion of the disk is made up of dense layers of collagen fibers and fibrocartilage. The collagen fibers in any one layer are parallel and angled around 60° to 65° to the axis of the spine, with the tilt alternating in successive layers.[34,50] Because of the orientation of the fibers, tensile strength is provided to the disk by the annulus when the spine is distracted, rotated, or bent. This structure helps restrain the various spinal motions as a complex ligament. The annulus is firmly attached to adjacent vertebrae, and the layers are firmly bound to one another. Fibers of the innermost layers blend with the matrix of the nucleus pulposus. The annulus fibrosus is supported by the anterior and posterior longitudinal ligaments.

***Nucleus pulposus.*** The central portion of the disk is a gelatinous mass that normally is contained within, but whose loosely aligned fibers merge with the inner layer of, the annulus fibrosus. It is located centrally in the disk except in the lumbar spine, where it is situated closer to the posterior border than the anterior border of the annulus. Aggregating proteoglycans, normally in high concentration in a healthy nucleus, have great affinity for water. The resulting fluid mechanics of the confined nucleus functions to distribute pressure evenly throughout the disk and from one vertebral body to the next under loaded conditions. Because of the affinity for water, the nucleus imbibes water when pressure is reduced on the disk and water is squeezed out under compressive loads. These fluid dynamics provide transport for nutrients and help maintain tissue health in the disk.

With flexion (forward bending) of a vertebral segment, the anterior portion of the disk is compressed, and the posterior is distracted. The nucleus pulposus generally does not move in a healthy disk but may have slight distortion with flexion, potentially to redistribute the load through the disk.[53] Asymmetrical loading in flexion results in distortions of the nucleus toward the contralateral posterolateral corner, where the fibers of the annulus are more stretched.[4]

***Cartilaginous end-plates.*** End-plates cover the nucleus pulposus superiorly and inferiorly and lie between the nucleus and vertebral bodies. Each is encircled by the apophyseal ring of the respective vertebral body. The collagen fibers of the inner annulus fibrosus insert into the end-plate and angle centrally, thus encapsulating the nucleus pulposus. Nutrition diffuses from the marrow of the vertebral bodies to the disk via the end-plates.[75]

## Intervertebral Foramina

The intervertebral foramina are between each vertebral segment in the posterior pillar; their anterior boundary is the intervertebral disk, the posterior boundary is the facet joint, and the superior and inferior boundaries are the pedicles of the superior and inferior vertebrae of the spinal segment. The mixed spinal nerve exits the spinal canal via the foramen along with blood vessels and recurrent meningeal or sinuvertebral nerves. The size of the intervertebral foramina is affected by spinal motion, being larger with

**TABLE 15.1**  Spinal Pathologies Related to Preferred Practice Patterns

| PATHOLOGY | PREFERRED PRACTICE PATTERNS AND ASSOCIATED IMPAIRMENTS[6] |
|---|---|
| • Postural stress, strain<br>• Abnormal posture | Pattern 4B—impaired posture |
| • Muscle strain, tear, contusion | Pattern 4C—impaired muscle performance |
| • Acute low back or cervical pain | Pattern 4E—impaired joint mobility, motor function, muscle performance, and ROM associated with localized inflammation |
| • Degenerative disk disease (DDD), disk herniation<br>• Degenerative joint disease (DJD), spondylosis<br>• Rheumatoid arthritis<br>• Radiculopathy, nerve root lesions, sciatica<br>• Spinal stenosis<br>• Segmental instability<br>• Spondylolistheses<br>• Sprains, strains | Pattern 4F—impaired joint mobility, motor function, muscle performance, ROM, and reflex integrity associated with spinal disorders |
| • Compression fracture | Pattern 4G—impaired joint mobility, muscle performance, and ROM associated with fracture |
| • Spondylosis with myelopathy<br>• Intervertebral disk disorders | Pattern 5H—impaired motor function, peripheral nerve integrity, and sensory integrity associated with nonprogressive disorders of the spinal cord |

forward bending and contralateral side bending and smaller with extension and ipsilateral side bending (see Fig. 15.2).

### Inert Structures: Influence on Movement and Stability

Osteoligamentous structures of the spine and their function in guiding movement and providing support to the spine are described in Chapter 14 and summarized in Table 14.1.

### Neuromuscular Function: Dynamic Stabilization

The function of global and core musculature and their neurological influence on postural control and movement of the spine are described in Chapter 14 and summarized in Table 14.3.

## SPINAL PATHOLOGIES AND IMPAIRED SPINAL FUNCTION

The relationship of common spinal pathologies to impairment-based diagnoses and preferred practice patterns are outlined in Table 15.1.

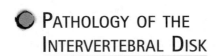

## PATHOLOGY OF THE INTERVERTEBRAL DISK

### Injury and Degeneration of the Disk

#### Definitions
Various authors have defined the terms herniation, protrusion, prolapse, and extrusion differently.[11,16,59,61,64,87] The following definitions are used in this text.

- **Herniation:** a general term used when there is any change in the shape of the annulus that causes it to bulge beyond its normal perimeter[61,64] (Fig. 15.4)
- **Protrusion:** nuclear material is contained by the outer layers of the annulus and supporting ligamentous structures
- **Prolapse:** frank rupture of the nuclear material into the vertebral canal.[11,59]
  - **Extrusion:** extension of nuclear material beyond the confines of the posterior longitudinal ligament or above and below the disk space, as detected on magnetic resonance imagine (MRI),[87] but still in contact with the disk[64]
  - **Free sequestration:** the extruded nucleus has separated from the disk and moved away from the prolapsed area[61,64]

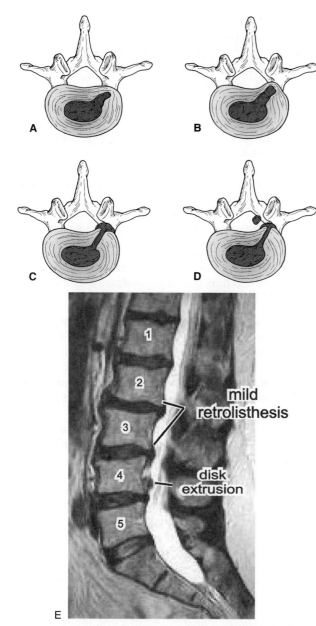

**FIGURE 15.4** Disk breakdown, showing (*A*) breakdown and compression of fibrous layers of the annulus and displacement of disk material; (*B*) radial fissures/tears with nuclear material bulging against the outer annulus; (*C*) extrusion of nuclear material through the outer annulus but still in contact with the disk; (*D*) sequestration of nuclear material beyond the annulus; and (*E*) magnetic resonance imaging (MRI) scan of a 61-year-old patient with low back pain and symptoms radiating into the leg. The scan demonstrates moderate multilevel degenerative disk disease of T12/L1 through L4/5 with mild retrolisthesis of L2 on L3 and L3 on L4. At the L4/5 level, note a small diffuse disk bulge with large paracentral disk extrusion dissecting cranially.

### Fatigue Breakdown and Traumatic Rupture
A decrease in the continuity and integrity of structure of the annulus fibrosus may occur with (1) repeated stress over time causing fatigue breakdown or (2) traumatic rupture.[3,4]

***Fatigue breakdown.*** Over time, the annulus breaks down as a result of repeated overloading of the spine in flexion with asymmetrical forward bending and torsional stresses.[3,4,24,51]

● With torsional stresses, the annulus becomes distorted, most obviously at the posterolateral corner opposite the direction of rotation. The layers of the outer annulus fibrosus lose their cohesion and begin to separate from each other.

● Each layer then acts as a separate barrier to the nuclear material. Eventually, radial tears occur, and there is communication of the nuclear material between the layers.[24]

● With repeated forward bending and lifting stresses, the layers of the annulus are strained; they become tightly packed together in the posterolateral corners, radial fissures develop, and the nuclear material migrates down the fissures.[3,4] Outer layers of annular fibers can contain the nuclear material so long as they remain a continuous layer.[3] After injury, there is a tendency for the nucleus to swell and distort the annulus. Distortion is more severe in the region where the annular fibers are stretched.[4,57] If the outer layers rupture, nuclear material may herniate through the fissures.

● Healing is attempted, but there is poor circulation in the disk. There may be self-sealing of a defect with nuclear gel or proliferation of cells of the annulus.[57] Any fibrous repair is weaker than normal and takes a long time because of the relative avascular status of the disk.

***Traumatic rupture.*** Rupture of the annulus can occur as a one-time event, or it can be superimposed on a disk where there has been gradual breakdown of the annular rings. This is seen most commonly in traumatic hyperflexion injuries.[4]

### Axial Overload
Axial overload (compression) of the spine usually results in end-plate damage or vertebral body fracture before there is any damage to the annulus fibrosus.[13,16]

### Age
Individuals are most susceptible to symptomatic disk injuries between the ages of 30 and 45 years. During this time the nucleus is still capable of imbibing water, but the annulus weakens owing to fatigue loading over time and therefore is less able to withstand increased pressures when there are disproportionately high stresses. The nuclear material may protrude into the tears of fissures, which most commonly are posterolateral and, with increased pressures, may bulge against the outer annular fibers, causing annular distortion; or the nuclear material may extrude from the disk through complete fissures in the annulus.[3,14,24,59]

### Degenerative Changes
Any loss of integrity of the disk from infection, disease, herniation, or an end-plate defect becomes a stimulus for degenerative changes in the disk.[34,45,60]

● Degeneration is characterized by progressive fibrous changes in the nucleus, loss of the organization of the rings of the annulus fibrosus, and loss of cartilaginous end-plates.[57]

● As the nucleus becomes more fibrotic, it loses its capacity to imbibe fluid. Water content decreases, and there is an associated decrease in the size of the nucleus.[60] Acute disk protrusions caused by a bulging nucleus pulposus against the annulus or extrusions of the nucleus through a torn annulus are rare in older people.

- It is possible to have protrusions of the annulus fibrosus without bulging from nuclear pressure. Myxomatous degeneration with annular protrusion has been demonstrated in disk lesions in older people.[101]

### Effect on Spinal Mechanics

Injury or degeneration of the disk affects spinal mechanics in general.[80] During the early stages there is increased mobility of the segment with greater than normal flexion/extension and forward and backward translation of the vertebral body, leading to segmental instability. Force distribution through the entire segment is altered, causing abnormal forces in the facets and supporting structures.[15,24,53]

## Disk Pathologies and Related Conditions

Disk herniation, tissue fluid stasis, diskogenic pain, and swelling from inflammation are conditions that may result from prolonged flexion postures, repetitive flexion microtrauma, or traumatic flexion injuries. Initially, symptoms may be exacerbated when attempting extension but then may be decreased when using carefully controlled extension motions. Several studies have documented that patients with a herniated nucleus pulposus who have symptom reduction with an extension approach to treatment respond favorably to conservative nonsurgical treatment.[5,51]

### Compression Fracture

Excessive axial compression loads usually cause end-plate or vertebral body fractures.[13,16] Flexion and axial loading usually cause increased pain. Pain may occur without nerve root involvement, although there may be referred pain in the extremities.

### Tissue Fluid Stasis

With sustained flexed postures in the spine, the disks, facet joints, and ligaments are placed under sustained loading. The intradiskal pressure increases, and there is compression loading on the cartilage of the facets and a distractive tension on the posterior longitudinal ligament and posterior fibers of the annulus fibrosus. Creep and fluid transfer occur. Sudden movement into extension does not allow for redistribution of the fluids and so increases the vulnerability of the distended tissue to injury and inflammation.[97] Symptoms may be similar to those described for disk lesions because they lessen with repeated extension motions and respond to treatment described in the management section (under Extension Bias) later in the chapter.

## Signs and Symptoms of Disk Lesions and Fluid Stasis

### Etiology of Symptoms

The disk is largely aneural; therefore not all disk protrusions are symptomatic.

*Pain.* Symptoms of pain arise from pressure of a swollen disk or swollen tissues against pain-sensitive structures (ligaments, dura mater, blood vessels around nerve roots) or from the chemical irritants of inflammation if there is herniated disk material.

*Neurological signs and symptoms.* Neurological signs arise from pressure against the spinal cord or nerve roots. The only true neurological signs and symptoms are specific motor weaknesses and specific dermatome sensory changes. Radiating pain in a dermatomal pattern, increased myoelectrical activity in the hamstrings, decreased straight-leg raising, and depressed deep tendon reflexes can also be associated with referred pain stimuli from spinal muscles, interspinous ligaments, the disk, and facet joints and therefore are not true signs of nerve root pressure.[16,48,67]

*Variability of symptoms.* Symptoms are variable depending on the degree and direction of the protrusion as well as the spinal level of the lesion.

- Posterior or posterolateral protrusions are most common. With a small posterior or posterolateral lesion, there may be pressure against the posterior longitudinal ligament or against the dura mater or its extensions around the nerve roots. The patient may describe a severe midline backache or pain spreading across the back into the buttock and thigh.
- A large posterior protrusion may cause spinal cord signs such as loss of bladder control and saddle anesthesia.
- A large posterolateral protrusion may cause partial cord or nerve root signs.
- An anterior protrusion may cause pressure against the anterior longitudinal ligament, resulting in back pain. There are no neurological signs.
- The most common levels of protrusion are the segments between the fourth and fifth lumbar vertebrae and between the fifth lumbar vertebra and sacrum, although a protrusion may occur at any level, including the cervical spine.

*Shifting symptoms.* Symptoms from a disk lesion may shift if there is integrity of the annular wall because the hydrostatic mechanism is still intact.[64,65]

*Inflammation.* Contents of the nucleus pulposus in the neural canal may cause an inflammatory reaction and irritate the dural sac, its nerve root sleeves, or the nerve roots. The symptoms may persist for extended periods and are not responsive to purely mechanical changes. The back pain may be worse than leg pain on the straight-leg raising test. Poor resolution of this inflammatory stimulus may lead to fibrotic reactions, nerve mobility impairments, and chronic pain.[63,89,91] Early medical intervention with anti-inflammatory agents is usually necessary.[91]

### Onset and Behavior of Symptoms from Disk Lesions

*Onset.* Onset is usually between 20 and 55 years of age but most frequently from the mid-thirties to forties. Except in cases of trauma, symptomatic onset in the lumbar spine is usually associated simply with bending, bending and lifting, or attempting to stand up after having been in a prolonged recumbent, sitting, or forward-bent posture. The person may or may not have the sensation of something tearing.[49,61,65] Although cervical disk lesions are not as prevalent, a prolonged flexed spinal position as in a forward head posture may lead to or exacerbate symptoms from a protrusion. Many patients have a predisposing history of a faulty flexion posture.

*Pain behavior.* Pain may increase gradually when the person is inactive, such as when sitting or after a night's rest. The patient often describes increased pain when attempting to get out of bed in the morning or when first standing up. Symptoms are usually aggravated with activities that increase the intradiskal pressure, such as sitting, forward bending, coughing, or straining or when attempting to stand after being in a flexed position. Usually, symptoms are lessened when walking except when the bulge is large or the nuclear material has prolapsed and moved beyond the confines of the annulus.[49,61,65]

*Acute pain.* When there is inflammation during the acute phase, pain is almost always present but varies in intensity, depending on the person's position or activity.

When there is a lumbar disk lesion, initially discomfort is noticed in the lumbosacral or buttock region. Some patients experience aching that extends into the thigh or leg. In the cervical spine, initially pain is noticed in the midscapular and shoulder area. Numbness or muscle weakness (neurological signs) are not noted unless the protrusion has progressed to a degree to which there is nerve root, spinal cord, or cauda equina compression.

### Objective Clinical Findings in the Lumbar Spine

N O T E : The following information relates to a contained posterior or posterolateral nuclear protrusion in the lumbar spine.[49,65] The impairments are summarized in Box 15.1.

- The patient usually prefers standing and walking to sitting.
- The patient may have a decrease in or loss of lumbar lordosis and may have some lateral shifting of the spinal column.
- Forward bending is limited. When repeating the forward-bending test, the symptoms increase or peripheralize. *Peripheralization* means the symptoms are experienced farther down the leg (Fig. 15.5).
- Backward bending is limited; when repeating the backward-bending test, the pain lessens or centralizes. *Centralization* means that the symptoms recede up the leg or become localized to the back. If the protrusion cannot be mechanically reduced, backward bending peripheralizes or increases the symptoms.
- If there is a *lateral shift* of the spinal column, backward bending increases the pain. If the lateral shift is first corrected, repeated backward bending lessens or centralizes the pain (see Figs. 15.8 and 15.9 in the management section of this chapter).
- Testing passive lumbar flexion in the supine position (double knees-to-chest) and passive extension in the prone position (press-ups) usually produces signs similar to those of the standing tests, but results may not be as dramatic because gravity is eliminated.
- Pain between 30° and 60° of straight-leg raising is considered positive for interference of dural mobility but not pathognomonic for a disk protrusion.[49,98]
- Contained nuclear protrusion can be influenced by movement because the hydrostatic mechanism is still intact. A complete tear of the outer layers of the annulus disrupts the hydrostatic mechanism, so the herniated or prolapsed nuclear material cannot be influenced by movement.[64] Anti-inflammatory intervention by a physician is important during the acute phase. Patients with disk extrusions may respond to conservative measures owing to resolution of the inflammation and resorption of the disk material.[87]

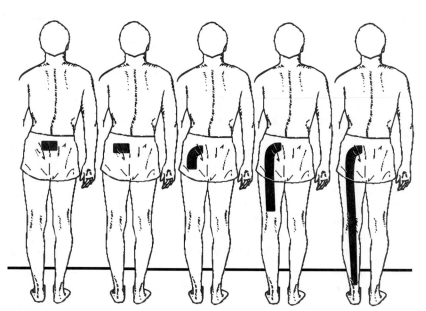

FIGURE 15.5 Examples of peripheralization and centralization of lower-quarter symptoms. Viewing the images left to right illustrates peripheralization of symptoms; from right to left illustrates centralization.

> **BOX 15.1    Summary of Common Impairments Related to Disk Protrusions in the Lumbar Spine**
>
> - Pain, muscle-guarding
> - Flexed posture and deviation away from (usually) the symptomatic side
> - Neurological symptoms in dermatome and possibly myotome of affected nerve roots
> - Increased symptoms (peripheralization) with sitting, prolonged flexed postures, transition from sit to stand, coughing, straining
> - Limited nerve mobility, such as straight-leg raising (usually between 30° and 60°)
> - Peripheralization of symptoms with repeated forward-bending (spinal flexion) tests

### Objective Clinical Findings in the Cervical Spine

- Findings are similar to those in the lumbar spine except they are displayed in the respective dermatomes and myotomes of the cervical nerve roots.
- Initially, the patient may present with a faulty forward head posture and may hold the head in a guarded side-bent or rotated position away from the symptomatic side.
- Cervical flexion peripheralizes the symptoms; neck retractions (axial extension) followed by extension may centralize the symptoms of a contained nuclear bulge.
- There may be nerve mobility impairments in the upper extremity.
- Traction may relieve the symptoms.

 ## PATHOMECHANICAL RELATIONSHIPS OF THE INTERVERTEBRAL DISK AND FACET JOINTS

### Three-Joint Complex

The disk and facets make up a three-joint complex between two adjoining vertebrae and are biomechanically interrelated. Asymmetrical disk injury affects the kinematics of the entire unit plus the joints above and below, resulting in asymmetrical movements of the facets, abnormal stresses, and eventually cartilage degeneration.[81] As the disk degenerates, there is a decrease in both water content and disk height. The vertebral bodies approximate, and the intervertebral foramina and spinal canal narrow.[15,16]

### Initial Changes

Initially, there is increased slack with increased mobility and translation in the spinal segment.[61] Opposition of the facet surfaces changes, and the capsules are strained, resulting in irritation, swelling, and muscle spasm.

### Altered Muscle Control

Altered joint receptor function negatively affects muscle recruitment in swollen joints.[94] Pain has also been cited as a factor for altered and diminished recruitment patterns in the stabilizing muscles of the spine.[38,39,42] Increasing shear forces from poor mid-range stabilization places increased stresses on the osteoligamentous support structures, which is thought to contribute to segmental hypermobility or instability.[25]

### Progressive Bony Changes

Eventually, with the repeated irritation due to the faulty mechanics, there are progressive bony changes in the facet and vertebral body margins. Osteophyte formation along the facets and spondylitic lipping and spurring along the vertebral bodies occur, and hypomobility develops.[53,68] These changes lead to additional narrowing of the associated foramina and spinal canal. In the cervical spine, the uncovertebral joints thicken, roughen, and distort.[86]

## Related Pathologies

### Segmental (Clinical) Instability

*Segmental instability* has been described as poor control in the neutral zones within the physiological range of spinal movement because of a decrease in the capacity of the neuromuscular stabilizing system to control the movement.[25,81] Clinically, patients demonstrate difficulty moving in the mid-ranges of spinal motion and may demonstrate shifting or fluctuation in movement. (See section on Pathomechanics of Spinal Instability in this chapter.)

### Stenosis

*Stenosis* is narrowing of a passage or opening. In the spine, stenosis is any compromise of the space in the spinal canal (central stenosis), nerve root canal, or foramen (lateral stenosis); it be congenital or acquired. The narrowing may be caused by soft tissue structures such as a disk protrusion, fibrotic scars, or joint swelling or by bony narrowing as with spondylitic osteophyte formation or spondylolisthesis. With progression, neurological symptoms develop. Extension exacerbates the symptoms.[74]

### Neurological Symptoms—Radiculopathy

Spinal nerve root or spinal cord symptoms occur.

- When protrusion of the disk compresses against the cord or nerve roots
- When there is decreased disk height due to degenerative changes[82] or excessive translation of the vertebra from shear forces[61] resulting in decreased foraminal space
- When there is an inflammatory response due to trauma, degeneration, or disease with accompanying edema and stenosis
- When a facet joint subluxes and the nerve root becomes impinged between the tip of the superior articulating facet and the pedicle
- When spondylosis results in osteophytic growth on the articular facets or along the disk borders of the vertebral bodies that decreases spinal canal or intervertebral foraminal size
- When there is spondylolisthesis or when there is scarring or adhesion formation after injury or spinal surgery

## Dysfunction

The cycle of dysfunction caused by injury, pain, and muscle splinting leads to further restriction of movement, pain, and muscle splinting unless appropriate therapy is introduced. There are additional descriptions of facet joint pathologies in the following section.

# PATHOLOGY OF THE ZYGAPOPHYSEAL (FACET) JOINTS

## Facet Joint Characteristics

Facet joints are synovial articulations that are enclosed in a capsule and supported by ligaments; they respond to trauma and arthritic changes similar to any peripheral joint.

Various types of meniscoid-like structures or invaginations of the facet capsules are present in the zygapophyseal joints of the spine. They are synovial reflections containing fat and blood vessels. In some cases, dense fibrous tissue develops as a result of mechanical stresses.[9,10] Some people describe entrapment of these structures between the articulating surfaces with sudden or unusual movement as a source of pain and limited motion via tension on the well-innervated capsule.[52,96] Bogduk and colleagues described the *locked-back mechanism* as being extrapment of the meniscoids in the supracapsular or infracapsular folds, which then blocks the return to extension from the flexed position.[9,10] It is called an extrapment because the meniscoid fails to re-enter the joint cavity; consequently, it becomes a space-occupying lesion in the capsular folds, causing pain as it impacts against and stretches the capsules.

## Common Diagnoses and Impairments from Facet Joint Pathologies

The etiology of facet joint pathologies may be trauma, degenerative, or systemic pathologies. Box 15.2 summarizes the impairments and functional limitations.

### Facet Sprain/Joint Capsule Injury

There is usually a history of trauma, such as falling or a motor vehicle accident. The joints react with effusion (swelling), limited range of motion (ROM), and accompanying muscle guarding. The swelling may cause foraminal stenosis and neurological signs.

### Osteoarthritis, Degenerative Joint Disease, Spondylosis

- Usually there is a history of faulty posture, prolonged immobilization after injury, severe trauma, repetitive trauma, or degenerative changes in the disk.
- During the early stages of degenerative changes, there is greater play, or hypermobility/instability, in the three-joint complex. Over time, stress from the altered mechanics leads to osteophyte formation with spurring and lipping along the joint margins and vertebral bodies. Progressive hypomobility with bony stenosis results.

---

> **BOX 15.2 Summary of Common Impairments and Functional Limitations Related to the Facet Joint Pathology**
>
> - *Pain:* When acute, there is pain and muscle guarding with all motions; pain when subacute and chronic is related to periods of immobility or excessive activity.
> - *Impaired mobility:* Usually hypomobility and decreased joint play in affected joints; there may be hypermobility or instability during early stages.
> - *Impaired posture.*
> - *Impaired spinal extension:* Extension may cause or increase neurological symptoms due to foraminal stenosis; therefore, may be unable to sustain or perform repetitive extension activities without exacerbating symptoms.
> - *Any functional activity that requires flexibility or prolonged repetition of trunk motions,* such as repetitive lifting and carrying of heavy objects, may exacerbate symptoms in the arthritic spine.

---

- Usually, where there is hypomobility, compensatory hypermobility occurs in neighboring spinal segments.
- Pain may result from the stresses of excessive mobility or from stretch to hypomobile structures. Pain may also be a result of the encroachment of developing osteophytes against pain-sensitive tissue or of swelling and irritation because of excessive or abnormal mobility of the segments.
- The encroachment of osteophytes on the spinal canal and intervertebral foramina may cause neurological signs, especially with spinal extension and side bending.[16]
- The degenerating joint is vulnerable to facet impingement, sprains, and inflammation, as is any arthritic joint.
- In some patients, movement relieves the symptoms; in others, movement irritates the joints, and painful symptoms increase.

### Rheumatoid Arthritis

- Symptoms of rheumatoid arthritis (RA) can affect any of the synovial joints of the spine and ribs. There is pain and swelling.
- RA in the cervical spine presents special problems. There are neurological symptoms wherever degenerative change or swelling impinges against neurological tissue. There is increased fragility of tissues affected by RA, such as osteoporosis with cyst formation, erosion of bone, and instabilities from ligamentous necrosis. Most common of the serious lesions are atlantoaxial subluxation and C-4/5 and C-5/6 vertebral dislocations.[69]
- Pain or neurological signs originating in the spine may or may not be related to subluxation. Therefore, these signs should be used as a precaution whenever dealing with this disease because of the potential damage to the spinal cord.[69]
- X-ray examinations are important in ruling out instabilities; signs and symptoms alone are not conclusive.

PRECAUTION: Inappropriate movements of the spine in patients with RA, such as cervical manipulation, could be life-threatening or extremely debilitating because of the potential of subluxations and dislocations to cause damage to the cervical cord or vertebral artery.[69]

### Facet Joint Impingement (Blocking, Fixation, Extrapment)

With a sudden or unusual movement, the meniscoid of a facet capsule may be extrapped, impinged, or stressed, which causes pain and muscle guarding. The onset is sudden and usually involves forward bending and rotation.[9,52,97]

- There is loss of specific motions, and attempted movement induces pain. At rest, the individual has no pain.
- There are no true neurological signs, but there may be referred pain in the related dermatome.
- Over time, stress is placed on the contralateral joint and on the disk, leading to problems in these structures.

# PATHOLOGY OF MUSCLE AND SOFT TISSUE INJURIES: STRAINS, TEARS, AND CONTUSIONS

Common impairments and functional limitations are summarized in Box 15.3.

## General Symptoms from Trauma

Often more than one tissue is injured as a result of trauma. The extent of the tissue involvement may not be detectable during the acute phase.

---

| BOX 15.3 | Summary of Common Impairments and Functional Limitations Associated with Muscle and Soft Tissue Injuries |
|---|---|

**Acute Stage**
- Pain and muscle guarding
- Pain with contraction of the muscle or stretch on the muscle
- Interference with ADLs (rolling over, turning, sitting, sit to stand, standing, walking)

**Subacute and Chronic Stages**
- Impaired muscle performance
- Impaired mobility: may have contractures in muscle and related connective tissue or may have adhesions at site of tissue injury
- Impaired spinal control and stabilization during functional activities
- Impaired postural awareness
- Limited IADLs, work, and recreational activities (difficulty with repetitive or sustained postures, lifting, pushing, pulling, reaching, and holding loads)

---

- There is pain, localized swelling, tenderness on palpation, and protective muscle guarding regardless of whether the injured tissue is inert or contractile. Muscle guarding serves the immediate purpose of immobilizing the region. If the muscle contraction is prolonged, it results in the buildup of metabolic waste products and sluggish circulation. This altered local environment results in irritation of the free nerve endings so the muscle continues to contract and becomes the source of additional pain (see Fig. 10.1).
- Ligamentous strains cause pain when the ligament is stressed. If torn, there is hypermobility of the segment.
- As healing of the involved structures occurs, there may be adaptive shortening or scar tissue adhering to surrounding tissue and restricting tissue mobility and postural alignment.

## Common Sites of Lumbar Strain

A common site for injury in the lumbar region is along the iliac crest. This is where many forces converge around the attachment of the lateral raphe of the lumbodorsal fascia, quadratus lumborum, erector spinae, and iliolumbar ligament (see Fig. 14.16). Injury to this region frequently occurs with falls and with repeated loading of the region during lifting or twisting motions.

## Common Sites of Cervical Strain

Common injuries in the neck and upper thoracic region occur with flexion/extension trauma. Serious cervical trauma may result in vertebral fractures and spinal cord injury. Discussion of vertebral fractures and spinal cord injury is beyond the scope of this text.

*Extension injuries.* When the head rapidly accelerates into extension, if nothing stops it (such as a headrest in a car) the occiput is stopped by the thorax. The posterior structures, especially the joints, are compressed. The anterior structures (longus colli, suprahyoid, and infrahyoid muscles) are stretched. The mandible is pulled open, the condylar head of the temporomandibular joint translates forward, stressing the joint structures, and the muscles controlling jaw elevation are stretched (masseter, temporalis, internal pterygoid).

*Flexion injuries.* When the head rapidly accelerates into flexion and nothing stops it (such as the steering wheel or air bag in a car), the chin is stopped by the sternum. The mandible is forced posteriorly so the condylar head is forced into the retrodiskal pad in the joint. The posterior cervical muscles, ligaments, fasciae, and joint capsules are stretched.

## Postural Strain

Strain to the posterior cervical, scapular, and upper thoracic muscles and fasciae is common with postural stresses such as prolonged sitting at a computer terminal, drawing table, or desk. Structures in the low back region are strained with faulty standing and sitting postures. Postural stresses are described in detail in Chapter 14.

## Emotional Stress

Emotional stress is often expressed as increased tension in the posterior cervical or lumbar region.

## Functional Limitations/Disabilities

Impaired muscle function underlies most spinal problems that demonstrate pain or poor spinal control and stabilization during functional activities. When acute, muscle guarding interferes with basic activities such as rolling over, sitting, standing, and walking. With the subacute and chronic conditions, muscle impairments result in poor stabilization and spinal control in prolonged upright postures and activities. Proximal stability of the spine is imperative for most activities and needs to be addressed for improved function.

# PATHOMECHANICS OF SPINAL INSTABILITY

Spinal stability was defined and described in Chapter 14. The mechanical model of stability in which stability is maintained over the base of support by the guy wire function of the global and core musculature was reviewed, as was the functional model proposed by Penjabi and colleagues[78-80] in which stability is visualized as a three-legged stool that requires not only the active muscle function but also the passive osteoligamentous structures and neural control from the central nervous system to program muscle response for spinal stability. All three legs of the stool are necessary for stability; instability results when one (or more) of the legs does not function properly.

There are various grades of instability. Patients who have severe symptoms and radiographic evidence of excessive motion and who do not respond to conservative treatment become candidates for spinal fusion.[25] Clinical instability that can be managed by therapeutic exercise interventions is defined by an increase in the neutral zone.

## Neutral Zone

The neutral zone[78,79] is the area that is mid-range in the ROM of a spinal segment where no stress is placed on the passive osteoligamentous structures. In the spine, the neutral zone is relatively small (usually only several degrees of range is possible between any two vertebrae before the elastic zone of the inert tissues is reached) and is controlled by dynamic tension in the core musculature that attaches to each of the spinal segments. The neutral zone can be visualized as a ball lying on the bottom of a bowl.

The sides of the bowl represent the osteoligamentous structures that provide passive support of the spinal segment. When the ball is disturbed, it rolls back and forth and up against the sides of the bowl and eventually settles back in the middle. A deep bowl has a smaller region in which the ball can roll back and forth and therefore less motion or more stability; a shallow bowl has a larger region in which the ball can roll so there is greater displacement or more mobility (less stability) (Fig. 15.6 A&B). Muscles added to this visualization are depicted as bungie cords that are attached to the ball and go outward to the edges of the bowl; they help center the ball in the middle of the bowl when perturbations occur (Fig. 15.6C). In a structure where there is less stability (more segmental movement), the muscles have greater responsibility to maintain the neutral zone (ball in the middle of the bowl).

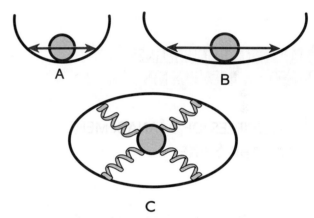

FIGURE 15.6 Neutral zone of a spinal segment depicted as a bowl, with the sides of the bowl representing the osteoligamentous tissues and the moving ball representing the segmental mobility. (A) In a deep bowl, when perturbations disturb the ball, there is little motion as the ball rolls back and forth and settles in the center of the bowl—representing stability. (B) In a shallow bowl, there is greater motion—representing greater segmental mobility or instability. (C) Viewing the bowl from above, bungee cords attached to the ball and the sides of the bowl represent the dynamic function of segmental muscles. Appropriately graded tension in the bungee cords stabilize the ball when perturbations disturb the unit.

*Neutral spine.* The term neutral spine is used clinically to define the mid-range of motion.

## Instability

If there is an increase in the neutral zone, the segment may show signs of instability.[25,78-80] More segmental movement may occur owing to disk degeneration, spondylolysis, spondylolisthesis, or ligamentous laxity; or it may be due to poor neuromuscular control of the core stabilizing muscles in maintaining the neutral zone because of fatigue, altered recruitment pattern, reflex inhibition from pain, or some pathology.[25,79,80,99] The individual may experience neck or back pain when aberrant movement occurs at the segment or stresses are imposed at the end of the range (relaxed postures for a period of time or sudden stress that the muscles cannot control).

**Focus on Evidence**_____

It has been shown that activation and function in the transversus abdominis (TrA) changes (delayed and more phasic) in patients with low back pain[40,41]; and there may be atrophy, structural change, and altered electromyographic (EMG) activity in the multifidus at the painful spinal level as well,[21,37,84] possibly indicating less effective stabilizing action from these muscles. Studies have also documented that training the core muscles for postural control and stability improves the long-term outcome in patient populations with acute[36] and chronic[77] low back pain as well as pelvic girdle pain following pregnancy.[95] In the cervical region, studies have documented that training the stabilizing function of the deep cervical musculature for postural control decreases the frequency and intensity of symptoms of cervical headaches.[46]

## MANAGEMENT GUIDELINES BASED ON IMPAIRMENTS

 ## PRINCIPLES OF MANAGEMENT FOR THE SPINE

At the time of a low back or cervical injury, impairments, functional limitations, and disabilities are not known. Usually 80% to 90% of acute injuries resolve within 1 month.[54] Disabilities are dependent on the extent of the injury. If it involves the spinal cord, levels of complete paralysis may occur. If it involves the nerve roots (also the cauda equina), varying degrees of sensory loss in specific dermatomes and muscle weakness in specific myotomes may occur, which may or may not interfere with the individual's daily personal and work-related activities. Upper-quarter nerve roots affect function of the arms and hands; lower-quarter nerve roots affect function of the lower extremities, especially during weight-bearing activities. Studies on chronic pain syndromes as a result of back injuries seem to conclude that the degree of disability is related to psychological, economic, and sociological factors and prior incidence of injury more than the actual tissues involved.[33,54] Nerve root involvement and pain provocation with active movements in several directions are more common in patients who develop chronic pain.[33] Discussion of treatment for spinal cord injuries and chronic pain syndromes is beyond the scope of this book.

### Examination and Evaluation

*History, systems review, and testing.* A history and systems review of the patient is conducted to rule out any serious conditions, to determine if the patient should be referred to another practitioner, or to determine if the

patient's condition is appropriate for physical therapy intervention. Then if it is safe, tests and measures are conducted to determine if the source of symptoms can be influenced by mechanical changes in position or movement and to establish a baseline of impairment and functional limitations measurements from which changes can be documented. Examination techniques and procedures are beyond the scope of this text, but a brief summary of concerns in the spinal area is listed to help focus on critical decisions prior to establishing an intervention strategy.

- *Serious "red flag" conditions related to orthopedic conditions* that should be referred to a physician for management include spinal cord symptoms and signs, recent trauma where spinal fracture or instabilities have not been ruled out, and serious pain (especially pain that awakens the individual) that cannot be explained mechanically.
- *Psychological distress* may interfere with a patient's recovery; therefore, referral to an appropriate professional may be indicated for a multidisciplinary approach in the patient's care.
- *Neurological symptoms* should be explored in an attempt to relate them to spinal cord, nerve root, spinal nerve, plexus, or peripheral nerve patterns. Causes of nerve root signs frequently seen by physical therapists include intervertebral disk protrusions; bony, soft tissue, or vascular stenosis in the spinal canal or intervertebral foramina; facet joint swelling; and nerve root tension from restricted mobility.
- *Pain patterns* should be explored to determine if they relate to a known musculoskeletal pattern or signal a medical condition. It should be recognized that pain is interpreted many ways and has various meanings for different people; therefore, the information is interpreted as only one factor when determining cause of the symptoms.

*Stage of recovery.* Time frames for each recovery stage vary depending on the reference used. In general, the acute stage usually lasts less than 4 weeks, the subacute stage is 4 to 12 weeks, and the chronic stage is greater than 12 weeks.[2] Chronic pain syndromes generally are conditions that extend beyond 6 months.

- *Acute inflammatory stage.* The patient experiences constant pain, and there are signs of inflammation. No position or movement completely relieves the symptoms. Medical intervention with anti-inflammatory medications is usually warranted.
- *Acute stage without signs of inflammation.* Symptoms are intermittent and related to mechanical deformation. There may be signs of nerve irritability when the nerve root or spinal nerve is compressed or placed under tension. The patient may be categorized into an extension bias, a flexion bias, or a non-weight-bearing bias based on the presenting posture, movement impairments, or positions of symptom relief. These categories are described in greater detail in the next section. Delitto and

associates[22] classified patients as being at this stage if they cannot stand longer than 15 minutes, sit longer than 30 minutes, or walk more than one-quarter mile without their status worsening.

- **Subacute stage.** Usually at this stage, certain movements and postures with some instrumental activities of daily living (IADLs) still provoke symptoms, such as lifting, vacuuming, gardening, and other activities requiring repetitive movement of loads so a basic lifestyle cannot fully be resumed. A more thorough examination is conducted to identify impairments that could be interfering with recovery.
- **Chronic stage.** When this stage is reached, emphasis is placed on returning the patient to high-level demand activities that require handling repetitive loads on a sustained basis over a prolonged period of time (from heavy material handling, to repetitive household activities that include lifting small children, to strenuous athletic activities).

***Diagnosis, prognosis, and plan of care.*** As mentioned in the introduction to this chapter, specific pathologies and medical diagnoses often do not guide the therapist when choosing appropriate treatment interventions, and that various systems of patient classification for treating musculoskeletal impairments and functional limitations are present in the literature.[2,22,23,27,64,85,92] In addition, validation studies supporting clinical prediction rules are available to assist the therapist in making decisions when developing and modifying interventions.[8,17,28,35,58] The material in the remainder of this chapter is organized to integrate impairment categories based on impaired posture, movement patterns, and diagnostic tests with pathological conditions that are described by the medical model in order to help the therapist choose an intervention strategy that best enhances the patient's recovery. The decisions concerning the approach to treatment are determined by the patient's responses to the examination maneuvers and the maneuvers that provide the greatest relief of symptoms. Adjustments in the intervention occur as the patient progresses through the healing process. The categories described in this and the following sections are summarized in Box 15.4.

 **Focus on Evidence**_____

Several validation and outcome studies have identified subgroups of patients who benefit from different approaches to therapeutic interventions.

- Long[58] identified patients with chronic low back pain as either centralizers (peripheral symptoms lessened or became more proximal) or noncentralizers as a result of repeated movement tests. Long concluded that those who were classified as centralizers had greater improvement in outcome measures (pain rating, return to work rate) than noncentralizers.
- Childs et al.,[17] in a multicenter randomized, controlled trial of 131 consecutive patients with low back pain, determined that patients most likely to benefit from

---

**BOX 15.4  Impairment-Based Diagnostic Categories That Direct Intervention**

**General—Stage of Recovery**
- Acute with inflammation (0–4 weeks).
- Acute without inflammation (0–4 weeks): intermittent symptoms with acute nerve root symptoms.
- Subacute (4–12 weeks).
- Chronic (> 12 weeks).
- Chronic pain syndrome (> 6 months).

**Non-Weight-Bearing Bias (Traction Syndrome[22])**
- Patient does not tolerate being upright for basic ADLs and IADLs.
- Movement testing makes symptoms worse.
- Traction (or other non-weight-bearing procedures) relieves symptoms.

**Extension Bias (Extension Syndrome[22])**
- Patient usually presents with flexed posture—a *lateral shift* may also be present.
- Extension tests decrease or centralize symptoms.
- Diagnosis may include intervertebral disk lesions, impaired flexed posture, fluid stasis.

**Flexion Bias (Flexion Syndrome[22])**
- Patient usually presents with flexed posture and is more comfortable when flexed.
- Extension tests exacerbate or peripheralize symptoms.
- Diagnoses may include spondylosis, stenosis, extension load injuries, swollen facet joints.

**Stabilization/Immobilization[22]**
- Patients present with hypermobile spinal segment(s); poor spinal stability (segmental or global).
- Diagnoses may include trauma, ligamentous laxity, spondylolysis, spondylolisthesis.

**Mobilization/Manipulation[22]**
- Restricted mobility in one or more spinal segments.

**Muscle and Soft Tissue Lesions**
- Patient usually presents with guarded posture or increased muscle tension.
- Diagnoses may include strains, tears, contusions, overuse.

---

spinal manipulation prior to stabilization exercises where those who met four of five of the following criteria: symptom duration less than 16 days, no symptoms distal to the knee, score less than 19 on a fear-avoidance measure, at least one hypomobile lumbar segment, and at least one hip with more than 35° internal rotation.

- Fritz et al.[28] reported that those who had positive tests for spinal hypomobility had more successful outcomes if manipulation was included in the interventions; and those with hypermobility were more successful if stabilization was included.
- Hicks et al.[35] determined that the patients most likely to benefit from stabilization exercises were those with lumbar segmental instability who met three or more of the

following criteria: positive prone instability test, aberrant motions during lumbar ROM, average straight-leg raise less than 91°, and age less than 40 years.

● Audrey et al.[8] studied 312 acute, subacute, and chronic patients with low back pain (with or without sciatica). They found significantly greater improvement in outcomes for individuals whose exercise interventions were matched with their directional preference (flexion, extension, or side glide/rotation) than those who undertook nondirectional exercises.

## General Guidelines for Managing Acute Spinal Problems: Protection Phase

Use of modalities and massage to decrease pain and swelling from acute symptoms is appropriate during the acute stage. It is also important that the patient becomes an active participant in his or her program. Kinesthetic training of neutral or functional spinal posture, nondestructive movements in the pain-free range, awareness and activation of core musculature, and basic functional training maneuvers are taught if they do not exacerbate the symptoms. Specific interventions for various impairments, specific biases, or syndromes and common pathologies in the spinal region are described in the remaining sections of this chapter. Specific techniques for kinesthetic training, core muscle activation, stabilization training, and functional training activities for the acute stage in the cervical and lumbar spinal regions are described in Chapter 16. Management guidelines for treating the patient with acute symptoms are summarized in Box 15.5. The following points are fundamental to all interventions.

### Patient Education

It is important to engage patients in all aspects of intervention, including information about anticipated progress and outcome, the healing time of inflamed tissues or reduction of symptoms due to nerve root pressure (if indicated), and precautions and contraindications.

### Symptom Relief or Comfort

If a patient is experiencing acute inflammation from a traumatic injury, there is constant pain; yet often an optimal position of comfort or symptom reduction can be determined in which there is the least amount of stress on the inflamed, irritated, or swollen region. The terms *functional position* or *functional range* are used to describe this position.[70] (*Neutral position* is mid-range.) The functional range may change for the individual as the tissues heal and the person gains mobility and strength in the region. Some pathological conditions typically tend to cause symptoms in one portion of the range and are relieved in another range.[70] The following terms, describing subcategories of diagnoses or syndromes, have been popularized based on the work of Morgan,[70] Saal et al.,[88,91] Delitto et al.,[22] and Fritz and George.[27]

***Extension bias—extension syndrome.*** The patient's symptoms are lessened in positions of extension (lordosis). Sustained flexed postures or repetitive flexion motions load the anterior disk region and facet joints, causing fluid redistribution from the compressed areas and swelling and creep in the distended areas. This is frequently the mechanism of symptom production with posterior or posterolateral intervertebral disk lesions or injury to the posterior longitudinal ligament. Whether the pathology is an injured disk or stressed and swollen tissues,

---

**BOX 15.5**
## MANAGEMENT GUIDELINES—Acute Spinal Problems/Protection Phase

**Impairments and Functional Limitations**
Pain and/or neurological symptoms
Inflammation
Inability to perform ADLs and IADLs
Guarded posture (prefers flexion, extension, or non-weight-bearing)

| Plan of Care | Intervention |
|---|---|
| 1. Educate the patient. | 1. Engage patient in all activities to learn self-management. Inform patient of anticipated progress and precautions. |
| 2. Decrease acute symptoms. | 2. Modalities, massage, traction, or manipulation as needed. Rest only for first couple days if needed. |
| 3. Teach awareness of neck and pelvic position and movement. | 3. Kinesthetic training: cervical and scapular motions, pelvic tilts, neutral spine. |
| 4. Demonstrate safe postures. | 4. Practice positions and movement and experience effect on spine. Provide passive support/bracing if needed. |
| 5. Initiate neuromuscular activation and control of stabilizing muscles. | 5. Core activation techniques: drawing-in maneuver, multifidus contraction. Basic stabilization: with arm and leg motions (passive support if needed, progress to active control). |
| 6. Teach safe performance of basic ADLs; progress to IADLs. | 6. Roll, sit, stand, and walk with safe postures. Progress tolerance to sitting > 30 minutes, standing > 15 minutes, and walking > 1 mile. |

repeated extension motions and positions relieve the symptoms by moving the fluid to reverse the stasis (these techniques are described in the sections on extension bias). Some patients present with a lateral shift, which usually requires correction before extension relieves the symptoms.[64-66]

***Flexion bias—flexion syndrome.*** The patient's symptoms are lessened in positions of spinal flexion and provoked in extension. This is often the case when there is compromise of the intervertebral foramen or spinal canal, as in bony spinal stenosis, spondylosis, and spondylolisthesis.

***Non-weight-bearing bias—traction syndrome.*** The patient's symptoms are lessened when in non-weight-bearing positions, such as when lying down or in traction. Symptoms also lessen when spinal pressure is reduced by leaning on the upper extremities (using arm rests to unweight the trunk), by leaning the trunk against a support, or when in a pool. The condition is considered *gravity sensitive*[12] because the symptoms worsen during standing, walking, running, coughing, or similar activities that increase spinal pressure. Often traction and aquatic therapy are the only interventions that minimize symptoms during the acute phase.

### Kinesthetic Awareness of Safe Postures and Effects of Movement

The patient is taught how to identify and assume the spinal position that is most comfortable and reduces the symptoms using pelvic tilts for lumbar positioning and head nods and chin tucks for cervical spine positioning. If necessary, corsets or cervical collars are used to provide support, and the patient is taught how to use *passive positioning* to help maintain the functional position during the acute stage (Box 15.6).

---

**BOX 15.6** | **Examples of Passive Positioning of the Lumbar Spine**

- *Supine:* Hook-lying flexes the lumbar spine; legs extended extends the spine. A pillow under the head flexes the neck; a small roll under the neck stabilizes a mild lordosis with the head neutral.
- *Prone:* Use of a pillow under the abdomen flexes the lumbar spine; no pillow extends the spine. To maintain the cervical spine in neutral alignment without rotation, a split table or a small towel roll placed under the forehead provides space for the nose so the patient does not turn the head.
- *Sitting:* Usually causes spinal flexion, especially if the hips and knees are flexed. To emphasize flexion, the feet are propped up on a small footstool; to emphasize extension, a lumbar pillow or towel roll is placed in the lowback region. To unweight the spine, the arms are placed on an armrest, or a reclining chair is used.
- *Standing:* Usually causes spinal extension; to emphasize flexion, one foot is placed on a small stool.

---

### Muscle Performance: Core Muscle Activation and Basic Stabilization

Whether the patient has a cervical or lumbar problem, as soon as tolerated the patient is taught how to activate the core muscles.

#### Lumbar Region—Core Muscle Activation

For the lumbar region, the *"drawing-in"* maneuver is used to activate the transversus abdominis and a gentle bulging contraction of the multifidus muscle. Facilitation techniques may be necessary, which are described in detail in the Core Activation section of Chapter 16.

#### Cervical Region—Core Muscle Activation

For the patient with cervical pain, gentle head nods and slight flattening of the cervical lordosis in the supine position are used for core activation of the longus colli and multifidus.

#### Basic Stabilization

Once the patient learns to activate the core muscles, simple upper and lower extremity motions with the spine stabilized are added to the intervention. *Passive prepositioning* is used if the patient is unable actively to maintain his or her functional position, as described in Box 15.6. For both cervical and lumbar problems, the patient is instructed first to do the drawing-in maneuver followed by gentle arm motions within a range that does not exacerbate symptoms. Leg motions require greater lumbopelvic control and are introduced if the patient is able to demonstrate pelvic control and the symptoms are not exacerbated with the movements. Suggestions for determining the exercise progressions are detailed in the Stabilization section of Chapter 16.

#### Basic Functional Movements

The patient is taught to perform simple movements for ADLs while protecting the spine in the functional position. These movements include rolling from prone to supine and reverse, lying to sitting and reverse, sitting to standing and reverse, and walking. Descriptions of these maneuvers are in the Functional Activities section of Chapter 16.

PRECAUTIONS: Review any special precautions for the condition with the patient. Condition-specific precautions are described in the remaining sections of this chapter.

### General Guidelines for Managing Subacute Spinal Problems: Controlled Motion Phase

When the signs and symptoms of the inflammatory process are under control and pain is no longer constant, the patient is progressed through a program of safe muscle endurance and strengthening exercises to prepare the tissue for functional activities and rehabilitation training. Functional activities that can be performed safely are resumed. Pain may still interfere with some daily activities, but it should no longer be constant. Poor neuromuscular control and stabilization, poor postural awareness and body mechanics,

## BOX 15.7
### MANAGEMENT GUIDELINES—Subacute Spinal Problems/Controlled Motion Phase

**Impairments and Functional Limitations**
Pain: only when excessive stress is placed on vulnerable tissues
Impaired posture/postural awareness
Impaired mobility
Impaired muscle performance: poor neuromuscular control of stabilizing muscles; decreased muscle endurance and strength
General deconditioning
Inability to perform IADLs for extended periods of time
Poor body mechanics

| Plan of Care | Intervention |
|---|---|
| 1. Educate the patient in self-management and how to decrease episodes of pain. | 1. Engage patient in all activities emphasizing safe movement and postures. Home exercise program. Ergonomic adaptation of work or home environment. |
| 2. Progress awareness and control of spinal alignment. | 2. Practice active spinal control in pain-free positions and with all exercises and activities. Practice posture correction. |
| 3. Increase mobility in tight muscles/joint/fascia. | 3. Joint mobilization/manipulation, muscle inhibition, self-stretching. |
| 4. Teach techniques to develop neuromuscular control, strength, and endurance. | 4. Progress stabilization exercises; increase repetitions and challenge. Initiate extremity-strengthening exercises in conjunction with core muscle activation. Initiate and progress dynamic trunk strengthening exercises. |
| 5. Develop cardiopulmonary endurance. | 5. Low to moderate intensity aerobic exercises; emphasize spinal bias. |
| 6. Teach techniques of stress relief/relaxation. | 6. Relaxation exercises and postural stress relief. |
| 7. Teach safe body mechanics and functional adaptations. | 7. Practice stable spine lifting, pushing/pulling, and reaching. Practice activities specific to desired outcome emphasizing spinal control, endurance, and timing. |

decreased flexibility and strength, and generalized deconditioning may be the underlying impairments at this stage. Intervention during this stage is critical because either the patient feels good and tends to overdo activities and reinjures the tissues, or the patient is fearful and does not adequately resume safe movements so impairments develop, leading to functional restrictions. Either extreme may slow down the recovery process.

Management guidelines for cervical and lumbar problems that require controlled motion interventions are summarized in Box 15.7. The specific techniques and progressions of intervention outlined here are described in detail in Chapter 16.

### Pain Modulation
At this stage, use of modalities to modulate pain is not recommended. Emphasis is placed on increasing patient awareness of posture, strength, mobility, and spinal control and their relationship to modulating pain.

### Kinesthetic Training
Kinesthetic training is progressed by using reinforcement techniques. Feedforward control of the core musculature, active control of the spinal position, and correct posture are reinforced in a variety of ways until activation and control become habitual. Kinesthetic training overlaps the stabilization exercises.

### Stretching/Mobilization
Decreased flexibility in joints, muscles, and fascia may restrict the patient's ability to assume normal spinal alignment. Manual techniques and safe self-stretching techniques are used to increase muscle, joint, and connective tissue mobility.

### Muscle Performance
Exercises are progressed with increased challenges for control, muscular endurance, and strength in the spinal stabilizing muscles; included are activities that increase control and strength in the extremity musculature in conjunction with spinal stabilization. If a patient continues to display a flexion or extension bias, exercises are adapted to emphasize that particular bias and prevent stresses in the symptom-producing direction. Detailed descriptions of principles and application of these exercises are in Chapter 16.

- Stabilization exercises are used to emphasize movement and resistance to the extremities while maintaining control of the spinal position. Increasing the time and number of repetitions is used to increase muscle endurance at each level of performance.
- Wall slides, partial squats, partial lunges, pushing, and pulling against resistance are used to strengthen the extremities to prepare for lifting, reaching, pushing, and pulling activities.

● When the patient learns effective spinal control with the core stabilizing muscles in a variety of stabilization exercise routines, dynamic trunk and neck strengthening exercises such as curl-ups, back extension, and cervical motions are introduced. Care is taken to monitor symptoms and modify any activities that exacerbate the problem.

## Cardiopulmonary Conditioning

Aerobic capacity is usually compromised after injury. It is important to guide the patient in the initiation of or safe return to an aerobic conditioning program. It may be necessary to help the patient identify activities that do not exacerbate spinal symptoms. Suggestions are included in Chapter 16.

## Postural Stress Management and Relaxation Exercises

It is common that patient's symptoms are exacerbated with sustained postural stresses such as sitting at a computer, talking on the phone (head tilted), or repetitive forward bending (shoe salesman); therefore analysis of work, home, or recreational postures and activities is a necessary component of the patient's program. The patient is then advised about methods to correct the sustained or repetitive postural stresses. In addition, frequent changes of position and movement through the pain-free ROMs should be encouraged. It may be necessary to teach the patient how to consciously relax tension in muscles to relieve stress. Relaxation exercises are described in Chapter 14.

## Functional Activities

Once the patient has learned spinal control and stabilization and has developed adequate flexibility and strength for specific tasks, components of the task are incorporated into the exercise program and then into the patient's daily lifestyle. Safe body mechanics are included in all aspects of care.

## General Guidelines for Managing Chronic Spinal Problems: Return to Function Phase

Patients who have been treated through the acute and subacute phases of healing with appropriately graded exercises should have minimal impairments that prevent or restrict daily activities. Individuals who must do heavy material handling (e.g., a manual laborer, firefighter, caregiver of small children or patients) or who participate in high-demand sports activities may require additional rehabilitative training to return safely to these high-demand activities and to avoid further injury. Impairments in strength, endurance, neuromuscular control, and skill are related to the functional goals of the individual. At this stage, conditioning and spinal control during high-intensity and repetitive activities are emphasized. Any underlying impairments that interfere with the desired outcomes must be remediated. Management guidelines for return to function are summarized in Box 15.8. Suggestions for progressing exercise intervention techniques from the subacute through chronic stages are described in Chapter 16.

---

## BOX 15.8
### MANAGEMENT GUIDELINES—Chronic Spinal Problems/Return to Function Phase

**Impairments and Functional Limitations**

Pain: only when excessive stress is placed on vulnerable tissues in repetitive or sustained nature for prolonged periods
Poor neuromuscular control and endurance in high-intensity or destabilized situations
Flexibility and strength imbalances
Generalized deconditioning
Inability to perform high-intensity physical demands for extended periods of time

| Plan of Care | Intervention |
|---|---|
| 1. Emphasize spinal control in high-intensity and repetitive activities. | 1. Practice active spinal control in various transitional activities that challenge balance. |
| 2. Increase mobility in tight muscles/joints/fascia. | 2. Joint mobilization/manipulation, muscle inhibition, self-stretching. |
| 3. Improve muscle performance; dynamic trunk and extremity strength, coordination, and endurance. | 3. Progress dynamic trunk and extremity resistance exercises emphasizing functional goals. |
| 4. Increase cardiopulmonary endurance. | 4. Progress intensity of aerobic exercises. |
| 5. Emphasize habitual use of techniques of stress relief/relaxation and posture correction. | 5. Motions and postures to relieve stress. Apply any ergonomic changes to work/home environment. |
| 6. Teach safe progression to high-level/high-intensity activities. | 6. Progressive practice using activity-specific training consistent with desired functional outcome, emphasizing spinal control, endurance, timing, and speed. |
| 7. Teach healthy exercise habits for self-maintenance. | 7. Engage patient in all activities and educate as to benefits of maintaining fitness level and safe body mechanics. |

# ● MANAGEMENT GUIDELINES— NON-WEIGHT-BEARING BIAS

During examination, some patients do not respond to extension, flexion, or even mid-range spinal positions or motions due to the acuity of or mechanical stimuli from their condition. The person is often more comfortable lying down and may have partial or full relief with a traction test maneuver to the painful region of the spine.

For these patients, use of traction procedures or unweighting the body in a pool may be the interventions of choice until the symptoms stabilize.

## Management of Acute Symptoms

### Traction

Various references have reported the benefits of traction.[16,32,62,83,93]

- Traction has the mechanical benefit of temporarily separating the vertebrae, causing mechanical sliding of the facet joints in the spine, and increasing the size of the intervertebral foramina. If done intermittently, this motion may help reduce circulatory congestion and relieve pressure on the dura, blood vessels, and nerve roots in the intervertebral foramina. Improving circulation may also help decrease the concentration of noxious chemical irritants due to swelling and inflammation.
- There may be a neurophysiological response via stimulation of the mechanoreceptors that may modulate the transmission of nociceptive stimuli at the spinal cord or brain stem level.

### Harness

Various unloading devices or body weight support systems may be used, such as partially suspending the patient in a harness while he or she performs ambulation on a treadmill or gentle extremity exercises.

### Pool

If a person is not fearful of being in a pool, supporting the individual with a buoyant life belt in deep water reduces the effects of gravity on the lumbar spine. If symptoms are reduced, it may be possible to begin and progress gentle stabilization exercises in this buoyant environment to meet some of the goals during the acute and subacute phases. Exercises can also be progressed by using the properties of water for resistance and stretching (see description of aquatic exercises in Chapter 9).

## Progression

As healing occurs, the patient should begin to tolerate weight bearing. After re-examination and assessment, identify the impairments and functional limitations. If a bias toward flexion or extension is determined or if there are areas of hyper- or hypomobility, plan the interventions accordingly.

# ● MANAGEMENT GUIDELINES— EXTENSION BIAS

Patients with an extension bias often assume a flexed posture or a flexed posture with lateral deviation of the trunk or neck, but during the examination sustained or repetitive extension maneuvers reduce or relieve their symptoms. These patients would benefit from early interventions that emphasize extension of the involved segments. The impairments may be due to a contained intervertebral disk lesion, fluid stasis, a flexion injury, or muscle imbalances from a faulty flexed posture. McKenzie[64-66] developed a method of categorizing these patients based on the extent of their pain and/or neurological symptoms. He also described the phenomena of peripheralization and centralization that accompany an expanding and receding lesion, frequently attributed to intervertebral disk lesions.

Many of the techniques that were originally described by McKenzie and May[65,66] to manage a patient with an acute disk lesion have been found to be beneficial in the management of patients who have a cluster of signs and symptoms that categorize them into the extension bias (extension syndrome) category.[26,27,58,88]

## Principles of Management

Because patients with signs and symptoms of a bulging intervertebral disk often fit into the "extension bias" category, a brief discussion of the response of the intervertebral disk is presented here.

### Effects of Postural Changes on Intervertebral Disk Pressure

Relative changes in posture and activities affect intradiskal pressure. When compared to the level of pressure when standing, intradiskal pressure is least when lying supine, increases by almost 50% while sitting with hips and knees flexed, and almost doubles if leaning forward while sitting.[45] Sitting with a back rest inclination of 120° and lumbar support 5 cm in depth provides the lowest load to the disk while sitting.[7,49] Therefore, sitting with the hips and knees flexed or leaning forward should be avoided when there is an acute disk lesion. If sitting is necessary, there should be support for the lumbar spine by reclining the trunk 120°.

### Effects of Bed Rest on the Intervertebral Disk

When a person is lying down, compression forces to the disk are reduced; and with time, the nucleus potentially can absorb more water to equalize pressures (imbibition). While lying down with the spine in flexion, the imbibed fluid accumulates posteriorly in the disk where there is greater space. Then, upon rising, body weight compresses the disk with the increased fluid, and intradiskal pressure greatly increases. The pain or symptoms from a disk protrusion are accentuated. To avoid exacerbating symptoms, absolute bed rest during the acute phase should be avoided. Bed rest during the first 2 days (when symptoms are highly irritable) may be needed to promote early healing, but it should be interspersed with short intervals of standing, walking, and appropriately controlled movement.[100]

### Effects of Traction on the Intervertebral Disk

Traction may relieve symptoms from a disk protrusion. It is proposed that separating the vertebral bodies may have the effect of placing tension on the annular fibers and posterior longitudinal ligament, thus have a flattening effect on the bulge; or it may decrease the intradiskal pressure.[62] If traction relieves symptoms, the time of application must be short because with the reduced pressure fluid imbibition may occur to equalize the pressure. Then, when the traction is released, the pressure increases and symptoms are exacerbated.

### Effects of Flexion and Extension on the Intervertebral Disk and Fluid Stasis

Rest in a slightly forward-bent position often lessens pain because of the space potential for the nucleus pulposus of the intervertebral disk. The patient may also deviate laterally to minimize pressure against a nerve root. Movement into extension initially causes increased symptoms. With acute disk lesions in which there is protective lateral shifting and lumbar flexion, techniques that cause lateral shifting of the spine opposite to the deviation followed by passive spinal extension (sustained or repetitive) to compress the protrusion mechanically have been found to relieve the clinical signs and symptoms in many patients.[51,65]

Patients experiencing pain due to fluid stasis after being in a sustained flexed posture also experience relief with movement into extension.

### Effects of Isometric and Dynamic Exercise

Isometric activities (resisted pelvic tilt exercises, straining, Valsalva maneuver) and active back flexion or extension exercises increase intradiskal pressures above normal. They therefore must be avoided during the acute stage of a disk lesion. Strong muscle contractions also exacerbate symptoms if a muscle has been injured. Therefore, active and resistive extension exercises are avoided during the acute stage.

### Effects of Muscle Guarding

Reflex muscle guarding or splinting often accompanies an acute disk lesion and adds to the compressive forces on the disk. Modalities and gentle oscillatory traction to the spine may help decrease the splinting.

## Indications, Precautions, and Contraindications for Interventions—Extension Approach

*Indications:* Extension is used if pain and/or neurological symptoms centralize (decrease of move more proximally) during extension testing maneuvers and peripheralize (worsen) during flexion. Extension is also indicated for flexed postural dysfunctions with limited range into extension.

---

**BOX 15.9  Contraindications to Specific Spinal Movements**

*Extension* of the spine is contraindicated[65]:

- When no position or movement decreases or centralizes the described pain
- When saddle anesthesia and/or bladder weakness is present (could indicate spinal cord or cauda equina lesion)
- When a patient is in such extreme pain that he or she rigidly holds the body immobile with any attempted correction

*Flexion* of the spine should be avoided:

- When extension relieves the symptoms
- When flexion movements increase the pain or peripheralize the symptoms

---

PRECAUTION: A patient with acute pain in the spinal region that is not influenced by changing the patient's position or by movement must be screened by a physician for signs of serious pathology.

CONTRAINDICATIONS: When there is a disk lesion, any form of exercise or activity that increases intradiskal pressure, such as the Valsalva maneuver, active pelvic tilt, or trunk-raising exercises, is contraindicated[65] during the protection phase of treatment. Any movement that peripheralizes the symptoms signals a movement that is contraindicated during the acute and early subacute period of treatment. Peripheralization with extension motions may indicate stenosis, a large lateral disk protrusion, or pathology in a posterior element[90] (Box 15.9).

## Techniques Using an Extension Approach in the Lumbar Spine

NOTE: These techniques are used only if the test movements have shown that the postures and movements used decrease the symptoms.[49,65] If no test movements decrease the symptoms, this mechanical approach to treatment should not be used.

### Management of Acute Symptoms

If symptoms are severe, bed rest is indicated with short periods of walking at regular intervals. Walking usually promotes lumbar extension and stimulates fluid mechanics to help reduce swelling in the disk or connective tissues. If the patient cannot stand upright, he or she should use crutches to help relieve the increased pressure of the forward-bent posture.[49]

If repeated flexion test movements increase the symptoms and if repeated extension test movements decrease or centralize the symptoms, all flexion activities should be avoided during the early phases of intervention. Treatment begins with the following maneuvers.

## Passive Extension

◉ *Patient position and procedure:* Prone. If the flexion posture is severe, place pillows under the abdomen for support. Gradually increase the amount of extension by removing the pillows and then progress by having the patient prop himself or herself up on the elbows, allowing the pelvis to sag (Fig. 15.7A). When propping, pillows placed under the thorax help take strain off the shoulders. Wait 5 to 10 minutes between each increment of extension to allow reduction of the water content and the size of the bulge. There should be an accompanying centralization of or decrease in symptoms. Progress to having the patient prop himself or herself up on the hands, allowing the pelvis to sag (Fig. 15.7B).

◉ If the sustained position of prone propping is not well tolerated, have the patient perform passive lumbar extension intermittently by repeating the *prone press-ups* (same end position as Fig. 15.7B) rather than just propping up.

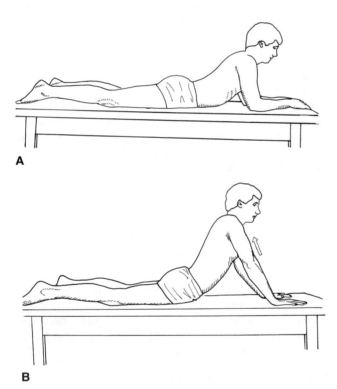

**A**

**B**

FIGURE 15.7 Passive lumbar extension is accomplished (*A*) by having the patient prop up on the elbows and (*B*) by propping on hands and allowing the pelvis to sag.

PRECAUTION: Carefully monitor the patient's symptoms. They should lessen peripherally (i.e., decreased foot and leg symptoms or decreased thigh and buttock symptoms) but may increase in the low back (centralize). If the symptoms progress down the lower extremity (peripheralize), immediately stop the exercises and reassess.[65]

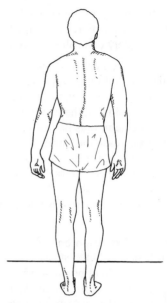

FIGURE 15.8 Patient with lateral shift of the thoracic cage toward the right. The pelvis is shifted toward the left.

## Lateral Shift Correction

If the patient has lateral shifting of the spine (Fig. 15.8), extension alone cannot reduce a nuclear protrusion of the disk until the shift is corrected. Once the shift is corrected, the patient must extend (as described above) to maintain the correction. Methods to correct the shift in various positions include the following.

◉ *Patient position and procedure:* Standing with flexed elbow against the side of the deviated rib cage. Stand on the side to which the thorax is shifted and place your shoulder against the patient's elbow. Then wrap your arms around the patient's pelvis on the opposite side and simultaneously pull the pelvis toward you while pushing the patient's thorax away (Fig. 15.9). This is a gradual maneuver. Continue with the lateral shifting if centralization of the symptoms occurs. If there is overcorrection, the pain and lateral shift may move to the contralateral side, which is corrected by shifting the thorax back. The purpose is to centralize the pain and correct the lateral shift. Once the shift is corrected, *immediately* have the patient backward-bend (Fig. 15.10). Again, allow time. Progress to passive extension with prone propping and prone press-ups as previously described.

◉ *Patient position and procedure:* Side-lying on the side to which the thorax is shifted. Place a small pillow or towel roll under the thorax. The patient remains in this position until the pain centralizes; he or she then rolls prone and begins passive extension with prone propping and prone press-ups.

◉ *Patient position and procedure:* Prone. Attempt to side-glide the thorax and pelvis toward the midline with manual pressure. The forces are in equal and opposite

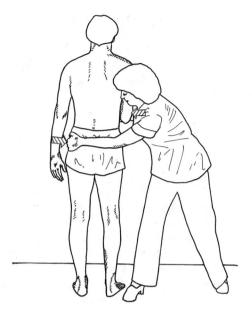

**FIGURE 15.9** A lateral gliding technique used to correct a lateral shift of the thorax is applied against the patient's elbow and thoracic cage as the pelvis is pulled in the opposite direction.

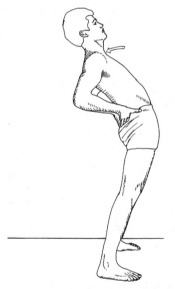

**FIGURE 15.10** Standing back bend.

directions. Once the symptoms centralize, instruct the patient to begin passive extension with prone propping and prone press-ups.

### Patient Education

- Help the patient recognize what positions and motions increase or decrease the pain or other symptoms by performing them under supervision.
- Instruct the patient to repeat the extension activities frequently, with lateral shift correction if necessary, during the first couple of days. For example:

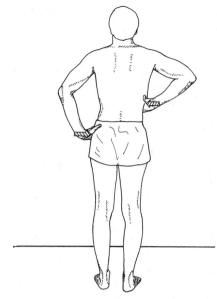

**FIGURE 15.11** Self-correction of a lateral shift.

- Teach *self-correction of the lateral shift.* The patient places the hand on the side of the shifted rib cage on the lateral aspect of the rib cage and places the other hand over the crest of the opposite ilium and then gradually pushes these regions toward the midline and holds (Fig. 15.11).
- Instruct the patient to correct the shift by side-lying or prone-lying as previously described.
- Caution the patient to stop the activity immediately if the pain worsens or peripheralizes during exercises.
- Instruct the patient to maintain an extended posture with passive support while the lesion is healing. For example, have the patient use a towel roll or lumbar pillow while sitting. This is especially important when riding in a car or sitting in a soft chair. When going to bed, have the patient pin a towel, folded lengthwise four times, around the waist.
- Instruct the patient to avoid flexion activities, lifting, or any other functions that increase intradiskal pressure while symptoms are acute.
- Teach safe movement patterns to protect the back as described in the guidelines for treating acute spinal problems (see Box 15.5).

### Lumbar Traction

Traction may be tolerated by the patient during the acute stage and has the benefit of widening the disk space and possibly reducing the nuclear protrusion by decreasing the pressure on the disk or by placing tension on the posterior longitudinal ligament.[93]

- Time of the traction should be short; osmotic forces soon equalize. However, upon release of the traction force, there could be an increase in disk pressure, leading to increased pain. Use less than 15 minutes of intermittent traction or less than 10 minutes of sustained traction.

- High poundage; more than half the patient's body weight is necessary for separating the lumbar vertebrae.
- If there is complete relief initially, often there is an exacerbation of symptoms later.

### Kinesthetic Training, Stabilization, and Basic Functional Activities

Once the patient learns to control the symptoms the following should be emphasized.

- Teach simple spinal movements in pain-free ranges using gentle pelvic tilts. The patient is taught to be aware of how far forward and backward he or she can rock the pelvis and move the spine without increasing the symptoms. The pelvic rocking is done in supine, sitting, hand-knee all-fours (quadruped), prone-lying, side-lying, and standing positions. It is important to stay within the patient's ability to control the symptoms. *Instruct the patient to finish all exercise routines with the pelvis tilted anteriorly and the spine in extension.*
- Teach the patient basic stabilization techniques utilizing the core trunk muscles while maintaining control of the extended spinal position and performing simple extremity motions. (These exercises are described in detail in the muscle performance section of Chapter 16.) It is important to caution against holding the breath and causing the Valsalva maneuver, which would excessively increase the intradiskal pressure.
- Encourage activities within the tolerance of the individual, such as walking or swimming.
- Initiate passive straight-leg raising with intermittent dorsiflexion and plantarflexion to maintain mobility in the nerve roots of the lumbar spine.

## Management When Acute Symptoms Have Stabilized

### Signs of Improvement

Improvement is noted with loss of spinal deformity, increased motion in the back, and negative dural mobility signs.[49] Loss of back pain with an increase in true neurological signs is an indication of worsening. The patient is tested to determine that the symptoms have stabilized; this is accomplished by performing repeated flexion and extension tests with the patient standing and then lying supine and prone, as done initially. The tests may be positive for dysfunction (restricted motion, tension) but should not cause peripheralization of the symptoms, as when the condition was acute.[65]

### Emphasis of Intervention

The emphases during this stage are *recovery of function, development of a healthy back care plan,* and *teaching the patient how to prevent recurrences* (see Box 15.7). Suggested exercises to correct the identified impairments are described in Chapter 16. The pain from adaptive shortening decreases as normal flexibility, strength, and endurance are restored.

In addition, teach the patient these principles.

- Following any flexion exercises, perform extension exercises, such as prone press-ups or standing back extension (see Figs. 15.7 and 15.10).

- If being in a prolonged flexed posture is necessary, interrupt the flexion with backward bending at least once every hour. Also, perform intermittent pelvic tilts.
- If symptoms of a protrusion develop and are felt, immediately perform press-ups in the prone position, anterior pelvic tilts in the quadruped position, or backward bending while standing to prevent progression of the symptoms.

## Techniques to Manage a Disk Lesion in the Cervical Spine

Disk lesions in the cervical spine are less common than in the lumbar spine. Often disk extrusions are an indication for surgery because of potential compromise of the spinal canal and pressure on the spinal cord.[87] Patients may present with peripheral neuropathy and forward-head posture without a diagnosis of disk pathology. Symptoms increase with activities and postures that increase flexion in the lower cervical and upper thoracic spine and decrease with extension in that region (axial extension or neck retraction).[1] Conservative management is similar to that in the lumbar spine and follows the same principles described in the previous section. Medical management includes pharmacological pain and inflammation control measures.

### Acute Phase

#### Passive Axial Extension (Cervical Retraction)

*Patient position and procedure:* Begin with the patient supine, with no pillow under the head or neck. Gently nod the patient's head, and allow the neck to flatten against the treatment table. If the neck is deviated or rotated to one side, moving the head and neck back toward the midline must be done first. This may require gentle progressive positioning and may take 10 to 20 minutes to accomplish.

*Progression:* Progress the retraction to hyperextension of the cervical spine and then progress to rotation. Use caution and carefully monitor the signs and symptoms; do not progress if symptoms peripheralize down the arm.

#### Patient Education

Teach the patient to retract his or her head and neck passively in the sitting position. The patient may gently push against the chin (caution not to push so hard as to cause joint compression of the temporomandibular joint) to direct the motion. This technique has been shown to improve the H-reflex amplitude and may be useful for improving mobility and decreasing symptoms of radiculopathy by decompressing nerve roots in the lower cervical spine.[1]

#### Traction

Cervical traction may relieve the patient's symptoms. As described for lumbar traction, during the acute phase sustained traction should be no longer than 10 minutes and intermittent traction no longer than 15 minutes in duration. The dosage is at an intensity that causes vertebral separation (at least 15 lb).

### Kinesthetic Training for Posture Correction

Instruct the patient in safe mechanics for maintaining the head position. During the acute phase, the patient may need to wear a cervical collar to immobilize the spine. It is important to help the patient identify the posture that centralizes the symptoms and to adjust the collar to maintain that position.

### Progression as Symptoms Stabilize

Follow the guidelines described in Box 15.5. The techniques are described in Chapter 16. Faulty cervical, thoracic, and scapular posture may be present. Emphasize kinesthetic training for postural awareness, stabilization exercises for postural control with emphasis on the scapular and shoulder muscles, environmental adaptations to reduce postural stresses, and functional activities with safe spinal mechanics.

## MANAGEMENT GUIDELINES— FLEXION BIAS

Patients may present with a flexed posture and be unable to extend because of increased neurological symptoms and decreased mobility; these patients would benefit from early interventions that emphasize flexion of the involved segments to relieve symptoms. The patients may have a medical diagnosis of spondylosis or spinal stenosis, may have sustained an extension load injury, or may have swollen facet joints so symptoms increase with extension. The flexed position reduces or relieves the symptoms.

## Principles of Management

***Effect of position.*** Flexion widens the intervertebral foramina, whereas extension decreases the size of the foramina. Any compromise of the foraminal opening, such as encroachment from bony spurs or lipping or swollen tissue, reduces the space. The patient may describe intermittent nerve root symptoms (intermittent numbness or tingling) whenever the involved segment extends, indicating mechanical compression. Constant nerve root symptoms could be caused by inflammation and swollen tissue.

***Effect of traction.*** Traction has been demonstrated to widen the intervertebral foramina. Positioning the spine in flexion prior to the application of traction provides the greatest increased space.[16,32,62,83]

***Effect of trauma and repetitive irritation.*** Swelling in the facet joints from macrotrauma or microtrauma leads to a compromised foraminal space. With degeneration and increased mobility in a spinal segment, instability could be the cause of repetitive microtrauma leading to swelling and pain.

***Effect of meniscoid tissue.*** The meniscoid tissue of the joint capsule may become impinged with sudden movements. This blocks specific movements, such as extension

and side bending to the involved side. Manipulation and traction usually relieve the symptoms.

## Indications and Contraindications for Intervention—Flexion Approach

***Indications.*** Flexion is used if neurological and/or pain symptoms are eased with flexion and worsened with extension positions or motions.

CONTRAINDICATIONS: Extension and extension with rotation positions, motions, and exercises are contraindicated if neurological symptoms or pain worsen with these motions. Flexion exercises are contraindicated if neurological or pain symptoms peripheralize with flexion or repeated flexion maneuvers (see Box 15.9).

## Techniques Utilizing a Flexion Approach

In general, spinal flexion postures and exercises are taught following the guidelines described in Boxes 15.5, 15.7, and 15.8. The following suggestions should also be considered for special conditions.

### Management of Acute Symptoms

**Rest and Support**

- With acute joint symptoms, a cervical collar or lumbar corset may help provide rest to the inflamed or swollen facet joints.
- Support is also beneficial in the management of patients with RA or other disorders associated with hypermobility or instability.
- It is important to discontinue the use of such devices as the acute symptoms decrease so the muscles can learn dynamic control and to avoid dependence.

**Functional Position for Comfort**

- For flexion bias in the lumbar spine, the position is usually with the hips and knees flexed so the lumbar spine flexes.
- In the cervical spine, the position is toward axial extension (upper cervical flexion) with some flexion also in the lower cervical region.
- If there are neurological signs, the position provides maximal opening of the intervertebral foramina to minimize impingement of the nerve root.

**Cervical Traction**

- Gentle intermittent joint distraction and gliding techniques may inhibit painful muscle responses and provide synovial fluid movement in the joint for healing.
- Dosages must be very gentle (grade I or II) to avoid stretching the capsules and are best applied with manual techniques during the acute stage.
- With spondylosis or stenosis, if a patient does not have signs of acute joint inflammation but does have signs of nerve root irritation, stronger traction forces may be beneficial to cause opening of the intervertebral foramina, which helps relieve the pressure.

CONTRAINDICATION: If a patient has RA, traction and joint mobilizations in the spine are potentially dangerous because of ligamentous necrosis and vertebral instability; they therefore should not be performed.[71]

### Correction of Lateral Shift

If the patient has a lateral shift of the thoracic region along with symptom relief when in flexion, he or she may be taught self-correction.

*Patient position and procedure*: Standing with the leg opposite the shift on a chair so the hip is in about 90° of flexion. The leg on the side of the lateral shift is kept extended. Have the patient then flex the trunk onto the raised thigh and apply pressure by pulling on the ankle (Fig. 15.12).

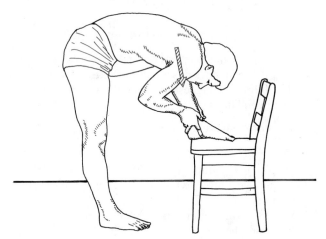

FIGURE 15.12 Self-correction of a lateral shift when there is deviation of the trunk as it flexes.

### Correction of Meniscoid Impingements

If there is entrapped synovial or meniscoid tissue in a facet joint that blocks motion into extension, release of the trapped meniscoid relieves the pain and the accompanying muscle guarding. The joint surfaces need to be separated and the joint capsules made taut.[51] General techniques include the following.

### Cervical Traction, Mobilization, Manipulation

Traction to the spine may be applied manually or mechanically. The patient can also be taught self-traction and positional traction techniques. Techniques of manual traction, self-traction, and positional traction with rotation are described in the stretching section of Chapter 16.

- Traction applied longitudinally along the axis of the spine has the effect of sliding the facets joint surfaces and thus places tension on the facet capsules.
- Traction with side bending and rotation of the spine has the effect of distracting the facet joint surfaces as well as placing tension on the capsules.
- See also the mobilization section later in this chapter

### Management When Acute Symptoms Have Stabilized

General guidelines for subacute and chronic spinal problems are summarized in Boxes 15.7 and 15.8. Specific emphasis when treating patients with mobility impairments due to hypomobile or hypermobile facet joints include:

- Hypomobile joints require stretching but not if the techniques stress a hypermobile region. Traction techniques may be effective if the hypermobile region is stabilized during stretching. For those trained in joint manipulation techniques, they are effective for selective facet joint stretching and have been found to be an effective part of a total treatment approach when there is instability in specific areas and restricted mobility in neighboring facet joints.[75]
- Emphasis is on developing dynamic stability through muscle control in the hypermobile regions while gaining mobility in the restricted regions.
- If there are bony changes and osteophytic spurs, the patient should avoid postures and activities of hyperextension, such as reaching or looking overhead for prolonged periods of time. Adaptations in the environment might include using a stepstool so reaching is at shoulder level. Postures and motions emphasizing flexion of the spine that increase the size of the intervertebral foramina are usually preferred.
- For patients with RA, emphasis is on stabilization and control. Because of the potential instabilities from necrotic tissue and bone erosion, subluxations and dislocations may cause damage to the spinal cord or vascular supply and be extremely debilitating or life-threatening.

## MANAGEMENT GUIDELINES— STABILIZATION

Patients with segmental instability—including hypermobility; ligamentous laxity; diagnoses such as spondylolysis, spondylolisthesis, or poor neuromuscular control of the core and stabilizing musculature—require interventions that improve stability. Some of the patients may have a history of trauma, repeated manipulations, or early signs of spondylosis. Mobility testing of the spinal segments reveals increased mobility at one or more segments. There may be decreased activity in the stabilizing musculature, particularly in response to postural perturbations, and there may be faulty respiratory patterns.

### Identification of Clinical Instability

Stress radiographs are typically used by the medical profession to identify instability. Those with more than 4 mm of translation or 10° of rotation are considered candidates for surgery.[25] Radiographs can identify problems only in the passive structures. To identify impairments in the musculature and the ability to control movement, techniques have been developed that specifically address core muscle activation and endurance and global muscle stabilization. The following may be used:

● *Quality of movement.* Observe spinal ROM (standing) and note if there is a catch or aberrant movement. Patients may demonstrate difficulty moving smoothly in the mid-ranges and demonstrate a shifting or fluctuation in movement.[28]

● *Control of core musculature.* In the lumbar region it is possible to palpate the transversus abdominis and multifidus muscles while the patient attempts to contract them. Devices to measure activation, such as using a biopressure feedback unit or ultrasound imaging, have been developed for both research and clinical usage[43] (see next section under Principles of Management as well as Chapter 16).

● *Control of the global musculature.* Several protocols have been developed to test the stabilizing function of the global musculature.[29,31,84] They primarily challenge the isometric holding capability of the anterior, posterior, and lateral trunk musculature under various loads.

## Principles of Management

### Passive Support
Braces or corsets may be necessary for external support to provide stability and reduce pain.[25] Ideally, these devices should be used in conjunction with training the core musculature for dynamic control.

### Core Muscle Activation
Activation of core musculature may not be automatic in patients with pain or instability. Techniques used to instruct patients in addition to verbal and tactile cues include use of a biofeedback pressure cuff (Chattanooga®) and ultrasound imaging. Ultrasound imaging is primarily used in research settings because of the cost of the units. The pressure cuff has been shown to have clinical relevance in providing immediate feedback to patients.[43] Use of the cuff for testing and instruction in core muscle activation of the cervical and lumbar regions is described in detail in the Muscle Performance section of Chapter 16.

Once the patient learns to activate the core muscles, emphasis is placed on sustaining the contraction over a period of time and on increasing the repetitions of the static hold to reinforce the postural function. These contractions are of low intensity to minimize the compressive activity of the global muscles.[30]

### Lumbar Region
Initially, the patient is taught to find and maintain a neutral spinal position (mid-range). The patient is then instructed in the "drawing-in maneuver" to activate the transversus abdominis and learns to contract the multifidus by bulging out the muscle. Gentle co-activation of the muscles of the perineum facilitates contraction of these core muscles.[73]

### Cervical Region
The patient is taught to activate the core musculature with gentle capital nodding and slight flattening of the cervical lordosis.[30]

### Progression of Stabilization Exercises

● Progressing from core muscle activation to general stabilization exercises using the global musculature emphasizes cervical and pelvic control while superimposing extremity motions. Included are weight-bearing activities such as wall slides, partial lunges, and partial squats, with emphasis on the "drawing-in" maneuver and spinal control in the neutral spinal position while doing the activities.

● Functional activities are incorporated into the stabilization exercise routines. The patient is encouraged to activate the core musculature consciously and maintain a neutral spinal position until it becomes habitual.

## MANAGEMENT GUIDELINES— MOBILIZATION

Some patients benefit from spinal manipulation during the early stages of intervention.[18,19] A clinical prediction validation study determined that those most likely to benefit from spinal manipulation presented with: (1) symptom duration of less than 16 days, with no symptoms distal to the knee; (2) at least one hypomobile lumbar segment; (3) at least one hip with more than 35° of internal rotation; and (4) a score of less than 19 on a fear-avoidance measure.[17] The lumbopelvic technique used in the validation study and a previous study by the same authors,[18] as well as an alternate technique,[19] are described below. The traction procedures described in the non-weight-bearing section earlier in this chapter may also be beneficial. Other manipulations are beyond the scope of this text.

### Management—Lumbar Spine

Following determination of a hypomobile segment in the lumbar spine, perform up to two attempts of the general manipulation followed by instruction in ROM exercises. This is repeated for two sessions, after which the patient is instructed in stabilization exercises and is progressed through treatment as summarized in Boxes 15.7 and 15.8.

*Patient position and procedure:* Supine. Stand on the side opposite the side of the symptoms and side-bend the patient toward the symptomatic side. Ask the patient to interlock the fingers behind the head. Rotate the upper torso toward you (away from the symptomatic side) by reaching across the elbows and placing one hand through the flexed elbow on the symptomatic side (Fig. 15.13A). A quick thrust is exerted against the anterior superior iliac spine on the symptomatic side in a posterior and inferior direction.[18]

*Alternate position and procedure:* Side lying with the symptomatic side upright. The patient's hands are crossed over the chest. Stand facing the patient and palpate the segment to be manipulated. Flex the top hip and knee until movement is detected at that segment; secure the position by placing the patient's foot in the popliteal fossa of the lower leg. Next, grasp the shoulder on which the patient is lying and slide it toward you, causing rotation of the upper trunk. Rotate until motion is detected at the identified segment. Place your upper arm through the patient's crossed arms and place your finger or thumb on the superior spinous process of the segment and the fingers of your lower hand under the inferior spinous process. Your forearm rests across the posterior aspect of the pelvis. Apply a thrust against the pelvis in an anterior direction (Fig. 15.13B).

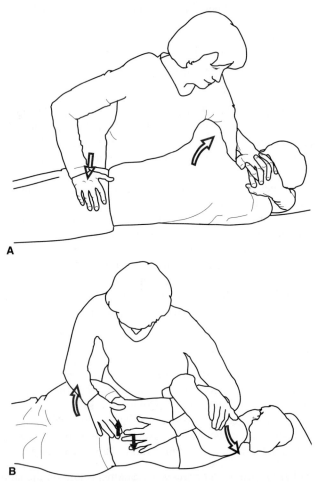

FIGURE 15.13 Rotation manipulation for restricted mobility in the lumbar spine: (A) *supine* (the trunk is side bent to the left and the thorax rotated to the right, creating right rotation) and (B) *side lying* (the pelvis is flexed and the thorax is rotated backward, creating left rotation).

## Management—Cervical Spine

Hypomobile spinal segments may add to stress of hypermobile segments and require a combined approach of mobilization/manipulation as well as stabilization exercises.[44,76] The reader is referred to several texts for instructions in specific examination and interventions using manipulation techniques.[47,93]

 MANAGEMENT GUIDELINES— SOFT TISSUE INJURIES

As previously described, symptoms in soft tissues, including muscles, can occur as a result of direct trauma (tears/contusions), strain from sustained or repetitive activities, or as a protective mechanism (guarding/spasm) from injury to joints or other tissues. General guidelines for management follow those presented previously and are summarized in Boxes 15.4, 15.7, and 15.8. In addition, specific considerations when treating muscle injury are described in this section.

### Management During the Acute Stage: Protection Phase

#### Pain and Inflammation Control
Use appropriate modalities and massage to control pain and inflammation. Passive support may be necessary to relieve the muscles from the job of supporting or controlling the injured part.

#### Cervical Region
Cervical collars provide passive support in the cervical region. The length of time a collar is worn during the day relates to the severity of the injury and the amount of protection required.

PRECAUTION: Collars often place the neck in a forward-head posture. This causes healing in a faulty position, which leads to future postural problems or painful syndromes. Usually, turning the collar around or cutting down the portion under the mandible allows the neck to assume correct alignment.

#### Lumbar Region
Corsets provide passive support of the lumbar region. As with the cervical region, the length of time that a corset is worn should be related to the amount of protection required. Some patients tend to become dependent on the corset and continue to wear it even after healing, when it no longer serves its intended purpose. After healing, it is better to strengthen the body's natural corset (deep abdominal muscles) and develop effective spinal mechanics (see Chapter 16).

#### Muscle Function
When evaluating muscle function, identify the functional position in which the patient has a decrease in the intensity of symptoms. With a muscle injury, this is often with the muscle in its shortened position. In this position, begin gentle muscle-setting techniques. Dosage is critical; resistance is minimal. Use only enough to generate a setting contraction.

#### Cervical Region

*Patient position and procedure:* Supine. Stand at the head of the treatment table, supporting the patient's head with your hands. Start with the guarding muscle in its shortened position. Ask the patient to hold as you apply gentle resistance (light enough to barely move a feather). Both the contraction and the relaxation should be gradual. There should be no neck movement or jerky resistance.

- If there has been muscle injury, the technique is repeated with the muscle kept in the shortened range for several days before beginning to lengthen it.
- As the muscle heals or if there is no muscle injury, progress the treatment by gradually lengthening the guarding muscle after each contraction and relaxation. Movement is performed only within the patient's pain-free range; no stretching is performed when there is muscle guarding.
- *Reverse muscle action.* These exercises are valuable for gentle muscle performance activity when neck motions cause pain and muscle guarding. The neck is not moved, but the muscles are called on to contract and relax. The motions include active scapular elevation, depression, adduction, and rotation. If symptoms are not exacerbated, active shoulder flexion, extension, abduction, adduction, and rotation are used to stimulate the stabilizing function of the cervical musculature.

**Lumbar Region**

*Patient position and procedure:* Prone, with arms resting at the side. Have the patient lift the head. This initiates a setting (stabilizing) contraction of the lumbar erector spinae muscles. A stronger contraction of the lumbar extensor muscles occurs if the head and thorax are extended. Alternate hip extension also causes a setting contraction of the lumbar extensor muscles.

- When there is muscle injury, the muscle is kept in this shortened range for several days.
- For progression as the muscle heals or if there is no muscle injury, gradually allow the muscle to elongate after each contraction by putting a pillow under the abdomen and then having the patient extend the thorax on the lumbar spine through a greater range. Elongation is performed only within tolerance during the early healing phase. There should be no increase in symptoms.

*Alternate position and procedure:* Supine. Have the patient press the head and neck into the bed, causing a setting contraction of the spinal extensors.

**Traction**

Gentle oscillating traction may reflexively inhibit the pain and help maintain synovial fluid and joint-play motion during the acute stage when the muscles do not allow full ROM. Gentle techniques are most effectively applied using manual traction. Position the part with the injured tissue in a shortened position and use a dosage less than that which causes vertebral separation.

PRECAUTION: Traction techniques may aggravate a muscle or soft tissue injury if the tissue is placed in a lengthened position during the setup or with a high dosage of pull during treatment.[70]

**Environmental Adaptation**

If there are activities or postures that caused the trauma or are continuing to provoke symptoms, identify the mechanism and modify the activity or environment to eliminate the potential of recurrence of the problem.

## Management in the Subacute and Chronic Stages of Healing: Controlled Motion and Return to Function Phases

Once acute symptoms are under control, re-examine the patient and determine the impairments and functional limitations. Refer to the general guidelines for management as presented in Boxes 15.7 and 15.8.

# ⬤ MANAGEMENT GUIDELINES— TEMPOROMANDIBULAR JOINT DYSFUNCTION

The function of the temporomandibular joint (TMJ) is closely related to the function of the upper cervical spine and posture. Because of this close relationship, a brief description of impairments and interventions related to the TMJ are included.

## Signs and Symptoms

Pain from a variety of sources is often cited as part of the temporomandibular joint (TMJ) syndrome.[55]

- Pain may occur locally in the TMJ, in the richly vascularized and highly innervated retrodiskal pad located in the posterior region of the joint or in the ear.
- Pain from muscle spasm or myofascial pain in the masseter, temporalis, or pterygoid internis or externis muscles may be described as a headache or facial pain.
- Tension in the muscles of the cervical spine may itself be painful or cause referenced pain from irritation of the greater occipital nerve that may be described as a tension headache.

## Etiology of Symptoms

Imbalance occurs between the head, jaw, neck, and shoulder girdle. Causes may be:

- Malocclusion, decreased vertical dimension of the bite, or other dental problems.
- Faulty joint mechanics from inflammation, subluxation of the meniscus (disk), dislocation of the condylar head, joint contractures, or asymmetrical forces from jaw and bite imbalances. Restricted motion results from periods of immobilization after reconstructive surgery or fracture of the jaw.

- Muscle spasm in the muscles of mastication, causing abnormal or asymmetrical joint forces. Muscle spasm can be the result of emotional tension, faulty joint mechanics, direct or indirect injury, or a postural dysfunction.
- Sinus problems, resulting in mouth breathing, which indirectly affects posture and jaw position.
- Forward-head posture resulting in retraction of the mandible, which places the anterior throat muscles in a lengthened position. Consequently, there is increased activity in the muscles that close the jaw to counter the changed forces. Extension of the head on the upper cervical spine places the muscles and soft tissue in the suboccipital region in a shortened position so they lose flexibility. Also, the nerves and joints in the upper cervical region become compressed or irritated.
- Sudden trauma such as a flexion/extension accident in which the jaw forcefully opens when the head whips back into hyperextension; a direct blow from an auto accident, boxing, a fall, or similar trauma.
- Sustained trauma associated with prolonged dental surgery in which the mouth is held open for a lengthy period of time may initiate symptoms in the TMJ or supporting tissue. Excessive stresses, such as biting or chewing on large pieces of hard food, may also traumatize the joints.

## Principles of Management

The approach to management depends on the cause. In simple cases in which posture, joint dysfunction, or muscle imbalances are the source of the problem, intervention with therapeutic exercise can directly address the problems. In many cases, a dental referral, otolaryngology referral, or psychological support may be necessary to deal with related pathology. A complete evaluation is necessary prior to the initiation of any treatment.

### Reduction of Pain and Muscle Guarding
Use modalities, massage, and relaxation techniques. In addition, the person should eat soft foods and avoid items requiring excessive jaw opening or firm biting and chewing motions.

### Fascial Muscle Relaxation and Tongue Proprioception and Control
The following are suggested techniques.

- Place the tip of the tongue on the hard palate behind the front teeth and draw little circles or letters on the palate. For additional stimulus, place a Lifesavor® between the tongue and palate; then follow the circular edge with the tip of the tongue.
- Place the tip of the tongue on the hard palate and blow air out to vibrate the tongue; making an "r r r r" sound.
- Fill the cheeks with air (mouth closed); then let the air out in a puff.
- Make a "clicking" sound with the tongue on the roof of the mouth. When doing so, the jaw drops open quickly and returns with the teeth slightly apart, and usually the tongue rests on the hard palate behind the front teeth. This is the resting position of the jaw and is also the first step in teaching relaxation exercises. (Relaxation exercises are described in Chapter 14.)

### Control of Jaw Muscles
First, teach recognition of the resting position of the jaw. The lips are closed, teeth slightly apart, and tongue resting lightly on the hard palate behind the front teeth. The patient should breathe in and out slowly through the nose, using diaphragmatic breathing.

- Teach control while opening and closing the jaw through the first half of the ROM. With the tongue on the roof of the mouth, the patient opens the mouth, trying to keep the chin in the midline. Use a mirror for visual reinforcement. The patient is also taught to lightly palpate the lateral pole of each condyle of the mandible bilaterally and to attempt to maintain symmetry between movement of the two sides when opening and closing the mouth.
- If the jaw deviates while opening or closing, have the patient practice lateral deviation to the opposite side. The lateral motion should not be excessive or cause pain.
- Progress to applying gentle resistance with the thumb against the chin. Do not overpower the muscles.

### Stretching Techniques
If there is restricted jaw opening, determine if it is from hypomobile tissues or a dislocated meniscus. Passive stretching and joint mobilization are used to stretch tight tissues. Joint distraction can be used to reposition a meniscus that is blocking opening.

#### Passive Stretching
Stretch to increase jaw opening if indicated. Begin by placing layered tongue depressors between the central incisors. The patient can gradually work to increase the amount of tongue depressors used until he or she can open approximately far enough to insert the knuckles of the index and middle fingers.

- Self-stretching is carried out by placing each thumb under the upper teeth and the index or middle fingers over the lower teeth and pushing the teeth open.

#### Joint Mobilization

*Patient position and procedures:* Supine or sitting, with the head supported and stabilized. Perform joint mobilization techniques with a gloved hand or hands. Determination of dosages and precautions for administration of mobilization techniques are described in Chapter 5.

- *Unilateral distraction* (Fig. 15.14A). Use the hand opposite the side on which you are working. Place your thumb in the patient's mouth on the back molars; the fingers are outside and wrapped around the jaw. The force is in a downward (caudal) direction.
- *Unilateral distraction with glide* (Fig. 15.14B). After distracting the jaw as described above, pull it in a

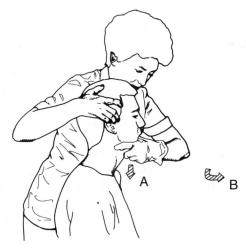

FIGURE 15.14 Unilateral mobilization of the temporomandibular joint. (*A*) Distraction is in a caudal direction. (*B*) Arrow indicates distraction with glide in a caudal, then anterior direction.

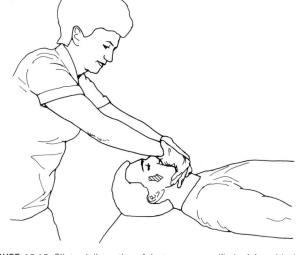

FIGURE 15.15 Bilateral distraction of the temporomandibular joint with the patient supine.

forward (anterior) direction with a tipping motion. The other hand can be placed over the TMJ to palpate the amount of movement.

● *Bilateral distraction* (Fig. 15.15). If the patient is supine, stand at the head of the treatment table. If the patient is sitting, stand in front of the patient. Use both thumbs, placing them on the molars on each side of the mandible. The fingers are wrapped around the jaw. The force from the thumbs is equal, in a caudal direction.

● *Self-mobilization.* Place cotton dental rolls between the back teeth and have the patient bite down. This distracts the condyles from the fossae in the joints.

### Reduction of Upper Quarter Muscle Imbalances
Identify flexibility and strength imbalances in the upper quarter. Stretch restricting postural muscles, teach relaxation, and then retrain for proper muscle control. Cervical and shoulder postural stretching and retraining exercises are described in Chapters 16 and 17, respectively.

## INDEPENDENT LEARNING ACTIVITIES

### ● Critical Thinking and Discussion

1. What are the functional differences between the way the cervical spine and lumbar spine are used in daily activities?
2. Explain how different individuals who sustain back injuries can experience different symptoms of radiating pain down the leg, numbness and tingling into the foot, deep aching down the leg, or no leg symptoms at all. What does each of these symptoms mean?
3. Explain why some people experience diminished symptoms and improved function if the emphasis of intervention is spinal extension, whereas others improve if the emphasis of intervention is spinal flexion.

### ● Laboratory Practice

1. Practice identifying cervical and lumbar spine positions when in the supine, prone, side-lying, sitting, and standing positions. Determine what is needed to change the position. For instance, if flexion is emphasized, what is needed to cause extension?

2. Identify and feel what happens to the various portions of the spine when moving from one position to another, such as rolling supine to prone and return, moving from supine to sit, moving from sit to stand and reverse.
3. Practice methods for developing gentle isometric muscle contractions that could be used during the acute phase of treatment for both the cervical and lumbar spines.

### ● Case Studies

CASE 1
A 45-year-old man sustained injuries in a rear-end collision 4 days ago (car hit him going approximately 45 mph while he was stopped at a stop light). He was in an older car without an air bag or properly positioned headrest, although he was wearing a seatbelt. Initially, he hit the headrest at the mid-cervical spine as his neck extended, and then his head flexed forward but did not hit anything. He has been cleared of cervical fractures or instability. Medical history is unremarkable; he is a social drinker and gave up smoking 5 years ago. He is an accountant and usually works long hours at a computer but has been

unable to work since the accident. He presents wearing a cervical collar and has a facial expression of distress. He states he has had difficulty sleeping because the pain wakes him whenever he moves.

Pain: constant posterior cervical pain, headaches, and pain radiating into the shoulder region bilaterally; intermittent tingling in the right thumb, index, and middle finger. Pain rated at 8/10 when at rest, 10/10 when attempting to move.

Positive findings: guarded forward-head posture. He is unwilling to move more than 10° into flexion or extension, 25° into side bending bilaterally; minimal rotation. Gentle traction to the head relieves the neurological symptoms. Palpation tenderness in upper trapezius and posterior cervical and anterior throat muscles bilaterally. Increased tenderness along facet margins of C-4/5, 5/6 and 6/7, right > left.

- Based on the above impairments and functional limitations, identify goals and interventions for this patient. Describe the techniques you would use and practice them on a laboratory partner.
- How long do you anticipate the patient will have these symptoms? At what point will you change your goals?

## CASE 2

Assume you did not see the patient described in case study 1 until 4 weeks after the accident. He no longer has constant pain and has returned to work. His complaints are an inability to sit at the computer for more than one-half hour before his hand starts to tingle. Numbness occurs after 1 hour of work. Headaches begin within 2 hours of work. Neck and shoulder pain is 6/10 by midday at which time he takes NSAIDs so he can continue working. Positive tests include forward-head posture with forward shoulders; decreased flexibility in the suboccipital muscles, anterior thorax, and internal rotators of the shoulder. Cervical flexion 75%, extension 50%, side bending and rotation 75% bilaterally. Sustained extension of the cervical spine causes tingling into the thumb, index, and middle finger of the right hand. Strength of scapular adductors and lateral rotators of the shoulder is 4/5; myotome testing is normal bilaterally.

- What are your goals and interventions for this patient at this stage?
- After studying the techniques described in Chapter 16, describe the techniques you would use with this patient and practice them on a laboratory partner.
- For each therapeutic exercise technique, practice progressions and determine how you would progress this patient so he could work without exacerbation of symptoms.

## CASE 3

A 55-year-old woman presents with early signs of degenerative joint disease of the lumbar spine. She has been an active runner since college. Occasionally, she has participated in aerobic dance classes. Her history is unremarkable. She has three grown children and had no complaints of back pain related to the pregnancies.

Current symptoms: intermittent periods of pain extending from the mid-lumbar spine, through the right buttock and posterior thigh. The pain begins 15 minutes into her running and progresses to an 8/10 by 25 to 30 minutes. She also complains of increased stiffness after sitting > 1 hour, standing > 15 minutes, and when waking in the morning and getting out of bed. She is a middle-school teacher and track coach for a girl's high school team.

Key findings: lordotic posture, with tight low back, hip flexors, and tensor fasciae latae. Strength of lower abdominals is 4/5. Forward bending of the spine increases tension in low back, repeated backward bending and prone press-ups increase buttock pain. Side bending is decreased 25%, with some discomfort with overpressure into right side bending.

- Based on these impairments and limitations, identify the irritability of the condition and determine goals and intervention.
- What are the most important factors to emphasize with this individual to help her manage her symptoms?
- After studying the exercises in Chapter 16, practice the techniques you would have this patient do. Also, practice how you would progress the techniques and what criteria you would use for progressions.

## CASE 4

A 42-year-old man presents with a medical diagnosis of herniated nucleus pulposus at the L5/S1 area. Present symptoms began 4 days ago when rising out of bed. He is a sedentary person who plays social golf on the weekends (rides in a cart) and is 50 lb overweight. He has had occasional episodes of low back pain over the past 15 years, but "nothing like this."

Medical history: smokes one pack of cigarettes per day and is on blood pressure medication. He describes the symptoms as a sharp pain beginning in the left buttock region and radiating down the back of the thigh; there is intermittent paresthesia along the lateral border of his foot, which is noticeable when sitting. He describes a considerable increase in symptoms when attempting to arise from bed, rise out of a chair, or whenever straining. He has been unable to walk because he cannot stand upright. On observation, you note that the patient is standing with a posterior pelvic tilt and forward-bend of the trunk, and the thorax is deviated to the right.

Examination maneuvers: all spinal flexion motions increase symptoms; side gliding of the thorax to the left followed by lumbar extension centralizes the symptoms primarily to buttock and low back pain.

- Based on this information, identify the impairments and functional limitations. What type of intervention should be used?
- Develop a sequence of treatment techniques that you would use during the first visit. Include instructions and precautions. Practice the techniques.

# REFERENCES

1. Abdulwahab, SS, Sabbahi, M: Neck retractions, cervical root decompression and radicular pain. J Orthop Sports Phys Ther 30(1):4, 2000.
2. Abenhaim, L, et al: The role of activity in the therapeutic management of back pain: report of the international Paris task force on back pain. Spine 25(4S):1S, 2000.
3. Adams, MA, Hutton, WC: Gradual disc prolapse. Spine 10(6):524, 1985.
4. Adams, MA, Hutton, WC: The effect of fatigue on the lumbar intervertebral disc. J Bone Joint Surg Br 65(2):199, 1983.
5. Alexander, AH, Jones, AM, Rosenbaum, DH: Nonoperative management of herniated nucleus pulposus: patient selection by the extension sign. Orthop Rev 21:181, 1992.
6. American Physical Therapy Association: Guide to Physical Therapist Practice, ed 2. Phys Ther 81:9–744, 2001.
7. Anderson, B, et al: The influence of backrest inclination and lumbar support on lumbar lordosis. Spine 4:52, 1979.
8. Audrey, L, Donelson, R, Fung, T: Does it matter which exercise? A randomized control trial of exercise for low back pain. Spine 29(23):2593–2602, 2004.
9. Bogduk, N, Engle, R: The menisci of the lumbar zygapophyseal joints: a review of their anatomy and clinical significance. Spine 9(5):454, 1984.
10. Bogduk, N, MacIntosh, JE: The applied anatomy of the thoracolumbar fascia. Spine 9:164, 1984.
11. Bogduk, N, Twomey, LT: Clinical Anatomy of the Lumbar Spine. Churchill-Livingstone, New York, 1987.
12. Bondi, BA, Drinkwater-Kolk, M: Functional stabilization training. Workshop notes, Northeast Seminars, October 1992.
13. Brinckmann, P: Injury of the annulus fibrosus and disc protrusions. Spine 11(2):149, 1986.
14. Burkart, S, Beresfore, W: The aging intervertebral disk. Phys Ther 59:969, 1979.
15. Butler, D, et al: Discs degenerate before facets. Spine 15:111, 1990.
16. Cailliet, R: Low Back Pain Syndrome, ed 4. FA Davis, Philadelphia, 1988.
17. Childs, JD, Fritz JM, et al: A clinical prediction rule to identify patients with low back pain most likely to benefit from spinal manipulation: a validation study. Ann Intern Med 141(12):920–928, 2004.
18. Childs, JD, Fritz, JM, et al: Clinical decision making in the identification of patients likely to benefit from spinal manipulation: a traditional versus an evidence-based approach. J Orthop Sports Phys Ther 33(5):259–275, 2003.
19. Cleland, JA, Fritz, JM, Whitman, JM, et al: The use of a lumbar spine manipulation technique by physical therapists in patients who satisfy a clinical prediction rule: a case series. J Orthop Sports Phys Ther 36(4):209–214, 2006.
20. Cloward, R: The clinical significance of the sino-vertebral nerve of the cervical spine in relation to the cervical disc syndrome. J Neurol Surg Psychiatry 23:321, 1960.
21. Danneels, LA, Coorevits, PL, Cools, AM, et al: Differences in electromyographic activity in the multifidus muscle and the iliocostalis lumborum between healthy subjects and patients with sub-acute and chronic low back pain. Eur Spine J 11:13–19, 2002.
22. Delitto, A, Erhard, RE, Bowling, RW: A treatment-based classification approach to low back syndrome: identifying and staging patients for conservative treatment. Phys Ther 75(6):470, 1995.
23. DeRosa, CP, Porterfield, JA. A physical therapy model for the treatment of low back pain. Phys Ther 72:261, 1992.
24. Farfan, HF, et al: The effects of torsion on the lumbar intervertebral joints: the role of torsion in the production of disc degeneration. J Bone Joint Surg Am 52(3):468, 1970.
25. Fritz, JM, Erhard, RE, Hagen, BF: Segmental instability of the lumbar spine. Phys Ther 78(8):889, 1998.
26. Fritz, JM: Use of a classification approach to the treatment of 3 patients with low back syndrome. Phys Ther 78(7):766–777, 1998.
27. Fritz, JM, George, S: The use of a classification approach to identify subgroups of patients with acute low back pain: interrater reliability and short-term outcomes. Spine 25(1):106–114, 2000.
28. Fritz, JM, Whitman, JM, Childs, JD: Lumbar spine segmental mobility assessment: an examination of validity for determining intervention strategies in patients with low back pain. Arch Phys Med Rehabil 86:1745–1752, 2005.
29. Gilleard, WL, Brown, MM: A electromyographic validation of an abdominal muscle test. Arch Phys Med Rehabil 75:1002–1007, 1994.
30. Grant, R, Jull, G, Spencer, T: Active stabilization training for screen based keyboard operators—a single case study. Aust Physiother 43(4):235–242, 1997.
31. Hagins, M, Adler, K, Cash, M, et al: Effects of practice on the ability to perform lumbar stabilization exercises. J Orthop Sports Phys Ther 29(9):546–555, 1999.
32. Harris, P: Cervical traction: review of literature and treatment guidelines. Phys Ther 57:910, 1977.
33. Hellsing, AL, Linton, SL, Kaluemark, M: A prospective study of patients with acute back and neck pain in Sweden. Phys Ther 74:116, 1994.
34. Hickey, DS, Hukins, DEL: Aging changes in the macromolecular organization of the intervertebral disc: an x-ray diffraction and electron microscopic study. Spine 7(3):234, 1982.
35. Hicks, GE, Fritz, JM, et al: Preliminary development of a clinical prediction rule for determining which patients with low back pain will respond to a stabilization exercise program. Arch Phys Med Rehabil 86:1753–1762, 2005.
36. Hides, JA, Jull, GA, Richardson, CA: Long-term effects of specific stabilizing exercises for first-episode low back pain. Spine 26:E243–E248, 2001.
37. Hides, JA, Stokes, MJ, et al: Evidence of lumbar multifidus muscle wasting ipsilateral to symptoms in patients with acute/subacute low back pain. Spine 19(2):165–172, 1994.
38. Hodges, PW, Moseley, GL: Pain and motor control of the lumbopelvic region: effect and possible mechanisms. J Electromyogr Kinesth 13:361–370, 2003.
39. Hodges, PW, Moseley, GL, et al: Experimental muscle pain changes feedforward postural responses of the trunk muscles. Exp Brain Res 151:262–271, 2003.
40. Hodges, PW, Richardson, CA: Altered trunk muscle recruitment in people with low back pain with upper limb movement at different speeds. Arch Phys Med Rehabil 80(9):1005, 1999.
41. Hodges, PW, Richardson, CA: Delayed postural contraction of transversus abdominis in low back pain associated with movement of the lower limb. J Spinal Disord 11(1):46, 1998.
42. Hodges, PW, Richardson, CA: Contraction of the abdominal muscles associated with movement of the lower limb. Phys Ther 77(2):132, 1997.
43. Hodges, P, Richardson, C, Jull, G: Evaluation of the relationship between laboratory and clinical tests of transversus abdominis function. Physiother Res Int 1(1):30–40, 1996.
44. Hoving, JL, Koes, BW, et al: Manual therapy, physical therapy, or continued care by a general practitioner for patients with neck pain. Ann Intern Med 136:713–722, 2002.
45. Jensen, G: Biomechanics of the lumbar intervertebral disc: a review. Phys Ther 60:765, 1980.
46. Jull, G, Trott, P, Potter, H, et al: A randomized controlled trial of exercise and manipulative therapy for cervicogenic headache. Spine 27(17):1835–1834, 2002.
47. Kaltenborn, FM: The Spine—Basic Evaluation and Mobilization Techniques. Olaf Norlis Bokhandel, Oslo, 1993.
48. Kellegren J: Observations on referred pain arising from muscle. Clin Sci 3:175, 1983.
49. Kessler, R: Acute symptomatic disk prolapse. Phys Ther 59:978, 1979.
50. Klein, JA, Hukins, DWL: Collagen fiber orientation in the annulus fibrosus of intervertebral disc during bending and torsion measured by x-ray diffraction. Biochim Biophys Acta 719:98, 1982.
51. Kopp, JR, et al: The use of lumbar extension in the evaluation and treatment of patients with acute herniated nucleus pulposus. Clin Orthop 202:211, 1986.
52. Kos, J, Wolf, J: Intervertebral menisci and their possible role in intervertebral blockage [translated by Burkart, S]. Bull Orthop Sports Med Sect Am Phys Ther Assoc 1(3):8, 1976.
53. Krag, MH, et al: Internal displacement distribution from in vitro loading of human thoracic and lumbar spinal motion segments: experimental results and theoretical predictions. Spine 12:1001, 1987.
54. Krause, N, Ragland, DR: Occupational disability due to low back pain: a new interdisciplinary classification based on a phase model of disability. Spine 19:1011, 1994.

55. Kraus, SL: TMJ Craniomandibular Cervical Complex: Physical Therapy and Dental Management. Clinical Education Associates, Atlanta, 1986.
56. Levangie, P, Norkin, C: Joint Structure and Function: A Comprehensive Analysis, ed 3. FA Davis, Philadelphia, 2001.
57. Lipson, SJ, Muir, H: Proteoglycans in experimental intervertebral disc degeneration. Spine 6(3):194, 1981.
58. Long, AL: The centralization phenomenon: its usefulness as a predictor of outcome in conservative treatment of chronic low back pain (a pilot study). Spine 20(23):2513–2521, 1995.
59. Lundon, K, Bolton, K: Structure and function of the lumbar intervertebral disk in the health, aging, and pathologic conditions. J Orthop Sports Phys Ther 31(6):291, 2001.
60. Lyons, G, Eisenstein, SM, Sweet, MBI: Biochemical changes in intervertebral disc degeneration. Biochim Biophys Acta 673:443, 1981.
61. MacNab, I: Backache. Williams & Wilkins, Baltimore, 1977.
62. Matthews J: The effects of spinal traction. Physiotherapy 58:64, 1972.
63. McCarron, RF, et al: The inflammatory effect of nucleus pulposus: a possible element in the pathogenesis of low-back pain. Spine 12:760, 1987.
64. McKenzie, R, May, S: The Lumbar Spine: Mechanical Diagnosis and Therapy, Vol 1, ed 2. Spinal Publications, Waikanae, New Zealand, 2003.
65. McKenzie, R, May, S: The Lumbar Spine: Mechanical Diagnosis and Therapy, Vol 2, ed 2. Spinal Publications, Waikanae, New Zealand, 2003.
66. McKenzie, R: Manual correction of sciatic scoliosis. N Z Med J 89:22, 1979.
67. Mooney, V, Robertson, J: The facet syndrome. Clin Orthop 115:149, 1976.
68. Mooney, V: The syndromes of low back disease. Orthop Clin North Am 14(3):505, 1983.
69. Moneur, C, Williams, HJ: Cervical spine management in patients with rheumatoid arthritis. Phys Ther 68:509, 1988.
70. Morgan, D: Concepts in functional training and postural stabilization for the low-back injured. Top Acute Care Trauma Rehabil 2:8, 1988.
71. Murphy, MJ: Effects of cervical traction on muscle activity. J Orthop Sports Phys Ther 13:220, 1991.
72. Nachemson, A: Recent advances in the treatment of low back pain. Int Orthop 9:1, 1985.
73. Neuman, P, Gill, V: Pelvic floor and abdominal muscle interaction: EMG activity and intra-abdominal pressure. Int Urogynecol J 13:125–132, 2002.
74. Nowakowski, P, Delitto A, Erhard, RE: Lumbar spinal stenosis. Phys Ther 76:187, 1996.
75. Ogata, K, Whiteside, LA: Nutritional pathways of the intervertebral disc. Spine 6(3):211, 1981.
76. Olson, KA, Dustin, J: Diagnosis and treatment of cervical spine clinical instability. J Orthop Sports Phys Ther 31(4):194, 2001.
77. O'Sullivan, PB, Twomey, LT, Allison, GT: Altered abdominal muscle recruitment in patients with chronic low back pain following a specific exercise intervention. J Orthop Sports Phys Ther 27(2):114–124, 1998.
78. Panjabi MM: The stabilizing system of the spine. Part I. Function, dysfunction, adaption, and enhancement. J Spinal Disord 5:383–389, 1992.
79. Panjabi MM: The stabilizing system of the spine. Part II. Neutral zone and instability hypothesis. J Spinal Disord 5:390–396, 1992.
80. Panjabi, MM, Lydon, C, Vasavada, A, et al: On the understanding of clinical instability. Spine 19:2642–2650, 1994.
81. Penjabi, MM, Krag, MH, Chung, TQ: Effects of disc injury on mechanical behavior of the human spine. Spine 9:707, 1984.
82. Porter, RW, Hibbert, C, Evans, C: The natural history of root entrapment syndrome. Spine 9:418, 1984.
83. Pellechia, GL: Lumbar traction: a review of the literature. J Orthop Sports Phys Ther 20:263, 1994.
84. Richardson, C, Hodges, PW, Hides, J: Therapeutic Exercise for Lumbopelvic Stabilization, ed 2. Churchill Livingstone, Edinburgh, 2004.
85. Riddle, DL: Classification and low back pain: a review of the literature and critical analysis of selected systems. Phys Ther 78(7):709, 1998.
86. Russell, EJ: Cervical disk disease. Radiology 177(2):313, 1990.
87. Saal, JS, Saal, JA, Yurth, EF: Nonoperative management of herniated cervical intervertebral disc with radiculopathy. Spine 21(16):1877, 1996.
88. Saal, JA: Dynamic muscular stabilization in the non-operative treatment of lumbar pain syndromes. Orthop Rev 19:691, 1990.
89. Saal, JS, et al: High levels of inflammatory phospholipase A2 activity in lumbar disc herniations. Spine 15:674, 1990.
90. Saal, JA, Saal, JS: Nonoperative treatment of herniated lumbar intervertebral disc with radiculopathy; an outcome study. Spine 14:431, 1989.
91. Saal, JA, Saal, JS, Herzog, RJ: The natural history of lumbar intervertebral disc extrusions treated non-operatively. Spine 15:683, 1990.
92. Sahrmann, SA: Diagnosis and Treatment of Movement Impairment Syndromes. Mosby, St. Louis, 2002.
93. Saunders, HD, Ryan, RS: Spinal traction. In Evaluation Treatment and Prevention of Musculoskeletal Disorders. Vol 1. Spine, ed 4. Saunders Group, Chaska, MN, 2004, p 301.
94. Spencer, JD, Hayes, KC, Alexander, IJ: Knee joint effusion and quadriceps reflex inhibition in man. Arch Phys Med Rehabil 65:171, 1984.
95. Stuge, B, Laerum, E, et al: The efficacy of a treatment program focusing on specific stabilizing exercises for pelvic girdle pain after pregnancy. Spine 29(4):351–359, 2004.
96. Taylor, JR, Twomey, LT: Age changes in lumbar zygapophyseal joints. Spine 11(7):739, 1986.
97. Twomey, LT: A rationale for the treatment of back pain and joint pain by manual therapy. Phys Ther 72:885, 1992.
98. Urban, L: The straight-leg-raising test: a review. J Orthop Sports Phys Ther 2:117, 1981.
99. Van Dieen, JH, Cholewicki, J, Radeboid, A: Trunk muscle recruitment patterns in patients with low back pain enhance the stability of the lumbar spine. Spine 28(8):834–841, 2003.
100. Waddell, G: A new clinical model for the treatment of low back pain. Spine 12:632, 1987.
101. Yasuma, T, et al: Histological development of intervertebral disc herniation. J Bone Joint Surg Am 68(7):1066, 1986.

# The Spine: Exercise Interventions

The basic anatomy, spinal mechanics, posture, pathomechanics, common pathologies, and management guidelines related to the spine were presented in Chapters 14 and 15. The management guidelines were outlined based on stages of healing as well as subgroupings based on impairments and movement disorders. Chapter 16 is a continuation of this material in which the techniques of intervention using therapeutic exercise for management of neck and trunk impairments are described.

This chapter is divided into six main sections. The first section describes the underlying concepts and approaches to exercise interventions. Each of the remaining five sections describes elements of physical function for the neck and trunk. The topics covered in these sections include exercises for kinesthetic awareness, mobility/flexibility, muscle performance (including stability, muscle endurance, and strength), cardiopulmonary endurance, and functional activities. Stress relief and relaxation principles and techniques, an important component of total rehabilitation, are covered in detail in Chapter 14.

## BASIC CONCEPTS OF SPINAL MANAGEMENT WITH EXERCISE

It is important to recognize that even though the material in this chapter is presented in separate sections there is an overlap in the use of the techniques described in each section, and there are fundamental interventions basic to all exercise programs.

 ## FUNDAMENTAL INTERVENTIONS

When patients seek treatment from a physical therapist, they come with different diagnoses, impairments, and functional limitations and are at different stages of tissue healing. Yet the treatment plan for each patient must begin with fundamental interventions in order to lay the foundation on which to build an effective therapeutic exercise program. *Fundamental interventions* are defined as exercises or skills that all patients with spinal impairments should learn regardless of their functional level at the time of examination and initial treatment. The interventions include basic kinesthetic training, basic spinal stabilization training, and functional training of basic body mechanics. These interventions are summarized in Box 16.1.

Once the fundamental skills are learned, exercise interventions then progress on a continuum at the level of the patient's abilities and willingness to learn. For example, a patient beginning treatment with chronic symptoms several months after the onset of symptoms must first become aware of and learn how to move the spine safely as well as learn what effects the various postures and movements have on symptoms (fundamental kinesthetic awareness). The patient must learn how to activate the core-stabilizing musculature and then how to use the core stabilizers with

---

**BOX 16.1  Fundamental Exercise Interventions for Spinal Rehabilitation**

These fundamental interventions are adapted or modified based on patient abilities and responses.

**Kinesthetic Training**
- Awareness and control of safe spinal motion: head nodding and pelvic tilts
- Awareness of neutral spinal position (if needed begin in the patient's spinal bias) while supine, prone, sitting, and standing
- Awareness of effects of activities of daily living (ADLs) and extremity motion on the spine (see Functional Training)

**Stabilization Training**
- *Core muscle* activation and sustained contraction
  - Cervical region: controlled axial extension with craniocervical flexion and lower cervical/upper thoracic extension
  - Lumbar region: drawing-in maneuver and multifidus muscle activation techniques
- *Global muscle* control of spinal posture with extremity loading
  - Passive support of spinal posture if needed; progress to active control
  - Coordinate core muscle activation with maintenance of a stable spine in neutral spinal position (or position of bias) with all arm and leg motions

**Functional Training (Basic Body Mechanics With Stable Spine)**
- Log roll supine to prone, prone to supine
- Transition from supine to side-lying to sitting and return
- Transition from sit to stand and return
- Walking

---

the global musculature to stabilize the spine against various extremity loading exercises (fundamental muscle performance). Finally, the patient must learn basic body mechanics (fundamental functional activities) in order to minimize stresses to the spine during daily activities before progressing to exercises that can be tolerated at the chronic stage of healing and returning to desired functional activities. The fundamental exercises are described in detail preceding the exercise progressions in each of the respective sections of this chapter. The principles of management are similar for the cervical and lumbar spinal regions, and many of the same techniques may be used or modified for both regions.

 ## PATIENT EDUCATION

Patient education is a component of every goal and intervention. It encompasses several ideas. First, the patient is a participant in identifying the desired outcomes; education as to potential outcomes is part of this process. Second, the patient may need to be educated about limitations at each stage of healing so as not to become concerned that the acute symptoms will be forever disabling or so as not to "overdo" exercises and activities during the early subacute phase and cause exacerbation of symptoms. The patient may then need to be challenged to progress beyond perceived limitations during the later stages of recovery.

To ensure that each individual develops control over and learns how to manage the symptoms and any impairments, it is important that the patient is engaged in all activities at each stage of recovery and is not just a passive recipient of "treatment." The patient needs instruction in how safely to progress self-management beyond the time spent under professional supervision so he or she can reach the maximum level of functional return.

Finally, the patient needs instruction in prevention. This includes safe ways to exercise, safe body mechanics for return to high-intensity activities, modification of the work and home environment, and activities to minimize stresses.

## ⬤ GENERAL EXERCISE GUIDELINES

Therapeutic exercise is an important intervention in the management of impairments in the spinal region. Although this text does not deal with specific examination techniques, it is critical to emphasize the importance of identifying each patient's impairments and functional limitations, as well as the stage of tissue healing or stage or rehabilitation, in order to establish a baseline for the initiation of intervention techniques and to measure progress toward the outcome goals. In many cases, tissue healing, stages of rehabilitation, and functional expectations parallel one another (Table 16.1).

In general, the following elements of physical function are used in all intervention programs for spinal problems. These five areas are listed in Table 16.2 with interventions for each stage of rehabilitation. The interventions are described in detail in the remaining sections of this chapter. Prior to developing an exercise program, it is important that the reader has knowledge of various spinal pathologies and the special precautions and con-

| TABLE 16.1 | Spinal Rehabilitation | |
|---|---|---|
| Stage of Tissue Healing | Stage of Rehabilitation | Functional Expectations |
| Acute | Early training protection phase | Control symptoms; ADL if possible |
| Subacute | Basic training/controlled motion phase | IADL and limited work |
| Chronic | Intermediate to advanced training/ return to function phase | Return to work, recreation, sports |

The sequence of rehabilitation parallels the stages of healing and functional outcome expectations.

traindications (see Chapter 15) so each patient can safely achieve his or her maximum potential.

### Kinesthetic Awareness

One of the fundamental interventions for spinal rehabilitation is to develop patient awareness of safe spinal positions and spinal movement as well as what effect the supine, prone, side-lying, sitting, and standing positions have on the spine. Awareness of what postures make the symptoms better or worse and identifying the neutral spinal position or position of bias are important in helping patients manage their symptoms. Awareness and control of spinal posture and movement is progressed and incorporated into all the exercises described in the remaining sections of this chapter and underlie exercises for the extremities as well.

### Mobility/Flexibility

Stretching and flexibility exercises as well as mobilization techniques to increase mobility of restricting tissues are used so the patient can assume effective alignment of the spine when exercising to improve muscle performance and functional outcomes. For patients who fit the manipulation subcategory (described in Chapter 15), manipulation may be indicated during the early intervention period and then followed with stretching exercises.

### Muscle Performance

In the spine, muscle performance involves not only strength, power, and endurance but also stability. Activation of the core-stabilizing muscles and exercises to develop spinal control in the global stabilizing muscles are fundamental for developing spinal stability. Emphasis is placed on awareness of muscle contraction and control of spinal position while moving the extremities. Exercises are then progressed to challenge the holding capacity of the stabilizing muscles, emphasizing muscle endurance, balance, and strength. Once the individual learns effective stabilization and management of symptoms, dynamic neck and trunk strengthening exercises are initiated. Most people are familiar with trunk curls, "crunches," and back lifts. The emphasis of therapeutic exercise is safe execution of the exercises combined with respect of the biomechanics of the spine. The choice of exercises should be with the functional outcome goals in mind and integrated with the principles discussed in the Functional Activities section.

### Cardiopulmonary Endurance

Aerobic conditioning exercises are initiated as soon as the patient tolerates repetitive activity without exacerbating symptoms. Emphasis is placed on using safe spinal postures while exercising. Aerobic activity increases the patient's feeling of well-being and improves cardiovascular and pulmonary fitness. Principles of aerobic conditioning are detailed in Chapter 4 and summarized in this chapter along with suggestions for safe application of aerobic exercises when there are spinal impairments.

## Functional Activities

Fundamental functional activities include training the basic body mechanics of rolling, supine to sit, sit to stand, walking, and reverse. These activities are coordinated with kinesthetic training and core muscle activation and stabi-lization exercises. When the patient is able, stabilization exercises, muscle endurance, and strengthening exercises are integrated with skills for body mechanics (lifting, pushing, pulling, carrying), safe work habits (ergonomic adaptations), and effective recreational or sport activities to meet the goals of the individual.

### TABLE 16.2 Intervention for Each Stage of Rehabilitation

| Stages of Rehabilitation Intervention | Early Training/Protection Phase Maximum to moderate protection of injured area, pathologically involved tissues, or painful region | Basic Training/Controlled Motion Phase Moderate to minimum protection | Intermediate to Advanced Training/Return to Function Phase Minimum to no protection |
|---|---|---|---|
| *Kinesthetic awareness* • Proprioception training of safe movement and postures | • Pelvic tilt / cervical retraction: passive —> active assist —> active in comfortable positions.* • Awareness of what makes symptoms better vs. worse* • Learn neutral spine (or bias)* | • Active spinal control in supine, prone, quadruped, sitting, standing • Dynamic maintenance of pain-free position with activities | Habitual use of neutral spine in all functional activities |
| *Mobility/flexibility* • Move, stretch, manipulate restricting tissues | • Movement to relieve fluid stasis. • Trunk stretching: only in pain-relieving positions. • Extremity stretching: stretch U/LE if no stress to the spine. • Mobilization: grades I and II • Manipulation if indicated (see text) | • Gentle spinal movement into painful range • Stretch U/LE muscles in position of spinal comfort (bias) • Mobilization: progress to grade III | • Move into painful ranges to stretch and mobilize as indicated for range of spine and extremities |
| *Muscle performance* • Stabilization training (core muscles for segmental stability, global muscles for general stability) • Muscle endurance • Strength and power | • Activation of core musculature.* • Stabilization exercises with extremity loading (use of passive positioning with pillows, splints, corsets if necessary)* | • Stabilization exercises with extremity loading (active control of spine position); emphasize muscle endurance • Low-intensity dynamic spinal exercises | • Stabilization with transitional motions, and functional activities; emphasize strength • Perturbation training • Progression to dynamic trunk strengthening |
| *Cardiopulmonary Endurance* • Aerobic training | • Only if tolerated with maximum protection in position of comfort | • Low to moderate intensity with moderate to minimal protection. • Use activities that emphasize spinal bias | High intensity (target heart rate), multiple times per week |
| *Functional Activities* • Body mechanics • Skill in home, community, work, recreation, sport activities | • Safe postures for recumbent, sitting, and standing* • Stable-spine techniques while rolling over, moving supine to sit, sit to stand* | • Strengthen U/LE while stabilizing spine • Stable spine body mechanics • Environmental and ergonomic adaptations | • High-intensity functional activities. • Endurance and strengthening activities that replicate return to desired activities • Practice prevention |

Conscious activation of core and global muscles with spine in neutral position in all stabilization exercises and activities.

*Fundamental interventions for all patients.

## KINESTHETIC AWARENESS

*Goal.* to develop proprioception of spinal positioning, safe movement, and postural control.

## ELEMENTS OF KINESTHETIC TRAINING—FUNDAMENTAL TECHNIQUES

### Position of Symptom Relief

The patient must learn how to move the spine and find the range or position in which symptoms are minimized. The position of symptom relief is called the *position of bias* or *the resting position*. The *neutral* spine position is midrange; the patient may or may not feel most comfortable in that position initially. See Chapter 15 for a discussion on spinal bias as it relates to relief of symptoms and common pathologies.

#### Cervical Spine

*Patient position and procedure:* Begin supine; progress to sitting and other functional postures as tolerated.

- Passively move the head and neck with gentle nodding motions of the head into flexion and extension, side bending, and/or rotation to find the most comfortable position for the patient. If necessary prop the head and neck with pillows.
- Describe the mechanics of what you are doing to the patient.
- Have the patient identify the change in symptoms as movement occurs in and out of the position of bias.
- Have the patient practice moving into and out of that position to develop control.
- If the patient cannot maintain this position while sitting and standing, wearing a cervical collar may be appropriate during the acute stage.

#### Lumbar Spine

*Patient position and procedure:* Begin supine or hook-lying, then sitting, standing, and quadruped.

- Teach the patient to move his or her pelvis into an anterior and posterior pelvic tilt (PT) through the range that is comfortable.
- Once the patient has moved the pelvis and spine through a safe range of motion (ROM), instruct him or her to find the position of greatest symptom relief.
- If active movement and control is not possible, teach *passive positioning* (see Box 15.6). Have the patient assume each of the following positions, and draw the association between the spinal position and what is felt. While supine, passively position the pelvis in posterior PT by placing the lower extremities in the hook-lying

position or anterior tilt by gently pulling on the extended legs or placing a small roll under the lumbar spine. Sitting encourages spinal flexion; if extension is more comfortable, instruct the person to use a lumbar pillow for support. Standing usually causes spinal extension; if flexion is desired, instruct the person to place one foot up on a stool while standing.

### Effects of Movement on the Spine

Once the functional spinal position is determined, it is important for the patient to feel and learn what motions make the symptoms better or worse. In general, movement of the extremities away from the trunk (shoulder flexion and abduction, hip extension and abduction) causes spinal extension; movement of the extremities toward the trunk (shoulder extension and adduction, hip flexion and adduction) causes spinal flexion.

- Have the patient find the neutral or functional spine position (bias); then move the arms and then the legs to feel the effect on the spine. Control of the spinal position is emphasized; have the patient practice the arm and leg motions and attempt to maintain control of the spinal position. These motions are the same as the basic stabilization exercises and are described in detail in the muscle performance section.
- If the patient cannot maintain control or the symptoms are made worse, he or she requires passive support or passive positioning when initiating the stabilization exercises.

### Integration of Kinesthetic Training With Stabilization Exercises and Fundamental Body Mechanics

Once awareness of safe positions and movement is learned, teach the patient the fundamental stabilization techniques for developing neuromuscular control of the position (Muscle Performance section), and teach the fundamental body mechanics of rolling, moving supine to sit, sit to stand, and ambulation (Functional Activities section).

## 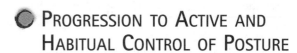 PROGRESSION TO ACTIVE AND HABITUAL CONTROL OF POSTURE

Awareness and control of posture is described in detail in Chapter 14 (see General Management Guidelines for Impaired Posture and Box 14.1). The use of reinforcement techniques (verbal, visual, tactile) are described, as are activities to train cervical, scapular, thoracic, and lumbopelvic alignment and control. It is important to reinforce the relationship between faulty posture and the development of painful symptoms and to identify if there is a need for postural support (temporary or long term).

Integrate the awareness of posture and control of the spinal segments into all stabilization exercises, aerobic conditioning, and functional training activities. Observe the patient as greater challenges to activities are performed and, if necessary, provide reminders to find the neutral spinal position and to initiate contraction of the stabilizing muscles prior to the activity. For example, when reaching overhead, help the patient become aware of the need to contract the abdominal muscles to maintain a neutral spine position and not allow the spine to extend into a painful or unstable range until the stabilization becomes habitual. This principle is also incorporated into body mechanics, such as when going from picking up and lifting to placing an object on a high shelf, or into sport activities when reaching up to block or throw a ball.

## MOBILITY/FLEXIBILITY

**Goal.** To increase ROM of specific structures that affect alignment and mobility in the neck and trunk.

In general, stretching is contraindicated in the region of inflamed tissue. However, if there are postures that relieve symptoms but are difficult to assume because of tissue restriction or fluid stasis, stretching or repetitive movement into the restricted range may be appropriate. For example, lumbar extension has been shown to relieve symptoms of fluid stasis or a disk lesion (see Chapter 15), yet a patient may not be able to get into an extended posture because of flexed postural dysfunction or swollen tissue. Prone propping and press-ups may stretch the tight tissue or may compress and massage swollen disk material or fluid stasis to reduce symptoms (see Fig. 15.7).

Another situation in which acute symptoms may be relieved with stretching is with acute nerve root irritation from bony spurs or lipping in an arthritic spine. Reducing pressure on the nerve roots with a stretch traction force, which widens the intervertebral foramina or with procedures that realign the spine in its optimal spinal position may relieve the symptoms.[1]

Decreased mobility in structures in the upper and lower extremities that restrict normal postural alignment may be stretched or mobilized if the techniques do not stress the area of inflammation.

Stretching is done on a continuum. Critical judgment is used to determine the intensity and duration of stretch based on proximity to the healing tissue and the integrity and tolerance of the tissue. Principles of stretching for impaired mobility are described in Chapter 4. Joint mobilization and manipulation techniques may be used to stretch hypomobile facet joint capsules or realign subluxed facets. A general manipulation technique for restricted spinal mobility is described under Management Guidelines—Restricted Mobility in Chapter 15. Other spinal manipulations are beyond the scope of this text.

If indicated, the patient is also taught general stress-relieving movements to reduce fluid stasis after being in prolonged postures. These movements are described in Chapter 14 in the section Management of Impaired Posture.

## CERVICAL AND UPPER THORACIC REGION—STRETCHING TECHNIQUES

### Techniques to Increase Thoracic Extension

#### Self-Stretching

● *Patient position and procedure:* Hook-lying, with the hands behind the head and the elbows resting on the mat. To increase the stretch, place a pad or rolled towel lengthwise under the thoracic spine between the scapulae. Segmental breathing (see Chapter 25) can also be used by having the patient start with the elbows together in front of the face and then inhaling as the elbows are brought down to the mat; holding; then exhaling as the elbows are brought together again.

● *Patient position and procedure:* Hook-lying, with both arms elevated overhead. The patient attempts to keep the back flat on the mat while inhaling and expanding the anterior thorax.

● *Patient position and procedure:* Supine, with a foam roll placed longitudinally down the length of the spine. If the patient cannot balance on the roll or experiences tenderness along the spinous processes from pressure, tape two foam rolls together. The patient elevates both arms overhead in a "touchdown" position and allows gravity to apply the stretch force (Fig. 16.1A). The patient then abducts and laterally rotates both shoulders so the hands are facing the ceiling (Fig. 16.1B). This

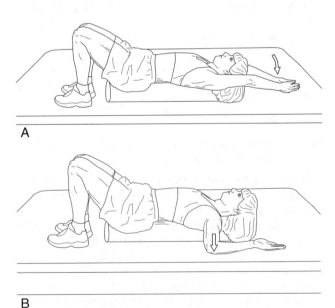

A

B

FIGURE 16.1 Foam roll stretch to increase flexibility of anterior thorax. (A) In the "touchdown" position the shoulder extensors are also stretched. (B) With the shoulders abducted and laterally rotated, the pectoralis major and other internal rotators are also stretched. For a less intensive stretch, use a rolled towel placed longitudinally under the spine.

position also stretches the pectoralis major and subscapularis muscles. Breathing exercises can be added to mobilize the ribs.

- *Patient position and procedure:* Sitting on a firm, straight-back chair with the hands behind the head or held abducted and externally rotated 90°. The patient then brings the elbows out to the side as the scapulae are adducted and the thoracic spine is extended (head held neutral, not flexed). To combine with breathing, have the patient inhale as he or she takes the elbows out to the side and exhale as the elbows are brought in front of the face (Fig. 16.2).

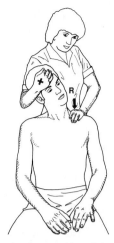

FIGURE 16.3 Unilateral active stretching of the scalenus muscles. The patient first performs axial extension, then side-bends the neck opposite and rotates it toward the tight muscles. The therapist stabilizes the head and upper thorax as the patient breathes in, contracting the muscle against the resistance. As the patient relaxes, the rib cage lowers and stretches the muscle.

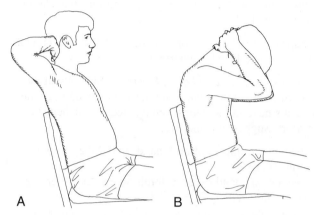

FIGURE 16.2 (*A*) A stretch is applied to the pectoralis muscles and anterior thorax during inspiration, and (*B*) the patient brings the elbows together to facilitate expiration.

## Techniques to Increase Axial Extension (Cervical Retraction)— Scalene Muscle Stretch

NOTE: Because the scalene muscles are attached to the transverse processes of the upper cervical spine and the upper two ribs, they either flex the cervical spine or elevate the upper ribs when they contract bilaterally. Unilaterally, the scalenes side-bend the cervical spine to the same side and rotate it to the opposite side.

### Manual Stretching

*Patient position and procedure:* Sitting. The patient first performs axial extension (tucks the chin and straightens the neck) and then side-bends the neck opposite and rotates it toward the tight muscles. Stand behind the patient and stabilize the upper ribs with one hand over the top of the rib cage on the side of tightness and stabilize the head with the other hand around the side of the patient's head and face, holding the head against your trunk (Fig. 16.3). The patient inhales and exhales; stabilize the ribs with a downward pressure as the patient inhales again. Repeat. This is a gentle, hold–relax stretching maneuver.

### Self-Stretching

*Patient position and procedure:* Standing next to a table and holding onto its underside. The patient positions the head in axial extension, side-bend opposite, and rotation toward the same side as the muscle being stretched. Have the patient stabilize the head by placing the opposite hand on the back of the occipital region. To stretch, he or she leans away from the table, inhales, exhales, and holds the stretch position.

## Techniques to Increase Upper Cervical Flexion—Short Suboccipital Muscle Stretch

### Manual Stretching

- *Patient position and procedure:* Sitting. Identify the spinous process of the second cervical vertebra and stabilize it with your thumb or with the second metacarpophalangeal joint (and the thumb and index finger around the transverse processes). Have the patient slowly nod, doing just a tipping motion of the head on the upper spine (Fig. 16.4). Guide the movement by placing the other hand across the patient's forehead.
- *Patient position and procedure:* Supine. Sit on a stool at the head of the treatment table with your forearms resting on the table. One hand stabilizes the C2 vertebra by grasping the transverse processes between the proximal portions of the thumb and index finger; the other hand supports the occiput. Nod the patient's head with the hand under the occiput to take up the slack of the suboccipital muscles; then ask the patient to roll the eyes upward. This causes a gentle isometric contraction of the

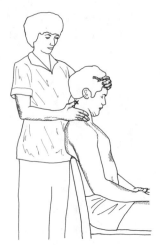

**FIGURE 16.4** Stretching the short suboccipital muscles. The therapist stabilizes the second cervical vertebra as the patient slowly nods the head.

suboccipital muscles. After holding 6 seconds, ask the patient to roll the eyes downward. As the suboccipital muscles relax, take up the slack by passively nodding the head through any new range. Only motion between the occiput and C2 should occur. The contraction is gentle in order to not cause overflow into the multisegmental erector spinae and upper trapezius muscles.

### Self-Stretching

*Patient position and procedure:* Supine or sitting. Instruct the patient to nod the head, bringing the chin toward the larynx until a stretch is felt in the suboccipital area. Putting light pressure under the occipital region with the palm of your hand while tipping the patient's head forward reinforces the motion.

## Techniques to Increase Scapular and Humeral Muscle Flexibility

Shoulder girdle posture is directly related to cervical and thoracic posture. Techniques to increase flexibility in the shoulder and scapular muscles are described in Chapter 17. Of primary importance are the pectoralis major (see Figs.

17.30 to 17.32), pectoralis minor (see Fig. 17.33), levator scapulae (see Figs. 17.34 and 17.35), and shoulder internal rotator muscles (see Fig. 17.26).

## Traction as a Stretching Technique

### Manual Traction—Cervical Spine

Traction techniques can be used for the purposes of stretching the muscles and the facet joint capsules and widening the intervertebral foramina.[47] The value of manual traction is that the angle of pull, head position, and placement of the force (via specific hand placements) can be controlled by the therapist; thus the force can be specifically applied with minimum stress to regions that should not be stretched.

*Patient position:* Supine on a treatment table. The patient should be as relaxed as possible.

*Therapist position and hand placement:* Standing at the head of the treatment table, supporting the weight of the patient's head in the hands. Hand placement depends on comfort. Suggestions include:

- Placing the fingers of both hands under the occiput (Fig. 16.5A).
- Placing one hand over the forehead and the other hand under the occiput (Fig. 16.5B).
- Placing the index fingers around the spinous process above the vertebral level to be moved. This hand placement provides a specific traction only to the vertebral segments below the level at which the fingers are placed. A belt around the therapist's hips can be used to reinforce the fingers and increase the ease of applying the traction force (Fig. 16.5C).

*Procedure:* Vary the patient's head position in flexion, extension, side bending, and side bending with rotation until the tissue to be stretched is taut; then apply a traction force by assuming a stable stance and leaning backward in a controlled manner. If a belt is used, the force is transmitted through the belt. The force is usually applied intermittently with smooth and gradual building and releasing of the traction force. The intensity and duration are usually limited by the therapist's strength and endurance.

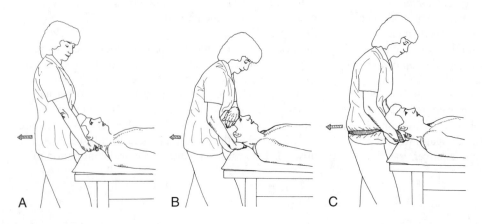

A      B      C

**FIGURE 16.5** Manual cervical traction: (*A*) with the fingers of both hands under the occiput; (*B*) with one hand over the frontal region and the other hand under the occiput; and (*C*) using a belt to reinforce the hands for the traction force.

## Positional Traction—Cervical Spine

The value of using positional traction is that the primary traction force can be isolated to a specific facet. This may be beneficial when selective stretching is necessary as when the segment above or on the contralateral side is hypermobile and should not be stretched.

*Patient position:* Supine, lying on the treatment table.

*Therapist position:* Standing at the head of the treatment table, supporting the patient's head in the hands. Determine the segment that is to receive most of the traction force and palpate the spinous process at that level.

*Procedure:* Flex the head until motion of the spinous process just begins at the determined level. Support the head with folded towels at that level of flexion. Then side-bend the head away from the side to be distracted until movement of the spinous process is felt at the desired level. Finally, rotate the head a few degrees toward the side to be distracted. Adjust the towel support to maintain this position for low-intensity, sustained traction stretch to that facet joint and surrounding soft tissue.[39]

## Self-Traction—Cervical Spine

*Patient position and procedure:* Sitting or lying down. Have the patient place his or her hands behind the neck with the fingers interlocking; the ulnar border of the fingers and hands are under the occiput and mastoid processes. The patient then gives a lifting motion to the head. The head may be placed in flexion, extension, side bending, or rotation for more isolated effects. He or she may apply the traction intermittently or in a sustained manner.

Positional traction can also be used for self-traction. The patient learns to assume the position determined by the therapist as described in the previous procedure.

NOTE: Various forms of mechanical traction can be used in the clinic and at home. The position, dosage, and duration of traction is determined by the therapist. Instruction for use of the equipment is not described in this text.

## Other Techniques for Increasing Mobility

***Inhibition techniques.*** Inhibition techniques, as described in Chapter 5, can be used on any muscle group or with any motion. Suggested position for the patient is supine, with the therapist standing at the head end of the treatment table supporting the patient's head in the hands. The intensity of resistance should be very gentle and applied smoothly.

***Joint mobilization/manipulation.*** Joint mobilization/ manipulation techniques can be used by those trained in the principles and maneuvers. Specific spinal techniques for the cervical and thoracic spinal area are not described in this text.

# MID AND LOWER THORACIC AND LUMBAR REGIONS— STRETCHING TECHNIQUES

## Techniques to Increase Lumbar Flexion

PRECAUTION: If flexion of the spine causes a change in sensation or causes pain to radiate down an extremity, reassess the patient's condition to determine if flexion is contraindicated.

### Assisted Stretching

*Patient position and procedure:* Cross-sitting. Have the patient place the hands behind the neck, adduct the scapulae, and extend the thoracic spine. This locks the thoracic vertebrae. Have the patient then lean the thorax forward onto the pelvis, flexing only at the lumbar spine. Stabilize the pelvis by pulling back on the anterior-superior iliac spines (Fig. 16.6).

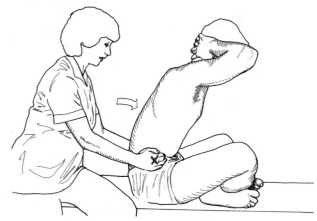

FIGURE 16.6 Stretching the lumbar spine with the patient stabilizing the thorax in extension and the therapist stabilizing the pelvis.

### Self-Stretching

- *Patient position and procedure:* Hook-lying. Have the patient first bring one knee and then the other toward the chest, clasp the hands around the thighs, and pull them to the chest, elevating the sacrum off the mat (Fig. 16.7). The patient should not grasp around the tibia; it places stress on the knee joints as the stretch force is applied.
- *Patient position and procedure:* Quadruped (on hands and knees). Have the patient perform a posterior pelvic tilt without rounding the thorax (concentrate on flexing the lumbar spine, not the thoracic spine), hold the position, then relax (Fig. 16.8A). Repeat; this time bring the

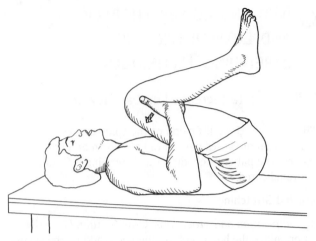

FIGURE 16.7 Self-stretching the lumbar erector spinae muscles and tissues posterior to the spine. The patient grasps around the thighs to avoid compression of the knee joints.

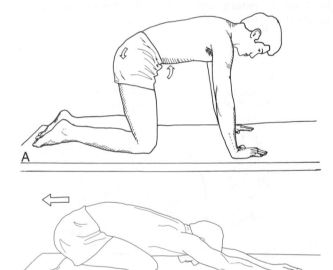

FIGURE 16.8 Stretching of the lumbar spine. (*A*) The patient performs a posterior pelvic tilt without rounding the thorax. (*B*) The patient moves the buttocks back over the feet for a greater stretch.

hips back to the feet, hold, and then return to the hands and knees position (Fig. 16.8B). This also stretches the gluteus maximus, quadriceps femoris, and shoulder extensor muscles.

## Techniques to Increase Lumbar Extension

PRECAUTION: Do not perform if extension causes a change in sensation or causes pain to radiate down an extremity (see Chapter 15).

### Self-Stretch

- *Patient position and procedure:* Prone, with hands placed under the shoulders. Have the patient extend the

elbows and lift the thorax up off the mat but keep the pelvis down on the mat. This is a *prone press-up* (Fig. 16.9A). To increase the stretch force, the pelvis can be strapped to the treatment table. This exercise also stretches the hip flexor muscles and soft tissue anterior to the hip.
- *Patient position and procedure:* Standing, with the hands placed in the low-back area. Instruct the patient to lean backward (Fig. 16.9B).
- *Patient position and procedure:* Quadruped (hands and knees). Instruct the patient to allow the spine to sag, creating lumbar extension. This, alternated with posterior pelvic tilts, can also be used to teach the patient how to control pelvic motion.

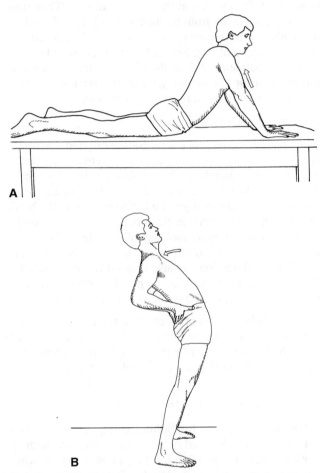

FIGURE 16.9 Self-stretching of the soft tissues anterior to the lumbar spine and hip joints with the patient (*A*) prone (using a press-up) and (*B*) standing.

## Techniques to Increase Lateral Flexibility in the Spine

Stretching techniques to increase lateral flexibility are used for intervention when there is asymmetrical flexibility in side bending as well as in the management of scoliosis. It is important to note that stretching has not been shown to correct or halt progression of structural scoliosis. If these exercises are used for patients with structural scoliosis, they may be beneficial in gaining some flexibility prior to surgical fusion of the spine for correcting a scoliotic deformity. They may also be used to regain flexibility in the frontal plane when muscle or fascial tightness is present with postural dysfunction. All of the following exercises are designed to stretch hypomobile structures on the concave side of the lateral curvature.

When stretching the trunk, it is necessary to stabilize the spine either above or below the curve. If the patient has a double curve, one curve must be stabilized while the other is stretched.

● *Patient position and procedure:* Prone. Stabilize the patient at the iliac crest (manually or with a belt) on the side of the concavity. Have the patient reach toward the knee with the arm on the convex side of the curve while stretching the opposite arm up and overhead (Fig. 16.10). Instruct the patient to breathe in and expand the rib cage on the side being stretched.

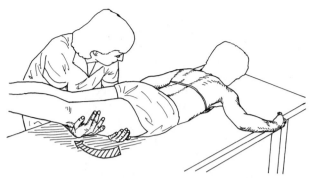

FIGURE 16.11 Stretching hypomobile structures on the concave side of a left lumbar curve. The patient stabilizes the upper trunk and thoracic curve as the therapist passively stretches the lumbar curve.

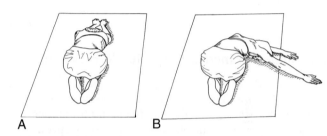

FIGURE 16.12 (*A*) Heel-sitting to stabilize the lumbar spine. (*B*) Hypomobile structures on the concave side of a right thoracic curve are stretched by having the patient reach the arms overhead and then walk the hands toward the convex side.

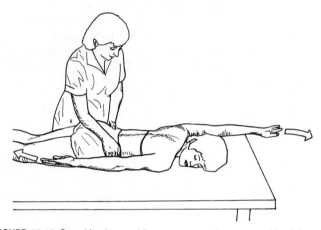

FIGURE 16.10 Stretching hypomobile structures on the concave side of the thoracic curve. Illustrated is a patient with a right thoracic left lumbar curve. The therapist stabilizes the pelvis and lumbar spine while the patient actively stretches the thoracic curve.

● *Patient position and procedure:* Prone. Have the patient stabilize the upper trunk (thoracic curve) by holding onto the edge of the mat table with the arms. Lift the hips and legs and laterally bend the trunk away from the concavity (Fig. 16.11).
● *Patient position and procedure:* Heel-sitting. Have the patient lean forward so the abdomen rests on the anterior thighs (Fig. 16.12A); the arms are stretched overhead bilaterally, and the hands are flat on the floor. Then have the patient laterally bend the trunk away from the concavity by walking the hands to the convex side of the curve. Hold the position for a sustained stretch (Fig. 16.12B).
● *Patient position and procedure:* Side-lying on the convex side of the curve. Place a rolled towel at the apex of the curve, and have the patient reach overhead with the top arm. Stabilize the patient at the iliac crest. Do not allow

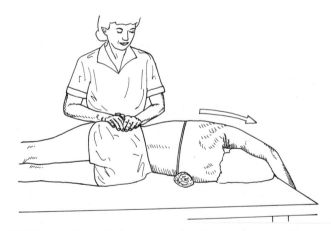

FIGURE 16.13 Stretching tight structures on the concave side of a right thoracic curve. The patient is positioned side-lying with a rolled towel at the apex of the convexity. The lumbar spine is stabilized by the therapist.

the patient to roll forward or backward during the stretch. Hold this position for a sustained period of time (Fig. 16.13).
● *Patient position and procedure:* Side-lying over the edge of a mat table with a rolled towel at the apex of the curve and the top arm stretched overhead. Stabilize the iliac crest. Hold this head-down position as long as possible (Fig. 16.14).

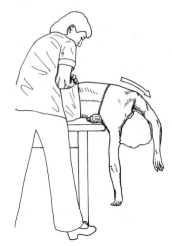

**FIGURE 16.14** Side-lying over the edge of a mat table to stretch hypomobile structures of a right thoracic scoliosis. The therapist stabilizes the pelvis.

## Techniques to Increase Hip Muscle Flexibility

Hip muscles have a direct effect on spinal posture and function because of their attachment on the pelvis. It is important that they have adequate flexibility for proper pelvic and spinal alignment. See Chapter 20 for specific stretching techniques of hip musculature.

## Traction as a Stretching Technique

### Manual Traction—Lumbar Spine

Manual traction is not as easily applied in the lumbar region as in the cervical region. At least one-half of the body weight of the patient must be moved, and the coefficient of friction of the part to be moved also must be overcome to cause vertebral distraction and stretching. It is helpful to place the patient on a split-traction table for ease in moving and stretching the spine.

*Patient position:* Supine or prone. Stabilize the thorax with a harness that is secured to the head end of the table or have an assistant stabilize the patient by standing at the head of the table and holding the patient's arms. Position the patient so there is maximal stretch on the hypomobile tissue.

- To stretch into extension, extend the hips.
- To stretch into flexion, flex the hips.
- To stretch into side bending, move the lower extremities to one side.

*Therapist position and procedures:* Position yourself so effective body mechanics and body weight can be used.

- If the lower extremities are extended to emphasize spinal extension, exert the pull at the ankles.
- If the lower extremities are flexed to emphasize spinal flexion, drape the legs over your shoulders and exert the stretch force with your arms wrapped across the patient's thighs. As an alternative, place a pelvic belt with straps around the patient and manually pull on the straps.

### Positional Traction—Lumbar Spine

The value of positional traction is that the primary traction force can be directed to the side on which symptoms occur, or it can be isolated to a specific facet and is therefore beneficial for selective stretching.[39]

*Patient position:* Side-lying, with the side to be stretched uppermost. A rolled blanket is placed under the spine at the level where the traction force is desired; this causes side bending away from the side to be treated and therefore an upward gliding of the facets (Fig. 16.15A).

*Therapist position:* Standing, at the side of the treatment table facing the patient. Determine the segment that is to receive most of the traction force and palpate the spinous processes at that level and the level above.

*Procedure:* The patient relaxes in the side-bent position. Rotation is added to isolate a distraction force to the desired level. Rotate the upper trunk by gently pulling on the arm on which the patient is lying while simultaneously palpating the spinous processes with your other hand to determine when rotation has arrived at the level just above the joint to be distracted. Then flex the patient's uppermost thigh, again palpating the spinous processes until flexion of the lower portion of the spine occurs at the desired level. The segment at which these two opposing forces meet now has maximum positional distraction force (Fig. 16.15B).

N O T E : Mechanical traction units can provide considerable stretch force to the tissues of the thoracic and lumbar spine. Positioning considerations are as described for manual traction. Instructions for use of the equipment are not part of this text.

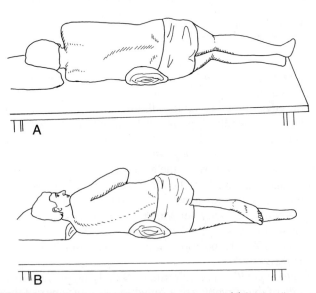

**FIGURE 16.15** Positional traction for the lumbar spine. (*A*) Side bending over a 6- to 8-inch roll causes longitudinal traction to the segments on the upward side. (*B*) Side-bending with rotation adds a distraction force to the facets on the upward side.

## MUSCLE PERFORMANCE: STABILIZATION, MUSCLE ENDURANCE, AND STRENGTH TRAINING

***Goals.*** To (1) activate and develop neuromuscular control of core and global spinal stabilizing muscles to support the spine against external loading; (2) develop endurance and strength in the muscles of the axial skeleton for functional activities; and (3) develop control of balance in stable and unstable situations.

This section is divided into two main sections. The first section presents principles and techniques of stabilization exercises for the cervical and lumbar spinal regions with a subsection on core muscle activation and a subsection on global muscle stabilization. The second section presents principles and techniques of general isometric, dynamic, and functional exercises for the neck and trunk.

### ● STABILIZATION TRAINING— FUNDAMENTAL TECHNIQUES AND PROGRESSIONS

"Proximal stability for distal mobility," a well known phrase, is an underlying principle of intervention with therapeutic exercise. The primary functions of the muscles of the trunk are to provide the stabilizing force so upright posture can be maintained against a variety of forces that disturb balance and to provide a stable base so the muscles of the extremities can execute their function efficiently and without undue stress to the spinal structures. Several studies have demonstrated altered or delayed neuromuscular recruitment patterns in the deep (core) stabilizing muscles of the lumbar spine during active movement in individuals with low back pain.[15,18,19,38] Results of other studies have shown improved ability to recruit these muscles with specific training[37] and improved outcomes compared with individuals not receiving the training.[14,37,38] Studies have also demonstrated improved outcomes in patients with cervical pain and cervicogenic headaches with recruitment of the deep stabilizing musculature in the cervical spine in conjunction with total trunk stabilization.[24,32]

The functions of the deep (core) segmental musculature and the superficial (global) spinal musculature were identified and described in Chapter 14. Both muscle systems are necessary for spinal stability and function. Therefore, one of the primary areas of emphasis during rehabilitation after spinal problems is recruiting the core muscles and training them to respond along with the global musculature to various forces and demands imposed on the spine to improve coordination of their overall function. Activation of the stabilizing musculature is then reinforced when progressing to muscular endurance and strengthening exercises, when performing aerobic exercises, and when practicing functional activities throughout the rehabilitative

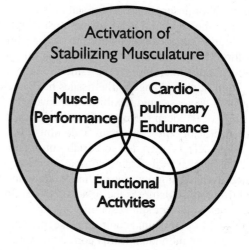

FIGURE 16.16 Exercises to improve muscle performance, cardiopulmonary endurance, and functional activities are integrated over a background of activating the core and global spinal stabilizing musculature.

process with the anticipation that muscle activation for stabilization will become automatic during all daily activities and functional challenges (Fig. 16.16).

Stabilization training follows the basic principles of learning motor control first by developing awareness of muscle contractions and spinal position, then by developing control in simple patterns and exercises and progressing to complex exercises, and finally by demonstrating automatic maintenance of spinal stability and control in a progression of simple functional activities to complex and unplanned situations.[48] Many of the exercises can be used to accomplish more than one purpose; and there is definite overlap with kinesthetic training and functional training. The choice and progression of exercises described in each of the sections relies on clinical judgment of the patient's response and attainment of goals, not on a strict, time-based protocol or days from injury. The ability of the patient to control the spine in a neutral or nonstressful position is paramount for all the exercises.

There is considerably more research on muscle function and its stabilization action in the lumbar spine. The cervical spine requires more mobility to position the head, yet relies on the thoracic and lumbar spinal regions to provide a base for stability and postural control. Even though there are unique anatomical considerations in the cervical spine, there is overlap between stabilization training for cervical and lumbar problems.

### Guidelines for Stabilization Training

It is important to understand and use the principles and progression of stabilization training for effective instruction.[6,34,44-46,51] The following guidelines are summarized in Box 16.2.

1. *Kinesthetic training* for awareness of safe motion and positions must precede stabilization training. The functional range and functional position in which symptoms

are minimal or absent are used for stabilization exercises.[34] When the condition is not acute, most people find the mid-range (the neutral position) to be their functional position. It is important to recognize that this position or range is not static; nor is it the same for every person. In addition, it may change as the tissues heal, nociceptive stimuli decrease, and flexibility improves.[34]

2. *Activation* of the deep (core) stabilizing muscles of the trunk, specifically the transversus abdominis (TrA) and multifidus (Mf), is often delayed or absent in patients with back pain.[15,19,38] Learning conscious activation of these core-stabilizing muscles without contracting the global trunk musculature is the first step in developing habitual activation for spinal stability in patients with pain related to poor spinal control and segmental instability. Once the individual learns correct activation of the core stabilizers with the drawing-in maneuver, this maneuver is used prior to all exercises and activities to develop the early activation and stabilizing function and eventually automatic feedforward stabilization from the muscles.[20] A study involving 42 subjects demonstrated that it is possible to alter abdominal muscle activation consciously and automatically with specific exercises.[37] In the cervical region the deep cervical flexors, the longus colli and cervicis, and the deep cervical and upper thoracic extensors are activated to stabilize the cervical spine in a neutral spinal position (axial extension with mild lordosis).

3. *Extremity motions* are added to the stabilization program to reinforce core muscle activation and coordinate core muscle activity with the global stabilizing musculature. Loading via the extremities increases the stabilizing challenge to the musculature. The patient positions the spine in the neutral position (using pelvic tilt motions in the lumbar region and gentle head nodding in the cervical region), performs the drawing-in maneuver, and then begins moving one or several extremities while maintaining the neutral position. Extremity motions are performed within the tolerance of the trunk or neck muscles to control the neutral or functional position. This is called *dynamic stabilization* because the stabilizing forces in the spinal area must respond to the changing forces coming from the extremities. Exercises that require stabilization against transverse plane rotational forces on the pelvis more consistently activate the oblique abdominal and deep spinal stabilizers than sagittal plane resistive forces.[43]

4. Once control of the position is established and the patient can activate the stabilizing muscles, repetitions of extremity motions are increased, and resistance is applied to the extremities to increase *muscular endurance and strength*. The intent is to challenge the trunk muscles to stabilize against these increased forces yet stay within their tolerance and ability to control the spinal position. Repetitions also help develop *habit*; therefore, it is important to use careful instructions and provide feedback. Fatigue is determined by the inability of the trunk or neck muscles to stabilize the spine in its functional position. For example:

- Begin at a resistance force that the patient can repeat for 30 to 60 seconds; progress the repetitions to 3 minutes.
- Progress by adding resistance to or increasing the lever arm of the extremities; initially reduce the time and again progress to doing the new activity for 1 to 3 minutes.
- Another way to develop endurance in the trunk muscles is to begin exercising at the most difficult level for that patient, then shift to simpler levels of resistance as fatigue begins in order to keep moving. It is important that the patient does not lose control of the functional position.

5. Alternating isometric contractions between antagonists and rhythmic stabilization of the trunk muscles against manual resistance also enhance stabilizing contractions. When performed while sitting and standing, the alternating contractions and co-contractions also develop control of balance.

6. *Transitional stabilization* develops as the patient moves from one position to another in conjunction with extremity motions. This requires graded contractions and adjustments between the trunk flexors and extensors and requires greater awareness and concentration.[6,34] For example, any motion of the arms or legs away from the trunk tends to cause the spine to extend. The abdominals (trunk flexors) must contract to maintain control of the functional spinal position. This occurs, for example, when lifting a load from the floor to overhead. Then, as the arms or legs move anteriorly toward the center of gravity, the spine tends to flex, which requires the extensors to contract to maintain the functional position (as would occur when lowering a weight to the floor). Greater concentration on maintaining the functional spinal position is necessary when doing more advanced functional activities.

7. *Perturbation* (balance) training, exercising against destabilizing forces or on unstable surfaces, develops neuromuscular responses to improve balance.

## Deep Stabilizing (Core) Muscle Activation and Training

The function of the core musculature (TrA and Mf in the lumbar spine and longus colli and other deep musculature in the cervical spine) is described in Chapter 14, and the results of impaired function in these muscles are described in Chapter 15. Techniques for activation of the core musculature are described in this section.

### ◉ Focus on Evidence

Methods for testing and training activation of the core musculature have been developed and used in both research and clinical settings.[40] Placement of fine-wire electrodes with ultrasound guidance has provided valuable information regarding the muscle function and recovery in research settings,[20,21] and ultrasound imaging has provided a valuable tool for biofeedback in training.[13,16,17,53] As of this date, use of ultrasound biofeedback imaging has been

**Guidelines for Stabilization Training: Principles and Progression**

1. Begin training awareness of safe spinal motions and the neutral spine position or bias.
2. Have patient learn to activate the deep (core) stabilizing musculature while in the neutral position.
3. Add extremity motions to load the global musculature while maintaining a stable neutral spine position (dynamic stabilization).
4. Increase repetitions to improve holding capacity (endurance) in the stabilizing musculature; increase load (change lever arm or add resistance) to improve strength while maintaining a stable neutral spine position.
5. Use alternating isometric contractions and rhythmic stabilization techniques to enhance stabilization and balance with fluctuating loads.
6. Progress to movement from one position to another in conjunction with extremity motions while maintaining a stable neutral spine (transitional stabilization).
7. Use unstable surfaces to improve the stabilizing response and improve balance.

prohibitively expensive to use clinically for training activation of the core musculature. As an alternative device, a pressure biofeedback unit (Stabilizer™; © 2006 Encore Medical, L.P.) has been developed and has been shown to have clinical usage in training activation and control of the core musculature of the trunk and neck.[22,49]

## Cervical Musculature

In the cervical region, the goal is to activate and control the muscles that control axial extension (cervical retraction). This requires capital flexion, slight flattening of the cervical lordosis, and flattening of the upper thoracic kyphosis (Fig. 16.17).

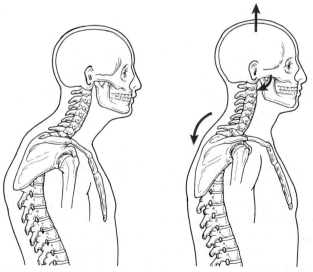

FIGURE 16.17 Axial extension (cervical retraction) involves the motions of capital flexion and extension of the lower and upper thoracic spine toward extension, resulting in slight flattening of the cervical lordosis.

## Deep Neck Flexors: Activation and Training

*Patient position and procedure:* Supine. For craniocervical flexion and gentle axial extension, teach the patient to perform slow, controlled nodding motion of the head on the upper cervical spine ("yes" motion). Once able to activate the motion, the Stabilizer™ may be used to monitor the amount of cervical flattening and measure the muscular endurance for holding the contraction (Fig. 16.18).

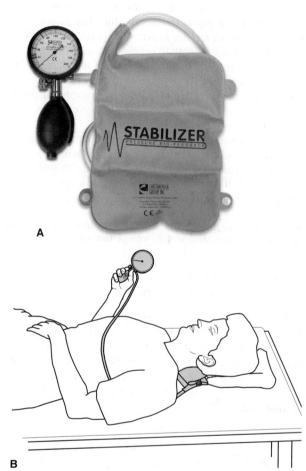

**B**

FIGURE 16.18 (A) The Stabilizer™ pressure biofeedback unit (© 2006 Encore Medical, L.P.) is used to provide visual feedback to the patient while training for core muscle activation. (B) Stabilizer folded into thirds under the cervical spine to test and train capital flexion with neutral spine axial extension.

The protocol for use of the Stabilizer™ is summarized in Box 16.3.

 **Focus on Evidence**

Jull et al.[25] reported that the controlled performance of upper cervical flexion increases the pressure in the Stabilizer™ to 30 mmHg and that the test–retest reliability of the craniocervical flexion test (conducted on 50 asymptomatic subjects 1 week between tests) was an ICC of 0.81 for the activation score and 0.93 for the performance index (see Box 16.3).

- Place the folded Stabilizer™ pressure biofeedback unit (folded into thirds) under the upper cervical spine and inflate to 20 mmHg.
- Instruct the patient to nod and increase pressure on the cuff to 22 mmHg and hold the pressure steady.
- If the patient is successful (i.e., can hold the position with minimal superficial muscle activity), have him or her relax and repeat the flexion, this time increasing pressure to 24 mmHg. Repeat this incremental activation up to 30 mmHg (total 10 mmHg increase).
- The final pressure is the one at which the patient can hold steady.
- Muscle endurance (holding or tonic capacity) of the deep neck flexors is measured by the number of 10-second holds (up to 10) at the final pressure.

    A performance index can be used to document an objective measure. Multiply the pressure increase by the number of times the patient can repeat the 10-second holds—with 100 reflecting the holding of a 10-mmHg increase for 10 repetitions.[25]

Adapted from the instruction manual that accompanies the Stabilizer™ © 2006 Encore Medical, L.P., with permission.

### Lower Cervical and Upper Thoracic Extensor Activation and Training

*Patient position and procedure:* Prone with forehead on the treatment table and arms at the sides. Have the patient lift the forehead off the treatment table, keeping the chin tucked and eyes focused on the table to maintain the neutral spinal position (reinforces the craniocervical flexion motion learned in the supine position). Lifting the head is a small motion (Fig. 16.19).

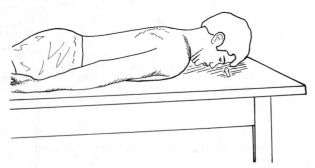

FIGURE 16.19 Axial extension (cervical retraction) exercises.

### Progression

Once the patient learns to activate the core musculature and assume the neutral posture in the cervical spine, practice throughout the day is encouraged. Core muscle activation is then coordinated with stabilization training using the global musculature and upper extremity loading. Extremity motions are added and used to stimulate muscu-

lar endurance as well as strengthen the stabilizing musculature in the spine. Global stabilization exercises are described in the section Global Muscle Training for Stabilization.

### Lumbar Musculature

Three techniques for abdominal muscle activation have been described and used in clinical practice: the drawing-in maneuver; abdominal bracing; and posterior pelvic tilt (Fig. 16.20). Studies are showing that each technique differs in the stabilization activity of the abdominal and multifidus muscles.[42] Research has demonstrated that the drawing-in maneuver is more selective in co-activating the transversus abdominis and multifidus muscles than the abdominal bracing and posterior pelvic tilt techniques.[22,42] The drawing-in maneuver also functions to increase intra-abdominal pressure by inwardly displacing the abdominal wall. Because of this, the drawing-in maneuver is recommended for stabilization training; the other two methods are also described, primarily so the reader can recognize the differences.

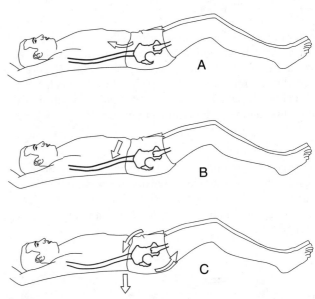

FIGURE 16.20 Three methods to activate the stabilizing musculature in the lumbar spine. (*A*) Drawing-in maneuver where the patient hollows the abdominal region ("draws" the belly button toward the spine). (*B*) Abdominal bracing where setting the abdominal muscles results in flaring laterally around the waist. (*C*) Posterior pelvic tilt where the pelvis is actively tilted posteriorly and the lumbar spine flattens.

### Drawing-In Maneuver (Abdominal Hollowing Exercise) for Transverse Abdominis Activation

*Patient positions:* Training may be easiest in the quadruped position in order to use the effects of gravity on the abdominal wall. Hook-lying (with knees 70° to 90° and feet resting on an exercise mat), prone-lying, or semireclined positions may be used if more comfortable for the patient. It is important to progress training to sitting and standing as soon as possible for functional activities.

*Procedure:* Teach the patient using demonstration, verbal cues, and tactile facilitation. Explain that the muscle encircles the trunk; and when activated, the waistline draws inward (see Fig. 16.20A). Palpation of the muscle is possible just distal to the anterior superior iliac spine (ASIS) and lateral to the rectus abdominis (Fig. 16.21). When the internal oblique (IO) contracts, a bulge of the muscle is felt; when the TrA contracts, flat tension is felt. The goal is to activate the TrA with minimal or no contraction of the IO. This is a gentle contraction.

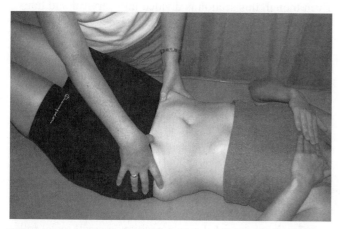

FIGURE 16.21 Palpation of the transversus abdominis muscle just distal to the ASIS and lateral to the rectus abdominis muscle. It feels like a tense sheet (a bulge is the internal oblique) when performing a gentle drawing-in maneuver.

Have the patient assume a neutral spinal position and attempt to maintain it while gently drawing in and hollowing the abdominal muscles.[40] Instruct the patient to breathe in, breath out, then gently draw the belly button in toward the spine to hollow out the abdominal region. When done properly there are no substitute patterns; that is, there is minimal to no movement of the pelvis (posterior pelvic tilting), no flaring or depression of the lower ribs, no inspiration or lifting of the rib cage, no bulging out of the abdominal wall, and no increased pressure through the feet.

If a patient has difficulty activating the TrA, the following two feedback techniques have been shown to assist with learning.[11,26,41,42]

- **Pressure biofeedback for clinical testing and visual feedback.** With the patient prone, the Stabilizer™ is placed horizontally under the abdomen (centered under the navel). Inflate the Stabilizer™ to 70 mmHg. Have the patient perform a drawing-in maneuver, as described above. A decrease of 6 to 10 mmHg during the drawing-in maneuver (without substitutions) indicates proper activation of the deep abdominal muscles. The dial on the unit is large and easily read by the patient for immediate feedback.
- **Biofeedback with surface electrodes.** Surface electrodes placed over the rectus abdominis and external obliques

**BOX 16.4 Testing and Training Core Muscle Activation (Transversus Abdominis) in the Lumbar Spine**

- Patient is prone lying.
- Place the Stabilizer™ pressure biofeedback unit horizontally under the abdomen with the lower edge just below the anterior superior iliac spines (ASIS) (navel at center of unit).
- Inflate to 70 mmHg and instruct the patient to perform the drawing-in maneuver.
- If done properly, the pressure drops 6 to 10 mmHg.
- See if the patient can maintain the pressure drop for up to 10 seconds.
- Muscle endurance (holding or tonic capacity) of the transversus abdominis (TrA) is measured by the number of 10-second holds (up to 10).

Adapted from the instruction manual that accompanies the Stabilizer™ © 2006 Encore Medical, L.P., with permission.

(near its attachment on the eighth rib) may be used in conjunction with the inflatable cuff. There should be minimal to no activation of these muscles if the drawing-in maneuver is done correctly.

As with the cervical spine, the Stabilizer™ can be used not only to train activation of the TrA but also to measure control for a period of time as well as number of repetitions. The protocol is summarized in Box 16.4.

**Abdominal Bracing**
In contrast to the drawing-in maneuver, abdominal bracing occurs by setting the abdominals and actively flaring out laterally around the waist (see Fig. 16.20B). There is no head or trunk flexion, no elevation of the lower ribs, no protrusion of the abdomen, and no pressure through the feet. The patient should be able to hold the braced position while breathing in a relaxed manner. This technique has been taught for a number of years as the method to stabilize the spine; and it has been shown to activate the oblique abdominal muscles consistent with their global stabilization function.[42]

**Posterior Pelvic Tilt**
Pelvic tilt exercises (see Fig. 16.20C) principally activate the rectus abdominis muscle, which is used primarily for dynamic trunk flexion activity. It is not considered a core spinal stabilization muscle; therefore, it is not emphasized in the training for stabilization.[42] It is used mostly to teach awareness of movement of the pelvis and lumbar spine. It is activated when the patient explores his or her lumbar ROM with pelvic tilts to find the neutral position or functional spinal range.

**Multifidus Activation and Training**

*Patient position and procedure:* Prone or side-lying. Place your palpating digits (thumbs or index fingers) immediately lateral to the spinous processes of the lumbar spine

(Fig. 16.22). Palpate each spinal level so comparisons in the activation of the multifidus (Mf) muscle can be made between each segment as well as from side to side. Instruct the patient to "swell the muscle" out against your digits. Palpate for consistency of muscle contraction at each level. Facilitation techniques include using the drawing-in maneuver and gently contracting the pelvic floor muscles (as in Kegel's exercises, described in Chapter 23). In the side-lying position, facilitate by gently applying manual resistance to the thorax or pelvis to activate the rotation function of the Mf.

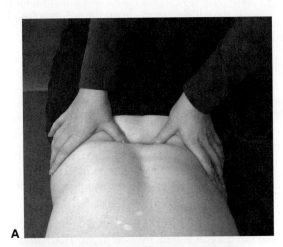

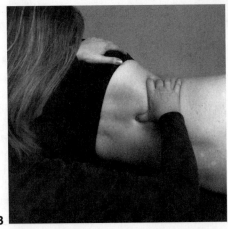

FIGURE 16.22 Palpation of the multifidus muscle lateral to the spinous processes in the lumbar spine, (A) bilaterally in the supine position and (B) unilaterally in the side-lying position.

The patient may be taught to self-palpate an Mf contraction in the following manner. Sit and rock the pelvis to find the neutral position. With the fingers or thumbs placed along the lumbar spinous processes, lean forward a couple degrees. The Mf is thus activated. Differentiate the Mf contraction from tension in the aponeurosis of the global erector spinae.

**Progression**

Once the patient learns to activate the core musculature, practice throughout the day is encouraged. Core muscle activation is then coordinated with stabilization training using the global musculature and extremity loading. Extremity motions are added and used to stimulate muscle endurance as well as strengthen the trunk muscles. Global stabilization exercises are described in the next section.

## Global Muscle Stabilization Exercises

Even though this section is divided into cervical and lumbar regions, many of the same exercises may be used for impairments in either region because of the functional relationships of the entire axial skeleton.

### Stabilization Exercises for the Cervical Region

**Stabilization with Progressive Limb Loading**
In general, stabilization exercises begin in the recumbent position and progress to sitting, sitting on a large gym ball, standing with the back supported against a wall, and finally standing without support.

- Begin all exercises with gentle craniocervical nods and axial extension to the neutral spinal position. During the early phases of training, if the patient has difficulty maintaining a neutral spinal position, a small towel roll may be placed under the neck for passive support.
- Initially, the only resistance load comes from simple upper extremity movements. When the patient can perform multiple repetitions of the upper extremity motions, resistance is added with handheld weights or elastic resistance.
- The principles of muscle endurance and strengthening described in Chapter 6 are used to challenge the spinal stabilizing musculature.
- Table 16.3 summarizes limb-loading exercises that emphasize the flexor muscles, and Figure 16.23 illustrates the basic exercise progression in the supine position.

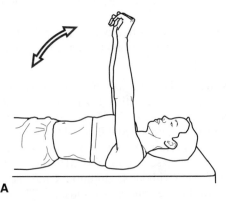

FIGURE 16.23 Limb loading for basic stabilization progression of cervical musculature in the supine position. Maximum protection phase: (A) shoulder flexion to 90°;

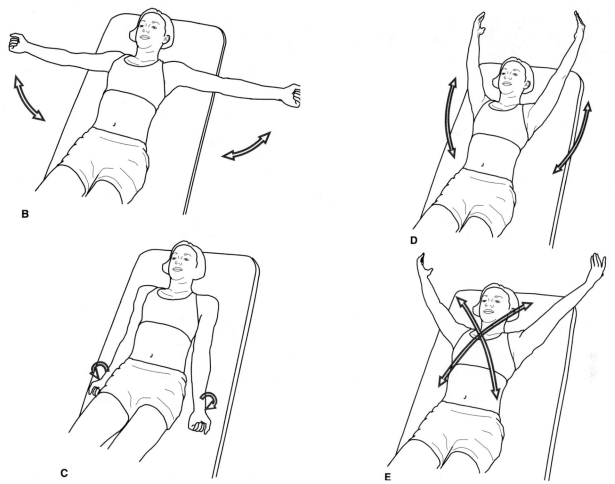

FIGURE 16.23 (continued) (*B*) shoulder abduction to 90°; (*C*) shoulder external rotation arms at the side. Moderate protection phase: (*D*) shoulder flexion and abduction to end range; (*E*) diagonal patterns.

---

**TABLE 16.3** **Cervical Stabilization with Progressive Limb Loading—Emphasis on Cervical Flexors**

| *Instructions*: Determine amount of support needed and amount of protection. Begin each exercise with axial extension to the neutral spinal position and maintain it while exercising; increase extremity repetitions, then increase resistance before progressing to a new challenge. | | *Maximum Support* ⟵—————————————⟶ *Minimum Support* | | | |
|---|---|---|---|---|---|
| | | *Supine* | *Sitting* (sitting on ball for less stability) | *Standing with wall support* | *Standing with no support* |
| **Core Activation** | | Gentle craniocervical flexion/axial extension hold 10 seconds × 10 repetitions | | | |
| **Minimum limb loading** ↕ **Maximum limb loading** | *Maximum to moderate protection* | Shoulder flexion to 90° | | | |
| | | Shoulder abduction 90° | | | |
| | | Shoulder external rotation with arms at sides | | | |
| | *Moderate to minimum protection* | Shoulder flexion to end of range | | | |
| | | Shoulder abduction combined with external rotation to end of range | | | |
| | | Diagonal patterns | | | |
| | *Minimum to no protection* | Reaching forward, outward, upward in functional patterns | | | |
| | | Standing, no support: pushing/pulling and lifting activities | | | |

**TABLE 16.4**  Cervical Stabilization with Progressive Limb Loading—Emphasis on Cervical and Thoracic Extensors

| *Instructions:* Determine amount of support needed and amount of protection. Begin each exercise with axial extension to the neutral spinal position and maintain it while exercising; increase extremity repetitions, then increase resistance before progressing to a new challenge. | | *Maximum Support* ⟵――――――――――⟶ *Minimum Support* | | | |
|---|---|---|---|---|---|
| | | Prone forehead on treatment table—lift forehead off table (Fig. 16.19) | Quadruped over padded stool or gym ball—maintain eyes focused on floor | Standing back supported by wall (ball behind head for less stability) | Standing, no support |
| *Core activation—gentle craniocervical flexion/axial extension* | | Lift forehead off exercise mat; hold 10 seconds × 10 repetitions | | | |
| **Minimum limb loading** ⬍ **Maximum limb loading** | *Maximum to moderate protection* | Arms at side: laterally rotate shoulders and adduct scapulae | | | |
| | | Arms in 90/90 position (abducted and laterally rotated), horizontally abduct shoulders and adduct scapulae | | | |
| | *Moderate to minimum protection* | Elevate shoulder in full flexion | | | |
| | | Arms abducted to 90° and laterally rotated, elbows extended: horizontally abduct shoulders and adduct scapulae | | | |
| | | Upper extremity diagonal patterns | | | |
| | *Minimum to no protection* | Standing: reaching forward, outward, upward in functional patterns | | | |
| | | Standing, no support: pushing/pulling and lifting activities | | | |

⦿ Table 16.4 summarizes limb-loading exercises that emphasize the lower cervical/upper thoracic extensor muscles, and Figure 16.24 illustrates a basic exercise progression in the prone position.

It is important to note that these exercises do not isolate the flexors or extensors, but that the designation is primarily for emphasis due to the effects of gravity.

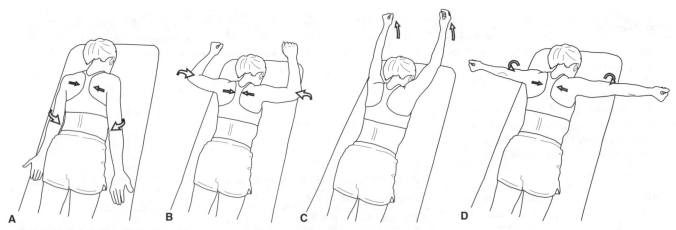

**FIGURE 16.24** Limb loading for basic stabilization progression of cervical musculature in prone position. Maximum protection phase: (*A*) arms at side, shoulder lateral rotation, and scapular adduction; (*B*) arms at 90/90, horizontal abduction, and scapular adduction. Moderate protection phase: (*C*) shoulder elevation full range, (*D*) shoulders 90° with lateral rotation and elbow extended, horizontal abduction, and scapular adduction.

## Variations and Progressions in the Stabilization Program

Remind the patient to find and maintain the neutral spinal position when doing these exercises.

- *Extremity loading.* During the early phases of training, limit shoulder flexion to 90° flexion and abduction. Once the patient can maintain stability and symptoms are not provoked, greater challenges occur with elevating the upper extremity full ROM. Unilateral upper extremity motion requires greater control than bilateral motion because the activity is asymmetrical.
- *External resistance.* Tables 16.3 and 16.4 summarize progressions based on position changes. In addition, use of resistance loads (free weights or elastic resistance) adds to the stabilizing challenge. Even though external resistance applied through the extremities has the benefit of increasing strength in the extremity musculature, the primary goal is to increase the stabilizing response of the cervical musculature. Therefore, any loss of the neutral spinal posture or increase in cervical symptoms signals the need to decrease the intensity of the resistance force.
- *Unstable surfaces.* Use of a ball while sitting (Fig. 16.25A), when in the quadruped position (Fig. 16.25B), or when standing supporting the ball between the head and the wall (Fig. 16.25C) provides an unstable surface that challenges the muscles to respond to perturbations.

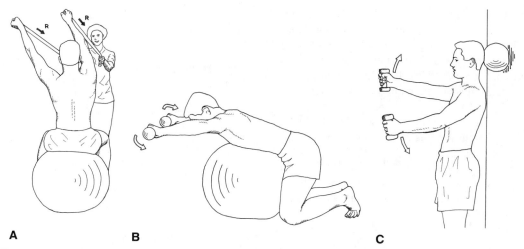

FIGURE 16.25 Unstable surfaces provide increased challenges to the cervical stabilizing musculature, requiring greater control. Examples include performing upper extremity motions, such as diagonal patterns, (A) while sitting on a gym ball, (B) while quadruped over a gym ball, and (C) while pressing a ball against the wall. Use of external resistance is also illustrated.

- *Muscular endurance and strength.* Determine the maximum level of resistance tolerated by the cervical-stabilizing musculature and that does not reproduce symptoms. Decrease the intensity and have the patient exercise with multiple repetitions at that level (20 to 30 repetitions or for 1 minute). Resistance can then be added for strengthening (decrease the number of repetitions) at that level before progressing to endurance training at the next level.

### Integration of Stabilization Exercises and Posture Training

Good postural alignment of the neck begins with the pelvis and lumbar spine and moves on up to the scapular and thoracic regions. The thorax must be lifted up from the pelvis and scapula retracted in a comfortable position for the cervical spine to assume an efficient position of axial extension (cervical retraction). Therefore, begin with lumbopelvic control if necessary and develop thoracic extension and scapular retraction. While the patient is performing the extremity motions to develop stability, reinforce good scapulohumeral alignment. It is important to remember that strengthening alone does not correct faulty posture and therefore to utilize reinforcement techniques and environmental adaptations that are discussed in Chapter 14.

### Progression of Isometric and Dynamic Strengthening in Conjunction with Functional Activities

When the patient demonstrates good cervical stabilization and response to various upper extremity resistance changes, isometric and dynamic exercises are integrated into the program. These are described in the Isometric and Dynamic Exercise section following this section.

## Stabilization Exercises for the Lumbar Region

### Stabilization with Progressive Limb Loading

Once the patient learns to activate the core-stabilizing muscles in the lumbar region, explain that prior to each exercise the patient is to find the neutral spinal position, perform the drawing-in maneuver, and then maintain control while applying an exercise load with extremity motions. The drawing-in maneuver develops the pattern of setting the deep abdominal and multifidus muscles in a feedforward pattern and then trains their holding capacity in coordination with the global muscles.[11,26] If the patient cannot control the position, preposition him or her using pillows, supports, or corsets

- To improve the holding capacity of the stabilizing muscles, increase the amount of time the patient does the exercises. It is important that no exercise is continued if the patient cannot maintain the stable position. If the deep abdominals cannot stabilize, substitute patterns in the superficial muscles override the deep muscle activation.
- The Stabilizer™ Pressure Bio-Feedback unit may be used for feedback during this early training (see Box 16.5 for guidelines).
- Table 16.5 summarizes basic limb loading exercises in the supine position that emphasize the abdominal muscles, and Figures 16.26 and 16.27 illustrate the exercise progression.

| BOX 16.5 | Instructions for use of Stabilizer™ for Stabilization Training with Leg Loading |
|---|---|

*Patient position*: Supine, hook lying.

- Place the three-chamber pressure cell under the lumbar spine horizontally across low back area.
- Position the spine in neutral.
- Inflate the pressure cell to a baseline of 40 mmHg.
- Draw in the abdominal wall without moving the spine or pelvis.
- Pressure should remain at 40 mmHg (±10 mmHg) while performing the lower extremity loading exercises.

Adapted from the instruction manual that accompanies the Stabilizer™ © 2006 Encore Medical, L.P., with permission.

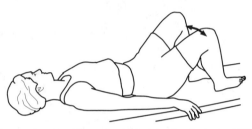

**FIGURE 16.26** Bent-leg fall out. Level 2 limb loading for basic stabilization of the abdominal muscles in the supine position. This requires control to prevent pelvic rotation; stability is assisted by the opposite lower extremity while hook-lying.

| TABLE 16.5 | Basic Lumbar Stabilization with Progressive Limb Loading—Emphasis on Abdominals |
|---|---|

| **Instructions:** Patient position hook lying (knees 90°). Place pressure cuff under lumbar spine and inflate to 40 mmHg. Begin each exercise with drawing-in maneuver to activate core muscles. Determine level at which patient can maintain pressure constant (stable pelvis) while performing either A, B, or C limb load activity. For endurance, decrease load and perform repetitive motion for 1 minute or longer. For strength, progress load. | | *Progressive Limb Loading* ⟶ | | |
|---|---|---|---|---|
| | | A. Lift bent leg to 90° hip flexion | B. Slide heel to extend knee | C. Lift straight leg to 45° |
| **Minimum external support** | *Level 1: core activation* | Draw in and hold 10 seconds | | |
| **Maximum external support** | *Level 2:* | Opposite LE on mat; bent leg fall out | | |
| | *Level 3: A, B, or C* | Opposite LE is on table | | |
| | *Level 4: A, B, or C* | Hold opposite LE @ 90° of hip flexion with UE | | |
| | *Level 5: A, B, or C* | Hold opposite LE @ 90° of hip flexion (no UE assistance) | | |
| **Minimum external support** | *Level 6: A, B, or C* | Bilateral LE movement | | |

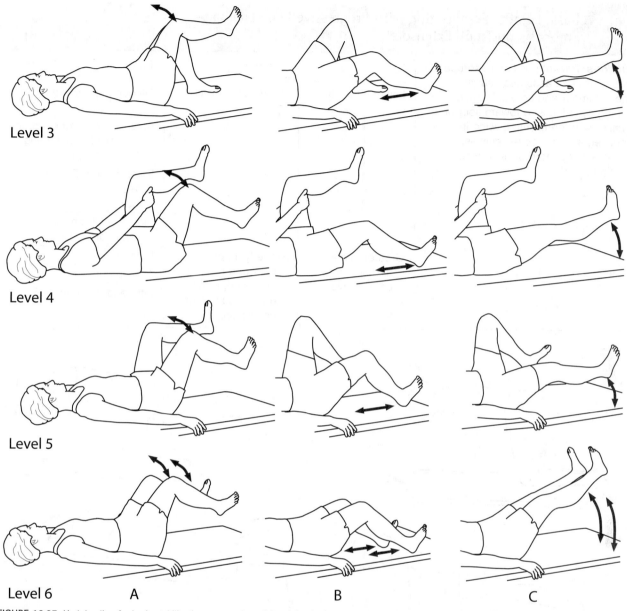

**FIGURE 16.27** Limb loading for basic stabilization progression of the abdominal muscles in the supine position, levels 3 to 6. Level 3, stability assisted by opposite extremity in hook-lying position; level 4, stability assisted by patient holding opposite leg at 90°; level 5, stability challenged by patient actively holding opposite leg at 90°; level 6, stability challenged with both lower extremities moving. (*A*) Bent leg lift to 90°. (*B*) Heel slide to extend knee. (*C*) Straight-leg lift to 45°.

Table 16.6 summarizes limb-loading exercises in the quadruped and prone positions that emphasize the extensor muscles, and Figure 16.28 illustrates a basic exercise progression. Performance of extremity loading in the prone position places a greater compressive load on the lumbar spine[4,33] and is not possible if there are hip flexion contractures; therefore, extension exercises are initiated in the quadruped position so the lumbar spine can more easily be positioned in neutral and the patient can learn control. If the patient cannot bear weight on the extremities or maintain balance in the quadruped position, use a padded stool or gym ball for additional support. It is important to maintain the cervical spine in its neutral position during these exercises. The patient should be able to align the head and focus the eyes on the floor. As the exercises progress, there is greater challenge on co-activation of all of the stabilizing musculature.

**TABLE 16.6**  Basic Lumbar Stabilization with Progressive Limb Loading—Emphasis on Trunk Extensors

**Instructions:** Patient position quadruped or prone. Patient assumes neutral spine in lumbar and cervical regions (keeping eyes focused toward floor or exercise mat), performs drawing-in maneuver, and moves extremities. Motions are repeated or alternated from side to side.

| | Position | Load |
|---|---|---|
| Lower intensity | Quadruped position | Flex one upper extremity (UE) |
| | | Extend one lower extremity (LE) by sliding it along the exercise mat |
| | | Extend one (LE) and lift 6–8 inches off exercise mat |
| | | Flex one UE and extend contralateral LE |
| Greater intensity and spinal compression | Prone lying position—near end of range of motion, requiring greater control of neutral spine | Extend one LE |
| | | Extend both LE |
| | | Lift head, arms and LE |

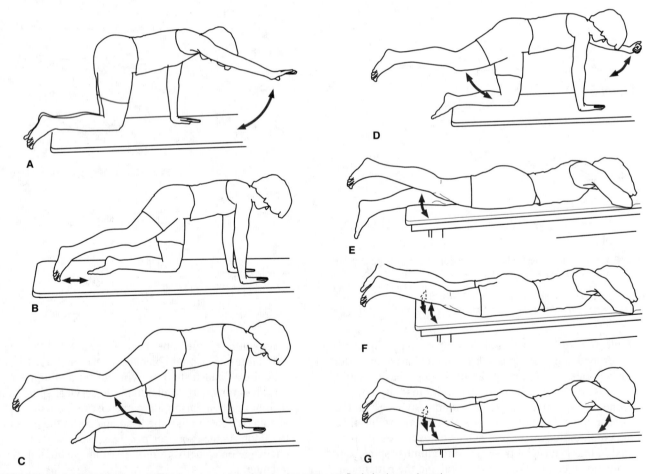

FIGURE 16.28 Limb loading for basic stabilization progression of the lumbar extensors. Begin in the quadruped position and progress the intensity by (A) flexing one UE, (B) extending one LE with a leg slide, (C) extending one LE by lifting it off the mat, (D) flexing one UE while extending contralateral LE and then alternate to opposite extremities. Progress to prone: (E) extending one LE, (F) extending both LE, and (G) lifting head, arms, and trunk.

**Focus on Evidence**

The exercise progressions described in Table 16.5 are adapted from several research studies that investigated the reliability, validity, and sensitivity to change one exercise level with abdominal muscle stabilizing ability using lower-limb loading.[10,11,23] The exercise progressions described in Table 16.6 are adapted from electromyography (EMG) studies that documented extensor activity with limb loading in the quadruped and prone-lying positions.[4,33]

## Variations and Progressions in the Stabilization Exercise Program

For all exercises, reinforce the importance of first finding the neutral spine (cervical and lumbar regions), performing the drawing-in maneuver, and then maintaining the neutral spine while superimposing any extremity motions. It is critical to instruct the patient to stop the exercises (or decrease the intensity) as soon as there is a sense that there is loss of control of the stable spinal position. It is important not to progress the patient beyond what he or she is able to control in order to develop the proper muscle response. The emphasis is first on improving the static holding capacity (endurance) of the trunk muscles followed by strengthening. Endurance training of the trunk extensor muscles is related to decreased pain and improving function during the early stages of recovery in patients with subacute low back pain.[8]

● *Emphasis on muscle endurance.* Determine a level of exercise that the patient can perform for several repetitions while maintaining a stable spine in the neutral position. Have the patient exercise at that level with the goal of increasing the number of repetitions or the time. Once the patient can perform repetitions for 1 minute, add weights, decrease the repetitions, and emphasize strength. Progress to the next level of difficulty for muscular endurance.

● *Use of external props.* Use of the Stabilizer™ pressure biofeedback unit to help the patient with learn control while doing the abdominal stabilization exercises was described earlier (see Box 16.5). For exercises in the quadruped position, if the patient has difficulty controlling the trunk rotation, use a prop such as a dowel rod placed along the spine. Have the patient attempt to keep it balanced while performing the arm and leg exercises (Fig. 16.29). It may be helpful to cue the patient to not shift his or her weight as the extremity is moved—this is difficult to do but is effective in bringing in the stabilizing trunk muscles.

● *Extremity loading.* Boxes 16.5 and 16.6 identify a progression of exercises in supine and quadruped/prone positions with extremity loading. Initially have the patient do the motions repetitively; then progress to

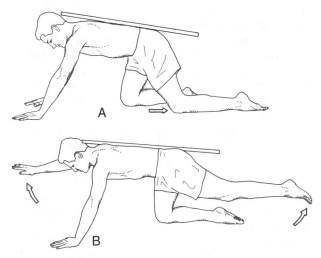

FIGURE 16.29 Balancing a rod on the back while doing quadruped exercises provides reinforcement that the trunk is not twisting. (A) Single leg slides. (B) Lifting the opposite arm and leg simultaneously, then alternating extremities.

alternating the extremities or moving all four extremities simultaneously (Fig. 16.30). This requires the stabilizing musculature to adjust to the shifting loads. Motions begin in the sagittal plane and then progress to the transverse plane and diagonal patterns (unilateral and bilateral), where movement away from the midline adds a rotational component and increases the challenge to the stabilizing musculature.

● *External resistance.* Use weights, elastic resistance, or pulleys for strengthening. Several suggestions are

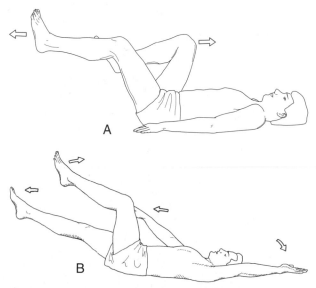

FIGURE 16.30 (A) Alternating lower extremity motions with the "modified bicycle" or (B) reciprocal and alternating patterns using the upper and lower extremities simultaneously require a strong controlling action in the abdominals.

illustrated in Figures 16.31, 16.32, and 16.33. Even though the extremities benefit from the exercises, the primary purpose is to improve performance in the stabilizing muscles of the trunk; therefore, when signs of fatigue occur, such as poor control of spinal stability (seen as movement of the pelvis or lumbar spine), reduce the intensity or stop the exercise and allow recovery.

- *Position changes.* Apply the extremity-loading exercises in the sitting (supported then unsupported), kneeling, and standing positions. Also use modified bridging to challenge the stabilizing function of the trunk musculature. Exercises such as wall slides and partial lunges and bridging with extremity motions use the extremities and trunk during weight bearing and prepare the muscles for functional activities. These exercises are described in the final section under Functional Activities

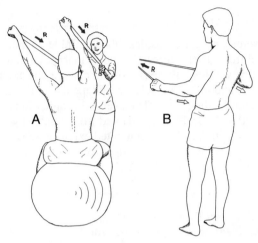

FIGURE 16.33 Using elastic resistance to train and strengthen the back extensor muscles to stabilize in the upright position (*A*) diagonal patterns while sitting on an unstable surface and (*B*) while standing.

but also serve the purpose of challenging the stabilizing muscles.

- *Unstable surfaces.* Use a large gym ball, foam roller, or wobble board to challenge the patient's balance and develop the stabilizing musculature. A variety of positions can be used, such as sitting upright on the ball with the feet on the floor, lying supine with the trunk on the ball and feet on the floor or with the feet on a low mat. If a foam roller is used, the patient is supine, with the roller placed longitudinally along the spine. Examples are shown in Figures 16.34 and 16.35. Secure elastic or pulley resistance in front of the patient at various heights and have him or her do pulling motions (see Fig. 16.33A).

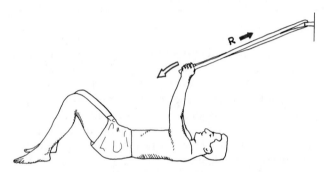

FIGURE 16.31 Developing the stabilizing action of the abdominal muscles by using pull-down activities against a resistive force from pulleys or elastic bands. This exercise can also be done sitting or standing to increase the challenge to the muscles in less stable positions.

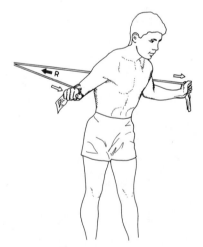

FIGURE 16.32 Using elastic resistance to train and strengthen the abdominal muscles in the upright position. The drawing-in maneuver to set the stabilizing muscles precedes the movement of the arms forward against the resistance.

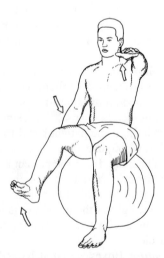

FIGURE 16.34 Strength, balance, and coordination are required to maintain spinal stabilization while sitting on a gym ball and moving the extremities. This activity is progressed by adding weights to the extremities.

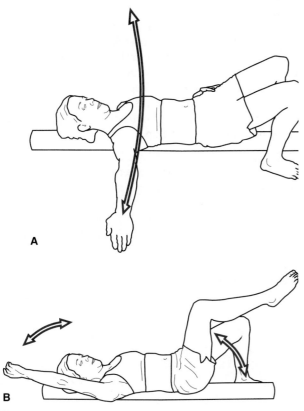

FIGURE 16.35 Activation of the core and global trunk muscles occur to maintain balance on a foam roll while the extremities move in various planes: for example (*A*) shoulder horizontal abduction/adduction and (*B*) ipsilateral hip and shoulder flexion/extension.

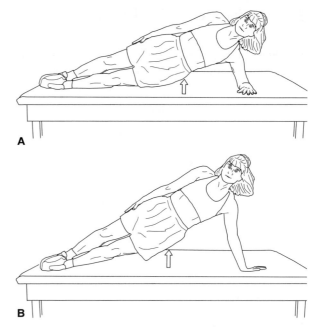

FIGURE 16.36 Quadratus lumborum stabilization training using closed-chain side-propping (*A*) on the elbow and knee and (*B*) on the hand and foot.

**Quadratus Lumborum—Stabilization Exercises**
The quadratus lumborum has been identified as an important stabilizer of the spine in the frontal and transverse planes.[33] Strongest activation of this muscle occurs with the side propping position. The external obliques are also activated in this position.[33]

*Patient position and procedure:* Begin side-lying. Have the patient prop up on the elbow and then lift the pelvis off the mat, supporting the lower body with the lateral side of the knee on the downward side. The position can be maintained for an isometric hold or performed intermittently (Fig. 16.36A). Progress by having the patient support the upper body with the hand (with the elbow extended) and lateral aspect of the foot on the downward side (Fig. 16.36B).

**Progression to Dynamic Exercises**
When the patient has developed control, endurance, and strength in the stabilizing muscles in weight-bearing and non-weight-bearing positions, *dynamic trunk strengthening* exercises are initiated at a low intensity (see following section). The emphasis is on control and safety.

As the patient returns to his or her instrumental activities of daily living (IADLs) and limited work activities,

instruct him or her to incorporate the core activation and stabilization techniques into the activities.

## ISOMETRIC AND DYNAMIC EXERCISES

Isometric exercises may be considered stabilizing exercises, as there is little or no movement of the spinal segments. They are included in this section with dynamic exercises, however, because of the method of application of the resistive force; that is, the resistive force is applied directly to the axial skeleton rather than through limb loading, as described in the spinal stabilization section. The decision to use the isometric exercises described in this section must be based on the goals of intervention. The exercises may be combined with the stabilization exercises in a home exercise program.

Dynamic exercises with spinal movement are introduced into the patient's exercise program when the patient demonstrates effective core and global stabilization techniques and has developed endurance in the stabilizing musculature. Dynamic exercises should not be a substitute for stabilization exercises. Because of the load imposed on the spine, they may exacerbate the patient's symptoms if introduced prior to effective stabilization and control. They are important in the total rehabilitation of the individual with neck or low back pain, as dynamic muscle endurance and strength is required for many daily activities as well as manual labor and athletic performance.

## Exercises for the Cervical Region

### Isometric Exercises—Self-Resistance

The intensity of the isometric exercises can be from light to strong, depending on the patient's symptoms and tolerance.

*Patient position and procedure:* Sitting.

● ***Flexion.*** Have the patient place both hands on the forehead and press the forehead into the palms in a nodding fashion while not moving (Fig. 16.37A).

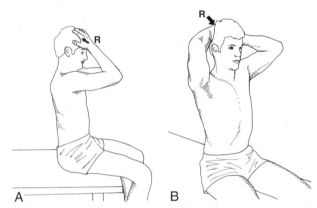

**FIGURE 16.37** Self-resistance for isometric (*A*) cervical flexion and (*B*) axial extension.

● ***Side bending.*** Have the patient press one hand against the side of the head and attempt to side-bend, as if trying to bring the ear toward the shoulder but not allowing motion.
● ***Axial extension.*** Have the patient press the back of the head into both hands, which are placed in the back, near the top of the head
● ***Rotation.*** Have the patient press one hand against the region just superior and lateral to the eye and attempt to turn the head to look over the shoulder but not allowing motion.

### Isometric Resistance Activities

● *Patient position and procedure:* Standing with a basketball-sized inflatable ball between the forehead and a wall. Have the patient keep the chin tucked and not go into a forward-head posture. The patient maintains the functional position while superimposing arm motions. Progress by adding weights to the arm motions.
● *Patient position and procedure:* Supine with the head over the edge of the mat, the neck maintained in a neutral functional position, and no support to the head. The patient must be able to keep the neck in its safe, functional position to perform this advanced stabilization exercise. He or she holds the position as tolerated. Progress by adding arm motions, then adding weights to the arm motions as tolerated.

### Dynamic Cervical Flexion

Often with faulty forward-head postures, the patient substitutes using the sternocleidomastoid (SCM) muscles to lift the head when getting up from the supine position rather than the overstretched, weak, deep cervical flexors. To correct this muscle imbalance, begin training capital flexion as described in the stabilization section (core muscle activation). For home exercise, emphasize "curling" the head and neck, not lifting the head up.

*Patient position and procedure:* Supine. If the patient cannot tuck the chin and curl the neck to lift the head off the mat, begin with the patient on a slant board or large wedge-shaped bolster under the thorax and head to reduce the effects of gravity (Fig. 16.38). Have the patient practice tucking the chin and curling the head up. Use assistance until the correct pattern is learned. Progress by decreasing the angle of the board or wedge and then adding manual resistance if the patient does not substitute with the SCM.

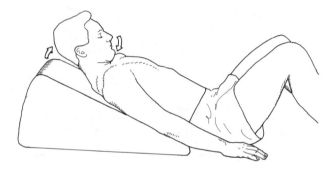

**FIGURE 16.38** Training the short cervical flexors while de-emphasizing the sternocleidomastoid for cervical flexion to regain a balance in strength for anterior cervical stabilization.

### Manual Resistance—Cervical Muscles

*Patient position and procedures:* Supine. Stand at the head end of the treatment table, supporting the patient's head for each exercise.

● Place one hand on the patient's head to resist opposite the motion. Do not resist against the mandible lest force be transmitted to the temporomandibular joint. Resistance is given to isolated muscle actions or to general ROMs, whichever best gains muscle balance and function.
● Isometric resistance can be applied with the head in any desired position before applying resistance. Avoid jerking the neck when applying or releasing the resistance by gradually building up the intensity, telling the patient to match your resistance, holding, and then gradually releasing and asking the patient to relax.

### Intermediate and Advanced Training

As the patient progresses in the rehabilitation program, greater challenges to the musculature to stabilize and

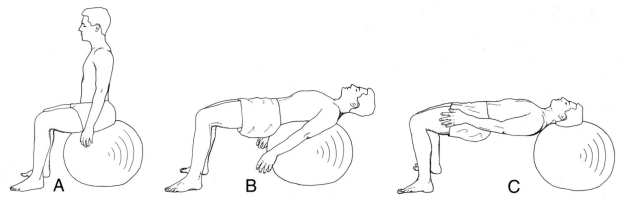

**FIGURE 16.39** Advanced exercises for strengthening the cervical and upper thoracic flexors and extensors as stabilizers. Begin by (A) sitting on a large gym ball, then (B) walking forward while rolling the ball up the back. With the ball behind the mid-thoracic area, the cervical flexors must stabilize. Continue walking forward until the ball is (C) under the head; the cervical extensors now must stabilize. Walk back and forth between the two positions (B and C) to alternate control between the flexors and extensors. Progress by adding arm motions or arm motions with weights to increase resistance.

control motion are emphasized, especially for those individuals returning to work, sports, or recreational activities that place greater demands on the cervical structures.

**Transitional Stabilization for the Cervical and Upper Thoracic Regions**

● *Patient position and procedure:* Standing with a basketball-size inflatable ball between the head and the wall. Have the patient roll the ball along the wall, using the head. This requires the patient to turn the body as he or she walks along.
● *Patient position and procedure:* Sitting on a large gym ball. Have the patient walk the feet forward so the ball rolls up the back and the thorax is resting on the ball (Fig. 16.39 A&B). The head and neck are maintained in neutral position, and the cervical flexors are emphasized. Have the patient then walk the ball farther so it is under the head. The extensors are now emphasized (Fig. 16.39C). The patient walks the feet forward and backward, alternating stabilization between the flexors and extensors. Progress to advanced training by adding arm motions and then arm motions with weights in each of the positions.

N O T E : This activity requires considerable strength in the cervical extensors to support the body weight and should be performed only with advanced training with patients who have been properly progressed to tolerate the resistance.

**Functional Exercises**
Design exercises that simulate patient-specific functional activities. Identify what activities stress that individual's neck and have the patient practice modifications of those activities with the spine kept in neutral position. Include pushing, pulling, reaching, and lifting (see Functional

Training section later in this chapter). Challenge the patient with increased repetitions and weight and in patterns that replicate functional demands.

## Exercises for the Thoracic and Lumbar Regions

### Alternating Isometric Contractions and Rhythmic Stabilization

*Patient positions and procedures:* Begin with the patient supine in the most stable position. Progress to sitting on a stable surface, sitting on an unstable surface such as a large gym ball, kneeling, and then standing. Sitting, kneeling, and standing require stabilizing action in the hip, knee, and ankle musculature, respectively, as well as the spinal muscles. Apply resistance directly against the patient's shoulders or pelvis, against a rod that is held by the patient (see Fig. 17.41), or against the patient's arms.

● Have the patient find the neutral spine position and then activate the stabilizing muscles with the drawing-in maneuver prior to applying the resistive force. Then instruct the patient to "meet my resistance" while applying a force to stimulate isometric contractions. Apply the resistance in alternating directions at a controlled speed while the patient learns to maintain a steady position.
● Initially, provide verbal cues, such as "hold against my resistance, but do not overpower me. Feel your abdominal muscles contracting. Now I'm pulling in the opposite direction. Match the resistance and feel your back muscles contracting."
● Progress by shifting the directions of resistance without the verbal cues and then by increasing the speed.
● Begin with alternating resistance in the sagittal plane; progress to side-to-side and then transverse plane resist-

ance. Isometric resistance to trunk rotation (transverse plane resistance) has been shown to be the most effective in stimulating the oblique abdominals, transversus abdominis, and deep spinal extensor muscles.[43]

 Alternating resistance to pelvic rotation can also be done by having the patient assume a modified bridge position. Apply resistance directly to the pelvis to stimulate rotation while the patient isometrically holds the pelvis and spine in a stable position.

## Dynamic Strengthening—Abdominal Muscles

N O T E : Dynamic exercises of the trunk musculature are not initiated until late during the rehabilitation process and not until after the patient has learned to activate the drawing-in maneuver automatically for stabilization in all functional activities.

No one abdominal exercise challenges all of the abdominal muscles[33]; therefore, a variety of exercises should be included in the patient's exercise program to include the entire region.

### ◉ Focus on Evidence_____

EMG studies have looked at abdominal muscle recruitment with various abdominal exercises.[3,29,33,54] In summary:

- Curl-ups (various types) recruit primarily the rectus abdominis, with low activity in the obliques, transversus abdominis, and psoas.
- Sit-ups (straight-leg and bent-knee) show high rectus and external oblique activity, high psoas activity, and high low-back compression. Heel press sit-ups increase psoas activity.
- Hanging-leg raises show high external oblique and high spinal compression.
- Supine single-leg lifts show negligible global abdominal muscle activity (opposite lower extremity provides stability). These exercises are primarily used early in the stabilization exercise routines to train the deep stabilizing muscles under progressive extremity loading.
- Supine bilateral-leg lifts show increased activity in the RA, EO, and IO during the first part of the range of hip flexion and increased load on the spine.
- Curl-ups on a labile surface doubled the activity of the rectus abdominis and increased the activity of the external obliques fourfold compared with curl-ups on a stable surface.[54]

*Rectus abdominis.* There is no clinically significant selective difference between the upper and lower rectus abdominis function.[29] Both portions contract strongly in all trunk curl-type and leg lift exercises.[29,33]

*External obliques.* External obliques contract strongest in sit-ups and diagonal sit-ups to the opposite side.[32]

*Internal obliques.* Internal obliques contract strongest in diagonal sit-ups to the same side and horizontal side propping (see Fig. 16.36).[33]

## Trunk Flexion

*Patient position:* Supine or hook-lying with the lumbar spine neutral. McGill[33] suggested supporting the low back with the hands to maintain slight lordosis. The spine should not be allowed to go into an increased lordosis during the exercise—this indicates weakness of the abdominals and consequently lifting of the trunk occurs from hip flexor action only.[27] When training the abdominals, curl-up exercises should be performed at a slow, controlled rate to activate the stabilizing function of the abdominals.[55]

P R E C A U T I O N S : Patients with conditions such as intervertebral disk lesions or osteoporosis should not do dynamic trunk flexion exercises because of the increased intra-abdominal pressure and increased compression forces on the vertebral bodies. Similarly, if a patient experiences pain with trunk flexion, these exercises should not be done. Use the stabilization exercises, as described in the previous section, with the spine maintained in a neutral position (slight lordosis).

### *Procedures*

***Curl-ups.*** First, instruct the patient to perform the drawing-in maneuver to cause a stabilizing contraction of the abdominal muscles (see section on Stabilization Training—Core Muscle Activation) and then lift the head. Progress by lifting the shoulders until the scapulae and thorax clear the mat, keeping the arms horizontal (Fig. 16.40). A full sit-up is not necessary because once the thorax clears the mat the rest of the motion is performed by the hip flexor muscles.

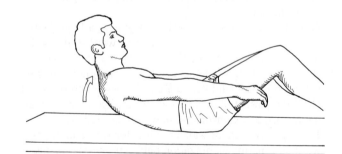

FIGURE 16.40 The curl-up exercise to strengthen the abdominal muscles. The thorax is flexed on the lumbar spine. The arms are shown in the position for least resistance. Progress by crossing the arms across the chest and then behind the head.

 Further progress the difficulty of the curl-up by having the patient change the arm position from horizontal to folded across the chest and then to behind the head.

 During all these activities, the low back should not arch; if it does, reduce the progression until the abdominals are strong enough to maintain lumbar flexion.

***Curl-downs.*** If the patient is unable to perform the curl-up, begin with curl-downs by having the patient start in the hook-sitting or long-sitting position and lower the trunk only to the point where he or she can maintain a flat low back and then return to the sitting position.

● Once the patient can curl-down full range, reverse and perform a curl-up.

***Diagonal curl-ups.*** Have the patient reach one hand toward the outside of the opposite knee while curling up; then alternate. Reverse the muscle action by bringing one knee up toward the opposite shoulder; then repeat with the other knee. Diagonal exercises emphasize the oblique muscles.

***Double knee-to-chest.*** To emphasize the lower rectus abdominis and oblique muscles, have the patient set a posterior pelvic tilt; then bring both knees to the chest and return. Progress the difficulty by decreasing the angle of hip and knee flexion (Fig. 16.41).

***Pelvic lifts.*** Have the patient begin with the hips at 90° and knees extended; then lift the buttocks upward off the mat (small motion). The feet move upward toward the ceiling (Fig. 16.42). The patient should not push against the mat with the hands.

***Bilateral straight-leg raising***

● Have the patient begin with legs extended; then perform a posterior pelvic tilt followed by flexing both hips, keeping the knees extended. If the pelvis and spine cannot be kept stable, the knees should be flexed to a degree that allows control.

● If the hips are abducted before initiating this exercise, greater stress is placed on the oblique abdominal muscles.

PRECAUTION: The strong pull of the psoas major causes shear forces on the lumbar vertebrae. Also this bilateral straight-leg raise (SLR) causes increased spinal compression loads. If there is any low-back pain or discomfort, especially with spinal hypermobility or instability, this exercise should not be performed even if the abdominals are strong enough to maintain a posterior pelvic tilt.

***Bilateral straight-leg lowering.*** Bilateral straight-leg lowering can be performed if the bilateral SLR is difficult. Have the patient begin with the hips at 90° and knees extended; then lower the extremities as far as possible while maintaining stability in the lumbar spine (should not increase the lordosis), followed by raising the legs back to 90°. See precaution under the bilateral SLR exercise.

**Trunk Flexion (Abdominals)—Sitting or Standing**

*Patient position and procedures:* Sitting or standing. Pulleys or elastic material are secured at shoulder level behind the patient. Progress the resistance as the patient's abdominal strength increases.

● Have the patient hold the handles or ends of the elastic material with each hand and then flex the trunk, with emphasis on bringing the rib cage down toward the pubic bone and performing a posterior pelvic tilt, rather than flexing at the hips (Fig. 16.43).

● Have the patient perform diagonal motions by bringing one arm down toward the opposite knee with emphasis on moving the rib cage down toward the opposite side of the pelvis. Repeat the diagonal motion in the opposite direction.

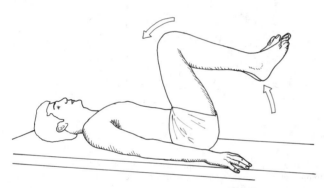

FIGURE 16.41 Strengthening the abdominal muscles by flexing the hip and pelvis on the lumbar spine. The legs are shown in the position for least resistance. Progress by decreasing the angle of hip flexion until the legs can be lifted with the knees extended, as in the pelvic lift.

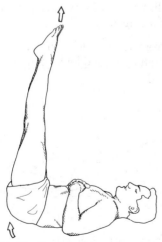

FIGURE 16.42 Pelvic lifts. Elevating the legs upward toward the ceiling by raising the buttock off the floor emphasizes strengthening the lower abdominal muscles.

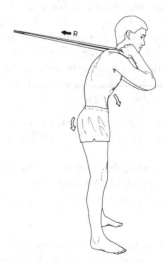

FIGURE 16.43 Standing trunk flexion against elastic material to strengthen the abdominal muscles. The patient performs a posterior pelvic tilt and approximates the ribs toward the pubis.

## Trunk Flexion (Abdominals)—Unstable Surfaces

Patients with chronic, unilateral low back pain have been shown to have impaired balance.[2] Use of unstable surfaces, such as a gym ball (Fig. 16.44) or a balance board, while doing abdominal curl-up exercises has been shown to increase activity in the internal and external obliques and the rectus abdominis.[49] The presumption is that these muscles generate increased activity to maintain balance on the unstable surfaces. Other suggestions include balancing on a foam roll or a biomechanical ankle platform system (BAPS) board while performing arm and leg activities or curl-up exercises.

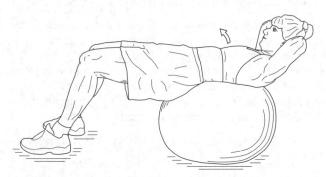

FIGURE 16.44 Curl-ups on an unstable surface. The unstable surface increases activity in the oblique and rectus abdominis muscles.

## Dynamic Strengthening—Erector Spinae and Multifidus Muscles

 **Focus on Evidence**

Strengthening the extensor muscles and an improved extensor/flexor ratio has been found to be important in decreasing symptoms in patients with chronic low back pain (LBP).[52] Lee et al.[28] determined that the trunk extensor/flexor ratio is a sensitive parameter for predicting LBP. After following 67 asymptomatic individuals for 5 years, they found an increased incidence of LBP in those who had lower extensor than flexor muscle strength. Danneels et al.[9] demonstrated that intensive lumbar resistance training (isometric or dynamic) is necessary to develop paravertebral muscle strength and bulk. The following is a summary of specific exercise outcomes studies.

- Prone arch, isometric trunk extension, and isometric leg extensions: high activity in both the multifidus and erector spinae.[36]
- Isolated training of multifidus: requires a low-intensity focus, as described in the stabilization section—techniques for core muscle activation.[40]

Resistance can be applied to any of the following recumbent exercises by having the patient hold weights in the hands or by strapping weights around the patient's legs.

## Extension Exercises in Prone Position

PRECAUTIONS: Extension exercises in the prone position are performed at the end of the ROM in spinal extension and therefore may not be appropriate for individuals with symptoms from conditions such as arthritis or nerve root compression. Patients with spondylosis or other flexion bias conditions or patients who develop symptoms under loaded conditions (e.g., with disk lesions) may experience increased symptoms and therefore should not do dynamic end-range extension exercises. If symptoms occur, modify the positioning toward more neutral spinal positions, such as the quadruped position, and emphasize stabilization with isometric holds rather than moving into full extension (see Figs. 16.28, 16.29, and 16.33).

***Thoracic elevation.*** Begin with the arms at the side, progress to behind the head or reaching overhead as strength improves. Have the patient tuck in the chin and lift the head and thorax. The lower extremities must be stabilized (Fig. 16.45).

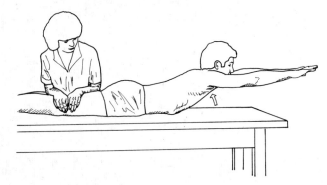

FIGURE 16.45 Strengthening the back extensors with the arms in position to provide maximal resistance. Additional resistance can be provided by holding weights in the hands.

***Leg lifts.*** Initially have the patient lift only one leg, alternate with the other leg, and finally lift both legs and extend the spine. Stabilize the thorax by having the patient hold onto the side of the treatment table.

***"Superman."*** Progress the extension exercises by having the patient lift both upper and lower extremities simultaneously (Fig. 16.46).

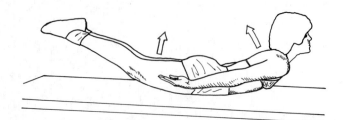

FIGURE 16.46 Strengthen the trunk and hip extensors by lifting the trunk and legs off the mat simultaneously. Greater resistance can be provided by abducting the shoulders to 90° or by elevating them to 180° ("Superman").

## Extension Exercises Sitting or Standing

***Elastic resistance or weighted pulleys.*** Secure pulleys or elastic resistance in front of the patient at shoulder level. Have him or her hold onto the ends of the material or handles and extend the spine (Fig. 16.47).

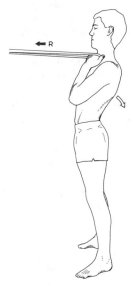

FIGURE 16.47 Using elastic resistance for concentric eccentric back extension.

For trunk rotation, use a pulley or elastic resistance secured under the foot or to a stable object opposite to the side being exercised. Have the patient pull against the resistance, extending and rotating the back. Change the angle of pull of the resistance to recreate functional patterns specific to the patient's needs (Fig. 16.48).

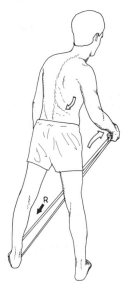

FIGURE 16.48 Rotation with extension strengthens the back extensors in functional patterns.

## Trunk Side Bending (Lateral Abdominals, Erector Spinae, Quadratus Lumborum)

Trunk side-bending exercises are used for general strengthening of the muscles that side-bend the trunk.

 **Focus on Evidence**_____

McGill[33] identified the quadratus lumborum as one of the most important stabilizers of the spine and documented the isometric horizontal side support as an effective exercise to strengthen this muscle (see discussion in the stabilization section and Figure 16.36).

_____

Side-bending exercises are also used if there is scoliosis, although exercise alone has not been shown to halt or change the progression of a structural scoliosis curve. Exercise in conjunction with other methods of correction, such as bracing, is often employed.[5,7] When there is a lateral curve, the muscles on the convex side are usually stretched and weakened. The following exercises are described for use as strengthening exercises on the side of the convexity, although they may be used bilaterally for symmetrical strengthening.

Stabilization exercises for spinal control, as previously described, may be beneficial for strengthening and conditioning when there is scoliosis.

● *Patient position and procedure:* Standing. Place elastic resistance under the foot or have the patient hold a weight in the hand on the side of the concavity; then have him or her side-bend the trunk in the opposite direction.

● *Patient position and procedure:* Side-lying on the concave side of the curve with the apex at the edge of the table or mat so the thorax is lowered. If you have access to a split table with one end that can be lowered, begin with the apex of the curve at the bend of the table. Have the patient place the lower arm folded across the chest and upper arm along the side of the body and side-bend the trunk up against gravity. Progress by having the patient clasp both hands behind the head (Fig. 16.49). Stabilization of the pelvis and lower extremities must be provided.

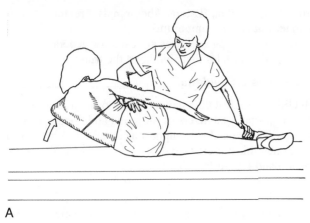

A

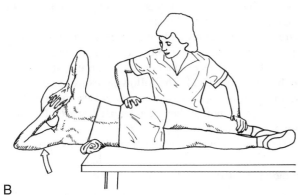

B

FIGURE 16.49 (A, B) Antigravity strengthening of the lateral trunk musculature. There is less resistance if the top arm is at the side and the bottom arm
is folded across the chest.

## CARDIOPULMONARY ENDURANCE

***Goal.*** To develop cardiopulmonary fitness for overall
endurance and well-being.

Aerobic conditioning exercises provide many benefits
for the patient with spinal symptoms. The activity not only
improves cardiopulmonary endurance but stimulates feelings of well-being and relief of symptoms.[35] Chapter 7
describes cardiopulmonary conditioning principles and
procedures. Specific precautions and suggestions for medical conditions are also explained. For patients recovering
from spinal injuries, surgery, or postural dysfunction, aerobic exercises may be initiated once signs of inflammation
no longer exist. Begin with low to moderate intensity and
work with the patient to choose activities that do not place
added stress on the recovering spinal structures. If a particular spinal bias has been identified (see Chapter 15),
choose aerobic exercises that emphasize that spinal bias.
A brief summary of the principles is reviewed in Box 16.6.
Guidelines for safe application of common conditioning
exercises when there are spinal impairments are described
in this section.

---

**BOX 16.6    Summary of Aerobic
                Conditioning Principles**

1. Establish the target heart rate and maximum heart rate.
   - The maximum heart rate is generally 220 minus the
     individual's age or may be the symptom-limiting heart
     rate (the rate at which cardiovascular symptoms
     appear).
   - Target heart rate is between 60% and 80% of the max-
     imum heart rate.
2. Perform warm-up exercises for 10 to 15 minutes, includ-
   ing active movements of the neck and trunk.
3. Individualize the program of exercise.
   - Select activities that emphasize the patient's spinal
     bias if necessary (see information in the text).
   - Not all people are at the same fitness level and there-
     fore cannot perform the same exercises. Any one exer-
     cise has the potential to be detrimental if attempted by
     someone not able to execute it properly.
   - To avoid overuse syndromes to structures of the mus-
     culoskeletal system, appropriate equipment, such as
     correct footwear, should be used for biomechanical
     support with weight-bearing exercises.
4. Increase the pace of the activity to reach the target heart
   rate and maintain it for 20 to 30 minutes.
5. Cool down for 5 to 10 minutes with slow, total body,
   repetitive motions and stretching activities.
6. Frequency of aerobic exercise should be three to five
   times per week.
7. Always stay within the tolerance of the individual.
   Overuse commonly occurs when there is an increase in
   time or effort without adequate rest (recovery) time
   between sessions. Increase repetitions or time by no
   more than 10% per week.[30] If pain begins while exercising, heed the warning and reduce the stress.

---

## COMMON AEROBIC EXERCISES AND EFFECTS ON THE SPINE

Some aerobic exercises place the spine in end-range positions. They are reviewed so the reader understands why
some activities may be inappropriate for patients with specific conditions. If modifications are possible, they should
be considered.

### Cycling

Road bikes place the thoracolumbar spine in flexion and
the upper cervical spine in hyperextension. Use this exercise for patients who have a flexion bias in the lumbar
region so long as there are no upper cervical symptoms.
Modifications include using a bike that positions the body
in a more upright posture, such as a mountain bike or

hybrid bike. Many stationary bikes also position the individual in upright postures and therefore are less likely to precipitate cervical problems.

## Walking and Running

The upright posture emphasizes normal spinal curves, and lumbar extension is emphasized with walking and running (terminal stance). Emphasize the importance of identifying the neutral spine, activating the drawing-in maneuver, and stabilizing the spine while walking or running. Because conscious control is not possible during the entire exercise time, coach the patient to check his or her posture and muscle control frequently, such as each time he or she is crossing an intersection, or when passing another individual, or if symptoms develop in the spinal region. Walking or running with the cervical spine in retraction (axial extension) and the scapulae comfortably adducted, along with a rhythmic arm swing, reinforces cervical stabilization. Easy access to treadmills, tracks, or roads and trails make these activities popular. Running is a high-impact activity and may not be tolerated by individuals with intervertebral disk lesions or degenerative joint conditions.

## Stair Climbing

Commercial devices that replicate stepping with various grades of resistance are used for strengthening and aerobic conditioning. Regular steps can also be used for aerobic conditioning. This activity requires pelvic control of the reciprocating lower extremities because lifting the leg on one side emphasizes spinal flexion while the contralateral lower extremity and spine are extending. Coach the patient to maintain the neutral spine with the stabilizing muscles against the rotational forces.

## Cross–Country Skiing and Ski Machines

Cross-country skiing, whether out in the cold or on a commercial machine, is a high-intensity aerobic activity. The kicking motion that accompanies the backward motion of the leg emphasizes spinal extension. It is important to coach the patient to maintain the neutral spine and contract the stabilizing abdominal muscles.

## Swimming

When swimming, the breaststroke emphasizes extension in the cervical and lumbar spinal regions when taking a breath. Coach the patient to not extend the neck full range but to keep it neutral and lift the head out of the water as a "solid" unit with the thorax just enough to clear the mouth for the breath.

The freestyle stroke may exacerbate cervical problems because of the repetitive cervical rotation while taking a breath; this stroke also emphasizes lumbar extension with the flutter kick. Teach the patient to breathe using a "log-roll" technique where the whole body rolls toward one side while breathing and then rolls back to the face-down position for the stroke. This requires good spinal stabilization.

The backstroke emphasizes spinal extension via kicking the lower extremities and the arm motions. The butterfly stroke moves the spine through a full ROM; emphasis is placed on controlling the range with the stabilizing muscles.

## Upper Body Ergometry Machines

Ergometry machines provide upper extremity resistance and can also be used for aerobic training. Forward motions emphasize spinal flexion and shoulder girdle protraction; backward motions emphasize spinal extension and shoulder girdle retraction. Coach the patient to assume the neutral spinal posture and use the stabilizing muscles prior to and during the use of the ergometer to enhance postural responses. If the machine can be used standing, progression to the standing position stimulates a total body response.

## Step Aerobics and Aerobic Dancing

Stepping is similar to using stairs or a stair machine except for the jumping and bouncing that is usually added to the more advanced step aerobic programs.

Dancing moves take on many forms, and classes are taught that address various fitness levels and age groups. If possible, review safe movement patterns and help the patient recognize the safe limits of his or her spinal range and abilities.

## "Latest Popular Craze"

People like variety and may be attracted to charismatic and energetic figures who demonstrate "new" workout techniques and routines or new exercise machines. Patients may ask for advice as to the value of the activities and techniques. Knowledge and skill in analyzing the biomechanics of the activity and the forces that are imposed through the spine should be used to provide advice about exercise safety. End-of-range postures and high-velocity stresses (such as vigorous kicking and ballistic motions) may be damaging to vulnerable tissues in the spine and should not be attempted by patients recovering from spinal problems.

## FUNCTIONAL ACTIVITIES

***Goal.*** To progress to independence safely.

NOTE: Achieving the maximum level of independence underlies all the goals of therapeutic exercise. The patient develops core and global stability; develops flexibility, muscle endurance, and strength; learns how exercise and posture correction relieves stress; and develops cardiopulmonary endurance—all to be able to function safely in daily activities, including work, recreation, and athletic pursuits.

# EARLY FUNCTIONAL TRAINING—FUNDAMENTAL TECHNIQUES

Early functional training consists of teaching basic maneuvers needed for ADLs such as how to roll over safely, go from lying down to sitting (and reverse), and go from sitting to standing (and reverse). These techniques follow the early kinesthetic training instruction in which the patient learns to find his or her neutral spine and experiences the effect that simple arm and leg motions have on the spine, as well as early muscle performance training in which the patient learns how to activate the core musculature for segmental stabilization. If the examination reveals problems with basic ADL activities, the following are included in the early training program.

*Rolling.* Rolling with a neutral spine requires that the patient first find the neutral spine, perform the drawing-in maneuver, and then roll the trunk as a unit.

- It may be helpful to suggest that the patient "imagine a solid rod connecting the shoulders and pelvis so as not to twist" or suggest that he or she "roll like a log."
- Encourage the patient to use the arms and top leg to assist the roll.

*Supine to sit/sit to lying down.* Have the patient use the log roll maneuver (as described above) to roll from supine to side-lying while simultaneously flexing the hips and knees and pushing up with the arms.

- Help the patient focus on stabilizing the trunk with commands such as "push up your trunk as if it is a board; do not allow it to twist or bend."
- The reverse is practiced by coaching the patient to lower oneself to the side-lying position as a unit first onto the elbow and then shoulder. Once down, the patient can roll to supine or prone-lying using the log-roll technique

*Sit to stand/stand to sit.* The patient's level of function dictates how much assistance from the upper extremities is needed to accomplish "sit to stand" or "stand to sit." If the hip and knee extensors are not strong enough to elevate the body, the patient requires a chair with armrests so there is some leverage for pushing up; alternatively, an elevated seat may be necessary.

- To use the stable spine technique, instruct the patient to find the neutral spine by rolling the pelvis forward and backward, activate the drawing-in maneuver, and then bend forward at the hips while maintaining the neutral spine position.
- Help the patient focus on the hip motion while keeping the spine "solid like a board." The reverse is also practiced.

*In and out of a car.* Getting in and out of a car is often symptom-provoking for patients with low back pain. Once

sit to stand can be safely performed, have the patient practice the following.

- Approach the open car door and seat with the back toward the seat; stabilize the spine in its neutral position with the drawing-in maneuver, then bend at the hips and sit down.
- Once seated, flex both hips and knees and pivot the whole body around as a unit, maintaining a stable spine.
- When exiting a car, keep both knees together and pivot the legs and trunk outward as a unit. Once the feet are on the ground, bend at the hips and elevate the trunk as a unit.

*Walking.* For some patients walking may provoke symptoms.

- Remind the patient to use the neutral spine and drawing-in maneuvers to stabilize the spine while walking.
- It is not possible to maintain conscious control for long, so remind the patient to check the spinal posture and reactivate the drawing-in maneuver whenever the symptoms recur.

# PREPARATION FOR FUNCTIONAL ACTIVITIES—BASIC EXERCISE TECHNIQUES

Once the patient has learned to manage his or her symptoms and the symptoms of inflammation diminish, exercises are initiated that prepare the extremities and trunk for functional activities such as safely lifting, carrying, pushing, pulling, and reaching in various directions. In the subacute or controlled motion phase of rehabilitation, emphasis is placed on strengthening the extremities in functional patterns while maintaining a stable spine. The patient should be able to perform IADLs and limited work activities at this stage. Evaluate the patient's performance and modify what he or she is doing to include safe spinal postures and correct stabilization. Use the activities in this section to prepare for or advance the patient's function.

Many of the strengthening exercises described in the extremity chapters are appropriate to use in preparation for functional training. With postural problems and recovery from back or neck injuries, it is critical to emphasize the neutral (functional) spinal posture before and during total body exercises. Many of the stabilization and movement patterns described earlier in this chapter can also be progressed in intensity, repetitions, speed, and coordination to prepare for return to functional activities.

## Weight-Bearing Exercises

### Modified Bridging Exercises
Modified bridging exercises require stabilization with the trunk flexor and extensor muscles in conjunction with strengthening the gluteus maximus and quadriceps muscles in preparation for lifting activities. The abdominals function with the gluteus maximus to control the pelvic tilt, and

the lumbar extensors stabilize the spine against the pull of the gluteus maximus.

*Patient position and procedures:* Begin with the patient hook-lying. Have the patient concentrate on maintaining the neutral spinal position while raising and lowering the pelvis (flexing and extending at the hips) (see Fig. 20.21). Hold the bridge for isometric control.

- Alternate arm motions; progress by adding weights to the hands.
- Alternate lifting one foot and then the other by marching in place (Fig. 16.50A); progress by extending the knee as each leg is lifted. When the patient tolerates greater resistance, add ankle weights and coordinate with arm motions (Fig. 16.50B).
- Abduct and adduct the thighs without letting the pelvis sag. Progress by placing the feet on a stool, chair, or large gym ball and repeating the bridging activities.

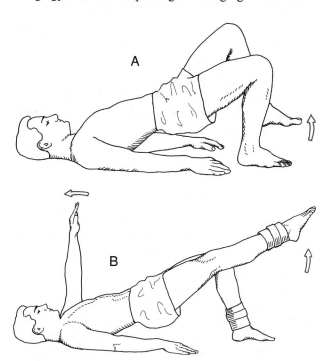

FIGURE 16.50 Holding a bridge to develop trunk control and gluteus maximus strength while superimposing extremity motions by (A) marching in place and (B) progressing to extending the extremities. Adding weights to the arms or legs requires greater strength and control.

## Push-Ups with Trunk Stabilization

Push-ups use the body weight to strengthen the triceps and shoulder girdle musculature in preparation for pushing activities. The trunk musculature must stabilize against the pull of the shoulder girdle musculature as well as control the neutral spinal position as the body is raised and lowered.

*Patient positions and procedures:* Standing facing a wall or prone-lying with hands placed against the wall or floor in front of the shoulders. Remind the patient to find and maintain the neutral spinal position while performing the exercise.

- These exercises may begin as wall push-ups if the patient is not strong enough to push up from the floor.
- Prone-lying on the floor the patient may push up with the pivot point being the knees or may perform full body push-ups with the pivot point being the feet.
- To challenge the patient on an unstable surface, he or she begins prone on a large gym ball. Have the patient walk forward with the hands on the floor until just the thighs are supported by the ball, maintain a stable spinal posture, and perform push-ups with the arms. To progress, walk out farther with the hands until just the legs are supported by the ball (Fig. 16.51).

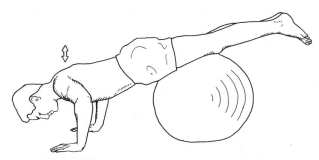

FIGURE 16.51 Push-up activities with the lower extremities balanced on a gym ball for strengthening the arms and developing trunk control.

## Wall Slides

Wall slides develop strength in the hip and knee extensor muscles to prepare the lower extremities for squatting activities and training in safe body mechanics.

*Patient position and procedure:* Standing with the back to a wall and the spine held in its neutral position. Place a towel behind the back so it slides easier along the wall. The exercise is more challenging if a large gym ball is placed between the back and the wall (Fig. 16.52). Have

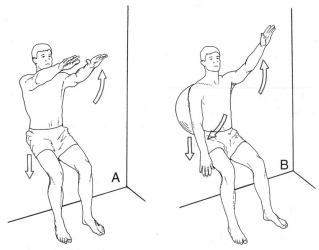

FIGURE 16.52 Wall slides/partial squats to develop lower extremity strength and coordinate with trunk stability in preparation for training body mechanics. (A) The back sliding down a wall, with bilateral arm motion for added resistance. (B) Rolling a gym ball down the wall, with antagonistic arm motion to develop coordination.

the patient slide his or her back down the wall into a partial squat and hold the position for isometric strengthening of the hip and knee extensors or move up and down for concentric/eccentric strengthening.

● Superimpose arm motions such as alternating or bilateral shoulder flexion/extension.
● Use handheld weights to add resistance for upper and lower extremity strengthening.

### Partial Lunges and Partial Squats

Partial lunges and squats are described in Chapters 20 and 21. They are beneficial for strengthening total body movement in preparation for learning body mechanics. If necessary, begin by having the patient balance by holding onto the side of a treatment table or other stable object and then progress to balancing with a cane (see Fig. 20.23). Once able to perform multiple repetitions without holding on, add weights to the upper extremities for resistance. Progress by adding arm motions that are synchronized with the leg motions, such as reaching forward and downward to develop coordination and control.

### Walking Against Resistance

Secure a weighted pulley or elastic resistance around the patient's pelvis with a belt, or the patient can hold the handles. Have the patient walk forward, backward, or diagonally against the resistive force. Emphasis is placed on spinal control (see Fig. 20.25).

   Progress by having the patient push and pull weighted objects, such as a cart or a box on a table. Place emphasis on maintaining a stable spinal position while the extremities are loaded (see Figs. 17.56 and 18.20A).

## Transitional Stabilization Exercises

Exercises that cause movement into spinal flexion and extension challenge the patient to control the neutral spine position. The patient learns to stabilize the spine against alternating trunk motions.

### Quadruped Forward/Backward Shifting

*Patient position and procedure:* Quadruped. Have the patient rock back to rest the buttocks on the heels, then shift the body forward onto the hands in the press-up position. The patient concentrates on controlling the pelvis in its neutral position rather than allowing full spinal flexion when shifting toward the heels or full spinal extension when shifting forward toward the press-up position.

### Squatting and Reaching

*Patient position and procedure:* Begin standing. Have the patient reach downward while partially squatting. The tendency is for the spine to flex, so have the patient concentrate on maintaining a neutral spinal position with the spinal extensors. The patient then stands up and reaches overhead. This causes the spine to extend, so have the patient concentrate on using the trunk flexors to stabilize in

the neutral position. Progress by lifting and reaching with weights while controlling the neutral posture of the spine.

### Shifting Weight and Turning

Have the patient practice shifting weight forward/backward and side to side while maintaining the neutral spinal position and absorbing the forces with the hip and knee muscles. Practice turning using small steps and rotating at the hips rather than the back. Instruct the patient to imagine two rigid poles connecting each shoulder to each hip that do not allow the spine to twist. Even though some movement in the spine occurs, the activity helps the patient focus on a stable spine rather than rotating full range. Progress by using weights and having the patient lift, turn, and then place the weight at a new location.

## ◑ BODY MECHANICS AND ENVIRONMENTAL ADAPTATIONS

### Principles of Body Mechanics— Instruction and Training

When teaching safe body mechanics it is advisable to not overwhelm the patient with too many instructions. Most people "know" they are to lift with their legs rather than their back, but still have faulty techniques. Initiate training by suggesting that the patient find his or her neutral spine, perform the drawing-in maneuver then lift. Observe the technique they use and suggest modifications if needed. Squatting is often taught as the preferred method, yet not all patients are able to squat if they have impairments such as knee pain or weakness. Under some circumstances, an individual may be more stable lifting with a lunge technique rather than the squat technique.

### Lumbar Spine Position

The position of the lumbar spine, whether it is flexed, extended, or in mid-range, raises several issues. Of the three postures, lifting with a neutral spinal posture provides greater stability of the spine[12] and uses both the ligamentous and muscular system for stabilization and control.[50] After a back injury, the preferred lifting posture may have to be adapted, depending on the type of injury and the response of the tissues when stressed.[50]

***Spinal flexion.*** When lifting with a flexed lumbar spine (posterior pelvic tilt), support for the spine is primarily from inert structures (ligaments, lumbodorsal fasciae, posterior annulus fibrosus, and facets); there is little muscle activity.

● Flexion occurs when stooping to the floor. Some have suggested that it may also be the posture of choice for a patient who has injured the back muscles because the muscles are "quiet" when the spine is in flexion.[50]
● Lifting with the lumbar spine in flexion may pose some problems. When lifting slowly with a flexed spine, the load is maintained on the ligaments, and creep of the

inert tissues occurs; this increases the chance of injury if the tissue is already weakened. In addition, with the muscles lengthened and relaxed, they may be at an unfavorable length–tension relationship to respond quickly with appropriate force to resist a sudden change in load. There is greater chance of ligamentous strain when a person lifts with a flexed spine.[22]

*Spinal extension.* When lifting with an extended (lordotic) lumbar spine, the muscles supporting the spine are more active than when flexed, which increases the compressive forces on the disk. Also, the facets are approximated (close-pack position). This posture relieves stress on the ligaments; but for an individual whose back muscles are in poor condition and fatigue quickly, this posture may jeopardize the spine when repeated lifts are performed because the ligaments are not providing support.[32]

### Load Position

Reinforce the concept of lifting and carrying objects as close to the center of gravity as possible.

● Have the patient practice carrying objects close to his or her center of gravity and draw attention to the feel of balance and control, as well as less stress on the neck and back, compared to the feel when carrying objects in more stressful positions. Point out that, when lifting, the closer the object is held to the center of gravity, the less stress is placed on the supporting structures.
● Have the patient practice shifting the load from side to side and turning. Have the patient practice turning with hip rotation and minimal trunk rotation. The action should be directed by the legs while the spine is kept stable.
● Replicate the mechanics of the patient's job setting and practice safe mechanics.

## Environmental Adaptations

Ergonomic assessment and modification of the home and working environments are necessary to correct stresses as well as prevent future recurrence of symptoms.

### Home, Work, and Driving Considerations

● Chairs and car seats should have lumbar support to maintain slight lordosis. Use a towel roll or lumbar pillow if necessary.
● Chair height should allow knees to flex to take tension off the hamstring muscles, support the thighs, and allow the feet to rest comfortably on the floor.
● Arm rests should be used if prolonged sitting is required in order to take the stress off shoulders and the cervical spine.
● Desk or table height should be adequate to keep the person from having to lean over the work.
● Work and driving habits should allow frequent changing of posture. If normally sedentary, the patient should get up and walk every hour.

### Sleeping Environment

● The mattress needs to provide firm support to prevent any extreme stresses. If it is too soft, the patient sags and stresses ligaments; if it is too firm, some patients cannot relax.
● Pillows should be of a comfortable height and density to promote relaxation but should not place joints in an extreme position. Foam rubber pillows tend to cause increased tension in muscles because of the constant resistance they provide.
● Whether the person should sleep prone, side-lying, or supine is something that must be analyzed for each individual patient. Ideally, a comfortable posture is one that is in the mid-range and that does not place stress on any supporting structure. Pain that is experienced when waking up in the morning is often related to sleeping posture; if this is the case, listen carefully to the patient's description of postures when sleeping and see if it relates to the pain. Then attempt to modify the sleep position accordingly. Remind the patient that it takes several weeks to change habits.

## INTERMEDIATE TO ADVANCED EXERCISE TECHNIQUES FOR FUNCTIONAL TRAINING

As the patient learns spinal control while doing the exercises, repetitions are increased to develop muscular endurance, and resistance is added to develop strength. If speed and balance are required, they are emphasized. By this stage it is recognized that the individual already knows the basic spinal stabilization techniques and is habitually assuming the neutral spinal position and activating the drawing-in maneuver. Reinforce the importance of this when doing the following exercises. It is also recognized that the patient should be able to control greater spinal ROM without experiencing symptoms. Adapt the exercises to replicate return to work or sport-related activities. Examples follow.

## Repetitive Lifting

The ability to do repetitive lifting throughout the workday is necessary for many jobs and may result in symptom recurrence. To prepare for returning to work, progressively increase the repetitions of lifting activities the patient must do to improve muscle endurance. Marras and Granta[31] demonstrated that with repetitive lifting (over a 5-hour period) subjects had a significant change in their lifting pattern and in the muscle recruitment patterns so there was a decrease in spine stabilization (decreased compression) and an increase in anterior/posterior shear in the lumbar spine. To reduce the risk of recurrence of low-back disorders, a patient needs to learn to monitor these changes and be conscious of correcting faulty patterns. Help the patient modify and adapt the stable spine body mechanics that were initiated under basic techniques to replicate the type of lifting he or she will be doing at home or on the job. Include variations in the lifting tasks to prepare for unexpected situations.

## Repetitive Reaching

Repetitive reaching requires that the patient learn to assume a comfortable stride and then practice shifting his or her weight forward and backward on the lower extremities rather than bending forward and backward with the spine. Preparatory exercises should include partial lunging forward, sideways, and backward. During practice have the patient use a weight comparable to that in the real-life situation and go through the action on a repetitive basis, concentrating on spinal control and resting only when control is no longer possible.

## Repetitive Pushing and Pulling

Repetitive pushing and pulling require strong upper extremities and a stable spine. Preparatory activities should include pushing and pulling against elastic resistance or pulley resistance set at heights that replicate the work environment. Progress to pushing and pulling a weighted cart or a weighted box across a table. Reinforce the importance of activating the spinal stabilizers.

## Rotation or Turning

Turning with a load is a component of most work activity. A person may rotate the spine to reach around to place a load to the side or behind. Rotation may create an unstable situation or may be damaging to the spinal structures. Therefore, it is important to take the rotation out of turning. Have the patient practice a "stable spine turn," which requires motion and control in the hips, or taking steps into the direction of the turn rather than twisting and rotating the back.

## Transitional Movements

Most functional activities require *transitional motions*, such as reaching downward to pick up something (spinal flexion), then reaching overhead to place it on a high shelf (spinal extension). In sports activities the activity may require moving quickly from a forward-bent position to an extended position with arms overhead (such as dribbling a basketball, then shooting). Set up drills that replicate the speed and movements of the desired outcome; have the patient practice moving through the patterns while attempting to maintain control of his or her functional spinal position and range.

## Transfer of Training

Ideally, each patient is progressed through rehabilitation to the level of being able to *transfer skills* learned to closely related but new situations. Provide variable learning opportunities from simple to complex and then help the patient analyze successful adaptations to each new experience. (See Figure 1.6 and accompanying text in Chapter 1 for examples of how to vary tasks from simple to complex.)

# ● EDUCATION FOR PREVENTION

Education occurs on a continual basis. Before discharge, review the following relationships of posture and pain with the patient.

- When experiencing pain or the recurrence of symptoms, check posture. Avoid any one posture for prolonged periods.
- If sustained postures are necessary, take frequent breaks and perform appropriate ROM exercises at least every half hour. Finish all exercises by assuming a well balanced posture.
- Avoid hyperextending the neck or being in a forward-head posture or forward-bent position for prolonged periods. Find ways to modify a task so it can be accomplished at eye level or with proper lumbar support.
- If in a tension-producing situation, perform conscious relaxation exercises.
- Use common sense and follow good safety habits.

Develop and progress a safe home exercise program.

- Teach flexibility, muscle endurance, and strengthening exercises appropriate for the patient to maintain ROM, muscle endurance, and strength.
- Address any misconceptions the patient may have about exercise.

Reinforce the importance of maintaining cardiopulmonary endurance and its effect on managing symptoms.

## INDEPENDENT LEARNING ACTIVITIES

### ● Critical Thinking and Discussion

1. Observe a homemaker or worker doing an activity that requires pushing, pulling, reaching, lifting, or some other repetitive pattern. Analyze what component motions are part of the total pattern and decide if strength, range, endurance, balance, or coordination (or a combination) is necessary in the upper extremities, lower extremities, and trunk. Decide what is necessary to make the spine safe while doing this activity and design an exercise program that encompasses all the components.

2. Go to a health club or exercise class and observe how individuals are performing the exercises. Note the activities that cause stress to the spine. How would you modify each exercise? Consider safe use of the equipment, safe biomechanics, and appropriate instruction for the audience. Can you tell the purpose of each exercise (strength, stretch, endurance)? Are the directions appropriately given for the level of participants?

### ● Laboratory Practice

1. With a laboratory partner practice the kinesthetic training techniques and core muscle activation techniques for the cervical spine and the lumbar spine until you become proficient at performing them and recognizing when they are done correctly. Then practice teaching them to a family member or friend and see how well they understand what they are to do.

2. Practice the progression of spinal stabilization exercises described in the muscle performance section. Start at the easiest level and progress the leg and arm movements until you feel you are at your maximum resistance for stabilization. After resting, time yourself for 1 minute, beginning at the most difficult level of movement. The idea is to keep the spine stable during the entire minute. If you begin to feel you are losing control, decrease the amount of extremity resistance (e.g., going from moving both lower extremities in a reciprocal pattern to moving just one extremity while the other is on the floor). This can also be done for 3 minutes. Were you able to meet the challenge yet keep the spine stable? Did you feel your stabilizing muscles "working?"

3. Practice doing wall slides, partial squats, and partial lunges with a stable spine. When you can do the squat comfortably with a stable spine, practice lifting a box from the floor to table height, then from the floor to shoulder height, then place it on a shelf at each height. Feel what is happening to your spine. Then repeat the maneuvers with a stable spine, and see if you can control the spinal position with the drawing-in maneuver. When you can do the lunge comfortably, practice lifting small objects from the floor with a lunging technique and stable spine. Finally, practice lifting objects from the floor and turning (using legs and hips to change direction, not spinal rotation) to place the objects on a table or shelf. Feel what is happening to the spine and repeat the activities with a stable spinal posture.

### ● Case Studies

Review the cases described in Chapter 14 and 15 and modify your answers based on information you studied in this chapter.

## REFERENCES

1. Abdulwahab, SS: Treatment based on H-reflexes testing improves disability status in patients with cervical radiculopathy. Int J Rehabil Res 22(3):207, 1999.
2. Alexander, KM, Kinney LaPier, TL: Differences in static balance and weight distribution between normal subjects and subjects with chronic unilateral low back pain. J Orthop Sports Phys Ther 28(6):378, 1998.
3. Andersson, EA, Nilsson, J, et al: Abdominal and hip flexor muscle activation during various training exercises. Eur J App Plysiol 75:115–123, 1997.
4. Arokoski, JP, Valta, T, et al: Back and abdominal muscle function during stabilization exercises. Arch phys Med Rehabil 82(8):1089–1098, 2001
5. Blount, WP, Moe, JH: The Milwaukee Brace. Williams & Wilkins, Baltimore, 1980.
6. Bondi, BA, Drinkwater-Kolk, M: Functional stabilization training. Workshop notes, Northeast Seminars, October 1992.
7. Cassella, MC, Hall, JE: Current treatment approaches in the nonoperative and operative management of adolescent idiopathic scoliosis. Phys Ther 71:897, 1991.
8. Chok, B, et al: Endurance training of the trunk extensor muscles in people with subacute low back pain. Phys Ther 79(11):1033, 1999.
9. Danneels, LA, Cools, AM, Vanderstraeten, GG, et al: The effects of three different training modalities on the cross-sectional area of the paravertebral muscles. Scand J Med Sci Sports 11:335–341, 2001.
10. Gilleard, WL, Brown, JM: An electromyographic validation of an abdominal muscle test. Arch Phys Med Rehabil 75:1002–1007, 1994.
11. Hagins, M, et al: Effects of practice on the ability to perform lumbar stabilization exercises. J Orthop Sports Phys Ther 29(9):546, 1999.
12. Hart, DL, Stobbe, TJ, Jaraiedi, M: Effect of lumbar posture on lifting. Spine 12:22, 1987.
13. Henry, SM, Westervelt, KC: The use of real-time ultrasound feedback in teaching abdominal hollowing exercises to healthy subjects. J Orthop Sports Phys Ther 35(6):338–345, 2005.
14. Hides, JA, Jull, GA, Richardson, CA: Long-term effects of specific stabilizing exercises for first-episode low back pain. Spine 26(11):E243–E248, 2001.
15. Hides, JA, Richardson, CA, Gwendolen, AJ: Multifidus muscle recovery is not automatic after resolution of acute, first-episode low back pain. Spine 21(23):2763, 1996.
16. Hides, JA, Richardson, CA, et al: Ultrasound imaging in rehabilitation. Aust J Physiother 41:187–193, 1995.
17. Hides, JA, Richardson, CA, Jull, GA: Use of real-time ultrasound imaging for feedback in rehabilitation. Manual Ther 3:125–131, 1993.
18. Hodges, PW, Richardson, CA: Transversus abdominis and the superficial abdominal muscles are controlled independently in a postural task. Neurosci Lett 265:91–94, 1999.
19. Hodges, PW, Richardson, CA: Delayed postural contraction of transversus abdominis in low back pain associated with movement of the lower limb. J Spinal Disord 11(1):46, 1998.

20. Hodges, PW, Richardson, CA: Contraction of the abdominal muscles associated with movement of the lower limb. Phys Ther 77(2):132, 1997.

21. Hodges, PW, Richardson, CA: Feedforward contraction of transversus abdominis is not influenced by the direction of arm movement. Exp Brain Res 114:362–370, 1997.

22. Hodges, PW, Richardson, CA, Jull, G: Evaluation of the relationship between laboratory and clinical tests of transversus abdominis function. Physiother Res Int 1(1):30, 1996.

23. Hubley-Kozey, CL, Vezina, MJ: Muscle activation during exercises to improve trunk stabaility in men with low back pain. Arch Phys Med Rehabil 83:1100–1108, 2002.

24. Jull, G, Trott, P, et al: A randomized controlled trial of exercise and manipulative therapy for cervicogenic headache. Spine 27(17):1835–1843, 2002.

25. Jull, G, Barrett, C, et al: Further clinical clarification of the muscle dysfunction in cervical headache. Cephalalgia 19:179–185, 1999.

26. Jull, GA, Richardson, CA: Rehabilitation of active stabilization of the lumbar spine. In Twomy, LT, Taylor, JR (eds) Physical Therapy of the Lumbar Spine, ed 2. Churchill Livingstone, New York, 1994.

27. Kendall, F, McCreary, E, Provance, PG: Muscles: Testing and Function, ed 4. Williams & Wilkins, Baltimore, 1993.

28. Lee, FH, Hoshino, Y, Nakamura, K, et al: Trunk muscle weakness as a risk factor for low back pain. Spine 24(1):54–57, 1999.

29. Lehman, GJ, McGill, SM: Quantification of the differences in electromyographic activity magnitude between the upper and lower portions of the rectus abdominis muscle during selected trunk exercises. Phys Ther 81(5):1096–1101, 2001.

30. Lubell, A: Potentially dangerous exercises: are they harmful to all? Phys Sports Med 17:187, 1989.

31. Marras, WS, Granata, KP: Changes in trunk dynamics and spine loading during repeated trunk exertions. Spine 22(21):2564, 1997.

32. McDonnell, KM, Sahrmann, SA, Van Dillen, L: A specific exercise program and modification of postural alignment for treatment of cervicogenic headache: a case report. J Orthop Sports Phys Ther 35(1):3–15, 2005.

33. McGill, SM: Low back exercises: evidence for improving exercise regimens. Phys Ther 78(7):754, 1998.

34. Morgan, D: Concepts in functional training and postural stabilization for the low-back injured. Top Acute Care Trauma Rehabil 2:8, 1988.

35. Nachemson, A: Recent advances in the treatment of low back pain. Int Orthop 9:1, 1985.

36. Ng, JK, Richardson, CA: EMG study of eretor spinae and multifidus in two isometric back extension exercises. Aust J Physiother 40:115–121, 1994.

37. O'Sullivan, PT, Twomey, L, Allison, GT: Altered abdominal muscle recruitment in patients with chronic back pain following a specific exercise intervention. J Orthop Sports Phys Ther 27(2):114, 1998.

38. O'Sullivan, P, Twomey, L, Allison, G, et al: Altered patterns of abdominal muscle activation in patients with chronic low back pain. Aust Physiother 43(2):91, 1997.

39. Parris, S: Spinal Dysfunction: Etiology and Treatment of Dysfunction Including Joint Manipulation. Manual of Course Notes, Atlanta, 1979.

40. Richardson, C, Hodges, P, Hides, J: Therapeutic Exercise for Lumbopelvic Stabilization: A Motor Control Approach for the Treatment and Prevention of Low Back Pain, ed 2. Churchill Livingstone, Philadelphia, 2004.

41. Richardson, C, Jull, G: An historical perspective on the development of clinical techniques to evaluate and treat the active stabilising system of the lumbar spine. Aust J Physiother Monogr 1:5, 1995.

42. Richardson, C, Jull, G, et al: Techniques for active lumbar stabilisation for spinal protection: a pilot study. Aust J Physiother 38:105, 1992.

43. Richardson, C, Toppenberg, R, Jull, G: An initial evaluation of eight abdominal exercises for their ability to provide stabilisation for the lumbar spine. Aust J Physiother 36:6, 1990.

44. Robinson, R: The new back school prescription: stabilization training. Part I. Occup Med 7:17, 1992.

45. Saal, JA: The new back school prescription: stabilization training. Part II. Occup Med 7:33, 1992.

46. Saal, JA: Dynamic muscular stabilization in the non-operative treatment of lumbar pain syndromes. Orthop Rev 19:691, 1990.

47. Saunders, HD, Ryan, RS: Spinal traction. In Saunders, HD, Ryan, RS (eds) Evaluation, Treatment and Prevention of Musculoskeletal Disorders, ed 4. Vol. 1. Spine. Saunders Group, Chaska, MN, 2004.

48. Stevans, J, Hall, KG: Motor skill acquisition strategies for rehabilitation of low back pain. J Orthop Sports Phys Ther 28(3):165, 1998.

49. Storheim, K, Bo, K, Pederstad O, Jahnsen R: Intra-tester reproducibility of pressure biofeedback in measurement of transversus abdominis function. Physiother Res Int 7(4):239–249, 2002.

50. Sullivan, MS: Back support mechanisms during manual lifting. Phys Ther 69:38, 1989.

51. Sweeney, T: Neck school: cervicothoracic stabilization training. Occup Med 7:43, 1992.

52. Takemasa, R, Yamamoto, H, Tani, T: Trunk muscle strength in and effect of trunk muscle exercises for patients with chronic low back pain. Spine 20(23):2522–2530, 1995.

53. Teyhen, DS, Miltenberger, CE, Deiters, HM, et al: The use of ultrasound imaging of the abdominal drawing-in maneuver in subjects with low back pain. J Orthop Sports Phys Ther 35(6):346–355, 2005.

54. Vera-Garcia, FJ, Grenier, SG, McGill, SM: Abdominal muscle response during curl-ups on both stable and labile surfaces. Phys Ther 80(6):564, 2000.

55. Wohlfahrt, D, Jull, G, Richardson, C: The relationship between the dynamic and static function of abdominal muscles. Aust J Physiother 39:9, 1993.

# The Shoulder and Shoulder Girdle

The design of the shoulder girdle allows for mobility of the upper extremity. As a result, the hand can be placed almost anywhere within a sphere of movement, being limited primarily by the length of the arm and the space taken up by the body. The combined mechanics of its joints and muscles provide for and control the mobility. When establishing a therapeutic exercise program for impaired function of the shoulder region, as with any other region of the body, the unique anatomical and kinesiologic features must be taken into consideration as well as the state of pathology and functional limitations imposed by the impairments. This chapter is divided into three major sections. The first section briefly reviews the structure and function of the shoulder girdle complex. The second section describes common disorders and guidelines for conservative and postsurgical management. The last section describes exercise techniques commonly used to meet the goals of treatment during the stages of tissue healing and phases of rehabilitation.

## STRUCTURE AND FUNCTION OF THE SHOULDER GIRDLE

The shoulder girdle has only one bony attachment to the axial skeleton (Fig. 17.1). The clavicle articulates with the sternum via the small sternoclavicular joint. As a result, considerable mobility is allowed in the upper extremity. Stability is provided by an intricate balance between the scapular and glenohumeral muscles and the structures of the joints in the shoulder girdle.

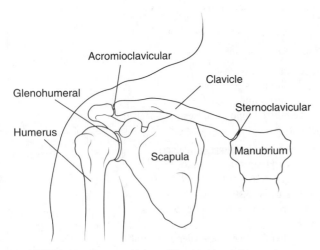

FIGURE 17.1 Bones and joints of the shoulder girdle complex.

## JOINTS OF THE SHOULDER GIRDLE COMPLEX

There are three synovial joints (glenohumeral, acromioclavicular, sternoclavicular) and two functional articulations (scapulothoracic, suprahumeral) that make up the shoulder girdle complex.

### Synovial Joints

#### Glenohumeral Joint

The glenohumeral (GH) joint is an incongruous, ball-and-socket (spheroidal) triaxial joint with a lax joint capsule. It is supported by the tendons of the rotator cuff and the glenohumeral (superior, middle, inferior) and coracohumeral ligaments (Fig. 17.2). The concave bony partner, the glenoid fossa, is located on the superior-lateral margin of the scapula. It faces anteriorly, laterally, and upward, which provides some stability to the joint. A fibrocartilagenous lip, the glenoid labrum, deepens the fossa for greater congruity and serves as the attachment site for the capsule. The convex bony partner is the head of the humerus. Only a small portion of the head comes in contact with the fossa at any one time, allowing for considerable humeral movement and potential instability.[133]

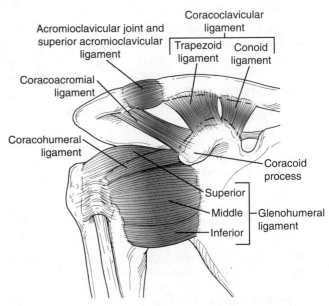

FIGURE 17.2 Ligaments of the glenohumeral and acromioclavicular joints.

### Arthrokinematics

According to the convex-concave theory of joint motion (see Chapter 5), with motions of the humerus (physiologi-

## BOX 17.1    Summary of Joint Arthrokinematics of the GH Joint

| Physiological Motion of the Humerus | Roll | Slide |
|---|---|---|
| Flexion | Anterior | Posterior |
| Horizontal adduction | Anterior | Posterior |
| Internal rotation | Anterior | Posterior |
| Extension | Posterior | Anterior |
| Horizontal abduction | Posterior | Anterior |
| External rotation | Posterior | Anterior |
| Abduction | Superior | Inferior |

cal motions) the convex head rolls in the same direction and slides in the opposite direction in the glenoid fossa (Box 17.1).

 **Focus on Evidence**

Of interest and apparent contradiction of this theory, one study reported that through the mid-range of the arc of passive motion there is minimal displacement of the humeral head. However, beyond mid-range the overall displacement of the head in normal joints is anterior with shoulder flexion and posterior with shoulder extension.[69] This cadaveric study demonstrated that the integrity of the capsular ligamentous system influenced the displacement and that both hyper- and hypomobility of the capsule changed the overall

displacement of the humeral head with passive range of motion (ROM).

In another study, Howel et al.,[84] using radiographs, measured humeral head displacement in normal and unstable shoulders. These investigators reported posterior displacement of the humeral head during end-range horizontal abduction with the humerus at 90° and in full external rotation in normal subjects, yet anterior displacement in subjects with anterior instability. These studies support the importance of joint mobility testing to examine restricted accessory motions to determine if interventions with joint mobilization techniques should be used and the direction of the mobilization force, rather than just using the convex-concave rule, to determine the direction of mobilizations.

### Stability

Static and dynamic restraints provide joint stability (Table 17.1).[31,44,162,199,202] The structural relationship of the bony anatomy, ligaments, and glenoid labrum and the adhesive and cohesive forces in the joint provide static stability. The tendons of the rotator cuff blend with the ligaments and glenoid labrum at their sites of attachment so when the muscles contract they provide dynamic stability by tightening the static restraints (Fig. 17.3). The coordinated response of the muscles of the cuff and tension in the ligaments provide varying degrees of support depending on the position and motion of the humerus.[151,162,184] In addition, the long head of the biceps and the long head of the

## TABLE 17.1    Static and Dynamic Stabilizers of the Scapula and Glenohumeral Joint

| Description | Static Stabilizers | Dynamic Stabilizers |
|---|---|---|
| **Scapula** | | |
| Weight of upper extremity creates downward rotation and forward tipping moment on the scapula | • Cohesive forces of subscapular bursa | Upper trapezius and serratus anterior middle trapezius and rhomboids |
| **Glenohumeral joint** | | |
| In dependent position: if scapula is in normal alignment, weight of arm creates an adduction moment on the humerus | • Superior capsule and suprahumeral ligament are taut<br>• Adhesive and cohesive forces of synovial fluid and negative joint pressure hold surfaces together<br>• Glenoid labrum deepens fossa and improves congruency | Rotator cuff, deltoid, and long head of biceps brachii |
| When the humerus is elevating and the scapula is rotating upward | • Tension placed on static restraints by the rotator cuff<br>• Glenohumeral ligaments provide inferior translation of humeral head | Rotator cuff and deltoid; elbow action brings in two-joint muscle support<br>• Long head of biceps stabilizes against humeral elevation<br>• Long head of triceps stabilizes against inferior translation |

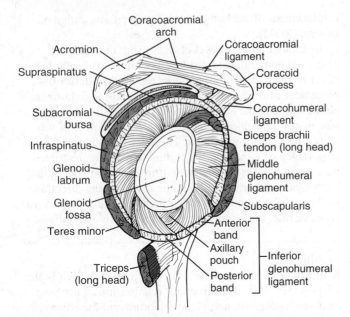

FIGURE 17.3 Lateral aspect of the glenoid fossa (interior view), showing attachments of the glenoid labrum, capsule, ligaments, and their relationship to the rotator cuff and long head of the biceps brachii musculature.

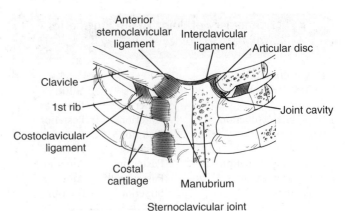

Sternoclavicular joint

FIGURE 17.4 Ligaments of the sternoclavicular joint.

triceps brachii reinforce the capsule with their attachments and provide superior and inferior shoulder joint support, respectively, when functioning with elbow motions.[96] The long head of the biceps in particular stabilizes against humeral elevation[96] and contributes to anterior stability of the glenohumeral joint by resisting torsional forces when the shoulder is abducted and externally rotated.[11,151] Neuromuscular control, including movement awareness and motor response, underlies coordination of the dynamic restraints.[199,202]

## Acromioclavicular Joint

The acromioclavicular (AC) joint is a plane, triaxial joint that may or may not have a disk. The weak capsule is reinforced by the superior and inferior AC ligaments (see Fig. 17.2). The convex bony partner is a facet on the lateral end of the clavicle. The concave bony partner is a facet on the acromion of the scapula.

### Arthrokinematics

With motions of the scapula, the acromial surface slides in the same direction in which the scapula moves because the surface is concave. Motions affecting this joint include upward rotation (the scapula turns so the glenoid fossa rotates upward), downward rotation, winging of the vertebral border, and tipping of the inferior angle.

### Stability

The AC ligaments are supported by the strong coracoclavicular ligament. No muscles directly cross this joint for dynamic support.

## Sternoclavicular Joint

The sternoclavicular (SC) joint is an incongruent, triaxial, saddle-shaped joint with a disk. The joint is supported by the anterior and posterior SC ligaments and the interclavicular and costoclavicular ligaments (Fig. 17.4). The medial end of the clavicle is convex superior to inferior and concave anterior to posterior. The joint disk attaches to the upper end. The superior-lateral portion of the manubrium and first costal cartilage is concave superior to inferior and convex anterior to posterior.

### Arthrokinematics

The motions of the clavicle occur as a result of the scapular motions of elevation, depression, protraction (abduction), and retraction (adduction) (Box 17.2). Rotation of the clavicle occurs as an accessory motion when the humerus is elevated above the horizontal position and the scapula upwardly rotates; it cannot occur as an isolated voluntary motion.

### Stability

The ligaments crossing the joint provide static stability. There are no muscles crossing the joint for dynamic stability.[41]

## Functional Articulations

### Scapulothoracic Articulation

Normally there is considerable soft tissue flexibility, allowing the scapula to slide along the thorax and participate in all upper extremity motions.

### Motions of the Scapula

Motions of the scapula are:

| BOX 17.2 | Summary of Arthrokinematics of the SC Joint | | |
|---|---|---|---|
| **Physiological Motion of the Clavicle** | | **Roll** | **Slide** |
| Protraction | | Anterior | Anterior |
| Retraction | | Posterior | Posterior |
| Elevation | | Superior | Inferior |
| Depression | | Inferior | Superior |

- Elevation, depression, protraction (abduction), and retraction (adduction), seen with clavicular motions at the SC joint (Fig. 17.5 A&B). They are also component motions when the humerus moves.
- Upward and downward rotation, seen with clavicular motions at the SC joint and rotation at the AC joint, occurs concurrently with motions of the humerus (Fig. 17.5C). Upward rotation of the scapula is a necessary component motion for full ROM of flexion and abduction of the humerus.
- Winging and tipping, seen with motion at the AC joint concurrently with motions of the humerus (Fig. 17.5D). Winging is a transverse plane motion where the medial border lifts away from the rib cage; it normally occurs with horizontal adduction of the humerus. Forward tipping of the scapula occurs in conjunction with internal rotation and extension of the humerus when reaching the hand behind the back.

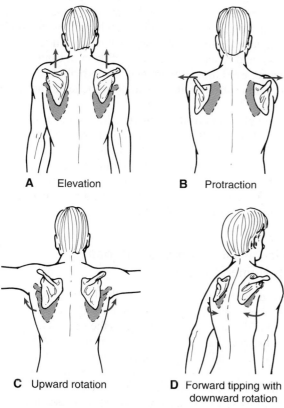

**A** Elevation    **B** Protraction

**C** Upward rotation    **D** Forward tipping with downward rotation

FIGURE 17.5 Scapular motions. (*A*) Elevation occurs with clavicular elevation at the SC joint when shrugging. (*B*) Protraction (abduction) occurs with clavicular abduction at the SC joint when reaching forward. (*C*) Upward rotation occurs with clavicular rotation at the SC and AC joints when flexing and abducting the shoulder. (*D*) Forward tipping (along with downward rotation) occurs at the AC joint when extending and internally rotating the shoulder.

## Scapular Stability

***Postural relationship.*** In the dependent position, the scapula is stabilized primarily through a balance of forces. The weight of the arm creates a downward rotation, abduction, and forward tipping moment on the scapula. The

downward rotation is balanced by the dynamic support of the upper trapezius and serratus anterior. The forward tipping and abduction is balanced by the dynamic support of the rhomboids and middle trapezius[98,163] (see Table 17.1).

***Active arm motions.*** With active arm motions, the muscles of the scapula function in synchrony to stabilize and control the position of the scapula so the scapulohumeral muscles can maintain an effective length–tension relationship as they function to stabilize and move the humerus. Without the positional control of the scapula, the efficiency of the humeral muscles decreases. The upper and lower trapezius with the serratus anterior upwardly rotate the scapula whenever the arm abducts or flexes, and the serratus anterior abducts (protracts) the scapula on the thorax to align the scapula during flexion or pushing activities. During arm extension or during pulling activities, the rhomboids function to downwardly rotate and adduct (retract) the scapula in synchrony with the latissimus dorsi, teres major, and rotator cuff muscles. These stabilizing muscles also eccentrically control acceleration motions of the scapula in the opposite directions.[135]

***Faulty posture.*** With a faulty scapular posture, muscle length and strength imbalances occur not only in the scapular muscles but also in the humeral muscles, altering the mechanics of the glenohumeral joint. A forward tilt of the scapula (seen with a forward head posture and increased thoracic kyphosis) is associated with decreased flexibility in the pectoralis minor, levator scapulae, and scalenius muscles and weakness in the serratus anterior or trapezius muscles. This scapular posture changes the posture of the humerus in the glenoid, which assumes a relatively abducted and internally rotated position with respect to the scapula (Fig. 17.6). The glenohumeral internal rotators may become less flexible, and external rotators may weaken, affecting the mechanics of the joint.

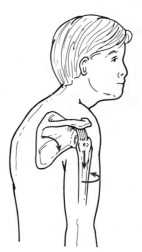

FIGURE 17.6 Faulty forward head, thoracic kyphosis, and shoulder girdle posture results in a forward tilt and downward rotation of the scapula with relative abduction and internal rotation of the humerus when the arm is in a dependent position.

**Focus on Evidence**

A study by Borstad and Ludewig,[19] which looked at the effect of pectoralis minor resting length on scapular kinematics in subjects without shoulder pain, documented that those individuals with a short pectoralis minor (n = 25) had greater scapular internal rotation (protraction) and less posterior tipping during arm elevation in flexion, abduction, and scaption than those with a longer pectoralis minor (n = 25), thus providing evidence for altered pectoralis minor muscle length and altered scapular movement. In a related study by the same author,[20] a correlation between the postural impairments of increased thoracic kyphosis, scapular internal rotation and forward tipping, and decreased pectoralis minor length was found to be significant, thus further supporting the relationship between muscle length and posture.

### Suprahumeral (Subacromial) Space

The coracoacromial arch, composed of the acromion and coracoacromial ligament, overlies the subacromial/subdeltoid bursa, the supraspinatus tendon, and a portion of the muscle (Fig. 17.7).[98] These structures allow for and participate in normal shoulder function. Compromise of this space from faulty muscle function, faulty postural relationships, faulty joint mechanics, injury to the soft tissue in this region, or structural anomalies of the acromion lead to impingement syndromes.[19,27,30,99,103,113] After a rotator cuff tear, the bursa may communicate with the glenohumeral joint cavity.[44]

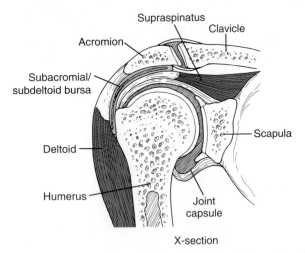

FIGURE 17.7 The supraspinatus and subacromial/subdeltoid bursa lie in the suprahumeral space.

 **SHOULDER GIRDLE FUNCTION**

### Scapulohumeral Rhythm

Motion of the scapula, synchronous with motions of the humerus, allows for 150° to 180° of shoulder ROM into

flexion or abduction with elevation. The ratio has considerable variation among individuals but is commonly accepted to be 2:1 (2° of glenohumeral motion to 1° of scapular rotation) overall motion. During the setting phase (0° to 30° abduction, 0° to 60° flexion), motion is primarily at the glenohumeral joint, whereas the scapula seeks a stable position. During the mid-range of humeral motion, the scapula has greater motion, approaching a 1:1 ratio with the humerus; later in the range, the glenohumeral joint again dominates the motion.[39,98,170]

- During humeral elevation, the synchronous motion of the scapula allows the muscles moving the humerus to maintain an effective length–tension relationship throughout the activity and helps maintain congruency between the humeral head and fossa while decreasing shear forces.[39,98,170]
- Muscles causing the upward rotation of the scapula are the upper and lower trapezius and the serratus anterior. Weakness or complete paralysis of these muscles results in the scapula being rotated downward by the contracting deltoid and supraspinatus as abduction or flexion is attempted. These two muscles then reach active insufficiency, and functional elevation of the arm cannot be reached, even though there may be normal passive ROM and normal strength in the shoulder abductor and flexor muscles.[170]
- During elevation of the humerus, the pectoralis minor is lengthened as the scapula upwardly rotates, retracts, and tips posteriorly. Restricted scapular movement during humeral elevation from a shortened pectoralis minor results in patterns similar to those seen in patients with impingement symptoms and could be a risk factor for development of the syndrome.[19]

## Clavicular Elevation and Rotation With Humeral Motion

It is commonly accepted that initially the first 30° of upward rotation of the scapula occurs with elevation of the clavicle at the SC joint. Then, as the coracoclavicular ligament becomes taut, the clavicle rotates 38° to 55° about its longitudinal axis, which elevates its acromial end (because it is crank-shaped). This motion allows the scapula to rotate an additional 30° at the AC joint.[98] Loss of any of these functional components decreases the amount of scapular rotation and thus the ROM of the upper extremity.

 **Focus on Evidence**

A recent three-dimensional study of clavicular motion during humeral flexion, scaption, and abduction to 115° using surface electromagnetic sensors on 30 asymptomatic subjects and 9 individuals with shoulder pathology documented 11° to 15° of clavicular elevation, 15° to 29° of retraction, and 15° to 31° of posterior long axis rotation, showing similar patterns but different ranges from previously reported studies.[104] Ranges of clavicular motion above 115° were not reliable owing to movement of the clavicle under the skin.[104]

## External Rotation of the Humerus With Full Elevation

During abduction of the arm in the frontal plane, for the greater tubercle of the humerus to clear the coracoacromial arch, the humerus must externally rotate as it is elevated above the horizontal. Weak or inadequate external rotation results in impingement of the soft tissues in the suprahumeral space, causing pain, inflammation, and eventually loss of function.

## Internal Rotation of the Humerus With Full Elevation

Medial rotation begins at around 50° of passive shoulder flexion when all structures are intact.[136] With full range of shoulder flexion and elevation, the humerus medially rotates 90°, and the medial epicondyle faces anteriorly.[17,18,136]

- As the arm elevates above the horizontal position in the sagittal plane, the anterior capsule and ligaments become taut, causing the humerus to rotate medially. The bony configuration of the posterior aspect of the glenoid fossa contributes to the inward rotation motion of the humerus as the shoulder flexes.[170] Most of the shoulder flexor muscles are also medial rotators of the humerus.[170]
- The infraspinatus and teres minor stabilize the humeral head against the inward rotating forces, helping to maintain alignment and stability of the head in the fossa. Weakness in these muscles may contribute to excessive anterior translation and instability.[31]

## Elevation of the Humerus Through the Plane of the Scapula—Scaption

The plane of the scapula is described as 30° anterior to the frontal plane. Motion of the humerus in this plane is popularly called *scaption*[181,198] or scapular plane abduction.[42] In this range there is less tension on the capsule, and greater elevation is possible than with pure frontal or sagittal plane elevation. Neither internal nor external rotation of the humerus is necessary to prevent greater tubercle impingement during elevation in scaption.[42,181] Many functional activities occur with the shoulder oriented in this plane.

## Deltoid—Short Rotator Cuff and Supraspinatus Mechanisms

- Most of the force of the deltoid muscle causes upward translation of the humerus; if unopposed, it leads to impingement of the soft tissues in the suprahumeral space between the humeral head and the coracoacromial arch.

- The combined effect of the short rotator muscles (infraspinatus, teres minor, subscapularis) causes stabilizing compression and downward translation of the humerus in the glenoid.
- The combined actions of the deltoid and short rotators result in a balance of forces that abduct the humerus and control the humeral head.
- The supraspinatus muscle has a significant stabilizing, compressive, and slight upward translation effect on the humerus; these effects, combined with the effect of gravity, lead to abduction of the arm.
- Interruption of function leading to fatigue or poor coordination of any of these muscles can cause microtrauma and eventual dysfunction in the shoulder region.

# ⬤ REFERRED PAIN AND NERVE INJURY

For a detailed description of referred pain patterns, peripheral nerve injuries in the shoulder, thoracic outlet syndrome, and complex regional pain syndromes (including reflex sympathetic dystrophy) and their management, see Chapter 13.

## Common Sources of Referred Pain in the Shoulder Region

### Cervical Spine

- Vertebral joints between C3 and C4 or between C4 and C5
- Nerve roots C4 or C5

### Referred Pain from Related Tissues

- Dermatome C4 is over the trapezius to the tip of the shoulder.
- Dermatome C5 is over the deltoid region and lateral arm.
- Diaphragm: pain perceived in the upper trapezius region.
- Heart: pain perceived in the axilla and left pectoral region.
- Gallbladder irritation: pain perceived at the tip of shoulder and posterior scapular region.

## Nerve Disorders in the Shoulder Girdle Region

***Brachial plexus in the thoracic outlet.*** Common sites for compression are the scalene triangle, costoclavicular space and under the coracoid process, and pectoralis minor muscle.[102]

***Suprascapular nerve in the suprascapular notch.*** This injury occurs from direct compression or from nerve stretch, such as when carrying a heavy book bag over the shoulder.

***Radial nerve in the axilla.*** Compression occurs from continual pressure, such as when leaning on axillary crutches.

## MANAGEMENT OF SHOULDER DISORDERS AND SURGERIES

To make sound clinical decisions when managing patients with shoulder disorders, it is necessary to understand the various pathologies, surgical procedures, and associated precautions and to identify presenting impairments, functional limitations, and possible disabilities. In this section, common pathologies and surgeries are presented and are related to corresponding preferred practice patterns (groupings of impairments) described in the *Guide to Physical Therapist Practice*[2] (Table 17.2). Conservative and postoperative management of these conditions are described in this section.

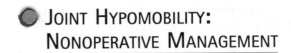

## JOINT HYPOMOBILITY: NONOPERATIVE MANAGEMENT

### Glenohumeral Joint

Restricted mobility of the glenohumeral joint may occur as a result of pathology such as rheumatoid arthritis or osteoarthritis, from prolonged immobilization, or from unknown causes (idiopathic frozen shoulder). Associated impairments in mobility and muscle performance also occur in the muscles and other connective tissues in the area.

### Related Pathologies and Etiology of Symptoms

***Rheumatoid arthritis and osteoarthritis.*** These disorders follow the clinical picture described in Chapter 11.

---

**TABLE 17.2    Shoulder Pathologies/Surgical Procedures and Preferred Practice Patterns**

| PATHOLOGY/SURGICAL PROCEDURE | PREFERRED PRACTICE PATTERNS AND ASSOCIATED IMPAIRMENTS[2] |
|---|---|
| • Abnormal posture (protracted scapula, kyphosis, forward head) | • Pattern 4B—Impaired posture |
| • Arthritis (osteoarthritis, rheumatoid arthritis, traumatic arthritis)<br>• Synovitis<br>• Postimmobilization arthritis (stiff shoulder)<br>• Idiopathic frozen shoulder<br>• Adhesive capsulitis<br>• Joint instability, subluxation, dislocation (nontraumatic/recurrent)<br>• Rotator cuff syndrome and allied disorders<br>• Labral lesion | • Pattern 4D—Impaired joint mobility, motor function, muscle performance, and range of motion (ROM) associated with connective tissue dysfunction |
| • Arthritis—acute stage<br>• Acute impingement syndrome (tendinitis, bursitis)<br>• Acute capsulitis<br>• Acute rotator cuff tear<br>• Traumatic shoulder dislocation | • Pattern 4E—Impaired joint mobility, motor function, muscle performance, and ROM associated with localized inflammation |
| • Fractures (proximal humerus, clavicle, scapula) | • Pattern 4G—Impaired joint mobility, muscle performance, and ROM associated with fracture |
| • Total shoulder replacement<br>• Hemireplacement arthroplasty<br>• Resurfacing and interposition arthroplasties<br>• Resection arthroplasty (distal clavicle) | • Pattern 4H—Impaired joint mobility, motor function, muscle performance, and ROM associated with joint arthroplasty |
| • Subacromial decompression procedures (bursectomy, acromioplasty, distal clavicular resection)<br>• Rotator cuff repair<br>• Capsulorrhaphy (capsular shift)<br>• Electrothermally-assisted arthroscopic capsulorrhaphy<br>• Capsulolabral reconstruction<br>• Fracture stabilization with internal fixation<br>• Joint débridement<br>• Synovectomy<br>• Arthrodesis | • Pattern 4I—Impaired joint mobility, motor function, muscle performance, and ROM associated with bony or soft tissue surgery |
| • Thoracic outlet syndrome (brachial plexus), suprascapular, axillary, median, ulnar, or radial nerve entrapment or injury in the shoulder girdle region. | • Pattern 5F—Impaired peripheral nerve integrity and muscle performance associated with peripheral nerve injury |

***Traumatic arthritis.*** This disorder occurs in response to a fall or blow to the shoulder or to microtrauma from faulty mechanics or overuse.

***Postimmobilization arthritis or stiff shoulder.*** This disorder occurs as a result of lack of movement or secondary effects from conditions such as heart disease, stroke, or diabetes mellitus.

***Idiopathic frozen shoulder.*** This disorder, which is also called *adhesive capsulitis* or *periarthritis,* is characterized by the development of dense adhesions, capsular thickening, and capsular restrictions, especially in the dependent folds of the capsule, rather than arthritic changes in the cartilage and bone, as seen with rheumatoid arthritis or osteoarthritis. The onset is insidious and usually occurs between the ages of 40 and 60 years; there is no known cause (primary frozen shoulder), although problems already mentioned in which there is a period of pain and/or restricted motion, such as with rheumatoid arthritis, osteoarthritis, trauma, or immobilization, may lead to a frozen shoulder (secondary frozen shoulder). With primary frozen shoulder, the pathogenesis may be a provoking chronic inflammation in musculotendinous or synovial tissue such as the rotator cuff, biceps tendon, or joint capsule.[41,66,122,125] Consistent with this is a faulty posture and muscle imbalance predisposing the suprahumeral space to impingement and overuse syndromes.[1]

## Clinical Signs and Symptoms

***Glenohumeral joint arthritis.*** The following characteristics are associated with glenohumeral (GH) joint pathologies that lead to hypomobility.

- *Acute phase.* Pain and muscle guarding limit motion, usually external rotation and abduction. Pain is frequently experienced radiating below the elbow and may disturb sleep. Joint swelling is not detected owing to the depth of the capsule, although tenderness can be elicited by palpating in the fornix immediately below the edge of the acromion process between the attachments of the posterior and middle deltoid.
- *Subacute phase.* Capsular tightness begins to develop. Limited motion is detected, consistent with a capsular pattern (external rotation and abduction are most limited, and internal rotation and flexion are least limited). Often, the patient feels pain as the end of the limited range is reached. Joint-play testing reveals limited joint play. If the patient can be treated as the acute condition begins to subside by gradually increasing shoulder motion and activity, the complication of joint and soft tissue contractures can usually be minimized.[117,122]
- *Chronic phase.* Progressive restriction of the GH joint capsule magnifies the signs of limited motion in a capsular pattern and decreased joint play. There is significant loss of function with an inability to reach overhead, outward, or behind the back. Aching is usually localized to the deltoid region.

***Idiopathic frozen shoulder.*** This clinical entity follows a classic pattern*.

- *"Freezing."* Characterized by intense pain even at rest and limitation of motion by 2 to 3 weeks after onset. These acute symptoms may last 10 to 36 weeks.
- *"Frozen."* Characterized by pain only with movement, significant adhesions, and limited GH motions, with substitute motions in the scapula. Atrophy of the deltoid, rotator cuff, biceps, and triceps brachii muscles occurs. This stage lasts 4 to 12 months.
- *"Thawing."* Characterized by no pain and no synovitis but significant capsular restrictions from adhesions. This stage lasts 2 to 24 months or longer. Some patients never regain normal ROM.

Some references indicate that spontaneous recovery occurs, on average, 2 years from onset,[66] although others have reported long-term limitations without spontaneous recovery.[156] Inappropriately aggressive therapy at the wrong time may prolong the symptoms.[15] Management guidelines are the same as for acute (maximum protection during the freezing stage), subacute (controlled motion during the frozen stage), and chronic (return to function during the thawing state) joint pathology described in this section.

## Common Impairments

- Night pain and disturbed sleep during acute flares
- Pain on motion and often at rest during acute flares
- Mobility: decreased joint play and ROM, usually limiting external rotation and abduction with some limitation of internal rotation and elevation in flexion
- Posture: possible faulty postural compensations with protracted and anteriorly tipped scapula, rounded shoulders, and elevated and protected shoulder
- Decreased arm swing during gait
- Muscle performance: general muscle weakness and poor endurance in the glenohumeral muscles with overuse of the scapular muscles leading to pain in the trapezius and posterior cervical muscles
- Guarded shoulder motions with substitute scapular motions

## Common Functional Limitations/Disabilities

- Inability to reach overhead, behind head, out to the side, and behind back; thus, having difficulty dressing (such as putting on a jacket or coat or women fastening undergarments behind their back), reaching hand into back pocket of pants (to retrieve wallet), reaching out a car window (to use an ATM machine), self-grooming (such as combing hair, brushing teeth, washing face), and bringing eating utensils to the mouth
- Difficulty lifting weighted objects, such as dishes into a cupboard
- Limited ability to sustain repetitive activities

---

*See references 41, 66, 122, 125, 153, 189

## Glenohumeral Joint Hypomobility: Management—Protection Phase

See general guidelines for management when symptoms are acute in Chapter 10 and Box 10.1.

### Control Pain, Edema, and Muscle Guarding

● The joint may be immobilized in a sling to provide rest and minimize pain.

● Intermittent periods of passive or assisted motion within the pain free/protected ROM and gentle joint oscillation techniques are initiated as soon as the patient tolerates movement in order to minimize adhesion formation.

### Maintain Soft Tissue and Joint Integrity and Mobility

● *Passive range of motion* (PROM) in all ranges of pain-free motion (see Chapter 3). As pain decreases, the patient is progressed to active ROM with or without assistance using activities such as rolling a small ball or sliding a rag on a smooth table top in flexion, abduction, and circular motions. Be sure the patient is taught proper mechanics and avoids faulty patterns, such as scapular elevation or a slumped posture.

● *Passive joint distraction and glides, grade I and II* with the joint placed in a pain-free position (see Chapter 5).

● *Pendulum (Codman's) exercises* are techniques that use the effects of gravity to distract the humerus from the glenoid fossa.[30,34] They help relieve pain through gentle traction and oscillating movements (grade II) and provide early motion of joint structures and synovial fluid. No weight is used during this phase of treatment (see Fig. 17.22).

PRECAUTION: If there is increased pain or irritability in the joint after use of these techniques, either the dosage was too strong or the techniques should not be used at this time.

CONTRAINDICATION: Stretching (grade III) techniques. If there are mechanical restrictions causing limited motion, appropriate stretching can be initiated only *after* the inflammation subsides.

● *Gentle muscle setting* to all muscle groups of the shoulder, including scapular and elbow muscles because of their close association with the shoulder. Instructions are given to the patient to gently contract a group of muscles while slight resistance is applied—just enough to stimulate a muscle contraction. It should not provoke pain. The emphasis is on rhythmic contracting and relaxing of the muscles to help stimulate blood flow and prevent circulatory stasis.

### Maintain Integrity and Function of Associated Areas

● Reflex sympathetic dystrophy (complex regional pain syndrome type I) is a potential complication after shoulder injury or immobility. Therefore special attention is given to the hand with additional exercises, such as having the patient repetitively squeeze a ball or other soft object.

● The patient is advised of the importance of keeping the joints distal to the injured site as active and mobile as possible. The patient or family member is taught to perform ROM exercises of the elbow, forearm, wrist, and fingers several times each day while the shoulder is immobilized. If tolerated, active or gentle resistive ROM is preferred to passive ROM for a greater effect on circulation and muscle integrity.

● If edema is noted in the hand, instruct the patient to elevate the hand, whenever possible, above the level of the heart.

NOTE: Conditions in which there is potentially a prolonged acute/inflammatory stage, such as with rheumatoid arthritis and during the freezing stage of idiopathic frozen shoulder, it is critical to teach the patient active-assistive exercises to maintain muscle and joint integrity and as much mobility as possible without exacerbating the symptoms.

## GH Joint Hypomobility: Management—Controlled Motion Phase

When symptoms are subacute, follow the guidelines as described in Chapter 10, Box 10.2, emphasizing joint mobility, neuromuscular control, and instructions to the patient for self-care.

NOTE: For normal shoulder joint mechanics, there must be good scapular posture and control, and the humerus must be able to externally rotate. To avoid suprahumeral impingement, passive stretching above 90° should be avoided until there is adequate glenohumeral external rotation. With a traumatic injury that involves the AC or SC joints, these joints tend to become hypermobile with improper stretching. Care should be taken to provide stabilization to the scapula and clavicle so as not to stretch these joints when mobilizing the glenohumeral joint.

### Control Pain, Edema, and Joint Effusion

● *Functional activities.* It is important to carefully monitor increasing activities. If the joint was splinted, the amount of time the shoulder is free to move each day is progressively increased.

● *Range of motion.* ROM is progressed up to the point of pain, including all shoulder and scapular motions. The patient is instructed in the use of self-assistive ROM techniques, such as the wand exercises or hand slides on a table.

PRECAUTION: With increased pain or decreased motion, the activity may be too intense or the patient may be using faulty mechanics. Reassess the technique and modify it if faulty joint mechanics exist.

### Progressively Increase Joint and Soft Tissue Mobility

● *Passive joint mobilization techniques.* Stretch grades (grade III sustained or grade III and IV oscillation) using techniques that focus on the restricting capsular tissue at the end of the available ROM are used to increase joint capsule mobility[89,127,187] (see Box 17.1 and Figs. 5.15 through 5.20 in Chapter 5). End-of-range techniques include rotating the humerus and then applying either a grade III distraction or a grade III glide to stretch the restrictive capsular tissue or adhesions (see Figs. 5.17, 5.21, and 17.20).

Use a grade I distraction with all gliding techniques. If the joint is highly irritable and gliding in the direction of restriction is not tolerated, glide in the opposite direction. As pain and irritability decrease, begin to glide in the direction of restriction.[89]

### ● Focus on Evidence

Evidence supporting joint mobilization techniques is limited. A multiple-subject case study, using seven subjects with adhesive capsulitis of the glenohumeral joint (mean disease duration 8.4 months, range 3–12 months) treated with end-range mobilization techniques twice a week for 3 months, showed increased active and passive range and increased capacity of the joint capsule at the end of treatment and at the 9-month follow-up. No control groups were used; therefore the natural course of the disease could not be excluded as the explanation for improvement.[187]

A follow-up study by the same author randomly assigned 100 subjects with stage II adhesive capsulitis to a group receiving high-grade mobilization techniques (end-range stretching using Maitland grade III or IV) or a group receiving low-grade mobilization techniques (Maitland grade I or II in nonstressful positions). After 3 months of treatment, both groups exhibited clinically significant improvement, with the group receiving the high-grade mobilization techniques showing greater improvement than the low-grade mobilization group. Because there was no control group, natural progression could not be ruled out.[188]

● Pendulum exercises can also be used for joint stretching by adding a cuff weight to the wrist or a weight to the hand to cause a grade III joint distraction force (see Fig. 17.22). To direct the stretch force to the glenohumeral joint, stabilize the scapula against the thorax manually or with a belt.

PRECAUTION: Carefully monitor the joint reaction to the mobilization stretches; if irritability increases, vigorous stretching should not be undertaken until the chronic stage of healing.

● *Self-mobilization techniques.* The following self-mobilization techniques may be used for a home program.
  • CAUDAL GLIDE. *Patient position and procedure:* Sitting on a firm surface and grasping the fingers under the edge. The patient then leans the trunk away from the stabilized arm (Fig. 17.8).
  • ANTERIOR GLIDE. *Patient position and procedure:* Sitting with both arms behind the body or lying supine supported on a solid surface. The patient then leans the body weight between the arms (Fig. 17.9).
  • POSTERIOR GLIDE. *Patient position and procedure:* Prone, propped up on both elbows. The body weight shifts downward between the arms (Fig. 17.10).

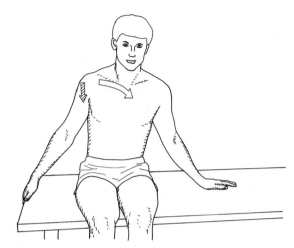

FIGURE 17.8 Self-mobilization. Caudal glide of the humerus occurs as the person leans away from the fixed arm.

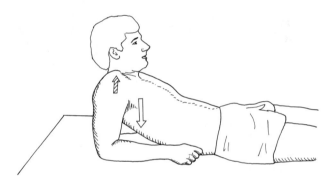

FIGURE 17.9 Self-mobilization. Anterior glide of the humerus occurs as the person leans between the fixed arms.

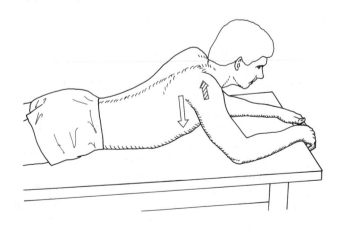

FIGURE 17.10 Self-mobilization. Posterior glide of the humerus occurs as the person shifts his weight downward between the fixed arms.

● *Manual stretching.* Manual stretching techniques are used to increase mobility in shortened muscles and related connective tissue.

● *Self-stretching exercises.* As the joint reaction becomes predictable and the patient begins to tolerate stretching, self-stretching techniques are taught (see Figs. 17.24 through 17.29 in the exercise section).

### Inhibit Muscle Spasm and Correct Faulty Mechanics

Muscle spasm may lead to a faulty deltoid–rotator cuff mechanism and scapulohumeral rhythm when the patient attempts abduction (Fig. 17.11). The head of the humerus may be held in a cranial position in the joint, making it difficult and/or painful to abduct the shoulder because the greater tuberosity impinges on the coracoacromial arch. In this case, repositioning the head of the humerus with a caudal glide is necessary before proceeding with any other form of shoulder exercise. The patient also needs to learn to avoid "hiking the shoulder" when abducting or flexing the arm. The following techniques may address these problems and faulty mechanics. See also mobilization with movement techniques in the next section.

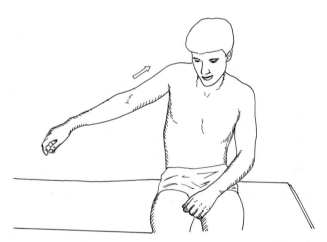

FIGURE 17.11  Poor mechanics with patient hiking the shoulder while trying to abduct the shoulder, thus elevating rather than depressing the humeral head.

● Gentle joint oscillation techniques to help decrease the muscle spasm (grade I or II).

● Sustained caudal glide joint techniques to reposition the humeral head in the glenoid fossa.

● Protected weight bearing, such as leaning hands against a wall or on a table, to stimulate co-contraction of the rotator cuff and scapular stabilizing muscles. If tolerated, gentle rocking forward/backward and side to side requires the muscles to begin controlling motion. Because weight bearing causes joint compression, the benefits of intermittent compression stimulates synovial fluid motion. Techniques are progressed within the tolerance of the joint.

● External rotation exercises to help to depress the humeral head (see Fig. 17.50).

### Improve Joint Tracking

Mobilization with movement (MWM) techniques may assist with retraining muscle function for proper tracking of the humeral head.[116]

● *Shoulder MWM for painful restriction of shoulder external rotation* (Fig. 17.12).

• *Patient position:* Supine lying with folded towel under the scapula; the elbow is near the side and flexed to 90°. A cane is held in both hands.

• *Therapist position and procedure:* Stand on the opposite side of the bed facing the patient and reach across the patient's torso to cup the anteromedial aspect of the head of the humerus with reinforced hands. Apply a pain-free graded posterolateral glide of the humeral head on the glenoid. Instruct the patient to use the cane to push the affected arm into the previously restricted range of external rotation. Sustain the movement for 10 seconds and repeat in sets of 5 to 10. It is important to maintain the elbow near the side of the trunk and ensure that no pain is experienced during the procedure. Adjust the grade and direction of the glide as needed to achieve pain-free function.

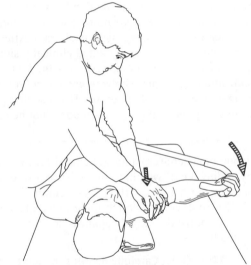

FIGURE 17.12  Mobilization with movement (MWM) to improve external rotation. A posterolateral glide is applied to the humeral head while the patient pushes the arm into the end-range of external rotation with a cane.

● *Shoulder MWM for painful restriction of internal rotation* and inability to reach the hand behind the back (Fig. 17.13).

• *Patient position:* Standing with a towel draped over the unaffected upper trapezius and affected hand at current range of maximum pain-free position behind back. The patient's hand on the affected side grasps the towel behind the back.

• *Therapist position and procedure:* Stand facing the patient's affected side. Place the hand closest to the patient's back high up in the axilla with the palm facing outward to stabilize the scapula with an upward

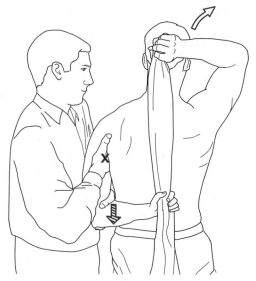

FIGURE 17.13 MWM to improve internal rotation. An inferior glide is applied to the humerus while the patient pulls the hand up the back with a towel.

and inward pressure. With the hand closest to the patient's abdomen hook the thumb in the cubital fossa and grasp the lower humerus to provide an inferior glide. Your abdomen is in contact with the patient's elbow to provide an adduction force to the arm. Have the patient pull on the towel with the unaffected hand to draw the affected hand up the back while the mobilization force is being applied in an inferior direction. Ensure that no pain is experienced during the procedure. Adjust the grade and direction of glide as needed to achieve pain-free function. Maximal glide should be applied to achieve end-range loading.

● *Shoulder MWM for painful arc or impingement signs.* If impingement signs are present in addition to the capsular restrictions, the MWM active elevation technique may be appropriate; see description in the impingement section and Figure 17.17

### Improve Muscle Performance

● Any faulty postures or shoulder girdle mechanics the patient displays when moving the upper extremity in various functional patterns should be identified and exercises to correct the muscle imbalances initiated. Stabilization, flexibility, and strengthening exercises for the shoulder-girdle musculature are described in the last section of this chapter. Emphasis is on developing control in the weak musculature. As the patient learns to activate the weak muscles, progress to strengthening functional patterns of motion.

● Exercises to manage faulty spinal posture are described in Chapter 16.

● Once proper mechanics are restored, the patient should perform active ROM of all shoulder motions daily and return to functional activities to the extent tolerated.

### GH Joint Hypomobility: Management—Return to Function Phase

For joint impairments in the chronic stage, follow the guidelines described in Chapter 10, Box 10.4.

**Progressively Increase Flexibility and Strength**

● Stretching and strengthening exercises are progressed as the joint tissue tolerates. The patient should be actively involved in self-stretching and strengthening by this time, so emphasis during treatment is on correct mechanics, safe progressions, and exercise strategies for return to function.

● If capsular tissue is still restricting ROM, vigorous manual stretching and joint mobilization techniques are applied.

**Prepare for Functional Demands**

If the patient is involved in repetitive heavy lifting, pushing, pulling, carrying, or reaching, when joint range and strength allow, exercises are progressed to replicate these demands. See the last section of this chapter for suggestions.

### GH Joint Management—Postmanipulation Under Anesthesia

Occasionally, no progress is made, and the physician chooses to perform manipulation under anesthesia. Following this procedure, there is an inflammatory reaction and the joint is treated as an acute lesion. If possible, joint-play and passive ROM techniques are initiated while the patient is still in the recovery room. Surgical intervention with incision of the dependent capsular fold may be used if the adhesions are not broken with the manipulation. Postoperative treatment is the same with the following considerations.[125]

● The arm is kept elevated overhead in abduction and external rotation during the inflammatory reaction stage; treatment principles progress as with any joint lesion.

● Therapeutic exercises are initiated the same day while the patient is still in the recovery room, with emphasis on internal and external rotation in the 90° (or higher) abducted position.

● Joint mobilization procedures are used, particularly a caudal glide, to prevent readherence of the inferior capsular fold.

● When sleeping, the patient may be required to position the arm abducted for up to 3 weeks after manipulation.

## Acromioclavicular and Sternoclavicular Joints

### Related Pathologies and Etiology of Symptoms

***Overuse Syndromes.*** Overuse syndromes of the AC joint are frequently arthritic or post-traumatic conditions. The causes may be from repeated stressful movement of the joint with the arm at waist level, such as with grinding, packing assembly, and construction work,[67] or repeated diagonal extension, adduction, and internal rotation motions, as when spiking a volleyball or serving in tennis.

***Subluxations or Dislocations.*** Subluxations or dislocations of either joint are usually caused by falling against the shoulder or against an outstretched arm. In the AC joint, the distal end of the clavicle displaces posteriorly and superiorly on the acromion; the ligaments supporting the AC joint may rupture.[124] Clavicular fractures may result from the fall.[124] After trauma and associated overstretching of the capsules and ligaments of either joint, hypermobility is usually permanent because there is no muscle support to restrict movement.

***Hypomobility.*** Decreased clavicular mobility may occur with sustained faulty postures involving clavicular and scapular depression or retraction. Restricted mobility may contribute to a thoracic outlet syndrome (TOS) with a compromise of space for the neuromuscular bundle as it courses between the clavicle and first rib (described in Chapter 13).

### Common Impairments

- Pain localized to the involved joint or ligament
- Painful arc with shoulder elevation
- Pain with shoulder horizontal adduction or abduction
- Hypermobility in the joints if trauma or overuse is involved
- Hypomobility in the joints if sustained posture or immobility is involved
- Neurological or vascular symptoms if TOS is present

### Common Functional Limitations/Disabilities

- Limited ability to sustain repeated loaded movements related to forward/backward motions of the arm, such as with grinding, packing, assembly, and construction work.[67]
- Inability to reach overhead without pain.
- Inability to serve effectively at tennis or spike a volleyball.
- See also limitations/disabilities from TOS if present (see Chapter 13).

### Nonoperative Management of AC or SC Joint Strain or Hypermobility

- Rest the joint by putting the arm in a sling to support the weight of the arm.
- Cross-fiber massage to the capsule or ligaments.
- ROM to the shoulder and grade II traction and glides to the glenohumeral joint to prevent glenohumeral restriction.
- Instructions in self-application of cross-fiber massage if joint symptoms occur after excessive activity.

### Nonoperative Management of AC or SC Joint Hypomobility

Joint mobilization techniques are used to increase joint mobility (see Figs. 5.22 through 5.24).

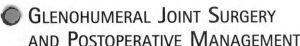

# GLENOHUMERAL JOINT SURGERY AND POSTOPERATIVE MANAGEMENT

Severe deterioration of one or both surfaces of the GH joint, causing significant pain and loss of upper extremity function, or an acute or nonunion fracture of the proximal humerus often must be addressed with surgical intervention. Underlying pathologies, causing advanced joint destruction, include late-stage osteoarthritis (OA), rheumatoid arthritis (RA), traumatic arthritis, cuff tear arthropathy, and osteonecrosis (avascular necrosis) of the head of the humerus as the result of a fracture of the anatomical neck of the humerus or long-term use of steroids for systemic disease.

The most common surgical procedure used to treat advanced shoulder joint pathology is *glenohumeral arthroplasty,* often simply referred to as *shoulder arthroplasty.*[36] In rare situations, *arthrodesis* (surgical ankylosis) of the GH joint may have to be selected as an alternative to arthroplasty or as a salvage procedure.[109]

The goals of these surgical procedures and postoperative rehabilitation are to (1) relieve pain, (2) improve shoulder mobility or stability, and (3) restore or improve strength and functional use of the upper extremity. The extent to which these goals are achieved is predicated on the patient's participation in postoperative rehabilitation, the distinguishing features and severity of the underlying pathology, the prosthetic design and surgical techniques, the integrity of the rotator cuff mechanism and other soft tissues, and the age, overall health, and anticipated activity level of the patient.[36,109,161,168]

## Glenohumeral Arthroplasty

Arthroplasty of the GH joint falls into several categories, the most common of which are *total shoulder replacement arthroplasty,*[109,119,161,168] in which the glenoid and humeral surfaces are replaced (Fig. 17.14), and *hemireplacement arthroplasty (hemiarthroplasty),* in which one surface, the humeral head, is replaced.[6,57,109,121,161] Other categories of shoulder arthroplasty include interpositional and resurfacing arthroplasties, which involve less extensive removal of bone.[109,161,168,182]

### Indications for Surgery

The following impairments associated with these pathologies are widely accepted indications for GH arthroplasty.*

- The primary indication is persistent and incapacitating pain (at rest or with activity) secondary to GH joint destruction.

---

*See references 6, 36, 47, 108, 109, 119, 121, 161, 168, 173, 174, 195.

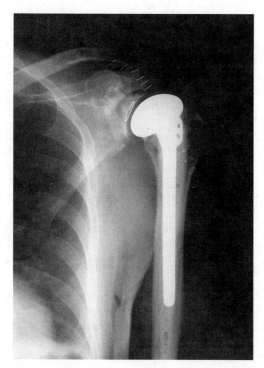

FIGURE 17.14 Postoperative anterior-posterior view of the shoulder showing a Neer II type of cemented humeral prosthesis and a nonmetal backed polyethylene glenoid. *(From Tovin, BJ, Greenfield, BH: Evaluation and Treatment of the Shoulder—An Integration of the Guide to Physical Therapist Practice. FA Davis, Philadelphia, 2001, p 266, with permission.)*

**Designs of Prosthetic Implants for Total Shoulder Replacement**

**Unconstrained**
- Anatomical design with a small, shallow glenoid component combined with a stemmed humeral component
- The most frequently used prosthetic design
- Provides the greatest freedom of shoulder motion but no inherent stability
- Indicated when the rotator cuff mechanism is intact or can be repaired to provide dynamic stability to the GH joint

**Semiconstrained**
- A larger glenoid component that is hooded or cup-shaped
- Some degree of joint stability inherent in the design
- Indicated when erosion of the glenoid fossa can be compensated for by reaming the fossa and rotator cuff function; although deficient preoperatively, can be improved by repair

**Reversed ball and socket**
- Small humeral socket that slides on a larger ball-shaped glenoid component
- Couples some degree of stability with mobility for rotator cuff-deficient shoulders that cannot be repaired
- Provides an alternative to standard semiconstrained and total shoulder replacement (TSR) and hemiarthroplasty

**Constrained**
- Fixed fulcrum, ball-in-socket designs with congruency of the glenoid and humeral components
- Greatest amount of inherent joint stability but less mobility than less constrained designs
- Once thought to be an alternative to hemiarthroplasty for the selected patient with a deficient rotator cuff or cuff tear arthropathy or chronic/recurrent GH joint dislocation after a previous TSR
- Rarely used today owing to high rate of loosening or failure of the components

⊙ Secondary indications include loss of shoulder mobility or stability and upper extremity strength leading to inability to perform functional tasks with the involved upper extremity.

## Procedures

### Background

***Implant design, materials, and fixation.*** Since the pioneering work of Neer during the 1960s and 1970s[119,121] and many other investigators,[28] prosthetic designs and surgical techniques for replacing the shoulder joint have continued to evolve. The designs of current-day total shoulder replacement (TSR), composed of a high-density polyethylene glenoid component (usually all plastic) and a modular humeral component made of an inert metal, closely approximate the biomechanical characteristics of the human shoulder.[206]

Fixation of the prosthetic components is achieved with a press fit, bio-ingrowth, or cement. The type of fixation selected by the surgeon depends on the component (glenoid or humeral), the underlying pathology, and the quality of the bone stock. Cement fixation is most often necessary in patients with osteoporosis.[†]

[†]See references 36, 108, 109, 173, 206.

The designs of total shoulder replacements, ranging from *unconstrained* to *semiconstrained* (including *reverse ball-and-socket*) to *constrained,* provide varying amounts of mobility and stability of the GH joint. Box 17.3 summarizes the characteristics of each of these designs.[36,108,109,159,161,168,182]

NOTE: The description of constrained designs is included in Box 17.3 for historical purposes and for a comparison with less constrained designs. Because of the high rate of complications that occurred with constrained designs, these implant systems are rarely, if ever, used today.[36,109]

***Selection of procedure.*** Controversy exists over the specific criteria for selection of TSR versus hemiarthroplasty, but in general it depends on the etiology and severity of the joint deterioration and the condition of the periarticular soft tissues, particularly the rotator cuff mechanism.[109,169] Several examples that follow underscore the complexity of the clinical decision-making process involved in the choice of operative procedure and prosthetic design.

In patients with late-stage primary OA, the most common pathology associated with shoulder arthroplasty, the GH joint typically exhibits loss or thinning or the articular cartilage of the head of the humerus and the posterior portion of the glenoid fossa. In addition, the rotator cuff is intact in approximately 90% to 95% of these patients, making them good candidates for either TSR or hemiarthroplasty.[36,108,139,159,161,168] However, opinions vary on whether selection of an unconstrained TSR yields results that are better than or equal to hemiarthroplasty for shoulders with these characteristics.[36,109,134,161,171]

Chronic synovitis, asssociated with RA and other types of synovium-based arthritis, tends to erode periarticular soft tissues in addition to the articular surfaces of a joint. As a consequence, a rupture or full-thickness tear of a rotator cuff tendon (typically the supraspinatus) develops in 25% to 40% of these patients and a rupture of the biceps tendon in an even greater percentage.[57,159,168,173,182] If the soft tissues can be repaired and their functions improved, a semiconstrained TSR (standard or possibly a reverse ball-and-socket design) that may include bone grafting at the glenoid to improve prosthetic fixation may be indicated. If an effective cuff repair cannot be achieved or if there is insufficient bone stock owing to osteoporosis for fixation of a glenoid implant, hemiarthroplasty is usually the procedure of choice.[57,109,159,161,169,173,182]

Hemiarthroplasty is often used when the articular surface and underlying bone of the humeral head have deteriorated but the glenoid fossa is reasonably intact, as seen with osteonecrosis of the head of the humerus.[36,109,168,169] A patient with severe, chronic pain and loss of function as the result of a massive, irreparable cuff tear and subsequent development of a *cuff tear arthropathy* is typically a candidate for hemiarthroplasty.[57,159,212] (The term "cuff tear arthropathy," first used by Neer, refers to deterioration and eventual collapse of the head of the humerus, an infrequent but debilitating long-term result of a primary, massive and irreparable tear of the rotator cuff.[109,159,195]) Chronic deficiency of the rotator cuff mechanism leads to superior migration of the head of the humerus in the glenoid fossa. If a glenoid component is inserted under these conditions, the superior migration creates an incongruous articulation that accentuates the risk of loosening and premature wear of the glenoid implant.[35,73,159]

### Operative Procedures

Total shoulder replacement and hemiarthroplasty are open surgical procedures performed with the patient in a semi-reclining position. The operative procedure involves the following components*: anterior approach using a deltopectoral incision that extends from the AC joint to the deltoid

---

*See references 6, 36, 57, 109, 161, 168.

insertion for adequate surgical exposure; release (tenotomy) of the subscapularis tendon from its proximal attachment on the lesser tuberosity; anterior capsulotomy; exposure of the humeral head for a humeral osteotomy; and preparation of the humeral canal for insertion of the prosthetic implant. The glenoid fossa is débrided and for a TSR is precisely contoured so the glenoid implant can be placed flush within the fossa.

Reconstruction and balancing of soft tissues is critical for optimal function after TSR and hemiarthroplasty. "Balancing" refers to the intraoperative lengthening or tightening of soft tissues to restore as near-normal resting tension in the tissues as possible, particularly in the rotator cuff, biceps, and deltoid muscle-tendon units.

Concomitant procedures that may be necessary during shoulder arthroplasty include:

- Repair of a deficient rotator cuff if the quality of the cuff tissue is sufficient
- Repair (reattachment) of the subscapularis and lengthening (medial advancement or Z-plasty) if a contracture significantly limits external rotation
- Capsular plication and tightening for chronic subluxation or dislocation (usually posterior) of the GH joint
- Anterior acromioplasty for a history of impingement syndrome
- Bone graft of the glenoid if bone stock is insufficient for fixation of the glenoid implant

After implantation of the prosthetic component(s) and repair of soft tissues but before closure of the skin incision, the shoulder is passively moved through all planes of motion to visually evaluate the stability of the prosthetic joint and the integrity of the repaired soft tissues. This determines the anatomical ROM possible after surgery and how aggressive the postoperative program can be.[36,109]

### Complications

Complications that can occur after a wide variety of orthopedic surgeries are summarized in Chapter 12 (see Box 12.6). Although the incidence of intraoperative and postoperative complications after current-day arthroplasty is low, even a single complication can adversely affect the functional outcome. The incidence of complications tends to be higher in patients with a deficient rotator cuff mechanism, osteoporosis, and a preoperative history of chronic GH joint instability.[72] Aside from medical complications, such as infection or a deep vein thrombosis, complications specific to shoulder arthroplasty are noted in Box 17.4.[35,72]

### Postoperative Management

N O T E : Effective patient education and close communication among the therapist, surgeon, and patient are the basis of an effective and safe rehabilitation program individualized to address the specific surgical procedures used to meet the unique needs of each patient.

### Special Considerations

*Integrity of the rotator cuff.* Regardless of the underlying cause of late-stage glenohumeral arthritis, the goals,

**Complications Specific to Glenohumeral Arthroplasty**

**Intraoperative**
- Insufficient lengthening of a tight subscapularis muscle-tendon unit
- Intraoperative damage to the axillary or suprascapular nerves, affecting the deltoid and supraspinatus/infraspinatus muscles, respectively
- Fracture of the humerus

**Soft Tissue-Related Postoperative Complications**
- Re-tearing a repaired rotator cuff mechanism
- Postoperative disruption of the repaired subscapularis (detached from the lesser tuberosity for the surgical approach and reattached medially on the cut surface of the neck of the humerus)
- Chronic instability of the GH joint
- Progressive erosion of the articular surface of the glenoid fossa (after hemiarthroplasty)

**Implant-Related Postoperative Complicatons**
- After TSR mechanical (aseptic) loosening or premature wear or fracture of the polyethylene glenoid implant
  - Most often seen in a rotator cuff-deficient shoulder
  - Due to excessive stresses at the bone–prosthesis interface
  - Low incidence with unconstrained designs but higher with early-generation constrained designs
- Loosening of the humeral prosthesis after hemiarthroplasy

components, and rate of progression of a rehabilitation program after TSR or hemiarthroplasty are influenced by the pre- and postoperative integrity of the rotator cuff mechanism. A deficient rotator cuff compromises the dynamic stability and kinematics of the GH joint, as demonstrated by upward riding of the humeral head leading to increased shear forces at the joint during active elevation of the arm.[43] The rehabilitation program for a patient with an intact rotator cuff prior to shoulder arthroplasty can be progressed more rapidly than the program for a patient with coexisting rotator cuff deficiency requiring a concomitant cuff–tendon repair at the time of shoulder arthroplasty. The postoperative program for a patient with an irreparable rotator cuff or a tenuous repair due to poor tendon quality must be progressed even more cautiously.[43,47,92,109,161,195]

If the rotator cuff was intact prior to surgery, the emphasis of postoperative rehabilitation is to restore shoulder mobility and functional use of the arm as soon as possible while protecting soft tissues as they heal. In contrast, with an irreparable rotator cuff, a tenuous repair, or a preoperative history of recurrent GH dislocation, rehabilitation must place greater emphasis on improving or maintaining joint stability for functional use of the arm than on increasing shoulder mobility.[43,47,51,92,109]

***Intraoperative ROM.*** In the operating room before closing the incision, the surgeon determines the extent of shoulder

ROM available, particularly elevation and external rotation, that does not place undue stress on periarticular soft tissues or compromise GH joint stability. Subsequent goals for safe, stable postoperative ROM are based on these measurements. For a patient with an unconstrained TSR and sufficient postoperative shoulder stability (static and dynamic), the goal at the conclusion of rehabilitation is to achieve active ROM equal to intraoperative ROM—ideally, 140° to 150° of shoulder elevation and 45° to 50° of external rotation.[43,109] For a patient with more constrained TSR, a deficient rotator cuff mechanism, or capsuloligamentous laxity, intraoperative ROM is typically less, and postoperative goals focus more on developing dynamic stability and less on shoulder mobility.

***Posture.*** Many patients undergoing shoulder arthroplasty are elderly. Therefore, the postural changes associated with aging[95] (increased thoracic kyphosis and scapular protraction) cause malalignment (excessive downward rotation) of the glenoid fossa, which predisposes the patient to shoulder impingement and pain particularly during overhead shoulder motions. Accordingly, it is important to emphasize an erect sitting or standing posture during elevation of the arm and to incorporate spinal extension and scapular retraction exercises into the postoperative program.

**Immobilization and Postoperative Positioning**
At the close of the surgical procedure the operated arm is placed in some type of shoulder immobilizer, usually a sling or sometimes a splint, to protect reattached and repaired soft tissues and for comfort.[6,36,109,159,168,174] Early postoperative positioning that protects the operated shoulder is detailed in Box 17.5.

Initially, the sling or splint is removed only for exercise and bathing. A patient who did not require repair of

**Positioning After Shoulder Arthroplasty: Early Postoperative (Maximum Protection) Phase**

**Supine**
- Arm immobilized in sling, which is worn continuously
  - Elbow flexed to 90°
  - Forearm and hand resting on abdomen
- Arm supported at the elbow on a folded blanket or pillow slightly away from the side and anterior to the midline of the trunk
  - Forward flexion (10° to 20°), slight abduction, and internal rotation of the shoulder
  - Head of bed elevated about 30°

**Sitting**
- Arm supported in sling or resting on a pillow in the patient's lap or on the armrest of a chair

**With Tenuous Rotator Cuff Repair**
- In some cases if a sling does not provide adequate protection of a repaired cuff, an abduction splint must be worn

the rotator cuff is weaned from the sling during the day as quickly as possible to prevent postoperative stiffness. However, a patient who underwent a cuff repair or other soft tissue reconstruction may need to wear a sling or splint while out in crowded areas or during sleep for approximately 4 to 6 weeks to protect the repaired tissues until sufficient healing has occurred.[23,26,36,43,47,48,92,109,174]

### Exercise

The guidelines for progression of exercises during each phase of rehabilitation after shoulder arthroplasty (TSR or hemiarthroplasty) presented in this section are drawn from the limited number of published protocols available, all of which are based on clinical experience rather than evidence from controlled studies and none of which has been shown to be more effective than another.[*] Also, almost all of these protocols are time-based, with few criteria reported for advancing a patient from one phase of rehabilitation to the next.

Recently, however, several resources have suggested such criteria.[37,47,195] Criteria from these resources are identified for the phases of rehabilitation after shoulder arthroplasty described below. It is important to note that these criteria and suggested timelines for progression of exercises and functional activities are typically adjusted for each patient based on periodic evaluations of the patient's status and ongoing communication between the therapist and the surgeon.

N O T E : The exercise guidelines in this section are for patients *without* preoperative rotator cuff deficiency and who *did not* undergo a cuff repair during TSR or hemiarthroplasty. For a complete picture, modifications in guidelines are noted throughout this section for patients with a poor quality rotator cuff mechanism. Remember, pain relief is the primary goal of shoulder arthroplasty, with improvement in functional mobility a secondary goal. Although improvements in surgical techniques and implant technology now allow more accelerated progression of postoperative rehabilitation than several decades ago, it is still important to proceed judiciously during each phase of rehabilitation to avoid excessive muscle fatigue or irritation or any damage of the healing soft tissues.

### Exercise: Maximum Protection Phase

The maximum protection phase of rehabilitation begins on the first postoperative day and extends for up to 6 weeks. The emphasis of this first phase is patient education, pain control, and initiation of ROM exercises to prevent adhesions and restore shoulder mobility as early as possible to the ranges achieved during surgery. Early motion is permissible after uncemented and cemented shoulder arthroplasty.

While the patient is hospitalized (usually for 3 to 4 days after surgery), patient education includes reviewing early postoperative precautions and teaching the initial exercises in the patient's home program. Precautions during the first 6 weeks after surgery, when protection of soft

---

*See references 23, 26, 37, 43, 47, 91, 92, 95, 109, 174, 195.

---

tissues as they heal is crucial, are summarized in Box 17.6. A patient's adherence to these precautions is of the utmost importance during this phase of rehabilitation.

***Goals and interventions.*** The first phase of rehabilitation includes the following.[23,26,37,43,47,48,91,92,109,174]

● *Control pain and inflammation.*
- Use of a sling or splint for comfort.
- Use of prescribed analgesic and anti-inflammatory medication.
- Use of cryotherapy, especially after exercise.

● *Maintain mobility of adjacent joints.*
- Active movements of the neck and scapula (while wearing the shoulder immobilizer and after it can be removed for exercise) to maintain normal motion and minimize muscle guarding and spasm. Incorporate "shoulder rolls" by elevating, adducting, and then relaxing the scapulae to reinforce an erect posture of the trunk. Emphasize active scapular retraction and spinal extension.
- Active ROM of the hand, wrist, and elbow when the arm can be removed from the sling.

● *Restore shoulder mobility.*
- Passive or therapist-assisted shoulder motions *within the safe limits determined during surgery*. With the patient lying supine and the arm slightly away from the side of the trunk on a folded towel and the elbow flexed, perform forward elevation of the arm in the plane of the scapula to tolerance, external rotation to no more than 30° to 45°, and internal rotation until the forearm rests on the chest.
- Pendulum (Codman's) exercises with the elbow flexed (for a shorter moment arm). Encourage the patient to periodically remove the sling and gently swing the arm during ambulation at home.
- Later during this phase, progress to *self-assisted* shoulder ROM (elevation and rotation) in the *supine position* initially by assisting with the sound hand and later using a wand or dowel rod. Add horizontal abduction to neutral and adduction across the chest holding a wand.
- Self-assisted shoulder ROM in a *sitting* position or *standing* with a wand by performing "gear shift" exercises (see Fig. 17.23), resting the arm on a table and sliding it forward (see Fig. 17.25), or use of an overhead rope-pulley system to lessen the weight of the arm. Remind the patient to maintain an erect trunk when performing assisted shoulder motions while seated or standing.
- Self-assisted reaching movements (to the nose, forehead, or over the head as comfort allows) to simulate functional movements.
- In selected patients, transition to *active* (unassisted) shoulder ROM is often possible by 4 weeks.
- Functional activities with the elbow at waist level, such as hand to face and writing, are permissible.

● *Minimize muscle inhibition, guarding, and atrophy.*
- Gentle muscle-setting of shoulder musculature (excluding the internal rotators) with the elbow flexed and the shoulder in the plane of the scapula or neutral. Teach these exercises prior to discharge from the hospital by having the patient practice isometrically contracting the muscles of the *sound* shoulder. Postpone setting exercises (light isometrics) of the operated shoulder until about 4 to 6 weeks after surgery.

- Scapular stabilization exercises in non-weight-bearing positions. Target the serratus anterior and trapezius muscles.

NOTE: For a patient who underwent repair of a large tear or rupture of a rotator cuff tendon or other soft tissue reconstruction, it may not be permissible to begin ROM exercises immediately after surgery. When the sling or splint can be removed for exercise, perform only passive or assisted ROM throughout the first phase of rehabilitation. The range of shoulder elevation and external rotation initially permitted may be less than for shoulders that did not require cuff repair. Postpone active (unassisted), antigravity ROM and light isometrics until the next phase (until about 6 weeks postoperatively, when repaired soft tissues are reasonably well healed).

**Exercise: Moderate Protection/Controlled Motion Phase**
Although suggested timelines vary from one resource to another, the moderate protection/controlled motion phase of rehabilitation, which typically begins at about 4 to 6 weeks and extends to at least 12 to 16 weeks or longer postoperatively, focuses on gradually establishing active (unassisted) control, dynamic stability, and strength of the shoulder while continuing to increase ROM.[23,26,43,47,91,92,109,174,195]

*Criteria for progression.* Criteria to advance to the second phase of rehabilitation are:

● ROM: At least 90° of passive elevation, at least 45° degrees of external rotation, and 70° of internal rotation in the plane of the scapula with minimal pain[195] or *almost* full, passive shoulder motion based on intraoperative measurements with little to no pain.[37,92]
● When testing the subscapularis, no tendon pain during resisted, isometric internal rotation.[37]
● Ability to perform most waist-level activities of daily living (ADLs) without pain.[92]

PRECAUTIONS: During this phase of rehabilitation, although it is safe to place increasing stresses (stretching or resistance) on periarticular soft tissues, it is important to do so gradually so as not to irritate these tissues, which are continuing to heal. Therefore, continue with short but frequent exercise sessions (preceded by application of heat and followed by cold) and avoid vigorous stretching or resistance exercises or overuse of the involved shoulder during functional activities.

*Goals and interventions.* The goals and exercises for this next phase of rehabilitation are as follows.

● *Continue to increase passive ROM of the shoulder.*
- Transition from passive or assisted ROM to low-*intensity, pain-free* stretching in all anatomical and diagonal planes of motion to achieve full, intraoperative ROM.
- Gentle joint mobilization techniques for specific capsular restriction.

- To increase shoulder elevation: arm-sliding exercises on the surface of a table and wall-climbing exercises, emphasizing overhead reaching.
- To increase external rotation: With the arm at the side, elbow flexed to 90°, and grasping a doorframe, rotate the trunk away from the involved arm.
- To increase shoulder extension and internal rotation: Add wand exercises behind the back. (This exercise also involves scapular winging and tipping, both necessary for reaching behind the back.)
- To increase horizontal adduction: Cross-body stretch with arm at shoulder level.

◉ ***Develop active control and dynamic stability and improve muscle performance (strength and endurance) of the shoulder.***
- Continue or gradually transition to *active* shoulder ROM exercises, avoiding antigravity abduction until the patient can initiate the movement without first shrugging the operated shoulder.
- Scapular and GH joint stabilization exercises (alternating isometrics and rhythmic stabilization) in a variety of positions initially in non-weight-bearing positions, progresing to light weight bearing.
- Pain-free, low-intensity (submaximal) resisted isometrics of shoulder muscles, including the subscapularis or any other repaired muscle-tendon units.
- Dynamic resistance exercises for the scapula and shoulder musculature (from 0° to 90° of shoulder elevation) using light weights or light-grade elastic resistance. Begin in the supine position to support and stabilize the scapula. Progress to the sitting position. Place emphasis on improving control of the rotator cuff to prevent superior translation of the humerus during shoulder elevation.[166]
- Upper extremity ergometry with stationary ergometer or a portable reciprocal exerciser on a table. Emphasize progressive repetitions to increase muscular endurance.

### Exercise: Minimum Protection/ Return to Functional Activity Phase

The minimum protection/return to functional activity phase usually begins around 12 to 16 weeks postoperatively (depending on rotator cuff tissue quality and function) and typically extends for several more months.[47,92,195] There is a continued effort during this phase to restore full, active ROM for functional activities so long as there is adequate stability of the GH joint. Consequently, pain-free strengthening of the shoulder girdle for dynamic stability and functional use of the upper extremity for progressively more demanding tasks is the primary focus of this phase. For optimal results, the home exercise program may need to be continued for 6 months or longer, and functional and recreational activities may need to be modified.

***Criteria for progression***. To advance to the final phase of rehabilitation and gradually return to necessary and desired functional activities, a patient should meet the following criteria.

◉ Full, passive ROM of the shoulder (based on intraoperative ranges)[37,92] or at least 130° to 140° of pain-free, passive or assisted shoulder flexion and 120° of abduction.[195]
◉ In the plane of the scapula, at least 60° pain-free, passive external rotation and 70° internal rotation.[195]
◉ Active (unassisted), antigravity elevation of the arm to at least 100° to 120° in the plane of the scapula while maintaining joint stability and using appropriate shoulder mechanics, particularly no shoulder shrugging prior to elevating the arm.[195]
◉ Strength of rotator cuff and deltoid muscles: 4/5.[47,92]

***Goals and interventions***. Goals and activities for the final phase of rehabilitation include the following.[23,26,37,47,48,91,92,195]

◉ ***Continue to improve or maintain shoulder mobility.***
- End-range self-stretching.
- Grade III joint mobilization and self-mobilization, if appropriate.[23,26,37,92]

◉ ***Continue to improve active control and muscle performance of the shoulder.***
- Pain-free, low-load, high-repetition progressive resistive exercise (PRE) of shoulder musculature in anatomical and diagonal planes and in patterns of movement that replicate functional tasks throughout the available ROM. Position the patient in a variety of gravity-resisted positions.
- Closed-chain, resisted shoulder exercises, gradually increasing weight bearing through the upper extremity.
- Use of the involved upper extremity for lifting, carrying, pushing, or pulling activities against increasing loads.

◉ ***Return to most functional activities.***
- Use of the operated upper extremity for progressively more advanced functional activities.
- Recreational activities, such as swimming and golf are possible.
- Modification of high-demand, high-impact work-related or recreational activities to avoid imposing excessive forces on the GH joint that could lead to loosening or premature wear of prosthetic implants.

N O T E : For the patient whose rotator cuff was irreparable or continues to be significantly deficient because of a tenuous repair and who has limited but pain-free shoulder ROM, modification of the environment and use of assistive devices may be necessary for independence in functional activities.

### Outcomes

Over the past 30 years, as patient selection criteria, prosthetic designs, and surgical techniques have been refined, postoperative outcomes after shoulder arthroplasty have improved. As noted at the beginning of this section on glenohumeral arthroplasty, numerous resources suggest that outcomes after TSR or hemiarthroplasty are influenced by many factors, including the type and severity of the underlying pathology, the status of soft tissues (especially the rotator cuff mechanism and subscapularis), the type and quality of the surgical procedure(s) performed, and patient-related factors, such as participation in a postoperative rehabilitation program.[32,36,195] The outcomes most often measured in follow-up studies using a variety of quantitative scales are pain relief and other paramenters of quality of life, passive and active shoulder ROM, and the ability to perform functional activities.

Despite the emphasis in numerous resources that a patient's participation in postoperative rehabilitation is crucial for successful outcomes, there are no studies to support this opinion because all patients undergoing shoulder arthroplasty are given some form of postoperative exercise instruction. Furthermore, published protocols are routinely modified to meet the needs of individual patients and consequently have not been compared to determine if one protocol yields better outomes than another.[195]

*Pain relief.* A decrease in pain is the most dramatic result of glenohumeral arthroplasty. Almost all patients—regardless of the underlying pathology, the type of arthroplasty (TSR or hemireplacement), or the design of the prosthetic implants—report complete or substantial relief of shoulder pain and improved functional use of the arm.[36,108,109,117,119,121,130,134,171]

The extent of pain relief has been shown to be associated with the underlying cause(s) of glenohumeral arthritis. Neer et al.,[119] Matsen,[108] and more recently Norris and Iannotti[130] reported that 90% of patients with primary OA or osteonecrosis had complete or near-complete pain relief after TSR. Similar results have been reported for patients with OA who underwent hemi-arthroplasty.[101,109,121] Patients with RA or other synovium-based diseases also report substantial pain relief after TSR or hemiarthroplasty, although not quite to the extent reported by patients with OA or osteonecrosis.[36,159,182]

Whether TSR is more effective than hemiarthroplasty for pain relief has also been studied. In a prospective follow-up study over a mean of 4.3 years when patients with OA having TSR were compared to those having hemiarthroplasty, postoperative pain scores were reported to be similar in the two groups, with patients in the TSR group demonstrating more improvement because of a higher level of pain preoperatively.[134] In another study, patients with OA were randomly assigned to undergo either TSR or hemiarthroplasty and were evaluated postoperatively over a 24-month period. Results of this study indicated that both groups of patients reported significant pain relief and improvements in other quality-of-life parameters, with no significant differences between the TSR and hemiarthroplasty groups.[101] Whether TSR versus hemiarthroplasty is more effective for pain relief in patients with RA has not been clearly established.[109,182]

*ROM and functional use of the upper extremity.* Despite the emphasis placed on improving ROM and use of the arm for function activities during rehabilitation after shoulder arthroplasty, improvements in these outcomes are less predictable than pain relief, with the functional status improving more consistently than ROM.* In general, patients with primary OA or osteonecrosis demonstrate greater improvement in active ROM (forward elevation and shoulder rotation) than patients with RA, in part because of a higher incidence of cuff deficiency asociated with RA or the use of more constrained prosthetic designs.[159,182,195] For example, in patients with OA or osteonecrosis, the mean active forward elevation of the shoulder (reported in reviews of a number of studies) changed from 105° to 161°. In patients with RA means ranged from 75° to 105°.[171,195]

Significant improvement in functional status has been reported for patients with OA or osteonecrosis. Although functional improvement after arthroplasty has been reported for patients with RA, many studies used nonstandardized measurement tools, making it difficult to compare their results with those of other studies.[195] Regardless of the underlying pathology, resources agree that a well functioning rotator cuff mechanism is the basis for significant postoperative gains in active ROM and functional abilities.[36,168,195]

## Arthrodesis of the Shoulder

### Indications for Surgery
The following are generally accepted indications for arthrodesis of the GH joint.[109,145,146,196]

- Incapacitating pain (at rest or with movement)
- Gross instability of the GH joint
- Complete paralysis of the deltoid and rotator cuff muscles
- Severe joint destruction due to infection
- Failed shoulder arthroplasty in a young, active patient who is not a candidate for revision arthroplasty
- Sufficient compensatory scapular motion and strength of the serratus anterior and trapezius muscles

### Procedure
The GH joint is fused with pins and bone grafts in a position of 15° to 30° flexion and abduction and up to 30° to 45° internal rotation so the hand can reach the middle of the body or the mouth.[109,145,146,174,196] The shoulder is immobilized in a shoulder spica cast or a thoracobrachial (airplane) splint that extends across the elbow joint. The immobilizer is worn for 3 to 5 months.

### Postoperative Management
Place emphasis on maintaining mobility of peripheral joints (wrist and hand) while the shoulder and elbow are immobilized. If a splint with a hinged elbow joint is used, begin elbow flexion and extension when permis-

*See references 57, 109, 130, 134, 161, 171, 195.

sible, often as early as the day after surgery. After the immobilization device may be removed for exercise, begin active scapulothoracic ROM. Strengthen the scapulothoracic musculature to maximize control and stability of the scapula.

### Outcomes

A patient may expect to achieve 90° to 130° of active elevation of the arm because of scapulothoracic mobility.[109,145,146,196] After bony and soft tissue healing is complete, the shoulder is stable and pain-free for activities that require strength or weight bearing at the shoulder. Patients are able to bring the hand to the mouth, behind the head, and to the hip.[145,174,196] Over time, excessive stress may be placed on the AC joint, resulting in AC joint hypermobility and pain.[145,146,174]

## PAINFUL SHOULDER SYNDROMES (ROTATOR CUFF DISEASE, IMPINGEMENT SYNDROMES, SHOULDER INSTABILITIES): NONOPERATIVE MANAGEMENT

Mechanical compression and irritation of the soft tissues (rotator cuff and subacromial bursa) in the suprahumeral space (see Fig. 17.7) is called *impingement syndrome* and is the most common cause of shoulder pain.[99,105] Various etiologic factors have been identified and therefore have led to several classification systems, which are summarized in Box 17.7.

### Related Pathologies and Etiology of Symptoms

The cause of impingement is multifactoral, involving both structural and mechanical impairments. Impingement syndrome is often used as the diagnosis when the patient's signs and symptoms are related to pain with overhead reaching, a painful arc mid-range, and positive impingement tests. Other test results may more specifically identify the tissue involved, the faulty mechanics associated with the condition, or the degree of instability or injury. Symptoms that derive from impingement are usually brought on with excessive or repetitive overhead activities that load the shoulder joint, particularly in the mid-range. Impingement syndromes are generally classified as *primary* or *secondary*.

Other types of musculotendinous strain in the shoulder region may result from overuse or trauma, such as in the anterior pectoral region from racket sports or in the long head of the triceps and serratus anterior from impact trauma such as holding onto a steering wheel in an automobile accident.

---

### BOX 17.7 Categories of Painful Shoulder Syndromes

*Impingement syndromes and other painful shoulder conditions have varying etiologic factors and therefore can be categorized several ways.*

**Based on Degree or Stage of Pathology of the Rotator Cuff (Neer's Classification of Rotator Cuff Disease)[118]**
- *Stage I.* Edema, hemorrhage (patient usually < 25 years of age)
- *Stage II.* Tendinitis/bursitis and fibrosis (patient usually 25 to 40 years of age)
- *Stage III.* Bone spurs and tendon rupture (patient usually > 40 years of age)

**Based on Impaired Tissue[41]**
- Supraspinatus tendinitis
- Infraspinatus tendinitis
- Bicipital tendinitis
- Subdeltoid (subacromial) bursitis
- Other musculotendinous strains (specific to type of injury or trauma)
  - Anterior—from overuse with racket sports (pectoralis minor, subscapularis, coracobrachialis, short head of biceps strain)
  - Inferior—from motor vehicle trauma (long head of triceps, serratus anterior strain)

**Based on Mechanical Disruption and Direction of Instability or Subluxation**
- Multidirectional instability from lax capsule with or without impingement
- Unidirectional instability (anterior, posterior, or inferior) with or without impingement
  - Traumatic injury with tears of capsule and/or labrum
  - Insidious (atraumatic) onset from repetitive microtrauma
  - Inherent laxity

**Based on Progressive Microtrauma (Jobe's classification)[88]**
- *Group 1.* Pure impingement (usually in an older recreational athlete with partial undersurface rotator cuff tear and subacromial bursitis)
- *Group 2.* Impingement associated with labral and/or capsular injury, instability, and secondary impingement
- *Group 3.* Hyperelastic soft tissues resulting in anterior or multidirectional instability and impingement (usually attenuated but intact labrum, undersurface rotator cuff tear)
- *Group 4.* Anterior instability without associated impingement (result of trauma; results in partial or complete dislocation)

**Based on Degree and Frequency**
- Instability → subluxation → dislocation
- Acute, recurrent, fixed

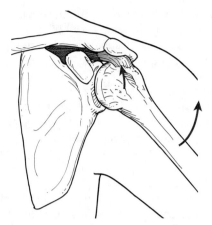

FIGURE 17.15 Decrease in the suprahumeral space during repetitive elevation activities lead to symptoms of impingement.

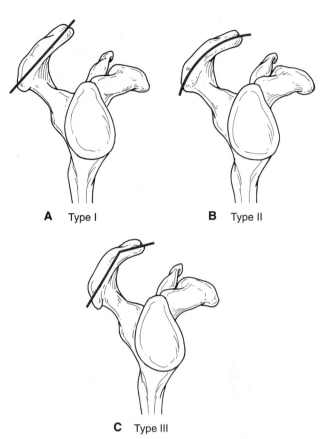

**A** Type I   **B** Type II

**C** Type III

FIGURE 17.16 Classifications of the acromion by shape: (*A*) type I (flat); (*B*) type II (curved); (*C*) type III (hooked).

## Primary Impingement—Rotator Cuff Disease

Primary impingement is believed to occur as a result of mechanical wear of the rotator cuff against the anteroinferior one-third of the acromion in the suprahumeral space during elevation activities of the humerus (Fig. 17.15). Encroachment may be the result of *intrinsic* or *extrinsic* factors.

*Intrinsic factors.* Intrinsic factors are those that are directly associated with encroachment of the subacromial space. They include vascular changes in the rotator cuff tendons, structural variations in the acromion, hypertrophic degenerative changes of the AC joint, or other trophic changes in the coracoacromial arch or humeral head. All of these factors decrease the suprahumeral space and often have to be dealt with surgically.[58,82,149]

Neer[120] first suggested that in patients undergoing surgery for impingement syndrome the size and shape of the structures that make up the coricoacromial arch are related to rotator cuff impingement. In later studies variations in the shape and thickness of the acromion were identified and classified. One such classification, based on the shape of the anteroinferior aspect of the acromion, identified three shapes: type I (flat), type II (curved), and type III (hooked) (Fig. 17.16). Rotator cuff pathology is often associated with type II and III, but not type I, acromial shapes.[1,115]

*Extrinsic factors.* Factors that result in decreased suprahumeral space and repetitive trauma to the soft tissues during elevation of the arm include posterior capsular tightness, poor neuromuscular control of the rotator cuff or scapular muscles, faulty scapulothoracic posture with muscle imbalances, or a partial or complete tear of the tissues in the suprahumeral space (incurred during a traumatic or degenerative situation).[74,99,103,105,118,167]

Neer described three pathological stages of impingement that demonstrate the potentially progressive nature of the pathology over time (see Box 17.7).[118] Other authors have identified chronic inflammation, possibly due to repetitive microtrauma in the joint region, as a stimulus for the development of frozen shoulder.[66,122,125]

### Tendinitis/Bursitis

Neer identified tendinitis/bursitis as a stage II impingement syndrome (see Box 17.7). The following sections describe specific pathological diagnoses and presenting signs and symptoms.

*Supraspinatus tendinitis.* With supraspinatus tendinitis, the lesion is usually near the musculotendinous junction, resulting in a painful arc with overhead reaching. Pain occurs with the impingement test (forced humeral elevation in the plane of the scapula while the scapula is passively stabilized so the greater tuberosity impacts against the acromion[74,118] or with the arm in internal rotation while flexing the humerus).[74] There is pain on palpation of the tendon just inferior to the anterior aspect of the acromion when the patient's hand is placed behind the back. It is difficult to differentiate tendinitis from subdeltoid bursitis because of the anatomical proximity.

*Infraspinatus tendinitis.* With infraspinatus tendinitis, the lesion is usually near the musculotendinous junction, resulting in a painful arc with overhead or forward motions. It may present as a deceleration (eccentric) injury due to overload during repetitive or forceful throwing activities. Pain occurs with palpation of the tendon just inferior to the posterior corner of the acromion when the patient horizontally adducts and laterally rotates the humerus.

***Bicipital tendinitis.*** With bicipital tendinitis, the lesion involves the long tendon in the bicipital groove beneath or just distal to the transverse humeral ligament. Swelling in the bony groove is restrictive and compounds and perpetuates the problem. Pain occurs with resistance to the forearm in a supinated position while the shoulder is flexing (Speed's sign) and on palpation of the bicipital groove.[106] Rupture or dislocation of this humeral depressor may escalate impingement of tissues in the suprahumeral space.[118,126]

***Bursitis (subdeltoid or subacromial).*** When acute, the symptoms of bursitis are the same as those seen with supraspinatus tendinitis. Once the inflammation is under control, there are no symptoms with resistance.

### Other Impaired Musculotendinous Tissues
The following are examples of other musculotendinous problems in the shoulder region.

◉ The pectoralis minor, short head of the biceps, and coracobrachialis are subject to microtrauma, particularly in racket sports requiring a controlled backward then a rapid forward swinging of the arm, as are the scapular stabilizers as they function to control forward motion of the scapula.[100]
◉ The long head of the triceps and scapular stabilizers are often injured in motor vehicle accidents as the driver holds firmly to the steering wheel on impact.
◉ A fall on an outstretched hand or against the shoulder may also cause trauma to the scapular stabilizers, which, if not properly healed, continue to cause symptoms whenever using the arm or when maintaining a shoulder posture.
◉ Injury, overuse, or repetitive trauma can occur in any muscle being subjected to stress.[129] Pain occurs when the involved muscle is placed on a stretch or when contracting against resistance. Palpating the site of the lesion causes the familiar pain.

### Secondary impingement—Shoulder Instability/Subluxation
Secondary impingement is used to describe symptoms resulting from faulty mechanics due to hypermobility or instability of the GH joint with increased translation of the humeral head. The instability may be *multidirectional* or *unidirectional*.

***Multidirectional instability.*** Some individuals have physiologically lax connective tissue causing excessive mobility in the joints of the body. In the GH joint, the humeral head translates to a greater degree than normal in all directions.[133,160,178] Many individuals, particularly those

involved in overhead throwing or lifting activities, have some inherent laxity or develop laxity of the capsule and instability from continually subjecting the joint to stretch forces.[58,88] A hypermobile joint may be satisfactorily supported by strong rotator cuff muscles; but once the muscles fatigue, poor humeral head stabilization leads to faulty humeral mechanics, trauma, and inflammation of the suprahumeral tissues.[88,114] This trauma is magnified with the rapidity of control demanded in the overhead throwing action.[58] Similarly, in individuals with poor rotator cuff muscle strength and function, the ligaments become stressed with repetitive use and hypermobility, resulting in impingement. With instability, the impingement of tissue in the suprahumeral space is the secondary effect.[58]

Hypermobility can cause problems in addition to impingement, such as subluxation, dislocation, or rotator cuff tendinitis, which with repetitive microtrauma can lead to degenerative changes including bone spurs, tendon rupture, or capsular restrictions and frozen shoulder. Jobe developed a classification system incorporating the progression of impingement and instability in the overhead athlete based on progressive microtrauma[88] (outlined in Box 17.7).

***Unidirectional instability with or without impingement.*** Unidirectional instability (anterior, posterior, or inferior) may be the result of physiologically lax connective tissue but is usually the result of trauma and usually involves rotator cuff tears. The tears can be classified as acute, chronic, degenerative, or partial- or full-thickness tears. Often there is damage to the glenoid labrum and tearing of some of the supporting ligaments.

***Traumatic tears or paralysis.*** Partial-thickness tears or full avulsion of the greater tubercle may occur in the elderly as the result of falling on an outstretched arm.[123] In young patients, trauma is usually associated with capsular injury, with or without labrum injury, resulting in instability. Dislocation of the humerus may occur with ensuing instability. The instability can lead to progressive degeneration and eventually tears in the supporting structures. Tears are associated with pain and most commonly weakness of shoulder abduction and external rotation.

◉ *Anterior instability* usually occurs with force against the arm when it is in an abducted and externally rotated position, and it frequently involves detachment of the anterior capsule and glenoid labrum (Bankart lesion). There may also be a fractured piece or flattening of the anterior lip of the glenoid.[68] Positive signs include apprehension, load and shift, and anterior drawer tests.[106,201]
◉ *Posterior instability* is the result of a forceful thrust against a forward-flexed humerus or fall on an outstretched arm. There is a positive posterior drawer sign.[106,201]
◉ *Inferior instability* is the result of rotator cuff weakness/paralysis and is frequently seen in patients with hemiplegia.[64] It is also prevalent in patients with multidirectional instability. This is detected with a positive sulcus sign.[106,201]

*Insidious (atraumatic) onset.* Neer has identified rotator cuff tears as a stage III impingement syndrome, a condition that typically occurs in persons over age 40 after repetitive microtrauma to the rotator cuff or long head of the biceps.[118] With aging, the distal portion of the supraspinatus tendon is particularly vulnerable to impingement or stress from overuse strain. With degenerative changes, calcification and eventual tendon rupture may occur.[58,132] Chronic ischemia caused by tension on the tendon and decreased healing in the elderly are possible explanations, although Neer stated that, in his experience, 95% of tears are initiated by impingement wear rather than by impaired circulation or trauma.[118]

## Common Impairments

Various impairments have been reported to be common in impingement syndromes, although it is not known if they are the cause or effect of the faulty mechanics.[31,103,105,135,192] A thorough examination of the cervical spine and shoulder girdle is necessary to differentiate signs and symptoms related to primary and secondary impingements or other causes of shoulder pain.[22,46,106]

### Impaired Posture and Muscle Imbalances
Increased thoracic kyphosis, forward head, abducted and forward-tipped scapula are often identified as related to impingement syndrome. Faulty scapular alignment may be one factor in decreasing the suprahumeral space and therefore leading to irritation of the rotator cuff tendons with overhead activities.[103] Faulty upper quadrant posture leads to an imbalance in the length and strength of the scapular and GH musculature and decreases the effectiveness of the dynamic and passive stabilizing structures of the GH joint.[202]

Typically with increased thoracic kyphosis, the scapula is protracted and tipped forward, and the GH joint is in an internally rotated posture. With this posture, the pectoralis minor, levator scapulae, and shoulder internal rotators are tight; and the lateral rotators of the shoulder and upward rotators of the scapula test weak and have poor muscular endurance. There is no longer the stabilizing tension on the superior joint capsule and coracohumeral ligament or compressive forces from the rotator cuff muscles. Consequently, the effect of gravity tends to cause an inferior force on the humerus. When reaching overhead, there is faulty scapular and humeral mechanics, resulting in faulty alignment of the scapula and altered function in the muscles controlling the scapula and GH joint.

### ⊙ Focus on Evidence

In a study which examined the kinematics of 52 subjects (26 without shoulder impairment and 26 with shoulder impingement), Ludewig and Cook[103] documented delayed upward rotation of the scapula during the 31° to 60° range of humeral elevation, incomplete backward tipping of the scapula, and excessive scapular elevation in individuals with impingement compared with those without shoulder impairments. This mechanical alteration may contribute to decreased clearance under the anterior acromion. They also documented decreased activation of the lower serratus anterior and overuse of the upper trapezius with scapular elevation, which was suggested as a possible compensation for the weak posterior tipping action of the serratus anterior.[103]

### Decreased Thoracic ROM
Thoracic extension is a component motion that is needed for full overhead reaching. Incomplete thoracic extension decreases the functional range of humeral elevation.

### Rotator Cuff Overuse and Fatigue
If the rotator cuff musculature or long head of the biceps fatigue from overuse, they no longer provide the dynamic stabilizing, compressive, and translational forces that support the joint and control the normal joint mechanics. This is thought to be a precipitating factor in secondary impingement syndromes when there is capsular laxity and increased need for muscular stability.[137] The tissues in the subacromial space may then become impinged as a result of faulty mechanics. There is also a relationship between muscle fatigue and joint position sense in the shoulder that may play a role in impaired performance in repetitive overhead activities.[33]

### Muscle Weakness Secondary to Neuropathy
Muscle weakness may be related to nerve involvement. Long thoracic nerve palsy has been identified as a cause of faulty scapular mechanics resulting from serratus anterior muscle weakness, leading to impingement in the suprahumeral region.[163]

### Hypomobile Posterior GH Joint Capsule
Tightness in the posterior GH joint capsule compromises the normal arthrokinematics and increases forces on the head of the humerus against the anterior capsule. Harryman et al.[69] demonstrated increased anterior translation in the humeral head when there is a tight posterior capsule.

### Summary of Common Impairments with Rotator Cuff Disease and Impingement Syndromes
Some, all, or none of the following may be present.

- Pain at the musculotendinous junction of the involved muscle with palpation, with resisted muscle contraction, and when stretched
- Positive impingement sign (forced internal rotation at 90° of flexion) and painful arc
- Impaired posture: thoracic kyphosis, forward head, and forward (anterior) tipped scapula with decreased thoracic mobility
- Muscle imbalances: hypomobile pectoralis major and minor, levator scapulae, and internal rotators of the GH joint; weak serratus anterior and lateral rotators
- Hypomobile posterior GH joint capsule
- Faulty kinematics with humeral elevation: decreased posterior tipping of scapula related to weak serratus anterior; scapular elevation and overuse of upper trapezius; and uncoordinated scapulohumeral rhythm

◎ With a complete rotator cuff tear, inability to abduct the humerus against gravity
◎ When acute, pain referred to the C5 and C6 reference zones

## Common Functional Limitations/Disabilities

◎ When acute, pain may interfere with sleep, particularly when rolling onto the involved shoulder.
◎ Pain with overhead reaching, pushing, or pulling.
◎ Difficulty lifting loads.
◎ Inability to sustain repetitive shoulder activities (such as reaching, lifting, throwing, pushing, pulling, or swinging the arm).
◎ Difficulty with dressing, particularly putting a shirt on over the head.

## Management: Painful Shoulder Syndromes (Without Dislocation)

N O T E : Even though symptoms may be "chronic" in terms of long standing or recurring, if there is inflammation the initial treatment priority is to get the inflammation under control.

### Management: Protection Phase

#### Control Inflammation and Promote Healing

◎ Modalities and low-intensity cross-fiber massage are applied to the site of the lesion. While applying the modalities, position the extremity to maximally expose the involved region.[42,45]
◎ Support the arm in a sling for rest.

#### Patient Education
The environment and habits that provoke the symptoms must be modified or avoided completely during this stage. The patient should be informed about the mechanics of the irritation and given guidelines for anticipated recovery with compliance.

#### Maintain Integrity and Mobility of the Soft Tissues

◎ Passive, active-assistive, or self-assisted ROM is initiated in pain-free ranges.
◎ Multiple-angle muscle setting and protected stabilization exercises are initiated. Of particular importance in the shoulder is to stimulate the stabilizing function of the rotator cuff, biceps brachii, and scapular muscles at an intensity tolerated by the patient.

P R E C A U T I O N : It is important to use caution with exercises during this stage to avoid the impingement positions. Often the mid-range of abduction, scaption with internal rotation, or an end-range position when the involved muscle is on a stretch (such as putting the hand behind the back) provokes a painful response.

#### Control Pain and Maintain Joint Integrity
Pendulum exercises without weights can be used to cause pain-inhibiting grade II joint distraction and oscillation motions (see Fig. 17.22 in the section on exercise).

### Develop Support in Related Regions
◎ Postural awareness and correction techniques are used. (See related information on interventions for impaired posture in Chapter 14.)
◎ Supportive techniques such as shoulder strapping or scapular taping, tactile cues, and mirrors can be used for reinforcement. Repetitive reminders and practice of correct posture is necessary throughout the day.

### Management: Controlled Motion Phase
Once the acute symptoms are under control, the main emphasis becomes use of the involved region with progressive, nondestructive movement and proper mechanics while the tissues heal. The components of the desired functions are analyzed and initiated in a controlled exercise program.[44,45,90,198,199] If there is a functional laxity in the joint, the intervention is directed toward learning neuromuscular control of and developing strength in the stabilizing muscles of both the scapula and glenohumeral joint.[29,90,93,162,181] If there is restricted mobility that prevents normal mechanics or interferes with function, mobilization of the restricted tissue is performed. Exercise techniques and progressions are described later in the chapter.

#### Patient Education
Patient adherence with the program and avoidance of irritating the healing tissues are necessary. The home exercise program is progressed as the patient learns safe and effective execution of each exercise.

#### Develop a Strong, Mobile Scar

◎ Manual therapy techniques such as cross-fiber or friction massage are used. The extremity is positioned so the tissue is on a stretch if it is a tendon or in the shortened position if it is in the muscle belly. The technique is applied to the tolerance of the patient.
◎ Following massage, the patient is instructed to perform an isometric contraction of the muscle in several positions of the range. The intensity of contraction should not cause pain.
◎ The patient should be taught how to self-administer the massage and isometric techniques.

#### Improve Postural Awareness
It is important to continue to reinforce proper postural habits. Tactile and verbal cues are used to increase patient awareness of scapular and cervical posture every time an exercise is performed, such as touching the scapular adductors and chin and reminding the patient to "pull the shoulders back" and "lift the head" while doing the shoulder exercises.

 **Focus on Evidence** _____

In a random placebo-controlled, crossover study of 120 subjects (60 with impingement and 60 without symptoms), changing posture resulted in a significant increase in ROM in flexion, abduction, and scaption; and the point in the range where symptoms were felt was significantly higher.

Thoracic and scapular taping had a positive influence in modifying posture; there was less forward head posture, smaller kyphosis, less lateral scapular displacement, less elevated and forward scapula position, and increased pain-free range of scaption compared with the measurements taken after placebo taping in both the symptomatic and asymptomatic groups.[99]

### Modify Joint Tracking and Mobility

Mobilization with movement (MWM) may be useful for modifying joint tracking and reinforcing full movement when there is painful restriction of shoulder elevation because of a painful arc or impingement[116] (see Chapter 5 for a description of principles).

● Posterolateral glide with active elevation (Fig. 17.17A)
*Patient position*: Sitting with the arm by the side and head in neutral retraction.
*Therapist position and procedure*: Stand on the side opposite the affected arm and reach across the patient's torso to stabilize the scapula with the palm of one hand. The other hand is placed over the anteromedial aspect of the head of the humerus. Apply a graded posterolateral glide of the humeral head on the glenoid. Request that the patient perform the previously painful elevation. Maintain the posterolateral glide mobilization throughout both elevation and return to neutral. Ensure that no pain is experienced during the procedure. Adjust the grade and direction of the glide as needed to achieve pain-free function. Add resistance in the form of elastic resistance or a cuff weight to load the muscle.

*Self-Treatment.* A mobilization belt provides the posterolateral glide while the patient actively elevates the affected limb against progressive resistance to end range (Fig. 17.17B).

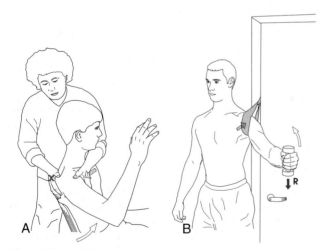

FIGURE 17.17 MWM to modify joint tracking and improve active elevation. A posterolateral glide is applied to the humeral head (A) manually or (B) with a belt for self-treatment, while the patient actively elevates the humerus. A weight is used to strengthen the muscles through the pain-free range.

### Develop Balance in Length and Strength of Shoulder Girdle Muscles

It is important to design a program that specifically addresses the patient's impairments. Typical interventions in the shoulder girdle include but are not limited to:

● *Stretch shortened muscles.* Shortened muscles typically include the pectoralis major, pectoralis minor, latissimus dorsi and teres major, subscapularis, and levator scapulae.
● *Strengthen and train the scapular stabilizers.* Scapular stabilizers typically include the serratus anterior and lower trapezius for posterior tipping and upward rotation and the middle trapezius and rhomboids for scapular retraction. It is important that the patient learns to avoid scapular elevation when raising the arm. Therefore, practice scapular depression when abducting and flexing the humerus.
● *Strengthen and train the rotator cuff muscles*, especially the shoulder lateral rotators.

### Develop Muscular Stabilization and Endurance

● Alternating isometric resistance is applied to the scapular muscles in *open-chain positions* (side-lying, sitting, supine), including protraction/retraction, elevation/depression, and upward/downward rotation so the patient learns to stabilize the scapula against the outside forces (see Fig. 17.36 and the exercise section).
● Scapular and glenohumeral patterns are combined using flexion, abduction, and rotation. Alternating isometric resistance is applied to the humerus while the patient holds against the changing directions of the resistance force (see Figs. 17.37, 17.38, and 17.41 in the exercise section).
● *Closed-chain stabilization* is performed with the patient's hands fixated against a wall, a table, or the floor (quadruped position) while the therapist provides a graded, alternating isometric resistance or rhythmic stabilization. Observe for abnormal scapular winging. If it occurs, the scapular stabilizers are not strong enough for the demand; so the position should be changed to reduce the amount of body weight (see Fig. 17.42 in the exercise section).
● *Muscular endurance* is progressed by increasing the amount of time the individual holds the pattern against the alternating resistance. The limit is reached when any one of the muscles in the pattern can no longer maintain the desired hold. The goal at this phase should be stabilization for approximately 3 minutes.

### Progress Shoulder Function

As the patient develops strength in the weakened muscles, it becomes important to develop a balance in strength of all shoulder and scapular muscles within the range and tolerance of each muscle. To increase coordination between scapular and arm motions, dynamically load the upper extremity within tolerance of the synergy with submaximal resistance. To improve muscular endurance, have the patient increase control from 1 minute to 3 minutes.

| BOX 17.8 | Patient Instructions to Prevent Recurrences of Shoulder Pain |

- Prior to exercise or work, massage the involved tendon or muscle; follow with isometric resistance and then with full ROM and stretching of the muscle.
- Take breaks from the activity if repetitive in nature. If possible, alternate the stressful, provoking activity with other activities or patterns of motion.
- Maintain good postural alignment; adapt seating or workstation to minimize stress. If sport-related, seek coaching in proper techniques or adapt equipment for safe mechanics.
- Prior to initiating a new activity or returning to an activity for which not conditioned, begin a strengthening and training program.

### Management: Return to Function Phase
Specificity of training toward the desired functional outcome begins as soon as the patient has developed control of posture and the basic components of the desired activities without exacerbating the symptoms. While working with the patient, continue to instruct him or her on how to progress the program when discharged as well as how to prevent recurrences. Suggestions are summarized in Box 17.8.

#### Increase Muscular Endurance
To increase muscular endurance, repetitive loading of the defined patterns is increased from 3 minutes to 5 minutes.

#### Develop Quick Motor Responses to Imposed Stresses

- The stabilization exercises are applied with increased speed.
- Plyometric training in both open-chain and closed-chain patterns is initiated if power is a desired outcome.

#### Progress Functional Training
Specificity of training progresses to an emphasis on timing and sequencing of events.

- Eccentric training is progressed to maximum load.
- Desired functional activities are simulated—first under controlled conditions, then under progressively challenged situations using acceleration/deceleration drills.
- The patient is involved in assessing performance in terms of safety, symptom provocation, postural control, and ease of execution and then practices adaptations to correct any problems.

## PAINFUL SHOULDER SYNDROMES: SURGERY AND POSTOPERATIVE MANAGEMENT

Surgical intervention is an option for painful shoulder syndromes when conservative management does not resolve

symptoms and improve a patient's function. For an individual with primary impingement as a result of structural variations in the acromion (see descriptions and Fig. 17.16 in the previous section), subacromial decompression may be performed. An individual with a partial- or full-thickness rotator cuff tear may require surgical repair. The subacromial decompression and rotator cuff repair surgeries and postoperative management are described in this section. Surgical repair and postoperative management due to instabilities and dislocations are described in a later section of this chapter.

### Subacromial Decompression and Postoperative Management

When pain and loss of functional mobility associated with primary impingement do not resolve sufficiently with nonoperative management, *subacromial decompression,* designed to increase the volume of the subacromial space and provide adequate gliding room for tendons, followed by postoperative rehabilitation is often warranted. Subacromial decompression, is commonly referred to as *anterior acromioplasty* or *decompression acromioplasty.* However, acromioplasty, which alters the shape of the acromion, is typically but not always one of the components of subacromial decompression.[111]

#### Indications for Surgery
The following are generally accepted indications for surgical management of impingement syndromes.*

- Pain during overhead activities and loss of functional mobility of the shoulder as the result of primary impingement that persists (typically for 3 to 6 months or longer) despite a trial of nonoperative interventions.
- Stage II (Neer classification) (see Box 17.7) impingement with nonreversible fibrosis or bony alterations of the subacromial compartment, calcific deposits in the cuff tendons, and symptomatic subacromial crepitus.
- Intact or minor tear of the rotator cuff.

NOTE: Patients who present with secondary impingement (GH joint hypermobility or instability associated with a partial- or full-thickness tear of the rotator cuff) are not candidates for surgical subacromial decompression alone. For these patients subacromial decompression is combined with concomitant repair of the cuff tear; otherwise the procedures inherent in subacromial decompression can worsen GH instability.[71,111,190]

#### Procedures

***Surgical approach.*** Subacromial decompression is performed using an arthroscopic or open approach. Although an open approach has been used successfully for many years,[75,117,120,149] the preferred procedure today in most cases is an arthroscopic approach.[53,190] Unlike a traditional open approach, in which the proximal attachment of the deltoid must be detached and then repaired prior to

*See references 1, 53, 71, 75, 111, 120, 149, 155, 190.

closure,[120] with an arthroscopic approach the deltoid remains intact, enabling the patient to regain functional use of the upper extremity more rapidly after surgery.

Another option, preferred by some surgeons to either a traditional open or arthroscopic decompression, is a "mini-open" approach, which involves splitting the deltoid insertion vertically rather than detaching it.[111] For the most part, the traditional open approach for subacromial decompression is now reserved for some patients with a massive rotator cuff tear who also are undergoing an open repair.

***Component procedures.*** There are several surgical procedures that can be performed for subacromial decompression depending on the pathology observed during examination of the shoulder prior to or during surgery.[1,53,67,71,111,131,155,190]

- Removal of the subacromial bursa (*bursectomy*), which is typically thickened (enlarged) by chronic inflammation.
- Release of the coricoacromial ligament, which is usually hypertrophied and may also be frayed, followed by complete or partial resection or recession.
- Resection of the anterior acromial protuberance and contouring the undersurface of the remaining portion of the acromion (*acromioplasty*) to enlarge the subacromial space (Fig. 17.18).
- Removal of any osteophytes at the AC joint and in some cases resection of the distal portion of the clavicle for advanced arthritis of the AC joint.

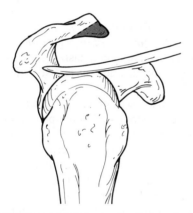

FIGURE 17.18 Arthroscopic acromioplasty showing the line of resection of the anterior acromion.

## Postoperative Management

The type of surgical approach used and the status of the rotator cuff significantly affect the progression of rehabilitation after subacromial decompression (acromioplasty). More often than not an arthrocopic approach is used. If the rotator cuff is intact preoperatively, rehabilitation after arthroscopic acromioplasty progresses quite rapidly because the shoulder musculature is left intact during the procedure. In contrast, if a repair of the rotator cuff is required in addition to acromioplasty or if the surgeon elects to use a mini-open or open approach, rehabilitation progresses at a slower rate to allow the repaired shoulder musculature adequate time to heal.

N O T E : The guidelines outlined in this section are for postoperative rehabilitation after *arthroscopic* subacromial decompression for a patient with primary shoulder impingement who has an *intact rotator cuff.* If subacromial decompression is combined with repair of the rotator cuff (arthroscopic, mini-open, or open approach), the guidelines presented in a later section of this chapter on rehabilitation after rotator cuff repair are appropriate.

### Immobilization

The shoulder is immobilized and supported in a sling with the arm positioned at the patient's side or in slight abduction, the shoulder is internally rotated, and the elbow is flexed to 90°. The sling is worn for comfort for 1 to 2 weeks but is removed for exercise the day after surgery.[111,190,200]

### Exercise

Exercise interventions after subacromial decompression target the same impairments common to rotator cuff impingement as do the exercises selected for a nonoperative program. These impairments and the associated pathomechanics of the shoulder girdle were discussed and summarized previously in this chapter. This information merits review to understand why specific exercises are included in the following postoperative rehabilitation program.

The suggested criteria and timelines for a patient to progress from one phase of rehabilitation to the next, as well as the goals, exercises, and activities in this section, are drawn from several published resources.[3,37,71,91,111,190,200] The exercises noted for each phase impose gradually increasing demands as soft tissues heal. In addition, patient education, emphasizing *prevention* of postures and movements that contribute to impingement and provoke pain, is woven throughout each phase of rehabilitation.

Because arthroscopic decompression often is performed on an outpatent basis, a patient must carry out the prescribed exercises at home with little supervision. Therefore, on the few visits the patient may have with a therapist, patient education is of the utmost importance for each phase of rehabilitation.

### Exercise: Maximum Protection Phase

The first phase of rehabilitation after arthroscopic decompression begins on the day after surgery and extends for 3 to 4 weeks. Emphasis is placed on pain control and immediate but comfortable assisted movement of the shoulder to prevent adhesions of the cuff tendons in the subacromial space. Attaining full or nearly full passive ROM of the operated shoulder (compared to the noninvolved shoulder) is a reasonable goal by 4 to 6 weeks postoperatively.[71]

Patient education begins immediately and is directed toward helping the patient recognize and prevent postures during exercise and ADL that contribute to symptoms. Active (unassisted) shoulder ROM is permissible as soon as motions are pain-free and proper scapulothoracic and glenohumeral control can be maintained. This may be possible as early as 2 weeks after arthroscopic decompression if the rotator cuff did not require repair and is functioning sufficiently.

***Goals and interventions.*** The following goals and exercises are indicated for the early stage of tissue healing.[1,3,37,71,111,200]

- ◎ ***Control pain and inflammation.***
  - Use of a sling when the arm is dependent.
  - Use of cryotherapy and prescribed anti-inflammatory medication.
  - Active ROM of the cervical spine and shoulder relaxation exercises.
- ◎ ***Prevent loss of mobility of peripheral joints.***
  - Active ROM of the elbow, wrist, and hand.
- ◎ ***Develop postural awareness and control.***
  - Active exercises of the scapula with emphasis on retraction.
  - Posture training, reinforcing an erect trunk (avoiding excessive thoracic kyphosis) for prevention of postures that can contribute to impingement symptoms during exercises and ADL.
- ◎ ***Restore pain-free shoulder mobility.***
  - Pendulum exercises for pain control and mobility.
  - Assisted shoulder ROM as tolerated by pain, initially guiding with the sound upper extremity and later a wand. Start in the supine position to provide additional stability to the scapula against the thorax and with the upper arm on a folded towel in slight abduction and flexion. Shoulder motions include elevating the arm in the plane of the scapula, forward flexion, abduction, rotation, and horizontal abduction and adduction. Progress to performing exercises in a semi-reclining position and then in a seated or standing position while maintaining thoracic extension.
  - Assisted shoulder extension in a standing position with a wand held behind the back.
  - Stretching the posterior shoulder structures in pain-free range using a cross-chest stretch into horizontal adduction. Postpone until next phase if painful.
  - Active ROM (unassisted) of the shoulder and scapula within pain-free ranges maintaining proper scapulothoracic and glenohumeral control; begin supine and progress to sitting. Active shoulder motions may be possible by 2 weeks postoperatively.
- ◎ ***Prevent reflex inhibition and atrophy of shoulder girdle musculature.***
  - *Pain-free,* low-intensity, multiple-angle isometrics of GH musculature with the arm supported and emphasis on the rotator cuff against minimal resistance. Begin submaximal isometrics a week or so postoperatively. Lightly resist with the uninvolved upper extremity. Focus on increasing repetitions more than resistance.[103,163]
  - Submaximal alternating isometric and rhythmic stabilization exercises for scapulothoracic muscles with the involved arm supported by the therapist. Target the scapular retractors and upward rotators.

### Exercise: Moderate Protection Phase

Exercises during the second phase of rehabilitation are directed toward attaining full, pain-free shoulder ROM and improving neuromuscular control and muscle performance (strength, muscular endurance) of the deltoid, rotator cuff, and scapular stabilizers. The patient may be ready to begin this phase of rehabilitation as early as 3 to 4 weeks postoperatively but more often by 4 to 6 weeks. This phase extends over a 4- to 6-week period or until the patient meets the criteria to progress to the next phase.

***Criteria for progression.*** Criteria to advance to the second phase include[37,71,91,111,200]:

- ◎ Minimal discomfort when the shoulder is unsupported; arm swing is comfortable during ambulation.
- ◎ Nearly complete, pain-free, *passive* ROM of the shoulder (full mobility of the scapula; at least 150° of shoulder elevation; full rotation).
- ◎ In the supine position, pain-free *active* elevation of the arm well above the level of the shoulder.
- ◎ Pain-free, *active* external rotation of the shoulder to about 45°.
- ◎ At least fair (3/5) and preferably good (4/5) muscle testing grade of shoulder musculature.

***Goals and interventions.*** The goals, exercises, and activities during the second (intermediate) phase of rehabilitation are[37,71,91,200]:

- ◎ ***Restore and maintain full, pain-free passive mobility of the shoulder girdle and upper trunk.***
  - Joint mobilization, emphasizing posterior and caudal glides of the humerus and scapulothoracic mobility.
  - Low-intensity self-stretching of range-limiting muscles that could restrict sufficient upward rotation of the scapula and rotation of the humerus necessary for full elevation of the arm overhead, specifically the levator scapulae, rhomboids, middle trapezius, latissimus dorsi, and pectoralis major and minor. Remember, shortening of these muscles contributes to impingement of soft tissues during overhead movements of the arm.
  - Self-stretching (cross-chest stretch) of the posterior deltoid and posterior capsule of the GH joint. These structures are usually tight in the presence of shoulder impingement. A tight posterior capsule causes excessive anterior translation and superior migration of the head of the humerus in the glenoid, which in turn causes impingement of soft tissues during overhead reach.[69]
  - Self-stretch of the upper trunk to increase thoracic extension by lying supine on a rolled towel placed vertically between the scapulae.
  - Use the gained ROM in exercises and functional movement patterns during ADL.
- ◎ ***Reinforce posture awareness and control.***
  - Through patient education, continue to incorporate an erect trunk into exercises and function activities.

○ **Develop dynamic stability, strength, endurance, and control of scapulothoracic and GH muscles.**

- Stabilization exercises against increasing resistance and in weight-bearing postures. If winging of the scapula occurs with weight bearing, provide manual support or decrease the imposed loads. Emphasize isolated strengthening of the serratus anterior and trapezius muscles.
- Upper extremity ergometry for muscular endurance. To avoid an impingement arc, initiate in a standing position rather than while seated.
- Dynamic strengthening exercises of isolated shoulder muscles against low loads (1- to 5-lb weight or light-grade elastic tubing), gradually increasing repetitions. Begin resisted elevation of the arm in the supine position to stabilize the scapula against the thorax; progress to sitting or standing.
- Use the involved arm for functional activities that involve light resistance.

N O T E : Target the upward rotators of the scapulothoracic joint (serratus anterior, upper and lower trapezius) and the rotator cuff muscles,[166] as well as the latissimus dorsi, teres major, and biceps brachii, which act as humeral head depressors and therefore oppose superior translation during active elevation of the arm. Initially perform resisted motions of the humerus below the level of the shoulder; later progress to overhead exercises if motions remain pain-free.

P R E C A U T I O N : Be certain the patient can perform active shoulder flexion and abduction against gravity without hiking the shoulder before progressing to resisted exercises above shoulder level.

### Exercise: Minimum Protection/ Return to Function Phase

The final phase of rehabilitation usually begins by 8 weeks postoperatively, at which time soft tissues are reasonably well healed and require little to no protection. Exercises continue until about 12 to 16 weeks postoperatively or until the patient has returned to full activity. Exercises are directed toward continuing to improve strength and endurance of the shoulder girdle muscles using isolated movements and those that simulate functional activities. Patients often see continued improvement in functional use of the operated upper extremity for 6 months postoperatively.[3]

The time necessary for full recovery and unrestricted activities depends largely on the level of demand of the anticipated activities. A patient wishing to return to competitive sports requires a more demanding progression of advanced exercises (e.g., plyometric training and sport-specific drills) than a sedentary individual.[37,200,203]

*Criteria for Progression.* The criteria that should be met to progress to the final phase of rehabilitation are[37,91,200]:

○ Negative impingement test.
○ Full, pain-free, active ROM of the shoulder without evidence of substitute motions.
○ Seventy-five percent or more strength of the shoulder musculature compared with the sound shoulder.[200]

*Goals and Interventions.* The goals, exercises, and activities during the final phase of rehabilitation after subacromial decompression and for the final phase of nonoperative management of primary impingement syndrome are similar. Refer to the information presented in the previous section of this chapter as well as other resources.[37,45,113,198,200,203]

### Outcomes

There appears to be no significant difference in the *long-term* results (pain-free ROM and return to desired functional activities) after either open or arthroscopic surgery for primary impingement syndrome with or without associated rotator cuff disease.[53,111,190] Based on the results of numerous outcome studies of open and arthroscopic procedures, 85% to 95% of patients report good to excellent results 1.0 to 2.5 years postoperatively.[1,71,111,190] In general, patients reporting the least satisfaction with their function after surgery are those who participate in high-demand athletic activities that involve overhead throwing and those with work-related injuries who are receiving workers' compensation.[111]

Follow-up studies have documented several advantages of an arthroscopic over comparable open surgical management of impingement syndrome. They include less postoperative pain; earlier restoration of full ROM and strength; earlier return to work (often as early as 1 week postoperatively); lower cost (shorter hospital stay or outpatient surgery); and a more favorable cosmetic result.[1,71,111,190]

Although exercises are routinely prescribed after subacromial decompression, the effectiveness of exercise has been the focus of very few studies. One prospective, randomized study carried out in Denmark looked at the effectiveness of a 6-week therapist-supervised exercise program compared to a self-managed program after arthroscopic subacromial decompression.[3] Patients in the therapist-supervised group received exercise instruction while in the hospital and then for a 1-hour therapy session once a week for 6 weeks after discharge from the hospital. Patients in the self-managed group received exercise instruction on one occasion prior to discharge from the hospital. Both groups received written instructions. At 6 weeks and 3, 6, and 12 months, all patients demonstrated improvement in all parameters tested. However, there were no significant diffferences between the two groups with the exception of one measurement. At 3 months postoperatively, the therapist-supervised group had a higher level of pain than the self-managed group. The authors concluded that initial, therapist-directed exercise instruction followed by a home-based, self-managed exercise program achieved rehabilitation goals as effectively as a therapist-supervised program.

## Rotator Cuff Repair and Postoperative Management

There are two broad categories of rotator cuff tears, defined by the depth of the tendon tear: partial-thickness and full-thickness tears. Either type may require surgical management. A *partial-thickness tear* extends inferiorly or superiorly through only a portion of the tendon from either the acromial (bursal) or humeral (articular) surface of the tendon. A *full-thickness tear* is a complete tear, which extends the entire depth of the tendon.[71,77,111]

### Indications for Surgery

The primary indications for surgical management of a rotator cuff tear confirmed by imaging are pain and impaired function as the result of the following.*

● Partial-thickness or full-thickness tears of the rotator cuff tendons resulting from repetitive microtrauma and chronic impingement, which lead to irreversible degenerative changes in soft tissues. Some patients with stage II lesions and most with stage III lesions (Neer classification[118]) who continue to be symptomatic and have functional limitations after a trial of nonoperative treatment are candidates for surgery.

● Acute, traumatic rupture (frank, full-thickness tear) of the rotator cuff tendons often combined with avulsion of the greater tuberosity, labral damage, or acute dislocation of the GH joint in individuals with no known history of cuff injury. Full-thickness, traumatic tears occur most often in young, active adults.

N O T E : Surgical repair is not indicated in patients who are asymptomatic despite the presence of a cuff tear confirmed by imaging.

### Procedures

Depending on the severity and location of a tear of one or more of the rotator cuff tendons, the extent of associated lesions, the onset of the tear (repetitive microtrauma or traumatic injury), the quality and mobility of the torn tissues, bone quality, patient-related considerations (age, health, activity level) and the surgeon's preference and experience, there are several operative options for repairing a torn rotator cuff.[71,72,111,190]

### Type of Repair

The type of cuff repair is typically classified by the surgical approach and techniques used. There are three categories of repair.

● *Arthroscopic approach.* The entire procedure is performed arthroscopically and requires only a few small incisions for port sites.[8,59,60,71,111,172,190,210]

● *Mini-open (arthroscopically assisted) approach.* There are two variations of this type of procedure, both of which involve arthroscopic subacromial decompression and a *deltoid-splitting* approach. In one variation only the subacromial decompression is performed arthroscopically, whereas in the other variation a portion of the cuff repair itself is also performed arthroscopically.[210] In both cases, an anterolateral incision is made at the acromion and is extended distally (either 1.5 or 3.5 cm but no more than 4 cm to avoid the axillary nerve) along the fibers of the deltoid insertion. The deltoid is split longitudinally between its anterior and middle portions to allow visualization of the cuff tear without detaching the deltoid from its proximal insertion.[56,111,138,180]

● *Traditional open approach.* An anterolateral incision is made that extends obliquely from the middle one-third of the inferior aspect of the clavicle, across the coracoid process, and to the anterior aspect of the proximal humerus. The proximal insertion of the deltoid must be detached and reflected for exposure of the operative field during an open subacromial decompression and cuff repair. After the cuff repair is complete, the deltoid is reattached to the acromion.† As arthroscopic and arthroscopically assisted repairs of the rototor cuff have advanced, the use of the traditional open approach has decreased.

### Components of a Rotator Cuff Repair

Regardless of the approach, subacromial decompression is performed (particularly for cuff tears associated with chronic impingement) before repair of the cuff is undertaken. After the tear is visualized through the approach selected, the margins of the torn tendon are débrided. The tendon is then released from any adherent soft tissues and mobilized for advancement and apposition to bone that has been prepared for sutures, followed by *tendon-to-bone* fixation. Depending on whether an arthroscopic or mini-open approach is used, fixation is accomplished by sutures and suture anchors, tacks, or staples.[56,59,71,111,179,190]

In addition to subacromial decompression, other concomitant procedures may be required.[71,111] For example, capsular tightening or labral reconstruction may be performed if unidirectional or multidirectional instability of the GH joint is present. Because degenerative changes in the tendon of the long head of the biceps brachii are often associated with chronic rotator cuff disease, a repair of this tendon may also be necessary.

### Selection of Surgical Procedures

The surgeon weighs many factors when determining which type of cuff repair is most appropriate for each patient. One such consideration is the severity of the tear, including thickness (partial or full), size, and number of tendons torn. Although there is some variability in the literature, there are four generally accepted categories that describe the longitudinal size of rotator cuff tears: *small* (1 cm or less), *medium* (1 to 3 cm), *large* (3 to 5 cm), and *massive* (more than 5 cm or a full-thickness tear of more than one tendon).[8,56,71,191]

If a small, *partial-thickness* cuff tear is managed surgically after failed nonoperative treatment, a fully arthroscopic approach typically is performed to débride the frayed margins of the torn tendon, coupled with a subacromial decompression procedure. However, the torn portion of the tendon may or may not be repaired.[8,71,111,172,179,190]

Two decades ago, primarily small and medium *full-thickness* cuff tears (≤ 1 to 3 cm) were managed with a fully arthroscopic approach.[60,71,111] With the evolution of arthroscopic techniques, an increasing number of large,

*See references 8, 12, 71, 77, 111, 138, 140, 167, 178, 190, 210.

†See references 12, 77, 97, 111, 140, 178.

full-thickness cuff tears and occasionally massive tears as well are managed with a fully arthroscopic approach.[190,210] However, variations of the mini-open (deltoid splitting) approach frequently are the surgeon's choice for repair of medium and large tears.[56,111,146,180] Even some massive tears (> 5 cm) are managed with a deltoid-splitting approach.[111,191] The traditional open approach, requiring detachment and repair of the deltoid, now primarily is reserved for repairs of multiple tendon tears associated with extensive injury to the shoulder or for use as a component of an open surgical procedure, such as total shoulder replacement arthroplasty.[56,111]

The location of the cuff tear, amount of retraction and mobility of a full-thickness tear, and the quality of the remaining tendon and underlying bone also influence the surgeon's selection of the type of cuff repair expected to be most effective.[71,111,179,190] Whereas small, medium, and large tears of the supraspinatus (the most frquently torn cuff tendon) or infraspinatus are routinely managed with arthroscopic or mini-open approaches, tears of the subscapularis are often managed with a traditional open approach.[56] If there is significant retraction and poor mobility of the torn tendon or poor tissue quality, many surgeons believe that a stronger repair can be achieved with an open procedure (mini-open or traditional) than with an arthroscopic repair.[71]

## Postoperative Management

After surgical repair of a torn rotator cuff tendon, there are many factors that influence decisions about the position and duration of immobilization, the selection and application of exercises, and the rate of progression of each patient's postoperative rehabilitation program. These factors and their potential impact are summarized in Table 17.3. Furthermore, these factors can affect postoperative outcomes.

There is little consensus reported in the literature or practiced in the clinical setting as to how and to what extent each of these factors, singularly or collectively, has an impact on the decisions made by the surgeon and the therapist about a patient's postoperative rehabilitation program. Hence, predetermined guidelines and protocols for postoperative management after rotator cuff repair are diverse and sometimes contradictory.* For example, some authors have pointed out that if deltoid detachment and repair are components of the surgery, as is necessary for a traditional open repair, deltoid strengthening exercises should be postponed for approximately 6 to 8 weeks postoperatively until the repaired deltoid has healed.[37,52,111] Yet another author suggested that rehabilitation should proceed similarly regardless of whether deltoid detachment was required so long as secure fixation of the deltoid was achieved.[71]

*See references 8, 24, 37, 50, 52, 56, 71, 111, 138.

| TABLE 17.3 | Factors that Influence Progression of Rehabilitation After Repair of the Rotator Cuff |
|---|---|
| Factors | Potential Impact on Rehabilitation |
| • Onset of injury | • Chronic impingement and atraumatic cuff deficiency → slower progression than after acute traumatic injury. |
| • Size and location of the tear | • Larger tears with more structures involved and probability of more extensive surgery → slower progression. |
| • Associated pathologies such as GH instability or fracture | • Associated pathologies often lengthen the period of immobilization → slower progression of exercises or the need for additional precautions. |
| • Preoperative strength and mobility of the shoulder | • Preexisting weakness and atrophy of the dynamic stabilizers or limited passive and active mobility of the shoulder → slower postoperative progression. |
| • Patient's general health | • Patient in poor health; history of smoking; history of inflammatory disease → slower progression. |
| • History of steroid injections or previous, failed cuff surgery | • Compromised bone and tendon tissue quality, which affects the security of the repair (fixation) → slower progression. |
| • Preinjury level of activity of postoperative goals | • Higher level goals require a more extended and advanced postoperative training program because of a higher risk of reinjury. |
| • Age of patient | • Older patient who has an insidious (chronic) onset and may have articular changes → slower progression. |
| • Type of approach | • Traditional open approach (with deltoid detachment and repair) → slightly slower progression than after an arthroscopic or arthroscopically assisted (mini-open/deltoid splitting) repair. |
| • Type of repair | • Tendon to tendon → slower progression than tendon to bone. |
| • Mobility (no excessive tension on the repaired tendon when arm at side) and integrity of the repair | • If mobility is inadequate → longer duration of exercise within a protected ROM during early rehabilitation. |
| • Patient's compliance with the program | • Lack of compliance (doing too much or too little) can affect outcome. |
| • Philosophy, skill, and training of the surgeon | • All have an impact that could → either slower or more accelerated progression. |

Given the diverse characteristics of patients undergoing repair of the rotator cuff and the variety of surgical options available, it is not surprising that no single postoperative program can be used for all patients or has been shown to yield better outcomes than another. Therefore, to meet each patient's needs and goals, a therapist can use published protocols or those developed at individual clinical facilities as general guidelines for postoperative management and can modify the guidelines based on ongoing examination of the patient's response to interventions and close communication with the surgeon.

Despite variations among postoperative programs, they share three common elements: (1) immediate or early postoperative motion of the GH joint; (2) control of the rotator cuff for dynamic stability; and (3) gradual restoration of strength and muscular endurance. The purpose of this section is to present *general* exercise guidelines that incorporate these elements into progressive phases of rehabilitation after arthroscopic or mini-open repair of a *full-thickness* cuff tear and to identify the differences in precautions and the progression of exercises for a traditional open procedure or differences based on the size and location of the tear and the quality of the repair.

N O T E : The goals, exercise interventions, and progression of rehabilitation after débridement rather than repair of a *partial-thickness* tear are comparable to postoperative management after subacromial decompression for cuff impingement presented in the previous section of this chapter.

### Immobilization

The position and duration of immobilization of the operated shoulder after rotator cuff repair are dependent on many factors, such as the severity and location of the tear and the type and quality of the repair. One of those factors, the size of the cuff tear, in part determines whether the patient's operated arm is supported in a sling (shoulder adducted, internally rotated, and elbow flexed to 90°) or in an abduction orthosis or pillow (shoulder elevated in the plane of the scapula approximately 45°, shoulder internally rotated, and elbow flexed). Some patients, using an abduction splint, initially may be required to have a family member support the operated arm in the 45° shoulder position when the splint is removed for exercise or dressing and even for bathing.

Table 17.4 summarizes the variations noted in the literature for fully arthroscopic and mini-open/deltoid-splitting approaches. Immobilization after a traditional open procedure that involves deltoid detachment and repair, is not included in Table 17.4 because of the variations in guidelines reported in the literature.[37,71,111,191]

The rationale for initially immobilizing the operated shoulder in abduction is based on two principles. (1) In the abducted position, the repaired cuff, as well as the reattached deltoid with an open approach, are held in a relaxed position, which reduces the possibility of reflexive muscle contractions that could disrupt the repairs. (2) Supporting the arm in abduction rather than adduction reduces tension on the tendons and therefore may improve blood flow to the repaired tendon(s).

### Exercise

Regardless of whether a patient undergoes a rotator cuff repair on an inpatient or outpatient basis, contact with a therapist for exercise instruction after surgery is usually limited to a few visits unless the patient does not progress satisfactorily. Therefore, the emphasis of a therapist's interaction with a patient must be placed on patient education for an effective and safe home-based exercise program. As with rehabilitation after arthroscopic subacromial decompression,[3] the extent of therapist-directed exercise after rotator cuff surgery also has been investigated.

### ● Focus on Evidence_____

In a randomized, controlled study by Roddey and colleagues,[150] two approaches to exercise instruction following arthroscopic repair of a full-thickness rotator cuff tear were compared, specifically in-person instruction by a therapist and video-based instruction. On the first postoperative day, both groups of patients (total 108) received one visit from the therapist for initial instruction in the postoperative program (sling use and passive shoulder exercises). Patients in both groups received written handouts about the home exercise program. In addition, patients in the video-instruction group received a video containing exercises for all phases of the rehabilitation program.

After discharge, patients in the video group saw the therapist four times (at 2, 6, 12, and 24 weeks) for evalua-

| TABLE 17.4 | Relationships of Type and Duration of Immobilization after Arthroscopic and Mini-Open Repair* to the Size of the Rotator Cuff Tear** |
|---|---|
| **Size of Tear** | **Type and Duration of Immobilization** |
| Small (≤ 1 cm) | Sling for 1–2 weeks; removal for exercise the day of surgery or 1 day postop |
| Medium to large (> 1 to 5 cm)† | Sling or abduction orthosis/pillow for 3–6 weeks; removal for exercise 1–2 days postop |
| Massive (> 5 cm)† | Sling or abduction orthosis/pillow for 4–8 weeks; removal for exercise 1–3 days postop |

*Fully arthroscopic and mini-open (arthroscopically assisted/deltoid splitting) approaches.

**Age of the patient, onset of the injury, and quality of repaired tissue also influence the position and duration of immobilization.

†A fully arthroscopic approach is not often used to repair massive cuff tears.

tion and an okay to advance to the next phase of rehabilitation, but they received all exercise instruction by watching the video at home. Patients in the other group also saw the therapist four times at identical intervals after discharge for follow-up evaluations and one-to-one instructions from the therapist on how to perform the exercises during the next phase of the home program. Between visits both groups had telephone access to their therapist for questions, and at 52 weeks all patients were evaluated a final time.

Results of this study indicated that there were no significant differences between the two groups in compliance with the exercise program and functional outcomes measured with a self-report instrument. The authors concluded that video-based exercise instruction was equally effective as therapist-directed exercise instruction. It is important to note that 30% of the patients dropped out of the study. The authors did not report whether these patients were progresssing well or if any of them left the study to seek individualized or more frequent therapy.

Goals and interventions for each phase of rehabilitation after arthroscopic or mini-open cuff repair follow. General guidelines for exercise and precautions after rotator cuff repair are summarized in Box 17.9. Precautions specific to a particular type of cuff tear or surgical procedure are also noted. The suggested timelines for each phase are general and must be adjusted based on factors already noted (see Table 17.3).

---

## BOX 17.9   General Exercise Guidelines and Precautions After Repair of a Full-Thickness Rotator Cuff Tear

### Early Shoulder Motion
- Perform passive or assisted shoulder ROM within *safe and pain-free ranges* based on the surgeon's intraoperative observation of the mobility and strength of the repair and the patient's comfort level during exercise.
- Only passive and no assisted ROM for 6 to 8 weeks after repair of a massive cuff tear or after a traditional open approach to prevent avulsion of the repaired deltoid.
- Initially perform passive and assisted shoulder ROM in the supine position to maintain stability of the scapula on the thorax.
- Minimize anterior translation of the humeral head and the potential for impingement. See that the humerus is positioned slightly anterior to the frontal plane of the body and in slight abduction
  - While at rest in the supine position support the humerus on a folded towel.
  - When the initiating passive or assisted shoulder rotation while lying supine, position the shoulder in slight flexion and approximately 45° of abduction.
  - When initiating assisted shoulder extension, perform the exercise in prone (arm over the edge of the bed) from 90° to just short of neutral. Later progress to exercises behind the back.
- When performing assisted or active exercises in the upright position (sitting or standing), be certain that the patient maintains an erect trunk posture to minimize the possibility of impingement.
- To ensure adequate humeral depression and avoid superior translation of the head of the humerus when beginning *active* elevation of the arm, restore strength in the rotator cuff, especially the supraspinatus and infraspinatus muscles, before dynamically strengthening the shoulder flexors and abductors.
- Do not allow *active* shoulder flexion or abduction until the patient can lift the arm without hiking the shoulder.

### Strengthening Exercises
- When beginning isometric resistance to scapulothoracic musculature, be sure to support the operated arm to avoid excessive tension in repaired GH musculature.
- Use low exercise loads; resisted motions should not cause pain.
- No weight-bearing (closed chain) exercises or activities for 6 weeks.
- Delay dynamic strengthening (progressive resistive exercise, or PRE) for a *minimum* of 8 weeks postoperatively for small, strong repair and for at least 3 months for larger tears.
  - If the supraspinatus was repaired, proceed cautiously when resisting external rotation.
  - If the subscapularis was repaired, proceed cautiously with resisted internal rotation.
- After an open repair, postpone isometric resistance exercises to the repaired deltoid and cuff musculature for *at least* 6 to 8 weeks unless advised otherwise.

### Stretching Exercises
- Avoid vigorous stretching, the use of contract–relax procedures or grade III joint mobilizations for at least 6 weeks and often for 12 weeks postoperatively to give time for the repaired tendon(s) to heal and become strong.
  - If the supraspinatus or infraspinatus was repaired, initially avoid end-range stretching into internal rotation.
  - If the subscapularis was repaired, initially avoid end-range stretching into external rotation.
  - If the deltoid was detached and repaired, initially avoid end-range shoulder extension, adduction, and horizontal adduction.

### Activities of Daily Living
- Wait until about 6 weeks after a mini-open or arthroscopic repair and 12 weeks after a traditional open repair before using the operated arm for light functional activities.
- After repair of a large or massive cuff tear, avoid use of operated arm for functional activities that involve heavy resistance (pushing, pulling, lifting, carrying heavy loads) for 6 to 12 *months* postoperatively.

### Exercise: Maximum Protection Phase

The priorities during the initial phase of rehabilitation are protection of the repaired tendon, which is at its weakest approximately 3 weeks after repair,[179] and prevention of the adverse effects of immobilization through early passive motion. In almost all instances, during the first few days after surgery the immobilization (sling or splint) is removed for brief sessions of passive or assisted ROM within limited (protected) and comfortable ranges (see Table 17.4).

The maximum protection phase extends for as little as 3 to 4 weeks after a fully arthroscopic or mini-open repair of small or medium tears or as long as 6 to 8 weeks after repair of large or massive tears. After a fully arthroscopic repair of a small or medium cuff tear, every effort is made to attain nearly full passive shoulder ROM, particularly elevation and external rotation, by 6 to 8 weeks postoperatively.[56,111,190]

*Goals and interventions.* The following goals and selected interventions combined with the appropriate use of pain medication are initiated during the maximum protection phase.[*]

◉ *Control pain and inflammation.*
  • Periodic use of ice.
  • Arm support for comfort.
  • Cervical spine ROM and shoulder relaxation exercises.
  • Grade I oscillations of the GH joint.
◉ *Prevent loss of mobility of peripheral joints.*
  • Assisted ROM of the elbow.
  • Active ROM of the wrist and hand.
◉ *Prevent shoulder stiffness/restore shoulder mobility.*
  • Pendulum exercises typically the first postoperative day or when the immobilizer may be removed for exercise.
  • Passive ROM of the shoulder within safe and pain-free ranges. Initially perform exercises in the supine position; begin with elevation of the arm and external rotation in the plane of the scapula.
  • Self-assisted ROM using the opposite hand or a wand for control by 1 to 2 weeks for patients with repairs of small to medium tears and about 2 weeks later for patients with repairs of large tears.
  • Active control of the shoulder with assistance as needed from therapist or family member. With the patient lying in the supine position, place the arm in 90° of shoulder flexion if pain-free. In this position the effect of gravity on the shoulder musculature is minimal. This position has been called the "balance point position" of the shoulder.[50] Help the patient control the shoulder while moving to and from the balance point position, making small arcs and circles with the arm.
  • Active shoulder ROM by the latter part of this phase for small tears and as symptoms permit, initially supine with the elbow flexed, later in a semi-reclining position with the elbow less flexed.

---
[*]See references 8, 24, 37, 50, 52, 56, 71, 111, 190, 191.

PRECAUTION: Use only passive and no assisted ROM for 6 to 8 weeks for a repair of a massive cuff tear or after a traditional open repair with deltoid detachment.[37,191]

◉ *Prevent or correct postural deviations.*
  • Posture training and exercises to prevent excessive thoracic kyphosis (see Chapters 14 and 16).
◉ *Develop control of scapulothoracic stabilizers.*
  • Active movements of the scapula.
  • Submaximal isometrics to isolated scapular muscles.[103] See that the operated arm is supported but not bearing weight to avoid excessive tension in repaired GH musculature.
  • Side-lying scapular protraction/retraction to emphasize control of the serratus anterior.
◉ *Prevent inhibition and atrophy of GH musculature.*
  • Low-intensity muscle-setting exercises (against minimal resistance). Setting exercises should not provoke pain in a healing cuff tendon. Begin as early as 1 to 3 weeks postoperatively depending on the size of the tear and quality of the repair.[37,50,52]

PRECAUTION: Recommendations for the safest position of the shoulder in which to begin isometric training of the GH musculature after cuff repair are inconsistent in the literature. One suggestion is to start in a position that creates minimal tension on the repaired cuff tendons (shoulder internally rotated and flexed and abducted to about 45° and elbow flexed).[52] Another option is to place the shoulder in 100° to 110° of flexion and 10° to 20° of horizontal abduction. In this position the deltoid creates a compression force on the head of the humerus into the glenoid fossa, thus diminishing the superior sheer forces generated by the deltoid than when the arm is in less flexion. As the strength of the cuff muscles improves during the later phases of rehabilitation, isometric activities can be performed with the arm positioned in less shoulder flexion.

### Exercise: Moderate Protection Phase

The focus of the second phase of rehabilitation is to begin to develop strength, endurance, and neuromuscular control of the shoulder while continuing to attain full or nearly full, pain-free shoulder motion. Emphasis is placed on developing control of the scapular stabilizers and rotator cuff muscles.

For a patient with a repair of a small or medium tear, this phase begins around 4 to 6 weeks postoperatively and extends an additional 6 weeks. For most patients, strengthening exercises typically begin around 8 weeks postoperatively. This phase may begin as late as 12 weeks for a patient with a repair of a large or masssive tear.

*Criteria for progression.* Criteria to advance to this phase are a well healed incision, minimal pain with assisted shoulder motions, and progressive improvement in ROM. The extent of improvement at just 6 weeks or so after surgery is dependent on factors such as the type and quality of the repair, the size of the tear, and preoperative ROM.

**Focus on Evidence**_____

In a descriptive study by Ellenbecker and colleagues,[50] patients (*n* = 37) with full-thickness cuff tears (small, medium, and large) but no concomitant lesions who had undergone a mini-open repair underwent physical therapy that emphasized early mobilization of the operated shoulder a mean of 10 times by 6 weeks after surgery. Investigators measured passive shoulder ROM at 6 weeks and active ROM and dynamic strength of shoulder musculature at 12 weeks and compared these measurements to those of the noninvolved limb.

At 6 weeks, mean values for passive flexion, abduction, and external and internal rotation (in 90° of abduction) of the operated shoulder approached those of the noninvolved shoulder: 154°, 138°, 74°, and 39°, respectively, in the operated shoulder compared to 156°, 164°, 91°, and 48°, respectively, in the noninvolved shoulder. Preoperative ROM was not reported in this study, nor were subjects divided into subgroups based on the size of the tear. However, the authors suggested that knowledge of short-term, objective measures of ROM and strength can assist a therapist in the clinical decision-making process, such as when to place more or less emphasis on restoring ROM or strength during a rehabilitation program. The ROM results of this study also demonstrate the value of early postoperative mobilization and to what extent return of shoulder mobility is possible just 6 weeks after mini-open rotator cuff repair.

_____

***Goals and interventions.*** The following goals and interventions are appropriate during this phase of rehabilitation.[8,24,37,50,52,56,111]

◉ ***Restore nearly complete or full, nonpainful, passive mobility of the shoulder.***
  • Self-assisted ROM with an end-range hold by means of wand or pulley exercises, in single plane and combined (diagonal) patterns. Add shoulder internal rotation, extension beyond neutral, and horizontal adduction.
  • Mobilization of the incision site if well healed to prevent adherence of the scar.

PRECAUTION: The use of passive stretching and grade III joint mobilizations, if initiated during this phase of rehabilitation, must be done *very cautiously*. Vigorous stretching is not considered safe for about 3 to 4 months, that is, until after the repaired tendons have healed and have become reasonably strong.[111]

◉ ***Increase strength and endurance and re-establish dynamic stability of the shoulder musculature.***
  • Active ROM of the shoulder continued or begun through gradually increasing but pain-free ranges. Continue to have the patient perform active elevation of the arm in the supine position until the motion can be initiated without first hiking the shoulder. When transitioning to an upright positions (sitting or

standing), reinforce the importance of maintaining an erect trunk during exercises.
  • Isometric and dynamic strengthening to key scapulothoracic stabilizers. First use alternating isometrics in non-weight-bearing positions. Progress to rhythmic stabilization during light upper extremity weight-bearing activities.
  • Submaximal multiple-angle isometrics of the rotator cuff and other GH musculature against gradually increasing resistance.
  • Dynamic strengthening and endurance training of the GH musculature within pain-free ranges against light resistance, such as light-grade elastic tubing or a 1- to 2-lb weight. Perform exercises below the level of the shoulder if pain is provoked with active movements above the shoulder.
  • Upper extremity ergometry at or just below shoulder level against light resistance to increase muscular endurance.
  • Use of the involved upper extremity for *light* (no-load or low-load) functional activities.

NOTE: Because weakness and atrophy of the rotator cuff were probably present prior to injury, strengthen the cuff muscles before dynamically strengthening the shoulder abductors and flexors.

**Exercise: Minimum Protection/ Return to Function Phase**
This final (advanced) phase usually begins no earlier than 12 to 16 weeks postoperatively for patients with strong repairs or at 16 weeks or later for a tenuous repair. This phase may continue until 6 months or more depending on the patient's expected functions during work-related or recreational activities.

If full ROM still has not been restored with assisted and active exercises, passive stretching of the GH musculature and joint mobilization (if not previously incorporated into the exercise program) is now initiated. Have the patient use the gained shoulder mobility in activities, such as gently swinging a golf club or tennis racket if the motions are pain-free. Advanced, task-specific strengthening activities dominate this phase of rehabilitation.

Patients generally are not allowed to return to high-demand activities for 6 months or possibly 1 year postoperatively depending on the patient's level of comfort, strength, and flexibility as well as the demands of the desired activities.

***Criteria for progression.*** Criteria to transition to the final phase of rehabilitation and gradually return to unrestricted activities include full, pain-free passive ROM, progressive improvement of shoulder strength and muscular endurance, and a stable GH joint.

***Goals and interventions.*** The goals and interventions during this final phase of rehabilitation are consistent with those previously discussed for late-stage nonoperative management of cuff disorders and for the final phase of rehabilitation after subacromial decompression. However, the progression of activities is more gradual, and the time frame for adhering to precautions is more extended.

## Outcomes

A considerable number of outcome studies of operative management of rotator cuff tears have been reported in the literature with follow-up ranging from less than 6 months to 5 years or more. Outcomes commonly measured, using a variety of instruments, are pain relief, shoulder ROM and strength, overall function, and patient satisfaction.

Comparable long-term outcomes have been reported after fully arthroscopic, mini-open (arthroscopically assisted), and traditional open repairs.[71] For example, after fully arthroscopic repair of full-thickness tears (mostly small or medium but some large or massive tears), overall outcomes of several studies were reported as good to excellent in 84%[59,60] and 92%[172] of patients followed for 2 to 3 years. These results are comparable to results reported for open repairs.[71,111] However, it has been shown that regardless of the type of operative repair performed the size of the cuff tear influences postoperative outcomes. For example, comparably favorable long-term functional outcomes and pain relief have been reported after mini-open and traditional open repairs of small to medium size, full-thickness tears (< 3 cm).[9,71,111] Outcomes are less favorable after repairs of large or massive tears.[111,191]

Other factors, such as the acuity or chronicity of the tear and the patient's age, also affect outcomes. Repairs of acute tears in young patients are more successful than repairs of similar-size tears associated with chronic cuff impingement and insufficiency in elderly patients (> 65 years).[67] The presence of fewer associated pathologies, such as a biceps tendon tear or cuff tear arthropathy, also are associated with better postoperative outcomes.[111]

*Pain relief*. Although the results of individual studies vary, a systematic review of the literature indicated that an average of 85% of patients who had undergone operative repair of the rotator cuff (arthroscopic, mini-open, or open), report satisfactory relief of pain. Pain relief after arthroscopic and mini-open repairs ranges between 80% and 92%.[157] This is comparable to results of previous studies of traditional open repairs, in which satisfactory pain relief was reported by 85% to 95% of patients.[70,77] The preoperative size of the tear has an impact on pain relief; specifically, patients with small and medium tears (≤ 3 cm) report a higher percentage of satisfaction with pain relief than patients with large or massive lesions.[70,111,157]

*Shoulder ROM.* Restrictions in preoperative ROM have an influence on postoperative ROM. In a prospective descriptive study of patients undergoing rotator cuff repair, the preoperative factor that most closely correlated with long-term limitation of shoulder ROM after surgery was the inability to place the hand behind the back.[183] Postoperative shoulder ROM also is associated with the size of the tear. For example, the results of one study showed that patients who had repairs of small to medium

tears had more active flexion and abduction than patients with large tears.[77]

As indicated in a study described earlier in this section of ROM measurements 6 and 12 weeks after mini-open repair of full-thickness cuff tears, passive ROM can approach near-normal (compared to the noninvolved shoulder) by 6 weeks postoperatively.[50]

*Strength.* As with ROM, the rate of recovery of shoulder muscle strength also appears to be associated with the size of the tear; that is, faster recovery occurs with small and medium tears than with large or massive tears. However, unlike recovery of ROM, near-complete restoration of shoulder muscle strength occurs gradually and may take a year after repair of small and medium tears. Recovery of strength after repair of large or massive tears is inconsistent.[111,157]

Although recovery of shoulder muscle strength occurs gradually throughout the first postoperative year, the most substantial gains are seen during the first 6 months.[111] In most cases, patients achieve 80% strength in the operated shoulder (compared to the noninvolved shoulder) by 6 months and 90% by 1 year.[152]

*Functional abilities*. It has been suggested that long-term functional outcomes correlate with the size of the tear, type of repair, tissue quality, and the integrity of the repair.[111] For example, patients who have undergone a mini-open repair return to functional activities about a month earlier than those who have had an open repair.[9] However, this outcome may be skewed by the fact that mini-open repairs are performed more often in younger patients with less severe tears.

Lastly, in a study of patients who presented with recurrence of a rotator cuff tear after repair, 80% of the patients had been reported to have good to excellent short-term functional outcomes, measured by objective criteria. This suggests that the evidence regarding whether there is a direct relationship between the integrity of the repair and the functional outcome is inconsistent.[70]

# ● SHOULDER DISLOCATIONS: NONOPERATIVE MANAGEMENT

With a dislocation there is complete separation of the articular surfaces of the glenohumeral joint caused by direct or indirect forces applied to the shoulder.[133] Instability (described in the section on painful shoulder syndromes) may be a predisposing factor to dislocation, especially with repetitive stressful overhead activities, as seen in some sports.[79]

## Related Pathologies and Mechanisms of Injury

### Traumatic Anterior Shoulder Dislocation

Anterior dislocation most frequently occurs when there is a blow to the humerus while it is in a position of external rotation and abduction. Stability normally is provided by the subscapularis, GH ligament, and long head of the biceps when in that position.[96,151,184] Poor integrity of any of these structures can predispose the joint to dislocation, or a significant blow to the arm may damage them along with the attachment of the anterior capsule and glenoid labrum (Bankart lesion depicted in Fig. 17.19). When dislocated, the humeral head usually rests in the subcoracoid region, rarely in the subclavicular or intrathoracic region. Traumatic anterior dislocation is usually associated with complete rupture of the rotator cuff. There may also be a compression fracture at the posterolateral margin of the humeral head (Hill-Sachs lesion also depicted in Fig. 17.19). Neurological or vascular injuries may occur during dislocations.[68] The axillary nerve is most commonly injured, but the brachial plexus or one of the peripheral nerves could be stretched or compressed.

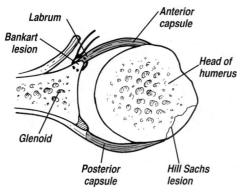

FIGURE 17.19 Lesions associated with traumatic anterior dislocation of the GH joint. A Bankart lesion is a fracture of the anterior rim of the glenoid with the attached labrum. The labrum is pulled away from the anterior glenoid along with a small piece of glenoid. A Hill-Sachs lesion is a compression fracture of the posterolateral humeral head, also may occur. (Adapted from Tovin, BJ, Greenfield, BH: Evaluation and Treatment of the Shoulder—An Integration of the Guide to Physical Therapist Practice. FA Davis, Philadelphia, 2001, p 295, with permission.)

### Traumatic Posterior Shoulder Dislocation

Traumatic posterior shoulder dislocation is less common. Most posterior dislocations are subacromial, although subglenoid or subspinous posterior dislocations do occur. The mechanism of injury is usually a force applied to the humerus that combines flexion, adduction, and internal rotation, such as falling on an outstretched arm.[164] The person complains of symptoms when doing activities such as push-ups, a bench press, or follow-through on a golf swing.[68]

### Recurrent Dislocation

With significant ligamentous and capsular laxity, unidirectional or multidirectional recurrent subluxations or dislocations may occur with any movement that reproduces the abduction and external rotation forces or the flexion, adduction, and internal rotation forces, causing significant pain and functional limitation. Some individuals can voluntarily dislocate the shoulder anteriorly or posteriorly without apprehension and with minimal discomfort.[133,164] The group in which the rate of recurrence after the first traumatic dislocation is highest is the younger population (< 30 years). Because they are more active and place

greater demands on the shoulder, longer immobilization (> 3 weeks) is advocated after dislocation than in the less than 30-year-old patient. Shorter immobilization (1 to 2 weeks) is advocated for older patients.[110,112]

## Common Impairments

- After an acute traumatic injury, symptoms resulting from tissue damage include pain and muscle guarding due to bleeding and inflammation.
- When a dislocation is associated with a complete rotator cuff tear, there is an inability to abduct the humerus against gravity, except the range provided by the scapulothoracic muscles.
- Asymmetrical joint restrictions/hypermobilities. With anterior instability, the posterior capsule may be tight; with posterior instability, the anterior capsule may be tight. After healing, there may be adhesions.
- With recurrent dislocations, the individual can dislocate the shoulder at will, or the shoulder may dislocate when doing specific activities. Instabilities, as described previously in this chapter, are present.

## Common Functional Limitations/Disabilities

- With rotator cuff rupture, inability to reach or lift objects to the level of horizontal, thus interfering with all activities using humeral elevation
- Possibility of recurrence when replicating the dislocating action
- With anterior dislocation, restricted ability in sports activities, such as pitching, swimming, serving (tennis, volleyball), spiking (volleyball)
- Restricted ability, particularly when overhead or horizontal abduction movements are required while dressing, such as putting on a shirt or jacket, and with self-grooming, such as combing the back of the hair
- Discomfort or pain when sleeping on the involved side in some cases
- With posterior dislocation, restricted ability in sports activities, such as follow-through in pitching and golf; restricted ability in pushing activities, such as pushing open a heavy door or pushing one's self up out of a chair or out of a swimming pool

## Closed Reduction of Anterior Dislocation

NOTE: Reduction manipulations should be undertaken only by someone specially trained in the maneuver because of the vulnerability of the brachial plexus and axillary blood vessels.

### Management: Protection Phase

#### Protect the Healing Tissue

- Activity restriction is recommended for 6 to 8 weeks in a young patient. If a sling is used, the arm is removed from the sling only for controlled exercise. During the first week, the patient's arm may be continuously immobilized because of pain and muscle guarding.

● An older, less active patient (> 40 years of age) may require immobilization for only 2 weeks.
● The position of dislocation must be avoided when exercising, dressing, or doing other daily activities

### ● Focus on Evidence_____

Traditionally, after acute anterior shoulder dislocation, immobilization (for various lengths of time) has been instituted. A clinical commentary that looked at outcomes from various studies found that the literature does not support use of a traditional sling for immobilizing the shoulder following primary anterior shoulder dislocation.[79] Still, it was noted that reports showed significantly better results (relative to redislocation) with activity restriction for 6 to 8 weeks in those < 30 years of age compared to activity restriction of less than 6 weeks.[79]

The commentary also summarized two studies that looked at positioning (magnetic resonance imaging with 18 patients and a cadavaric study). The study results supported positioning the humerus in adduction and external rotation (rather than internal rotation) for better approximation between the detached glenoid labrum (Bankart lesion) and the glenoid neck.[79]

### Promote Tissue Health

Protected ROM, intermittent muscle setting of the rotator cuff, deltoid, and biceps brachii muscles, and grade II joint techniques (with the humerus at the side or in the resting position) are initiated as soon as the patient tolerates them.

PRECAUTIONS: In order not to disrupt healing of the capsule and other damaged tissues after anterior dislocation, ROM into external rotation is performed with the elbow at the patient's side, with the shoulder flexed in the sagittal plane, and with the shoulder in the resting position (in the plane of the scapula, abducted 55° and 30° to 45° anterior to the frontal plane) but not in the 90° abducted position. The forearm is moved from in front of the trunk (maximal internal rotation) to 0° or possibly 10° to 15° external rotation.

CONTRAINDICATION: Extension beyond 0° is contraindicated.

### Management: Controlled Motion Phase

#### Provide Protection

The patient continues to protect the joint and avoid full return to unrestricted activity. If a sling is being used, the patient increases the time the sling is off. The sling is used when the shoulder is tired or if protection is needed.

#### Increase Shoulder Mobility

● Mobilization techniques are initiated using all appropriate glides except the anterior glide. The anterior glide

is *contraindicated* even though external rotation is necessary for functional elevation of the humerus. For a safe stretch to increase external rotation, the shoulder is placed in the resting position (abducted 55° and horizontally adducted 30°); it is then externally rotated to the limit of its range, after which a grade III distraction force is applied perpendicular to the treatment plane in the glenoid fossa (Fig. 17.20).
● The posterior joint structures are passively stretched with horizontal adduction self-stretching techniques.

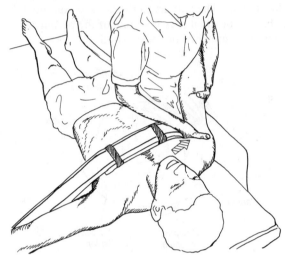

FIGURE 17.20 Mobilizing to increase external rotation when an anterior glide is contraindicated. Place the shoulder in resting position, externally rotate it, then apply a grade III distraction force.

### Increase Stability and Strength of Rotator Cuff and Scapular Muscles

Both the internal and external rotators need to be strengthened as healing occurs.[25] The internal rotators and adductors must be strong to support the anterior capsule. The external rotators must be strong to stabilize the humeral head against anterior translating forces and to participate in the deltoid-rotator cuff force couple when abducting and laterally rotating the humerus. Scapular stability is important for normal shoulder function and to maintain the scapula in normal alignment. The following exercises are initiated.

● *Isometric resistance* exercises with the joint positioned at the side and progressed to various pain-free positions within the available ranges.
● Partial weight-bearing and stabilization exercises.
● *Dynamic resistance,* limiting external rotation to 50° and avoiding the position of dislocation.
● At 3 weeks, supervised *isokinetic resistance* for internal rotation and adduction at speeds of 180° per second or higher.[7]
 • *Patient position and procedure:* Standing with the arm at the side or in slight flexion and elbow flexed 90°.

The patient performs internal rotation beginning at the zero position with the hand pointing anteriorly and moving across the front of the body. Progress to positioning the shoulder at 90° flexion; then perform the exercise from zero to full internal rotation. Do not position in 90° abduction.

● By 5 weeks, all shoulder motions are incorporated into exercises on isokinetic or other mechanical equipment except in the position of 90° abduction with external rotation.

### Management: Return to Function Phase

**Restore Functional Control**
The following are emphasized.

● A balance in strength of all shoulder and scapular muscles.
● Coordination between scapular and arm motions.
● Endurance for each exercise as previously described for shoulder instabilities.

As stability improves, progress to:

● Eccentric training to maximum load
● Increasing speed and control
● Simulating desired functional patterns for activity.

**Return to Maximum Function**

● It is important that the patient learns to recognize signs of fatigue and impingement and stays within the tolerance of the tissues.
● The patient can return to normal activities when there is no muscle imbalance, when good coordination of skill is present, and when the apprehension test is negative. Full rehabilitation takes 2.5 to 4 months.[7]

## Closed Reduction Posterior Dislocation

The management approach is the same as for anterior dislocation with the exception of avoiding the position of flexion with adduction and internal rotation during the acute and healing phases.

N O T E : During the *protection phase* a sling may be uncomfortable because of the adducted and internally rotated position, particularly if the sling elevates the humerus so the head translates in a superior and posterior direction. The patient may be more comfortable with the arm hanging freely in a dependent position while kept immobile.

When mobilization is allowed, begin joint mobilization techniques using all appropriate glides except the posterior glide. Posterior glide is *contraindicated.* If adhesions develop, preventing internal rotation, mobility can safely be regained by placing the shoulder in the resting position (abducted 55° and horizontally adducted 30°), internally rotating it to the limit of its range, and applying a grade III distraction force perpendicular to the treatment plane in the

glenoid fossa (same as in Fig. 17.20 but with the arm internally rotated).

## SHOULDER INSTABILITIES: SURGERY AND POSTOPERATIVE MANAGEMENT

Surgical stabilization procedures are often necessary to repair chronic, recurrent instabilities and acute traumatic lesions in the glenohumeral, acromioclavicular, and sternoclavicular joints to restore function. Background information on GH joint instabilities and injuries that frequently occur with dislocations to this joint was described in the previous sections on nonoperative management.

### Glenohumeral Joint Stabilization Procedures and Postoperative Management

If a reasonable trial of nonoperative management has not been successful in preventing recurrence of GH joint instability, surgical stabilization may be considered. Recurrent instability of traumatic origin responds more favorably to surgical management than atraumatic instabilities.[14,110] Young, active patients who have sustained an acute, traumatic, anterior dislocation for the first time may elect to undergo surgery without a prior course of rehabilitation because there is a particularly high rate of redislocation in this group after nonoperative management.[110,112]

 **Focus on Evidence**_____

In a small, prospective, randomized study[21] of young athletes who had sustained a first-time, acute, traumatic, anterior shoulder dislocation, one group of patients ($n = 14$) participated in a nonoperative rehabilitation program of immobilization and exercise and another group ($n = 10$) underwent arthroscopic stabilization (repair of a Bankart lesion) and postoperative rehabilitation (the same program as the nonoperative group followed). Over an average of 36 months, of the 12 nonoperatively managed patients who were available for follow-up 9 (75%) experienced recurrent instability, whereas of the 9 operatively managed patients available for follow-up only 1 (11.1%) experienced recurrent instability. Six of the nine nonoperatively treated patients who experienced recurrent instability subsequently had an open Bankart repair.

In another randomized study[94] of young patients (mean age 22 years) who sustained traumatic anterior dislocations, patients either participated in a trial of nonoperative management or underwent immediate arthroscopic stabilization. Over a 2-year period, 47% of the patients in the nonoperative goup but only 15% of the surgical group experienced recurrence of the dislocation. The results of these studies demonstrate that in this population of patients, early surgical stabilization followed by postoperative rehabilitation significantly reduces the incidence of recurrent instability compared to nonoperative management.

## Indications for Surgery

The following are common indications for surgical stabilization of the GH joint.[110,112,175,190,193]

- Recurrent episodes of GH joint dislocation or subluxation that impair functional activities.
- Unidirectional or multidirectional instability during active shoulder movements that causes apprehension about placing the arm in positions of potential dislocation, leading to compromised use of the arm for functional activities.
- Instability-related impingement (secondary impingement syndrome) of the shoulder.
- Significant inherent joint laxity resulting in recurrent involuntary dislocation.
- High probability of subsequent episodes of redislocation after an acute traumatic dislocation in young patients involved in high-risk (overhead), work-related, or sport activities.
- Dislocations associated with significant cuff tears or displaced tuberosity or glenoid rim fractures.
- Irreducible (chronic, fixed) dislocation.
- Failure to resolve the instability and restore function with nonoperative management.

## Procedures

Procedures designed to improve stability and prevent recurrent instability of the GH joint must balance stabilization of the joint with retention of near-normal, functional mobility. Stabilization procedures, which may involve the anterior, posterior, or inferior portions of the capsule, are performed today using either an arthroscopic or open approach depending on the type of lesion(s) present and type of procedure selected by the surgeon.[110,112,142,175,190] Open stabilization procedures are highly successful (low recurrence of dislocation) and have been considered the standard for years. However, with advances in arthroscopic techniques and methods of tissue fixation, the use and success of arthroscopic stabilization procedures has steadily increased.[190]

Recurrent anterior (unidirectional) dislocation is by far the most common form of GH instability managed with surgical stabilization.[112] In contrast, posterior or posteroinferior instabilities are less fequently managed with surgical stabilization.[142] This section provides a brief description of surgical procedures for anterior and other types of GH instability. The procedures can be organized into several categories.

***Bankart repair.*** A Bankart repair involves an open or arthroscopic repair of a Bankart lesion (detachment of the capsulolabral complex from the anterior rim of the glenoid) (see Fig. 17.19), which commonly accompanies a traumatic anterior dislocation. During the repair an anterior capsulolabral reconstruction is performed to reattach the labrum to the surface of the glenoid lip.‡

With an open repair, the humeral insertion of the subscapularis is detached (a takedown) or split longitudi-

nally for access to the lesion and capsule,[63,110,154,158] or occasionally access is achieved through the rotator cuff interval, which allows the subscapularis to remain intact.[110] If the subscapularis is detached, it is subsequently repaired after the labrum has been reattached. With an arthroscopic approach, multiple portal sites are used, and the subscapularis is not disturbed.[5,190] Repair of a Bankart lesion is combined with an anterior capsular shift if capsular redundancy is present.

With an open procedure the labrum is reattached with direct transglenoid sutures or suture anchors, whereas with an arthroscopic approach transglenoid sutures, suture anchors, or tacks are used.[79,190] Generally, more secure fixation is achieved with an open repair than with an arthroscopic repair, although in recent years advances in arthroscopic tissue fixation have improved.[190]

***Capsulorrhaphy (capsular shift).*** Capsulorrhaphy, which can be performed using either an open or arthroscopic approach, involves tightening the capsule to reduce capsular redundancy and overall capsule volume by incising, overlapping in a pants-and-vest manner (imbrication), and then securing the lax or overstretched portion of the capsule (plication) with direct sutures, suture anchors, tacks, or staples.* A capsular shift procedure is tailored to the direction(s) of instability: anterior, inferior, posterior, or multidirectional (anteroinferior or posteroinferior). For example, if a patient has recurrent anteroinferior (multidirectional) instability, an anterior or inferior capsular shift is performed in which the anterior or inferior portion of the capsule is incised, tightened by imbrication (plication), and resutured. Most capsular shift procedures are performed because of anterior instability.[13,110,112,207]

***Electrothermally assisted capsulorrhaphy.*** Electrothermally assisted capsulorrhaphy (ETAC) involves an arthroscopic approach that uses thermal energy (radiofrequency thermal delivery or nonablative laser) to shrink and tighten loose capsuloligamentous structures. The procedure—also referred to as a *thermal-assisted capsular shift* (TACS) or *thermocapsular shrinkage*—can be used alone but more often is used in conjunction with other arthroscopic procedures, such as repair of a glenoid tear, a capsular shift, débridement of a partial rotator cuff tear, or subacromial decompression.[51,55,110,114,177,185,190,204] It has been shown in animal and human cadaveric studies that thermal energy initially makes collagen fibrils more extensible; but as the collagen tissue of the capsuloligamentous structures heals, it shortens or "shrinks" thus causing a decrease in capsular laxity.[78,165] If one or more of the glenohumeral ligaments is detached or if rotator cuff lesions are detected that could be contributing to the instability, they are repaired arthroscopically prior to ETAC.

***Soft tissue transfers.*** Open transfer and realignment of the subscapularis tendon (*Putti-Platt* or *Magnuson-Stack* procedures) to stabilize the anterior capsule is rarely done today. This is because they have resulted in poor func-

---

‡See references 5, 79, 86, 93, 110, 154, 158, 190.

*See references 4, 65, 86, 110, 112, 142, 190, 207.

tional outcomes owing to significant loss of external rotation.[110,112]

***Bony procedures.*** Open transfer of the tip of the coracoid process to the anterior glenoid rim (with the short head of the biceps and the coracobrachialis still attached) to form a bony block *(Bristow procedure)* is of interest only from an historical perspective to understand how the management of recurrent anterior dislocation has evolved.[110,112] As with procedures involving transfer of the subscapularis, the Bristow procedure also resulted in significant loss of external rotation.

***Posterior capsulorrhaphy (posterior or posteroinferior capsular shift).*** Recurrent, involuntary posterior or posteroinferior instability (far less common than anterior instability), if treated surgically, can be managed with either an open or arthroscopic capsular shift to remove posterior and inferior redundancy of the capsule.[§] Additional soft tissue procedures may be necessary, such as repair of a posterior labral tear (reverse Bankart lesion) or in rare instances plication and advancement of the infraspinatus to reinforce the posterior capsule. Shoulders without an effective posterior glenoid can be surgically managed with capsulolabral augmentation[190] or occasionally with a glenoid osteotomy.[110,142]

Employing arthroscopic posterior stabilization, a capsular shift and repair of the posterior labrum can be accomplished with the shoulder musculature remaining intact.[141] For an open stabilization, a posterolateral incision is made, the deltoid is split, and the infraspinatus, teres minor, and posterior capsule are incised.[142,176] In some instances of traumatic multidirectional instability, anterior capsulorrhaphy is used to tighten the posterior capsule indirectly.[110,142,190]

***Repair of a SLAP lesion.*** A tear of the superior labrum is classified as a SLAP lesion (*superior labrum extending anterior to posterior*).[175,190,205] Some SLAP lesions are associated with a tear of the proximal attachment of the long head of the biceps and recurrent anterior instability of the GH joint. An arthroscopic repair involves débridement of the torn portion of the superior labrum, abrasion of the bony surface of the superior glenoid, and reattachment of the labrum and biceps tendon with tacks or suture anchors. Concomitant anterior stabilization is also performed if instability is present.

***Summary.*** Glenohumeral stabilization procedures may be performed with an open or arthroscopic approach for correcting unidirectional or multidirectional instabilities. Associated procedures, such as a repair of the glenoid labrum or rotator cuff, may also be required.

## Postoperative Management

### General Considerations
As with rehabilitation after repair of rotator cuff tears, guidelines for postoperative management after surgical sta-

bilization of the GH joint are based on many factors. These factors, all of which can influence the composition and progression of a postoperative program, are summarized in Table 17.5. Additional factors, such as the philosophy and training of the surgeon and a number of patient-related variables (general health, medications, preinjury functional status and postoperative goals, education, compliance) that affect rehabilitation after GH stabilization and rotator cuff repair already have been addressed (see Table 17.3).

The content in this section identifies *general* principles of management across three broad phases of postoperative rehabilitation after a variety of surgical stabilization and reconstruction procedures for recurrent unidirectional or multidirectional instabilities of the GH joint. These general guidelines cannot begin to address the many variations of rehabilitation programs recommended for specific stabilization procedures. However, many detailed protocols or case-based descriptions of rehabilitation programs for use after specific procedures and for specific types of shoulder instabilities and associated labral or rotator cuff lesions in various patient populations are available in the literature.[*]

Regardless of the type of instability or associated pathology or the type of surgical stabilization procedure, a postoperative rehabilitation program must be based on the findings of a comprehensive examination and is individualized to meet the unique needs of each patient. The focus of postoperative rehabilitation always is to restore pain-free shoulder mobility and a level of strength and endurance of the shoulder musculature, particularly the dynamic stabilizers, to meet the patient's functional needs *while preventing recurrence of shoulder instability.*

### Immobilization

***Position.*** The position in which the patient's shoulder is immobilized after surgery is determined by the *direction(s) of instability* prior to surgery. After surgical reconstruction for recurrent *anterior* or *anteroinferior* instability, the shoulder is immobilized in a sling or splint in adduction (arm at the side) or varying degrees of abduction and in internal rotation (forearm across the abdomen) with the arm slightly anterior to the frontal plane of the body.[86,110] After surgery for *posterior* or *posteroinferior* instability, the upper extremity is supported in an orthosis, and the shoulder is immobilized in the "handshake" position (neutral rotation to 10° to 20° of external rotaion, 20° to 30° of abduction, elbow flexed, and arm at the side or sometimes with the shoulder in slight extension).[54,110,142]

***Duration.*** The duration of immobilization—that is, the period of time before use of the immobilizer is *completely* discontinued—is determined by many factors, including the type of instability and procedure(s) performed and the surgeon's intraoperative assessment. This period ranges from 1 to 3 weeks to as long as 6 to 8 weeks. However, the period of *continuous* immobilization of the operated

---

[§]See references 14, 76, 80, 110, 141, 142, 175, 176, 190.

[*]See references 24, 37, 51, 79, 91, 128, 143, 185, 205, 211.

| TABLE 17.5 | Factors that Influence the Rehabilitation Program After Surgery for Recurrent Instability of the GH Joint |
|---|---|
| **Factors** | **Potential Impact on Rehabilitation** |
| • Onset of instability | • Capsular redundancy and greater risk of recurrent dislocation more often associated with atraumatic instability, which requires more conservative postoperative rehabilitation than stabilization of recurrent instability of traumatic origin.[110] |
| • Severity of associated lesions | • The more severe the underlying pathology, the slower the progression of rehabilitation. |
| • Previous failure of a surgical stabilization | • Slower progression after previous failed stabilization procedure surgery. |
| • Direction of instability | • Stabilization of anterior instability: more rapid advancement than after stabilization of posterior or multidirectional instabilities.[142] |
| • Type of surgical approach | • Less postoperative pain with arthroscopic procedure but rate of progression essentially the same after open and arthroscopic stabilization or procedures because rate of healing of repaired tissues is the same in both procedures. |
| • Type of procedure | • Electrothermally assisted capsulorrhaphy: slower progression than arthroscopic or open capsular tightening without thermal application.[51,185,144] Bony reconstruction: slower progression than after soft tissue reconstruction. |
| • Patient variables   • Tissue integrity   • Preoperative status of dynamic stabilizers   • Generalized joint laxity | • The progression of postoperative rehabilitation is conservative for the inactive patient with multidirectional atraumatic instability who has generalized joint laxity and poor preoperative strength of the dynamic (muscular) stabilizers. |

shoulder (before pendulum exercises or shoulder ROM can be initiated) is kept as short as possible but varies with the type of procedure. For example, after an anterior stabilization procedure, the immobilizer may need to be worn continuously for only a day to a few days but in some cases up to 1 to 2 weeks.[112] In contrast, repairs of posterior or multidirectional instabilities, which are associated with a higher recurrence of dislocation, usually require a longer period of immobilization than do repairs employing an anterior stabilization procedure.[110,142,176] After a posterior stabilization procedure, the shoulder may be continuously immobilized and ROM delayed for up to 6 weeks postoperatively.[91,142]

Time frames for immobilization vary based on other factors that influence all aspects of postoperative rehabilitation (see Table 17.5). For example, the duration of immobilization is usually shorter for an elderly patient than for a young patient because the elderly patient is more likely to develop postoperative shoulder stiffness than the younger patient. In contrast, a patient with generalized hyperelasticity or a younger patient involved in high-demand activities, who is likely to place excesive stresses on healing tissues, requires a longer period of immobilization to reduce the risk of redislocation.[110]

### Exercise

As with the position and duration of immobilization, the decisions of when the arm may be temporarily removed from the immobilizer (sling or splint) to begin shoulder exercises and to what extent specific shoulder motions are either permissible or must be limited are also based on many of the factors previously summarized (see Table 17.5).

N O T E : During the early weeks of rehabilitation after a surgical stabilization procedure, determination of what ranges fall within "safe" limits of motion is based on the extent of intraoperative ROM that was possible without placing excessive tension on the repaired, tightened, or reconstructed tissues. This information may be available in the operative report or should be communicated by the surgeon to the therapist prior to initiating postoperative exercises.

The overall goal of postoperative exercise is to develop strength and stability as well as mobility of the shoulder consistent with functional needs while preventing recurrence of instability. A sufficient rotator cuff is a fundamental necessity for functional shoulder stability and mobility. Patient education and, when possible, supervised exercise instruction are the means by which the goals of each phase of rehabilitation are achieved.

Rehabilitation after anterior stabilization (anterior capsular shift or Bankart repair) is similar after open and arthroscopic procedures. In both instances, there are precautions that must be heeded, particularly during the first 6 weeks after surgery while soft tissues are healing. During this time period after an open procedure, the anterior capsule and the detached and repaired subscapularis must be protected from excessive stresses. With an arthroscopic anterior stabilization, although the subscapularis remains intact, it is also necessary to protect the anterior capsule during the initial phase of rehabilitation because soft tissue fixation may not be as secure as the fixation used in an open procedure.

###  Focus on Evidence

In a 4-year follow-up study by Sachs and colleagues[158] of 30 patients who had sustained a traumatic anterior dislocation and had undergone an open Bankart repair (that included takedown and repair of the subscapularis tendon), only one factor measured postoperatively significantly correlated with the patients' perception of a succcessful outcome after surgery. That factor was the function of the subscapularis muscle postoperatively. Although only two patients (6.7%) reported recurrence of instability over the 4-year period, postoperative testing indicated that seven patients (23%) had incompetence of the subscapularis muscle. Specifically, the mean strength of the subscapularis in these patients was only 27%, whereas in the remaining patients, said to have a competently functioning subscapularis, the mean strength was 80% (both compared with the noninvolved shoulder). There was no significant loss of strength in other shoulder muscles in either group of patients.

Of the patients with a reasonably strong subscapularis at the 4-year follow-up, 91% reported good to excellent results determined by several measurement tools, and 100% indicated that in retrospect they would have the surgery again. However, among the patients with a substantially weak subscapularis, 57% reported good to excellent results but only 57% would undergo the surgery again. The investigators indicated that the results of their study suggested that the handling of the subscapularis tendon during the repair and protection of the subscapularis during the first few weeks after surgery were critical to shoulder function and then patients' perception of the success of an open Bankart repair. Although not noted by the investigators, emphasis on strengthening the internal rotators during the late phase of rehabilitation could also contribute to the success outcomes.

---

Precautions after arthroscopic or open anterior stabilization or reconstruction procedures are summarized in Box 17.10.[37,63,79,91,110,112,128,190] Precautions for thermally assisted capsular tightening,[51,55,144,185,204] posterior stabilization procedures,[54,91,141,142] and repair of a SLAP lesion[37,205] are noted in Box 17.11.

### Exercise: Maximum Protection Phase
The initial phase of rehabilitation extends for about 6 weeks after surgery, during which time protection of the tightened capsule or repaired or reconstructed structures, such as the labrum or the subscapularis, is necessary while minimizing the negative consequences of immobilization. How soon after surgery the immobilizer may be temporarily removed for exercises varies significantly and depends on a number of factors already discussed. Exercises may be initiated as soon as the day after surgery for selected

---

| BOX 17.10 | Precautions After Anterior Glenohumeral Stabilization and/or Bankart Repair* |
| --- | --- |

- Limit *ER, horizontal abduction,* and *extension* (shoulder positions that place stress on the anterior capsule) during first 6 weeks postoperatively.
  - After an arthroscopic stabilization, although the subscapularis is intact, to avoid pull-out of fixation, limit ER to 5° to 10° with the arm in slight abduction or at the side for the first 2 weeks.[37] Then gradually progress to 45° over the next 2 to 4 weeks with the shoulder in greater abduction. With a tenuous stabilization, may need to limit ER to only neutral for the first 4 to 6 postoperative weeks.[190]
  - After an open procedure involving subscapularis takedown and repair, limit ER to 0° (no ER past neutral), to no more than 30° to 45° or to the "safe" limits identified during the intraoperative assessment for 4 to 6 weeks.[37]
  - Postpone ER combined with full shoulder abduction for at least 6 weeks.[79]
- After an arthroscopic stabilization, progress forward flexion of the shoulder more cautiously than after an open stabilization.
- After bony procedures, delay passive or assisted ROM for 6 to 8 weeks to allow time for bone healing.[110,112]
- No vigorous passive stretching to increase end-range ER for 8 to 12 weeks after either arthroscopic or open procedure except for patients with hypoelastic tissue quality.[190]
- When stretching is permissible, avoid positioning the shoulder in abduction and external rotation during grade III joint mobilization procedures.
- After procedures with subscapularis detachment and repair, no *active* or *resisted* IR for 4 to 6 weeks; avoid lifting objects, especially if pushing the hands together is required.[37,63,79,128]
- Avoid activities involving positions that place stress on the anterior aspect of the capsule for about 4 to 6 weeks.
  - Avoid functional activities that require ER, especially if combined with horizontal abduction during early rehabilitation as when reaching to put on a coat or shirt.
  - Avoid upper extremity weight bearing particularly if the shoulder is extended, as when pushing up from the armrests of a chair.
- When dynamically strengthening the rotator cuff, maintain the shoulder in about 45° rather than 90° of abduction.

*Precautions apply primarily to early rehabilitation during the first 6 weeks after surgery except as noted. The allowable ROM during the initial phase of rehabilitation depends on the type of pathology, surgical procedure, the patient's tissue quality (degree of hyper- or hypo-elasticity), and the intraoperative evaluation of shoulder stability.

---

patients who have had an anterior stabilization procedure,[37] but more often are begun 1 to 2 weeks postoperatively.[91,128] ROM is delayed for a longer period of time after a thermally assisted stabilization,[51,55,144,185,204] a posterior stabi-

**BOX 17.11    Precautions After Additional Glenohumeral Stabilization Procedures**

**Thermally Assisted Capsular Tightening**
- Be extremely cautious with ROM exercises for the first 4 to 6 weeks postoperatively because collagen in the thermally treated capsuloligamentous structures is initially more extensible (more vulnerable to stretch) until it heals. Some patients may begin ROM within protected ranges the day after surgery, whereas others may be required to postpone ROM exercises entirely for 2 weeks or more.
- While sleeping, complete immobilization (sling and swarthe) for 2 weeks or more.
- Precautions for ROM depend on the direction of instability, patient's tissue quality (hyper- or hypoelastic), and the extent of concomitant surgical procedures necessary. For example, progress patients with congenital hyperelasticity more cautiously than those with hypoelasticity.

**Posterior Stabilization Procedure and/or Reverse Bankart Repair**
- Postpone all shoulder exercises or limit elevation of the arm to 90° and IR to neutral or no more than 15° to 20° and horizontal adduction to neutral (up to 6 weeks postoperatively).
- Restrict upper extremity weight bearing, particularly when the shoulder is flexed, to avoid stress to the posterior aspect of the capsule, for example during closed-chain scapulothoracic and GH stabilization exercises and functional activities, for at least 6 weeks postoperatively.
- Avoid resistance exercises that direct loads and place stress on the posterior capsule, such as bench press exercises and prone push-ups until late in the rehabilitation program, if at all.

**Repair of a SLAP Lesion**
- For SLAP lesions where the biceps tendon is detached, progress rehabilitation more cautiously than when the biceps remains intact.
  - Limit passive or assisted elevation of arm to 60° for the first 2 weeks and to 90° at 3 to 4 weeks postoperatively.
  - Perform only passive assisted humeral rotation with the shoulder in the plane of the scapula for the first 2 weeks (ER to only neutral or up to 15° and IR to 45°); during weeks 3 to 4, progress ER to 30° and IR to 60°.
- Avoid positions that create tension in the biceps, such as elbow extension with shoulder extension (as when reaching behind the back) during the first 4 to 6 weeks postoperatively.
- Postpone active contractions of the biceps (elbow flexion with supination of the forearm) for 6 weeks and resisted biceps exercises or lifting and carrying weighted objects until 8 to 12 weeks postoperatively depending on the extent and type of biceps repair; then progress cautiously.
- If the mechanism of injury was a fall onto the outstretched hand and arm causing joint compression, progress weight-bearing exercises gradually.
- If anterior instability is also present, follow precautions in Box 17.10.
- Avoid positions of abduction combined with maximum external rotation as this places torsion forces on the base of the biceps attachment on the glenoid.
  - Perform latissimus dorsi strengthening (pull-down exercises) in front of the body rather than behind the head.

---

lization procedure,[54,91,141,142] or repair of a SLAP lesion and torn biceps tendon[37,205] (see Box 17.11).

***Goals and interventions.*** The goals and exercises for the maximum protection phase are summarized in this section.[37,51,54,79,128,203,211]

◉ ***Control pain and inflammation.***
- Use of a sling for comfort when the arm is dependent or for protection when in public areas. While seated, remove the sling (if permissible) and rest the forearm on a table or wide armrest with the shoulder positioned in abduction and neutral rotation. (This position provides support but prevents prolonged internal rotation and potential contracture of the subscapularis and other internal rotators of the shoulder.)
- Use of cryotherapy and prescribed anti-inflammatory medication.
- Active ROM of the cervical spine and shoulder relaxation exercises.

◉ ***Prevent or correct posture impairments.***
- Emphasis on spinal extension and scapular retraction; avoid excessive thoracic kyphosis.

◉ ***Maintain mobility and control of structures proximal and distal to the shoulder.***
- Active ROM of the elbow, forearm, wrist, and fingers the day after surgery.
- Active scapulothoracic movements.

PRECAUTION: Initially, strengthen the scapular stabilizing muscles in open-chain positions to avoid the need for weight bearing on the operated upper extremity. When weight-bearing activities are initiated, be cautious about the position of the operated shoulder to avoid undue stress to the vulnerable portion of the capsule for about 6 weeks postoperatively.

◉ ***Restore shoulder mobility while protecting tightened or repaired tissues.***
- Pendulum exercises (nonweighted), usually for the first 2 weeks postoperatively.
- Self-assisted ROM, wand exercises for the GH joint, initially *within protected ranges* as early as 2 weeks or as late as 6 weeks postoperatively. Begin shoulder elevation in the supine position to stabilize the scapula; begin humeral rotation with the arm supported and the shoulder in a slightly abducted and flexed position.

- With an anterior stabilization, gradually progress to near-complete ROM (compared to the uninvolved shoulder) by 6 to 8 weeks except for external rotation and extension and horizontal abduction past neutral. With a posterior stabilization, progress forward flexion, horizontal adduction, and internal rotation cautiously.
- Progression to active shoulder ROM when motion can be performed without pain, apprehension, or use of substitute motions, such as hiking the shoulder to initiate abduction.
- Use of the operated arm for *unresisted, non-weight-bearing, waist-level* functional activities by 2 to 4 weeks postoperatively.

◎ *Prevent reflex inhibition and atrophy of GH musculature.*
- Multiple-angle, low-intensity isometric (muscle-setting) exercises (very gentle isometrics) of GH musculature as early as the first week or by 3 to 4 weeks postoperatively after some procedures.
- *Possible* initiation of dynamic exercises against *light* resistance (light-grade elastic) below shoulder level at 4 to 6 weeks. Emphasize the GH stabilizers.
- Be particularly cautious when applying resistance to musculature that has been torn or surgically detached, incised, or advanced and then repaired.

NOTE: In some cases, dynamic exercises against light resistance are delayed until the intermediate phase of rehabilitation (about 6 to 8 weeks postoperatively), when only moderate protection is necessary.

### Exercise: Moderate Protection Phase

The moderate protection phase of rehabilitation begins around 6 weeks postoperatively and continues until approximately 12 to 16 weeks. The focus is on always maintaining joint stability while achieving nearly full active (unassisted) ROM of the shoulder; continued development of neuromuscular control, strength, and endurance of scapulothoracic and GH musculature; and progressive use of the upper extremity through greater ROMs for functional activities.

*Criteria for progression.* Criteria to advance to the second phases of rehabilitation are a well healed incision, reasonable progress in ROM, minimal pain, and no sense of apprehension about instability with active motions.[37,51,79,91]

*Goals and interventions.* The goals and interventions for the intermediate phase of rehabilitation are as follows.[37,51, 79,91,203,211]

◎ *Regain nearly full, pain-free, active ROM of the shoulder.*
- Continuation of active ROM with the goal of achieving nearly full ROM by 12 weeks.
- Gains in ROM used in functional activities.
- As stability permits, stretching and grade III mobilization in positions that do not provoke instability. After

an anterior stabilization procedure for chronic (atraumatic) anterior instability, pay particular attention to increasing horizontal adduction, as the posterior structures are often tight preoperatively and continue to be tight postoperatively.

◎ *Continue to increase strength and endurance of shoulder musculature.*
- Alternating isometrics against increasing resistance with emphasis on the scapula and rotator cuff musculature.
- Dynamic (concentric and eccentric) resistance exercises initiated or progressed using weights and elastic resistance with emphasis on scapulothoracic and glenohumeral stabilizers. Begin in mid-range positions, progressing to end-range positions.
- *After anterior stabilization,* do not initiate dynamic strengthening of the internal rotators from full external rotation, particularly in the 90° abducted position. When strengthening the shoulder extensors, *do not extend the arm posterior to the frontal plane.* Accordingly, strengthen the shoulder extensors in the prone position with the arm over the side of the table or while standing and leaning forward with the hips flexed to approximately 90°. Use the same precaution when strengthening the horizontal abductors and adductors. In addition, maintain the shoulder in neutral rotation during horizontal abduction and adduction.
- *After a posterior stabilization* do not initially begin dynamic strengthening of the external rotators from full internal rotation.
- Dynamic strengthening in diagonal and simulated functional movement patterns.
- Upper extremity ergometry with a portable reciprocal exerciser on a table for muscular endurance. Include forward and backward motions.
- Progressive upper extremity weight bearing during strengthening and stabilization exercises.

### Exercise: Minimum Protection/ Return To Function Phase

Criteria to progress to the final phase of rehabilitation and the focus of exercises are similar to the criteria already discussed for rehabilitation after rotator cuff repair. This phase usually begins around 12 weeks postoperatively or as late as 16 weeks, depending on individual characteristics of the patient and the surgical stabilization procedure. Stretching should continue until ROM consistent with functional needs has been attained. Gains in ROM are possible for up to 12 months as collagen tissue continues to remodel. Resistance exercises to improve strength and endurance are progressed to replicate movements involved in functional activities, including positions of provocation of instability. Plyometric training is introduced and gradually progressed, particularly in patients intending to return to high-demand sports or work-related activities. Participation in desired work-related and sports activities often takes up to 6 months postoperatively.

PRECAUTIONS: Some patients may have permanent restrictions placed on functional activities that involve high-risk movements and that could potentially cause recurrence of the instability. After some anterior stabilization procedures, full external rotation (ER) in 90° of abduction may not be advisable or possible.[91]

## Outcomes

A successful postoperative outcome involves regaining the ability to participate in desired functional activities without a recurrence of instability of the GH joint. Follow-up studies measure subjective and objective outcomes, such as restoration of ROM and strength, recurrence of pain, apprehension of instability, ability to participate in desired activities, and general patient satisfaction. There is a wealth of follow-up studies describing various outcomes after stabilization procedures. However, most of the studies comparing the success of one surgical intervention with that of another are not randomized—understandably so because the surgeon's examination is the basis for determining which procedure is most appropriate and will most likely lead to successful results for each patient.

Although postoperative exercise (supervised or unsupervised) is consistently described as essential for optimal outcomes after stabilization surgery, no current, randomized studies were identified that compared the effectiveness of postoperative exercise programs after stabilization of the GH joint (method of instruction, content, rate of progression) for this review. As with surgical decisions, most postoperative rehabilitation programs are customized to meet each patient's needs, making comparison of outcomes difficult.

Results of surgery and postoperative rehabilitation are typically reported for specific pathologies, patient populations, and surgical stabilization procedures and are determined by means of a variety of outcome measures. Despite this, some generalizations can be made.

*Recurrence of instability*. As noted at the beginning of this section on stabilization procedures, recurrent instability of traumatic origin responds more favorably to surgical management than atraumatic instabilities.[14,110] In addition, the rate of recurrence of instability is substantially higher in young patients (≤ 30 or ≤ 40 years of age) or patients who return to high-demand, work-related activities or competitive overhead sports than less active, older patients (> 30 or > 40 years of age).[110,190]

The rates of redislocation after open and arthroscopic procedures have also been compared. Historically, recurrence rates after arthroscopic stabilization have been higher than after open stabilization.[38,110] For example, in a review of studies on anterior stabilization procedures, the mean redislocation rate after open stabilization (Bankart lesion repair) was 11% (range 4% to 23%), but after arthroscopic stabilization recurrence rates were 18% (range 2% to 32%) with transglenoid suture fixation and 17% (range 0% to 30%) with tack fixation.[79] In another review of recent studies, the rates of recurrence of anterior instability after an arthroscopic Bankart repair ranged from 8% to 17%.[190] The decreasing redislocation rates after arthroscopic procedures have been attributed to improvements in arthroscopic techniques. Today, arthroscopic stabilization has been shown, in many instances, to be equal to open stabilization for patients with unidirectional, anterior instability of the GH joint.[38,190,194] However, for multidirectional instabilities, results of follow-up studies after arthroscopic stabilization, although promising, are not yet equal to outcomes after open stabilization.[190]

Outcomes after stabilization procedures for anterior and posterior instabilities have also been compared. Surgical stabilization of a recurrent, unidirectional *anterior* instability has yielded more predictable results and lower rates of instability recurrence than stabilization of *posterior* or *multidirectional* instabilities.[14,110,142,190,207] The average rate of posterior instability recurrence (after arthroscopic stabilization) has been reported to be particularly high. One source reported a 30% to 40% rate of redislocation,[176] and another reported rates as high as 50%.[190] In contrast, after anterior stabilization procedures mean recurrence rates have been reported at 11% and 17% to 18%, respectively, for open and arthroscopic procedures.[79]

As the preoperative diagnosis has improved and the selection of appropriate candidates for surgery has gotten better, the recurrence of instability after posterior stabilization has decreased. In a study[141] with a mean follow-up of 39.1 months, the rate of recurrence of instability after posterior stabilization (arthroscopic approach) was only 12.1% (4 of 33 patients with a mean age of 25 years and a history of involuntary or voluntary dislocaton of the GH joint associated with acute traumatic and chronic repetitive microtrauma).

*Shoulder ROM*. Range of shoulder motion is another outcome often measured. Although it is possible to achieve full ROM postoperatively, after anterior stabilization procedures, full ER or horizontal abduction is sometimes not advisable or possible.[91] Likewise, some posterior stabilization procedures permanently limit full internal rotation (IR) and, to some extent, overhead elevation of the arm.[110]

After open anterior stabilization and Bankart repair, which usually requires detachment and repair of the subscapularis, a mean loss of 12° of ER has been reported.[61] It has been suggested that there is less loss of shoulder ER after arthroscopic procedures than after open procedures.[79] However, in a nonrandomized study that compared open and arthroscopic anterior stabilization procedures, both groups had some loss of ER (mean loss of 9° and 11°, respectively, in the arthroscopic and open groups), but these differences between groups were not significant.[38]

After an open GH stabilization for instability due to repetitive microtrauma, postoperative loss of shoulder ER is the most common reason athletes involved in overhead sports are unable to successfully return to competition. Loss of shoulder rotation is reported to be less after arthroscopic stabilization procedures, thus enabling a greater percentage of these athletes to return to competition.[144] Early follow-up of patients who have undergone thermally assisted capsular stabilization is encouraging,[55] but long-term outcomes are just becoming available. To date, the largest study of overhead athletes who underwent thermally assisted stabilization followed 130 patients for a mean of 29.3 months. Of these athletes, 113 (87%) returned to competition in a mean of 8.4 months. Although postoperative ROM was not reported, the implication was that the return of ROM after thermally assisted arthroscopic stabilization was sufficient for a high percentage of athletes being able to return to competition.

## Acromioclavicular and Sternoclavicular Joint Stabilization Procedures and Postoperative Management

### Acromioclavicular Joint Stabilization

Grade III instability (separation), in which the acromioclavicular (AC) and coricoclavicular ligaments are completely ruptured and the clavicle is acutely or chronically dislocated in a superior direction on the acromion, may be surgically reduced and stabilized with a variety of techniques.[124] Techniques for management of acute dislocations include primary stabilization of the AC joint with Kirschner wires, Steinman pins, screws, or most recently bioabsorbable tacks, sutures, or fiber wires. A muscle-tendon transfer that includes the tip of the coracoid process and the attached tendons of the coracobrachialis and short head of the biceps to the undersurface of the clavicle,[131] or use of the Weaver-Dunn procedure, which involves resecting the distal clavicle with coracoacromial (CA) ligament reconstruction (transferring the CA ligament from the acromion to the shaft of the distal clavicle) also can be performed.[124] Based on a small body of evidence in the literature, it appears the best results are achieved with primary AC and coracoclavicular stabilization procedures. Chronic AC dislocations, which are usually associated with degenerative changes of the AC joint, are most often managed with distal clavicle resection coupled with coracoclavicular stabilization.[131,148]

### Sternoclavicular Joint Stabilization

Although most sternoclavicular (SC) dislocations are managed nonoperatively, an acute posterior dislocation of the SC joint that cannot be successfully reduced with a closed maneuver or an SC joint that dislocates recurrently are managed surgically. Surgical reduction of a traumatic anterior dislocation is not recommended.[147] Surgical options for posterior SC dislocations include open reduction with repair of the stabilizing ligaments or resection of a portion of the medial clavicle and fixation of the remaining clavicle to the first rib or sternum with a soft tissue graft.[147,208]

### Postoperative Management

After surgical stabilization of either the AC or SC joint, the shoulder is immobilized in a sling or swarthe for up to 6 weeks.[40] Exercise interventions are directed at functional recovery as the signs of healing allow. No specific muscles cross the AC and SC joints, so scapular and glenohumeral strength is developed to provide indirect control.

During the first few weeks of immobilization, the patient is encouraged to perform active ROM of the wrist and hand. If the elbow is supported on a table, the patient is permitted to perform active ROM of the elbow and forearm. The operated extremity, if supported, may be used for light functional activities, such as holding a utensil or typing, but weight bearing and shoulder ROM are completely prohibited during the first 6 weeks.[40]

When the immobilization can be removed, restoration of shoulder and elbow mobility and neuromuscular control of the shoulder girdle are the focus of the exercise program to decrease the adverse effects of prolonged immobilization. Shoulder ROM (passive, progressing to assisted ROM to tolerance in the supine position to stabilize the scapula and minimize stress to the AC joint), active scapular motions, and light isometrics of the shoulder musculature are initiated. Stabilization exercises, dynamic strengthening of the shoulder and scapula musculature, and stretching to restore full ROM are gradually introduced and progressed, as graduated functional activities are integrated into the rehabilitation program.

## EXERCISE INTERVENTIONS FOR THE SHOULDER GIRDLE

## EXERCISE TECHNIQUES DURING ACUTE AND EARLY SUBACUTE STAGES OF TISSUE HEALING

During the *protection* and *early controlled motion* phases of management, when inflammation is present or just beginning to resolve and the healing tissues should not be stressed, early motion may be utilized to inhibit pain and muscle guarding and help prevent deleterious effects of complete immobilization. This section describes and summarizes techniques that may be used for these purposes. During the acute and early subacute stages, when motion in the shoulder itself is limited to allow tissues to begin to heal, it is also valuable to treat associated areas such as the cervical and thoracic spine, the scapulae, and the remainder of the upper extremity (elbow, wrist, and hand) to begin correcting faulty posture, relieve stresses to the shoulder girdle, and prevent fluid stasis in the extremity.

General guidelines for management during the acute stage are described in Chapter 10, and specific precautions for various pathologies and surgical interventions in the shoulder are identified throughout the second major section of this chapter. Early motion is usually passive ROM (PROM) and applied within pain-free ranges. When tolerated, active-assistive range of motion (A-AROM) is initiated.

### Early Motion of the Glenohumeral Joint

Manual PROM and A-AROM techniques are described in detail in Chapter 3. This section expands on self-assisted exercises.

## Wand Exercises

*Patient position and procedure:* Initiate A-AROM using a cane, wand, or T-bar in the supine position to provide stabilization and control of the scapula during the protection and early controlled motion phases. Motions usually included are flexion, abduction, flexion in the plane of the scapula (scaption), and rotation (Fig. 17.21A).

● If it is necessary to relieve stress on the anterior capsule, such as following surgical repair of the capsule or labrum, place a folded towel under the humerus to position the humerus anterior to the midline of the body when the patient performs internal or external rotation (Fig. 17.21B).

● When treating a shoulder impingement (primary or secondary), have the patient grasp the wand with the forearm supinated when flexing and abducting to emphasize external rotation.

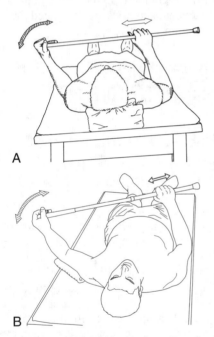

FIGURE 17.21 Self-assisted shoulder rotation using a cane (*A*) with the arm at the side and (*B*) in scaption. To relieve stress on the anterior capsule, elevate the distal humerus with a folded towel.

## Ball Rolling or Table Top Dusting

*Patient position and procedure:* Sitting with the arm resting on a table and hand placed on a 6- to 8-inch ball or towel and the shoulder in the plane of the scapula. Have the patient initiate gentle circular motions of the shoulder by moving the trunk forward, backward, and to the side, allowing the hand to roll the ball or "dust the table." As pain subsides, have the patient use the shoulder muscles to actively move the ball or cloth through greater ROMs.

## Wall (Window) Washing

*Patient position and procedure:* Standing with hand placed against a wall supporting a towel or a ball. Instruct the patient to perform clockwise and counterclockwise circular motions with the hand moving the towel or rolling the ball. Progress this activity by having the patient reach upward and outward as far as tolerated without causing symptoms.

## Pendulum (Codman's) Exercises

*Patient position and procedure:* Standing, with the trunk flexed at the hips about 90°. The arm hangs loosely downward in a position between 60° and 90° flexion or scaption (Fig. 17.22).

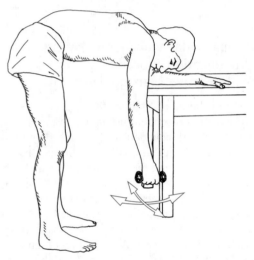

FIGURE 17.22 Pendulum exercises. For gentle distraction, no weight is used. Use of a weight causes a grade III (stretching) distraction force.

● A pendulum or swinging motion of the arm is initiated by having the patient move the trunk slightly back and forth. Motions of flexion, extension, and horizontal abduction, adduction, and circumduction can be done.[34] Increase the arc of motion as tolerated. This technique should not cause pain.

● If the patient cannot maintain balance while leaning over, have the patient hold on to a solid structure or lie prone on a table.

● If the patient experiences back pain from bending over, use the prone position.

● Adding a weight to the hand or using wrist cuffs causes a greater distraction force on the GH joint. Weights should be used only when joint stretching maneuvers are indicated late in the subacute and chronic stages—and then only if the scapula is stabilized by the therapist or a belt is placed around the thorax and scapula so the stretch force is directed to the joint, not the soft tissue of the scapulothoracic region.

PRECAUTIONS: If a patient gets dizzy when standing upright after being bent over, have the patient sit and rest. With increased pain or decreased ROM, the technique may be an inappropriate choice. Pendulum exercises are also inappropriate for a patient with peripheral edema.

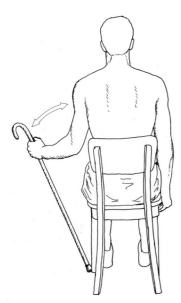

FIGURE 17.23 Gear shift exercise. Self-assisted shoulder rotation using a cane. Flexion/extension and diagonal patterns can also be done.

## "Gear Shift" Exercises

*Patient position and procedure*: Sitting with the involved arm at the side, holding a cane or wand with the tip resting on the floor to support the weight of the arm. Instruct the patient to move the pole forward and back, diagonally, or laterally and medially in a motion similar to shifting gears in a car with a floor shift (Fig. 17.23).

## Early Motion of the Scapula

PROM and A-AROM of the scapula are described in Chapter 3. During the acute phase, the side-lying position is usually more comfortable than prone-lying. If the patient can perform active scapular elevation/depression and protraction/retraction, use the sitting position.

## Early Neuromuscular Control

Frequently, the muscles of the rotator cuff are inhibited after trauma or surgery.[198] Initiate the following to stimulate activation and develop control in key muscles as soon as the patient tolerates it.

### Multiple-Angle Muscle Setting

Begin gentle multiple-angle muscle-setting exercises of the internal and external rotators in pain-free positions of humeral flexion or scaption. Activate the scapular and remaining GH muscles with gentle muscle-setting techniques in positions that do not exacerbate symptoms.

### Closed-Chain or Protected Weight Bearing

Have the patient lean onto his or her hands or elbows and gently move from side to side. This helps to seat the humeral head in the glenoid fossa and stimulate muscle action.

## ● EXERCISE TECHNIQUES TO INCREASE FLEXIBILITY AND RANGE OF MOTION

To regain neuromuscular control and function in the shoulder girdle, it may be necessary to increase flexibility in restricted muscles and fascia so proper shoulder girdle alignment and functional ranges are possible. The principles of muscle inhibition and passive stretching are presented in Chapter 4. Techniques to stretch tight joints in the shoulder girdle were discussed earlier in this chapter with reference to Chapter 5 (joint mobilization procedures). Specific manual and self-stretching techniques are described in this section.

### ● Focus on Evidence

In a recent randomized study of 20 subjects with impaired GH joint mobility, the experimental group underwent an intervention of soft tissue mobilization of the subscapularis, followed by contract–relax against manual resistance to the internal rotators, and then actively moved their extremity through the $D_2$ PNF pattern (flexion, abduction, and external rotation). The control group received no treatment; they rested for 10 minutes. Those who underwent the interventions had an immediate post-treatment increase in external rotation of $16.4° \pm 5.5°$ compared with $0.9° \pm 1.5°$ in the control group ($p < 0.0005$) and an increase in overhead reach of $9.6 \pm 6.2$ cm compared with $2.4 \pm 4.5$ cm in the control group ($p\ 0.009$).[62]

It is worth noting the immediate positive results in this study; but because long-term results were not determined, it is important to reinforce the need for follow-up self-stretching and ROM exercises in the patient's home exercise program.

## Self-Stretching Techniques

Teach the patient a low-intensity, prolonged stretch. Emphasize the importance of not bouncing at the end of the range.

### To Increase Horizontal Flexion/ Adduction—Cross-Chest Stretch

*Patient position and procedure*: Sitting or standing. Teach the patient to adduct the tight shoulder horizontally by placing the arm across the chest and then apply sustained overpressure to the adducted arm by pulling the arm toward the chest, being careful not to rotate the trunk (Fig. 17.24).

N O T E : This stretch is used when treating impingement syndromes to increase mobility in the structures of the posterior GH joint.

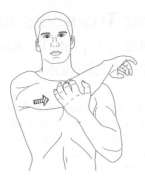

FIGURE 17.24 Self-stretching to increase horizontal adduction.

## To Increase Flexion and Elevation of the Arm

*Patient position and procedure*: Sitting with the involved side next to the table, forearm resting along the table edge, and elbow slightly flexed (Fig. 17.25A). Have the patient slide the forearm forward along the table while bending from the waist. Eventually the head should be level with the shoulder (Fig. 17.25B).

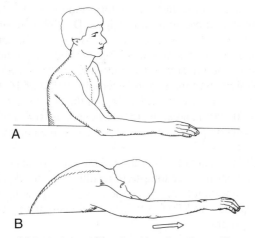

FIGURE 17.25 (*A*) Beginning and (*B*) end positions for self-stretching to increase shoulder flexion with elevation.

## To Increase External (Lateral) Rotation

● *Patient position and procedure*: Standing and facing a doorframe with the palm of the hand against the edge of the frame and elbow flexed 90°. While keeping the arm against the side or in slight abduction (held in abduction with a folded towel or small pillow under the axilla), have the patient turn away from the fixed hand (Fig. 17.26A).

● *Patient position and procedure*: Sitting at the side of a table with the forearm resting on the table and elbow flexed to 90°. Have the patient bend from the waist, bringing the head and shoulder level with the table (Fig. 17.26B).

PRECAUTION: Avoid the stretch position (illustrated in Figure 17.26B) if there is anterior GH instability.

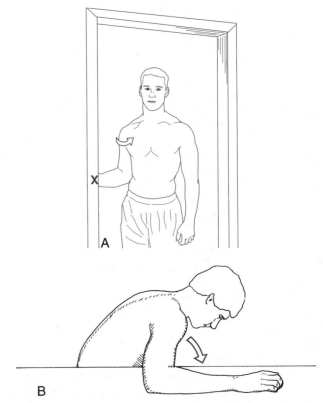

FIGURE 17.26 Self-stretching to increase lateral rotation of the shoulder (*A*) with the arm at the side using a doorframe and (*B*) with the arm in scaption using a table to stabilize the forearm.

## To Increase Internal Rotation

● *Patient position and procedure*: Standing facing a doorframe with the elbow flexed to 90° and the back of the hand against the frame. Have the patient turn his or her trunk toward the fixed hand.

● *Patient position and procedure*: Side-lying on the affected side, with the shoulder and elbow each flexed to 90° and arm internally rotated to end position. Have the patient then push the forearm toward the table with the opposite hand (Fig. 17.27).

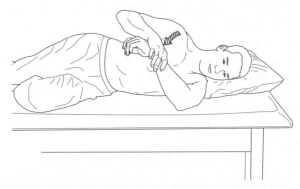

FIGURE 17.27 Self-stretching to increase internal rotation of the shoulder using a table to stabilize the humerus.

### To Increase Abduction and Elevation of the Arm

● *Patient position and procedure*: Sitting with the side next to a table, the forearm resting with palm up (supinated) on the table and pointing toward the opposite side of the table (Fig. 17.28A). Have the patient slide his or her arm across the table as the head is brought down toward the arm and the thorax moves away from the table (Fig. 17.28B).

● *Patient position and procedure*: Same as above with a folded towel or belt placed across the proximal humerus and held in the opposite hand. Have the patient pull downward on the towel to cause a caudal slide of the humeral head when in the end-range stretch position of abduction.

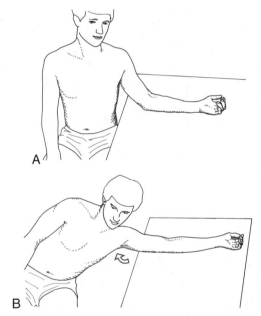

FIGURE 17.28 (A) Beginning and (B) end positions for self-stretching to increase shoulder abduction with elevation.

### To Increase Extension of the Arm

*Patient position and procedure*: Standing with the back to the table, both hands grasping the edge with the fingers facing forward (Fig. 17.29A). Have the patient begin to squat while letting the elbows flex (Fig. 17.29B).

P R E C A U T I O N : If a patient is prone to anterior subluxation or dislocation, this stretching technique should not be done.

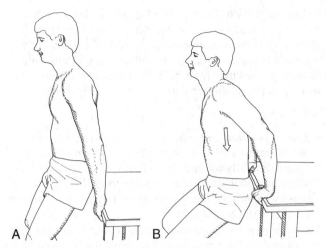

FIGURE 17.29 (A) Beginning and (B) end positions for self-stretching to increase shoulder extension.

### To Increase Internal Rotation, Extension, and Scapular Tipping (Towel or Wand Stretch)

*Patient position and procedure*: Sitting or standing. Instruct the patient to hold each end of a towel (or wand) with one arm overhead and the arm to be stretched behind the lower back, and then pull up on the towel with the overhead hand (see Fig. 17.13). This stretch is used to increase the ability to reach behind the back. It is a generalized stretch that does not isolate specific tight tissues. Before using it, each component of the motion should be stretched so no one component becomes the "weak link" in the chain.

P R E C A U T I O N : If a patient has anterior or multidirectional GH joint instability or has had recent anterior stabilization surgery to correct a dislocated shoulder, this exercise should not be done until late in the rehabilitation program, when the capsule is well healed, because it forces the head of the humerus against the anterior capsule.

## Manual and Self-Stretching Exercises for Specific Muscles

Manual stretching of specific multijoint muscles that affect alignment of the shoulder girdle are presented in this section along with self-stretching techniques for these muscles.

### To Stretch the Latissimus Dorsi Muscle

#### Manual Stretch

*Patient position and procedure*: Supine, with hips and knees flexed so the pelvis is stabilized in a posterior pelvic tilt. Provide additional stabilization to the pelvis with one hand, if necessary. With the other hand grasp the distal humerus and flex, laterally rotate, and partially abduct the shoulder to the end of the available range. Instruct the patient to contract into extension, adduction, and medial rotation while providing resistance for a hold–relax maneuver. During the relaxation phase, elongate the muscle (see Fig. 4.16B).

### Self-Stretch

● *Patient position and procedure*: Hook-lying with the pelvis stabilized in a posterior pelvic tilt and the arms flexed, laterally rotated, and slightly abducted overhead as far as possible (thumbs pointing toward floor). Allow gravity to provide the stretch force. Instruct the patient to not allow the back to arch.

● *Patient position and procedure*: Standing with back to a wall and feet forward enough to allow the hips and knees to partially flex and flatten the low back against the wall, with the arms in a "hold-up" position (abducted 90° and laterally rotated 90° if possible). Tell the patient to slide the back of the hands up the wall as far as possible without allowing the back to arch.

N O T E : This exercise is also used to strengthen the lower trapezius and serratus anterior as they upwardly rotate and depress the scapulae during humeral abduction.

### To Stretch the Pectoralis Major Muscles

#### Manual Stretch

*Patient position and procedure*: Sitting on a treatment table or mat, with the hands behind the head. Kneel behind the patient and grasp the patient's elbows (Fig. 17.30). Have the patient breathe in as he or she brings the elbows out to the side (horizontal abduction and scapular adduction). Hold the elbows at this end-point as the patient breathes out. No forceful stretch is needed against the elbows, because the rib cage is elongating the proximal attachment of the pectoralis major muscles bilaterally. As the patient repeats the inhalation, again move the elbows up and out to the end of the available range and hold as the patient breathes out. Repeat only three times in succession to avoid hyperventilation.

N O T E : Hyperventilation should not occur because the breathing is slow and comfortable. If the patient does become dizzy, allow time to rest; then reinstruct for proper technique. Be sure the patient maintains the head and neck in the neutral position, not forward.

### Self-Stretch

● *Patient position and procedure*: Standing, facing a corner or open door, with the arms in a reverse T or a V against the wall (Fig. 17.31). Have the patient lean the entire body forward from the ankles (knees slightly flexed).

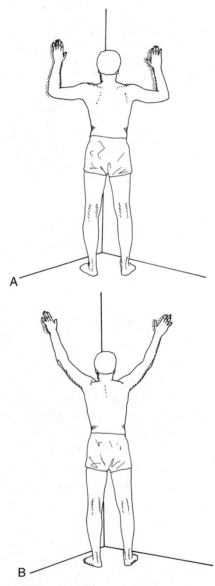

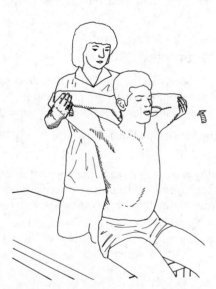

FIGURE 17.30 Active stretching of the pectoralis major muscle. The therapist gently pulls the elbows posteriorly while the patient breathes in and then holds the elbows at the end-point as the patient breathes out.

FIGURE 17.31 Self-stretching the pectoralis major muscle with the arms in a reverse T to stretch (*A*) the clavicular portion and in a V to stretch (*B*) the sternal portion.

The degree of stretch can be adjusted by the amount of forward movement.

● *Patient position and procedure*: Sitting or standing and grasping the wand with the forearms pronated and elbows flexed 90°. Have the patient then elevate the shoulders and bring the wand behind the head and shoulders (Fig. 17.32). The scapulae are adducted, and the elbows are brought out to the side. Combine with breathing by having the patient inhale as he or she brings the wand into position behind the shoulders; then exhale while holding this stretched position.

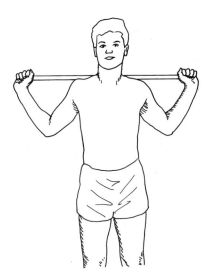

FIGURE 17.32 Wand exercises to stretch the pectoralis major muscle.

## To Stretch the Pectoralis Minor Muscle

*Patient position and procedure*: Sitting, place one hand posterior on the scapula and the other hand anterior on the shoulder just above the coracoid process (Fig. 17.33).

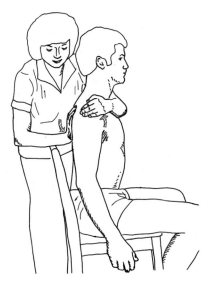

FIGURE 17.33 Active stretching of the pectoralis minor muscle. The therapist holds the scapular and coracoid process at the end-point as the patient breathes out.

As the patient breathes in, tip the scapula posteriorly by pressing up and back against the coracoid process while pressing downward against the inferior angle of the scapula; then hold it at the end-position while the patient breathes out. Repeat, readjusting the end-position with each inhalation and stabilizing as the patient exhales.

## To Stretch the Levator Scapulae Muscle

NOTE: The levator scapulae muscle attaches to the superior angle of the scapula and causes it to rotate downward and elevate; it also attaches to the transverse processes of the upper cervical vertebrae and causes them to backward bend and rotate to the ipsilateral side. To minimize stress to the cervical spine, it is recommended that the cervical spine and head be placed at end range and stabilized and that the stretch force be applied against the scapula.

### Manual Stretch

*Patient position and procedure*: Sitting with the head rotated opposite to side of tightness (looking away from the tight side) and forward bent until a slight pull is felt in the posterolateral aspect of the neck (in the levator muscle). The arm on the side of tightness is abducted, and the hand is placed behind the head to help stabilize it in the rotated position. Stand behind the patient and stabilize with one arm; place the other hand (same side as the tight muscle) over the superior angle of the scapula (Fig. 17.34). With the muscle now in its stretched position, have the patient breathe in, then out. Hold the shoulder and scapula down to maintain the stretch as the patient breathes in again (he or she contracts the muscle against the resistance of the fixating hand). To increase the stretch, press down against the superior angle of the scapula. This is not a forceful stretch but a gentle hold–relax maneuver. Do not stretch the muscle by forcing rotation on the head and neck.

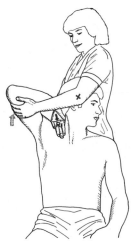

FIGURE 17.34 Stretching of the levator scapulae muscle. The therapist stabilizes the head and scapula as the patient breathes in, contracting the muscle against the resistance. As the patient relaxes, the rib cage and scapula depress, which stretches the muscle.

**Self-Stretch**

◉ *Patient position and procedure*: Standing with the head side bent and rotated away from the tight side and bent elbow against a wall. The other hand can be placed across the forehead to stabilize the rotated head. Instruct the patient to slide the elbow up the wall as he or she takes in a breath, then hold the position while exhaling (Fig. 17.35A).

◉ *Patient position and procedure*: Sitting with head side bent and rotated away from the tight side. To stabilize the scapula, have the patient reach down and back with the hand on the side of the tightness and hold onto the seat of the chair. The other hand is placed on the head to gently pull it forward and to the side in an oblique direction opposite the line of pull of the tight muscle (Fig. 17.35B).

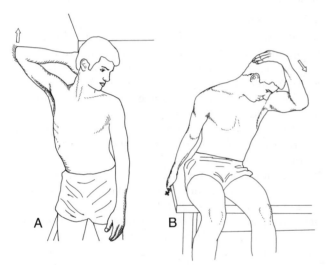

FIGURE 17.35 Self-stretching the levator scapulae muscle (*A*) using upward rotation of the scapula and (*B*) using depression of the scapula.

# ◉ EXERCISES TO DEVELOP AND IMPROVE MUSCLE PERFORMANCE AND FUNCTIONAL CONTROL

Developing control of the scapula and GH joint musculature is fundamental to correcting pathomechanics of the shoulder girdle and for improving strength, muscle endurance, power, and performance of functional activities. During observation of scapular alignment and movement, if excessive tipping, winging, or poorly coordinated scapu-

lohumeral rhythm during humeral elevation is identified, it is important to correct these faulty mechanics with properly chosen exercises. Insufficient stabilization and control of GH rotation and translation during humeral elevation likewise necessitate the selection of exercises that emphasize training the rotator cuff musculature. When designing an exercise program, the intensity and type of exercises must not exceed the capability of the healing tissues whether the cause of the impaired control is nerve injury, disuse, traumatic insult, overuse, instability, or surgery.

The exercises described in the following sections begin at the most simple or least stressful level and progress to more difficult levels for each type of exercise. They also progress from uniplanar or isolated muscle activity to more complex and functional patterns. Initially, choose exercises that help the patient focus on using correct muscles to counteract the identified impairments; then increase the challenge by emphasizing patterns of exercises that prepare the musculature to respond to functional demands.

No matter what the level of exercise, it is important to challenge patients at intensities they can meet so they can safely progress to more intense levels. Before teaching the resistance exercises and functional training activities presented in this section, it is important that the reader understands and knows how to apply the principles of resistance exercise and open- and closed-chain training described in Chapter 6. It is also important to know the principles of tissue healing described in Chapter 10 and the precautions for various shoulder pathologies and surgical interventions presented in this chapter. Because posture has a direct effect on the function of the shoulder girdle, refer to Chapters 14 and 16 for principles and exercises to correct postural impairments that might underlie faulty shoulder girdle mechanics. Box 17.12 summarizes a method of progressing an individual toward functional recovery.

## Isometric Exercises

Isometric exercises are applied along a continuum of very gentle to maximum contraction, and they are applied at varying muscle lengths and joint angles. Choice of the intensity, muscle length, or joint angle and the number of repetitions is based on strength, stage of recovery after injury or surgery, and/or the pathomechanics of the region.

### Scapular Muscles
*Patient position and procedure*: Side-lying, prone-lying, or sitting, with the arm supported if necessary. Resist elevation, depression, protraction, or retraction with pressure

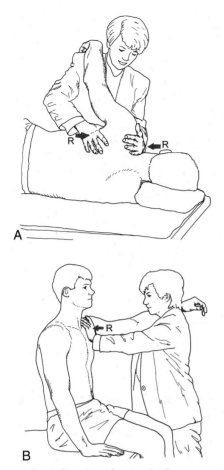

FIGURE 17.36 Isometric or dynamic manual resistance to scapular muscles. (*A*) Resistance to elevation/depression. (*B*) Resistance to protraction/retraction. Direct the patient to reach across the therapist's shoulder to protract the scapula while the therapist resists against the coracoid and acromion process. The other hand is placed behind the scapula to resist retraction.

directly on the scapula in the direction opposite the motion (Fig. 17.36).

***Depression (lower trapezius).*** Activation of the lower trapezius is emphasized when there is forward tipping and delayed upward rotation of the scapula often seen with impingement syndromes. Apply resistance against the inferior angle of the scapula (Fig. 17.36A).

***Protraction (serratus anterior).*** Activation of the serratus anterior is emphasized when there is scapular winging or when there is delayed or incomplete upward rotation of the scapula with GH elevation. Apply resistance against the axillary border of the scapula or coracoid process or indirectly against the humerus positioned in the plane of the scapula (Fig. 17.36B).

***Retraction (rhomboids and trapezius).*** Activation of the rhomboids and trapezius muscle groups is emphasized when the scapular posture is protracted (abducted), as typically seen with a forward head and increased kyphotic posture. Apply resistance against the medial border of the scapula.

### Multiple-Angle Isometrics to the GH Muscles

*Patient position and procedure*: Supine, sitting, or standing. If pain from joint compression occurs, apply a slight distractive force to the GH joint as resistance is applied.

***Internal and external rotation.*** Position the humerus at the patient's side in slight flexion, slight abduction, or scaption (plane of the scapula) and with the elbow flexed 90°. Apply resistance against the forearm as if turning a crank (Fig. 17.37).

---

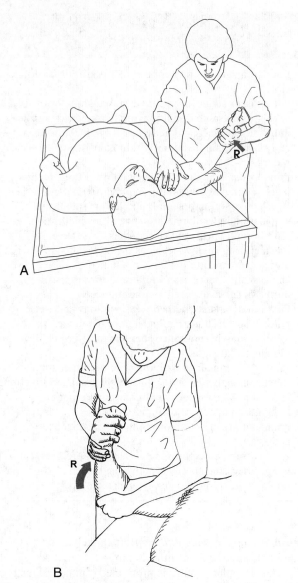

FIGURE 17.37 Isometric or dynamic resistance to shoulder rotation. (*A*) External rotation with the shoulder in the plane of the scapula. (*B*) Internal rotation with the shoulder at 90° abduction.

**Abduction.** Maintain the humerus neutral to rotation and resist abduction at 0°, 30°, 45°, and 60°. If there are no contraindications to motion above 90°, preposition the humerus in external rotation before elevating the humerus and resisting above 90° abduction.

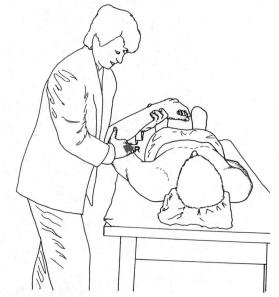

FIGURE 17.38 Isometric resistance in scaption. The shoulder is positioned between 30° and 60° degrees of scaption, and controlled manual resistance is applied against the humerus.

**Scaption.** Position midway between flexion and abduction and resist at various positions in the range, such as 30° and 60° in the plane of the scapula (Fig. 17.38).

**Extension.** Position the humerus at the side or in various positions of flexion and apply resistance against the humerus.

**Adduction.** Position the humerus between 15° and 30° abduction and apply resistance.

**Elbow flexion with the forearm supination.** Position the humerus at the side and neutral to rotation. Apply resistance to forearm flexion, causing tension in the long head of the biceps. Change the position of the shoulder into more flexion or extenson and repeat the isometric resistance to elbow flexion.

### Self-Applied Multiple-Angle Isometrics
Teach the patient how to independently apply isometric resistance using positions and intensities consistent with therapeutic goals. The patient can use the opposite hand (Fig. 17.39) or a stationary object such as a wall or door frame (Fig. 17.40).

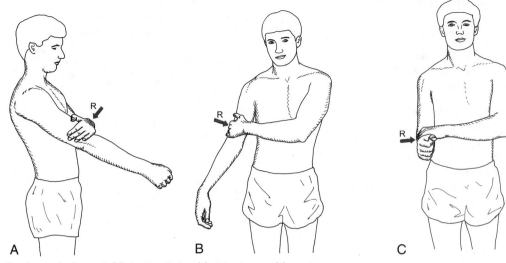

**FIGURE 17.39** Self-resistance for isometric (*A*) shoulder flexion, (*B*) abduction, and (*C*) rotation.

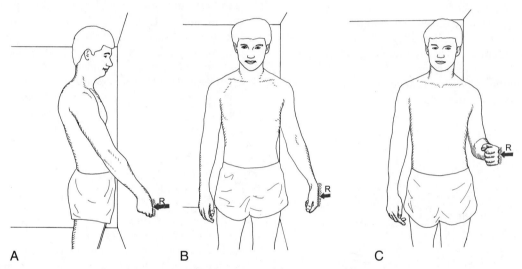

**FIGURE 17.40** Using a wall to provide resistance for isometric (*A*) shoulder flexion, (*B*) abduction, or (*C*) rotation.

## Stabilization Exercises

The application of alternating isometrics and rhythmic stabilization techniques (described in Chapter 6) is designed to develop strength and stability of proximal muscle groups in response to shifting loads. The shoulder girdle functions in both open- and closed-chain activities, and therefore the muscles should be trained to respond to both situations.

Begin training the scapular muscles so when the muscles of the GH joint need to contract they have a stable base (scapular stability). Initially, apply the alternating resistance slowly and command the patient to "hold" against the resistance. At the beginning of training it may also be necessary to tell the patient which way you are going to push to help the patient focus on the contracting muscles and alternating forces. As the patient learns to respond by contracting the proper muscles and stabilizing

the joints, increase the rapidity of the shifting resistance and decrease the verbal warning so the muscles learn to respond accordingly.

### Open–Chain Stabilization Exercises for the Scapular Muscles

Begin with the patient side-lying, with the affected extremity up. Drape the forearm of the involved extremity over your shoulder. The degree of shoulder flexion, scaption, or abduction can be controlled by your stance and the relative position of the patient. Progress to sitting with the patient's arm draped over your shoulder; apply resistance to all scapular motions in the same manner as described previously.

***Scapular elevation/depression.*** Place your top hand superiorly and the other hand inferiorly around the scapula to provide manual resistance (see Fig. 17.36A).

***Scapular protraction/depression.*** Place your top hand along the medial border and the other around the coracoid process to provide resistance (see Fig. 17.36B).

***Scapular upward and downward rotation.*** Place one hand around the inferior angle and the other hand around the acromion and coracoid process to provide resistance.

### Open–Chain Stabilization Exercises for the Shoulder Girdle

*Patient position and procedure*: Supine holding a rod or ball with elbows extended and shoulders flexed to 90°. Stand at the patient's head and grasp the rod; instruct the patient to hold against or match the resistance you provide. Push, pull, and rotate the rod in various directions (Fig. 17.41). Resistance can also be applied directly against the arm or forearm.

● If too much assistance is being given by the normal extremity, apply the stabilization technique to just the involved extremity.
● As the patient gains control, progress to sitting and then standing and have the patient hold the arm in various positions as the alternating resistance is applied. Observe the scapula to be sure there is good stabilization. If not, return to the exercises described above or decrease the intensity of resistance. Progress these exercises to functional patterns as strength and control improves.

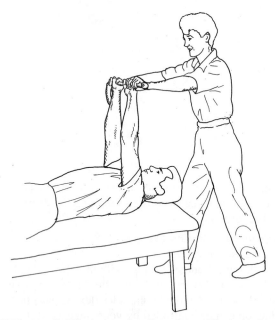

FIGURE 17.41 Stabilization exercises. The patient stabilizes with the shoulder girdle musculature (isometrically) against the resistance imposed by the therapist. Resistance to flexion/extension, abduction/adduction, and rotation is applied in a rhythmic sequence.

### Static Closed–Chain (Weight-Bearing) Stabilization Exercises

Weight bearing activates contraction of stabilizing muscles in proximal joints and may be a stimulus for improving fluid dynamics of the articular cartilage as described in Chapter 5. Early during the controlled motion phase of treatment (subacute stage), if the healing tissues tolerate it, it may be beneficial to initiate protected weight-bearing stabilization exercises. The amount and intensity of weight bearing and resistance is progressed as tissues heal.

N O T E :  If scapular winging is observed when the patient is weight bearing, do not progress these exercises until there is enough strength to stabilize the scapula against the rib cage.

 **Focus on Evidence**_____

Seeking an answer as to when upper extremity weight-bearing exercises could be included in an exercise program, Uhl and colleagues[186] analyzed the pectoralis major, anterior and posterior deltoid, supraspinatus, and infraspinatus with surface electromyography (EMG) in a progression of static exercises in 18 healthy subjects. Positions for isometric exercises included the prayer position (to simulate weight bearing against a wall), quadruped, tripod, pointer, push-up position (shoulders flexed to 90°), push-up position with feet elevated 18 inches (45 cm), and one-arm push-up position. There was a significant correlation between the increasing weight-bearing postures and increased muscular activity ($r = 0.97$, $p < 0.01$) in all the muscles. Also, the infraspinatus was the most active of the muscles tested in all positions except the prayer position (in which the pectoralis major was most active).

The authors suggested that the prayer and quadruped positions were appropriate for early rehabilitation owing to the low-activity level in all the muscles; that the tripod and pointer positions placed an intermediate demand on the infraspinatus and deltoid musculature; and that the push-up positions placed a high demand on the infraspinatus. They also concluded that the two-handed positions required less demand on the posterior deltoid but more load on the anterior deltoid and pectoralis muscles and that the one-arm push-up placed a high demand on all muscles except the supraspinatus.

---

● ***Scapular stabilization.***
*Patient position and procedure:* Side-lying on uninvolved side. Both the elbow and shoulder of the involved arm are flexed to 90°, with the hand placed on the table and bearing some weight. Resist the scapular motions of elevation/depression and retraction directly against the scapula; resist protraction by pushing against the elbow.

● **Protected weight bearing.**
*Patient position and procedure:* Sitting with forearms resting on thighs or a table; or standing with arms resting on a table. Apply a gentle resistance force against the shoulders and ask the patient to match the resistance and "hold." Alternate resisting in various directions.

● **Progression of closed-chain stabilization exercises.**
*Patient position and procedure:* Standing with shoulder at 90° and one or both hands leaning against a wall or on a ball (Fig. 17.42).

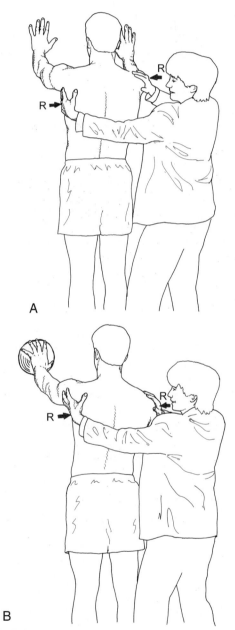

**A**

**B**

FIGURE 17.42 Closed-chain scapular and glenohumeral stabilization exercises. (*A*) Bilateral support in a minimal weight-bearing position with both hands against a wall. (*B*) Unilateral support on a less stable surface (ball). The therapist applies alternating resistance while the patient stabilizes against the resistance, or the therapist applies resistance as the patient moves from side to side.

Additional, more advanced progressions include having the patient in the "all-fours," or quadruped, position with hands on the floor, on a rocker or wobble board, or on a ball. The ball provides an unstable surface and requires greater neuromuscular control and balance reactions. Each of the positions can also be done with weight on only the involved upper extremity. Apply alternating resistance against the shoulders or trunk and ask the patient to "hold" against the force. Pressing forward against the trunk increases the effect of the body weight and requires the serratus anterior to stabilize more strongly against the additional force. As already noted, if the scapula wings, the resistance is either too strong and should be reduced, or the degree of weight bearing is excessive.

### Dynamic Closed-Chain Stabilization Exercises

Dynamic stabilization in weight-bearing positions requires the stabilizing muscles to maintain control of the scapula and GH joint while *moving the body weight* over the fixed extremity or extremities.

● *Patient position and procedure:* Standing with shoulders flexed 90° and hands supported against a wall, leaning hands on a table, or assuming a quadruped (all-fours) position. Have the patient shift his or her body weight from one extremity to the other (rock back and forth). Apply resistance against the shoulders (see Fig. 17.42).
● Progress by having the patient alternately lift one extremity and then the other, so one extremity bears the body weight and stabilizes against the shifting load. Apply manual resistance to the shoulders or strap a weight around each wrist.
● When the muscles are able to control and stabilize, progress to using unstable surfaces [such as a rocker board, biomechanical ankle platform system (BAPS) board, or ball]. Suggestions for more vigorous closed-chain activities are described in the following section.

## Dynamic Strengthening Exercises—Scapular Muscles

It is imperative that the proximal stabilizing muscles of the thorax, neck, and scapula function properly before initiating dynamic strengthening of the muscles that move the GH joint through the ROM to avoid faulty mechanics. Strengthening exercises can be done in both open- and closed-chain positions. Progress exercises with repetitions and resistance within the mechanical limits of the involved tissues.

Initially apply light resistance with multiple repetitions to develop dynamic control and muscular endurance. As control develops, progress to combined patterns of motion and training for muscle groups to function in a coordinated sequence. Begin with simple functional activities and progress to more complex and challenging activities. Both muscular endurance and strength are necessary for postural and dynamic control of activities.

**Focus on Evidence**_____

Two EMG studies analyzed exercises often used to strengthen the scapular muscles using either free weights or elastic tubing against maximum resistance.[49,81] The findings of these studies indicate the degree of activation of the trapezius and serratus anterior muscles during the following exercises.

● *Shoulder shrug, standing:* strongly activates the upper trapezius.
● *Full elevation of the arm above the head in the prone-lying position:* activates all three portions of the trapezius and serratus anterior when the shoulder is in line with the fibers of the lower trapezius.
● *External rotation in the prone-lying position with the shoulder positioned at 90° abduction and the elbow flexed 90°:* strongly activates the lower trapezius. This position is the "best exercise" to cause maximum depression of the scapula and isolation of the lower trapezius from the middle and upper portions.[49]
● *Horizontal abduction in the prone-lying position with the shoulder in external rotation:* activates the middle and lower trapezius.
● *Rowing action, seated or prone-lying:* emphasizes the middle trapezius over the upper and lower trapezius.
● *Diagonal exercises* (flexion, abduction, external rotation), and *shoulder abduction in the plane of the scapula above 120°,* standing resulting in upward rotation of the scapula: higher activity in the serratus anterior than in the trapezius.
● *Isolated protraction exercises:* do not activate the serratus anterior to as great a degree as upward rotation exercises.[49]

_____

### Scapular Retraction (Rhomboids and Middle Trapezius)
The following exercises are designed to isolate scapular retraction. Once the patient is able to retract the scapula against resistance, combine patterns with the GH joint to progress strength and functional patterns as described in the next sections.

● *Patient position and procedure*: Prone, sitting, and standing. Instruct the patient to clasp the hands together behind the low back. This activity should cause scapular adduction. Draw attention to the adducted scapulae and have the patient hold the adducted position of the scapulae while the arms are lowered to the sides. Have the patient repeat the activity without arm motion.
● *Patient position and procedure*: Prone with the arm over the edge of the table in a dependent position and a weight in the hand. Instruct the patient to pinch the scapulae together (Fig. 17.43). Progress this exercise to prone rowing and horizontal abduction against gravity (described below).

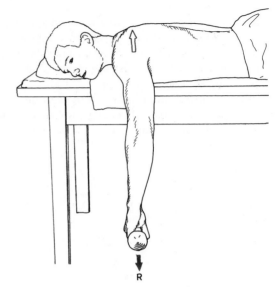

FIGURE 17.43 Scapular retraction against handheld resistance in the prone position.

_____

● *Patient position and procedure*: Sitting or standing with the shoulder flexed to 90° and elbows extended. Have the patient grasp each end of an elastic band or tubing that has been secured at shoulder level or a two-handled pulley that is at shoulder level, and pinch the scapulae together by pulling against the resistance.

### Scapular Retraction Combined with Shoulder Horizontal Abduction/Extension (Rhomboids, Middle Trapezius, Posterior Deltoid)

● *Patient position and procedure:* Prone with shoulders abducted 90°, elbows flexed, and forearms pointed vertically toward the floor. Instruct the patient to perform horizontal abduction with scapular retraction. This exercise can also be done with the elbows extended for greater resistance (Fig. 17.44). Progress this exercise by adding weights and then by having the patient perform the rowing motion standing or sitting in front of a length of elastic resistance that has been secured at shoulder level.

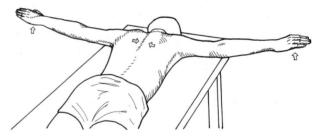

FIGURE 17.44 Horizontal abduction and scapular adduction exercises, with the arms positioned for maximal resistance from gravity. External rotation of the shoulders (thumbs pointing upward) emphasizes the middle and lower trapezius. To progress the exercise further, weights can be placed in the patient's hands.

● *Corner press-out.*
*Patient position and procedure:* Standing with the back toward a corner, shoulders abducted 90°, and elbows flexed. Instruct the patient to press the elbows into the walls and push the body weight away from the corner (Fig. 17.45).

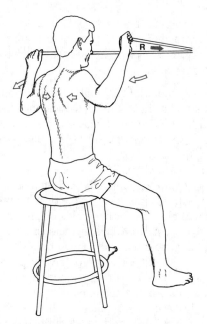

FIGURE 17.46 Combined scapular adduction with shoulder horizontal abduction and lateral rotation against resistance.

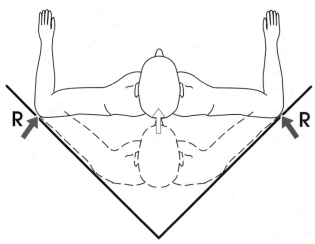

FIGURE 17.45 Corner press-outs to strengthen scapular retraction and shoulder horizontal abduction (view looking from above).

## Scapular Retraction and Shoulder Horizontal Abduction Combined with External Rotation (Rhomboids, Trapezius, Posterior Deltoid, Infraspinatus, Teres Minor)

● *Patient position and procedure*: Prone with shoulders abducted 90° and externally rotated 90° (90–90 position). The elbows can be flexed 90° (easier position) or extended (more difficult position). Instruct the patient to lift the arm a few degrees off the table. To do this correctly the scapulae must adduct simultaneously. Greater ROM can be used if these exercises are done on a narrow bench so the arm can begin in a horizontally adducted position.

● *Patient position and procedure*: Sitting or standing with shoulders in the 90–90 position. Secure the middle of a piece of elastic resistance in front of the patient slightly above the shoulders and have the patient grasp each end of the resistance. Then have the patient pull the hands and elbows back while simultaneously adducting the scapulae (Fig. 17.46).

## Scapular Protraction (Serratus Anterior)

● *Patient position and procedure*: Sitting or standing with shoulder flexed around 90° and elbow extended. Secure a piece of elastic resistance behind the patient at shoulder level or use a pulley system. Instruct the patient to "push" outward against the resistance without rotating the body (Fig. 17.47).

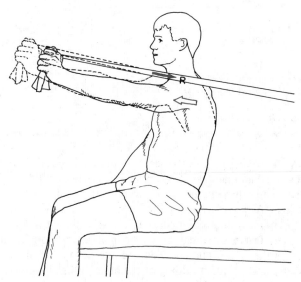

FIGURE 17.47 Scapular protraction; pushing against elastic resistance.

**N O T E :** According to a study by Ekstrom and colleagues,[49] isolated protraction exercises do not activate the serratus anterior as effectively as exercises that involve upward rotation of the scapula.

● *Patient position and procedure:* Supine with the arm flexed 90° and slightly abducted and the elbow extended. Place a light weight in the hand if resistance is tolerated and have the patient "push" the weight upward without rotating the body.

● ***Push-ups with a "plus."***
*Patient position and procedure:* Standing with arms against a wall, leaning on a table or lying prone. Have the patient place his or her hands directly in front or slightly to the side of the shoulders and push the trunk up (or away from the wall). Once full GH range is reached, instruct the patient to "give an extra push" to protract the scapulae. Progress the wall push-ups to table push-ups, then prone push-ups with knees as a fulcrum, and finally prone-lying push-ups, lifting the full body weight (Fig. 17.48). Add weight around the trunk if the patient is able to tolerate greater resistance.

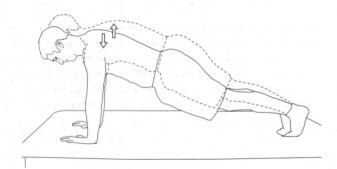

FIGURE 17.48 Push-ups with a "plus" to strengthen scapular protraction.

## Scapular Depression (Lower Trapezius, Lower Serratus Anterior)

● ***Shoulder rolls.***
*Patient position and procedure:* Sitting or standing. Ask the patient to roll the shoulders forward, up, and then around to the back so the scapulae are resting in the retracted and depressed position. Have the patient do this frequently throughout the day as part of a posture correction activity (see Chapter 14).

● *Patient position and procedure:* Sitting with elbow flexed. Provide manual resistance in an upward direction under the elbow, and ask the patient to push down into your hands. Caudal gliding of the humeral head may also occur (Fig. 17.49A).

● ***Scapular "push-ups."***
*Patient position and procedure:* Sitting or standing with both hands on blocks, on the armrests of a chair, or on parallel bars. Have the patient push down on the hands and lift the body (Fig. 17.49B).

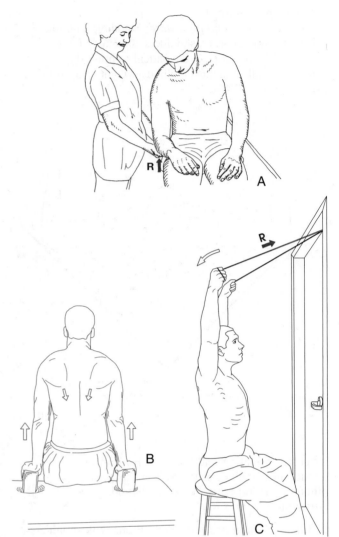

FIGURE 17.49 Exercises that emphasize the lower trapezius. (*A*) Shoulder girdle depression against manual resistance. (*B*) Closed-chain shoulder girdle depression using body weight for resistance. (*C*) Scapular depression with upward rotation of the scapula against elastic resistance (this also brings in the upper and middle trapezius and serratus anterior).

## Scapular Upward Rotation with Depression (Lower Trapezius, Serratus Anterior)

Scapular upward rotation with depression cannot be isolated from the humerus. The upward rotation action of the trapezius and serratus anterior require coordination with humeral elevation. As noted elsewhere in this chapter, a patient may substitute with scapular elevation, primarily using the upper trapezius, so this exercise draws attention to maintaining the scapula in depression while upwardly rotating.

● ***"Superman" motion.***
*Patient position and procedure:* Prone, with humerus elevated overhead. Ask the patient to barely lift the arm off the table. This end-range motion may not be possible for patients with restricted glenohumeral mobility or who have impingement syndrome.

*Patient position and procedure:* Sitting or standing if the patient has a tight shoulder and cannot do the "superman motion" lying prone. Secure elastic resistance overhead and instruct the patient to move the shoulder into greater flexion with scapular depression. The scapular depression is most important; it may be necessary to use tactile cues on the lower trapezius to help the patient focus on scapular depression, not scapular elevation (Fig. 17.49C).

*Patient position and procedure:* Standing with the back to the wall, heels away from the wall enough to comfortably do a posterior pelvic tilt and maintain the back flat against the wall. Begin with arms slightly abducted and externally rotated and the elbows flexed 90° (backs of the hands should be against the wall). Have the patient slide the hands and arms up the wall (abduction) as far as possible while maintaining the back flat against the wall.

## Dynamic Strengthening Exercises—Glenohumeral Muscles

Several EMG studies have investigated exercises commonly used to activate and strengthen shoulder muscles using either free weights or elastic resistance.[10,16,81,143] The findings of these studies indicate the extent of activation of the rotator cuff, deltoid, pectoralis major, and latissimus dorsi muscles under maximum load conditions during the following exercises.

- **Shoulder shrug:** causes highest activation in the subscapularis, trapezius, and latissimus dorsi; also activates the supraspinatus, infraspinatus, and serratus anterior.[81]
- **Middle-grip and narrow-grip seated rowing:** activates subscapularis.[81]
- **Wide grip seated rowing:** activates the infraspinatus and trapezius and to a lesser extent the supraspinatus.[81]
- **External rotation:** *in prone and side-lying positions and in the plane of the scapula:* activates the infraspinatus and teres minor.[10,16,143]
- **Internal rotation:** *movement across the body with arm at side and elbow flexed 90°* activates the subscapularis and pectoralis major.[81]
- **Forward punch:** causes highest activation in the supraspinatus and anterior deltoid; resistance also activates the pectoralis major and infraspinatus.[81]
- **Horizontal abduction at 100° with full external rotation:** activates the supraspinatus, middle and posterior deltoid.[143]

### Shoulder External Rotation (Infraspinatus, Teres Minor)
Position the arm at the patient's side or in various positions of abduction, scaption, or flexion. Flex the elbow to 90° and apply the resistive force at right angles to the forearm.

Be sure the patient rotates the humerus and does not extend the elbow. When the arm is positioned at the patient's side, a folded towel placed between the elbow and side of the rib cage reminds the patient to keep the elbow at the side and ensures proper technique. However, it does not significantly alter recruitment of the external rotators.[143] As indicated in the supporting evidence just presented, external rotation applied in the side-lying position (arm at side), prone-lying in the 90/90 position, and standing with the humerus in scaption (45° abduction, 30° horizontal adduction) produces the strongest contractions of these muscles compared with other external rotation exercises.[143]

- *Patient position and procedure*: Sitting or standing, using elastic resistance or a wall pulley in front of the body at elbow level. Have the patient grasp the elastic material or the pulley handle and rotate his or her arm outward (Fig. 17.50).
- *Patient position and procedure*: Side-lying on the normal side with the involved shoulder up and the arm resting on the side of the thorax with a rolled towel under the elbow. Have the patient use a handheld weight, cuff weight, or elastic resistance and rotate the arm through the desired ROM.
- *Patient position and procedure*: Prone on a treatment table, upper arm resting on the table with the shoulder at 90° if possible, elbow flexed with forearm over the edge of the table. Lift the weight as far as possible by rotating the shoulder, not extending the elbow (Fig. 17.50B).
- *Patient position and procedure*: Sitting with elbow flexed 90° and supported on a table so the shoulder is in the resting position (scaption). The patient lifts the weight from the table by rotating the shoulder (Fig. 17.50C).

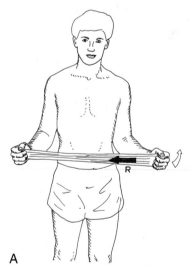

**FIGURE 17.50** Strengthening external rotation with (*A*) the arm at the side using elastic resistance

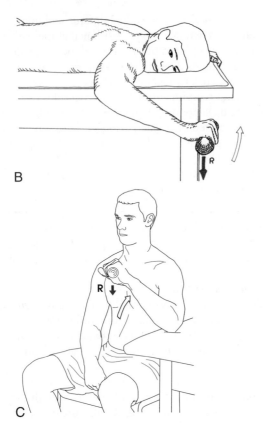

B

C

FIGURE 17.50 (continued) (*B*) prone with the arm at 90° using a free weight, and (*C*) sitting with the shoulder in scaption using a free weight.

## Shoulder Internal Rotation (Subscapularis)

Position the arm at the patient's side or in various positions of flexion, scaption, or abduction. The elbow is flexed to 90°, and the resistive force is held in the hand.

- *Patient position and procedure*: Side-lying on the involved side with the arm forward in partial flexion. Have the patient lift the weight upward off the table into internal rotation (Fig. 17.51).
- *Patient position and procedure*: Sitting or standing using elastic resistance or a pulley system with the line of force out to the side and at the level of the elbow. Have the patient pull across the front of the trunk into internal rotation.

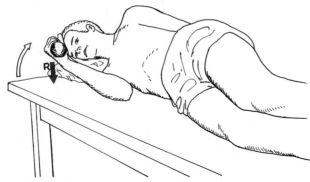

FIGURE 17.51 Resisted internal rotation of the shoulder using a hand-held weight. To resist external rotation, place the weight in the patient's upper hand.

## Shoulder Abduction and Scaption (Deltoid and Supraspinatus)

Abduction exercises are classically done with the humerus moving in the frontal plane. It is commonly accepted that most functional activities occur with the humerus 30° to 45° forward to the frontal plane where the arc of motion is more in line with the glenoid fossa of the scapula. Many abduction exercises can be adapted to be performed in scaption.

PRECAUTION: Teach the patient that whenever the shoulder elevates beyond 90° it must externally rotate to avoid impingement of the greater tubercle against the acromion. If the patient has impingement syndrome, limit the range to avoid the painful arc.

- ***Military press.***
  *Patient position and procedure:* Sitting, arm at the side in external rotation with elbow flexed and forearm supinated (thumb pointing posteriorly). Have the patient lift the weight straight up overhead (Fig. 17.52).

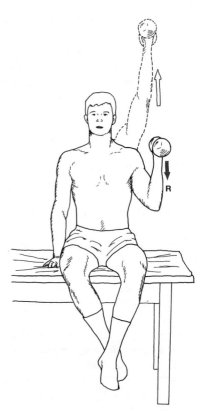

FIGURE 17.52 Military press-up. Beginning with the arm at the side in external rotation with elbow flexed and forearm supinated (thumb pointing posteriorward), the weight is lifted overhead.

*Patient position and procedure:* Sitting or standing with a weight in hand. Have the patient abduct the arm to 90° and then laterally rotate and elevate the arm through the rest of the range. This same motion can be performed with elastic resistance secured under the patient's foot, but be cautious in that the greater the elastic stretch, the greater the resistance. The patient may not be able to complete the ROM because of the increased resistance at the end of the range.

*Patient position and procedure:* Side-lying with involved arm uppermost. Have the patient lift a weight up to 90°. The greatest effect of the resistance is at the beginning of the range. At 90° all of the force is through the long axis of the bone.

● *"Full can" and "empty can."*

*Patient position and procedure:* Standing with the humerus either externally rotated (full can) or internally rotated (empty can). Have the patient raise the arm away from the side in the plane of the scapula, halfway between abduction and flexion (Fig. 17.53). Performing scaption with the humerus in various positions of rotation has the value of emphasizing each of the rotatory muscles of the cuff in their synergy with the supraspinatus and deltoid muscles.[106] Resistance is applied with a handheld weight or from elastic resistance secured under the patient's foot.

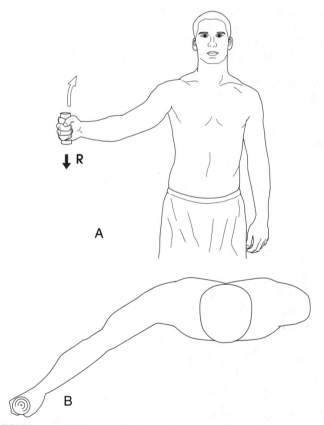

FIGURE 17.53 Abduction in the plane of the scapula (scaption). This is called the "full can" exercise because the shoulder is held in external rotation as if lifting a full can. (*A*) Front view. (*B*) Top view. If the shoulder is held in internal rotation, it is called an "empty can" exercise.

 **Focus on Evidence**_____

EMG studies have confirmed that no one exercise isolates the action of the supraspinatus muscle from the other rotator cuff or deltoid muscles.[107,181] The supraspinatus muscle is effectively activated in both the "empty can"[87,198] and "full can"[85,107,181] exercises. It also contracts strongly with the military press[181] and horizontal abduction with external rotation exercises.[16,107,209] These findings give the therapist several choices of exercises for strengthening the supraspinatus. Several authors,[45,83,85] as well as the authors of this text, have suggested that the "empty can" exercise (scaption with internal rotation of the humerus) should not be used for shoulder rehabilitation because it can cause impingement of the suprahumeral tissues, especially as the arm approaches and elevates above 90°. The "full can" position (scaption with external rotation) does not cause impingement.[45,85]

### Shoulder Flexion (Anterior Deltoid, Rotator Cuff, Serratus Anterior)

*Patient position and procedure:* Sitting, standing, or supine. If a free weight is used when supine, the greatest resistive force is at the beginning of the range; during standing, the greatest resistive force is when the shoulder is flexed 90°. Elastic resistance also can be used if secured under the patient's foot or a solid object.

### Shoulder Adduction (Pectoralis Major, Teres Major, Latissimus Dorsi)

*Patient position and procedure:* Sitting or standing with the arm abducted. Have the patient pull down against a pulley force or elastic resistance tied overhead. The greatest resistance is when the line of the resistive force is at right angles to the patient's arm.

### Shoulder Horizontal Adduction (Anterior Deltoid, Coracobrachialis, Pectoralis Major)

*Patient position and procedure:* Supine. Begin with one or both arms out to the side in horizontal abduction. Have the patient bring the arms forward into horizontal adduction until the arm or arms are vertical.

### Shoulder Extension (Posterior Deltoid, Latissimus Dorsi, Rhomboids)

● *Patient position and procedure:* Prone with the arm over the side of the table in 90° flexion. Have the patient lift the weight and extend the shoulder. Simultaneous elbow flexion while extending the shoulder is easiest (shortest lever arm); maintaining elbow extension while extending the shoulder is more difficult (longer lever arm).

● *Patient position and procedure:* Sitting or standing with the arm flexed. A pulley or elastic resistance is secured overhead. Have the patient pull down against the resistance into extension.

### Elbow Flexion (Biceps Brachii)

● *Biceps Curls.*

*Patient position and procedure:* Sitting or standing. Have the patient flex the elbow while holding a handheld weight and keeping the forearm supinated and the arm at the side or with the shoulder moving into slight extension (see Fig. 18.11).

N O T E : Because the biceps brachii is a two-joint muscle, the muscle not only serves to flex the elbow as its primary function, the long head assists the rotator cuff muscles by acting as an additional dynamic stabilizer of the GH joint by approximating the humeral head against the glenoid fossa and by depressing the head of the humerus as the arm elevates and the scapula upwardly rotates.[98] As such, the biceps brachii must be strengthened in a shoulder rehabilitation program.

### PNF (Diagonal) Patterns

Proprioceptive neuromuscular facilitation (PNF) patterns, as described in Chapter 6, utilize the entire upper extremity or address specific regions, such as the scapula. Apply resistance manually to emphasize specific muscles in the pattern by adjusting hand placement and resistance. Teach the patient exercises that utilize PNF patterns with weights or elastic resistance.

◉ **$D_1$ flexion pattern.**
*Patient position and procedure:* Standing. The arm begins in extension, internal rotation, and slight abduction. Have the patient bring the arm into flexion, adduction, and external rotation while holding a weight or pulling against elastic resistance that is secured under the foot.

◉ **$D_2$ flexion pattern.**
*Patient position and procedure:* Standing. The arm begins in extension, internal rotation, and slight adduction. Have the patient bring the arm into flexion, abduction, and external rotation while holding a weight or pulling against elastic resistance (Fig. 17.54).

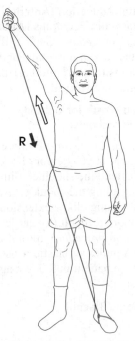

**FIGURE 17.54** Elastic resistance to the $D_2$ flexion pattern, emphasizing shoulder flexion, abduction, and external rotation using elastic resistance.

◉ **$D_1$ extension pattern.**
*Patient position and procedure:* Supine, standing, or sitting. The arm begins in flexion, adduction, and external rotation. Have the patient pull against elastic resistance that is secured above the head or against an overhead cable attached to a weighted pulley system with a combined extension, abduction, and internal rotation motion.

◉ **$D_2$ extension pattern.**
*Patient position and procedure:* Supine, standing, or sitting. The arm begins in flexion, abduction, and external rotation. Have the patient pull against elastic resistance that is secured above the head with combined extension, adduction, and internal rotation.

### Isokinetic Training

The principles of isokinetic training are discussed in Chapter 6. Early in an isokinetic exercise program have the patient use *submaximal* effort at slow speeds. During the advanced phase of rehabilitation, when tissues are reasonably well healed, have the patient perform maximum-effort concentric and eccentric exercises at medium to high speeds. Simulate functional patterns of movement if the equipment setup allows.

### Resisted Exercises Using Functional Movement Patterns

A variety of exercise devices can be used or modified for shoulder girdle strengthening that require coordination between the stabilizing and dynamic functions of the scapula and humerus. Some are considered closed-chain exercises in that the proximal segments move over the stabilized extremity, or there is pressure through the extremity causing approximation of the GH joint surfaces. The exercises may be used to accomplish several goals, such as improving strength, power, endurance (muscular and/or cardiovascular/pulmonary), balance, coordination, and skill.

◉ **Handwalking on a treadmill.**
*Patient position and procedure:* Kneeling at the end of a treadmill. The surface can be moving forward or backward. Have the patient "walk" with his or her hands while bearing weight through the shoulders.

◉ **ProFitter™.**
*Patient position and procedure:* Kneeling with one or both hands on the movable platform. The hands slide the platform from side to side. Change the position of the unit to obtain different angles of motion (Fig. 17.55).

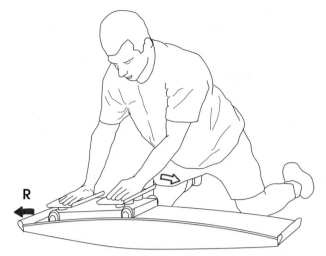

FIGURE 17.55 Advanced closed-chain exercise to resist the upper extremity using a ProFitter™ to provide an unstable, moving surface.

● **Stepping machine.**
*Patient position and procedure:* Kneeling with each hand on a step of the unit. The upper extremities do the climbing. Encourage the patient to use scapular protraction/retraction rather than elbow flexion/extension.

● **Rowing machine.**
*Patient position and procedure:* Long-sitting. Follow the instructions provided by the manufacturer if a commercial unit is used. Elastic resistance or a cable system on a pulley can be used to simulate a commercial rowing machine. Have the patient secure the elastic resistance under the feet or around a solid object, grasp the ends of the resistance, and pull backward in a rowing action with the arms. Also have the patient long-sit facing a cable system with the pulley at ground level. If there is just one cable, secure a bar to the cable and have the patient pull the bar toward his or her trunk in a rowing action.

● **"Lawnmower pull."**
*Patient position and procedure:* Standing with hips partially flexed and holding onto a table or chair for balance with the hand of the sound upper extremity. Have the patient reach diagonally across the midline and grasp a piece of elastic resistance that is secured under the foot of the sound side or attached to the floor. Then have the patient pull upward on the resistance as if starting a lawnmower. This may also be simulated with a free weight (see Fig. 18.18).

● **Upper body ergometry.**
*Patient position and procedure:* Sitting or standing in front of an ergometer with hands on the handles. Determine the arc of motion and the direction (forward or backward), speed, and time. This machine may be used for general warm-up, ROM, strengthening, or endurance training. Because tight or overused anterior

structures and weak or underused posterior structures tend to be the pattern with shoulder impairments, place emphasis on backward (retro) motions of the ergometer.

### Advanced Closed–Chain Stabilization and Balance Activities
*Patient position and procedure:* Quadruped on the floor with hands on an unstable surface such as a BAPS board, rocker board, wobble board, foam roll, or an 8- to 10-inch ball. Alternatively, have the patient assume a quadruped position with knees on a mat and hands on a large gym ball on the floor next to the mat. A variety of activities can then be done. For example, have the patient perform the following activities.

● Maintain a balanced posture as resistance is applied to the shoulders or trunk to disturb balance.
● Shift body weight from one hand to the other using an alternating protraction/retraction motion of the scapulae.
● Alternately flex each upper extremity so only one hand is balanced on the unstable surface.
● Perform push-ups and push-ups with a plus on the unstable surface.
● Increase speed of the above activities.

## Functional Activities

As soon as the patient develops control of scapular and humeral motions and the basic components of the desired activities without exacerbating the symptoms, initiate specificity of training toward the desired functional outcome by progressing the strengthening exercises to maximum resistance concentrically and eccentrically. Use the actual patterns and type of contraction required in the desired outcome and progress to the desired speed first in a controlled manner, then with less control.

An individual who has a sedentary lifestyle may require postural adaptations and ergonomic analysis of his or her home environment or workstation to change repetitive stress, whereas an athlete or industrial worker may require high-intensity exercises that develop endurance, power, and skill. Functional exercises may begin simply by having the patient unload a dishwasher and place the dishes on a low shelf using correct shoulder mechanics or washing windows using small circular motions. Body mechanics are incorporated into lifting, pushing, or pulling activities (Fig. 17.56). If catching and throwing or swinging a bat or golf club are necessary, total body patterns are practiced with the upper extremity exercises. Creativity in adapting exercises to meet progressive upper extremity challenges is a must. Basic principles to progress the patient during the return to function phase of therapy follow.

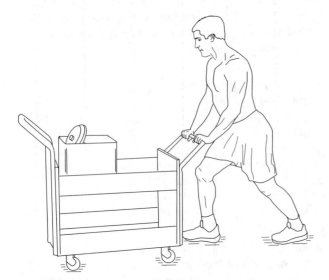

FIGURE 17.56 Functional exercise incorporating body mechanics.

### Endurance Training

Muscle and cardiopulmonary endurance are important for general health as well as for functioning throughout a workday. Utilize repetitive loading of each exercise for 3 to 5 minutes using patterns of motion that simulate work or functional activities. Principles of conditioning are discussed in Chapter 7. Have the patient maintain his or her target heart rate for 20 minutes with repetitive exercises.

### Eccentric Training

Eccentric exercises are high-intensity exercises and may be used for specific training. Because eccentric contractions tolerate greater resistance than concentric contractions, when loading resistance for eccentric training the patient is taught to assist the arm to the end of the shortened range of the muscles to be stressed; then the muscles control the return motion. This can be performed with elastic resistance, pulleys, or free weights first in single-plane motions and then progressed to simulated functional patterns.

### Plyometric Training

Initiate *stretch-shortening drills* in safe, controlled patterns with light resistance; then progress speed and resistance as tolerated. For example, toss a weighted ball such as a Plyoball® for the patient to reach for and catch and then immediately toss it back using the reciprocal pattern (Fig. 17.57). Progress to total body patterns, which include step

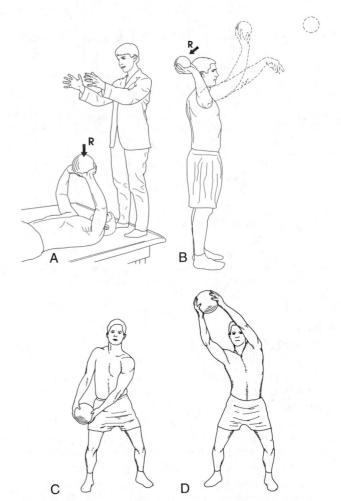

FIGURE 17.57 Plyometric activities catching and throwing a weighted ball (*A*) in a stable supine position, (*B*) in a standing position, (*C*) in a diagonal extension pattern, and (*D*) in a diagonal flexion pattern.

and throw and overhead pass activities. Spring-loaded rebounders and elastic tubing are commercially available so the patient can do the activity independently once the drills are learned.[197–199]

### Total Body Training

Increase *speed* with superimposed stresses to tolerance while simulating the desired activity. Assess the total body function while the desired activity is being carried out. Develop timing and sequencing of events that are consistent with the functional activity.

## INDEPENDENT LEARNING ACTIVITIES

### ● Critical Thinking and Discussion

1. Describe the functions and interrelationships of the scapulothoracic and GH musculature as dynamic stabilizers of the shoulder.
2. Which structures can restrict normal upward rotation of the scapula, and how does inadequate passive or active upward rotation of the scapula adversely affect elevation of the arm?
3. How does sitting or standing in a slumped posture (excessive thoracic kyphosis and forward head) with scapular abduction versus an erect posture with scapular adduction alter ROM of the shoulder?

4. Which mechanisms and structures could be sources of pain in primary impingement syndrome?

5. How are impingement and instability related to each other in secondary impingement syndrome?

6. A patient experienced a traumatic shoulder injury when falling down five cement steps 2 weeks ago. She now has a capsular pattern, decreased joint play, and muscle guarding with passive GH motions. She does not actively use the extremity because of pain. You observe edema in the hand. What potential complications could develop if left untreated? Design an exercise program for this patient at her present level of involvement. What would you teach the patient about her symptoms, impairments, and parameters for recovery?

7. An individual with a history of diabetes has developed a frozen shoulder. She has had shoulder discomfort for several months, but she did not seek treatment until 1 week ago when she was unable to wash or fix her hair with her left hand. Identify your intervention plan and instructions for this patient.

8. A new patient describes experiencing episodes of numbness and tingling in the hand with occasional periods of "puffiness." She reports that it is particularly annoying because it happens whenever she carries her briefcase or heavy purse with a shoulder strap. She also experiences pain at night and wakes up with her hand "having fallen asleep." What shoulder girdle problems could cause these symptoms? What is the probable cause of the symptoms? Create a scenario of objective findings, identify the impairment and functional goals, and outline a plan of intervention. What precautions are related to nerve pathologies?

9. During the early and middle stages of a rehabilitation program, what types of functional activities (ADL, work-related, or sport-related) should initially be avoided or modified for patients with a history of recurrent anterior dislocation of the GH joint? With recurrent posterior dislocation of the GH joint?

10. What criteria should patients with each of the following shoulder diagnoses meet before progressing to *overhead* exercises and functional activities: primary impingement syndrome; anterior GH instability; frozen shoulder; S/P rotator cuff repair?

## Laboratory Practice

1. With your partner, review and practice key tests and measurements that you might need to do to determine what is causing shoulder pain and/or diminished upper extremity function. What does each of those tests indicate?

2. Mobilize the scapula with manual techniques.

3. Mobilize the GH joint capsule with manual techniques; practice the mobilization with movement techniques for the shoulder.

4. Teach your partner a series of self-mobilization techniques for the GH joint capsule.

5. Using appropriate stabilization, manually stretch all major muscle groups of the shoulder.

6. Teach your partner effective self-stretching techniques for each of these muscle groups.

7. Practice a sequence of exercises to strengthen the muscles of the scapula using manual resistance (applied by the therapist). Use open-chain and closed-chain positions.

8. Teach your partner a progressive sequence of strengthening exercises that he or she could do in a home exercise program to develop stability and dynamic control of the scapula.

9. Teach your partner a progressive sequence of strengthening exercises that he or she could do in a home exercise program to develop strength, stability, and endurance of the GH muscles. Have your patient perform each exercise for a specified number of repetitions and at a specified level of resistance. Correct any faulty postures or motions as your partner executes each exercise. Watch for and teach your partner signs of fatigue and poor exercise technique.

10. Develop a series of functional activities to complement the self-stretching and self-strengthening exercise you have taught your partner.

## Case Studies

1. A patient referral states: Evaluate and treat shoulder pain S/P MVI. The patient describes shoulder pain whenever reaching overhead. She is a nurse and finds symptoms worsen whenever placing solutions on an IV pole, a frequent activity for her. She was the driver of the car in a head-on collision. Examination reveals painful resisted scapular protraction, elbow extension, and shoulder extension with pain on palpation of the long head of the triceps near its insertion on the inferior glenoid as well as pain in the serratus anterior in the axilla. Other impairments include weak rhomboids and lower trapezius muscles (4-/5).

   • Explain why these muscles would be injured in this type of accident.

   • Explain why this patient's job would perpetuate these symptoms.

   • Outline a treatment plan to manage the acute symptoms and initiate a therapeutic exercise program.

   • Identify a measurable functional outcome goal and interventions you would use to reach the goal.

   • As the patient's symptoms subside, how would you progress her exercise program?

2. Your patient describes pain whenever reaching overhead. He likes to play volleyball in a weekend league but otherwise has a sedentary lifestyle. On examination, you observe moderate atrophy in the infraspinous fossa, a protracted scapula, and thoracic kyphosis with forward head. You have him assume the quadruped position in anticipation of instruction in closed-chain rhythmic stabilization and scapular protraction exercises and note significant winging of the scapula.

   • Describe what muscles probably test weak with these observations.

- How would you change the quadruped exercise to develop control and strength in the involved muscles at a safe resistance level?
- Based on your assumptions of muscle involvement, develop an intervention plan for this patient that includes a home exercise program. Indicate parameters (frequency, repetitions), positions, safety, and progressions.

3. You have received a referral to "evaluate and treat" a 62-year-old patient who had undergone total shoulder arthroplasty for osteoarthritis 2 weeks ago. The patient has been wearing a sling to support and protect the operated shoulder but has been allowed to remove the sling for daily pendulum exercises and active ROM of the elbow, wrist, and hand.

- Prior to initiating your examination and developing an exercise program, what additional information would you like to find out from the surgeon?

- What information do you want to gather from the patient?
- What examination procedures would you wish to perform during the patient's initial visit?
- The patient's insurance, most likely, initially approves six visits. Develop, implement, teach, and then progress a series of exercises over a period of six visits with the patient.

4. Six months ago your patient underwent surgery for repair of a Bankart lesion and stabilization of the anterior capsule (capsular shift) after a traumatic anterior dislocation of the GH joint. The patient now has full ROM and 90% strength in the shoulder after a program of rehabilitation. Your patient wants to return to recreational sports, such as tennis, softball, and volleyball, but is apprehensive that the shoulder might dislocate during these activities. Design an advanced rehabilitation program to gradually return the patient to the desired recreational activities.

# REFERENCES

1. Altchek, DW, et al: Arthroscopic acromioplasty: technique and results. J Bone Joint Surg Am 72:1198, 1990.
2. American Physical Therapy Association: Guide to Physical Therapist Practice, ed 2. Phys Ther 81:9–744, 2001.
3. Anderson, NH, Sojbj, JO, Johannsen, HV, Sheppen, O: Self-training versus physiotherapist supervised rehabilitation of the shoulder in patients with arthroscopic subacromial decompression: a clinical randomized study. J Shoulder Elbow Surg 8:99–101, 1999.
4. Andrews, JR, Satterwhite, YE: Anatomic capsular shift. J Orthop Tech 1:151, 1993.
5. Arciero, RA, et al: Arthroscopic Bankart repair versus nonoperative treatment for acute, initial anterior shoulder dislocation. Am J Sports Med 22:589, 1994.
6. Arntz, CT, Jackins, S: Prosthetic replacement of the shoulder for the treatment of defects in the rotator cuff and the surface of the glenohumeral joint. J Bone Joint Surg Am 75:485–491, 1993.
7. Aronen, JG, Regan, K: Decreasing the incidence of recurrence of first-time anterior dislocations with rehabilitation. Am J Sports Med 12:283, 1984.
8. Arroyo, JS, Flatow, EL: Management of rotator cuff disease: intact and repairable cuff. In Iannotti, JP, Williams, GR (eds) Disorders of the Shoulder: Diagnosis and Management. Lippincott Williams & Wilkins, Philadelphia, 1999, p 31.
9. Baker, CL, Liu, SH: Comparison of open and arthroscopically-assisted rotator cuff repair. Am J Sports Med, 23:99, 1995.
10. Ballantyne, BT, O'Hare, SJ, Paschall, JL, et al: Electromyographic activity of selected shoulder muscles in commonly used therapeutic exercises. Phys Ther 73(10):668–692, 1993.
11. Bassett, RW, et al: Glenohumeral muscle force and movement mechanics in a position of shoulder instability. J Biomech 23:405, 1990.
12. Bigliani, LV, et al: Repair of rotator cuff tears in tennis players. Am J Sports Med 20(2):112–117, 1992.
13. Bigliani, LV, et al: Inferior capsular shift procedure for anterior-inferior shoulder instability in athletes. Am J Sports Med 22:578, 1994.
14. Bigliani, LV, et al: Shift of the posteroinferior aspect of the capsule for recurrent posterior glenohumeral instability. J Bone Joint Surg Am 77:1011, 1995.
15. Binder, AI, et al: Frozen shoulder: a long-term prospective study. Ann Rheum Dis 43:361, 1984.
16. Blackburn, TA, et al: EMG analysis of posterior rotator cuff exercises. Athletic Training 25:40, 1990.
17. Blakely, RL, Palmer, ML: Analysis of rotation accompanying shoulder flexion. Phys Ther 64:1214, 1984.
18. Blakely, RL, Palmer, ML: Analysis of shoulder rotation accompanying a proprioceptive neuromuscular facilitation approach. Phys Ther 66:1224, 1986.
19. Borstad, JD, Ludewig, PM: The effect of long versus short pectoralis minor resting length on scapular kinematics in healthy individuals. J Orthop Sports Phys Ther 35(4):227–238, 2005.
20. Borstad, JD: Resting position variables at the shoulder: evidence to support a posture-impairment association. Phys Ther 86(4):549–557, 2006.
21. Bottoni, CR, Wilckens, JH, DeBerardino, TM, et al: A prospective, randomized evaluation of arthroscopic stabilization versus nonoperative treatment of patients with acute traumatic, first-time shoulder dislocations. Am J Sports Med 30(4):576–580, 2002.
22. Boublik, M, Hawkins, RJ: Clinical examination of the shoulder complex. J Orthop Sports Phys Ther 18:379, 1993.
23. Brems, JJ: Rehabilitation following total shoulder arthroplasty. Clin Orthop 307:70, 1994.
24. Brewster, C, Schwar, DRM: Rehabilitation of the shoulder following rotator cuff injury or surgery. J Orthop Sports Phys Ther 18:422, 1993.
25. Brostrom, LA, et al: The effect of shoulder muscle training in patients with recurrent shoulder dislocations. Scand J Rehabil Med 24:11, 1992.
26. Brown, DD, Friedman, RJ: Postoperative rehabilitation following total shoulder arthroplasty. Orthop Clin North Am 29:535, 1998.
27. Brunet, ME, Haddad, RJ, Porche, EB: Rotator cuff impingement syndrome in sports. Physician Sports Med 10:87, 1982.
28. Burkhead, WZ, Buark, DA: History and development of prosthetic replacement of the glenohumeral joint. In Williams, GR, Yamaguchi, K, Ramsey, ML, Glatz, LM (eds) Shoulder and Elbow Arthroplasty. Lippincott, Williams & Wilkins, Philadelphia, 2005, pp 3–10.
29. Burkhead, WZ, Rockwood, CA: Treatment of instability of the shoulder with an exercise program. J Bone Joint Surg Am 74:890, 1992.
30. Cailliet, R: Shoulder Pain, ed 3. FA Davis, Philadelphia, 1991.
31. Cain, PR, et al: Anterior stability of the glenohumeral joint. Am J Sports Med 15:144, 1987.
32. Cameron, B, Glatz, L, Williams, GR: Factors affecting the outcome of total shoulder arthroplasty. Am J Orthop 30:613–623, 2001.
33. Carpenter, JE, Blasier, RB, Pellizzon, GG: The effects of muscle fatigue on shoulder joint position sense. Am J Sports Med 26:262, 1998.
34. Codman, EA: The Shoulder. Thomas Todd, Boston, 1934.
35. Cofield, RH, Chang, W, Sperling, JW: Complications of shoulder arthroplasty. In Iannotti, JP, Williams, GR (eds) Disorders of the Shoulder: Diagnosis and Management. Lippincott Williams & Wilkins, Philadelphia, 1999, p 571.

36. Cofield, RH, Hattrup, SJ, Sanchez-Sotelo, J, Steinmann, SP: Shoulder arthroplasty for arthritis. In Morrey, BF (ed) Joint Replacement Arthroplasty, ed 3. Churchill Livingstone, Philadelphia, 2003, pp 438–449.

37. Cohen, BS, Romeo, AA, Bach, BR: Shoulder injuries. In Brotzman, SB, Wilk, KE (eds) Clinical Orthopedic Rehabilitation, ed 2. Mosby, Philadelphia, 2003, pp 125–250.

38. Cole, BJ, L'Insalata, J, Irrgang, J, Werner, JJ: Comparison of arthroscopic and open anterior shoulder stabilization: a two- to six-year follow-up study. J Bone Joint Surg Am 82:1108–1114, 2000.

39. Culhan, E, Peat, M: Functional anatomy of the shoulder complex. J Orthop Sports Phys Ther 18:342, 1993.

40. Culp, LB, Romani, WA: Physical therapist examination, evaluation, and intervention following the surgical reconstruction of a grade III acromioclavicular joint separation. Phys Ther 86(6):857–869, 2006.

41. Cyriax, J: Textbook of Orthopaedic Medicine, ed 8. Vol 1. Diagnosis of Soft Tissue Lesions. Bailliere Tindall, London, 1982.

42. Cyriax, J: Textbook of Orthopaedic Medicine, ed 10. Vol 2. Treatment by Manipulation, Massage and Injection. Bailliere Tindall, London, 1980.

43. Dahm, DL, Smith, J: Rehabilitation and activities after shoulder arthroplasty. In Morrey, BF (ed) Joint Replacement Arthroplasty, ed 3. Churchill Livingstone, Philadelphia, 2005, pp 502–511.

44. Davies, GJ, Dickoff-Hoffman, S: Neuromuscular testing and rehabilitation of the shoulder complex. J Orthop Sports Phys Ther 18:449, 1993.

45. Davies, GJ, Durall, C: "Typical" rotator cuff impingement syndrome: it's not always typical. PT Magazine 8:58, 2000.

46. Donatelli, RA, Irwin, JP, Johanson, MA, Gonzales-King, BZ: Differential soft tissue diagnosis. In Donatelli, RA (ed) Physical Therapy of the Shoulder, ed 4. Churchill Livingstone, St. Louis, 2004, p 89.

47. Duralde, XA: Total shoulder replacements. In Donatelli, RA (ed) Physical Therapy of the Shoulder, ed 4. Churchill Livingstone, St. Louis, 2004, pp 529–545.

48. Edmonds, A: Shoulder arthroplasty. In Clark, GL, et al (eds) Hand Rehabilitation. Churchill Livingstone, New York, 1998, p 267.

49. Ekstrom, RA, Donatelli, RA, Soderberg, GL: Surface electromyographic analysis of exercises for the trapezius and serratus anterior muscles. J Orthop Sports Phys Ther 33(5):247–258, 2003.

50. Ellenbecker, TS, Elmore, E, Bailie, DS: Descriptive report of shoulder range of motion and rotational strength 6 and 12 weeks following rotator cuff repair using mini-open deltoid splitting techniques. J Orthop Sports Phys Ther 36(5):326–335, 2006.

51. Ellenbecker, TS, Mattalino, AJ: Glenohumeral joint range of motion and rotator cuff strength following arthroscopic anterior stabilization with thermal capsulorrhaphy. J Orthop Sports Phys Ther 29:160, 1999.

52. Ellenbecker, TS: Etiology and evaluation of rotator cuff pathologic conditions and rehabilitation. In Donatelli, RA (ed) Physical Therapy of the Shoulder, ed 4. Churchill Livingstone, St. Louis, 2004, p 337.

53. Ellman, H: Arthroscopic subacromial decompression. In Welsh, RP, Shephard, RJ (eds) Current Therapy in Sports Medicine, Vol 2. BC Decker, Toronto, 1990.

54. Engle, RP, Canner, GC: Posterior shoulder instability: approach to rehabilitation. J Orthop Sports Phys Ther 10(12):70–78, 1989.

55. Fanton, G, Thabit, G: Orthopedic uses of arthroscopy and lasers. Orthopedic Knowledge. Update Sports Medicine, American Academy of Orthopedic Surgeons, Rosemont, IL, 1994.

56. Fealy, S, Kingham, TP, Altchek, DW: Mini-open rotator cuff repair using a two-row fixation technique outcomes analysis in patients with small, moderate and large rotator cuff tears. Arthroscopy 18:665–670, 2002.

57. Fenlin, JM, Friedman, B: Shoulder arthroplasty: massive cuff deficiency. In Iannotti, JP, Williams, GR (eds) Disorders of the Shoulder: Diagnosis and Management. Lippincott Williams & Wilkins, Philadelphia, 1999, p 559.

58. Fu, FH, Harner, CD, Klein, AH: Shoulder impingement syndrome: a critical review. Clin Orthop 269:162, 1991.

59. Gartsman, GM, Hammerman, SM: Full-thickness tears: arthroscopic repair. Orthop Clin North Am 28:83, 1997.

60. Gartsman, GM, Khan, M, Hammerman, SM: Arthroscopic repair of full thickness tears of the rotator cuff. J Bone Joint Surg Am 80:832, 1998.

61. Gill, T, Micheli, J, Gebhard, F, et al: Bankart repair for anterior instability of the shoulder. J Bone Joint Surg Am 79:850–857, 1997.

62. Godges, JJ, Mattson-Bell, M, et al: The immediate effects of soft tissue mobilization with proprioceptive neuromuscular facilitation on glenohumeral external rotation and overhead reach. J Orthop Sports Phys Ther 33(12):713–718, 2003.

63. Greis, PE, Dean, M, Hawkins, RJ: Subscapularis tendon disruption after Bankart reconstruction for anterior instability. J Shoulder Elbow Surg 5:219, 1996.

64. Griffin, JW: Hemiplegic shoulder pain. Phys Ther 66:1884, 1986.

65. Gross, RM: Arthroscopic shoulder capsulorrhaphy: does it work? Am J Sports Med 17:495, 1989.

66. Grubbs, N: Frozen shoulder syndrome: a review of literature. J Orthop Sports Phys Ther 18:479, 1993.

67. Guidotti, TL: Occupational repetitive strain injury. Am Fam Physician 45:585, 1992.

68. Haig, SV: Shoulder Pathophysiology Rehabilitation and Treatment. Aspen Publishers. Gaithersburg, MD, 1996.

69. Harryman, DT, et al: Translation of the humeral head on the glenoid with passive glenohumeral motion. J Bone Joint Surg Am 72:1334, 1990.

70. Harryman, DT II, et al: Reports of the rotator cuff: correlation of functional results with integrity of the cuff. J Bone Joint Surg Am 73:982, 1991.

71. Hartzog, CW, Savoie, FH, Field, LD: Arthroscopic acromioplasty and arthroscopic distal clavicle resection, mini-open rotator cuff repair: Indications, techniques, and outcome. In Iannotti, JP (ed) The Rotator Cuff: Current Concepts and Complex Problems. American Academy of Orthopedic Surgeons, Rosemont, IL, 1998, p 25.

72. Hattrup, SJ: Rotator cuff repair: relevance of patient age. J Shoulder Elbow Surg 4:95, 1995.

73. Hattrup, SJ: Complications in shoulder arthroplasty. In Morrey, BF (ed) Joint Replacement Arthroplasty, ed. 3, Churchill Livingstone, Philadelphia, 2003, pp 521–542.

74. Hawkins, RJ, Abrams, JS: Impingement syndrome in the absence of rotator cuff tear (stages 1 and 2). Orthop Clin North Am 18:373, 1987.

75. Hawkins, RJ, et al: Acromioplasty for impingement with an intact rotator cuff. J Bone Joint Surg Br 70(5):795–797, 1988.

76. Hawkins, RJ, Koppert, G, Johnston, G: Recurrent posterior instability (subluxation) of the shoulder. J Bone Joint Surg Am 66:169, 1984.

77. Hawkins, RJ, Misamore, GW, Hobeika, PE: Surgery for full-thickness rotator cuff tears. J Bone Joint Surg Am 67:1349–1355, 1985.

78. Hayashi, K, Markel, M, et al: The effect of nonablative laser energy on joint capsular properties: an in vitro mechanical study using a rabbit model. Am J Sports Med 23:482, 1995.

79. Hayes, K, Callanan, M, Walton, J, et al: Shoulder instability: management and rehabilitation. J Orthop Sports Phys Ther 32(10):497–509, 2002.

80. Hernandez, A, Drez, D: Operative treatment of posterior shoulder dislocation by posterior glenoidplasty, capsulorrhapy and infraspinatus advancement. Am J Sports Med 14:187, 1986.

81. Hintermeister, RA, Lange, GW, Schultheis, JM, et al: Electromyographic activity and applied load during shoulder rehabilitation exercises using elastic resistance. Am J Sports Med 26(2):210–220, 1998.

82. Ho, CP: Applied MRI anatomy of the shoulder. J Orthop Sports Phys Ther 18:351, 1993.

83. Horrigan, JM, et al: Magnetic resonance imaging evaluation of muscle usage associated with three exercises for rotator cuff rehabilitation. Med Sci Sports Exerc 31:1361, 1999.

84. Howell, SM, Galinet, BJ, et al: Normal and abnormal mechanics of the glenohumeral joint in the horizontal plane. J Bone Joint Surg Am 70:227, 1988.

85. Itoi, E, et al: Which is more useful, the "full can test" or the "empty can test," in detecting the torn supraspinatus tendon? Am J Sports Med 27:65, 1999.

86. Jobe, FW, Giangarra, CE, et al: Anterior capsulolabral reconstruction of the shoulder in athletes in overhead sports. Am J Sports Med 19:428, 1991.

87. Jobe, FW, Moynes, DR: Delineation of diagnostic criteria and a rehabilitation program for rotator cuff injuries. Am J Sports Med 10:336, 1982.

88. Jobe, FW, Pink, M: Classification and treatment of shoulder dysfunction in the overhead athlete. J Orthop Sports Phys Ther 18:427, 1993.

89. Kaltenborn, F: Manual Mobilization of the Joints; The Kaltenborn Method of Joint Examination and Treatment, ed 5. Vol 1. The Extremities, Olaf Norlis Bokhandel, Oslo, 1999.

90. Kamkar, A, Irrgang, JJ, Whitney, SI: Nonoperative management of secondary shoulder impingement syndrome. J Orthop Sports Phys Ther 17(5):212–224, 1993.

91. Kelley, MJ, Leggin, BG: Shoulder rehabilitation. In Iannotti, JP, Williams, GR (eds) Disorders of the Shoulder: Diagnosis and Management. Lippincott Williams & Wilkins, Philadelphia, 1999, p 979.

92. Kelley, MJ, Leggin, BG: Rehabilitation. In Williams, GR, Yamaguchi, K, Ramsey, ML, Galatz, LM (eds) Shoulder and Elbow Arthroplasty. Lippincott, Williams & Wilkins, Philadelphia, 2005, pp 251–268.

93. Kennedy, K: Rehabilitation of the Unstable Shoulder. Sportsmedicine Performance and Research Center. WB Saunders, Philadelphia, 1993.

94. Kirkley, A, Griffin, S, Richards, C, et al: Prospective randomized clinical trial comparing effectiveness of immediate arthroscopic stabilization versus immobilization and rehabilitation in first traumatic anterior dislocations of the shoulder. Arthroscopy 15:507–514, 1999.

95. Kosmahl, EM: The shoulder. In Kauffman, TL (ed) Geriatric Rehabilitation Manual. Churchill Livingstone, New York, 1999, p 99.

96. Kumar, VP, Satku, K, Balasubramaniam, P: The role of the long head of the biceps brachii in the stabilization in the head of the humerus. Clin Orthop 244:172, 1989.

97. Kunkel, SS, Hawkins, RJ: Open repair of the rotator cuff. In Andrews, JR, Wilk, KE (eds) The Athlete's Shoulder. Churchill Livingstone, New York, 1994.

98. Levangie, PM, Borstead, JD: The shoulder complex. In Levangie, PM, Norkin, CC (eds) Joint Structure and Function: A Comprehensive Analysis, ed 4. FA Davis, Philadelphia, 2005.

99. Lewis, JS, Wright, C, Green, A: Subacromial impingement syndrome: the effect of changing posture on shoulder range of movement. J Orthop Sports Phys Ther 35(2):72–87, 2005.

100. Litchfield, R, et al: Rehabilitation for the overhead athlete. J Orthop Sports Phys Ther 18:433, 1993.

101. Lo, IK, Litchfield, RB, Griffin, S, et al: Quality-of-life outcome following hemiarthroplasty or total shoulder arthroplasty in patients with osteoarthritis: a prospective randomized trial. J Bone Joint Surg Am 87(10):2178–2185, 2005

102. Lord, J, Rosati, JM: Thoracic outlet syndromes, Vol 23. Ciba, Summit, NJ, 1971.

103. Ludewig, PM, Cook, TC: Alterations in shoulder kinematics and associated muscle activity in people with symptoms of shoulder impingement. Phys Ther 80:276, 2000.

104. Ludewig, PM, Behrens, SA, Meyer, SM, et al: Three-dimensional clavicular motion during arm elevation: reliability and descriptive data. J Orthop Sport Phys Ther 34(3):140–149, 2004.

105. Lukasiewics, AC, McClure, P, et al: Comparison of 3-dimensional scapular position and orientation between subjects with and without shoulder impingement. J Orthop Sports Phys Ther 29:574, 1999.

106. Magee, DJ: Orthopedic Physical Assessment, ed 4. WB Saunders, Philadelphia, 2002.

107. Malanga, GA, et al: EMG analysis of shoulder positioning in testing and strengthening the supraspinatus. Med Sci Sports Exerc 28:661, 1996.

108. Matsen, FA: Early effectiveness of shoulder arthroplasty for patients who have primary degenerative disease. J Bone Joint Surg Am 78:260, 1996.

109. Matsen, FA, Rockwood, CA, Wirth, MA, et al: Glenohumeral arthritis and its management. In Rockwood, CA, Matsen, FA, Wirth, MA, Lippitt, SB (eds) The Shoulder, Vol 2, ed 3. Saunders, Philadelphia, 2004, pp 879–1007.

110. Matsen, FA, Titelman, RM, Lippitt, SB, et al: Glenohumeral instability. In Rockwood, CA, Matsen, FA, Wirth, MA, Lippitt, SB (eds) The Shoulder, Vol 2, ed 3. Saunders, Philadelphia, 2004, pp 655–794.

111. Matsen, FA, Titelman, RM, Lippitt, SB, et al: Rotator cuff. In Rockwood, CA, Matsen, FA, Wirth, MA, Lippitt, SB (eds) The Shoulder, Vol 2, ed 3. Saunders, Philadelphia, 2004, pp 795–878.

112. Matthews, LS, Pavlovich, LJ: Anterior and anteroinferior instability: diagnosis and management. In Iannotti, JP, Williams, GR (eds) Disorders of the Shoulder. Lippincott Williams & Wilkins, Philadelphia, 1999, p 251.

113. McClure, PW, Bailker, J, Neff, N, et al: Shoulder function and 3-dimensional kinematics in people with shoulder impingement syndrome before and after a 6-week exercise program. Phys Ther 84(9):832–848, 2004.

114. Meister, K, Andrews, JR: Classification and treatment of rotator cuff injuries in the overhand athlete. J Orthop Sports Phys Ther 18:413, 1993.

115. Miller, MD, Flatlow, EL, Bigliani, LU: Biomechanics of the coricoacromial arch and rotator cuff: Kinematics and contact of the subacromial space. In Iannotti, JP (ed) The Rotator Cuff: Current Concepts and Complex Problems. American Academy of Orthopedic Surgeons, Rosemont, IL, 1998, p 1.

116. Mulligan, BR: Manual Therapy "NAGS," "SNAGS," "MWM's" etc, ed 4. Plane View Press, Wellington, 1999.

117. Neer, CS: Surgery in the shoulder. In Kelly, WH, Harris, ED, Ruddy, S, Sledge, CB (eds) Surgery in Arthritis. WB Saunders, Philadelphia, 1994, p 754.

118. Neer, CS: Impingement lesions. Clin Orthop 173:70, 1983.

119. Neer, CS, Watson, KC, Stanton, FJ: Recent experiences in total shoulder replacement. J Bone Joint Surg Am 64:319–337, 1982.

120. Neer, CS: Anterior acromioplasty for the chronic impingement syndrome in the shoulder: a preliminary report. J Bone Joint Surg Am 54:41, 1972.

121. Neer, CS: Replacement arthroplasty for glenohumeral osteoarthritis. J Bone Joint Surg Am 56:1, 1974.

122. Nevaiser, RJ, Nevaiser, TJ: The frozen shoulder: diagnosis and management. Clin Orthop 223:59, 1987.

123. Nevaiser, RJ: Ruptures of the rotator cuff. Orthop Clin North Am 18:387, 1987.

124. Nevaiser, RJ: Injuries to the clavicle and acromioclavicular joint. Orthop Clin North Am 18:433, 1987.

125. Nevaiser, TJ: Adhesive capsulitis. Orthrop Clin North Am 18:439, 1987.

126. Nevaiser, TJ: The role of the biceps tendon in the impingement syndrome. Orthop Clin North Am 18:383, 1987.

127. Nicholson, GG: The effects of passive joint mobilization on pain and hypomobility associated with adhesive capsulitis of the shoulder. J Orthop Sports Phys Ther 6:238, 1985.

128. Nixon, RT, Lindenfeld, TN: Early rehabilitation after a modified inferior capsular shift procedure for multidirectional instability of the shoulder. Orthopedics 21:441, 1998.

129. Noonan, TJ, Garrett, WE: Injuries at the myotendinous junction. Clin Sports Med 11:783, 1992.

130. Norris, TR, Iannotti, JR: Functional outcome after shoulder arthroplasty for primary osteoarthritis: a multicenter study. J Shoulder Elbow Surg 11(2):130–135, 2002.

131. Nuber, GW, Bowen, MK: Disorders of the acromioclavicular joint: pathophysiology, diagnosis and management. In Iannotti, JP, Williams, GR (eds) Disorders of the Shoulder. Lippincott Williams & Wilkins, Philadelphia, 1999, p 739.

132. O'Brien, M: Functional anatomy and physiology of tendons. Clin Sports Med 11:505, 1992.

133. O'Brien, SJ, Warren, RF, Schwartz, E: Anterior shoulder instability. Orthop Clin North Am 18:385, 1987.

134. Orfaly, RM, Rockwood, CA, Esenyel, CZ, Wirth, MA: A prospective functional outcome study of shoulder arthroplasty for osteoarthritis with an intact rotator cuff. J Shoulder Elbow Surg 12: 214–221, 2003.

135. Paine, RM, Voight, M: The role of the scapula. J Orthop Sports Phys Ther 18:386, 1993.

136. Palmer, ML, Blakely, RL: Documentation of medial rotation accompanying shoulder flexion: a case report. Phys Ther 66:55, 1986.

137. Payne, LZ, Deng, XH, et al: The combined dynamic and static contributions to subacromial impingement: a biomechanical analysis. Am J Sports Med 25:801, 1997.

138. Pollock, RG, Flatow, LL: Full-thickness tears: mini-open repair. Orthop Clin North Am 28:169, 1997.

139. Post, M, Grinblat, E: Preoperative clinical evaluation. In Friedman, RJ (ed) Arthroplasty of the Shoulder. Theime Medical, New York, 1994, p 41.

140. Post, M, Morrey, BE, Hawkins, RJ (eds) Surgery of the Shoulder. Mosby Year-Book, St. Louis, 1990

141. Provencher, MT, Bell, SJ, Menzel, KA, Mologne, TS: Arthroscopic treatment of posterior shoulder instability: results in 33 patients. Am J Sports Med 33(10):1463–1471, 2005.

142. Ramsey, ML, Klimkiewicz, JJ: Posterior instability: diagnosis and management. In Iannotti, JP, Williams, GR (eds) Disorders of the Shoulder: Diagnosis and Management. Lippincott Williams & Wilkins, Philadelphia, 1999, p 295.

143. Reinold, MM, Wilk, KE, Fleisig, GS, et al: Electromyographic analysis of the rotator cuff and deltoid musculature during common shoulder external rotation exercises. J Orthop Sports Phys Ther 34(7):385–394, 2004.

144. Reinold, MM, Wilk, KE, Hooks, TR, et al: Thermal-assisted capsular shrinkage of the glenohumeral joint in overhead athletes: a 15- to 47-month follow-up. J Orthop Sports Phys Ther 33(8):455–467, 2003.

145. Richards, RR: Redefining indications for and problems of shoulder arthrodesis. In Warner, JJP, Iannotti, JB, Gerber, C (eds) Complex and Revision Problems in Shoulder Surgery. Lippincott-Raven, Philadelphia, 1997.

146. Richards, RR: Glenohumeral arthrodesis. In Iannotti, JP, Williams, GR (eds) Disorders of the Shoulder: Diagnosis and Management. Lippincott Williams & Wilkins, Philadelphia, 1999, p 501.

147. Rockwood, CA, Wirth, MA: Disorders of the sternoclavicular joint. In Rockwood, CA, Matsen, FA (eds) The Shoulder, Vol 1, ed 3, Saunders, Philadelphia, 2004, p 597.

148. Rockwood, CA, Williams, GR, Young, DC: Disorders of the acromioclavicular joint. In Rockwood, CA, Matsen, FA (eds) The Shoulder, Vol 1, ed 3. Saunders, Philadelphia, 2004, p 521.

149. Rockwood, CA, Lyons, FR: Shoulder impingement syndrome: diagnosis, radiographic evaluation, and treatment with a modified Neer acromioplasty. J Bone Joint Surg Am 75:409, 1993.

150. Roddey, TS, Olsen, SL, Gartsman, GM, et al: A randomized controlled trial comparing 2 instructional approaches to home exercise instruction following arthroscopic full-thickness rotator cuff repair surgery. J Orthop Sports Phys Ther 32(11):548–559, 2002.

151. Rodosky, MW, Harner, CD: The role of the long head of the biceps muscle and superior glenoid labrum in anterior stability of the shoulder. Am J Sports Med 22:121, 1994.

152. Rokito, AS, et al: Strength after surgical repair of the rotator cuff. J Shoulder Elbow Surg 5:12, 1996.

153. Rose, BS: Frozen shoulder. N Z Med J 98(792):1039, 1985.

154. Rowe, CR: Anterior glenohumeral subluxation/dislocation: the Bankart procedure. In Welsh, RP, Shephard, RJ (eds) Current Therapy in Sports Medicine, Vol 2. BC Decker, Toronto, 1990.

155. Roye, RP, Grana, WA, Yates, CK: Arthroscopic subacromial decompression: two- to seven-year follow-up. Arthroscopy 11:301, 1995.

156. Rundquist, PJ, Ludewig, PM: Correlation of 3-dimensional shoulder kinematics to function in subjects with idiopathic loss of shoulder range of motion. Phys Ther 85(7):636–647, 2005.

157. Ruotolo, C, Nottage, WM: Surgical and nonsurgical management of rotator cuff tears. Arthroscopy 18:527–531, 2002.

158. Sachs, RA, Williams, B, Stone, ML, et al: Open Bankart repair: correlation of results with postoperative subscapular function. Am J Sports Med 33(10):1458–1462, 2005.

159. Safron, O, Seebauer, L, Iannotti, J: Surgical management of the rotator cuff tendon-deficient arthritic shoulder. In Williams, GR, Yamaguchi, K, Ramsey, ML, Galatz, LM (eds) Shoulder and Elbow Arthroplasty. Lippincott, Williams & Wilkins, Philadelphia, 2005, pp 105–114.

160. Schenk, T, Brems, JJ: Multidirectional instability of the shoulder: pathophysiology, diagnosis, and management. J Am Acad Orthop Surg 6:65, 1998.

161. Schenk, T, Iannotti, IP: Prosthetic arthroplasty for glenohumeral arthritis with an intact or repairable rotator cuff: indications, techniques and results. In Iannotti, JP, Williams, GR (eds) Disorders of the Shoulder: Diagnosis and Management. Lippincott Williams & Wilkins, Philadelphia, 1999, p 521.

162. Schieb, JS: Diagnosis and rehabilitation of the shoulder impingement syndrome in the overhand and throwing athlete. Rheum Dis Clin North Am 16:971, 1990.

163. Schmitt, L, Snyder-Mackler, L: Role of scapular stabilizers in etiology and treatment of impingement syndrome. J Orthop Sports Phys Ther 29:31, 1999.

164. Schwartz, E, et al: Posterior shoulder instability. Orthop Clin North Am 18:409, 1987.

165. Selecky, MT, Vangsness, CT, et al: The effects of laser-induced collagen shortening on the biomechanical properties of the inferior glenohumeral ligament complex. Am J Sports Med 27:168, 1999.

166. Sharkey, NA, Marder, RA: The rotator cuff opposes superior translation of the humeral head. Am J Sports Med 23:270, 1995.

167. Simon, ER, Hill, JA: Rotator cuff Injuries: an update. J Orthop Sports Phys Ther 10(10):394–398, 1989.

168. Smith, CA, Williams, GR: Replacement arthroplasty in glenohumeral arthritis: intact or repairable rotator cuff. In Williams, GR, Yamaguchi, K, Ramsey, ML, Galatz, LM (eds) Shoulder and Elbow Arthroplasty. Lippincott, Williams & Wilkins, Philadelphia, 2005, pp 75–103.

169. Smith, KL, Matsen, FA: Total shoulder arthroplasty versus hemi-arthroplasty—current trends. Orthop Clin North Am 29(3):491–506, 1998.

170. Smith, LK, Weiss, EL, Lehmkuhl, LD: Brunnstrom's Clinical Kinesiology, ed 5. FA Davis, Philadelphia, 1996.

171. Sperling, JW, Cofield, RH: Results of shoulder arthroplasty. In Morrey, BF (ed) Joint Replacement Arthroplasty, ed 3. Churchill Livingstone, Philadelphia, 2003, p 511–520.

172. Tauro, JC: Arthroscopic rotator cuff repair: analysis of technique and results in 2- and 3-year follow-up. Arthroscopy 14:45–51, 1998.

173. Thomas, BJ, Amstuts, HC: Shoulder arthroplasty for rheumatoid arthritis. Clin Orthop 269:125, 1991.

174. Thornhill, TS, Gall, V, Vermetle, S, Griffen, F: Shoulder surgery and rehabilitation. In Melvin, I, Gall, V (eds) Rheumatologic Rehabilitation Series. Vol 5. Surgical Rehabilitation. American Occupational Therapy Association, Bethesda, MD, 1999, p 37.

175. Tibone, JE, McMahon, PJ: Biomechanics and pathologic lesions in the overhead athlete. In Iannotti, JP, Williams, GR (eds) Disorders of the Shoulder: Diagnosis and Management. Lippincott Williams & Wilkins, Philadelphia, 1999, p 233.

176. Tibone, JE, Bradley, JP: The treatment of posterior subluxation in athletes. Clin Orthop 291:124, 1993.

177. Tibone, JE, et al: Glenohumeral joint translation after arthroscopic, nonablative thermal capsuloplasty with a laser. Am J Sports Med 26:495, 1998.

178. Tibone, JE, et al: Surgical treatment of tears of the rotator cuff in athletes. J Bone Joint Surg Am 68:887, 1986.

179. Ticker, JB, Warner, JP: Rotator cuff tears: principles of tendon repair. In Iannotti, JP (ed) The Rotator Cuff: Current Concepts and Complex Problems. American Academy of Orthopedic Surgeons, Rosemont, IL, 1998, p 17.

180. Timmerman, LA, Andrews, JR, Wilk, KE: Mini-open repair of the rotator cuff. In Wilk, KE, Andrews, JR (eds) The Athlete's Shoulder. Churchill-Livingstone, New York, 1994.

181. Townsend, H, et al: Electromyographic analysis of the glenohumeral muscles during a baseball rehabilitation program. Am J Sports Med 19:264, 1991.

182. Trail, IA: Replacement arthroplasty in synovial-based arthritis. In Williams, GR, Yamaguchi, K, Ramsey, ML, Galatz, LM (eds) Shoulder and Elbow Arthroplasty. Lippincott Williams & Wilkins, Philadelphia, 2005, pp 113–129.

183. Trenerry, K, Walton, J, Murrrell, G: Prevention of shoulder stiffness after rotator cuff repair. Clin Orthop 430: 94–99, 2005.

184. Turkel, SJ, et al: Stabilizing mechanisms preventing anterior dislocation of the glenohumeral joint. J Bone Joint Surg Am 61:1208, 1981.

185. Tyler, TF, Calabrese, GJ, Parker, RD, Nicholas, SJ: Electrothermally-assisted capsulorrhaphy (E.T.A.C.): a new surgical method for glenohumeral instability and its rehabilitation considerations. J Orthop Sports Phys Ther 30:390, 2000.

186. Uhl, TL, Carver, TJ, Mattacola, CG, et al: Shoulder musculature activation during upper extremity weight-bearing exercises. J Orthop Sports Phys Ther 33:109–117, 2003.

187. Vermeulen, HM, Obermann, WR, et al: End-range mobilization techniques in adhesive capsulitis of the shoulder joint: a multiple-subject case report. Phys Ther 80:1204, 2000.

188. Vermeulen, HM, Rozing, PM, Obermann, WR, et al: Comparison of high-grade and low-grade mobilization techniques in the management of adhesive capsulitis of the shoulder: randomized controlled trial. Phys Ther 86(3):355–368, 2006.

189. Wadsworth, CT: Frozen shoulder. Phys Ther 66:1878, 1986

190. Wahl, CJ, Warren, RF, Altchek, DW: Shoulder arthroscopy. In Rockwood, CA Jr, Matsen, FA III, Wirth, MA, Lippitt, SB (eds) The Shoulder, Vol 1, ed 3. Saunders, Philadelphia, 2004, pp 283–353.

191. Warner, JJP, Gerber, C: Treatment of massive rotator cuff tears: posterior-superior and anterior-superior. In Iannotti, JP (ed) The Rotator Cuff: Current Concepts and Complex Problems. American Academy of Orthopedic Surgeons, Rosemont, IL, 1998, p 59.

192. Warner, JP, Micheili, LJ, et al: Scapulothoracic motion in normal shoulders and shoulders with glenohumeral instability and impingement syndrome: a study using Moire's topographic analysis. Clin Orthop 285:191, 1992.

193. Warner, JP: Treatment options for anterior instability: open vs. arthroscopic. Operative Tech Orthop 5:233, 1995.

194. Weiss, KS, Savoie, FH: Recent advances in arthroscopic repair of traumatic anterior glenohumeral instability. Clin Orthop 400:117–122, 2002.

195. Wilcox, KB, Arslanian, LE, Millett, PJ: Rehabilitation following total shoulder arthroplasty. J Orthop Sports Phys Ther 35(12):821–835, 2005.

196. Wilde, AH, Brems, JJ, Bounphrey, FRS: Arthrodesis of the shoulder: current indications and operative technique. Orthop Clin North Am 18:463–472, 1987.

197. Wilk, KE, et al: Stretch-shortening drills for the upper extremities: theory and clinical application. J Orthop Sports Phys Ther 17(5):225–239, 1993.

198. Wilk, KE, Arrigo, C: An integrated approach to upper extremity exercises. Orthop Phys Ther Clin North Am 1:337, 1992.

199. Wilk, KE, Arrigo, C: Current concepts in the rehabilitation of the athletic shoulder. J Orthop Sports Phys Ther 18:365, 1993.

200. Wilk, KE, Andrews, JR: Rehabilitation following arthroscopic subacromial decompression. Orthopedics 16:349, 1993.

201. Wilk, KE, Andrews, JR, Arrigo, CA: The physical examination of the glenohumeral joint: emphasis on the stabilizing structures. J Orthop Sports Phys Ther 25:380, 1997.

202. Wilk, KE, Arrigo, CA, Andrews, JR: Current concepts: the stabilizing structures of the glenohumeral joint. J Orthop Sports Phys Ther 24:364, 1997.

203. Wilk, KE, Meister, K, Andrews, JR: Current concepts in the rehabilitation of the overhead throwing athlete. Am J Sports Med 30(1):136–151, 2002.

204. Wilk, KE, Reinold, WM, Dugas, JR, Andrews, JR: Rehabilitation following thermal-assisted capsular shrinkage of the glenohumeral joint: current concepts. J Orthop Sports Phys Ther 32(60):268–287, 2002.

205. Wilk, KE, Reinold, MM, Dugas, JR, et al: Current concepts in the recognition and treatment of superior labral (SLAP) lesions. J Orthop Sports Phys Ther 35(5):273–291, 2005.

206. Williams, GR, Iannotti, JP: Biomechanics of the glenohumeral joint: Influence on shoulder arthroplasty. In Iannotti, JP, Williams, GR (eds) Disorders of the Shoulder: Diagnosis and Management. Lippincott Williams & Wilkins, Philadelphia, 1999, p 471.

207. Wirth, MA, Blatter, G, Rockwood, CA: The capsular imbrication procedure for recurrent anterior instability of the shoulder. J Bone Joint Surg Am 78:246, 1996.

208. Wirth, MA, Rockwood, CA: Disorders of the sternoclavicular joint: pathophysiology, diagnosis, and management. In Iannotti, JP, Williams, GR (eds) Disorders of the Shoulder: Diagnosis and Management. Lippincott Williams & Wilkins, Philadelphia, 1999, p 763.

209. Worrell, TW, et al: An analysis of supraspinatus EMG activity and shoulder isometric force development. Med Sci Sports Exerc 24:744, 1992.

210. Yamaguchi, K, Levine, WN, Marra, G, et al: Transitioning to arthroscopic rotator cuff repair: the pros and cons. J Bone Joint Surg Am 85:144–155, 2003.

211. Zazzali, MS, Vad, VB, Harrera, J, et al: Shoulder instability. In Donatelli, RA (ed) Physical Therapy of the Shoulder, ed 4. Churchill Livingstone, St. Louis, 2004, pp 483–504.

212. Zuckerman, JD, Scott, AJ, Gallagher, MA: Hemiarthroplasty for cuff tear arthropathy. J Shoulder Elbow Surg 9(3):169–172, 2000.

# The Elbow and Forearm Complex

A freely mobile but strong and stable elbow complex is required for normal upper extremity function. The design of the elbow and forearm adds to the mobility of the hand in space by shortening and lengthening the upper extremity and by rotating the forearm. The muscles provide control and stability to the region as the hand is used for various activities, from eating, dressing, and grooming; to pushing, pulling, turning, lifting, throwing, catching, and reaching for objects; to coordinated use of equipment, tools, and machines.[33,43,55,59,67] Most activities of daily living require a 100° arc of flexion and extension at the elbow, specifically between 30° and 130°, as well as 100° of forearm rotation, equally divided between pronation and supination.[55,56] Tasks such as drinking and eating primarily require elbow flexion, whereas a task such as reaching to tie shoelaces requires substantial elbow extension.

Injury or disease of bony, articular, or soft tissue structures of the elbow and forearm can cause pain and compro-

557

mised mobility, strength, stability, and functional use of the upper extremity. Loss of active or passive elbow flexion interferes with grooming and eating, whereas loss of elbow extension restricts a person's ability to push up from a chair or reach out for objects. In general, loss of terminal flexion of the elbow contributes to greater limitation of function than loss of terminal extension.[55]

The anatomical and kinesiologic relationships of the elbow and forearm are outlined in the first section of this chapter. Chapter 10 presents information on principles of soft tissue healing and management; the reader should be familiar with that material before proceeding with establishing a therapeutic exercise program to improve function of the elbow and forearm.

## STRUCTURE AND FUNCTION OF THE ELBOW AND FOREARM

The distal end of the humerus has two articular surfaces: the trochlea, which articulates with the ulna, and the capitulum, which articulates with the head of the radius (Fig. 18.1). Flexion and extension occur between these two joint surfaces. The radius also articulates with the radial notch on the ulna and is called the proximal radioulnar joint. This joint participates in pronation and supination along with the distal radioulnar joint. The capsule of the elbow encloses the humeroulnar, humeroradial, and proximal radioulnar articulations. The distal radioulnar joint is structurally separate from the elbow complex even though its function is directly related to the proximal radioulnar joint.

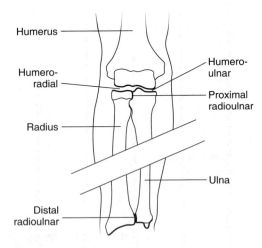

FIGURE 18.1 Bones and joints of the elbow and forearm.

## JOINTS OF THE ELBOW AND FOREARM

There are four joints involved in elbow and forearm function: the humeroulnar, humeroradial, proximal radioulnar, and distal radial ulnar joints.

### Elbow Joint Characteristics and Arthrokinematics

The elbow is a compound joint with a lax joint capsule, supported by two major ligaments—the medial (ulnar) and lateral (radial) collateral—which provide medial and lateral stability, respectively.[13,37,59,67]

#### Humeroulnar Articulation

**Characteristics.** The humeroulnar (HU) articulation is a modified hinge joint. The medially placed hourglass-shaped trochlea at the distal end of the humerus is convex. It faces anteriorly and downward 45° from the shaft of the humerus. The concave trochlear fossa, on the proximal ulna, faces upward and anteriorly 45° from the ulna (see Fig. 5.27). The primary motion at this articulation is flexion and extension

**Arthrokinematics.** During flexion/extension the concave fossa slides in the same direction in which the ulna moves, so with elbow flexion the fossa slides around the trochlea in an anterior and distal direction. With elbow extension, the fossa slides in a posterior and proximal direction.

There is also slight medial and lateral sliding of the ulna, allowing for full elbow range of motion (ROM); it results in a valgus angulation of the joint with elbow extension and a varus angulation with elbow flexion. When the bone moves in a medial/lateral direction, the trochlear ridge provides a convex surface, and the trochlear groove provides a concave surface—so with varus the ulna slides in a lateral direction and with valgus the ulna slides in a medial direction.

The arthrokinematics are summarized in Box 18.1.

#### Humeroradial Articulation

**Characteristics.** The humeroradial (HR) articulation is a hinge-pivot joint. The laterally placed, spherical capitulum at the distal end of the humerus is convex. The concave bony partner, the head of the radius, is at the proximal end of the radius. Flexion/extension and pronation/supination occur at this articulation.

| BOX 18.1 | Summary of Joint Arthrokinematics of the Elbow and Forearm Joints | | |
|---|---|---|---|

| Physiological Motion | Roll | Slide |
|---|---|---|
| *Humeroulnar articulation* | *Motion of ulnar joint surface* | |
| Flexion | Anterior | Distal/anterior |
| Extension | Posterior | Proximal/posterior |
| *Humeroradial articulation* | *Motion of radial joint surface* | |
| Flexion | Anterior | Anterior |
| Extension | Posterior | Posterior |
| *Forearm varus* | *Motion of proximal forearm* | |
| | Medial | Lateral |
| *Forearm valgus* | *Motion of proximal forearm* | |
| | Lateral | Medial |
| *Proximal radiounlar joint* | *Motion of rim of radial head* | |
| Pronation | Anterior | Posterior (dorsal) |
| Supination | Posterior | Anterior (volar) |
| *Distal radioulnar joint* | *Motion of distal radial joint surface* | |
| Pronation | Anterior | Anterior |
| Supination | Posterior | Posterior |

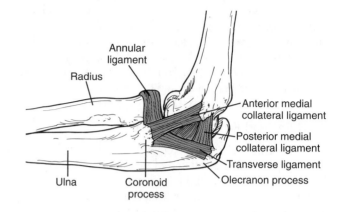

**A**      Medial aspect

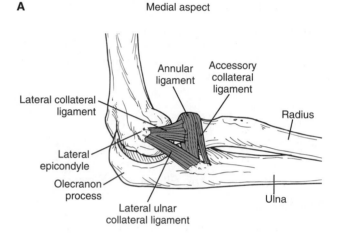

**B**      Lateral aspect

FIGURE 18.2 (A) The three parts of the medial (ulnar) collateral ligament are shown on the medial aspect of the right elbow. The musculature and joint capsule have been removed to show the ligament's attachments. (B) The lateral collateral ligament complex includes the lateral (radial) collateral ligament, lateral ulnar collateral ligament, and annular ligament. The musculature and joint capsule have been removed to show the ligaments' attachments. *(From Norkin, with permission.)*

*Arthrokinematics.* As the elbow flexes and extends, the concave radial head slides in the same direction as the bone motion so with elbow flexion the concave head slides anteriorly and with elbow extension it slides posteriorly. With pronation and supination of the forearm, the radial head spins on the capitulum (see Box 18.1).

### Ligaments of the Elbow

***Medial (ulnar) collateral ligament.*** The medial collateral ligament complex consists of bundles of fibers that may be differentiated into anterior, posterior, and transverse portions (Fig. 18.2A). Various portions of the ligament are taut in different ROMs, providing medial support to the elbow against valgus stresses and limiting end-range elbow extension. The ligament also keeps the joint surfaces in approximation.[59,67] Activities such as throwing and golfing impose significant stresses to the medial collateral ligament complex.

***Lateral (radial) collateral ligament.*** The lateral collateral ligament complex, a fan-shaped ligament on the lateral surface of the elbow, is composed of the lateral collateral ligament, the lateral ulnar collateral ligament, and the annular ligament.[59] This complex provides stability to the lateral aspect of the elbow against varus forces and prevents posterior translation of the radial head (Fig. 18.2B).

## Forearm Joint Characteristics and Arthrokinematics

Both the proximal and distal radioulnar joints are uniaxial pivot joints that function together to produce pronation and supination (rotation) of the forearm.[13,37,59,67]

### Proximal (Superior) Radioulnar Articulation

The proximal radioulnar (RU) articulation is within the capsule of the elbow joint but is a distinct articulation.

*Characteristics.* The convex rim of the radial head articulates with the concave radial notch on the ulna and the annular ligament. This ligament encircles the rim of the radial head and stabilizes it against the ulna. The primary motion is pronation/supination.

***Arthrokinematics.*** As the forearm rotates into pronation and supination, the convex rim of the radial head slides opposite the bone motion, so with pronation the head slides posteriorly (dorsally) on the radial notch and with supination it slides anteriorly (volarly). It also slides in the annular ligament (see Fig. 18.2), and the proximal surface spins on the capitulum (see Box 18.1).

### Distal (Inferior) Radioulnar Articulation

***Characteristics.*** The distal RU joint is an anatomically separate joint at the distal end of the radius and ulna. The concave ulnar notch on the distal radius articulates with the convex notch on the head of the ulna. It, along with the proximal RU joint, participates primarily in pronation/supination.

***Arthrokinematics.*** As the forearm rotates, the concave radius slides in the same direction as the physiological motion. It slides anterior (volar) with pronation and posterior (dorsal) with supination (see Box 18.1).

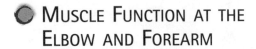

# MUSCLE FUNCTION AT THE ELBOW AND FOREARM

## Primary Actions at the Elbow and Forearm

### Elbow Flexion

***Brachialis.*** The brachialis is a one-joint muscle that inserts close to the axis of motion on the ulna, so it is unaffected by the position of the forearm or the shoulder; it participates in all flexion activities of the elbow.[13,59,67]

***Biceps brachii.*** The biceps is a two-joint muscle that crosses both the shoulder and elbow and inserts close to the axis of motion on the radius, so it also acts as a supinator of the forearm. It functions most effectively as a flexor of the elbow between 80° and 100° of flexion. For the optimal length–tension relationship, the shoulder extends to lengthen the muscle when it contracts forcefully for elbow and forearm function.[13,59,67]

***Brachioradialis.*** With its insertion a great distance from the elbow on the distal radius, the brachioradialis mainly functions to provide stability to the joint. However, it also participates as the speed of flexion motion increases and a load is applied with the forearm from mid-supination to full pronation.[13,59,67]

### Elbow Extension

***Triceps brachii.*** The long head of the triceps brachii crosses both the shoulder and elbow; the other two heads are uniaxial. The long head functions most effectively as an elbow extensor if the shoulder simultaneously flexes. This maintains an optimal length–tension relationship in the muscle.[59,67]

***Anconeus.*** The anconeus muscle stabilizes the elbow during supination and pronation and assists in elbow extension.[59,67]

### Forearm Supination

***Supinator.*** The proximal attachment of the supinator at the annular and lateral collateral ligaments may function to stabilize the lateral aspect of the elbow. Its effectiveness as a supinator is not affected by the elbow position as is the biceps brachii.[69]

***Biceps brachii.*** The biceps muscle acts as a supinator if the elbow simultaneously flexes or if resistance is given to supination when the elbow is in extension.[10]

***Brachioradialis.*** The brachioradialis contributes to pronation and supination only as an accessory muscle when resistance is provided to the motion.[10] It cannot function alone as a rotator or stabilizer of the forearm joints when other forearm muscles are paralyzed.[67]

### Forearm Pronation

***Pronator teres.*** The pronator muscle pronates as well as stabilizes the proximal radioulnar joint and helps approximate the humeroradial articulation.[59]

***Pronator quadratus.*** The pronator quadratus is a one-joint muscle and is active during all pronation activities.

## Relationship of Wrist and Hand Muscles to the Elbow

Many muscles that act on the wrist and hand are attached on the distal portion (epicondyles) of the humerus. This allows for movement of the fingers and wrist, whether the forearm is in pronation or supination. The muscles provide stability to the elbow but contribute little to motion at the elbow. The position of the elbow affects the length–tension relationship of the muscles during their actions on the wrist and hand.[59]

***Wrist Flexor Muscles.*** Originating on the *medial epicondyle* are the flexor carpi radialis, flexor carpi ulnaris, palmaris longus, and flexor digitorum superficialis and profundus.

***Wrist Extensor Muscles.*** Originating on the *lateral epicondyle* are the extensor carpi radialis longus and brevis, extensor carpi ulnaris, and extensor digitorum.

# REFERRED PAIN AND NERVE INJURY IN THE ELBOW REGION

For a detailed description of referred pain patterns and injuries to the peripheral nerves coursing through the elbow and forearm region, see Chapter 13. Table 13.1 in Chapter 13 summarizes the muscle involvement and functional loss that occurs with each of the nerve injuries.

## Common Sources of Referred Pain into the Elbow Region

Symptoms referred from the C5, C6, T1, and T2 nerve roots cross the elbow region but are not usually isolated in the elbow.

## Nerve Disorders in the Elbow Region

*Ulnar nerve.* The ulnar nerve courses posteromedial to the olecranon process in the cubital tunnel, which is the most common site for compression of this nerve in the elbow region.

*Radial nerve.* The radial nerve pierces the lateral muscular septum anterior to the lateral epicondyle and passes under the origin of the extensor carpi radialis brevis and then divides into a superficial and deep branch. Entrapment of the deep branch may occur under the edge of the extensor carpi radialis brevis, or injury may occur with a radial head fracture. The superficial branch may receive direct trauma as it courses along the lateral aspect of the radius.

*Median nerve.* The median nerve courses the elbow region deep in the cubital fossa, medial to the tendon of the biceps and brachial artery, where it is well protected. The nerve then progresses between the ulnar and humeral heads of the pronator teres muscle and dips under the flexor digitorum profundus muscle. Entrapment may occur between the heads of the pronator muscle, mimicking carpal tunnel syndrome.

## MANAGEMENT OF ELBOW AND FOREARM DISORDERS AND SURGERIES

In order to make sound clinical decisions when treating patients with elbow and forearm disorders with conservative interventions or after surgery, it is necessary to understand the various pathologies, surgical procedures, and associated precautions and to identify presenting impairments, functional limitations, and possible disabilities. In this section pathologies and surgical procedures are presented and related to the corresponding preferred practice patterns (groupings of impairments) described in the *Guide to Physical Therapist Practice*[3] (Table 18.1). Conservative and postoperative guidelines for managing these conditions are described in this section.

**TABLE 18.1** Elbow and Forearm Pathologies/Surgical Procedures, and Preferred Practice Patterns

| PATHOLOGY/SURGICAL PROCEDURE | PREFERRED PRACTICE PATTERN AND ASSOCIATED IMPAIRMENTS[3] |
|---|---|
| • Arthritis (rheumatoid arthritis, traumatic arthritis, osteoarthritis)<br>• Postimmobilization arthritis (stiff joint)<br>• Joint instability (subluxation, dislocation)<br>• Overuse syndromes (lateral epicondylitis, medial epicondylitis)<br>• Myositis ossificans (heterotopic bone formation) | • Pattern 4D—impaired joint mobility, motor function, muscle performance, and ROM associated with connective tissue dysfunction |
| • Acute arthritis<br>• Acute "pulled elbow," distal subluxation of radius | • Pattern 4E—impaired joint mobility, motor function, muscle performance, and ROM associated with localized inflammation |
| • Fracture (nondisplaced distal humerus, proximal radius, proximal ulna fractures—closed reduction) | • Pattern 4G—impaired joint mobility, muscle performance, and ROM associated with fracture |
| • Total elbow arthroplasty—linked and unlinked<br>• Excision of the radial head with prosthetic implant<br>• Interposition arthroplasty | • Pattern 4H—impaired joint mobility, motor function, muscle performance, and ROM associated with joint arthroplasty |
| • Open reduction and internal fixation of displaced/comminuted elbow fracture-dislocations<br>• Resection of the radial head without implant<br>• Synovectomy<br>• Ligament repair/reconstruction<br>• Capsulotomy<br>• Arthrodesis | • Pattern 4I—impaired joint mobility, motor function, muscle performance, and ROM associated with bony or soft tissue surgery |
| • Median, ulnar, or radial nerve entrapment or injury in the elbow/forearm region | • Pattern 5F—impaired peripheral nerve integrity and muscle performance associated with peripheral nerve injury |

# JOINT HYPOMOBILITY: NONOPERATIVE MANAGEMENT

## Related Pathologies and Etiology of Symptoms

Pathologies such as rheumatoid arthritis (RA), juvenile rheumatoid arthritis (JRA), and degenerative joint disease (DJD) as well as acute joint reactions after trauma, dislocations, or fractures affect this joint complex. Postimmobilization contractures and adhesions develop in the joint capsule and surrounding tissues any time the joint is immobilized in a cast or splint. This typically occurs after dislocations and fractures of the humerus, radius, or ulna. The reader is referred to Chapter 11 for background information on arthritis and fractures.

## Common Impairments

*Acute stage.* When symptoms are acute, joint effusion, muscle guarding, and pain restrict elbow flexion and extension, and there is usually pain at rest. If pronation and/or supination are restricted after an acute injury, other conditions such as fracture, subluxation, or dislocation may be present.[20] These conditions require medical intervention.

*Subacute and chronic stages.* A capsular pattern usually exists in the subacute or chronic stages. Elbow flexion is more restricted than extension. There is a firm end-feel and decreased joint play. In long-standing arthritis at the elbow, pronation and supination also become restricted with a firm end-feel and decreased joint play in the proximal RU joint.[20] Arthritis in the distal RU joint results in pain on overpressure.

## Common Functional Limitations/Disabilities

- Difficulty turning a doorknob or key in the ignition
- Difficulty or pain with pushing and pulling activities, such as opening and closing doors
- Restricted hand-to-mouth activities for eating and drinking and hand-to-head activities for personal grooming and using a telephone
- Difficulty or pain with pushing self up from a chair
- Inability to carry objects with a straight arm
- Limited reach

## Joint Hypomobility: Management— Protection Phase

See guidelines for management related to the stages of tissue healing in Chapter 10, Box 10.1.

### Educate the Patient

- Inform the patient regarding the anticipated length of acute symptoms and teach methods of joint protection and how to modify activities of daily living (ADL). For example, the patient should avoid activities that involve lifting or pushing off with the involved upper extremity.
- Instruct the patient to avoid excessive fatigue by performing exercises frequently during the day but limiting the number of repetitions during each bout (set) of exercises.

### Reduce Effects of Inflammation or Synovial Effusion and Protect the Area

- Immobilization in a sling provides rest to the part, but complete immobilization can lead to joint hypomobility, contractures, and limited motion; therefore, frequent periods of controlled movement within a pain-free range should be performed.

N O T E : Often the elbow is immobilized in 90° flexion. The position of relative extension (20° to 30° flexion) is used to prevent or treat ulnar neuropathy by preventing positions that could aggravate the ulnar nerve already at risk in the cubital tunnel because of joint swelling. The somewhat extended position and use of a posterior splint bubbled out around the cubital tunnel deepen the cubital tunnel, thereby reducing pressure on the ulnar nerve.[11]

- Gentle grade I or II distraction and oscillation techniques in the resting position may inhibit pain and move synovial fluid for nutrition in the involved joints (see Chapter 5 for principles of application and techniques).

### Maintain Soft Tissue and Joint Mobility

- Passive or active-assistive ROM within limits of pain, including flexion/extension and pronation/supination
- Multiple-angle muscle setting of elbow flexors, extensors, pronators, and supinators and wrist flexors and extensors in pain-free positions

### Maintain Integrity and Function of Related Areas

- Shoulder, wrist, and hand ROM and activities should be encouraged within the tolerance of the individual.
- If edema develops in the hand, the arm should be elevated whenever possible and distal-to-proximal massage techniques applied.

## Joint Hypomobility: Management— Controlled Motion Phase

If joint hypomobility exists, ROM is increased by utilizing joint mobilization techniques as well as passive stretching and muscle inhibition techniques following the principles described in Chapters 4 and 5. Box 18.2 highlights several important precautions if joint restrictions are related to trauma.

### Increase Soft Tissue and Joint Mobility

Initiate stretching cautiously and note the joint and tissue response. Vigorous stretching should not be undertaken until the chronic stage of healing. As noted in Box 18.2, high-intensity stretching of the elbow flexors is contraindicated following trauma because of the potential for development of heterotopic bone formation.

● *Passive joint mobilization techniques.* Because several articulations are involved with each motion at the elbow, it is important to identify which of the articulations have reduced joint play prior to applying grade III sustained or grade IV oscillation techniques. See Figures 5.28 through 5.33 and their descriptions in Chapter 5 for specific techniques to use. Progress each technique by positioning the joint at the end of its available range before applying the mobilization technique.

To progress joint mobility in the terminal ranges of flexion and extension, it may be necessary to emphasize the accessory motions of varus and valgus, respectively. This is accomplished with medial and lateral gliding techniques or with a varus or valgus physiological stretch at the elbow.

● *Mobilization to reduce a "pushed elbow."* Proximal subluxation of the radius may result from falling on an outstretched hand. The radial head is pushed proximally in the annular ligament and impinges against the capitulum. This injury sometimes accompanies a fracture of the distal radius (Colles' fracture) or scaphoid and is not identified as an impairment until after the fracture has healed and the cast is removed. It is often overlooked because there is considerable soft tissue and joint restriction caused by the period of immobilization. Bilateral palpation of the joint spaces reveals the decreased space on the involved side. There may be limited flexion or extension of the elbow, limited wrist flexion, and limited pronation.

*Technique.* If acute (and no fracture), distal traction is applied to the radius to reposition the radial head. If chronic, repetitive stretching with sustained grade III distal traction to the radius is necessary (see Fig. 5.29) in addition to the soft tissue stretching and strengthening techniques needed for increasing motion.

● *Manipulation to reduce a "pulled elbow."* Distal subluxation of the radius is usually seen as an acute injury in children and is sometimes labeled "tennis elbow" when it occurs in adults. It occurs as a result of a forceful pull on the hand such as would occur when a child jerks away from a parent or caregiver or a person tries to pick up a heavy object with a jerking motion on the handle. The force causes the radius to move distalward with respect to the ulna. The head of the radius is unable to slide proximally in the annular ligament when supination is attempted, resulting in the person holding the forearm in pronation. Supination is either restricted, or the patient guards against the motion.

*Technique.* A quick compressive manipulation with supination is applied to the radius (see Fig. 5.31) to reposition the radial head. If it is an initial injury, there may be soft tissue trauma from the injury, which is treated with cold and compression.

● *Manual stretching and self-stretching.* Use manual stretching and inhibition techniques to increase the flexibility of any periarticular tissues that are restricting mobility. Use of a cuff weight placed around the distal forearm with the patient carefully positioned for an effective stretch provides a low-intensity, long-duration stretch and is an alternative to manual passive stretching (see Fig. 18.7 in the exercise section). If elbow ROM does not steadily improve after acute symptoms have subsided, the patient may need to begin wearing an adjustable, dynamic splint that applies a low-intensity stretch force over an extended period of time. These stretching interventions are described in Chapter 4.

● *Home instructions.* Teach the patient self-stretching maneuvers followed by active exercise that utilize the new range. Suggestions are provided in the last section of this chapter.

### Improve Joint Tracking of the Elbow

A mobilization with movement (MWM) technique consisting of a lateral glide combined with the active movement of flexion or extension and pain-free passive overpressure may improve articular surface tracking by allowing the muscles to move the joint in a painfree manner.[51] (Refer to the principles of MWM in Chapter 5.)

*Technique.* *Patient position and maneuver*: Supine with elbow either flexed or extended to the end of the available range. A mobilization belt is secured around the proximal forearm and your hips. Stabilize the distal humerus at the olecranon process with one hand and support the forearm with the other. Apply a gentle lateral glide to the proximal ulna with the belt by moving your hips. Have the patient produce an active elbow flexion or extension movement and apply a passive overpressure stretch at the end of the range (Fig. 18.3). This should not elicit any pain.

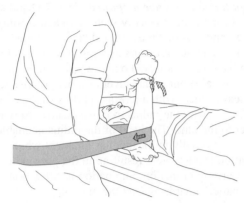

FIGURE 18.3 Mobilization with movement (MWM) to improve elbow flexion. A lateral glide is applied to the proximal ulna while the patient actively flexes, followed by a passive end-range stretch.

### Improve Muscle Performance and Functional Abilities

Initiate active and light resistance exercises in open- and closed-chain positions to develop control, muscular endurance, and strength in the muscles of the elbow and forearm. As the patient improves, adapt the exercises to progress toward functional activities. Specific exercises are described in the exercise section of this chapter. Include the shoulder girdle, wrist, and hand in the exercise program as their flexibility and strength has an influence on the recovery of elbow function.

## Joint Hypomobility: Management— Return to Function Phase

### Improve Muscle Performance

Progress self-stretching and strengthening exercises as the joint tissue tolerates. Teach the patient safe progressions and exercise strategies that promote return to function. Use exercises that replicate the repetitions and demands of daily activities, such as pushing, pulling, lifting, carrying, and gripping, to prepare the joints and muscles for specific tasks. Chronic arthritic conditions may require modification of high-load activities to minimize deforming stresses.

### Restore Functional Mobility of Joints and Soft Tissues

If restrictions remain, use vigorous manual or mechanical stretching and joint mobilization techniques.

## 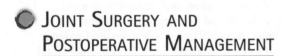 JOINT SURGERY AND POSTOPERATIVE MANAGEMENT

Intra-articular or extra-articular surgical intervention is often necessary for management of severe fractures or dislocations that affect the joints of the elbow and surrounding soft tissues. These injuries may require open reduction with internal fixation or arthroscopic or open excision of bone fragments. In adults, the most common fracture in the elbow region is a fracture of the head and neck of the radius. This type of fracture accounts for approximately one-third of all elbow fractures.[9] This injury usually occurs when a person falls on an outstretched hand when the elbow is extended, causing a posterior dislocation and fracture of the radial head coupled with injury of elbow ligaments.[26]

If the proximal radius is displaced and the radial head fracture is comminuted, either open or occasionally arthroscopically assisted reduction with internal fixation or a radial head excision (resection) with or without prosthetic implant is a surgical option.[26,45,49,50] It has been suggested that rigid internal fixation (screws or plate fixation) of radial head fractures is indicated in the young, active adult, whereas excision of the radial head is more appropriate for the low-demand patient or if the fracture is severely comminuted and fixation is not possible.[34] Box 18.3 summarizes the advantages and disadvantages of surgical options for management of displaced fractures of the radial head. Radial head fractures are relatively uncommon in children. When they do occur, closed reduction is preferred.[68]

---

**BOX 18.3**    **Surgical Options for Displaced Fractures of the Radial Head**

**Open Reduction and Internal Fixation**
- *Advantages:* Achieves stabilization and fixation of multiple fracture fragments with normal or near-normal alignment; ability to repair significant ligamentous damage; early postoperative motion permissible unless reconstruction of ligaments required
- *Disadvantages:* Extensive soft tissue disruption and arthrotomy required; not amenable to nonreconstructible fractures and less practical than radial head excision for severely comminuted fractures

**Arthroscopic or Arthroscopically Assisted Reduction and Internal Fixation**
- *Advantages:* Allows arthroscopic evaluation of the joint and débridement of fracture debris; if fully arthroscopic, no arthrotomy, less soft tissue disturbance, less postoperative pain, better cosmetic outcome
- *Disadvantages:* Limited to reduction and fixation of no more than two-part displaced fractures; not appropriate for radial neck fractures; if fully arthroscopic, fixation techniques more technically difficult (e.g., use of percutaneous screw fixation) than open procedure

**Excision of the Radial Head**
- *Advantages:* Only option for severely comminuted, nonreconstructible fractures; no potential for mechanical blockage of joint motion from malalignment of fracture fragments or internal fixation; early ROM permissible
- *Disadvantages:* Requires arthrotomy; may compromise joint stability if a prosthetic implant is not used

Early-stage or long-standing joint disease (RA, JRA, post-traumatic arthritis) associated with synovial proliferation and destruction of articular surfaces of the elbow joints and leading to pain, limitation of motion, and impaired upper extremity function also may need to be managed with extra-articular or intra-articular surgery. For example, with early-stage RA in which synovial proliferation is present but joint surfaces are still in good condition, *arthroscopic* or *open synovectomy* is the procedure of choice for relief of pain if medications have not controlled the disease.[14,36,40] Occasionally, advanced arthritis is managed surgically by *interposition arthroplasty* (only in the young patient on a selective basis),[18,62] *resection of the radial head* with or without prosthetic implant and concomitant synovectomy,[17,25,50] or *arthrodesis.*[62] However, today the most common surgical procedure used to manage severe destruction of the elbow joint is *total elbow arthroplasty.*[14,17,18,25,41,51,62] Table 18.2 summarizes how the severity of joint disease and the extent of soft tissue involvement influence the choice of surgical procedure for the elbow complex.[14,18,25]

The goals of surgery and postoperative rehabilitation of the elbow joint complex include[18,54] (1) relief of pain, (2) restoration of bony alignment and joint stability, and (3) sufficient strength and ROM to allow functional use of the elbow and upper extremity. Surgical procedures done to relieve pain and improve elbow stability tend to be more successful than procedures done solely to increase ROM. Heterotopic bone formation, which leads to joint stiffness, is often a complication of elbow fractures, dislocations, and elbow joint surgery.[47] Therefore, the single goal of improving ROM is rarely an indication for surgery.[18,45]

## Excision of the Radial Head

### Indications for Surgery

- Severe comminuted fractures of the distal humerus or fracture-dislocations of the head of the radius that cannot be reconstructed and held in place with internal fixation[16,45,49]

- Chronic synovitis and mild deterioration of the articular surfaces associated with arthritis of the humeroradial and proximal radioulnar joints resulting in joint pain at rest or with motion, possible subluxation of the head of the radius, and significant loss of upper extremity function[18,25,50]

***Contraindication to surgery:*** Excision of the radial head is contraindicated in the growing child.[68]

### Procedure

### Background

***Selection of procedure.*** Depending on the integrity of the ligaments and stability of the joint, with a radial head excision procedure the head of the radius may or may not be replaced with a prosthetic implant. The use of a prosthetic implant is indicated when there is clinical instability of the elbow as the result of disruption of the supporting ligaments.[25,49,50]

***Implant design and material.*** Radial head implants originally were flexible and made of silicone (Silastic material).[18,50] However, this material is no longer used because it has been associated with fatigue failure, particulate debris, and the development of adverse biological reactions, specifically inflammatory arthrosis (synovitis) of the humeroulnar joint.[72] Today, rigid, modular (two-piece) implants, made of metal (cobalt-chrome and titanium), ceramics, or ultra-high molecular weight polyethylene, are being used and investigated.[30,49,50] However, the optimal radial head implant has yet to be designed and fabricated.

### Overview of Operative Procedure
A lateral triceps-sparing incision at the elbow and forearm is made into the joint (arthrotomy) just anterior to the lateral collateral ligament. The radial head is exposed, and a radial osteotomy is performed at the level of the annular ligament to resect the head. When exposing the operative field, effort is made not to detach intact ligaments. A concomitant synovectomy is done if proliferative synovitis is present (typically seen in RA and JRA).

| TABLE 18.2 Severity of Elbow Joint Disease and Selection of Surgical Procedure | |
|---|---|
| **Severity of Joint Disease** | **Selection of Surgical Procedure** |
| • Mild synovitis: joint surfaces normal or minimally deteriorated; osteoporosis | • Nonoperative/medical management |
| • Moderate synovitis; some loss of articular cartilage; narrowing of joint space but joint contour maintained | • Arthroscopic synovectomy or resection of the radial head with synovectomy |
| • Moderate to severe synovitis; loss of articular cartilage; loss of joint space; intact collateral ligaments | • Resurfacing total elbow arthroplasty or, possibly in a growing child, an interpositional arthroplasty |
| • Severe synovitis; destruction of articular cartilage; complete loss of joint space (bone-to-bone articulation); significant joint instability; bone loss; ankylosis | • Semiconstrained total elbow arthroplasty |

If an implant is to be inserted, the medullary canal of the radius is prepared to accept the stem of the prosthesis. If the elbow is unstable, ligamentous structures are repaired. If the lateral ulnar collateral ligament (LUCL) is insufficient, it may be reinforced with a palmaris longus autograft or allograft. To prevent injury to the ulnar nerve or if symptoms of compression are present, ulnar nerve transposition is also performed.[25,49,50]

### Postoperative Management

The goals and interventions, the rate of progression, and the length of the rehabilitation program, as well as final outcomes, are highly dependent on the extent of damage to soft tissues from injury or chronic inflammation, the integrity of repaired soft tissues particularly the supporting ligaments of the elbow complex, the philosophy of the surgeon, and the patient's expectations of the surgery and response to treatment.[44,78]

### Immobilization

The elbow is immobilized continuously in a well-padded posterior resting splint in a position of 90° of flexion and mid-position of the forearm after surgery.[49,50] When elbow motion is permissible (often as early as 1 to 3 days after surgery or longer if significant reconstruction of ligaments was necessary), the splint is removed for exercise but is replaced after exercise and worn at night for an extended period of time to protect healing tissues. If the stability of the elbow is in question, the patient may need to wear a dynamic (hinged) splint for ROM exercises.

### Exercise: Maximum Protection Phase

*Goals and interventions.*[9,44,49,50,78] The first phase of rehabilitation focuses on patient education that emphasizes wound care, control of pain and peripheral edema, and exercises to offset the adverse effects of immobilization while protecting repaired soft tissues that maintain the stability of the elbow. The arm is elevated for comfort and to control edema distally.

◉ *Maintain mobility of unoperated joints.* Active ROM exercises of the shoulder, wrist, and hand immediately after surgery.
◉ *Maintain mobility of the elbow and forearm.* When permitted, have the patient remove the splint several times daily for self-ROM (passive or active-assisted) of the elbow and forearm within pain-free ranges. Active ROM is allowed within a week after exercises are initiated. As noted previously, some patients must wear a hinged splint for additional stability during ROM exercises.

PRECAUTION: Some specific motions initially may need to be restricted to prevent excessive stress on recon-

structed ligaments. Restrictions vary depending on the extent of ligament disruption and which ligaments were repaired. For example, if the lateral collateral complex was repaired, supination is limited to 20° during the early weeks of rehabilitation.[26]

◉ *Minimize muscle atrophy.* Submaximal, pain-free, multiple-angle setting exercises of elbow and forearm musculature.

### Exercise: Moderate and Minimum Protection Phases

*Goals and interventions.*[9] The intermediate phase of rehabilitation begins when wound healing is satisfactory and active movements of the elbow are relatively pain-free. This phase and the final phase of rehabilitation are characterized by continued efforts to restore nearly full or at least sufficient ROM for functional activities while maintaining stability of the elbow. Exercises to improve upper extremity strength and muscular endurance and use of the involved elbow for light functional activities are introduced and progressed.

NOTE: Some surgeons and therapists prefer to improve strength and endurance solely through ADL, that is, without the use of specific resistance exercises.[44,49,50]

◉ *Increase ROM,* particularly if contractures were noted preoperatively.
  • Gentle (low-intensity) manual stretching or self-stretching using inhibitory elongation techniques.
  • Grade II joint mobilization techniques initially, followed by grade III mobilizations after 6 weeks when the joint capsule is well healed.

CONTRAINDICATION: When applying joint mobilization techniques, do not perform valgus/varus stretches in terminal extension/flexion, particularly if the radial head was not replaced with a prosthetic implant or if the integrity of the supporting ligaments and stability of joints are questionable.

  • Low-load, long-duration, dynamic splinting or alternating use of static splints in maximum flexion and extension.
◉ *Improve functional strength and muscular endurance.*
  • Low-load resistance exercises (maximum 1 to 2 lb), emphasizing high repetitions.
  • Use of the operated upper extremity for *light* ADL.

PRECAUTION: Be certain the patient knows to avoid using the involved upper extremity for moving or holding heavy objects.

## Outcomes

The anticipated outcomes after resection of the radial head for a severely displaced and comminuted fracture or advanced arthritis are a stable elbow and pain-free movement (flexion/extension and pronation/supination) within functional ranges.[26,49,50] Short-term postoperative results of excision arthroplasty with and without implant are similar with regard to relief of pain and functional motion. However, patients with preoperative instability necessitating an implant and those with a tenuous repair of ligamentous structures have less satisfactory results than those with a stable elbow. If preexisting contractures exists, ROM does not necessarily improve.

Some patients may develop complications causing elbow pain, such as a slight increase (about 5° to 10°) in valgus laxity of the elbow, without complaints of instability during functional activities if ligaments are intact. Others may develop pain and instability. In a recent study,[31] posterolateral rotary instability was identified associated with a deficient lateral ulnar collateral ligament was identified at a mean of 44 months in only 16.6% of patients (7 of 42) who reported lateral elbow pain and a sense of instability or weakness after radial head resection (without implant). Another complication, slight proximal migration of the radius, may occur if resection does not include implantation of a prosthetic radial head. This complication may or may not be associated with wrist pain.[49]

Most long-term studies of excision with prosthetic implant have evaluated the results of procedures using flexible components made of silicone, which, as previously noted, have been shown to be associated with material fatigue or inflammatory responses and have led to premature failure. Short-term outcomes after current-day procedures, using rigid implants, are promising, but long-term reults are not yet available.[50] In patients with chronically active arthritis, synovitis eventually recurs necessitating another synovectomy or a total elbow arthroplasty. Regardless of the underlying pathology, patients who have undergone excision of the radial head with or without a prosthetic implant must permanently refrain from high-demand or high-impact, work-related or recreational activities.[44]

## Total Elbow Arthroplasty

### Indications for Surgery

Since the early use of total elbow arthroplasty (TEA) several decades ago,[21] the indications for this procedure have broadened considerably as the design of prosthetic implants and surgical techniques have evolved. The following are currently accepted indications for TEA.

- Severe joint pain and articular destruction of the humeroulnar and humeroradial joints, resulting in loss of functional use of the upper extremity.[18,25,62] Underlying conditions managed with total elbow arthroplasty include RA (by far the most common pathology),[19,25,26,28,41,48,51,53] JRA,[17] and post-traumatic degenerative arthritis.[19,52,65]
- Gross instability of the elbow.[26,35,63]
- Acute intra-articular, comminuted fractures[16,19] and nonunion fractures of the distal humerus.[48,54]
- Failed interposition arthroplasty or radial head resection.[64]
- Marked bilateral limitation of motion of the elbows.[18,19,48]

Absolute and relative contraindications for total elbow arthroplasty are identified in Box 18.4.[19,25,41,51] It is important to note, however, with the exception of active infection there is lack of agreement as to which contraindications are absolute versus relative.

---

**BOX 18.4  Contraindications to Total Elbow Arthroplasty**

**Absolute**
- The presence of active (acute or subacute) infection
- Inadequate control (paralysis) of elbow musculature, particularly the elbow flexors

**Relative**
- Irreparable supporting ligaments
- Inadequate control of elbow extensors
- Heterotopic ossification or pain-free ankylosis
- Insufficient bone stock
- A young patient, particularly one who needs to lift heavy loads

---

### Procedure

#### Background

The complex structural relationships among the HU, HR, and proximal RU joints have made developing a prosthetic elbow joint a challenging task. Since the first cemented total replacement of the elbow in 1972,[21] incremental improvements in design, materials, fixation, and surgical technique have contributed to increasingly predictable and successful outcomes.[18,62] Elbow replacement systems include a humeral and an ulnar implant (Fig. 18.4), and some designs also include replacement of the head of the radius.[41,48,51]

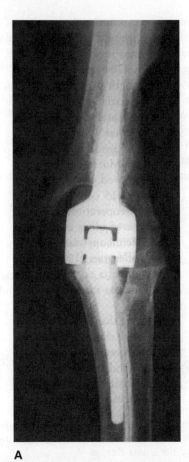

**A**

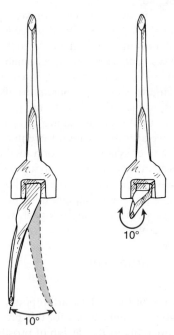

***Implant design and selection considerations***. Early designs were *hinged (linked, articulated)* and *fully constrained* metal-to-metal humeral and ulnar implants that allowed only flexion and extension of the elbow joint.[18,51,62] These designs made no allowances for normal varus and valgus and rotational movements, and hence the implants rapidly loosened at the bone–cement interface. Metal fatigue at the linkage of the prosthetic components and joint dislocation were also common complications.[7,18,29,62] As more accurate information about the biomechanical characteristics of the elbow joint became known, the design of prosthetic replacements evolved. In addition to an arc of flexion and extension, contemporary designs provide 5° to 10° of varus and valgus and a small degree of rotation (Fig. 18.5).[51]

The designs of total elbow replacement can be classified into two broad categories: *linked* (articulated) and *unlinked* (nonarticulated).[7] Rather than being fully constrained, as the early components were, linked humeral and ulnar implants are now loosely constrained and, as such, are referred to as *semiconstrained* designs.[28,48,51,65] Designs classified as unlinked are composed of two separate, nonarticulated implants and are often called *resurfacing* replacements.[7,19,24,41] The most recent advance in implant design is the *hybrid* prothesis, which can be inserted as either a linked or unlinked replacement system. Use of a hybrid replacement enables the surgeon to determine the

**B**

FIGURE 18.4 (*A*) Anteroposterior and (*B*) lateral radiographs following placement of a Conrad-Morrey (linked/semiconstrained) total elbow arthroplasty. *(From Field and Savoié,[26] with permission.)*

FIGURE 18.5 A linked, semiconstrained design is characterized by varus-valgus and axial rotation tolerances of several degrees at the articulation. *(From Morrey, BF [ed] The Elbow and Its Disorders, ed 3. WB Saunders, Philadelphia, 2000, p 617, with permission from the Mayo Clinic Foundation.)*

more appropriate design based on intraoperative observations and evaluation.[7]

The criteria for use of a linked or unlinked TEA is based in part on the characteristics of these designs with respect to stability. Linked designs derive inherent stability from one or two pins, which couple the humeral and ulnar components.[48] In addition, some semiconstrained designs have an anterior flange to enhance joint stability and decrease the risk of posterior dislocaion.[51] Unlinked implant systems, although sometimes referred to as non-constrained,[44] actually have varying degrees of constraint built into their designs based on the degree of congruency of the articulating surfaces.[19,24,41] The less constraining the articular surfaces of the implants, the more reliant the replacement system is on the surrounding soft tissues, particularly the collateral ligaments, for joint stability.

Overall, linked designs, because of their inherent stability, are considered appropriate for use with a broader spectrum of patients, including those with unstable elbows, than unlinked designs. Although both linked and unlinked designs derive some degree of stability from the supporting capsuloligamentous structures and elbow musculature, the integrity of these soft tissues is far more critical for successful use of unlinked than linked designs.[7,44,48]

In addition to considerations related to stability, the etiology and extent of joint destruction, the degree of deformity, the quality of the available bone stock, and the training and experience of the surgeon are factors that influence the type of replacement system used.

*Materials and fixation.* A stemmed titanium humeral component that has a cobalt-chrome alloy articulating surface interfaces with a high-density polyethylene articulating surface of a stemmed ulnar component.[7,18] Currently, prosthetic components are cemented in place with polymethylmethacrylate, an acrylic cement. Some designs also have a porous-coated extramedullary flange for osseous ingrowth. To date, all-cementless fixation has not yet been developed for total elbow arthroplasty.[18,62] Despite improvements in fixation, loosening of the implants at the bone–cement interface continues to be a cause of failure of elbow arthroplasty.[8]

### Overview of Operative Procedure

The following is a brief overview of typical elements involved in a TEA.[19,41,48,51,52,65] A longitudinal incision is made at the posterior aspect of the elbow, either slightly lateral or medial to the olecranon process. The distal attachment of the triceps is typically detached and reflected (*triceps-reflecting approach*) or split longitudinally and retracted along the midline (*triceps-splitting approach*).[51] The more recently developed *triceps-sparing approach* is used occasionally. It involves incisions on the medial and lateral aspects of the elbow joint. This approach preserves

the attachment of the triceps tendon on the olecranon but makes insertion of the implants more technically difficult.[8]

As the procedure progresses, the ulnar nerve is isolated, temporarily displaced, protected throughout the procedure, and possibly transposed. Ligaments and other soft tissues are released as necessary; the posterior aspect of the capsule is incised and retracted; and the joint is dislocated. In preparation for the implants, small portions of the distal humerus and proximal ulna are resected. Depending on the status of the radial head, the integrity of the collateral ligaments, and the design of the prosthesis, the head of the radius may or may not be resected. Then the intramedullary canals of the humerus and ulna and possibly the radius are prepared, and the components are inserted and cemented in place. The available ROM and stability of the prosthetic joint is checked intraoperatively. The capsule and any ligaments that had ruptured prior to surgery or were released during the procedure are repaired to the extent possible or necessary based on the design of the prosthesis and the quality of the structures. The extensor mechanism, if detached or split, is securely reattached or meticulously repaired.

### Complications

Although the incidence of complications has steadily declined over the past few decades as selection of patients, prosthetic design, and surgical technique have improved, complications after TEA continue to occur more frequently than after total hip, knee, or shoulder arthroplasty.[8] Complications are categorized as intraoperative, early postoperative (before 6 weeks), and late postoperative (after 6 weeks).[61]

Intraoperative complications, such as fracture and component malposition, can occur with TEA and significantly affect short- and long-term outcomes. In addition to infection, which is a concern after any surgery, early complications, including joint instability, wound healing problems, and triceps insufficiency, are of particular concern during the early and intermediate phases of rehabilitation. These complications also can occur several months or even years later, as can fracture, aseptic (biomechanical) loosening of the prosthetic implants over time at the bone–cement interface, and mechanical failure or premature wear of the components. Another complication, ulnar neuropathy, either transient or permanent, can occur intraoperatively or during the early weeks after surgery.[8,29,61]

It is important for a therapist to be familiar with the incidence and possible causes of complications after TEA in order to effectively structure and progress a postoperative rehabilitation program that decreases at least some of the risk factors associated with these complications. The incidence and characteristics of selected complications (joint instability, triceps insufficiency, prosthetic loosening) after TEA and factors that contribute to these complica-

## BOX 18.5    Analysis of Three Potential Complications after Total Elbow Arthroplasty

### Joint Instability

- *Incidence.* One of the more common complications after TEA; predominantly a problem in unlinked arthroplasty,[8] higher incidence with prior radial head resection.[64] Rates of instability in unlinked implants reported at 4% to 15% (mean 8%)[41] and in linked implants at 0% to 14% (mean 3.5%).[28,38,65]
- *Characteristics.* Early or late dislocation or subluxation of the prosthetic elbow; associated with pain and loss of function.
  - Disruption of a repaired LCL → posterolateral, rotary, and varus instability; disruption of a repaired MCL → posteromedial and valgus instability.
  - Disruption of triceps mechanism → diminished dynamic compressive forces across the joint.
- *Contributing factors.* Excessive release or inadequate or failed soft tissue repair → deficient static or dynamic stabilizers (possibly due to inadequate postoperative immobilization and excessive postoperative stresses across the elbow, particularly during the early postoperative period before soft tissue repairs have healed), malpositioning of implants, and long-term polyethylene wear of the ulnar component increase the risk of instability.[8,41,61]

### Triceps Insufficiency

- *Incidence.* Primarily occurs after surgical approaches that disrupt the triceps mechanism; occurs in both linked and unlinked arthroplasty, usually during the first postoperative year. Examples of rates of occurance in retrospective studies reported at 1.8% of 887 elbows,[15] 4% of 78 elbows,[28] and 11% of 28 elbows.[38] Higher risk in patients with previous elbow surgery before TEA.[15]

- *Characteristics.* Partial or complete rupture, or avulsion, of the extensor mechanism (during the early or late postoperative period) → weakness (particularly in terminal extension), often posterior elbow pain, and difficulty with pushing activities and overhead functions, such as combing one's hair.
- *Contributing factors.* Occasionally postoperative trauma but most commonly a failed surgical reattachment or repair of a poor quality tendon; premature or excessive ROM or loads on the extensor mechanism during early rehabilitation or during long-term functional use of the arm.[41]

### Implant Loosening

- *Incidence.* Occurs in linked more than unlinked implants. Overall rates are low but remain higher than after hip, knee, and shoulder arthroplasty.[61] The more constrained the design, the greater the risk of loosening.
  - Rate of clinical loosening of contemporary implants up to a 6-year follow-up has been reported to range from 0% to 6%.[29,38,53,65]
  - Rates of 0% reported in patients with RA over a mean follow-up of 3.8 years[53] and in patients with post-traumatic arthritis with a mean follow-up of 5 years.[65]
  - The incidence of radiologic loosening is consistently higher than clinical loosening (where the patient becomes symptomatic).
- *Characteristics.* Aseptic (biomechanical) loosening, a late complication, occurs at the bone–cement interface; clinical loosening associated with pain. Excludes loosening caused by infection.[8]
- *Contributing factors.* Inadequate cementing technique, implant malpositioning, and lack of adherence to postoperative activity modification. High-load, high-impact activities place patient at higher risk of loosening.

---

tions are summarized in Box 18.5.[8,29,61] Precautions to reduce the risk of these and other complications are addressed in the following section on postoperative management.

### Postoperative Management

The overall goal of rehabilitation after total elbow arthroplasty is to achieve pain-free ROM of the elbow joints as well as strength of the upper extremity sufficient for functional activities while minimizing the risk of early or late postoperative complications. This goal is best achieved with an individualized rehabilitation program based on a thorough examination of each patient's postoperative status.

### Immobilization

Immediately after surgery a soft compression dressing is applied, and the arm is elevated to control peripheral edema. A well padded posterior or anterior splint is used to immobilize the elbow to maintain stability and protect structures as they heal.

*Position.* The position of immobilization varies based on a number of factors, including the surgical approach, the implant design, and which soft tissues were repaired and require protection.[6,19,25,44] If, for example, a triceps-reflecting approach was used for a linked TEA, the position typically selected is full or almost full elbow extension to protect the reattached triceps tendon and a neutral position of the forearm.[6,19,48,51] In contrast, with an unlinked TEA, which typically requires repair of the lateral ligament complex because of preoperative damage or release for operative exposure of the joint, the position of immobilization is a moderate degree of flexion with limitation of full forearm supination to lessen stress on the repaired ligaments.[6,61] If a patient had a significant preoperative elbow flexion contracture that was surgically released, an anterior splint may be selected with the elbow placed in the available amount of extension. An extended position is also indicated if symptoms of ulnar neuropathy are present to alleviate pressure in the cubital tunnel.[48,51,61]

***Duration.*** The period of continuous immobilization after surgery, which is kept as short as possible to avoid stiffness, also varies widely, ranging from 1 to 2 days to several weeks. This time period depends on the design of the prosthesis, the surgical approach, the integrity of ligamentous structures, wound healing, and intraoperative observations by the surgeon. In general, unlinked/resurfacing designs, which have little inherent stability, require a longer period of immobilization than linked/semicontrained designs.[8,25,44]

If there is increased risk of delayed wound healing because of poor skin quality or a patient's history of diabetes, smoking, or use of steroids, the elbow may be continuously maintained in extension for 10 to 14 days postoperatively to limit stress on the posterior incision.[48,51,61] Even after it is permissible to remove the splint for exercise or self-care, the patient is advised to continue to wear the splint at night for protection for up to 6 weeks.[6,44] If there was a preoperative flexion contracture, an adjustable splint that maintains the elbow in extension is worn periodically during the day for a prolonged stretch, and a static (resting) splint is worn at night to hold the arm in a comforably extended postion. This regimen may be followed for 8 to 12 weeks postoperatively to prevent recurrence of the contracture.[44,48,51]

## Exercise

The progression of a postoperative exercise program after a TEA varies considerably based on many factors. Key factors and their impact on postoperative rehabilitation are identified in Table 18.3.[6,19,44,78] The rehabilitation process proceeds most rapidly when a triceps-sparing approach has been used to insert a linked replacement in a patient whose incision is healing well. On the other end of the spectrum, in which rehabilitation must progress most cautiously, is the use of a triceps-reflecting approach for an unlinked replacement requiring release and repair of the lateral ligament complex in a patient with poor skin quality.

Just as the progression of exercise is based on the unique features of each patient's surgery, precautions are determined in a similar manner. It is particularly important for the therapist to know the status of repaired soft tissues to incorporate the necessary precautions into the exercise program. Information in the operative report and close communication with the surgeon are the best sources for these details. Specific precautions for exercise and functional use of the operated upper extremity are summarized in Box 18.6.[6,44,48,78] Patient education about these precautions should occur throughout the rehabilitation program. A patient's adherence to precautions ensures more positive outcomes and lessens the likelihood of short- or long-term postoperative complications related to exercise and use of the operated arm for functional activities.

### Exercise: Maximum Protection Phase

***Goals and interventions.*** The focus during the first phase of rehabilitation, which extends approximately over a 4-week period, includes control of inflammation, pain, and edema with use of medication as needed, application of cold (often with a Cryocuff®) and regular elevation of the operated arm. Emphasis is also placed on careful inspec-

| TABLE 18.3 | Factors That Influence the Progression of Exercise After Total Elbow Arthroplasty |
|---|---|
| **Factors** | **Impact on Rehabilitation** |
| • Design of prosthesis: linked/semicontrained vs. unlinked/resurfacing | • Earlier ROM and use of the operated upper extremity for light ADL with linked/semiconstrained replacements, which typically do not require ligament repair for joint stability<br>• More protected, controlled motion during exercise and delayed use for ADL with unlinked/resurfacing replacements, which typically require repair of supporting ligaments for stability |
| • Surgical approach: triceps-sparing vs. triceps-splitting or triceps-reflecting | • Initial postoperative ROM permissible through a greater range of flexion and earlier active antigravity elbow extension, low-load resistance exercise, and light ADL with triceps-sparing approach |
| • Preoperative and postoperative status of supporting ligaments of the elbow | • Earlier and less protected motion during exercise, less protected use during ADL, and less time in splint during the day and at night if ligaments were intact preoperatively and did not undergo a release and repair during arthroplasty |
| • Wound healing | • Longer duration of immobilization of the elbow in an extension splint or delayed end-range flexion if posterior skin quality is poor and healing of the incision is likely to be delayed |
| • Ulnar neuropathy | • May require extended immobilization in an extension splint or delay of exercises to regain elbow flexion |
| • Surgical release of elbow flexion contracture | • May require use of extension splint at night for a prolonged period of time |

| BOX 18.6 | Specific Precautions After Total Elbow Arthroplasty |
|---|---|

### ROM Exercise

- Perform ROM exercises only within the arc of motion achieved during surgery.
- To reduce postoperative stress on a repaired triceps mechanism, avoid end-range flexion during assisted ROM and active, antigravity elbow extension for 3 to 4 weeks.
- If elbow stability is questionable after an unlinked TEA, limit full extension of the elbow and rotation of the forearm, particularly supination past neutral, to avoid overload on repaired lateral ligaments for 4 weeks. With an unlinked replacement, the greatest risk of instability is when the elbow is extended beyond 40° to 50°.[6]
- If symptoms of ulnar nerve compression are noted, avoid prolonged positioning or stretching into end-range flexion.[2,11]

### Strengthening Exercises

- Postpone resisted elbow extension for 6 weeks (or as long as 12 weeks) if a triceps-reflecting approach was used.
- When strengthening the shoulder, apply resistance above the elbow to eliminate stresses across the elbow joint.
- Weight training using moderate and high loads is not appropriate after TEA.

### Functional Activities

- Avoid moving or carrying objects with the operated extremity for 6 weeks.
- If the triceps mechanism was detached and repaired, avoid pushing motions for at least 6 weeks, including propelling a wheelchair, pushing up from a chair, and using a walker, crutches (other than forearm platform design), or a cane.
- If an unlinked replacement was implanted, do not lift weighted objects during daily tasks with the elbow extended to avoid shear forces across the lateral ligament repair, which could contribute to postero-lateral instability.
- Limit repetitive lifting to 1 lb for the first 3 months, 2 lb for the first 6 months, and no more than 5 lb thereafter. Never lift more than 10 to 15 lb in a single lift.[6,19,41,44,51]
- Do not participate in recreational activities, such as golf and tennis, that place high loads or impact across the elbow.

tion of the wound, protection of repaired soft tissues as they begin to heal, and early ROM exercises to offset the adverse effects of immobilization without jeopardizing the stability of the prosthetic joint. Assisted ROM as tolerated and within the ranges achieved intraoperatively typically is initiated 2 to 3 days after linked TEA and a few days later after unlinked TEA if the elbow is stable.[6,44,78]

NOTE: If there was significant preoperative instability of the elbow or if the repair of ligaments released during surgery is in question, ROM typically is delayed for more than a week; and when it is initiated, the patient may need to wear a hinged splint for 4 to 5 weeks that allows only flexion and extension and restricts rotation of the forearm.[6,44]

The goals and exercise interventions during this first phase include the following.[6,19,22,41,44,48,51,78]

- **Maintain mobility of the shoulder, wrist, and hand.**
  - Active ROM of these regions during the immediate postoperative period. This is particularly important for the patient with RA or JRA involving these joints.
- **Regain motion of the elbow and forearm.**
  - After a linked TEA or if the elbow is stable after an unlinked TEA, start with gentle self-assisted elbow flexion/extension and pronation/supination with the elbow comfortably flexed and the forearm in mid-position, progressing to active ROM as tolerated. As acute symptoms subside, have the patient maintain the end-range position to apply a very low-intensity stretch.
  - If the triceps mechanism was reflected and repaired, limit assisted flexion to 90° to 100° for the first 3 to 4 weeks to avoid excessive stretch on the repaired triceps tendon. Perform active elbow flexion/extension in a seated or standing, rather than supine, position for the same time frame to avoid antigravity extension, which also could cause excessive stress to the reattached triceps mechanism and subsequent insufficiency.[6,19,44] While sitting and standing, elbow extension is gravity-assisted; extension is controlled by an eccentric contraction of the elbow flexors.
  - If a linked replacement was implanted using a triceps-sparing approach, there is little to no risk of early postoperative instability or disruption of the triceps mechanism. Therefore, active ROM in all planes of motion is permissible immediately.

NOTE: It is important to point out that some sources recommend that after linked arthroplasty involving a triceps-reflecting approach—and if secure reattachment of the triceps tendon was achieved—ROM exercises progress as tolerated without restrictions.[26,51]

- **Minimize atrophy of upper extremity musculature.**
  - Gentle, pain-free muscle-setting exercises of elbow musculature (against no resistance) while in the splint and, later, multiple-angle setting exercises when the splint can be removed.
  - Low-intensity, isometric resistance exercises of the shoulder, wrist, and hand.
  - Use of the hand for light functional activities as early as 1 to 2 week postoperatively if a linked replacement was inserted but several weeks later after an unlinked TEA.[48,51]

**Exercise: Moderate and Minimum Protection Phases**

By about 4 to 6 weeks postoperatively soft tissues have healed sufficiently to withstand increasing stresses. By 12 weeks, barring complications, only minimum protection is necessary; and a patient typically can resume most functional activities with some imposed restrictions (see Box 18.6). However, the recommended timeline for return to a reasonably full level of activity varies from 6 weeks[19,41,48] to 3 to 4 months.[6,22,44]

*Goals and interventions.* The focus of rehabilitation during the intermediate and final phases is to improve ROM to the extent achieved intraoperatively, regain strength and endurance of elbow musculature, and use the operated arm for gradually demanding functional activities. However, these goals must be reached without disrupting repaired soft tissues and compromising the stability of the prosthetic elbow. Strength and muscular endurance usually continues to improve up to 6 to 12 months postoperatively by cautious use of the operated arm for functional activities.

Patient education, especially with regard to the resumption of functional activites, is ongoing until the patient is discharged from therapy. The following goals and interventions are added during the moderate and minimum protection phases of rehabilitation.[6,22,44]

◉ *Increase ROM of the elbow.*

N O T E : It is the opinion of the authors that use of joint mobilization techniques to increase ROM of the elbow or forearm is inappropriate after TEA, particularly with linked implants or if the stability of the elbow is questionable. If selected as a stretching technique, it should be implemented only after specific consultation with the surgeon to determine its appropriateness. It is a more prudent choice to forego full motion than to jeopardize the stability of the joint.

- Low-intensity manual self-stretching.
- Low-load, long-duration dynamic splinting,[12,32,44] as described and illustated in Chapter 4 (see Fig. 4.13), or alternating use of static splints, each fabricated in maximum but comfortable extension and flexion.

P R E C A U T I O N S : Emphasize end-range extension before end-range flexion to protect the posterior capsule and the triceps mechanism. If symptoms of cubital tunnel syndrome are present (aching along the medial forearm and hand, paresthesia, or hyperesthesia due to compression or entrapment of the ulnar nerve), avoid prolonged or repeated end-range positioning or stretching to increase elbow flexion.[2,11]

◉ *Regain functional strength and muscular endurance of the operated extremity.*

N O T E : Some sources advocate progressive use of the operated upper extremity to regain strength and muscular endurance rather than an exercise program.[26,41,48,51]

- Resisted, multiple-angle isometric exercises at 5 weeks if not initiated previously.
- *Light* ADL (initally < 1 lb of weight) performed with the arm positioned along the side of the trunk and the elbow flexed. If a triceps-reflecting approach was used, incorporate activities that require elbow flexion before elbow extension. Initially modify activities to avoid those that require lifting with the elbow extended and pushing motions, such as pushing up from a chair or using a walker, axillary crutches, or a cane.
- Dynamic, open-chain resistance exercises no earlier than 6 weeks and often later using a light-weight (1 lb) or light-grade elastic resistance. Emphasize gradually increasing repetitions rather than resistance.
- Repetitive lifting during exercise and functional activities limited to 1 lb for the first 3 months and 2 lb for the next 3 months. Permanently limit repetitive lifting to no more than 5 lb and a single lift to no more than 10 to 15 lb.[6,19,41,44,48,51] Refer to Box 18.5 for additional restrictions to strengthening exercises and functional activities.
- Low-load, closed-chain activities, such as wall push-ups after 6 weeks or later (when the triceps mechanism and posterior capsule have healed).
- Upper extremity ergometry.

C O N T R A I N D I C A T I O N S : High-load progressive resistive exercise (PRE), heavy lifting during home- and work-related activities, and recreational activities that place high loads or impact on the upper extremities (e.g., racquet and throwing sports or golf) are not allowed after TEA. These activities must be permanently avoided to reduce the risk of complications, such as elbow instability, implant loosening, and polyethylene wear.[6,22,41,44,51]

**Outcomes**

Although the results of the early use of TEA during the 1970s were quite unsatisfactory, improvements in prosthetic design and fixation, surgical techniques, postoperative management, and criteria for patient selection have made this procedure an important treatment option for pain relief, improving physical function, and preventing eventual disability. Relatively recent long-term studies of patients with RA, for example, have indicated that the "survival rate" (the point at which revision arthroplasty is necessary) of contemporary implants is 94% at a mean of 7.6 years[38] and 92.4% at a minimum of 10 years[28] after linked arthroplasty and 87% at a mean of 12 years[71] and 90% at 16 years[70] after unlinked arthroplasty. These rates are dramatically better than those for the early, constrained implants in which upward of 70% failed within 10 years and are even better than the 82% survival rate of 5.5 years reported in an analysis of studies published worldwide from 1986 to 1992.[29] For the best long-term results, a patient must be selective in the type of work-related or recreational activities performed, modifying some activities and eliminating those that impose high loads and high impact on the elbow.

Outcomes typically are assessed by a combination of patient self-report instruments that address pain relief, function, and quality of life (e.g., the Patient Related Elbow Evaluation form), and physician-administered tools (e.g., the American Shoulder and Elbow Surgeons Questionnaire, which also includes measurements of ROM, strength, and specific shoulder and elbow functions).[5] Because of the variety of tools used, comparison among studies is often difficult.

As noted at the beginning of this discussion on TEA, although the indications have broadened over the past three decades, elbow arthroplasty continues to be used most frequently in patients with RA followed by patients with post-traumatic arthritis. Follow-up studies of patients with these and other underlying pathologies who have undergone linked or unlinked TEA indicate an overall high rate of patient satisfaction, with 80% to 100% of patients reporting "good" or "excellent" results after linked[16,28,38,63,65] and unlinked[24,41] TEA.

*Pain relief.* Complete or nearly complete relief of pain is the most consistently positive and predictable outcome after elbow arthroplasty, occurring in more than 85% to 95% of patients.[17,28,41,63]

***ROM and functional use of the upper extremity.*** Improvements in elbow ROM after TEA are less significant than relief of pain. In addition, maintaining stability of the prosthetic elbow postoperatively is a higher priority than gaining full ROM. However, results of most studies of linked[28,38,52,65] and unlinked[24,70,71,76] arthroplasty indicate some increase in the arc of elbow extension/flexion and forearm rotation in patients with late-stage post-traumatic,[52,65] rheumatoid,[24,28,38,70,71] and juvenile[17] arthritis. Anecdotal evidence suggests that most gains are achieved within 6 to 12 weeks but occasionally up to 6 months postoperatively. Patients with little active movement of the elbow because of preoperative instability have exhibited marked improvement of active motion postoperatively.[35,63]

Many resources suggest or report supporting preoperative and postoperative data to show that greater improvement occurs in elbow flexion than extension after TEA.[19,24,38,41,65,70,71] Some typical examples of the arc of extension/flexion achieved after TEA are 30° to 135°,[24] 26° to 131°,[28] 19° to 140°,[38] and 27° to 131°.[65] Remember that arcs of 100° (from 30° to 130° of extension/flexion and 50° each of pronation/supination) are necessary for most functional activities.[55,56] Therefore, in all of these studies functional ROM for extension and flexion was achieved.

It is important to note that when reviewing the literature for this summary of outcomes there were no studies found that compared outcomes after different approaches to rehabilitation.

# MYOSITIS OSSIFICANS

The terms *myositis ossificans* and *heterotopic* or *ectopic bone formation* are often used interchangeably to describe the formation of bone in atypical locations of the body. Some references[33,45,47] use the term myositis ossificans to denote only ossification of muscle. More often, the term is used generally to characterize heterotopic bone formation in the muscle-tendon unit, capsule, or ligamentous structures. In this text, the terms myositis ossificans and heterotopic bone formation are used synonymously.

## Etiology of Symptoms

Although not a common phenomenon, the sites most frequently involved are the elbow region and thigh. In the elbow, heterotopic bone formation most often develops in the brachialis muscle or joint capsule as the result of trauma, such as a comminuted fracture of the radial head, a fracture-dislocation (supracondylar or radial head fracture) of the elbow, or a tear of the brachialis tendon.[20,33,47,49] Patients with neurological impairments, specifically traumatic brain injury or spinal cord injury, and patients with burns to the extremities are also prone to develop this complication.[47] It may also develop as the result of aggressive stretching of the elbow flexors after injury and a period of immobilization.[20]

Myositis ossificans is distinguished from traumatic arthritis of the humeroulnar joint in that passive extension is more limited than flexion, resisted elbow flexion causes pain, flexion is limited and painful when the inflamed muscle is pinched between the humerus and ulna, and resisted flexion in mid-range causes pain in the brachialis muscle. Palpation of the distal brachialis muscle is tender.[20,33] After the acute inflammatory period, heterotopic bone formation is laid down in muscle between, not within, individual muscle fibers or around the joint capsule within a 2- to 4-week period. This makes the muscle extremely firm to touch. Although this condition can permanently restrict elbow motion, in most cases the heterotopic bone, to a large extent, is reabsorbed over several months, and motion usually returns to near normal.[45]

## Management

Massage, passive stretching, and resistive exercise are contraindicated if the brachialis muscle is implicated after trauma. The elbow should be kept at rest in a splint, which should be removed only periodically during the day for active, pain-free ROM. Rest should continue until the bony mass matures and then resorbs. Surgical excision of heterotopic bone from muscle or TEA, if the capsule is also involved, is necessary only in rare instances.[45,47]

# OVERUSE SYNDROMES: REPETITIVE TRAUMA SYNDROMES

Overuse can occur in any muscle in the elbow region, including the flexors and extensors of the elbow, but it most commonly occurs in the muscles attached to the lateral or medial epicondyles in response to repetitive stressful wrist motions. Problems anterior or posterior to the elbow are frequently caused by excessive extension or flexion strain in sporting activities.[4]

## Related Pathologies

Medial and lateral epicondylitis commonly occurs with repetitive activities of the wrist and hand. Other repetitive trauma in the elbow includes distal biceps tendonitis, triceps tendonitis, and olecranon bursitis.

### Lateral Epicondylitis (Tennis Elbow)

With lateral epicondylitis, there is pain in the common wrist extensor tendons along the lateral epicondyle and radiohumeral joint with gripping activities. Activities such as the backhand stroke in tennis, requiring firm wrist stability, or repetitive work tasks such as computer keyboarding or pulling weeds in a garden, which requires repeated wrist extension, can stress the musculotendinous unit and cause symptoms. The highest incidence is in the musculotendinous junction of the extensor carpi radialis brevis.[20,23,33,60] Symptoms also occur when the annular ligament is stressed.

Positive tests of provocation include palpation tenderness on or near the lateral epicondyle, pain with resisted wrist extension performed with the elbow extended, pain with resisted middle finger extension performed with the elbow extended, and pain with passive wrist flexion with elbow extended and forearm pronated.[20,58,75]

N O T E : Pulled elbow, pushed elbow, rotated elbow, radial head fracture, pinched synovial fringe, meniscal lock, radial tunnel syndrome, tendinosis,[39] and periosteal bruise are also possible sources of pain at the elbow and are sometimes erroneously called tennis elbow.[42]

### Medial Epicondylitis (Golfer's Elbow)

Medial epicondylitis involves the common flexor/pronator tendon at the tenoperiosteal junction near the medial epicondyle. It is associated with repetitive movements into wrist flexion such as swinging a golf club, pitching a ball, or work-related grasping, shuffling papers, and lifting heavy objects. Concomitant ulnar neuropathy is often an associated finding.[27,33]

Positive tests of provocation include palpation tenderness on or near the medial epicondyle, pain with resisted wrist flexion performed with the elbow extended, and pain with passive wrist extension performed with the elbow extended.

## Etiology of Symptoms

The most common cause of epicondylitis is excessive repetitive use or eccentric strain of the wrist or forearm muscles. The result is microdamage and partial tears, usually near the musculotendinous junction when the strain exceeds the strength of the tissues and when the demand exceeds the repair process. With continued irritation, chronic inflammation develops.

Inflammation of the periosteum may develop with formation of granulation tissue and adhesions.[60] Recurring problems are seen because the resulting immobile or immature scar is redamaged when returning to activities before there is sufficient healing or mobility in the surrounding tissue.

## Common Impairments

- Gradually increasing pain in the elbow region after excessive activity of the wrist and hand.
- Pain when the involved muscle is stretched or when it contracts against resistance.
- Decreased muscle strength and endurance for the demand.
- Decreased grip strength, limited by pain.
- Tenderness with palpation at the site of inflammation, such as over the lateral or medial epicondyle, head of the radius, or in the muscle belly.

## Common Functional Limitations/Disabilities

- Inability to participate in provoking activities, such as racket sports, throwing, or golf
- Difficulty with repetitive forearm/wrist tasks, such as sorting or assembling small parts, typing on a keyboard or using a mouse, gripping activities, using a hammer, turning a screwdriver, shuffling papers, or playing a percussion instrument

## Nonoperative Management of Overuse Syndromes: Protection Phase

### Decrease Pain, Edema, or Spasm

- *Immobilization.* Rest the muscles by immobilizing the wrist in a splint such as a cock-up splint, where the elbow and fingers are free to move.
- *Avoid provoking activities.* Instruct the patient to avoid all aggravating activities, such as strong or repetitive gripping actions.
- *Cryotherapy.* Use ice to help control edema and swelling.

### Develop Soft Tissue and Joint Mobility

- *Multiple-angle muscle setting (low-intensity isometrics).* Have the patient remove the splint several times a day and perform gentle multiple-angle setting techniques to the involved muscle followed by pain-free ROM.

◉ *Technique for wrist extensor muscles.*
*Patient position and procedure:* Sitting with the elbow flexed, forearm pronated and resting on a table, and the wrist in extension. Begin with gentle isometric contractions with the wrist extensors in the shortened position. Resist wrist extension, hold the contraction to the count of 6, relax, and repeat several times; then move the wrist toward flexion and repeat the isometric resistance. Do not move into the painful range or provide resistance that causes a painful contraction.

When full wrist flexion is obtained without pain in the lateral epicondyle region, progress by placing the elbow in greater degrees of extension and repeat the isometric resistance sequence to the wrist extensors. Progress until gentle resistance can be applied to the wrist extensors in the position of elbow extension and wrist flexion. It may take several weeks to reach this position.

◉ *Technique for wrist flexor muscles.*
*Patient position and procedure:* Sitting with the elbow flexed, forearm resting on a table, and the wrist in flexion. Begin with gentle isometric contractions with the wrist flexors in the shortened position. Resist wrist flexion, hold the contraction to the count of 6, relax, and repeat several times; then move the wrist toward extension and repeat the isometric resistance. Do not move into the painful range or provide resistance that causes a painful contraction.

When full wrist extension is obtained without pain in the medial epicondyle region, progress by placing the elbow in greater degrees of extension and supination and repeat the isometric resistance sequence to the wrist flexors. As stated above, it may take several weeks to reach the full range of elbow extension, forearm supination, and wrist extension and to be able to tolerate gentle resistance.

◉ *Cross-fiber massage.* Apply gentle cross-fiber massage within tolerance at the site of the lesion. Teach the patient to self-administer the submaximal isometric and cross-fiber massage techniques in a home exercise program.

### Maintain Upper Extremity Function

◉ *Active ROM.* Have the patient perform ROM to joints not immobilized to maintain the integrity of the rest of the upper extremity.
◉ *Resistive exercises*. Have the patient perform shoulder and scapular ROM exercises with the resistance applied proximal to the elbow.

## Nonoperative Management: Controlled Motion and Return to Function Phases

N O T E : Progress to this stage when signs of inflammation are under control.

### Increase Muscle Flexibility and Scar Mobility

◉ *Manual stretching techniques.* Use agonist contraction, hold–relax, and passive stretching techniques to elongate the tight muscle to the end of its range (principles for application of these techniques are described in Chapter 4). Use an intensity of muscle contraction and stretch that causes a stretching sensation but not increased pain. For both the wrist flexors and wrist extensors, the elbow must be extended. Then, to stretch the wrist extensors, pronate the forearm, flex and ulnarly deviate the wrist, and flex the fingers. To stretch the wrist flexors, supinate the forearm, extend and radially deviate the wrist, and extend the fingers.
◉ *Self-stretching techniques.* The patient may use a wall (see Fig. 18.10) and slide the hand along the wall until a stretch force is experienced, or the patient may use the opposite hand to apply the stretch force. These techniques are described in the self-stretching section later in the chapter.
◉ *Cross-fiber (friction) massage.* Palpate to localize the scar, then apply pressure and cross-fiber massage. Increase the intensity of massage as the inflammation decreases.

### Restore Joint Tracking of the RU Joint

◉ *Mobilization with movement (MWM).* Mobilization with movement techniques are used to restore normal tracking of the radius on the capitulum so the forearm muscles can be strengthened without painful symptoms.[57] Several researchers have reported decreased pain and increased grip strength during or shortly after MWM at the elbow.[46,73,74] One researcher observed decreased shoulder rotation in patients with lateral epicondylalgia and demonstrated significant improvement in shoulder range after MWM at the elbow. He proposed that the mechanism was mediated neurophysiologically.[1] Refer to Chapter 5 for principles of application. The following techniques are used if the patient experiences pain when making a fist or with resisted wrist extension.
*Patient position and procedure:* Supine with the forearm pronated. Place a mobilization belt around the patient's proximal forearm and across your shoulders and stabilize the distal humerus with one hand. Apply a lateral glide to the forearm through the belt and then have the patient do repeated wrist extension against manual resistance applied by your other hand (Fig. 18.6A).
*Alternative method:* Apply the lateral glide force against the proximal forearm with your distal hand and have the patient do repeated gripping by squeezing a ball or inflatable bulb (Fig. 18.6B). Both the lateral glide force and the muscle contraction must be pain-free.
◉ *Self-mobilization:* The patient stands with the humerus of the involved elbow stabilized against a doorframe and the forearm in the opening and then applies lateral glide force against the proximal forearm with the contralateral hand. The patient then does repetitive gripping or squeezing against a resistive force such as a pneumatic bulb or squeezable ball (Fig. 18.6C).

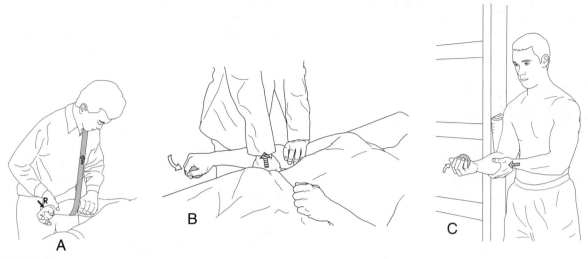

FIGURE 18.6 MWM for lateral epicondylitis. Lateral glide is applied to the proximal forearm (*A*) with resistance added to wrist extension, (*B*) with patient squeezing a ball to bring in the wrist extensors, and (*C*) self-treatment.

## Improve Muscle Performance and Function

- **Isometrics.** Progress the isometric exercises by applying resistance in various pain-free positions.
- **Dynamic exercise.** Progress the exercises to using free weights and elastic resistance through pain-free ranges. Initially use low-intensity resistance with multiple repetitions for muscular endurance, then progress to more intense resistance to strengthen the muscles in preparation for functional demands.
- **Functional patterns.** As flexibility and strength improve and the pain is under control, incorporate functional training utilizing functional patterns into the exercises. Emphasize control of the resistance through the pattern. If pain or deviation of the pattern with substitute motions occurs, have the patient rest before resuming additional repetitions.
- **General strengthening and conditioning.** Incorporate any unused or underused part of the extremity or trunk into the training program prior to returning to the stressful activity.
- **Simulation.** Exercises simulating the desired activity are progressed from slow, controlled motions to high speeds with low resistance to improve timing (see Fig. 18.21).
- **Plyometric exercises.** Add plyometrics to the program if the patient's goals include returning to sport activities or occupational activities that require elbow and forearm power. Suggestions include:
  - Bouncing a tennis ball on a short-handled racket; progress to a long-handled racket.
  - Rapid eccentric/concentric elbow and forearm motions with an elastic resistance.
  - Rapid chest passes or overhead passes using a weighted plyometric ball.
- **Activity modification.** It may be necessary to modify the patient's activity or technique before returning to the stressful activity. For example, it may require taking tennis lessons to correct improper tennis techniques, adapting use of a hammer or other equipment if used, or making ergonomic modifications of a computer workstation.[23,33,58,60,75]

## Patient Education

- Education includes advice and techniques on prevention, recognition of provoking factors, and identification of warning symptoms.
- Teach the patient how to reduce the overload forces that caused the problem and retrain the patient in proper techniques.[23,33,58]
- In addition to exercises, include home instructions on the application of friction massage and stretching the involved muscle prior to using it.

## ⦿ Focus on Evidence

In a descriptive study of 60 subjects with lateral epicondylalgia who were followed for 6 months after initiating physical therapy intervention, Waugh et al.[75] reported that 80% of the participants continued to improve but only 33% had complete resolution of symptoms. The therapy intervention consisted of 8 weeks of ultrasound, deep transverse friction massage, and a stretching/strengthening program for the wrist extensor muscles; 37% of the participants also received treatment for the cervical spine or shoulder. Altogether, 50% continued with some form of therapeutic intervention after the initial 8 weeks. Those with poorer outcomes had repetitive work duties, with 92% of the repetitive duties involving computer work. This study also reported that women who have positive cervical signs as well as repetitive job duties involving computer usage had a poorer prognosis. This was observed at both 8 weeks and 6 months. Ergonomic recommendations for postural adaptations when using a computer included having forearm support, smooth movements, and relaxed shoulders.[75]

N O T E : Additional information on ergonomic recommendations for computer workstations are described in Chapter 14.

# EXERCISE INTERVENTIONS FOR THE ELBOW AND FOREARM

## ● EXERCISE TECHNIQUES TO INCREASE FLEXIBILITY AND RANGE OF MOTION

Prior to initiating a muscle stretching program, be sure the joint capsule is not restricting motion. Techniques to increase joint play in the elbow and forearm articulations are discussed earlier in the chapter. Principles and techniques for applying joint mobilization techniques are presented in Chapter 5.

In addition to the description of principles and techniques of stretching presented in Chapter 4, manual, mechanical, and self-stretching techniques directed to the elbow are described in this section. When teaching the patient self-stretching, emphasize the importance of maintaining a low-intensity, prolonged stretch and not bouncing at the end of the range.

## Manual, Mechanical, and Self-Stretching Techniques

### To Increase Elbow Extension

N O T E : Of the three muscles that flex the elbow, only one, the biceps brachii, crosses two joints (the elbow and the shoulder). Therefore, techniques to fully elongate the biceps brachii must be done with the shoulder extended.

### Mechanical Stretch—Mild Flexion Contracture

*Patient position and procedure*: Supine with the arm supported on the treatment table and a folded towel under the distal humerus as a fulcrum. Place a cuff weight around the distal forearm. Position the forearm in pronation, midposition, and then supination to affect each of the flexor muscles. Have the patient stabilize the proximal humerus with the other hand or place a sandbag or belt across the proximal humerus to stabilize it. Instruct the patient to maintain the stretch for an extended period of time.[77]

### Mechanical Stretch—Dynamic Splinting

Apply a low-intensity, long-duration mechanical stretch force with a dynamic splint to reduce a long-standing elbow flexion contracture by affecting the soft tissue properties of creep and stress-relaxation.[12,32]

### Manual Stretch—Biceps Brachii

*Patient position and procedure*: Prone with the elbow in end-range but comfortable extension and forearm in pronation. Stabilize the scapula and passively extend the shoulder.

### Mechanical Stretch—Biceps Brachii

*Patient position and procedure*: Supine with a cuff weight around the distal forearm. The elbow is in extension and the forearm is in pronation. Have the patient stabilize the proximal humerus with the opposite hand and then place the arm over the side of the table. Allow the elbow and shoulder to extend as far as possible and sustain the stretch position for an extended period of time (Fig. 18.7A).

### Self-Stretch—Biceps Brachii

*Patient position and procedure*: Standing at the side of a table. Have the patient grasp the edge of the table and walk forward, causing shoulder extension with elbow extension (Fig. 18.7B). It is important to note that this stretching position does not include forearm pronation.

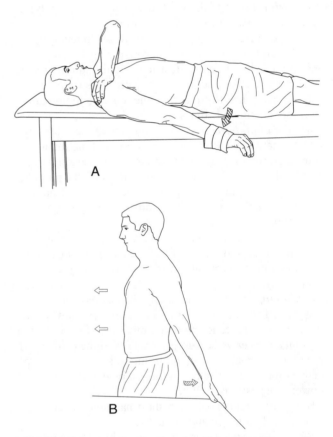

FIGURE 18.7 Self-stretching the biceps brachii musculotendinous unit includes stretching the long head across the shoulder joint (A) supine and (B) standing.

## To Increase Elbow Flexion

### Self-Stretch—Mild Extension Contracture

● *Patient position and procedure*: Prone-lying and propped up on elbows with forearms resting on the exercise mat. Have the patient lower the chest as far as elbow flexion allows and maintain the position as long as tolerated.
● *Patient position and procedure*: Sitting with elbow flexed as far as possible. Have the patient press against the distal forearm with the opposite hand to provide the stretch force into flexion.

### Self-Stretch Long Head of Triceps

*Patient position and procedure*: Sitting or standing. Have the patient flex the elbow and shoulder as far as possible. The other hand can either push on the forearm to flex the elbow, or push the shoulder into more flexion (Fig. 18.8). Hold the stretch position as long as tolerated.

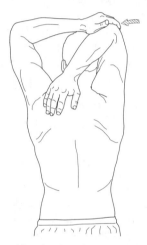

FIGURE 18.8 Self-stretching the triceps brachii musculotendinous unit includes stretching the long head across the shoulder joint.

### To Increase Forearm Pronation and Supination

*Patient position*: Sitting with the elbow flexed to 90° and the elbow resting on a padded table or stabilized against the side of the trunk.

### Self-Stretch to Increase Pronation

Have the patient grasp the dorsal surface of the involved forearm so the heel of the uninvolved hand is against the radius just proximal to the wrist and so the fingers wrap around the ulna. Then have the patient pronate the forearm and sustain the stretch as long as tolerated. The force is applied against the radius so there is no trauma to the wrist.

### Self-Stretch to Increase Supination

Have the patient place the heel of the uninvolved hand against the volar aspect of the involved radius just proxi-

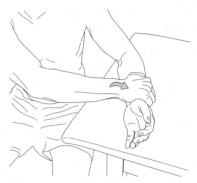

FIGURE 18.9 Self-stretching the forearm into supination. It is important that the stretch force is against the radius, not the hand.

mal to the wrist, supinate the forearm, and sustain the stretch as long as tolerated (Fig. 18.9).

## Self-Stretching Techniques—Muscles of the Medial and Lateral Epicondyles

### To Stretch the Wrist Extensor Muscles (From the Lateral Epicondyle)

● *Patient position and procedure*: Sitting or standing with the elbow extended and forearm pronated. While holding this position have the patient ulnarly deviate the wrist and flex the wrist and fingers; then apply a gentle stretch force against the dorsum of the hand. The patient should feel a stretching sensation along the lateral epicondyle or proximal forearm.
● *Patient position and procedure*: Standing with elbow extended, forearm pronated, and back of the hand against a wall (fingers pointing down). Have the patient then slide the back of the hand up the wall[66] (Fig. 18.10). For additional stretch have the patient actively flex the fingers.

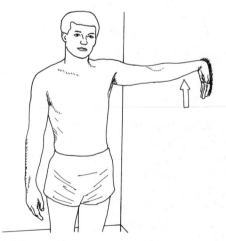

FIGURE 18.10 Self-stretching of the muscles of the lateral epicondyle.

### To Stretch the Wrist Flexor Muscles (from the Medial Epicondyle)

● *Patient position and procedure*: Sitting or standing with the elbow extended and forearm supinated. While holding this position have the patient radially deviate and extend the wrist and apply a gentle stretch force with the other hand against the palm of the hand. A stretch sensation should be felt along the medial epicondyle or proximal forearm.

● *Patient position and procedure*: Standing with the elbow extended and forearm supinated. Have the patient place the palm of the hand against a wall, fingers pointing down, and then move the hand up the wall until a stretch sensation is felt in the wrist flexor muscles.[66]

# ● EXERCISES TO DEVELOP AND IMPROVE MUSCLE PERFORMANCE AND FUNCTIONAL CONTROL

In addition to the conditions already described in this chapter, imbalances in length and strength of muscles crossing the elbow and forearm can be the result of a variety of causes, such as nerve injury or after surgery, trauma, disuse, or immobilization. Appropriate exercises to develop neuromuscular control, increase strength, and improve endurance for return to functional activities can be selected from the following exercises as well as the techniques described in Chapter 6.

For patients with elbow impairments, exercises for the regions above (shoulder girdle) and below (wrist and hand) should also be incorporated into the therapeutic program to prevent complications and restore proper function in the entire upper quarter. The general principles of managing acute soft tissue lesions are discussed in Chapter 10. The exercises described in this section are for use during the controlled motion and return to function phases of intervention when tissues are in the subacute and chronic stages of healing and require only moderate to minimum protection.

## Isometric Exercises

### Multiple-Angle Isometric Exercises
Use manual or mechanical resistance at various positions throughout the available ROM of elbow flexion and extension and forearm rotation. Isolate the key musculature. Apply resistance at the distal forearm, not at the hand, to avoid forces across the wrist joints.

### Angle-Specific Training
During isometric exercises emphasize joint positions that simulate use of the elbow for anticipated functional activities. For example, to simulate carrying large boxes close to the chest, strengthen the elbow flexors in a 70° to 90° position with the forearm in mid-position.

### Endurance
Emphasize holding objects for extended periods of time to increase muscular endurance.

### Alternating Isometrics and Rhythmic Stabilization

#### Open-Chain Exercises
Use alternating isometric contractions by means of manual resistance between antagonists at multiple angles of elbow flexion/extension and forearm pronation/supination. Stabilize the humerus and apply the resistance against the forearm.

Once the patient has learned to respond to the resistance at various elbow and forearm positions and at varying speeds of alternation, progress to alternating isometrics using total upper extremity patterns.

#### Closed-Chain Exercises
Patient positions include standing with hands on a wall or a table, in the quadruped position, or in the prone push-up position (with knees as fulcrum or toes as fulcrum). Have the patient hold the desired elbow position and apply alternating isometrics and rhythmic stabilization by means of manual resistance against the shoulders and trunk.

## Dynamic Strengthening and Endurance Exercises

Many muscles that cross the elbow joint are multijoint muscles, such as the biceps, long head of the triceps, and wrist flexors and extensors. It is particularly important to consider the position of the shoulder and forearm during resistance training at the elbow.[67] Dynamic strengthening and endurance activities for the *prime movers* of the elbow, forearm, and wrist using manual or mechanical resistance are noted in this section. Combined patterns of motion during open- and closed-chain activities are described in the next section.

### Elbow Flexion
Muscles include the biceps brachii, brachialis, and brachioradialis.

● *Patient position and procedure*: Sitting or standing, with the humerus at the side of the chest (arm perpendicular to the floor). Have the patient hold a weight or grasp a piece of elastic resistance material (secured under the foot or to the floor), and flex and extend the elbow. This strengthens the elbow flexors concentrically and eccentrically throughout the available ROM to simulate functional lifting and lowering. Perform this motion with the forearm supinated, pronated, and in mid-position.

● *Patient position and procedure*: Supine or prone, with the humerus supported on the treatment table. When the patient is supine, the resistive force from a free weight or gravity has a greater effect on the muscles near end-range extension and has little to no effect as the elbow reaches 90°. To provide resistance with the patient prone with the forearm over the side of the bed, a pulley sys-

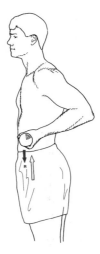

FIGURE 18.11 Resisting elbow flexion with emphasis on the biceps brachii. The shoulder extends as the elbow flexes with the forearm in supination. This combined action lengthens the proximal portion of the musculotendinous unit across the shoulder while it contracts to move the elbow, thus maintaining a more optimal length–tension relationship through a greater ROM.

tem or elastic resistance is necessary to provide resistance to the elbow flexors.

● *Patient position and procedure*: Standing or sitting while holding a weight with the forearm supinated. Have the patient extend the shoulder as the elbow flexes (Fig. 18.11). This combined motion elongates the biceps brachii over the shoulder as the muscle is shortening to move the elbow and thus most efficiently maintains optimal length for development of maximum tension in the *biceps*. This combined motion develops control for carrying objects at the side.

### Elbow Extension
Muscles include the triceps and anconeus.

● *Patient position and procedure*: Prone, humerus abducted to 90° and supported on a rolled towel on a treatment table. Have the patient extend the elbow while holding a weight or pulling against elastic resistance. This position strengthens the elbow extensors from only 90° of flexion to terminal extension.

● *Patient position and procedure*: Supine with the shoulder flexed 90°, holding a weight in the hand. Have the patient begin with the elbow flexed and the weight either at the ipsilateral or contralateral shoulder (external or internal rotation of the shoulder); then extend and flex the elbow (lift and lower the weight) to strengthen the elbow extensors concentrically and eccentrically. To help maintain the shoulder in a stable position, have the patient stabilize the humerus in the 90° position with the opposite hand.

### Long Head of Triceps with Elbow Extension
*Patient position and procedure*: Sitting or standing with the arm held overhead (shoulder flexed) and elbow flexed so the weight is near the shoulder (Fig. 18.12). Have the

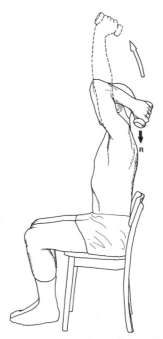

FIGURE 18.12 Resisting elbow extension, beginning with the long head of the triceps brachii on a stretch.

patient lift the weight overhead and then lower the weight for a concentric and eccentric contraction. The patient may support the humerus with the opposite hand. Perform this exercise only if the patient has sufficient control of the shoulder.

### Pronation and Supination
Muscles of pronation are the pronator teres and quadratus; muscles of supination are the supinator and biceps brachii. *Patient position*: Sitting or standing with the elbow flexed to 90°. When sitting, the forearm may be on a table for support.

● *Free weights.* When using a free weight to strengthen the pronators and supinators, the weight must be placed to one side or the other of the hand (Fig. 18.13). If a person holds a dumbbell with weight equal on each side of the hand, one side of the weight is assistive and the other is resistive, in essence canceling out the resistive force. Note also the position of the thumb for each exercise so it is not lifting the bar. The weight can also be turned through a downward arc by placing the resistance on the ulnar side of the hand.

● *Elastic resistance.* Have the patient grasp one end of the elastic resistance with the normal hand, or secure it by standing on it. Have the patient grasp the other end with the involved extremity and turn the forearm against the resistance. For greater resistance, secure the end of the resistance around the end of a short rod and have the patient pull against the resistance force.

● *Functional activity.* Have the patient stand facing a doorknob with the arm kept at the side and the elbow

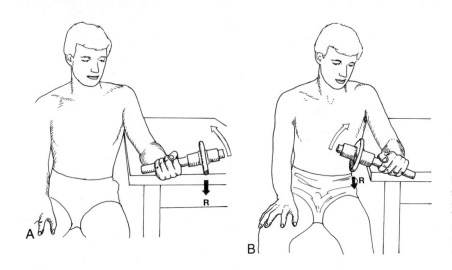

FIGURE 18.13 Mechanical resistance exercise using a small bar with asymmetrically placed weights for strengthening (A) forearm pronators and (B) supinators. The bar can also be rotated through a downward arc to affect the other half of the range for each muscle by placing the weight on the ulnar side of the hand.

flexed to 90° to avoid substituting with shoulder rotation. Have the patient turn the knob.

### Wrist Flexion and Extension

Wrist flexion involves muscles of the medial epicondyle; extension involves muscles of the lateral epicondyle.

● *Free weights.* Patient position and procedure: Sitting, with forearm resting on a table and hand over the edge of the table holding a small weight. When the forearm is pronated, resistance is against the wrist extensors (Fig. 18.14); when supinated, the resistance is against the wrist flexors. Elastic resistance can be applied by secur-

ing a loop of material under the patient's foot and holding the other end in the hand.

● *Wrist roller.* Patient position and procedure: Sitting or standing, with the elbows flexed or extended and the forearms pronated or supinated. Tie a 2- to 4-ft cord to the middle of a short rod; secure a weight to the other end of the cord. Have the patient hold each end of the rod and with an alternating wrist action, turn the rod causing the cord to wind around the rod and elevate the weight. The weight is then lowered with a reverse motion (Fig. 18.15).

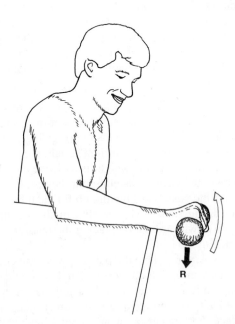

FIGURE 18.14 Mechanical resistance exercise using a handheld weight for strengthening the muscles of the lateral epicondyle (wrist extensors).

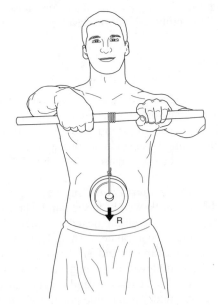

FIGURE 18.15 Wrist roller exercise to strengthen grip and develop muscles of the lateral epicondyle. This exercise requires stabilization in the shoulder girdle and elbow muscles. The elbows may be flexed or the forearms supinated to emphasize the elbow flexors or muscles of the medial epicondyle, respectively.

## Functional Exercises

**N O T E :** Because the elbow primarily functions during activities that also involve the shoulder and hand, use combined patterns that strengthen the entire upper extremity. Be careful that substitute motions do not occur to compensate for a weak link in the chain. Include exercises to progressively improve strength, power, and endurance. Isokinetic exercises may also be used to address specific patterns of motion.

### Diagonal Patterns

***PNF patterns against manual or mechanical resistance.***
Use unilateral or bilateral diagonal (proprioceptive neuromuscular facilitation, or PNF) patterns as described in Chapter 6. Use manual resistance, free weights, elastic resistance, a weight-pulley system, or an isokinetic dynamometer to provide the resistance as the patient moves through the diagonal patterns. Gradually increase resistance, speed (if appropriate with the choice of equipment), and repetitions.

### Combined Pulling Motions

Elbow flexors are used in pulling, lifting, and carrying activities in open- and closed-chain activities. These upper extremity actions also require strength in the scapular retractors, shoulder extensors, and wrist and hand musculature. Many of the exercises that are described for the shoulder in Chapter 17 also involve resisted elbow flexion and therefore can be used to strengthen muscle groups during pulling motions. Additional suggestions include:

- Bilateral pull-ups against elastic resistance (Fig. 18.16)

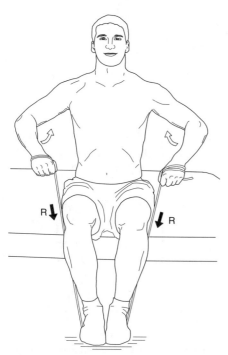

FIGURE 18.16 Bilateral pull-ups against elastic resistance.

- Closed-chain chin-ups or modified pull-ups on an overhead bar (Fig. 18.17)

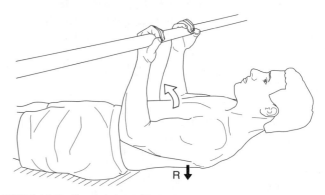

FIGURE 18.17 Closed-chain modified chin-ups using top half of body weight for resistance to strengthen the elbow flexors. This exercise may be performed in a bed with an overhead trapeze.

- Bilateral or unilateral rowing motions, such as using a rowing machine or simulating starting a lawn mower (Fig. 18.18)

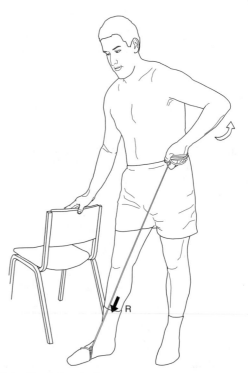

FIGURE 18.18 Simulation of a "lawn mower pull" for functional strengthening of the upper extremity.

- Pulling a variety of weighted objects with one or both arms, emphasizing elbow flexion and proper body mechanics.

### Combined Pushing Motions

The triceps muscle is involved in pushing motions. Pushing also involves variations of shoulder flexion and scapular protraction or depression so muscles controlling these motions are functioning with the triceps. Many of the exercises described in Chapter 17 for the shoulder also involve resisted elbow extension and may be used to strengthen muscles groups used in pushing patterns. Additional suggestions include:

● Military press (see Fig. 17.52).
● Bench press.
● Upper extremity ergometry (see Fig. 6.54).
● Wall push-ups, semiprone or prone push-ups (Fig. 18.19A).
● Push-ups from a chair or on parallel bars (Fig. 18.19B).

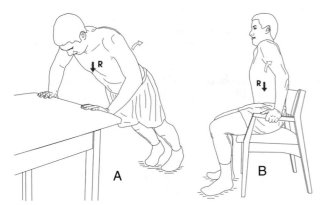

**FIGURE 18.19** Closed-chain strengthening of the triceps. *(A)* Modified push-ups. *(B)* Seated push-ups.

● Stepping/stair-climbing machine with hands on the "steps." Emphasize elbow extension.
● Pushing a variety of weighted objects with one or both arms using dynamic elbow extension (Fig. 18.20).

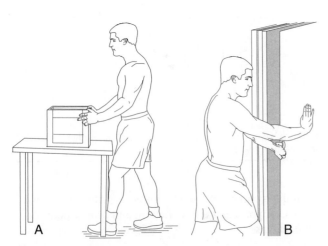

**FIGURE 18.20** Strengthening the triceps with pushing activities. *(A)* Pushing weighted objects across a table. *(B)* Depressing a door handle and pushing open a door.

### Stretch-Shortening Drills (Plyometrics)
Suggestions for increasing power using plyometric exercises[77]:

● Have the patient perform elbow flexion and extension exercises against elastic resistance, emphasizing rapid reversal between eccentric and concentric motions.
● Use a weighted ball and have the patient catch and then quickly throw it back. Emphasize elbow motions with overhead passes, chest passes, and lateral passes.
● Have the patient bounce a tennis ball on a racket with the forearm pronated and with it supinated.

### Simulated Tasks and Activities
Determine the component motions of the patient's desired functional activities as well as occupational or recreational tasks. Have the patient simulate these motions and practice the entire task. Activities could involve lifting, lowering, carrying, pushing, pulling, twisting, turning, catching, throwing, or swinging. For example, if the patient is recovering from repetitive trauma to the muscles of the lateral epicondyle ("tennis elbow"), have the patient practice the various strokes using a wall pulley (Fig. 18.21). Impose controlled forces to challenge the patient by increasing the time or repetitions, speed, or resistance.[77]

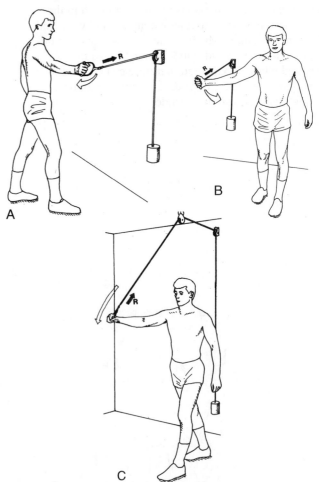

**FIGURE 18.21** Mechanical resistance exercise using wall pulleys to simulate tennis swings. *(A)* Backhand stroke. *(B)* Forehand stroke. *(C)* Serve.

# INDEPENDENT LEARNING ACTIVITIES

## ● Critical Thinking and Discussion

1. Differentiate between the etiology, signs and symptoms, and management of lateral and medial epicondylitis. Note the similarities and differences.
2. Develop, compare, and contrast the postoperative management after two types of total elbow arthroplasty: (1) a semiconstrained implant/triceps-reflecting approach and (2) a resurfacing implant/triceps-splitting approach.
3. The goal is to increase muscle performance and function in the elbow flexors that are currently functioning at a 3/5 strength level and endurance of four repetitions. Identify exercises that could be used at each increment of strength, including exercises for strength, endurance, power, control, stability, and function. Identify parameters for progression of each exercise and any precautions.
4. Do the same sequence of analysis and identification to increase muscle performance and function of the elbow extensors.
5. Analyze the following household, occupational, or sports-related activities. Identify the components and sequence of motions related to each of these motor tasks; pay particular attention to elbow and forearm motions during these tasks. Design a sequence of upper extremity exercises and simulated activities that could be incorporated into a late-stage rehabilitation program to prepare a patient to return to the desired task after an elbow injury.
   • Housecleaning
   • Gardening
   • Grocery store stocking
   • Carpentry
   • Volleyball
   • Tennis
   • Throwing sports

## ● Laboratory Practice

1. Apply mobilization techniques to a laboratory partner to increase the following elbow and forearm motions: mid- and end-range elbow flexion; mid- and end-range elbow extension; forearm pronation and supination (proximal and distal articulations).

2. Demonstrate passive stretching and hold–relax techniques to elongate the following muscles that cross the elbow: brachialis, brachioradialis, biceps, long head of the triceps, extensor communis digitorum, flexor carpi ulnaris, flexor carpi radialis.
3. Using the following pieces of resistance equipment demonstrate at least two methods (setups) to strengthen the elbow flexors/extensors and forearm rotators: free weights, weight-pulley system, and elastic resistance. Then demonstrate a progressive sequence of resistance exercise to strengthen the same muscle groups using self-resistance (body weight or manual resistance).

## ● Case Studies

1. Describe the mechanical problem causing impairments in the elbow and forearm in the following scenario and what techniques could be used for intervention. A patient is referred to you 4 weeks after sustaining a fracture of the distal radius with immobilization in a cast following a fall on an outstretched hand. She has limited elbow, forearm, and wrist motions. On palpation you note a decreased space between the lateral aspect of the head of the radius and capitellum as well as decreased joint play at all articulations of the elbow, forearm, and wrist.
2. A 15-year-old patient with a 5-year history of polyarticular JRA just underwent open synovectomy and excision of the head of the radius with implant for late-stage joint disease of the elbow. Prior to surgery, the patient had severe pain in the elbow region, lacked full elbow flexion/extension and forearm rotation, and had limited use of the arm for functional activities. Continuous passive motion (CPM) was implemented during the patient's hospitalization (3 days). On the day prior to discharge the patient was referred to physical therapy for a home program. Design an exercise program for this teenager. Prioritize and describe each exercise you want the patient to do for the first week at home. Outline a program of exercises for later use in the rehabilitation process. The patient plans to return to school within a week of discharge from the hospital. Indicate whether you recommend outpatient therapy; if so, indicate the frequency and duration; justify the need for this recommendation.

# REFERENCES

1. Abbott, JH, Patla, CE, Jensen, RH: Manual therapy to the elbow affects shoulder range of motion in subjects with lateral epicondylalgia. In Singer, KP (ed) Proceedings of the 7th Scientific Conference of the IFOMT, Perth, Australia, November 2000, p 11.
2. Aiello, B: Ulnar nerve compression. In Clark, GL, et al (eds): Hand Rehabilitation, ed. 2. Churchill Livingstone, New York, 1998, p 213.
3. American Physical Therapy Association: Guide to Physical Therapist Practice, ed 2. Phys Ther 81:9–744, 2001.
4. Andrews, JR, Whiteside, JA: Common elbow problems in the athlete. J Orthop Sports Phys Ther 17:289, 1993.
5. Angst, F, John, M, Pap, G, et al: Comprehensive assessment of clinical outcomes and quality of life after total elbow arthroplasty. Arthritis Rheum 53:73–82, 2005.
6. Antuna, SA: Rehabilitation after elbow arthroplasty. In Williams, GR, Yamaguchi, K, Ramsey, ML, Galatz, LM (eds) Shoulder and Elbow

Arthroplasty. Lippincott Williams & Wilkins, Philadelphia, 2005, pp 475–484.

7. Armstrong, AD, King, GJW, Yamaguchi, K: Total elbow arthroplasty design. In Williams, GR, Yamaguchi, K, Ramsey, ML, Galatz, LM (eds) Shoulder and Elbow Arthroplasty. Lippiincott Williams & Wilkins, Philadelphia, 2005, pp 297–312.

8. Armstrong, AD, Galatz, LM: Complications of total elbow arthroplasty. In Williams, GR, Yamaguchi, K, Ramsey, ML, Galatz, LM (eds) Shoulder and Elbow Arthroplasty. Lippincott Williams & Wilkins, Philadelphia, 2005, pp 459–473.

9. Barenholtz, A, Wolff, A: Elbow fractures and rehabilitation. Orthop Phys Ther North Am 10(4):525–539, 2001.

10. Basmajian, JV: Muscles Alive: Their Functions Revealed by Electromyography, ed 4. Williams & Wilkins, Baltimore, 1979.

11. Blackmore, SM, Hotchkiss, RN: Therapist's management of ulnar neuropathy at the elbow. In Hunter, JM, Mackin, EJ, Callahan, AD (eds) Rehabilitation of the Hand: Surgery and Therapy, ed. 4. Mosby-Year Book, St. Louis, 1995, p 665.

12. Bonutti, PM, et al: Static progressive stretch to re-establish elbow range of motion. Clin Orthop 303:128, 1984.

13. Bowling, RW, Rockar, PA: The elbow complex. In Malone, TR, McPoil, TM, Niyz, AJ (eds) Orthopedic and Sports Physical Therapy, ed 2. CV Mosby, St. Louis, 1997, p 379.

14. Buckwalter, JA, Ballard, WT: Operative treatment of rheumatic disease. In Klippel, JH (ed) Primer on the Rheumatic Diseases, ed. 12. Arthritis Foundation, Atlanta, 2001, pp 613–623.

15. Celli, A, Arash, A, Adams, RA, Morrey, BF: Triceps insufficiency following total elbow arthroplasty. J Bone Joint Surg Am 87(9): 1957–1964, 2005.

16. Cobb, TK, Morrey, BF: Total elbow arthroplasty as primary treatment for distal humeral fractures in elderly patients. J Bone Joint Surg Am 79:826, 1997.

17. Connor, PM, Morrey BF: Total elbow arthroplasty in patients who have juvenile rheumatoid arthritis. J Bone Joint Surg Am 80:678, 1998.

18. Cooney, WP: Elbow arthroplasty: historical perspective and current concepts. In Morrey, BF (ed) The Elbow and Its Disorders, ed 3. WB Saunders, Philadelphia, 2000, p 583.

19. Cresswell, T, Stanley, D: Unlinked elbow arthroplasty. In Williams, GR, Yamaguchi, K, Ramsey, ML, Galatz, LM (eds) Shoulder and Elbow Arthroplasty. Lippincott Williams & Wilkins, Philadelphia, 2005, pp 333–345.

20. Cyriax, J: Textbook of Orthopaedic Medicine, ed 8. Vol 1. Diagnosis of Soft Tissue Lesions. Bailliere Tindall, London, 1982.

21. Dee, R: Total replacement arthroplasty of the elbow for rheumatoid arthritis. J Bone Joint Surg Br 54:88, 1972.

22. Edmonds, A: Elbow arthroplasty. In Clark, GL, et al (eds) Hand Rehabilitation, ed 2. Churchill Livingstone, New York, 1998, p 287.

23. Ellenbecker, TS, Mattalino, A: The Elbow in Sport—Injury, Treatment and Rehabilitation. Human Kinetics, Champaign IL, 1997.

24. Ewald, FC, et al: Capitellocondylar total elbow replacement in rheumatoid arthritis: long-term results. J Bone Joint Surg Am 75:498, 1993.

25. Ferlic, DC: Rheumatoid arthritis in the elbow. In Green, DP, Hotchkiss, RM, Peterson, WC (eds) Green's Operative Hand Surgery, Vol 2, ed 4. Churchill Livingstone, New York, 1999, p 1740.

26. Field, LD, Savoié, FH, III: Master Cases: Shoulder and Elbow Surgery. Thieme, New York, 2003.

27. Gebel, GT, Morrey, BF: Operative treatment of medial epicondylitis: influence of concomitant ulna neuropathy at the elbow. J Bone Joint Surg Am 77:1065, 1995.

28. Gill, DR, Morrey, BF: The Coonrad-Morrey total elbow arthroplasty in patients who have rheumatoid arthritis: a 10 to 15 year follow-up study. J Bone Joint Surg Am 80:1327, 1998.

29. Gschwend, N, Simmen BR, Matejovsky, Z: Late complications in elbow arthroplasty. J Shoulder Elbow Surg 5:86, 1996.

30. Gupta, GG, Lucas, G, Hahn DL: Biomechanical and computer analysis of radial head prostheses. J Shoulder Elbow Surg 6:37, 1997.

31. Hall, JA, McKee, MA: Posterolateral rotary instability of the elbow following radial head resection. J Bone Joint Surg Am 87(7): 1571–1579, 2005.

32. Hepburn, G, Crivelli, K: Use of elbow dynasplint for reduction of elbow flexion contractures: a case study. J Orthop Sports Phys Ther 5:259, 1984.

33. Hertling, D, Kessler, RM: Management of Common Musculoskeletal Disorders, Physical Therapy Principles and Methods (ed 3). Lippincott Williams & Wilkins, Philadelphia, 1996.

34. Hotchkiss, RN: Displaced fractures of the radial head: internal fixation or excisions? J Am Acad Orthop Surg 5:1, 1997.

35. Inglis, AE, Inglis AE Jr, Friggie, MM, Asnis, L: Total elbow arthroplasty for flail and unstable elbows. J Shoulder Elbow Surg 6:29, 1997.

36. Jerosch, J, Schroder, M, Schneider, T: Good and relative indications for elbow arthroscopy: a retrospective study on 103 patients. Arch Orthop Trauma Surg 117:246, 1998.

37. Kapadji, IA, Kandel, MJ: The Physiology of the Joints, Vol. I, ed 5. Churchill-Livingstone, Edinburgh, 1997.

38. Kelly, EV, Coghlan, J, Bell, S: Five- to thirteen-year follow-up of the GBS III total elbow arthroplasty. J Shoulder Elbow Surg 13:434–440, 2004.

39. Kraushaar, BS, Nirschl, RP: Tendinosis of the elbow (tennis elbow): clinical features and findings of histological, immunohistochemical and electron microscopy studies. J Bone Joint Surg Am 81(2):259, 1999.

40. Lee, BP, Morrey BF: Synovectomy of the elbow. In Morrey, BF (ed) The Elbow and Its Disorders, ed 3. WB Saunders, Philadelphia, 2000, p 708.

41. Linscheid, RL, Morrey, BF: Resurfacing elbow replacement arthroplasty. In Morrey, BF (ed) Joint Replacement Arthroplasty, ed 3. Churchill Livingstone, Philadelphia, 2003, pp 303–315.

42. Lutz, FR: Radial tunnel syndrome: an etiology of chronic lateral elbow pain. J Orthop Sports Phys Ther 14:14, 1991.

43. Magee, DJ: Orthopedic Physical Assessment, ed 4. WB Saunders, Philadelphia, 2002.

44. Manning-Kloos, S, Nestor, BJ: Elbow surgery and rehabilitation. In Melvin, J, Gall, V (eds) Rheumatologic Rehabilitation Series. Vol 5. Surgical Rehabilitation. American Occupational Therapy Association, Bethesda, 1999, p 13.

45. Mercier, LR: Practical Orthropedics, ed 4. CV Mosby, St. Louis, 1995.

46. Miller, J: Mulligan concept—management of "tennis elbow." Orthop Div Rev May/June:45, 2000.

47. Morrey, BF: Ectopic ossificans about the elbow. In Morrey, BF (ed) The Elbow and Its Disorders, ed 3. WB Saunders, Philadelphia, 2000, p 437.

48. Morrey, BF: Linked arthroplasty. In Williams, GR, Yamaguchi, K, Ramsey, ML, Galatz, LM (eds) Shoulder and Elbow Arthroplasty. Lippincott Williams & Wilkins, Philadelphia, 2005, pp 475–484.

49. Morrey BF: Radial head fracture. In Morrey BF (ed) The Elbow and Its Disorders, ed 3. WB Saunders, Philadelphia, 2000, p 341.

50. Morrey, BF: Radial head prosthetic replacement. In Morrey, BF (ed) Joint Replacement Arthroplasty, ed 3. Churchill Livingstone, Philadelphia, 2003, pp 294–302.

51. Morrey, BF: Semiconstrained total elbow replacement: indications and surgical technique. In Morrey, BF (ed) Joint Replacement Arthroplasty, ed 3. Churchill Livingstone, Philadelphia, 2003, pp 316–328.

52. Morrey, BF, Adams, RA, Bryan, RS: Total replacement for post-traumatic arthritis of the elbow. J Bone Joint Surg Br 73:607, 1991.

53. Morrey, BF, Adams, RA: Results of semiconstrained replacement for rheumatoid arthritis. In Morrey, BF (ed) Joint Replacement Arthroplasty, ed 3. Churchill Livingstone, Philadelphis, 2003, pp 329–337.

54. Morrey, BF, Adams, RA: Semiconstrained elbow for distal humeral nonunion. J Bone Joint Surg Br 77:67, 1995.

55. Morrey, BF, An, K: Functional evaluation of the elbow. In Morrey, BF (ed) The Elbow and Its Disorders, ed 3. WB Saunders, Philadelphia, 2000, p 74.

56. Morrey, BE, Askew, LI, An, KN, et al: A biomechanical study of normal functional elbow motion. J Bone Joint Surg Am 63:872–876, 1981.

57. Mulligan, BR: Manual Therapy "NAGS," "SNAGS," "MWM'S" etc. (ed 4). Plane View Press, Wellington, 1999.

58. Nerschl, R, Sobel, J: Conservative treatment of tennis elbow. Phys Sportsmed 9.6:43, 1981.

59. Norkin, CC: The elbow complex. In Levangie, PK, Norkin, CC (eds) Joint Structure and Function: A Comprehensive Analysis. FA Davis, Philadelphia, 2005, pp 273–304.

60. Noteboom, T, et al: Tennis elbow: a review. J Orthop Sports Phys Ther 19:357, 1994.

61. O'Driscoll, SW: Complications of total elbow arthroplasty. In Morrey, BF (ed) Joint Replacement Arthroplasty, ed 3. Churchill Livingstone, Philadelphia, 2003, pp 352–378.
62. Ramsey, ML: The history and development of total elbow arthroplasty. In Williams, GR, Yamaguchi, K, Ramsey, ML, Galatz, LM (eds) Shoulder and Elbow Arthroplasty. Lippincott Williams & Wilkins, Philadelphia, 2005, pp 271–278.
63. Ramsey, ML, Adams, RA, Morrey, BF: Instability of the elbow treated with semiconstrained total elbow arthroplasty. J Bone Joint Surg Am 81:38, 1999.
64. Schemitsch, EH, Ewald, FC, Thornhill, TS: Results of total elbow arthroplasty after excision of the radial head and synovectomy in patients who had rheumatoid arthritis. J Bone Joint Surg Am 78:1541, 1996.
65. Schneeberger, AG, Adams, R, Morrey, BF: Semiconstrained total elbow replacement for the treatment of post-traumatic osteoarthrosis. J Bone Joint Surg Am 79:1211, 1997.
66. Sheon, R, Moskowitz, R, Goldberg, V: Soft tissue rheumatic pain: recognition, management, prevention. Lea & Febiger, Philadelphia, 1982.
67. Smith, LK, Weiss, EL, Lehmkuhl, LD: Brunnstrom's Clinical Kinesiology, ed 5. FA Davis, Philadelphia, 1996.
68. Stans, AA, Wedge, JH: Fractures of the neck of the radius in children. In Morrey, BF (ed) The Elbow and Its Disorders, ed 3. WB Saunders, Philadelphia, 2000, p 236.
69. Stroyan, M, Wilk, KE: The functional anatomy of the elbow complex. J Orthop Sports Phys Ther 17:179, 1993.
70. Tanaka, N, Kudo, H, Iwano, K, et al: Kudo total elbow arthroplasty in patients with rheumatoid arthritis. J Bone Joint Surg Am 83:1506–1513, 2001.
71. Trail, IA, Nuttall, D, Stanley, JK: Survivorship and radiological analysis of the standard Souter-Strathclyde total elbow arthroplasty. J Bone Joint Surg Br 81:80–84, 1999.
72. Vander-Wilde, RS, et al: Inflammatory arthrosis of the ulnohumeral joint after failed silicone radial head implant. J Bone Joint Surg Br 76:78, 1994.
73. Vicenzino, B, Buratowski, S, Wright, A: Preliminary study of the initial hypoalgesic effect of a mobilisation with movement treatment for lateral epicondylalgia. In Singer, KP (ed) Proceedings of the 7th Scientific Conference of the IFOMT. Perth, Australia, November 2000, p 460.
74. Vicenzino, B, Wright, A: Effects of a novel manipulative physiotherapy technique on tennis elbow: a single case study. Manual Ther 1:30, 1995.
75. Waugh, EJ, Jaglal, SB, Davis, AM: Computer use associated with poor long-term prognosis of conservatively managed lateral epicondylalgia. J Orthop Sports Phys Ther 34(12):770–780, 2004.
76. Weiland, AJ, et al: Capitellocondylar total elbow replacement. J Bone Joint Surg Am 71:217, 1989.
77. Wilk, KE, Arrigo, C, Andrews, JR: Rehabilitation of the elbow in the throwing athlete. J Orthop Sports Phys Ther 17:305, 1993.
78. Wilk, KE, Andrews, JR: Elbow injuries. In Brotzman, SB, Wilk, KE (eds) Clinical Orthopedic Rehabilitation, ed 2. Mosby, Philadelphia, 2003, pp 85–123.

# The Wrist and Hand

The wrist is the final link of joints that positions the hand for functional activities. It has the significant function of controlling the length–tension relationship of the multiarticular muscles of the hand as they adjust to various activities and grips.[5] The hand is a valuable tool through which we control and manipulate our environment and express ideas and talents. It also has an important sensory function of providing feedback to the brain.

This chapter is divided into three major sections. The first section briefly reviews the rather complex structure and function of the wrist and hand—information that is important to know in order to effectively treat hand problems. The second section describes common disorders and guidelines for conservative and postoperative management. The last section describes exercise techniques commonly used to meet the goals of treatment during the stages of tissue healing and phases of rehabilitation.

## STRUCTURE AND FUNCTION OF THE WRIST AND HAND

The bones of the wrist consist of the distal radius, scaphoid (S), lunate (L), triquetrum (Tri), pisiform (P), trapezium (Tm), trapezoid (Tz), capitate (C), and hamate (H). Five metacarpals and 14 phalanges make up the hand and the five digits (Fig. 19.1).

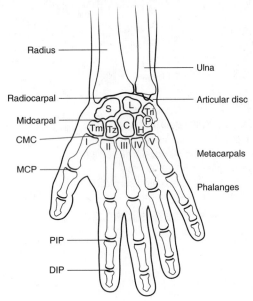

FIGURE 19.1 Bones of the wrist and hand complex.

 JOINTS OF THE WRIST AND HAND

### Wrist Joint—Characteristics and Arthrokinematics

The distal radioulnar (RU) joint is not part of the wrist joint, although pain and impairments in this forearm articulation are often described by the patient as wrist pain. Its structure and function are described in Chapter 18.

The wrist joint is multiarticular and is made up of two compound joints. It is biaxial, allowing flexion (volar flexion), extension (dorsiflexion), radial deviation (abduction), and ulnar deviation (adduction). Stability is provided by numerous ligaments: the ulnar and radial collateral, the dorsal and volar (palmar) radiocarpal, the ulnocarpal, and the intercarpal.

The pisiform is categorized as a carpal and is aligned volar to the triquetrum in the proximal row of carpals. It is not part of the wrist joint per se but functions as a sesamoid bone in the flexor carpi ulnaris tendon.

### Radiocarpal Joint

***Characteristics.*** The radiocarpal (RC) joint is enclosed in a loose but strong capsule that is reinforced by the ligaments shared with the midcarpal joint. The biconcave articulating surface is the distal end of the radius and radioulnar disk (discus articularis); it is angled slightly volarward and ulnarward. The biconvex articulating surface is the combined proximal surface of the scaphoid, lunate, and triquetrum. The triquetrum primarily articulates with the disk. These three carpals are bound together with numerous interosseous ligaments.

***Arthrokinematics.*** With motions of the wrist, the convex proximal row of carpals slides in the direction opposite the physiological motion of the hand. The arthrokinematics are summarized in Box 19.1.

### Midcarpal Joint

***Characteristics.*** The midcarpal joint is a compound joint between the two rows of carpals. It has a capsule that is also continuous with the intercarpal articulations. The combined distal surfaces of the scaphoid, lunate, and triquetrum articulate with the combined proximal surfaces of the trapezium, trapezoid, capitate, and hamate.

***Arthrokinematics.*** The articulating surfaces of the capitate and hamate are, in essence, convex and slide on the concave articulating surfaces of a portion of the scaphoid, lunate, and triquetrum so with flexion and extension, as well as radial and ulnar deviation, their combined surfaces slide opposite the physiological motion.

The articulating surfaces of the trapezium and trapezoid are concave and slide on the convex distal surface of the scaphoid so with flexion and extension their combined surfaces slide in the same direction as the physiological motion. Because the trapezoid is bound to the capitate, they cannot slide in opposite directions during radial and ulnar deviation. The trapezii (the trapezium and trapezoid) therefore slide in a dorsal direction on the scaphoid during radial deviation and in a volar direction during ulnar deviation.[59]

Physiological motions of the wrist result in a complex motion between the proximal and distal row of carpals. Because the concave trapezii slide in a dorsal direction on the scaphoid and the convex capitate and hamate slide in a volar direction on the lunate and triquetrum during extension and radial deviation, the resulting motion is a supination twist of the distal row on the proximal row. A pronation twist occurs during flexion and ulnar deviation as the trapezii slide volarly and the capitate and hamate slide dorsally.[5]

These arthrokinematic relationships are summarized in Box 19.1.

### Hand Joints—Characteristics and Arthrokinematics

#### Carpometacarpal Joints of Digits 2 through 5

***Characteristics.*** The carpometacarpal (CMC) joints are enclosed in a common joint cavity and include the articulations of each metacarpal with the distal row of carpals and the articulations between the bases of each metacarpal.

## BOX 19.1    Arthrokinematics of the Wrist and Hand Joints

| Physiological Motion | Roll | Slide |
|---|---|---|
| **Radiocarpal joint: motion of proximal row of carpals** | | |
| *Flexion of wrist* | *Volar* | *Dorsal* |
| *Extension of wrist* | *Dorsal* | *Volar* |
| *Radial deviation* | *Radial* | *Ulnar* |
| *Ulnar deviation* | *Ulnar* | *Radial* |
| **Midcarpal joints: motion of distal row of carpals** | | |
| *Flexion of wrist* | *Volar* | *C and H dorsal* |
| | | *Tm and Tz volar* |
| *Extension of wrist* | *Dorsal* | *C and H volar* |
| | | *Tm and Tz dorsal* |
| *Radial deviation* | *Radial* | *C and H ulnar* |
| | | *Rm and Tz dorsal* |
| *Ulnar deviation* | *Ulnar* | *C and H radial* |
| | | *Tm and Tz volar* |
| **Carpometacarpal joints of digits 2–5: motion of proximal phalanx** | | |
| *Flexion (increased arch)* | *Volar* | *Volar* |
| *Extension (decreased arch)* | *Dorsal* | *Dorsal* |
| **Carpometacarpal joint of thumb: motion of 1st metacarpal** | | |
| *Flexion* | *Ulnar* | *Ulnar* |
| *Extension* | *Radial* | *Radial* |
| *Abduction* | *Volar* | *Dorsal* |
| *Adduction* | *Dorsal* | *Volar* |
| **Metacarpophalangeal joints of digits 2–5: motion of phalanx** | | |
| *Flexion* | *Volar* | *Volar* |
| *Extension* | *Dorsal* | *Dorsal* |
| *Abduction* | *Away from center of hand* | |
| *Adduction* | *Toward center of hand* | |
| **Interphalangeal joints and MCP joint of thumb: motion of phalanx** | | |
| *Flexion* | *Volar* | *Volar* |
| *Extension* | *Dorsal* | *Dorsal* |

The joints of digits 2, 3, and 4 are plane uniaxial joints; the joint of digit 5 is biaxial. They are supported by transverse and longitudinal ligaments. The fifth metacarpal is most mobile, with the fourth being the next most mobile. Flexion of the metacarpals and additional adduction of the fifth contribute to cupping (arching) of the hand, which improves the ability of the hand to grasp objects of various sizes. Extension of the metacarpals contributes to flattening of the hand, which improves the ability to release objects.

***Arthrokinematics.*** The proximal surfaces slide in a volar direction with flexion and in a dorsal direction with extension motions in the hand (see Box 19.1).

### Carpometacarpal Joint of the Thumb (Digit 1)

***Characteristics.*** The CMC joint of the thumb is a saddle-shaped (sellar) biaxial joint between the trapezium and base of the first metacarpal. It has a lax capsule and wide range of motion (ROM), which allows the thumb to move away from the palm of the hand for opposition in prehension activities.

***Arthrokinematics.*** For flexion/extension of the thumb (components of opposition/reposition, respectively), occurring in the frontal plane, the surface of the trapezium is convex and the base of the metacarpal is concave; therefore, its surface slides in the same direction as the angulating bone. For abduction/adduction, occurring in the sagittal plane, the trapezium surface is concave and the metacarpal is convex; therefore, the surface of the metacarpal slides in the opposite direction of the physiological motion (see Box 19.1).

### Metacarpophalangeal Joints of Digits 2 through 5

***Characteristics.*** The metacarpophalangeal (MCP) joints are biaxial condyloid joints. Each joint is supported by a volar and two collateral ligaments. The collaterals become taut in full flexion and prevent abduction and adduction in this position.

*Arthrokinematics.* The distal end of each metacarpal is convex and the proximal phalanx concave. The proximal surface of the proximal phalanx rolls and slides in the same direction as the physiological motion (see Box 19.1).

### Interphalangeal Joints and MCP Joint of the Thumb

*Characteristics.* There is a proximal (PIP) and distal (DIP) interphalangeal joint for each digit, 2 through 5. The thumb has only one interphalangeal joint, although the MCP joint of the thumb is uniaxial and therefore functions similarly to the IP joints. The MCP joint of the thumb differs in that it is reinforced by two sesamoid bones on the volar surface, which improve the leverage of the flexor pollicis brevis muscle. Each of these joints is a uniaxial hinge joint.

The capsule of each joint is reinforced with collateral ligaments, which are taut in extension. Going radial to ulnar in digits 2 through 5, there is increasing flexion/extension range in the joints. This allows for greater opposition of the ulnar fingers to the thumb and also causes a potentially tighter grip on the ulnar side of the hand.

*Arthrokinematics.* The articulating surface at the distal end of each phalanx is convex; the articulating surface at the proximal end of each phalanx is concave. Therefore, the proximal surface of each phalanx rolls and slides in the same direction as the physiological motion (see Box 19.1).

## ● HAND FUNCTION

### Muscles of the Wrist and Hand

The complex function of the hand occurs as a result of an intricate balance and control of forces between the extrinsic and intrinsic muscles of the wrist and hand. The muscles are depicted in Figure 19.2.

### Length–Tension Relationships

The position of the wrist controls the length of the extrinsic muscles of the digits. As the fingers or thumb flex, the wrist must be stabilized by the wrist extensor muscles to prevent the flexor digitorum profundus and flexor digitorum superficialis or the flexor pollicis longus from simultaneously flexing the wrist. As the grip becomes stronger, synchronous wrist extension lengthens the extrinsic flexor tendons across the wrist and maintains a more favorable overall length of the musculotendinous unit for a stronger contraction.

For strong finger or thumb extension, the wrist flexor muscles stabilize or flex the wrist so the extensor digitorum communis, extensor indicis, extensor digiti minimi, or extensor pollicis longus muscles can function more efficiently. In addition, there is ulnar deviation; the flexor and extensor carpi ulnaris muscles are both active as the hand opens.[69]

### Extensor Mechanism

Structurally, the extensor hood (extensor expansion) is made up of the extensor digitorum communis tendon, its connective tissue expansion, and fibers from the tendons of the dorsal and volar interossei and lumbricales (Fig. 19.3).[5] Each structure that is a part of the hood has an effect on the extensor mechanism.

● An isolated contraction of the extensor digitorum produces clawing of the fingers (MCP hyperextension with IP flexion from passive pull of the extrinsic flexor tendons, also called the hook position).

● PIP and DIP extension occurs concurrently and can be caused by the interossei or lumbrical muscles through their pull on the extensor hood.

● There must be tension in the extensor digitorum communis tendon for there to be interphalangeal extension. This occurs either by active contraction of the muscle, causing MCP extension concurrently as the intrinsic muscles contract, or by stretch of the tendon, which occurs with MCP flexion.

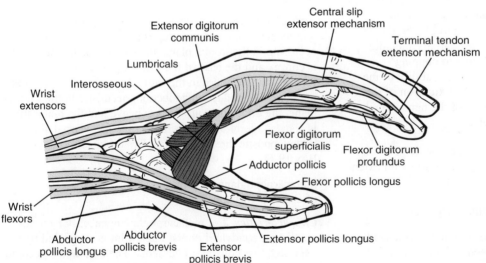

FIGURE 19.2 The extrinsic and intrinsic muscles of the wrist and hand create a balance of forces that affect hand function.

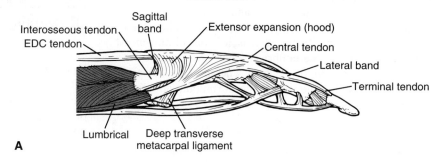

**Lateral view**

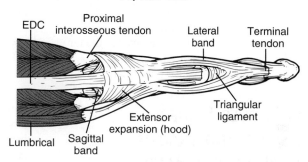

**Superior view**

**FIGURE 19.3** Anatomical structures of the extensor mechanism: (*A*) lateral view and (*B*) dorsal view. See text for description of functional relationships.

### Control of the Unloaded (Free) Hand

Anatomical factors, muscular contraction, and viscoelastic properties of the muscles influence finger motion.[5,69]

- When only the extrinsic muscles contract, clawing motions occur in the digits.
- Closing motions can occur only with extrinsic muscle contractions but also require the viscoelastic force of the biarticular interossei.
- Opening motions require synergistic contraction of the extrinsic extensor and the lumbrical muscles.
- Reciprocal motion of MCP flexion and IP extension is caused by the interossei. The lumbrical removes the viscoelastic tension from the profundus tendon and assists IP extension.

## Grips and Prehension Patterns

The nature of the intended activity dictates the type of grip used.[5,68,69,82]

### Power Grips

***Description.*** Power grips involve clamping an object with partially flexed fingers against the palm of the hand and with counter pressure from the adducted thumb. Power grips are primarily isometric functions. The fingers are flexed, laterally rotated, and ulnarly deviated. The amount of flexion varies with the object held. The thumb reinforces the fingers and helps make small adjustments to control the direction of the force.

Varieties include cylindrical grip, spherical grip, hook grip, and lateral prehension.

***Muscle control.*** The muscles primarily function with isometric contractions[5,108]

- Extrinsic finger flexors provide the major gripping force.
- The extensor digitorum provides a compressive force to the MCP joints, which increases stability and also provides a balancing force for the flexors.
- Interossei rotate the first phalanx for positioning to compress the external object and also flex the MCP joint.
- Lumbricales do not participate in the power grip (except the fourth).
- The thenar muscles and adductor pollicis provide compressive forces against the object being gripped.

### Precision Patterns

***Description.*** Prehension patterns involve manipulating an object that is not in contact with the palm of the hand between the opposing abducted thumb and fingers. The muscles primarily function isotonically. The sensory surfaces of the digits are used for maximum sensory input to influence delicate adjustments. With small objects, precise handling occurs primarily between the thumb and index finger. Varieties include pad-to-pad, tip-to-tip, and pad-to-side prehension.

***Muscle control.*** The primary dynamic function of the muscles includes the following.[5,108]

● Extrinsic muscles provide the compressive force to hold the objects between the fingers and thumb.

● For manipulation of an object, the interossei abduct and adduct the fingers, the thenar muscles control movement of the thumb, and the lumbricales help move the object away from the palm of the hand. The amount of participation of each muscle varies with the amount and direction of motion.

### Combined Grips

*Description.* Combined grips involve digits 1 and 2 (and sometimes 3) performing precision activities, whereas digits 3 through 5 supplement with power.

*Pinch.* Pinch requires holding an object between the thumb and index or middle finger, as in precision handling, but may require primarily an isometric hold. Compression between the thumb and fingers is provided by the thenar eminence muscles, the adductor pollicis, the interossei, and extrinsic flexors. The lumbricales also participate.[5]

## MAJOR NERVES SUBJECT TO PRESSURE AND TRAUMA AT THE WRIST AND HAND

For a detailed description of peripheral nerve injuries and entrapments in the wrist and hand region, as well as complex regional pain syndromes (including reflex sympathetic dystrophy) and their management, see Chapter 13.

### Nerve Disorders in the Wrist

*Median nerve.* The most common site for compression of the median nerve is the carpal tunnel.

*Ulnar nerve.* The most common site for compression of the ulnar nerve is in the ulnar tunnel (Guyon's canal).

### Referred Pain and Sensory Patterns

The hand is the terminal point for the C6, C7, and C8 nerve roots coursing through the median, ulnar, and radial nerves (see Figs. 13.5, 13.6, and 13.7). Injury or entrapment of these nerves may occur anywhere along their course, from the cervical spine to their termination. What the patient perceives as pain or a sensory disturbance in the hand may be from injury of the nerve anywhere along its course, or the pain may derive from irritation of tissue of common segmental origin such as the zygapophyseal facet joints of the spine. For treatment to be effective, it must be directed to the source of the problem, not to the site where the patient perceives the pain or sensory changes. Therefore, a thorough history is taken and examination of the entire upper quarter must be done, including the cervical spine when referred pain patterns or sensory changes are reported by the patient.[36,72]

## MANAGEMENT OF WRIST AND HAND DISORDERS AND SURGERIES

To make sound clinical decisions when treating patients with wrist and hand disorders, it is necessary to understand the various pathologies, surgical procedures, and associated precautions and to identify presenting impairments, functional limitations, and possible disabilities. In this section, common pathologies and surgeries are presented and are related to corresponding preferred practice patterns (groupings of impairments) described in the *Guide to Physical Therapist Practice*[2] (Table 19.1). Conservative and postoperative management of these conditions are also described in this section.

## JOINT HYPOMOBILITY: NONOPERATIVE MANAGEMENT

Pathologies such as rheumatoid arthritis (RA) and degenerative joint disease (DJD) affect the joints of the wrist and hand and may have a significant effect on the functional abilities of an individual as a result of pain, impaired mobility, and potential joint deformities. Impaired joint, tendon, and muscle mobility also occurs any time joints are immobilized due to fractures, trauma, or surgery. Chapter 11 describes the etiology and general guidelines for management of impairments due to these joint pathologies. This section focuses on specific interventions for the wrist and hand.

### Common Joint Pathologies and Associated Impairments

#### Rheumatoid Arthritis

The following is a summary of signs and symptoms and resulting impairments typically seen in the wrist and hand with RA.[3,13,74,83,90]

*Acute stage.* There is pain, swelling, warmth, and limited motion from synovial inflammation (synovitis) and tissue proliferation, most commonly in the MCP, PIP, and wrist joints bilaterally. There is also inflammation (tenosynovitis) and synovial proliferation in the extrinsic tendons and tendon sheaths. In addition:

● Progressive muscle weakness and imbalances in length and strength between agonists and antagonists and between intrinsic and extrinsic muscles occur.

● Carpal tunnel syndrome may occur in conjunction with tenosynovitis due to compression of the median nerve from the swollen tissue.

● General systemic as well as muscular fatigue occurs.

*Advanced stages.* Joint capsule weakening, cartilage destruction, bone erosion, and tendon rupture, as well as imbalances in musculotendinous forces, lead to joint instabilities, subluxations, and deformities (Fig. 19.4). Typical deformities and the pathomechanics in the hand include:

**TABLE 19.1  Wrist and Hand Pathologies/Surgical Procedures and Preferred Practice Patterns**

| PATHOLOGY/SURGICAL PROCEDURE | PREFERRED PRACTICE PATTERN AND ASSOCIATED IMPAIRMENTS[2] |
|---|---|
| • Arthritis (osteoarthritis, rheumatoid arthritis, post-traumatic arthritis)<br>• Synovitis<br>• Postimmobilization arthritis (stiffness)<br>• Tendon adhesions | Pattern 4D—Impaired joint mobility, motor function, muscle performance, and ROM associated with connective tissue dysfunction |
| • Acute arthritis<br>• Acute sprain, tendonitis | Pattern 4E—Impaired joint mobility, motor function, muscle performance, and ROM associated with localized inflammation |
| • Interposition arthroplasty (flexible silicone spacer, soft tissue implant)<br>• Total joint replacement arthroplasty | Pattern 4H—Impaired joint mobility, motor function, muscle performance, and ROM associated with joint arthroplasty |
| • Synovectomy and tenosynovectomy<br>• Repair, reconstruction, or transfer of a ruptured or lacerated tendon<br>• Soft tissue release (capsule, ligament, or tendon)<br>• Open reduction and internal fixation of a fracture or fracture-dislocation<br>• Bone resection (distal styloidectomy of the ulna, proximal row carpectomy)<br>• Arthrodesis | Pattern 4I—Impaired joint mobility, motor function, muscle performance, and ROM associated with bony or soft tissue surgery |
| • Carpal tunnel syndrome (median nerve)<br>• Tunnel of Guyon syndrome (ulnar nerve) | Pattern 5F—Impaired peripheral nerve integrity and muscle performance associated with peripheral nerve injury. |

- *Volar subluxation of the triquetrum on the articular disk and ulna.* The extensor carpi ulnaris tendon displaces volarly and causes a flexor force at the wrist joint.
- *Ulnar subluxation of the carpals.* This causes radial deviation of the wrist.
- *Ulnar drift of the fingers and volar subluxation of the proximal phalanx.* There is stretching or rupture of the collateral ligaments at the MCP joints and a bowstringing effect from the extrinsic tendons.[13]

- *Swan-neck deformity.* Laxity of the PIP joint with an overstretched palmar plate and bowstringing of the lateral bands of the extensor hood result in hyperextension of the PIP and flexion of the DIP joints (Fig. 19.5A). Tight or overactive interossei muscles pulling on the extensor tendon reinforces the hyperextension of the hypermobile PIP joints, and increased passive tension in the flexor digitorum produndus tendon causes flexion of the DIP joint.
- *Boutonnière deformity.* Rupture of the central band (central slip) of the extensor hood results in the lateral bands of the extensor apparatus (extensor hood) slipping in a volar direction to the PIP joint, causing PIP flexion and DIP extenison (Fig. 19.5B).

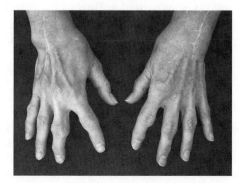

FIGURE 19.4 Joint deformities seen in the hand of a patient with rheumatoid arthritis. Note the hypertrophy of the IP joints, rheumatoid nodules, and volar subluxation of the triquetrum. This patient had fusion of the wrist joints due to pain and complete destruction of the joints, which has helped prevent the deforming bowstringing effect of the extrinsic tendons on the MCP joints. *(Courtesy of Turtle Services Limited, www.turtleserviceslimited.org/.)*

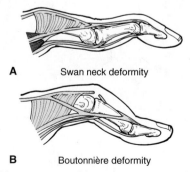

**A**    Swan neck deformity

**B**    Boutonnière deformity

FIGURE 19.5 (*A*) Swan-neck and (*B*) Boutonnière deformities. See text for description of the pathomechanics.

● *Zigzag deformity of the thumb.* Muscle imbalances and ligamentous laxity lead to metacarpal dislocation of the thumb and deformities similar to swan-neck or boutonnière deformity. Tightness in the adductor pollicis contributes to deformities in the thumb.[83]

### Osteoarthritis and Post-traumatic Arthritis

Age and repetitive joint trauma lead to degenerative cartilaginous and bony changes in susceptible joints. Osteoarthritis (OA) most commonly involves the trapezioscaphoid articulation, CMC joint of the thumb, and DIP joints of the digits, although the effects of trauma can occur in any joint.

Post-traumatic arthritis can develop in any joint of the wrist or hand as the result of a severe intra-articular fracture or fracture-dislocation. At the wrist, for example, deficiency of the scapholunate interosseus ligament, as the result of a severe wrist sprain, can alter joint alignment, which can cause articular degeneration over time. In the fingers, the PIP joint is a common site of articular fracture and subsequent joint degeneration.

The following is a summary of signs and symptoms and resulting impairments commonly seen in OA or post-traumatic arthritis.[123]

*Acute stage.* During the early stages of OA the symptoms include achiness and feelings of stiffness, which abate with movement. Following stressful activities or trauma, joint swelling, warmth, and restricted and painful motion occur.

*Advanced stages.* With degeneration there is capsular laxity resulting in hypermobility or instability; with progression, contractures and limited motion develop. Affected joints may become enlarged or sublux (Fig. 19.6). Limitation of both flexion and extension with a firm capsular end-feel develops in the affected joints. There is general muscle weakness, weak grip strength, and poor muscular endurance. Pain may also be a limiting factor in pinch and gripping activities.

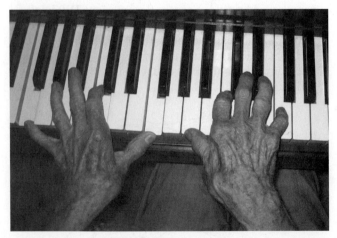

FIGURE 19.6 Advanced stages of osteoarthritis in the hands of an 86-year-old pianist. Note the carpometacarpal joint subluxation at the base of each thumb. Atrophy of the first dorsal interossei as well as nodules and joint enlargements are apparent, but the individual is still functional.

PRECAUTION: After trauma, the therapist must be alert to signs of a fracture in the wrist or hand because small bone fractures may not show on radiographs for up to 2 weeks. Signs include swelling, muscle spasm when passive motion is attempted, increased pain when the involved bone is stressed (e.g., deviation toward the involved bone), and tenderness on palpation over the fracture site.[36,77]

### Postimmobilization Hypomobility

Immobilization may be necessary following a fracture, surgery, or trauma; or it may be used to rest a part when an individual sustains repetitive stress. Impairments and functional limitations may occur from the lack of motion and muscle contraction, including:

● Decreased ROM and decreased joint play with firm end-feel and pain on overpressure.
● Tendon adhesions. This is a significant complication if there was any inflammation in a tendon or its sheath.
● Decreased muscle performance including muscle weakness, weak grip strength, decreased flexibility, and decreased muscle endurance.

## Common Functional Limitations/ Disabilities with Joint Pathologies

When joint pathology is acute, many prehension activities are painful, interfering with activities of daily living (ADL and IADL), such as dressing, eating, grooming, and toileting or almost any functional activity that requires gripping and fine-finger dexterity, including writing and typing.

Depending on which joints are involved, the amount of restricted movement and residual weakness, fatigue, or dexterity loss, and the type of grip or amount of precision handling required, functional loss may be minor or significant.

## Joint Hypomobility: Management— Protection Phase

General guidelines for managing acute joint lesions are described in Chapter 11, with special concerns for patients with RA and OA summarized in Boxes 11.2 and 11.4, respectively.

### Control Pain and Protect Joints

*Patient education.* Teach the patient how to protect involved joints and control pain with activity modification, ROM exercises, and appropriate use of a splint.

*Pain management.* In addition to physician-prescribed medications or nonsteroidal anti-inflammatories and modalities, gentle grade I or II distraction and oscillation techniques may inhibit pain and move synovial fluid for nutrition in the involved joints.

*Splinting.* Use a splint to rest and protect the involved joints. Instruct the patient to remove the splint for brief periods of nonstressful motion throughout the day.

## BOX 19.2   Joint Protection in the Wrist and Hand

*Purpose.* Performance of daily activities with minimal pain, stress to joints, and energy expenditure. Most of these principles are applicable to any arthritic problem in the hand but are especially important in the hand affected by rheumatoid arthritis.[90,91]

*Respect pain.* Monitor activities; stop when fatigue or discomfort begins to develop. Modify or discontinue any activity or exercise that causes pain that lasts longer than 1 hour after stopping the activity.

*Maintain strength and ROM.* Integrate exercises into daily activities.

- Look for early signs of muscle tightness in the intrinsic muscles. If tight, initiate stretching. One cause of swanneck deformity is tight interossei muscles pulling on the extensor tendon, leading to hyperextension of hypermobile PIP joints.
- Strengthen radial deviation of the MP joints of the fingers to counter the ulnar drifting of the fingers that occur in many functional activities.

*Balance activity level and rest.* More rest than normal is required during the active phases of the disease of RA.

Conserve energy and perform activities in the most economic way or do the most important activities first.

*Avoid deforming positions or one position for prolonged periods.*

*Avoid using strong grasping activities that facilitate the deforming force.* Typical joint deformities with RA include radial deviation and extension of the wrist and ulnar deviation and volar subluxation of the MP joints. Adaptive suggestions include:

- Open jars with the left hand or with an assistive device.
- Cut food with the blade of the knife protruding from the ulnar side of the hand.
- Stir food with spoon on the ulnar side of the hand.
- Build up the handles of eating utensils.
- Use stronger, larger joints whenever feasible. For example, carry items in a shoulder bag or over the forearm or with two hands rather than with one hand.
- Avoid twisting or wringing motions with the fingers. Press water out of a rag by opposing the palms of both hands together.

*Activity modification.* Analyze the patient's daily activities and recommend adaptations or assistive devices to minimize repetitive or excessive stresses on the joints. This is particularly important for patients with chronic arthritic disorders to prevent repetitive trauma and to minimize joint-deforming forces. Examples are summarized in Box 19.2.

### Maintain Joint and Tendon Mobility and Muscle Integrity

*Passive, assistive, or active ROM.* It is important to move the joints as tolerated because immobility of the hand quickly leads to muscle imbalance and contracture formation or further articular deterioration. Aquatic therapy is an effective method of combining nonstressful, non-weight-bearing exercises with therapeutic heat.

*Tendon-gliding exercises.* Have the patient perform full motion in the uninvolved joints and as much motion as possible in the involved joints to prevent adhesions between the long tendons or between the tendons and their synovial sheaths.[50] Tendon-gliding exercises are described in the exercise section of this chapter.

*Multiple-angle muscle setting exercises.* Do gentle isometrics to all wrist and hand musculature. Resistive ROM exercises are usually not tolerated if there is joint effusion or inflammation; therefore isometric resistance within the tolerance of pain, is performed.

### Joint Hypomobility: Management—Controlled Motion and Return to Function Phases

With joint pathology, increase ROM by utilizing joint mobilization techniques to stretch the capsule[93] as well

as passive stretching and muscle inhibition techniques to elongate the periarticular connective tissue and musculotendinous units following the principles described in Chapters 4 and 5. It is also critical to determine if scar tissue has formed in the long tendon sheaths in the hand, and, if so, attempt to re-establish smooth tendon gliding. Tendon gliding techniques are described in the Exercise Intervention section of this chapter.

### Increase Joint Play and Accessory Motions

*Joint mobilization techniques.* Determine which of the articulations of the distal RU, wrist, hand, or digits are restricted because of decreased joint play, and apply grade III sustained or grade IV oscillation techniques to stretch the capsules. See Figures 5.33 through 5.43 for mobilizing restricted joints of the distal forearm, wrist, hand, and digits.

PRECAUTIONS: For patients with RA, modify the intensity of joint mobilization and stretching techniques that are used to counter any restrictions. This is necessary because the disease process and steroid therapy weaken the tensile quality of the connective tissue, and consequently they are more easily torn.

*Unlock a subluxated ulnomeniscal-triquetral joint.* The mechanism of the dysfunction is not clear, but some patients describe locking in the wrist and an inability to supinate the forearm. The meniscus may be displaced and be the cause of the blocked motion. The following techniques may free up the motion.

- Apply a volar glide to the ulna on a stabilized triquetrum (similar to Fig. 5.38).

● *Self-mobilization.* Have the patient grasp the distal ulna with the fingers of the opposite hand, place the thumb on the palmar surface of the triquetrum just medial to the pisiform, and then press with the thumb, causing a dorsal glide of the triquetrum on the radioulnar disk and ulna (Fig. 19.7).

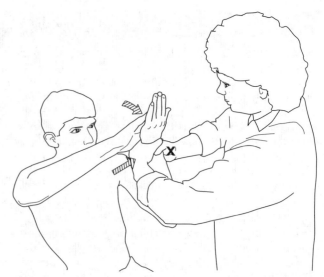

FIGURE 19.8 Mobilization with movement (MWM) to increase wrist flexion or extension. Apply a lateral glide while the patient actively flexes or extends the wrist and then applies a passive stretch force with the other hand at the end of the range.

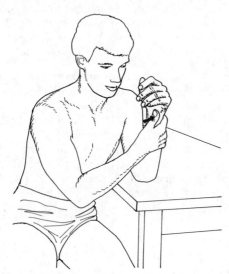

FIGURE 19.7 Self-mobilization of the ulnomeniscal-triquetral (UMI) joint.

### Improve Joint Tracking and Pain-Free Motion

Mobilization with movement (MWM) techniques may be applied to increase ROM and/or decrease the pain associated with movement.[78] (The principles of MWM are described in Chapter 5.)

*MWM of the wrist.* Have the patient seated with the elbow flexed and forearm supinated (patient's palm facing towards his or her face); stabilize the distal radius with your hand placed around the lateral aspect of the forearm. Apply a pain-free lateral glide to the proximal row of carpals utilizing the web space of your other hand. Have the patient then perform active wrist extension or flexion to the end of the available range, and with his or her free hand apply a passive stretch at the end of the range (Fig. 19.8).

An internal or external rotation of the carpals relative to the radius may need to be combined with the glide to achieve pain-free, end-range loading.

The intercarpal joint may require specific anterior-posterior gliding of one proximal row of carpals relative to its distal row neighbor combined with active physiologic motion to the end of the range. The mobilization and movement are pain-free. While holding the mobilization force, ask the patient to do repetitive gripping activities or resisted wrist motions.

*MWM of the MCP and IP joints of the digits.* Medially or laterally glide the involved phalanx in a painless direction, then have the patient actively flex or extend the finger and apply a pain-free, end-range stretch. Internal or external rotation of the more distal phalanx may be required in conjunction with the medial or lateral glide to achieve painless end-range overpressure.[78]

### Improve Mobility, Strength, and Function

Carefully examine the multijoint and intrinsic muscles for restricted motion due to contractures or adhesions and poor movement patterns due to weakness or imbalances in strength. Stretching, tendon gliding, and strengthening exercises are described in the exercise sections of this chapter. Utilize techniques that specifically address the impairments the patient has. Once range is gained, it is critical that the patient uses the new range with active ROM and functional activities.

*Neuromuscular control and strength.* Progress exercises with controlled and nondestructive forces to increase strength and muscle balance between antagonists and progress endurance training. With pathological joints, use caution when applying weights so as not to stress the joints beyond the capability of the stabilizing tissues.

*Functional activities.* Develop exercises that prepare the patient for functional activities. Consider prehension patterns that are required for the patient's job, recreational, and daily activities. Include exercises that require coordination and fine finger dexterity.

*Conditioning exercises.* Initiate physical conditioning exercises using activities that do not provoke joint symptoms, such as aquatic exercises or cycling.

*Joint protection.* Reinforce use of joint protection techniques as summarized in Box 19.2.

## Focus on Evidence

In a systematic literature review of randomized, controlled trials of adult patients with RA, the reviewers concluded that there is evidence to support the idea that low-intensity therapeutic exercise is beneficial for reducing pain and improving functional status (including hand grip strength) in patients with RA, whereas high-intensity exercise programs may exacerbate symptoms.[87]

# JOINT SURGERY AND POSTOPERATIVE MANAGEMENT

Long-standing RA, OA, or post-traumatic arthritis that affects the joints and soft tissues of the wrist and hand can lead to chronic pain, instability and deformity of joints, restricted ROM, loss of strength in the hand, and impaired function of the upper extremity. When nonoperative management is not sufficient, surgical intervention coupled with individually designed and carefully supervised postoperative rehabilitation is indicated to improve and restore function.

Some of the more common surgical options for management of arthritis are listed in Box 19.3. Refer to Table 19.1 to see the groupings of impairments typically associated with each of these surgeries.

Soft tissue procedures, such as synovectomy, tenosynovectomy for chronic tenosynovitis of the extensor and flexor tendons of the wrist, repair of ruptured tendons, capsulotomy or release of other soft tissues for correcting

---

**BOX 19.3  Surgical Intervention for RA or DJD of the Wrist and Hand**

**Soft Tissue Procedures**
- Synovectomy
- Tenosynovectomy
- Tendon repair, graft, or transfer/realignment
- Nerve decompression
- Capsuloligamentous reconstruction
- Contracture release
  - Capsulectomy/capsulotomy
  - Tendon release
- Soft tissue arthroplasty

**Joint and Bony Procedures**
- Excision/resection arthroplasty
  - Styloidectomy
  - Proximal row carpectomy
- Tendon interposition/trapezial resection arthroplasty
- Interposition, flexible implant arthroplasty
- Total joint arthroplasty
- Arthrodesis

---

a deformity, or muscle balancing of the wrist or finger joints are employed independently or concomitantly when articular surfaces of the involved joints remain reasonably intact.[16,20,37,50,132,133] If joint deterioration is significant, resection arthroplasty, such as resection of the distal ulna (Darrach procedure) or proximal row carpectomy, arthrodesis, or implant arthroplasty, performed in conjunction with soft tissue repair or reconstruction, are surgical options for advanced joint deterioration.[12,16,20]

Some procedures are selected to relieve pain and others to minimize or delay further deformity. For example, if medical management of RA of the wrist does not adequately control synovitis, tenosynovectomy is performed to remove proliferated synovium from tendon sheaths and prevent erosion or rupture of tendons before significant deformity and loss of active control of the wrist and fingers occur.[132] If rupture occurs, tendon repairs and transfers can improve function of the hand and delay or prevent subluxation and dislocation of joints or fixed deformities.[50,51]

Partial or complete arthrodesis of the wrist or arthrodesis of an individual joint of a digit, such as the CMC joint of the thumb, are procedures that yield predictable and durable results. Fusion corrects deformity and gives the patient stability and relief of pain with only some compromise of function despite the loss of joint motion.[49,50,80] If fusion is inappropriate and pain-free functional mobility is necessary, implant arthroplasty, either interposition arthroplasty or total joint replacement, are possible options. In many instances, a combination of joint and soft tissue procedures is indicated.[10,11,16,30] For the most part, however, arthroplasty is reserved for the patient who requires only low-demand use of the hand.

The goals of surgery and postoperative management of advanced arthritis and associated deformities of the wrist and hand include[10,16,57,95,121] (1) relief of pain, (2) restoration of normal or sufficient function of the wrist and hand, (3) correction of instability or deformity, (4) restoration of ROM, and (5) improved strength of the wrist and fingers for functional grasp and pinch.

A discussion of several types of arthroplasty and general guidelines for postoperative management follow. Information on surgical management and postoperative rehabilitation of tendon repairs and transfers associated with RA is then outlined. Given the complexity of hand rehabilitation, suggested phase-specific guidelines for exercise, founded on principles of tissue healing, must be individualized for each patient and determined by the patient's level of participation in the rehabilitation process and response to exercise.

Successful outcomes are contingent upon close communication among the surgeon, therapist, and patient or patient's family. An effective postoperative rehabilitation program combines early, supervised therapy with patient education and progresses to long-term self-management by the patient. Although rehabilitation is deemed essential after each of the surgical interventions covered in this section, postoperative protocols vary and have not been compared for each type of procedure, making it difficult to suggest that there is one best approach to postoperative management.

## Wrist Arthroplasty

Although arthrodesis of the wrist continues to be the most common surgical intervention for late-stage RA of the wrist, arthroplasty has become an acceptable alternative, particularly for patients with arthritis and impaired mobility of other joints of the extremities. Although wrist arthrodesis has not been shown to limit upper extremity function in daily living activities in patients with post-traumatic arthritis of the wrist but without arthritis of other upper extremity joints, it is thought that loss of wrist motion may adversely affect functions such as personal care in patients with RA who also have impaired mobility of other upper extremity joints.[131] For these patients, wrist arthroplasty—total joint replacement or flexible implant (interposition) arthroplasty—is an option that provides relief of symptoms while retaining some wrist mobility.

### Indications for Surgery

The following are common indications for arthroplasty of the wrist.[10,12,16,95,119]

- Severe pain in the wrist region as the result of deterioration of the articular surfaces of the distal radius, carpals, and distal ulna from chronic arthritis (usually RA, but also OA and post-traumatic arthritis) that compromises hand and upper extremity function.
- Deformity and marked limitation of the wrist that causes muscle-tendon imbalances of the digits.
- Subluxation or dislocation of the radiocarpal joint.
- Appropriate for *low-demand* upper extremity functional needs.
- Appropriate for patients with bilateral wrist involvement where arthrodesis of both wrists would limit rather than improve overall function.
- Also appropriate for patients with significant stiffness of the ipsilateral shoulder, elbow, or finger joints in whom unilateral arthrodesis of the wrist would further limit rather than improve functional use of the upper extremity.

Box 19.4 identifies some absolute and relative contraindications to wrist arthroplasty and arthroplasty of the joints of the fingers and thumb.[10–12,16]

### Procedures

***Implant designs, materials, and fixation.*** Because partial or total arthrodesis of the wrist is often considered the procedure of choice (not just a salvage procedure) for patients with severe pain and instability of the wrist[49,80] and because resection arthroplasty of the distal radius and proximal row carpectomy[37] are also suitable options that relieve pain but retain some mobility of the wrist, the use of joint replacement surgery for patients with late-stage arthritis of the wrist has been somewhat limited.[20] Never-

---

**BOX 19.4    Contraindications to Arthroplasty of the Wrist or Digits**

**Absolute**
- Active infection
- Expected high-demand use of the hand (e.g., manual labor) or high-impact sport activities (e.g., tennis and volleyball)
- Inadequate motor control of the wrist or hand as the result of neurological damage
- Rupture of the radial wrist extensors
- Limited ROM without pain

**Relative**
- Severe and irreparable deformity of the wrist or digits
- Rupture of multiple extensor tendons of the digits
- Inadequate, poor quality bone stock
- Need for ambulation aids (e.g., crutches or a walker) that place significant forces across the wrist and hand
- Compromised immune system

---

theless, designs of implants and operative techniques for arthroplasty of the wrist have gradually evolved.

During the late 1960s, Swanson first used a one-piece, uncemented, double-stemmed, flexible ("hinged") implant made of silicone for the radiocarpal joint, primarily for use in patients with RA.[119,122] The prosthesis, which is inserted between the distal radius, through the capitate, and into the intramedullary canal of the third metacarpal (after a proximal row carpectomy), is designed to act as a *dynamic spacer* to maintain joint alignment during healing. Over time the implant becomes encapsulated, forming a new fibrous capsule.[12,119,122] Although the procedure provides pain relief and some degree of stability and ROM (approximately a 60° arc of flexion/extension and a total of 10° of radial and ulnar deviation), its use has been associated with a high rate of failure as the result of excessive wear of the prosthesis or cystic changes in bone and eventual fracture or loosening of the prosthesis.[10–12,16] It has also been suggested that as a silicone implant gradually wears (abrades), and it may give rise to *particulate synovitis* (silicone synovitis).[58] Design changes have been made to reinforce the silicone implant with bone-shielding devices (titanium grommets) to improve the long-term durability of the prosthesis.[10,12,119] Development of flexible materials as alternatives to silicone is also being investigated.[119] Despite improvements, with the increased use of rigid implants for wrist arthroplasty, flexible interposition implant arthroplasty now plays a limited role, with its use reserved for the low-demand, older (> 60 years) patient with RA.[16]

Numerous designs of total wrist replacement arthroplasty (Fig. 19.9) have been developed and consistently refined over the past few decades, making arthroplasty available not only to patients with late-stage joint disease but also those with severe deformity and collapse of the wrist joint.[10,11,76] Total wrist arthroplasty typically involves inserting a two-piece system with elliptical (convex-

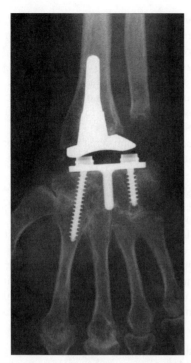

FIGURE 19.9 Total wrist arthroplasty. *(From Wadsworth C, Steyers C, Adams B: Postoperative Management of the Wrist and Hand. Independent Study Course 15.2. Postoperative Management of Orthopedic Surgeries. Orthopedic Section, APTA, La Crosse, WI, 2005:25, with permission.)*

concave) surfaces that are loosely constrained or non-constrained. Components are made of rigid materials (cobalt-chrome or titanium and high-density polyethylene). The implants are sometimes porous-coated along the stems for bio-ingrowth,[96] and a combination of cement and screws is employed for additional fixation.[10,12,16] Most total wrist systems are designed to allow a combined 90° arc of flexion and extension.

***Operative procedures.*** Total wrist arthroplasty requires a longitudinal incision along the dorsal aspect of the wrist in line with the third metacarpal.[10–12,16] Concomitant *dorsal clearance* (synovectomy of the wrist and tenosynovectomy of the extensor tendons) is often necessary. The retinaculum is incised and reflected, and the digital extensor tendons are retracted for access to the joint capsule.

The distal portions of the radius and ulna, some of the carpals, and a small portion of the proximal aspect of the third and often the second and fourth metacarpals are resected. The rigid, stemmed prosthetic components are then tightly fit into the reamed intramedullary canals of the necessary metacarpals and the distal radius.[10,11,50] In patients with instability and subluxation of the radiocarpal joint, capsule and ligament reconstruction is typically performed to improve wrist stability. Soft tissue balancing is critical for satisfactory results.

After closure of the dorsal incision, the hand is placed in a long-arm or short-arm bulky compression dressing and elevated several days postoperatively to control edema.

## Postoperative Management

### Immobilization
After total wrist replacement, the wrist is continuously immobilized in a neutral position for several days to 2 weeks. After the bulky, postoperative dressing is removed, the wrist and forearm are placed in a short-arm volar wrist splint with the wrist positioned in about 10° to 15° extension. The splint allows full finger ROM and opposition of the thumb. The timeframe for removal of the splint for exercise varies from 1 to 4 weeks, depending on the extent of soft tissue reconstruction and bone stock qualtiy.[11,16,70,96]

If a concomitant repair of the extensor tendons was performed, the immobilizer is fitted with outriggers that have elastic slings to hold the fingers in extension. Even after wrist exercises are initiated, the immobilizer is worn for protection between exercise sessions. A static resting splint is worn at night for 6 to 8 weeks postoperatively.[51]

Generally, flexible implant arthroplasty requires a longer period of immobilization than total wrist replacement, with a duration as short as 3 to 4 weeks or as long as 6 to 8 weeks, to allow time for encapsulation of the prosthetic spacer to occur.[48,119]

### Exercise
As with arthroplasty of other large or small joints, the goals and progression of exercise during each successive phase of rehabilitation after wrist arthroplasty (both total wrist or interposition arthroplasties) are based on the stages of soft tissue healing. The stability of the wrist always takes precedence over restoration of wrist mobility. If concomitant extensor tendon repairs were also done, the guidelines and timeframe for exercise are adjusted and special precautions are taken, as discussed in a later section of the chapter on repair of extensor tendon ruptures in RA.

For protection of the wrist after arthroplasty, precautions, identified in Box 19.5, must be incorporated into postoperative exercises and functional activities during and after rehabilitation.[70,118]

### Exercise: Maximum and Moderate Protection Phases
The focus of rehabilitation during the maximum protection phase is to control pain and peripheral edema, protect the

---

**BOX 19.5** **Precautions After Wrist Arthroplasty**

- Avoid weight bearing on the operated hand during transfers, ambulation with assistive devices, or other daily living activities.
- If ambulation aids are required because of lower extremity joint involvement, use forearm-support crutches or walker.
- Avoid functional activities that place more than 5- to 10-lb loads on the wrist.
- Wear a wrist splint for additional protection during functional activities.
- Permanently refrain from high-impact vocational or recreational activities, such as heavy labor or racquet sports.

wrist, and prevent stiffness of the rest of the upper extremity. When the immobilizer can be removed for wrist exercises, protection of the wrist is still essential.

The emphasis during the moderate protection (controlled motion) phase, which typically begins about 4 to 8 weeks postoperatively, is to gradually restore active control and mobility of the digits, wrist, and forearm motion without jeopardizing wrist stability.[11,48,57,70,119]

◉ *Maintain and later improve mobility of unoperated joints.*
- Begin active ROM exercises of the digits, elbow, and shoulder while the wrist is immobilized and the use of the hand is restricted.
- Around 6 weeks postoperatively, if there was limitation of finger mobility preoperatively, selectively use low-load, dynamic finger splint(s) during the day or gentle passive stretching *initially with the wrist maintained in a neutral position* to increase mobility for a sufficient level of hand function.
- Grade II and possibly grade III joint mobilizations are appropriate if the joints of the digits are not inflamed.

◉ *Restore control and mobility of the wrist.*
- Include active ROM, emphasizing wrist extension more than flexion, and tendon-gliding exercises with the wrist in neutral (see Fig. 19.17A–E).

P R E C A U T I O N S : Postpone radial and ulnar deviation if wrist stability is questionable.[57] When performing radial and ulnar deviation, avoid wrist flexion with ulnar deviation (the position of wrist deformity).

◉ *Regain use of wrist, finger, and thumb musculature.*
- Start with gentle setting exercises and progress to low-intensity, isometric resistance exercises of the wrist and finger musculature.
- After total wrist arthroplasty, begin to use the hand for light (minimum-load) functional activities around 6 to 8 weeks.[96]
- After flexible implant arthroplasty, this may be delayed until about 12 weeks postoperatively.[119]

### Exercise: Minimum Protection/ Return to Function Phase

During the minimum protection phase, which usually does not begin until 8 to 12 weeks postoperatively, regaining sufficient strength and muscular endurance of the entire upper extremity for appropriate functional activities is the priority.[70] In the wrist, emphasize strengthening the wrist extensors more so than the wrist flexors. Patient education focuses on incorporating joint protection during functional activities (refer to Box 19.2). Use of a cock-up resting splint is advisable at night, particularly if a wrist flexion contracture persists. Although 15° of wrist extension is preferable for a strong functional grasp, the use of manual stretching procedures to increase wrist extension is not consistently advocated so as not to compromise wrist stability.[119]

◉ *Regain functional strength of the hand and wrist.*
- Transition to low-intensity dynamic resistance (about 1 lb) exercises of the hand and wrist.[70]
- Emphasize simulated functional movement patterns, such as various types of grasping activities, being certain to reinforce principles of joint protection.[91] If not previously initiated, begin to use the hand for light functional activities.
- By 12 weeks after total wrist arthroplasty or flexible implant arthroplasty, the patient may use the hand for most low-load functional activities.[48,96]

◉ *Increase ROM of the wrist to a functional level.*
- Continue active ROM and gentle stretching exercises as dictated by the stability of the wrist.
- Use low-load dynamic splinting of the wrist, emphasizing wrist extension to at least 15°.
- In patients who exhibit significant postoperative stiffness of the wrist soon after surgery, stretching activities may be initiated earlier than during the minimum protection phase, possibly at 6 weeks postoperatively.[48]

### Outcomes

A successful outcome after wrist arthroplasty gives the patient a stable, pain-free wrist with functional ROM. Postoperative outcomes typically measured are pain relief, use of the hand for functional activities, wrist and forearm ROM, and grip strength. Instruments, such as the Disabilities of the Arm, Shoulder and Hand (DASH) questionnaire and the Patient-Rated Wrist Evaluation, are used to assess pain, function, and satisfaction.[79]

*Pain relief.* Barring complications, short- and long-term relief of pain after flexible implant arthroplasty[61,112,119] and total wrist arthroplasty[10,11,16] is a consistent finding. For example, in a retrospective study that followed 14 patients (12 with RA) with arthritis of the wrist, who underwent 17 primary semiconstrained total wrist replacements, preoperatively 88% of wrists (15/17) were ranked as being moderately to severely painful. Postoperatively, all wrists were less painful, with 15 ranked as pain-free and 2 mildly painful.[96] Another author indicated that about 75% of patients experience complete pain relief after total wrist arthroplasty.[16]

In a long-term study, patients with RA who underwent Swanson silicone wrist arthroplasty were followed for a minimum of 10 years (mean follow-up 15 years) and reported "good" or "very good" outcomes, primarily due to adequate pain relief.[61]

*Wrist and forearm ROM, strength, and function*. Improvement in ROM is less predictable than pain relief. ROM of the wrist achieved postoperatively is usually about 15° to 30° each of wrist flexion and extension, 5° to 10° each of radial and ulnar deviation, and at least a 100° arc of pronation and supination.[11,119] A functional level of active wrist ROM appears to be retained over an extended number of years. For example, 10 years or more after implantation of the Swanson silicone prosthesis, a group of patients (all with RA) in a follow-up study had 28°

flexion and 15° extension (i.e., a total flexion/extension arc of 43°).[61]

In studies comparing pre- and postoperative results of newer designs of total wrist arthroplasty, the postoperative ROM reported was even greater for most motions.[40,79,96] However, actual *improvements* in ROM after arthroplasty have[40] and have not[96] been statistically significant. As a point of interest, the results of biomechanical studies of normal individuals performing a variety of functional activities have indicated that no more than 35° each of wrist flexion and extension was used.[88,98]

Grip strength[96] and use of the operated hand for functional activities[40,79] routinely improve after wrist arthroplasty. Relief of pain has an obvious impact on hand function. Concomitant soft tissue repair, such as repair of ruptured tendons, also contribute to improved function. Furthermore, arthroplasty provides some additional length to the wrist, which in turn improves the length–tension relationship of the muscle-tendon units that cross the wrist.[10]

*Complications.* Complications rates have always been higher for wrist arthroplasty, particularly the early designs, than replacement arthroplasty of larger joints, such as the shoulder, hip, and knee.[11,12] One author has suggested that one in five wrist arthroplasties require revision within 5 years.[10] After flexible implant arthroplasty, prosthetic fracture rates 5 to 10 years postoperatively have been reported at 20%[50] and 22%.[110] Loosening of the distal component and dislocation are frequently reported complications associated with total wrist arthroplasty,[10,16] particularly the early designs.[76] Early results of recent modifications to implant designs appear to be decreasing the rate of loosening.[16,40,79,96]

Complications may require an alternative procedure or revision arthroplasty. If a silicone implant arthroplasty fails, total wrist replacement is still possible; if a total wrist arthroplasty fails because of mechanical loosening or component failure, revision arthroplasty and wrist arthrodesis are still viable alternatives.[10,12,49,80]

## Metacarpophalangeal Implant Arthroplasty

Arthroplasty of the MCP joints of fingers (digits 2 to 5), combined with necessary reconstruction of soft tissues, is the most common surgical procedure performed to manage impaired function and progressive deformity as the result of late-stage RA of the hand.[29,30] However, arthroplasty is also an option for patients with idiopathic OA and post-traumatic arthritis of the MCP joints.[30,94] For MCP arthroplasty to be successful, a patient must have intact extensor digitorum communis tendons, or repair of these tendons must be performed. The two procedures may be staged, one prior to the other, or performed simultaneously as determined by the surgeon. Other procedures to balance soft tissues must also accompany MCP arthroplasty for improved hand function postoperatively.[30,73,115]

If joints other than the MCP joints are involved, which is often the case in patients with RA, surgeries are carefully

sequenced. For example, if the wrist is involved, a radiolunate or total wrist arthrodesis for pain-free wrist stability in a functional position may be necessary prior to MCP arthroplasty. In contrast, a swan-neck deformity of a finger is managed with PIP fusion in 30° to 40° of flexion, but typically it is done after, not before, MCP arthroplasty.[30,118]

The goals of this surgery and postoperative management are to relieve pain, correct alignment of the fingers, improve active hand opening and grasp, and improve the cosmetic appearance of the hand.[73,118]

### Indications for Surgery

The following are common indications for arthroplasty of the MCP joint(s).[12,30,73,95,115,121]

- Pain at the MCP joint(s) of the hand and diminished hand function as the result of deterioration of the articular surfaces, usually because of RA but sometimes as the result of OA or post-traumatic arthritis.
- Instability, often coupled with volar subluxation, and deformity (flexion and ulnar drift) of the MCP joint(s) that cannot be corrected with soft tissue releases and reconstruction alone.
- Stiffness and decreased active ROM of the MCP joints, often associated with a deficient extensor mechanism, causing inability to open the hand to grasp large objects.
- Poor appearance of the hand.

### Procedures

*Implant design, materials, and fixation.* MCP joint arthroplasty is designed to provide a balance of stability and mobility to the MCP joints for patients with late-stage arthritis. There are several designs using different materials and methods of fixation that have evolved over the past few decades. Swanson developed a one-piece, flexible, double-stemmed prosthesis made of silicone (Fig. 19.10)

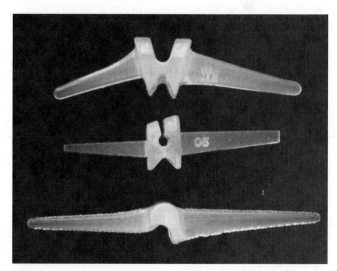

FIGURE 19.10 Lateral view of the three most common silicone-based implants: Neuflex (*top*), Avanta (*middle*), Swanson (*bottom*). Note that the Avanta and Swanson implants are of a 0° bend type. *(From Manuel, JLM, Weiss, A-PC: Silicone metacarpophalangeal joint arthroplasty. In Strickland JW, Graham, TJ [eds] Master Techniques in Orthopedic Surgery—The Hand, ed 2. Lippincott Williams & Wilkins, Philadelphia, 2005, p 393, with permission.)*

that is uncemented; it serves as a dynamic spacer and an internal joint mold as it becomes encapsulated during the healing process.[12,15,30,81,121] The implant maintains internal alignment of the joint during healing and allows early postoperative joint motion. As with radiocarpal flexible implants, the MCP silicone implant sometimes is reinforced with circumferential titanium grommets to minimize long-term component wear or fracture and the possibility of silicone synovitis.[121] Although the original Swanson implant has undergone some minor design changes, it has been a highly reliable design and remains the most widely used MCP implant for patients with RA.[30,115] The Swanson implant has also been used successfully in patients with OA[94] and post-traumatic arthritis.[30]

Other silicone implants have been developed as alternatives to the Swanson implant. One such design is the Neuflex implant (see Fig. 19.10), which is preformed in 30° of flexion to replicate the position of the MCP joints when the hand is at rest. The design is intended to improve ROM.[39,73]

Total MCP joint replacement, sometimes referred to as resurfacing arthroplasty, is an alternative to flexible implant arthroplasty.[30] Surface replacements typically are two-component, convex-concave designs made of either metal and high-density polyethylene or pyrolytic carbon with highly polished articular surfaces. The metal-plastic designs are usually cemented in place, but bio-ingrowth fixation is being investigated as an alternative. The pyrolytic carbon implants, because of the nature of the material, exclusively rely on bio-ingrowth fixation.[29,30]

Unlike the one-piece flexible implant designs, resurfacing replacements have little to no inherent stability and therefore must rely on intact or repairable collateral ligaments for joint stability. Consequently, MCP resurfacing arthroplasty is used less frequently in patients with RA—in whom there tends to be poor quality soft tissues as the result of long-standing inflammation and deformity, making it difficult to repair the collateral ligaments—than in patients with OA or post-traumatic arthritis, whose collateral ligaments are either intact or can be repaired. One resource suggests that a silicone implant is indicated if there is an extensor lag (lack of active extension) of the MCP joints > 60° and ulnar deviation > 45°.[30]

***Operative procedures.*** MCP arthroplasty and related soft tissue balancing involve the following procedures.[30,73,94,118,121] The involved MCP joints are approached by either a single, transverse incision over the dorsal aspect of the metacarpal heads or by double, longitudinal incisions made between the index and middle fingers and between the ring and little fingers. The joint capsule is exposed by carefully separating the extensor tendons, which are often ulnarly displaced, from the underlying capsule and longitudinally incising the extensor hood. The tendons are retracted; the ulnar and possibly the radial collateral ligaments, if intact, are reflected from the head of each metacarpal; and the dorsal aspect of the capsule is incised (capsulotomy). Every effort is made to preserve the radial collateral ligaments. A synovectomy is performed if necessary. If a sig-

nificant flexion contracture exists, the volar aspect of each capsule may also be incised to allow greater extension of the MCP joints.

The heads (distal aspect) of the metacarpals and proximal aspect of the first phalanges of the involved joints are excised, and the intramedullary canals of the metacarpals and proximal phalanges are widened to accept the prosthetic implants. After insertion of the implants, the ROM of the replaced joints is checked. The joint capsule, radial collateral ligament (if preserved), and extensor mechanism of each digit are repaired. The wound is then closed, and a bulky compression dressing and volar hand and forearm splint are placed on the hand. The hand is elevated to control edema.

### Postoperative Management

As with arthroplasty of the wrist or other joints of the digits, the postoperative rehabilitation program is founded on the principles of soft tissue healing and includes phase-specific goals and interventions, including the use of dynamic and/or static splinting and a supervised home exercise program.

General postoperative guidelines from a number of resources for a progression of exercises combined with the use of splints to maintain alignment and protect soft tissues as they heal are summarized in this section.[14,21,30,48,121,126] These guidelines must be individualized, based on the type of arthroplasty and soft tissue procedures performed and each patient's responses. Ongoing patient education and close communication with the surgeon are essential for effective outcomes. Postoperative rehabilitation continues for 3 to 6 months.

#### Immobilization

Initially, the wrist and hand are continuously immobilized in the bulky compression dressing and volar splint applied at the end of surgery, with the wrist positioned in neutral, the MCP joints in full extension and either neutral or slight radial deviation (opposite the position of deformity), and the distal joints (PIP and DIP) in slight flexion.[30,70,121] In some instances the splint extends only to the level of the PIP joints.[94] The bulky dressing is later replaced with a light compression dressing.

Continuous immobilization is not lengthy but varies with the type of arthroplasty, the type and quality of the soft tissue repairs, and the stability of the reconstructed joints. If only an MCP implant was performed, the hand remains immobilized for only a few days. If, in addition to the MCP arthroplasty, ruptured extensor tendons also were repaired or transferred, the hand remains immobilized longer to protect the tendons.[50,51]

***Dynamic splinting.*** When the compression dressing is removed, the hand is placed in a dynamic MCP extension splint with an outrigger (Fig. 19.11). The splint is worn to protect healing structures, maintain alignment (to prevent recurrent flexion and ulnar drift deformities at the MCP joints), and control and guide the range and plane of motion during exercises as soft tissues heal.[14,30,71,115,121,126,129]

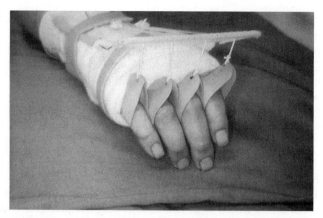

**FIGURE 19.11** A dynamic extension splint with rubber bands attached to a dorsal outrigger used after MCP arthroplasty permits active MCP flexion but at rest maintains the MCP joints in extension and sometimes slight radial deviation. *(Courtesy of Janet Bailey, OTR/L, CHT.)*

The dynamic splint holds the wrist in about 10° to 15° of extension and the MCP joints in full extension and slight radial deviation as well as supination of the index finger, but it does not control motion in the IP joints. Slings under the proximal phalanx of each finger with rubber bands attached to the outrigger of the splint hold the MCP joints in extension when the hand is at rest but still allow active flexion of the MCP joints within a functional range. The patient wears the dynamic splint throughout the day, including exercise sessions.

At 2 to 3 weeks, a dynamic MCP flexion splint may be indicated and worn intermittently or alternately during the day with the dynamic extension splint if sufficient MCP flexion has not yet been attained, particularly in digits 3, 4, and 5.[12,14,48,70,121,126,129] By 6 weeks, but sometimes as late as 12 weeks postoperatively, dynamic splinting is gradually discontinued unless an active extensor lag or a flexion or extension contracture of the MCP joints persists.[14,30,70,121,126,129]

***Static splinting.*** If a dynamic splint is worn during the day, at night the patient wears a volar static (resting splint), which holds the wrist in 15° of extension and the fingers in full or almost full extension. A block along the ulnar border of the splint prevents ulnar deviation of the fingers. If a flexion contracture or active extensor lag of the MCP joints is present, night splinting is often continued for 3 to 4 months or as long as a year.[12,14,70,118,126,129]

Although dynamic splinting is widely used after MCP arthroplasty, another option is the alternating use of two static splints, one that holds all of the finger joints in extension and another that holds the MCP joints in flexion and the PIP and DIP joints in almost full extension.[21] Each splint is worn for 24 hours at a time. During the day the splint is removed frequently for gentle assisted ROM exercises. Some clinicians suggest that static splints are as effective as dynamic splints and are easier and less expensive to fabricate and modify, easier for patients to apply, and less cumbersome to wear because there is no need for

the high-profile outrigger and rubber band suspension slings used in a dynamic splint.[21]

 **Focus on Evidence** _____

In a prospective study by Burr and colleagues[21] designed to investigate the effectiveness of the use of an alternating static splinting regimen combined with postoperative exercises as an alternative to dynamic splinting, 15 patients with RA who underwent 51 MCP silicone implant arthroplasties were followed for 19 months. The results indicated that there was a significant improvement in the mean total arc of active flexion/extension when the preoperative ROM of all MCP joints (27.6°) was compared to the postoperative ROM (47.2°) at 19 months. In addition, there was a significant improvement in the total arc of active MCP flexion/extension for each of the four fingers. The mean active MCP extension deficit also improved significantly from 50° before surgery to 18° postoperatively. The degree of ulnar deviation also improved, decreasing from 30.4° to 9.7°.

Although this study did not include a dynamic splint comparison group, the investigators compared their findings to the results of other studies over a similar period of follow-up in which dynamic splinting had been used and found that the two approaches to splinting yielded similar results.

_____

**Exercise**
Protected motion in a dynamic splint or out of a static splint is initiated as early as 3 to 5 days or as late as 10 to 14 days postoperatively when the bulky compression dressing is removed and splints have been fabricated.[12,14,21,30,70,118,121,126] Timeframes vary with the type of procedures performed, the underlying pathology, and the stability of the joint. Even after the bulky dressing is removed, exercise may be delayed for several weeks for a patient with poor quality soft tissue repairs and potential joint instability or delayed wound healing.

The involved MCP joints of patients with OA or post-traumatic arthritis usually are stable postoperatively. Therefore, MCP exercises typically are begun earlier and progressed more rapidly in these patients than is permissible for patients with RA, whose joints tend to be less stable as the result of long-standing tissue inflammation and deformities.[94]

A goal of a rehabilitation program, proposed by Swanson et al.,[121] is to achieve full or almost full active extension and about 45° to 60° of flexion of the MCP joints of the index and middle fingers, respectively, and 70° in the ring and little fingers in patients with RA. Greater ROM may be possible in the patient with OA, particularly in the index and middle fingers. In addition to improving the overall excursion of each reconstructed joint, another goal of exercise is to *elevate* the arc of active MCP motion to a more functional range—that is, to decrease or eliminate the active extension deficit while increasing flexion to improve hand opening and grasp.[21,52]

During the course of rehabilitation, active MCP flexion usually plateaus before active MCP extension, with flexion leveling off at about 3 to 4 months but extension often continuing to improve for up to a year.[21,38]

### Exercise: Maximum Protection Phase

For the first 4 to 6 weeks, the patient performs only assisted or active exercises and is not allowed to use the hand for functional activities. The focus of management is to protect healing structures while applying safe levels of stress to soft tissues to influence organized scar tissue formation and prevent adhesions through protected motion within limited ranges. Early motion also assists in controlling or reducing postoperative peripheral edema.

NOTE: Every effort should be made to obtain the desired degree of flexion, particularly in the ring and little fingers, by the end of the third week postoperatively, the time at which the reconstructed joint capsules become very tight. Otherwise, it becomes difficult to gain additional joint ROM.[48,121,126]

The following goals and exercises are emphasized during the maximum protection phase.[14,21,48,70,126,129]

● *Maintain mobility of the shoulder, elbow, and forearm.*
  • Perform active shoulder, elbow, and forearm ROM. This is particularly important for patients whose RA is affecting multiple joints of the body.
● *Improve functional ROM of the fingers and maintain gliding of tendons within their sheaths.*
  • Initiate active PIP and DIP flexion and extension, with the MCP joints held in extension by the dynamic splint. If static splinting is being used, remove the splint and teach the patient to manually stabilize the MCP joints in extension.
  • Perform active, pain-free MCP flexion initially with the IP joints in extension followed by extension of the MCP joints assisted manually or by the dynamic splint. The dynamic splint usually allows no more than 60° to 70° of MCP flexion.[70,126] Manually stabilize the IP joints in extension or temporarily splint them in extension with tape and tongue depressors during exercise sessions so the lumbricals act to flex the MCP joints. If multiple MCP joints have been replaced, which is usually the case in patients with RA, have the patient exercise one MCP joint at a time to be certain that flexion and extension increase in each of the MCP joints. If the patient is having difficulty actively flexing the MCP joint of the little finger, the fourth and fifth digits can be taped together some of the time to allow the ring finger to assist flexion of the little finger.[14,21,70,126]
  • If it is permissible to remove the splint for exercise, teach the patient how to perform active radial deviation of the MCP joints by placing the open hand palm-down on a table, stabilizing the dorsum of the hand with the opposite hand, and sliding ("walking") the fingers toward the thumb.[90,91]
  • Include active composite finger flexion and opposition of the thumb to each digit, emphasizing pad-to-pad pinch rather than lateral pinch.

PRECAUTIONS: During exercise, avoid lateral pressure of the thumb against the digits, which could contribute to recurrence of an ulnar deviation deformity of the fingers. Carefully observe the incision during MCP flexion, being certain to avoid excessive tension on the skin and delayed wound closure.

● *Prevent adhesions along the healed incision.*
  • Perform gentle mobilization of the scar when sutures have been removed.

### Exercise: Moderate and Minimum Protection Phases

The goal of the *moderate protection phase*, which begins at about 3 to 4 weeks or as late as 6 weeks postoperatively, is to achieve full *active* extension of the MCP joints (no extensor lag) and continue to increase active MCP flexion as early as possible during this phase of rehabilitation for functional use of the hand.[12,14,121,126,129]

Sometime after 3 or 4 weeks or by 6 weeks, it may be permissible to remove the dynamic extension splint for exercise if the MCP joints are stable. Very low-intensity strengthening exercises and light use of the hand for ADL also are initiated around 4 to 6 weeks. If the joints are stable and well aligned and there is sufficient MCP flexion and no active extension deficit, daytime splinting during general activity is gradually discontinued starting around 6 weeks or as late as 12 weeks if joint stability is in question.[14,21,30,70]

During the *minimum protection phase*, which begins around 8 to 12 weeks postoperatively, progressive strengthening of the wrist and hand musculature and increasing use of the hand for functional activities while reinforcing principles of joint protection are emphasized. In most instances, a patient is allowed full use of the hand for light to moderate functional tasks by 12 weeks postoperatively.

Goals and interventions during the moderate and minimum protection phases include the following.[14,21,30,70,118,121,126,129]

● *Continue to increase ROM and active control of the MCP joints.*
  • Have the patient continue active flexion exercises in the dynamic splint or with the static splint removed and even after daytime splinting is discontinued. Add gentle passive stretching, one finger at a time, to increase flexion.
  • Emphasize active MCP extension with the wrist in neutral and the IP joints flexed (the intrinsic minus/hook fist position of the hand) to reinforce the action of the extensor digitorum communis (EDC) muscle and minimize influence of the intrinsic finger extensors. This movement also promotes gliding of the extrinsic extensors in the tendon sheaths.
  • Reinforce end-range MCP extension by maintaining the extended position briefly with each repetition.
● *Restore ROM of the wrist.*
  • When the dynamic splint can be removed during exercise, initiate active ROM of the wrist, emphasizing wrist extension. Be sure that the fingers are relaxed during wrist motions.

◉ *Improve functional strength in the hand and wrist.*

- Have the patient begin isometric flexion and extension against submaximal manual resistance or a solid object at 6 to 8 weeks postoperatively. Then transition to resisted dynamic finger flexion and extension using a variety of exercise devices, such as a small spring-loaded hand exerciser or exercise putty.
- Include resisted radial deviation of the digits. For example, have the patient place the hand on a table palm-down and stabilize the dorsum of the involved hand with the opposite hand. Abduct the index finger against the resistance of a rubber band or push against a coffee cup and slide it across the table.[14]

◉ *Regain use of the hand for functional activities while protecting the operated joints to prevent recurrence of deformity.*

- Reinforce principles of joint protection and energy conservation through patient education (see Box 19.2). Emphasize avoidance of stresses on the fingers in an ulnar direction.
- Perform simulated functional grasping activities, beginning with light prehension activities. Use the hand for light to moderate functional activities by 8 to 12 weeks postoperatively.
- Modify activities of daily living that could contribute to deforming stresses on the MCP or other involved joints.[70,90,91] Consider use of a commercially fabricated, hand-based, digital alignment splint made of neoprene during heavier, more stressful activities.[14]

### Outcomes

A successful outcome provides the patient with pain-free, stable, properly aligned MCP joints combined with improved active extension of the digits while retaining or improving MCP flexion sufficient for functional grasp.[118] Of these outcomes, pain relief is the primary value of MCP arthroplasty.

*Pain relief and patient satisfaction.* Pain relief is excellent or good for most patients, and correction of a flexion/ulnar drift deformity is consistently sufficient after silicone implant arthroplasty and resurfacing arthroplasty. Both of these outcomes contribute to patient satisfaction because they improve hand function and the cosmetic appearance of the hand.[30]

*ROM and hand function.* As noted previously, approximately 70° of active flexion of the MCP joints of the ring and little fingers and 45° to 60° of flexion of the index and middle fingers, full active extension, and correction of ulnar drift of the fingers and pronation primarily of the index finger are considered an ideal overall result.[121]

This degree of mobility enables a patient to open the hand far enough to grasp large objects, touch the fingertips of the ulnar digits to the palm (which is necessary for grasping small objects), and touch the tips of the index finger and thumb for pinch. Less MCP flexion in the index and middle fingers is acceptable because limited motion of the MCP joints enhances stability and allows dexterity and pinch without compromising functional grasp.[12,121]

In an early follow-up study[15] of 28 patients with RA after 115 Swanson implant arthroplasties followed by a dynamic splinting program, the mean arc of active motion for all operated joints at 54 months was 43° (56° of flexion and a 13° active extension deficit). In a review of a number of short- and long-term studies of patients with various types of arthritis undergoing MCP arthroplasty, the postoperative range of MCP flexion/extension varied considerably from study to study, with the mean arc of active motion for all fingers reported to be 45° and a mean extensor lag of 15°.[30] In another review of studies in which only the Swanson silicone implant arthroplasty was used in patients with RA, the reviewers found that the mean postoperative arc of active motion was 50° with a range of flexion from 39° to 67° and an active extension deficit from 7° to 28°.[38] In the early study and in both reviews, the ROM outcomes are less than the potential ranges suggested by Swanson et al.[121] However, postoperative ROM was not reported for individual fingers in any of these studies.

When comparing pre- and postoperative mobility, the total range of flexion/extension may increase only to a small or moderate extent, but the arc of active motion postoperatively often is elevated and becomes more functional. For example, in an 8-year follow-up study of 901 Swanson silicone MCP implants in 294 patients with RA, the mean total active ROM was 40° preoperatively and 50° postoperatively, an increase of only 10°. However, the preoperative active MCP extension deficit was 40° but only 10° postoperatively, creating a more functional range of active MCP movement (an arc from 10° to 60° of flexion) for hand closing and opening.[52] Similar findings were reported in a follow-up study of two-piece, nonconstrained, pyrolytic carbon implants.[29] In this study the prosthetic joints were stable and pain-free, and the mean range of flexion/extension improved by just 13°, but the arc of motion was elevated by 16°.

Few studies have directly compared one type of prosthetic implant to another. However, a recent prospective, double-blind study of patients with RA, which followed patients for 2 years postoperatively, compared the results of two types of silicone implant, the Swanson and the Neuflex designs (see Fig. 19.10). The findings indicated that there was a significantly greater improvement in MCP flexion in patients who received the Neuflex design than in patients receiving the Swanson implant, but there was no significant difference in active MCP extension, ulnar deviation, or grip strength between the two groups.[39] Of interest in this study is that the Neuflex implant, which is pre-formed in 30° of flexion, did not adversely affect active MCP extension, which had been a concern of the investigators.

Although satisfactory improvement of MCP mobility is a predictable outcome after joint arthroplasty, grip and pinch strength do not seem to increase significantly or consistently, or they improve only modestly.[30]

*Complications.* Approximately 70% of MCP silicone implants survive 10 years before revision is necessary as the result of a number of complications.[30] However, some postoperative complications affect outcomes but do not necessitate additional surgery. Delayed wound healing is a short-term complication that may have an adverse effect on re-establishing adequate MCP flexion for functional grasp.[118]

As with the wrist, the most common long-term complication after silicone implant arthroplasty is fracture of the prosthesis,[12,118,121] whereas mechanical loosening is most common after metal-plastic arthroplasty.[29,30] It is believed that these long-term complications can be minimized with the practice of principles of joint protection by consistently avoiding heavy loads and deforming forces on the reconstructed joints.

## Proximal Interphalangeal Implant Arthroplasty

There are a number of joint and soft tissue procedures for managing arthritis and associated deformities of the PIP joints. They include soft tissue release and reconstruction for swan-neck and boutonnière deformities[118] and implant arthroplasty or arthrodesis when there is significant destruction of the articular surfaces.[1,12,50,66,120,121] Arthroplasty may or may not be preferable to arthrodesis to improve functional use of the hand.

In the ulnar digits, where mobility of the PIP joints is particularly important for functional grasp, arthroplasty may be the procedure of choice.[50] However, in the index finger where stability of the PIP joint is a necessity for many functional activities, arthrodesis is often preferable.[1,12,121] If the MCP and PIP joints are involved, as is often the case in patients with RA, the MCP joint is usually replaced, but the PIP joint deformity (usually a swan-neck deformity) is corrected by soft tissue reconstruction[121] or fusion.[1]

### Indications for Surgery

- PIP joint pain and destruction of the articular surfaces (with or without joint subluxation) secondary to OA or post-traumatic arthritis; less frequently indicated for RA.[1,12,70,120,121] In general, PIP implant arthroplasty is indicated for patients with *isolated* PIP involvement, particularly those who are free of MCP joint disease. Implant arthroplasty of contiguous joints (both the MCP and PIP joints) is not recommended.[12,120,121]
- Joint stiffness and decreased ROM that cannot be managed with nonoperative treatment or corrected with soft tissue reconstruction.[1,70]
- Only occasionally for isolated boutonnière deformity or swan-neck deformity[12,50,121] if fusion is not a viable option.

N O T E : Lateral stability of the PIP joint is necessary for a successful outcome.

### Procedure

***Implant design, materials, and fixation.*** The type of arthroplasty of the PIP joint selected by the surgeon depends on the underlying pathology, the extent of associated impairments and deformities, and the experience of the surgeon. As with the MCP joints, there are two categories of implant arthroplasty for the PIP joints: a one-piece, flexible silicone joint spacer[12,120,121] or a two-component (nonarticulated), minimally constrained, surface (total joint) replacement system made of metal and plastic or pyrolytic carbon.[1,66,118] The components of a surface replacement are secured by cement or press-fit fixation.

The silicone implant, designed by Swanson during the 1960s, remains in use today.[120,121] Two-piece, surface replacement systems, first developed during the late 1970s, have undergone many design changes and improvements.[1,12] A surface replacement design affords greater joint mobility than the one-piece silicone design but provides no inherent stability. Therefore, when PIP arthroplasty is deemed appropriate for patients with RA, who typically have compromised joint stability as the result of damage to periarticular soft tissues secondary to chronic synovitis, a one-piece silicone implant tends to be used to provide some stability to the joint. In contrast, surface replacement arthroplasty is used almost exclusively in patients with OA or post-traumatic arthritis because the collateral ligaments usually are intact or repairable.

***Operative procedures.*** For both types of arthroplasty, a curved, longitudinal incision is made along the dorsal aspect of the PIP joint. Occasionally, a volar (palmar) or lateral approach is used. Either a *central slip-sparing approach* (which leaves the central tendon intact) or, when there is significant joint deformity, a *central slip-splinting approach* (where the central tendon is incised longitudinally) is used. The collateral ligaments are preserved or detached and repaired after insertion of the implant(s) whenever possible.[1,9,66]

Portions of the head of the proximal phalanx and the base of the middle phalanx are resected. The intramedullary canals of the proximal and middle phalanges are reamed and prepared for the prosthetic implant(s), which is/are then inserted.

If necessary, the volar plate is released for a flexion contracture, and the extensor tendon mechanism is repaired. Then the joint capsule is repaired, the wound is closed, and a bulky compression dressing is placed on the hand. The hand is supported in a volar splint, which includes the forearm, and elevated in a sling above the level of the shoulder to minimize edema.

### Postoperative Management

**Immobilization**
When the surgical dressing is removed, a custom static splint and possibly a dynamic extension splint with an outrigger are fabricated. These are hand-based splints that leave the wrist free. The position of PIP joint immobilization varies with the type of preoperative deformity that existed and the type of soft tissue reconstruction performed. Recommended positions of the immobilization are summarized in Table 19.2.[1,12,121,127]

The duration of immobilization varies with the type of arthroplasty, whether extensor tendon or collateral ligament

| TABLE 19.2 | Position of Immobilization After PIP Arthroplasty | |
|---|---|---|
| **Preoperative Deformity** | **Postoperative Positioning in Splint** | |
| PIP flexion contracture | PIP extension | |
| Boutonnière deformity | PIP extension and slight DIP flexion | |
| Swan-neck deformity | −10° to 30° PIP flexion and full DIP extension | |

reconstruction of the fingers was part of the procedure, and the surgeon's philosophy.[1,12,50,70,121,127] Protective splinting with frequent sessions of assisted or active exercises continues during the day for at least 6 to 8 weeks postoperatively and is gradually eliminated by 12 weeks. Night splinting may continue for 3 to 6 months or up to a year to protect the repaired joint(s).

### Exercise

The sequence of exercises after PIP arthroplasty emphasizes early but protected motion of the operated and adjacent joints. The time frame for initiation of PIP exercises in the dynamic splint or out of the static splint varies from a few days[1,50,70] to 10 to 14 days[127] postoperatively based on the type and extent of impairments of the fingers preoperatively and the type of reconstructive procedures used. For example, after a *central slip-sparing approach* (extensor mechanism remains intact), ROM exercises are initiated as soon as the bulky dressing has been removed (1 to 3 days postoperatively). After a *central slip-splitting approach* in a joint with no associated swan-neck or boutonnière deformity, ROM exercises are begun several days to a week to 10 days later.

The goals of exercise during each phase of rehabilitation after PIP arthroplasty are similar to those already detailed in this chapter for rehabilitation after MCP arthroplasty. Only guidelines and precautions unique to PIP arthroplasty or procedures for associated correction of specific soft tissue deformities of the PIP joints are addressed in this section.

### Exercise: Maximum and Moderate Protection Phases

The primary goals of the maximum and moderate protection phases of rehabilitation after PIP arthroplasty are to control peripheral edema and restore functional mobility of the operated joint(s) without compromising the repair or reconstruction of soft tissues.

In most instances, the emphasis is to gradually increase PIP flexion by 10° to 15° per week[1] and to achieve approximately 70° of PIP flexion in the ring and little fingers, 60° in the middle finger, and at least 45° in the index finger with full or almost full PIP extension by the end of the moderate protection phase (by 6–8 weeks postoperatively).[17] Dynamic flexion splinting may be instituted if adequate flexion is not achieved with exercise alone.

The following guidelines for exercise are recommended.[12,50,70,120,121,127]

- ● ***Maintain mobility of the wrist, MCP and DIP joints.***
  - Immediately after surgery initiate active ROM of all joints not restricted by the bulky dressing.
- ● ***Restore ROM of the operated joints.***
  - Begin active PIP flexion in the dynamic splint or with the static splint removed and assisted flexion and extension of each PIP joint. Stabilize the MCP and DIP joints in neutral to direct motion to the PIP joint (promotes joint mobility and tendon gliding).

PRECAUTION: During ROM exercises avoid lateral stresses to the operated joints that could compromise the integrity of the collateral ligaments and joint stability.

- ● If a *boutonnière deformity* was corrected (which requires reconstruction of the extensor mechanism), follow the guidelines and precautions described in Box 19.6.[118,127]
- ● If a *swan-neck deformity* was corrected, follow the guidelines and precautions noted in Box 19.7.[50,118,127] A central slip-splitting approach is necessary for correcting a swan-neck deformity to allow the tension on the extensor mechanism to be adjusted and to allow greater excursion of the PIP joint into flexion.

### Exercise: Minimum Protection/ Return to Function Phase

The primary goal of the minimum protection phase shifts from restoration of functional ROM to improving strength

| BOX 19.6 | Postoperative Guidelines and Precautions after Correction of a Boutonnière Deformity |
|---|---|

**Exercise**
- Maintain as much extension as possible of the PIP joint through splinting and exercise for 3 to 6 weeks postoperatively. Remove the splint only for exercise and wound care.
- Initiate early DIP flexion exercises with the PIP joint stabilized in extension to maintain the length of the oblique retinacular ligament.
- Begin active or assisted PIP flexion/extension exercises by 10 to 14 days or sooner postoperatively. Stabilize the MCP joint in neutral (on a book or at the edge of a table) during PIP movements.
- Emphasize PIP extension and DIP flexion during exercise.

**Precautions**
- Avoid hyperextension of the DIP joint.
- Because correction of a boutonnière deformity requires a central slip splitting approach and repair of the extensor mechanism, avoid resisted exercises and stretching of the extensor mechanism of the PIP joint for 6 to 8 weeks or as long as 12 weeks postoperatively.

| BOX 19.7 | Postoperative Guidelines and Precautions after Correction of a Swan–Neck Deformity |

**Exercise**
- Maintain the PIP joint(s) in 10° to 20°[127] or 20° to 30°[50] of flexion and the DIP joint(s) in full extension with static digital splinting.
- Initiate active ROM exercises at the PIP and DIP joints several days[50] to 10 to 14 days[127] postoperatively.
- Perform DIP extension exercises with the PIP joint stabilized in slight flexion.
- Stabilize the DIP joint in neutral during PIP ROM exercises.
- Emphasize PIP flexion and DIP extension.

**Precautions**
- Limit PIP extension to 10° of flexion during exercise to avoid excessive stretch to the volar aspect of the capsule.
- Avoid extreme flexion of the DIP joint.

in the hand and wrist and gradually incorporating safe but progressive use of the hand into functional activities of daily living. This transition occurs around 6 to 8 weeks or as late as 12 weeks postoperatively. The status of the soft tissue repairs, particularly the extensor tendons, determines how early resisted exercises are initiated. For optimal results, rehabilitation may need to continue (through adherence to a home program) for 6 months or longer postoperatively.

As with MCP arthroplasty, low-intensity strengthening exercises can be performed with equipment specifically designed for hand rehabilitation, such as exercise putty, or through graded functional activities that involve resisted movements. Principles of joint protection (see Box 19.2) are integrated into daily living through patient education, with attention paid to continued avoidance of lateral stresses to the PIP joints.

**Outcomes**
After PIP joint arthroplasty, an optimal result provides the patient with a pain-free, mobile but stable and well-aligned joint for functional use of the hand.[1,9,12,120,121] Pain relief is the most consistent outcome after PIP arthroplasty.[1] Outcomes usually are better in patients with OA than in those with post-traumatic arthritis or RA and in fingers without preoperative deformity.[1]

Optimal ROM for functional use of the hand after arthroplasty of the PIP joint is 45° to 70° of active flexion (depending on the finger) and full or almost full active extension (no extensor lag). However, postoperative ROM reported in most studies is substantially less.[1] One surgeon[120] reported that the expected motion after flexible implant arthroplasty ranges from 0 to 10° extensor lag and 30° to 70° flexion but did not differentiate expected results for each finger. In a large follow-up series by Swanson et al.,[120] approximately two-thirds of

the replaced PIP joints had greater than 40° of motion. In a follow-up study after surface replacement arthroplasty primarily for OA, the average arc of motion was 47° (average 16° extensor lag and 63° of PIP flexion).[66]

If the extensor tendon mechanism is intact and a central slip-sparing approach is used, which allows early initiation of mobility exercises, approximately 10° more PIP flexion can be expected than if a central slip-splitting approach is used or repair of extensor tendons is required.[121] If a swan-neck deformity was corrected, a slight (up to 10°) flexion contracture at the PIP joint is acceptable to protect the volar aspect of the joint capsule and possibly avoid recurrence of the deformity.

Patients must continue to avoid forceful grasping and high-impact activities and must practice principles of joint protection for a lifetime to prevent common long-term complications, such as fracture of the implant.[1,127]

## Carpometacarpal Arthroplasty of the Thumb

Arthritis of the CMC joint, also called the trapeziometacarpal joint, of the thumb, leading to pain and stiffness, occurs with advancing age in women more often than men.[83] When this joint is involved, patients have difficulty with forceful grasp and pinch and wringing motions. If a patient remains symptomatic after a period of conservative management, including anti-inflammatory medications, splinting, activity modification, and exercise, one of several types of arthroplasty may be appropriate for relief of symptoms and improved function.[31]

### Indications for Surgery
The following are common indications for CMC arthroplasty of the thumb.[12,23,31,50,113,125]

- Disabling pain at the base of the thumb, specifically the CMC joint, as the result of osteoarthritis, post-traumatic arthritis, or RA. However, most CMC arthroplasties are performed for degenerative joint diseases and less often for synovium-based diseases.
- Dorsoradial instability (subluxation or dislocation) of the first metacarpal on the trapezium, leading to a hyperextension deformity at the MCP joint of the thumb.
- Stiffness and limited ROM (often an adduction contracture) of the thumb.
- Decreased pinch and grip strength because of CMC pain or subluxation.
- When arthrodesis of the CMC joint is inappropriate.

### Procedures

***Background and surgical options.*** The type of procedure selected depends on the degree of ligament laxity, the extent of destruction of the articular surfaces, the underlying pathology, and the expected demands that will be placed on the hands postoperatively.[31,113] Arthrodesis, rather than arthroplasty, is an option for patients who use the hand for high-demand occupational activities. However, for the patient whose activities place less stress on the hand, there are several soft tissue and bony procedures that relieve pain and restore joint stability but preserve functional mobility at the base of the thumb.[31,83] Retaining some CMC joint mobility is particularly important for the patient with RA, who typically has loss of mobility of other joints of the hand and wrist.[125]

Procedures for CMC arthroplasty fall into three broad categories: ligament reconstruction, trapezial resection/tendon interposition or suspension arthroplasty (usually with ligament reconstruction), and joint replacement arthroplasty (resurfacing or total joint replacement) of the CMC joint with prosthetic components that are cemented in place. Among these procedures, ligament reconstruction alone is used when there is pain and instability but little to no loss of articular cartilage.[31] One of the many variations of trapezial resection/tendon interposition arthroplasty is by far the most widely used approach to treatment when there is joint subluxation and loss of the joint space due to deterioration of articular cartilage.[9,12,23,31,50,64,113,125] Trapezial resection combined with ligament reconstruction but without tendon interposition also has been shown to be an effective surgical approach to treatment.[65]

Joint replacement arthroplasty (resurfacing arthroplasty or total joint arthroplasty) with rigid prosthetic components is an alternative to trapezial resection/tendon interposition arthroplasty for a few selected patients with CMC OA, who require improved pinch but do not need to use the hand for high-load, high-impact activities.[12,31,50] A patient must have good quality bone stock to be a candidate for joint replacement arthroplasty. If bone stock is poor, as often occurs in RA, cement fixation of the prosthetic components usually is not successful. Silicone implant arthroplasty, although considered a viable option in the past,[33] now is used infrequently because of the problems of joint dislocation and silicone wear.[9,31]

Because instability (hyperextension) and arthritis of the MCP joint are frequently associated with CMC arthritis, concomitant stabilization with a temporary K-wire or arthrodesis of the MCP joint is performed in addition to reconstruction of the CMC joint.[31,125]

*Operative overview.* For a tendon interposition arthroplasty, a dorsal incision is made at the base of the thumb, with careful attention paid to protecting the branches of the superficial radial nerve. The capsule is approached through the extensor tendons and incised longitudinally. All or a portion of the trapezium is resected (trapeziectomy), as is a small portion of the base of the first metacarpal. A tendon graft is harvested from a portion of the flexor carpi radialis, abductor pollicis longus, or palmaris longus and inserted into the trapezial space to act as a soft tissue spacer.[9,12,23,31,50,64,113,125] The anterior oblique ligament may also be reconstructed with a portion of the tendon graft; and the abductor pollicis longus, if not used for the tendon graft, may be imbricated or advanced to enhance joint stability and function of the abductor postoperatively.[50] The capsule and adjacent soft tissues are then repaired, and the wound is closed.

For a resurfacing arthroplasty, a dorsal approach is also used to reach the capsule through a longitudinal incision between the abductor pollicis longus and the extensor pollicis brevis. For a total joint replacement arthroplasty, a volar approach is often used.[31] After the capsule has been split longitudinally, portions of the distal trapezium and the base of the first metacarpal are resected. The trapezium and the intramedullary canal of the metacarpal are prepared, and the prosthetic components are inserted and cemented in place. The capsule is repaired; and as with soft tissue interposition arthroplasty, the abductor pollicis longus may be advanced to enhance joint stability. Joint stability and ROM are assessed prior to closure.

### Postoperative Management
The goal of rehabilitation is to develop sufficient mobility of the thumb for functional activities while maintaining joint stability for strong pinch and grasp. It may take up to a year after surgery for a patient to achieve optimal results.

### Immobilization
With all procedures, the thumb and hand are immobilized postoperatively in a bulky compression dressing and elevated for several days to a week to control edema.

After the postoperative dressing is removed, the hand is placed in a static, forearm-based thumb spica cast, which is later replaced with a removable splint, with the CMC joint immobilized in abduction (40° to 60°), the MCP joint in slight flexion, and the wrist in neutral to slight extension.[12,31,50,83,100] The IP joint of the thumb and the fingers are left free.

The length of time the CMC joint is continuously immobilized depends on the surgery. The time frame varies from just 7 to 10 days after total joint arthroplasty[31] to 3 to 5 weeks after ligament reconstruction/tendon interposition arthroplasty or resurfacing arthroplasty with prosthetic implants.[12,31,48,50,83,100,125]

At 3 to 6 weeks after surgery the splint is removed frequently during the day for exercise. From 8 to 12 weeks, as the patient uses the hand for functional activities, daytime splinting is gradually discontinued. Use of a night splint to stabilize the thumb continues for 8 to 12 weeks or until the joint is stable and essentially pain-free.[31,100,125]

### Exercise
Progression of exercises varies with the type of arthroplasty. Guidelines presented in this section are for *ligament reconstruction/tendon interposition arthroplasty*, still the most common form of CMC arthroplasty. Management guidelines unique to joint replacement arthroplasty are also noted. Precautions after CMC arthroplasty are summarized in Box 19.8.[31,83,100]

### Exercise: Maximum Protection Phase
The focus of the first 6 weeks of rehabilitation is control of pain and edema, maintaining ROM in nonimmobilized joints, and initiating protected motion of the CMC joint when it is permissible to remove the thumb spica splint for exercise.[31,83,100,125] The following are suggested goals and exercises.

| BOX 19.8 | Precautions after CMC Arthroplasty of the Thumb |
| --- | --- |

- Initially refrain from full CMC flexion with adduction (sliding the thumb across the palm to the base of the fifth finger) as this motion places excessive stress on the dorsal aspect of the capsule and ligament reconstruction. Be certain it is possible to oppose the thumb to each fingertip before attempting to touch the base of the fifth finger.
- When stretching to increase CMC abduction or extension, apply the stretch force to the metacarpal, not the first phalanx, to avoid hyperextension or compromise stability of the MCP joint. Follow the same precaution during light resistance exercises.
- Avoid forceful pinch and grasp for at least 3 months after surgery.
- Modify activities of daily living to limit heavy lifting. If occasionally heavy lifting is necessary, advise the patient to wear a protective splint.

◉ **Maintain mobility of the fingers and IP joint of the thumb.**
- During the period of continuous immobilization of the wrist and CMC and MCP joints of the thumb, have the patient perform active ROM of the fingers and the IP joint of the thumb.
◉ **Initiate protected mobility of the thumb and wrist.**
- When permissible, begin active, controlled ROM of the thumb within protected ranges and the wrist.
- After *tendon interposition arthroplasty*, protected ROM is not initiated until about 3 to 6 weeks after surgery to allow time for the reconstructed soft tissues to heal adequately.[31,48,83,100,125]
- After *total joint arthroplasty*, ROM may be initiated at about 1 week postoperatively because of the inherent stability of the cemented, ball-and-socket design prosthesis.[31] When it is permissible to remove the splint for exercise, begin active wrist ROM in all directions and CMC ROM with active abduction and extension; then add opposition and circumduction. Also include active MCP flexion and extension, being certain to stabilize the CMC joint.

**Exercise: Moderate and Minimum Protection Phases**

◉ **Re-establish functional mobility of the hand and wrist.**
- Continue active ROM exercises using gradually increasing ranges.
- At about 8 weeks, begin gentle self-stretching exercises or dynamic splinting if limitations in functional ROM persist.
◉ **Regain strength and functional use of the hand and wrist.**
- At about 8 weeks postoperatively initiate isometric exercises against light resistance, emphasizing abduction and extension.

- If the CMC joint is stable and pain-free, progress to dynamic resistance exercises to regain pinch and grasp strength.
- Between 8 and 12 weeks, gradually begin to use the hand for light ADL with the splint removed, such as buttoning and unbuttoning.[48,83,125]
- Incorporate principles of joint protection during strengthening exercises and ADL.
- Continue to increase use of the hand for light to moderate ADL over the next 4 to 6 weeks. A patient typically can return to light-duty work by 3 to 4 months and can resume most functional activities by 4 to 6 months.

### Outcomes

Most of the studies reported in the literature have investigated outcomes of trapezial resection/tendon interposition arthroplasty with very limited data reported on the results of joint replacement arthroplasty. A successful overall outcome after CMC arthroplasty, based on data from a variety of instruments that measure pain, ROM, hand function, patient satisfaction, and quality of life, is pain-free motion of the basal joint of the thumb and improved hand function, such as dexterity, pinch, and grasp.[12,23,31,113,125] The time required to achieve maximum benefit from the surgery is typically 6 to 12 months.[12,48,100]

Among the procedures available, trapezial resection/tendon interposition arthroplasty with or without ligament reconstruction yields the most predictable and successful outcomes.[31] In a review of tendon interposition arthroplasty, outcomes appear to be better when the procedure includes reconstruction of ligaments, possibly because the CMC joint is more stable with than without ligament reconstruction.[31]

**Pain relief and patient satisfaction.** Regardless of the type of CMC arthroplasty, the most consistent and predictable benefit of these procedures is relief of pain.[12,23,31,33,50,64,65] For example, in a review of outcomes of a number of studies for patients with OA who had undergone tendon interposition arthroplasty with or without ligament reconstruction, 94% of patients reported long-term relief of pain.[113] Although tendon interposition is designed to resurface the deteriorated joint to make motion more comfortable, in a prospective, randomized study of patients with OA investigators compared the results of trapezial resection and ligament reconstruction with and without the use of tendon interposition. They found that at a mean of 48 months after surgery, both groups had equally satisfactory pain relief.[65]

The patients' quality of life also improves after CMC arthroplasty. In a follow-up study of 103 patients with OA, who had primary tendon interposition arthroplasty, participants completed several standardized self-assessment questionnaires at a mean of 6.2 years after surgery.[4] In an overall rating, 79 of 103 reported their quality of life had improved greatly, and an additional 15 reported slight improvement.

***ROM and hand function.*** Active ROM of the thumb, particularly opposition, and dexterity usually improve after CMC arthroplasty. Increased abduction and extension widen the web space, making it easier to open the hand to grasp large objects. However, the results of some studies of ligament reconstruction/tendon interposition arthroplasty indicate that preoperative and postoperative ROM essentially is unchanged. Although data are limited, total joint arthroplasty is thought to produce the most improvement in ROM compared to other procedures.[31]

One author has observed that it is not uncommon for patients to experience discomfort in the region of the CMC joint for up to 1 year after surgery as structures heal.[48] Consequently, hand functions that require some degree of force production, such as pinch and grasp, improve only gradually. Most studies that follow patients for several years after surgery, however, indicate that measurements of pinch and grasp strength as well as performance of functional tasks improve significantly.[23,31] The most successful long-term functional outcomes have been reported for patients who use the hand primarily for low-demand activities. For example, after silicone implant arthroplasty, satisfactory results were reported for 80% of patients who typically used the hand for activities that placed only light to moderate loads on the thumb.[33]

***Complications.*** Complications vary with the type of CMC arthroplasty. Overall, however, the rate of complications is low, with inadequate pain relief or recurrence of joint instability the most common complications that necessitate revision arthroplasty. In a retrospective study of 606 primary tendon interposition-ligament reconstruction arthroplasties performed over a 16-year period, only 3.8% were known to have required a revision procedure for mechanically based pain.[32] Neuropathic pain can also develop after CMC arthroplasty. The pain may be caused by damage to or impingent of the radial nerve (radial sensory neuritis), carpal tunnel syndrome, or complex regional pain syndrome (reflex sympathetic dystrophy).[23,32]

For arthroplasties that include implantation of prosthetic components, loosening and dislocation are the most common complications. Loosening has been identified after silicone implant arthroplasty[33] as well as joint replacement arthroplasty.[31]

## Tendon Rupture Associated with RA: Surgical and Postoperative Management

### Background and Indications for Surgery

Ruptures of tendons of the hand are common in patients with chronic tenosynovitis of the tendons of the wrist and hand associated with RA. The actual site of the rupture may be in the wrist or the hand. When a tendon ruptures, there is a sudden loss of active control of one or more of the digits. Rupture of a single or multiple tendons is usually painless and occurs during unremarkable use of the hand.[9,50,51,132] Such ruptures are evidence of severely diseased tendons.

The extensor tendons are affected far more frequently than the flexor tendons. Extensor tendons that most often rupture, in order of frequency, are the common extensor tendons to the small and ring fingers and the extensor pollicis longus (EPL). The most common flexor tendon to rupture is the flexor pollicis longus (FPL).[50,51,95,132]

The causes of rupture include infiltration of proliferative synovium in the tendon sheaths into tendons, which subsequently weakens the affected tendon; abrasion and fraying of a tendon as it moves over a bony prominence roughened or eroded by synovitis; periodic use of local steroid injections over time; or ischemic necrosis caused by direct pressure from hypertrophic synovium, particularly at the dorsal retinaculum, that compromises blood supply to a tendon. Common sites of abrasion that affect the extensors are the distal ulna and Lister's tubercle and the volar aspect of the scaphoid where it contacts the flexor tendons.[5,9,50,51,132]

The indication for surgery is loss of function of the hand. Rupture of a single tendon, such as the extensor digiti minimi, may not impair a patient's function, whereas rupture of multiple tendons simultaneously or over a period of time may cause significant functional limitations and disability.

### Procedures

The surgical procedures available for treatment of tendon ruptures in RA vary depending on which tendon(s) has ruptured, the number of ruptured tendons, the location of the rupture, the condition of the tendon at the site of rupture, and the quality of the remaining intact tendons of the hand. Options include[9,50,51,95,132]:

- ***Tendon transfer.*** A tendon is removed from its normal distal attachment and attached at another site. For example, the extensor indicis proprius (EIP) can be transferred if the EPL has ruptured. A flexor tendon can also be transferred to the dorsal surface of the hand to act as an extensor if multiple extensor tendons have ruptured.
- ***Tendon graft reconstruction.*** A portion of another tendon that acts as a "bridge" is inserted between and sutured to the two ends of the ruptured tendon. The palmaris longus tendon is often selected as the donor tendon. A wrist extensor tendon may be selected if a wrist arthrodesis is performed at the time of the tendon reconstruction.
- ***Tendon anastomosis (side-to-side tenorrhaphy).*** The ruptured tendon is sutured to an adjacent intact tendon. This is a common option at the wrist for the finger extensor tendons.[132]
- ***Direct end-to-end repair.*** The two ends of the ruptured tendon are re-opposed and sutured together. This option is used only occasionally because the ends of the ruptured tendons in patients with RA usually are frayed. Therefore, a considerable portion of the frayed tendon(s) must be resected, which shortens the tendon, making it difficult to suture end-to-end.

Concomitant procedures in the rheumatoid hand include tenosynovectomy, removal of osteophytes from bony prominences, and ligament reconstruction or arthrodesis for instability. If late-stage MCP joint disease is also present and passive extension of the MCP joints is significantly limited, arthroplasty of the involved joints may also be indicated, either simultaneously with the tendon procedure or during two separate operations as determined by the surgeon. Without adequate joint mobility the transferred or reconstructed extensor tendons become adherent, resulting in a poor outcome.

## Postoperative Management

The guidelines described in this section apply only to management of tendon transfer, reconstruction, or repair of *extensor* tendons in the rheumatoid hand. As mentioned previously, rupture of extensor tendons occurs far more frequently than flexor tendon rupture. As with postoperative management for other surgeries described in this chapter, pain and edema control and exercises for the nonoperated extremities are always essential components of rehabilitation.

Tendon transfers and reconstruction are delicate procedures requiring ongoing communication between the therapist and surgeon and active involvement of the patient in the postoperative program. Therefore, patient education is woven into every phase of rehabilitation.

### Immobilization

A bulky compression dressing is applied to the hand and wrist at the close of extensor tendon surgery to control edema. The surgical compression dressing is removed after several days, and the wrist and hand are then immobilized in a volar splint. A forearm-based, static splint holds the wrist and digits in a position that minimizes stress to the transferred or reconstructed tendon(s).

For example, after side-to-side finger extensor transfer or extensor tendon reconstruction, the wrist and all fingers are immobilized in extension in the splint, but the thumb is free to move. After reconstruction of a ruptured EPL tendon or transfer of the EIP tendon to restore thumb extension, the wrist is immobilized in extension and the thumb in adduction, but the fingers are free to move.

Continuous immobilization of the wrist and digits is maintained for approximately 3 to 4 weeks to protect the healing tendons.[71,132] Daytime splinting is discontinued at about 12 weeks, but night splinting typically continues for 6 months or longer.

N O T E : Use of dynamic splinting and early mobilization (a few days after surgery) typically is not recommended for tendon reconstruction or transfers in the rheumatoid hand. Tissue healing is slower and the risk of re-rupture higher postoperatively for patients with long-standing, systemic disease (who likely have been treated periodically with corticosteroids) than in otherwise healthy patients who have sustained an acute laceration or rupture of a tendon in the hand.[43]

### Exercise

During each phase of postoperative rehabilitation after extensor tendon transfer or reconstruction, exercises are

---

| BOX 19.9 | Precautions after Extensor Tendon Transfers or Reconstruction in the Rheumatoid Hand |
|---|---|

- During the early phase of rehabilitation, do not initiate MCP extension from full, available MCP flexion to avoid excessive stretch on the operated tendon(s).
- Postpone stretching to increase MCP flexion if there is a deficit in active extension.
- Avoid activities or hand postures that combine finger flexion or thumb flexion and adduction with wrist flexion as this places extreme stress on the reconstructed or transferred extensor tendons. If a patient must use the hands for transfer activities, avoid weight bearing on the dorsum of the hand.
- Avoid vigorous grasping activities that could potentially overstretch or rupture the reconstructed or transferred extensor tendon(s).

---

progressed very gradually. Precautions during exercise and functional use of the hand are summarized in Box 19.9.

### Exercise: Maximum Protection Phase

During the first 6 weeks after surgery, the priorities of rehabilitation are edema control and protection of the transferred or reconstructed tendon(s), followed by carefully controlled mobility of the operated areas to prevent adherence of healing tissues. It is usually permissible to remove the protective splint for exercise at around 3 to 4 weeks. If tendon quality is poor and the security of the sutured tissues is in question, exercise may be delayed until about 6 weeks postoperatively. The goals and intervention during the first phase include the following.[51,71,132]

- *Maintain mobility of the elbow and forearm, unsplinted digits, and other involved joints.*
  - While the operated hand is immobilized, perform active ROM of all necessary joints.
- *Re-establish mobility and control of the repaired or transferred extensor muscle-tendon units.*
  - When the splint may be removed for exercise, initiate active wrist motions with the fingers relaxed.
  - Begin assisted MCP extension of each of the fingers or thumb with the wrist and IP joints of each digit stabilized in neutral.
  - Perform *place and hold* exercises by passively positioning the operated MCP joint first in a neutral and later in a slightly extended position. Have the patient briefly hold the position. This emphasizes end-range extension to prevent an extensor lag.
  - Progress to dynamic MCP extension with the wrist in neutral, initially from slight MCP flexion with the palm of the hand on a table and the fingers relaxed over the edge.

N O T E : To help a patient learn the new action of a transferred tendon, initially have the patient focus on the original action (function) of the muscle-tendon unit. For example, if the EIP was transferred to replace the action of the EPL of the thumb, have the patient think about extending the index finger when trying to actively extend the thumb. Use biofeedback or functional electrical stimulation (FES) to assist with the motor learning.[71]

● *Regain active flexion of the digits.*
- Initiate MCP flexion of the fingers by having the patient relax the EDC after active extension rather than actively flexing the fingers.
- Progress to active MCP flexion within a protected range with the wrist and PIP joints stabilized in neutral. With the wrist and MCP joints stabilized in extension, actively flex (hook fist/intrinsic minus position) and extend (straight hand position) the PIP joints. PIP flexion while in wrist and MCP extension prevents stiffness of the IP joints without placing a stretch on the repaired EDC.[45]

**Exercise: Moderate and Minimum Protection Phases**
By 6 to 8 weeks postoperatively, the transferred or reconstructed tendon can withstand greater imposed stresses. Use of the hand for light functional activities usually begins at this time. At about 8 weeks, daytime splinting is gradually decreased and is typically discontinued by 12 weeks postoperatively. Splint use during the day continues over a longer period of time if there is an extensor lag. Rehabilitation progresses as follows.

● *Continue to increase active mobility of the operated digits.*
- Add gentle passive stretching to increase MCP extension or flexion if one or both motions is restricted.
- Continue active MCP extension exercises to prevent an extensor lag or consider dynamic extension splinting if an extensor lag has developed and persists. If MCP extension to neutral is possible (no extensor lag), perform active MCP extension with the palm of the hand on a flat surface and extend each finger beyond neutral.
- With the wrist in neutral or slight extension, gradually increase MCP flexion by touching each fingertip to the palm of the hand (first straight and then full-fist positions) or the thumb to each fingertip and gradually to the base of the fifth finger. At 8 to 12 weeks institute dynamic flexion splinting intermittently during the day if grasp is significantly limited.
● *Regain strength, control, and functional use of the hand.*
- Incorporate active movements of the digits into manual dexterity and coordination activities that simulate functional activities. Remove the splint for functional activities that involve light grasp, such as picking up or holding light objects or folding clothing.
- Around 8 to 12 weeks add isometric and dynamic, *submaximal* resistance exercises to improve functional strength and endurance of the hand.
- Through ongoing patient education, reinforce principles of joint protection during functional use of the hand.

**Outcomes**
The results of surgical intervention and postoperative rehabilitation of ruptured tendons in the rheumatoid hand are highly dependent on the extent of involvement in the joints and soft tissues of the hand and wrist preoperatively. It is often difficult to differentiate postoperative functional improvement strictly as the result of a tendon transfer or reconstruction from procedures performed concurrently, such as joint arthroplasty or arthrodesis.

Barring complications, the most common of which is tendon re-rupture, a few generalizations can be made.[50,51,132] Patients with a recent rupture of a single tendon and who have full passive ROM of the affected joint realize an optimum postoperative outcome, which is full functional grasp and no extensor lag in the involved digit. The greater the number of tendon ruptures or associated impairments, such as joint contractures, fixed deformities, or joint instabilities, the poorer are the results.

## ● REPETITIVE TRAUMA SYNDROMES/ OVERUSE SYNDROMES

Disorders from cumulative or repetitive trauma in the wrist and hand lead to significant loss of hand function and lost work time.[8] The causes are related to repeated movements over an extended period of time. The resulting inflammation can affect muscles, tendons, synovial sheaths, and nerves. Diagnoses include carpal tunnel syndrome, trigger finger, de Quervain's disease, and tendinitis. Management of impairments related to carpal tunnel syndrome and nerve compression in the tunnel of Guyon are described in Chapter 13.

### Tenosynovitis, Tendinitis

#### Etiology of Symptoms
Inflammation results from continued or repetitive use of the involved muscle, from the effects of RA, from a stress overload to the contracting muscle (such as strongly gripping the steering wheel during a motor vehicle accident), or from roughening of the surface of the tendon or its sheath.

#### Common Impairments
● Pain whenever the related muscle contracts or whenever there is movement of another joint that causes gliding of the tendon through the sheath.
● Warmth and tenderness with palpation in the region of inflammation.
● In RA, synovial proliferation and swelling in affected tendon sheaths such as over the dorsum of the wrist or in the flexor tendons in the carpal tunnel.[44]
● Frequently, an imbalance in muscle length and strength or poor endurance in the stabilizing muscles. The fault may be more proximal in the elbow or shoulder girdle, thus causing excessive load and substitute motions at the distal end of the chain.

## Common Functional Limitations/Disabilities

Pain that worsens with the provoking activity of the fingers, thumb, or wrist, which may affect grip or repetitive hand motions.

## Management: Protection Phase

Follow the guidelines for acute lesions described in Chapter 10, with special emphasis on relieving the stress in the involved musculotendinous unit and maintaining a healthy environment for healing with nondestructive forces.

- Splint the related joints to rest the involved tendon.
- If the tendon is in a sheath, apply cross-fiber massage while the tendon is in an elongated position so mobility develops between the tendon and sheath.
- Perform multiangle muscle-setting techniques in pain-free positions followed by pain-free ROM.
- Instruct the patient in tendon-gliding exercises to prevent adhesions. (These are described in the exercise section of this chapter.)

## Management: Controlled Motion and Return to Function Phases

- Progress the intensity of massage, exercises, and stretching techniques.
- Assess the biomechanics of the functional activity provoking the symptoms and design a program to regain a balance in the length, strength, and endurance of the muscles. Frequently, problems arise because of poor stabilization or endurance in the shoulder or elbow.

### ⦿ Focus on Evidence

Backstrom[6] reported a case study on a patient diagnosed with deQuervain's disease of 2 months' duration in which mobilization with movement (MWM) was used in addition to physical agents, exercise, and transverse friction massage. Pain was markedly reduced from 6/10 to 3/10 (50%) by the third intervention, and by completion of 12 sessions it was 0 to 1/10. The author proposed that the subtle malalignments in the wrist joints associated with the overuse syndrome perpetuated the symptoms and that the MWM helped restore normal arthrokinematics. The MWM techniques used included active movements of the thumb and wrist while a passive radial glide of the proximal row of carpals was applied (similar to Fig. 19.8). The principles of MWM are described in Chapter 5.

# ⦿ TRAUMATIC LESIONS IN THE WRIST AND HAND

## Simple Sprain: Nonoperative Management

After trauma from a blow or a fall, an excessive stretch force may strain the supporting ligamentous tissue. There may be a related fracture, subluxation, or dislocation.

## Common Impairments

- Pain at the involved site whenever a stretch force is placed on the ligament
- Possible hypermobility or instability in the related joint if supporting ligaments are torn

## Common Functional Limitations/Disabilities

- With a simple sprain, pain may interfere with functional use of the hand for a couple of weeks whenever the joint is stressed. There is no limitation of function if a splint or tape can be worn to protect the ligament and the splint does not interfere with the task.
- With significant tears there is instability, and the joint may subluxate or dislocate with provoking activities, which requires surgical intervention.

## Management

Follow the guidelines in Chapter 10 for treating acute lesions with emphasis on maintaining mobility while minimizing stress to the healing tissue. If immobilization is necessary to protect the part, only the involved joint should be immobilized. Joints above and below should be free to move. This maintains mobility of the long tendons in their sheaths that cross the involved joint. Avoid positions of stress and activities that provoke the symptoms while healing. Cross-fiber massage to the site of the lesion may help prevent the developing scar from adhering and restricting motion.

# Lacerated Flexor Tendons of the Hand: Surgical and Postoperative Management

## Background and Indications for Surgery

Lacerations of the flexor tendons of the hand, which can occur in various areas (zones) along the volar surface of the fingers, palm, wrist, and distal forearm, are common and cause an immediate loss of hand function consistent with the tendons severed. The musculotendinous structures damaged depend on the location and depth of the wound. Damage to one or more tendons may be accompanied by vascular, nerve, and skeletal injuries, which can cause additional loss of function and complicate management. An acute rupture of a flexor tendon may also occur as the result of a closed traumatic injury to the hand.[35,116]

The volar surfaces of the forearm, wrist, palm, and fingers are divided into five zones; the thumb is divided into three zones. These zones are illustrated in Figure 19.12. The anatomical landmarks for each of the zones are described in Box 19.10.[35,53,75,105,116,117] Use of this system of classifying lacerations improves consistency of communication and can provide a basis for predicting outcomes.[79]

Knowledge of the complex anatomy and kinesiology of the hand is essential to understand the impairments and functional implications caused by damage to the flexor tendons in each of these zones. Box 19.11 identifies common impairments associated with damage in each of the zones.[35,47,75,89]

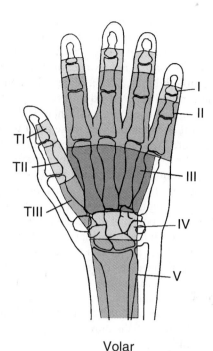

Volar

FIGURE 19.12 Flexor tendon zones; volar aspect of the hand and wrist.

Flexor tendons, when severed or ruptured, readily retract, thus requiring surgical intervention in most instances to restore function to the hand and prevent deformity. Repair and rehabilitation of lacerations in zone II, traditionally referred to as "no-man's land," pose a particu-

---

### BOX 19.10  Flexor Tendon Zones: Anatomical Landmarks

**Zones of the Fingers, Palm, Wrist, and Forearm**
- I—from the insertion of the FDP on the distal phalanx to just distal of the FDS insertion on the middle phalanx
- II—from the distal insertion of the FDS tendon to the level of the distal palmar crease (just proximal to the neck of the metacarpals)
- III—from the neck of the metacarpals, proximally along the metacarpals to the distal border of the carpal tunnel
- IV—the carpal tunnel (area under the transverse carpal ligament)
- V—area just proximal to the wrist (proximal edge of the carpal ligament) to the musculotendinous junction of the extrinsic flexors in the distal forearm

**Zones of the Thumb**
- T-I—from the distal insertion of the FPL on the distal phalanx of the thumb to the neck of the proximal phalanx.
- T-II—from the proximal phalanx, across the MCP joint to the neck of the first metacarpal.
- T-III—from the first metacarpal to the proximal margin of the carpal ligament.

---

### BOX 19.11  Consequences of Injury to the Volar Surface of the Hand, Wrist, and Forearm

- *Zone I.* Only one tendon, the FDP, can be severed as can the A-4 and A-5 retinacular pulleys, which are important for maintaining the mechanical advantage of the FDP for complete finger flexion (full fist).
- *Zone II.* FDS and FDP tendons, a double-layered synovial sheath and multiple annular pulleys (including A-1) of the flexor retinaculum (the fibrous sheath that approximates the tendons to the underlying bones and maintains them relatively close to the joints for full tendon excursion) can all be damaged. Inability to flex the PIP and DIP joints occurs if both tendons are severed. Potential damage to the vincula, the vascular structures that provide blood, and supplement nutrition derived from synovial diffusion can compromise tendon healing.
- *Zone III.* In addition to loss of the FDP and FDS, damage to lumbricales can disrupt MCP flexion.
- *Zone IV.* Damage in this zone (in the carpel tunnel) can affect all three extrinsic flexors of the digits—FDP, FDS, FPL—which disrupts finger and thumb flexion. Synovial sheath also sustains damage. Nerve injury frequently accompanies laceration in this zone.
- *Zone V.* Laceration in the forearm can cause major damage to flexor tendons of the digits and wrist, resulting in loss of wrist and digital flexion. The median and ulnar nerves and the radial and ulnar arteries also lie superficial in this zone.
- *Zones T-I and T-II.* Damage to the retinacular pulley system of the thumb, synovial sheath in addition to the FPL, and possibly the distal insertion of the FPB can occur; IP and MCP flexion are disrupted.
- *Zone T-III.* Potential damage to the thenar muscles.

---

lar challenge to hand surgeons and therapists. Because of the confined space in which the extrinsic flexors of the fingers lie and the limited vascular supply to the tendons in zone II, healing tissues in this area are prone to excursion-restricting adhesions. Scar tissue formation during the healing process can interrupt tendon-gliding in the synovial sheath and subsequently restrict ROM of the involved fingers. In zone IV (the carpal tunnel), the extrinsic flexor tendons of the digits (FDS, FDP, FPL) lie in close proximity to each other. An injury in this zone may lead to adherence of adjacent tendons to each other in the carpal tunnel and impairment of differential gliding between the tendons.

### Procedures

Many factors influence the type of surgical repair selected to manage a tendon injury.[35,53,75,105,115–117] Injury-related factors include the mechanism of injury; the type and location (zone) of the laceration; the extent of associated skin, vascular, nerve, and skeletal damage; and the time elapsed since the injury. Surgery-related factors include timing of the repair, the need for staging surgeries, and the hand surgeon's background and experience. Patient-related influences are the patient's age, health, and lifestyle. These factors also have a significant impact on rehabilitation and outcomes of a tendon repair.

**Types of repairs.** Surgical options for repair of lacerations or a closed rupture of flexor tendons can be classified by the *type* of procedure.[35,75,105,116]

- **Direct repair.** An end-to-end repair in which the tendon ends are re-opposed and sutured together.
- **Tendon graft.** An autogenous donor tendon (autograft), such as the palmaris longus, is sutured in place to replace the damaged tendon. This is necessary when the ends of the severed tendon(s) cannot be brought together without undue tension. Tendon grafts are performed in one or more stages depending on the severity, type, and location of injury.

A straight laceration usually lends itself well to a direct (end-to-end) repair, whereas a jagged laceration that frays the tendon may require a tendon graft.

**Timing of a repair.** Another method of classifying and describing tendon repairs is the *timing* of the repair, as related to the elapsed time since the injury. The timing of a repair after an acute tendon injury is critical because the severed ends of the tendon begin to soften and deteriorate quickly, and the proximal portion of the tendon retracts. These factors make it difficult to reattach the tendon with a strong repair at its normal length. However, only a tendon laceration associated with major damage to the vascular system is considered an emergency situation.[35,75,116] Although better outcomes are thought to occur if the repair is done within the first few days, a delay of up to 10 days yields results equal to those of an immediate repair. Delays beyond 2 weeks are associated with poorer outcomes.[35,116] If a repair must be delayed for more than 3 to 4 weeks, a direct repair is no longer possible, which necessitates a tendon graft.[35]

Categories of surgeries based on elapsed time include[17,35,55,75,105,116,117]:

- **Immediate primary repair.** A repair done within the first 24 hours after injury.
- **Delayed primary repair.** A repair performed up to 10 days after injury.
- **Secondary repair.** A repair done 10 days to 3 weeks after injury.
- **Late reconstruction.** Surgery performed well beyond 3 to 4 weeks, sometimes months after the injury.
- **Staged reconstruction.** Multiple separate surgeries performed over a period of weeks or months.[55] A staged reconstruction enables a surgeon to prepare an extensively damaged or scarred tendon bed months prior to a tendon graft so adhesions are less likely to develop.

A simple, clean, acute laceration of a tendon without associated injuries of the hand is most often managed with a *direct primary repair*, either immediate or delayed a few days.[35,116,117] However, if the wound is not clean, a *delayed primary repair* allows time for medical intervention to reduce the risk of infection. Lengthy delays that necessitate a *secondary repair* or *late reconstruction* are often associated with multiple injuries, such as extensive skin loss, fractures that cannot be stabilized immediately, or long-standing scarring and contractures. If there is damage to one or more of the tendon pulleys, these must be repaired before the lacerated tendon can be effectively repaired.

Of the multiple-stage reconstructions for extensive and complex flexor tendon injuries of the hand, the *Hunter two-stage reconstruction passive or active implant* is most widely known. During the first stage of this procedure, the scarred and adherent portions of the damaged flexor tendon are resected. A Hunter implant (rod) made of silicone is then secured in place to act as a tendon spacer around which a new sheath develops over a period of 3 months. In addition, a damaged retinacular pulley system is reconstructed, and any contractures are released during the first surgery. During the second phase, the implant is removed, and a donor tendon (graft) is drawn through the new sheath and sutured in place.[55]

**Overview of operative procedures.** Some general aspects of the many variations of operative procedures for primary flexor tendon injuries are described in this section.[35,75,79,115–117] However, careful review of a patient's operative report and close communication with the hand surgeon are necessary sources of specific details of each patient's surgery. For repair of lacerated finger tendons in zone II, for example, a volar, zigzag approach designed to avoid the lines of stress or a lateral incision may be elected by the surgeon, the former being the more common. When approaching the lacerated tendon, the incision is made between the annular pulleys to ensure optimal excursion. This approach preserves the function of these fibrous sheaths, which encircle the finger flexors and keep the tendons close to the joints (preventing bowstringing of the tendon).

For a direct repair after the tendon ends are located, prepared, and re-opposed, there are a number of delicate techniques for suturing the tendons.[35,75,103,107,115–117] Core sutures and epitendinous sutures are used to hold the tendon ends together. Suturing technique and the number of suture strands influence the initial strength of the repair and consequently the type and timing of motion allowable postoperatively.[35,75,105,115–117] A larger number of suture strands across the repair site (e.g., four or six strands instead of two) produces a proportionally stronger repair. Running, locked epitendinous sutures used in addition to core sutures appear to further increase the initial strength of the repair.[103,107]

Suturing technique must also address the vascular supply to the repaired tendon. Nonreactive sutures are placed in the nonvascular volar aspect of the tendon so as not to disturb the vincula, which lies in the dorsal aspect of the tendon and provides a blood supply to the tendon.[35,75,105,115–117] When present, as in zones II and IV, the synovial sheath is also repaired to re-establish circulation of synovial fluid, an important source of nutrition to the healing tendons.[115]

After all repairs have been completed, the incision(s) are closed, and the hand and wrist are immobilized in a bulky compression dressing and elevated to control edema. The compression dressing remains in place for 1 to 3 days. When the bulky surgical dressing is removed, it is replaced with a light compressive dressing and splint.

### Postoperative Management

***General considerations.*** After surgical intervention for a flexor tendon injury, a strong, well-healed tendon that glides freely is the cornerstone for restoring functional mobility and strength in the hand.[47,89,115–117] Every effort is made to prevent excursion-restricting adhesions from forming while simultaneously protecting the repaired tendon as it heals. Box 19.12 summarizes the factors that contribute to adhesion formation after tendon repair.[35,47,55,54,79,89,105,116]

Many of the same patient-related and injury-related factors, already noted, that a surgeon weighs when determining the most appropriate approach to surgical management for a patient's hand injury also influence the complex components and progression of postoperative rehabilitation. In addition, surgery-related factors, including the type and timing of the repair, suturing technique, strength of the tendon repair, and the need for concomitant operative procedures affect rehabilitation and eventual outcomes. Furthermore, therapy-related factors—in particular the timing of when therapy is initiated, the use of early or delayed mobilization procedures, the quality of splinting, the expertise of the therapist, and ultimately the quality and consistency of the patient's involvement in the rehabilitation process—influence outcomes.

Extensive research has been done on the process of tendon healing, the tensile strength of tendon repairs, adhesion formation, and tendon excursion and imposed stresses (loading) on a repaired tendon during digital motion. A number of sources provide an in-depth analysis and sum-

mary of basic and clinical studies, typically animal and cadaveric but some in vivo human studies, as they apply to rehabilitation.[25,35,47,54,55,89,105,115–117]

The purpose of this section is to examine and summarize current concepts and approaches to immobilization and exercise used in rehabilitation after flexor tendon injury and repair, rather than to put forth or ascribe to any one particular approach or protocol. Therapists treating patients after tendon repair must be familiar with the various postoperative protocols or guidelines used by referring hand surgeons and those described in the literature.

A therapist's knowledge of the underlying concepts in any protocol is essential for effective communication with the surgeon. A therapist's skill in applying and teaching exercise procedures is equally necessary for effective patient education and helping a patient achieve optimal functional outcomes. This knowledge enables a therapist to make sound clinical judgments to determine when progression of activities in a protocol preferred by a referring surgeon is safe or when activities must be adjusted based on each patient's responses. Remember, a regimented protocol is only safe and effective when there are no postoperative variables, a situation that certainly does not occur in the clinical setting.

***Approaches to postoperative management.*** There are two basic approaches to management after flexor tendon repair characterized by the timing and type of exercises in the program. They are categorized as *early controlled motion*, either passive or active, and *delayed motion*.

Numerous published protocols with considerable variability fall within these categories. Most current-day programs emphasize early controlled (protected) motion after surgery and include both passive and active exercises of the operated digit(s). Advances in surgical management (in particular, improved suturing technique) that establish a relatively strong initial tendon repair allow the use of early motion.

 **Focus on Evidence** _____

Tottenham and colleagues[128] studied 22 patients who underwent primary zone II flexor tendon repairs. Half of the patients began passive motion exercises of the operated fingers by the first 7 days after surgery, whereas the other half began passive motion 7 to 21 days postoperatively. The results of the study, based on several assessment measures of motion and function, indicated that there was a significant difference between groups, with all of the early motion group but only 75% of the delayed motion group achieving "excellent or good" results (i.e., 25% of the delayed motion group had only "fair or poor" results). The investigators noted that nonrandomization and the small size of the groups were limitations of their study.

---

Box 19.13 summarizes the rationale for early, but carefully graded, motion as soon as a day or two after tendon repair based on three to four decades of evidence derived

---

| BOX 19.12 | Factors that Contribute to Adhesion Formation After Tendon Injury and Repair |
|---|---|

- Location of the injury and repair: higher risk in zones II and IV; tendons glide in a closely confined area
- Extent of trauma: higher risk with extensive trauma and damage to associated structures
- Reduced blood supply, subsequent ischemia, and reduced nutrition to healing tendons
- Excessive handling of damaged tissues during surgery
- Ineffective suturing technique
- Damage or resection of components of the tendon sheath
- Prolonged immobilization after injury or repair, which prevents tendon-gliding
- Gapping of the repaired tendon ends associated with *excessive* stress to the healing tendon

---

**BOX 19.13    Rationale for Early Controlled Motion After Tendon Repair**

- Decreases postoperative edema.
- Maintains tendon-gliding and decreases the formation of adhesions that can limit tendon excursion and that consequently limit functional ROM. Gliding deteriorates by 10 days after repair when a tendon is immobilized.
- Increases synovial fluid diffusion for tissue nutrition, which increases the rate of tendon healing.
- Increases wound maturation and the tensile strength of the repaired tendon more rapidly than continuous immobilization by means of *appropriate-level* stresses achieved with early tendon motion. The repair site loses strength during the first 2 weeks after surgery.
- Decreases gap formation at the repair site, which in turn increases the tensile strength of the repair.

---

from scientific studies.[25,27,35,47,54,89,103,107,115–117] However, there are instances when a traditional, delayed motion approach must be used. Indications for prolonged (3 to 4 weeks) immobilization after tendon repair (and therefore delayed motion) are noted in Box 19.14.[17,33,86,89,105,115,116]

Key elements of early passive and active motion approaches and the delayed motion approach with regard to immobilization and selection and progression of exercises are presented in the following sections. More detailed descriptions of these approaches, as well as specific protocols, advocated by various practitioners and researchers, are available in many sources.*

With all approaches, the postoperative goals and interventions for pain reduction, edema control, and mainte-

---

*See references 17, 24, 25, 27, 35, 42, 44, 46–48, 63, 67, 79, 89, 103, 106, 107, 112, 114–117, 129.

---

**BOX 19.14    Indications for Use of Prolonged Immobilization and Delayed Motion After Flexor Tendon Repair**

- Patients who are unable to comprehend and actively participate in an early controlled motion exercise program. This includes:
  - Children less than 7 to 10 years of age
  - Patients with diminished cognitive capacity associated with head injury, developmental disability, or psychological impairment
- Patients who have the cognitive ability to understand and follow an early controlled motion program but who are unlikely to adhere to the program
  - The unmotivated patient
  - The overzealous, impatient individual with a history of a previously failed repair
- Patients in whom repair of other hand injuries or surgeries necessitates extended immobilization of the hand

---

nance of function in uninvolved regions (e.g., the elbow and shoulder) are consistent with management employing other operative procedures previously discussed in this chapter. Patient education is of the utmost importance for effective outcomes after hand surgery.

N O T E : Unless otherwise noted, the guidelines described in this section for immobilization and exercise are for injury and primary repair or one-stage tendon grafts of the FDS and/or FDP muscle-tendon units in zones I, II, and III. The guidelines are similar but not addressed for zones T-I and T-II of the thumb. Postoperative guidelines for multistage or late reconstructions are progressed in a similar but more cautious manner. Refer to other resources for this information.[55,89,105]

**Immobilization**
The duration, type, and position of immobilization must be considered.

***Duration of immobilization.*** With some exceptions previously noted (see Box 19.14) when prolonged immobilization (3 to 4 weeks) is necessary, the repaired tendon is continuously immobilized after surgery for up to 5 days while the bulky compression dressing is kept in place. This allows some time for postoperative edema to decrease.

***Type or method of immobilization.*** This usually depends on the preference of the hand surgeon and therapist, the approach to postoperative exercise, and the stage of tissue healing. If motion of the operated digit is to be delayed for 3 to 4 weeks, a cast or static splint provides the immobilization. Early controlled motion approaches require the fabrication of different types of customized splint.

There are three general types of splint used after flexor tendon repair: a static dorsal blocking splint[27,42,47,89,112,116]; a dorsal blocking splint with dynamic traction, originally proposed by Kleinert and colleagues[63,67] and subsequently modified and improved by clinicians and researchers[47,89,107,112]; and a dorsal tenodesis splint with a wrist hinge.[24,25,115–117] Descriptions of these static and dynamic splinting techniques for immobilization and/or exercise are noted in Box 19.15. Figure 19.13 shows an example of a dorsal blocking splint with dynamic traction. The splint allows active extension of the involved finger, and the elastic band passively returns the finger to a flexed position. (See Figure 19.14A for a depiction of a dorsal tenodesis splint.)

***Position of immobilization.*** The typical position of immobilization for repairs in zones I, II, and III is wrist and MCP flexion coupled with PIP and DIP extension. This position prevents full lengthening and undue stress on the repaired FDS and/or FDP tendons while minimizing the risk of IP flexion contractures. The recommended degrees of wrist and MCP flexion differ somewhat from one source to another. Recommended positions range from 10° to 45° of wrist flexion and from 40° to 70° of MCP flexion with the IP joints in full but comfortable extension.[24,25,27,35,42,47,89,112,115–117] The wrist typically is positioned in less flexion than the MCP joints. The trend over the years has been

## BOX 19.15 Static and Dynamic Dorsal Blocking Splints: Position and Use

### Static dorsal blocking splint
- Covers the dorsal surface of the entire hand and the distal forearm (the thumb is free).
- Positioned in wrist and MCP flexion and IP extension to avoid excessive tension on the repaired flexor tendon. The degrees of flexion vary with the philosophy of the surgeon or therapist and the approach (protocol) used.
- Straps across the volar aspect of the hand and forearm hold wrist and fingers in this position.
- Restricts wrist and MCP extension.
- Is worn during early phases of rehabilitation. Splint is loosened or removed for early exercises.
- Also worn as a protective night splint.

### Dorsal blocking splint with dynamic traction
- Allows early motion of the operated joint while the hand is in the splint.
- Elastic band (or nylon line with a rubber band) is attached to the nail of the operated finger (or all four fingers), pass-es under a palmar bar that acts as a pulley, and then attaches proximally at the wrist.
- At rest, the elastic band provides dynamic traction that holds the operated finger in flexion.
- Allows *active extension* of the IP joints to the surface of the dorsal splint.
- When PIP and DIP extensors relax, the tension from the elastic band pulls on the finger, causing *passive flexion*.

### Dorsal tenodesis splint with wrist hinge
- Worn *exclusively* for exercise sessions
- No dynamic traction with elastic bands.
- Allows full wrist flexion and limited (approximately 30°) wrist extension but maintains the MCP joints in at least 60° of flexion and the IP joints in full extension when the straps are secured.
- When the straps across the fingers are loosened during exercise, allows active wrist extension initially during passive IP flexion and later when finger flexion is maintained for several seconds by a static contraction of the IP flexors.

---

to fabricate splints in less wrist and MCP flexion than early protocols recommended to increase patient comfort and reduce the risk of carpal tunnel syndrome.[47,89]

Positioning after a zone IV repair typically is 70° MCP flexion and a neutral position of the wrist.[89]

#### Exercise—Early Controlled Motion Approaches
There are two basic approaches to the application of early, controlled motion to maintain tendon-gliding and prevent tendon adhesions after flexor tendon repair: early passive motion and early active motion. The way in which passive or active motion of the repaired tendon is achieved, however, varies among protocols.

***Early controlled passive motion.*** Historically, the use of early passive motion is based on the work of Duran and Houser[42] and that of Kleinert et al.[63,67] Both proposed early passive flexion of the IP joints within a protected range

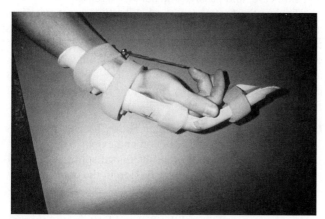

**FIGURE 19.13** A dorsal blocking splint with dynamic traction for early controlled motion after flexor tendon repair.

postoperatively but used different approaches to splinting and exercise. Duran advocated use of a static dorsal blocking splint and early removal of the splint or loosening of the stabilization straps for passive ROM exercise of the IP joints of the operated finger(s). Kleinert and colleagues[63,67] advanced use of a dorsal splint with dynamic traction, for early exercise (see Fig. 19.13). Within the confines of the splint, the patient performs *active extension* of the operated finger. The elastic band returns the finger to a flexed position with each repetition after the finger extensors relax, thus causing excursion of the repaired tendon without active tension in the finger flexors. A manual push into maximum DIP flexion may be added to increase passive flexion.

NOTE: When a dynamic traction splint is used during the day, a static splint is worn at night that holds the IP joints in neutral and the wrist and MCP joints in flexion to prevent IP flexion contractures.

These original passive motion protocols have been modified over the past three decades. Today, some surgeons and therapists use selected elements (splinting and/or exercise) of these passive motion approaches.[25,27,47,89,129] However, use of early *active* motion that imposes controlled stresses on the repaired tendon is gradually replacing passive motion approaches.[115]

***Early controlled active motion.*** The primary feature that distinguishes an early active motion from an early passive motion approach is the use of *minimum-tension, active contractions* of the repaired muscle-tendon units initiated during the acute stage of tissue healing, often by the first 24 to 48 hours but no later than 5 days postoperatively.[25,46,47,103,106,107,115–117] Some passive exercises also are incorporated into active regimens.

Based primarily on experimental studies using animal models, it is hypothesized that gentle stresses placed on a repaired tendon by means of a very low-intensity static or dynamic muscle contraction, which "pulls" the repaired tendon through its sheath, is a more effective method of creating tendon excursion (gliding) than "pushing" the tendon with passive motion.[46,47,54,105,107,115,116] Early active motion has become more widely accepted because stronger suturing techniques produce a repair that can withstand early, controlled stresses.

PRECAUTION: Proponents of early, active tendon mobilization caution that this approach is recommended only for primary tendon repairs, using the stronger four- and six-strand core and epitendinous suture techniques (in contrast to conventional, two-strand suturing) in carefully selected patients who have access to rehabilitation with an experienced hand therapist and who are most likely to adhere to the prescribed exercise and splinting regimen.[24,25,46,47,54,89,116,117]

There are two ways in which early active motion can be implemented. Both methods are founded on an analysis and application of evidence in the scientific literature on tendon repair and healing, tendon excursion, and imposed loading on repaired tendons.[103,106,107,115–117] One approach uses "place-and-hold" exercises by means of *static* muscle contractions to generate active tension of the finger flexors and impose controlled stress on the repaired tendon. (Place-and-hold exercises are described in the phase-specific exercises that follow.) This approach to early active motion is used in the Indiana protocol.[24,25,79,115–117] The other approach to early active motion, developed by Evans,[46,47] and others[103,106,107] uses *dynamic*, short-arc, minimum muscle tension exercises to impose initially low-intensity stresses on the healing tendon.

A recently developed conceptual model for the use of early active motion and application of progressive forces to the healing tendon after flexor tendon repair, proposed by Groth,[54] combines elements of both of the aforementioned approaches. In addition, in the rationale for this model Groth discusses the effects of each level of exercise on internal tendon loads and tendon excursion supported by key evidence from the literature when available. A unique feature of this model is that it is criterion-based, rather than time-based. By providing criteria for progressing exercises based on optimal tendon loading, this program provides a mechanism for an individualized sequence of exercises adjusted for each patient rather than using predetermined timelines for progression.

The model contains eight progressive levels of active exercises, from the least to the greatest levels of loading on the tendon. The sequence is preceded by warm-up exercises (slow, repetitive passive finger motions in protected ranges). As with other early active motion approaches, exercises are begun during the first few days after surgery and are progressed until conclusion of postoperative rehabilitation. Box 19.16 describes the eight-level sequence of exercises in Groth's conceptual model.[54]

Descriptions and a progression of early active exercises during maximum, moderate, and minimum protection

---

| **BOX 19.16** | **A Sequence of Exercises for Early Active Motion with Progressive Tendon Loading after Flexor Tendon Repair[54]** |

**Warm-up**
Warm-up exercises (passive finger motions within protected ranges) precedes each exercise session.

**Progressive Levels of Exercise***
- Level 1—place-and-hold finger flexion
- Level 2—active composite finger flexion
- Level 3—hook and straight fist finger flexion
- Level 4—isolated finger joint motion
- Level 5—continuation of levels 1–4 of exercise and discontinuation of protective splinting with introduction of gradually increasing use of the hand for functional activities
- Level 6—resisted composite finger flexion
- Level 7—resisted hook and straight fist exercises
- Level 8—resisted isolated joint motion.

*Note: Exercise sequence is from least to greatest tendon loading. Repetitions are highest at the lowest level of loading and least at the highest level of loading. Progression to next level occurs when specific criteria are met.

---

phases of rehabilitation after *zone I, II, or III flexor tendon repairs*, drawn from several resources, are presented in the following sections. Then, key features of a delayed motion approach to management are summarized.

**Exercise: Maximum Protection Phase**
The maximum protection phase begins 1 to 3 days postoperatively and continues for the first 3 to 5 weeks, the period of time when the tendon repair is weakest. The goals of this phase of rehabilitation are control of pain and edema and protection of the newly repaired tendon while imposing very low-level, controlled stresses on the tendon to maintain adequate tendon gliding and prevent adhesions that can restrict tendon excursion. Interventions in this phase include elevating the hand, splint use and care, wound management and skin care, and passive and active exercises.

During the first phase of rehabilitation, most exercises are performed in a static dorsal blocking splint or in a wrist tenodesis splint (Fig. 19.14A) specifically designed for exercise. With both types of splint, the stabilization straps are loosened to allow finger flexion. The following exercises are performed frequently during the day and continue for about the first 4 weeks.

- **Passive ROM exercises.** On an hourly basis perform passive MCP, PIP, and DIP flexion and extension of each individual joint to the extent the dorsal splint allows, followed by composite passive flexion in the confines of the splint. Composite flexion can include passive movements into full fist and straight fist positions.
- Independent motions of the PIP and DIP joints achieve *differential gliding* of the FDP and FDS tendons. For

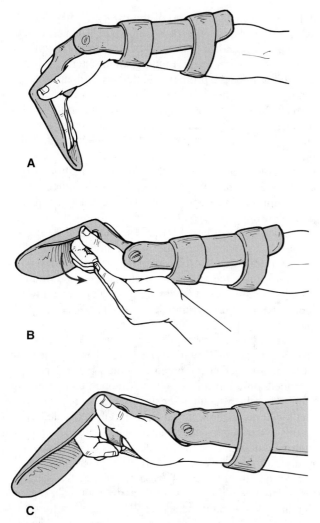

**FIGURE 19.14** Splinting and exercise for early active motion post-flexor tendon repair. (*A*) Following removal of the surgical compression dressing and fabrication of a static dorsal blocking splint, a tenodesis splint with a wrist hinge is fabricated. (*B*) The tenodesis splint allows full wrist flexion but limits wrist extension to 30°. During early movement of the fingers, the MCP joints are maintained in at least 60° of flexion as the IP joints are passively moved and placed in composite flexion. (*C*) Then the patient actively extends the wrist while maintaining the flexed finger position with a static muscle contraction and the least amount of tension possible in the finger flexors. *(From Strickland, JW: Flexor tendon injuries. In Strickland, JW, Graham, TJ [eds] Master Techniques in Orthopedic Surgery—The Hand, ed 2. Lippincott Williams & Wilkins, Philadelphia, 2005, p 262, with permission.)*

example, the DIP joint must be flexed and extended separately while each PIP joint is stabilized in flexion. In this way, as the DIP joint is passively extended, the FDP repair site glides distally, away from the FDS repair.[89,114]

PRECAUTION: It is essential to maintain the MCP joints in flexion during passive ROM of the IP joints to avoid excessive stretch of the repair site, which could cause gapping of the re-opposed tendon ends during IP extension.

● ***Place-and-hold exercises.*** Many programs initiate place-and-hold exercises of the repaired digit with the patient wearing either a dorsal blocking splint[46,47,107] or a tenodesis splint.[24,25,54,115–117] With the MCP joints in flexion, passively place the IP joints in a partially flexed position and have the patient hold the position independently for 5 seconds with a minimum static contraction of the finger flexors. If the patient is wearing a tenodesis splint, combine place-and-hold finger flexion with active wrist extension (Fig. 19.14 B&C). Have the patient relax and allow the wrist to passively flex and the digits to passively extend. Initially, have the patient practice this with the uninjured hand or use biofeedback to learn how to hold the position with a minimum of force production in the FDP and FDS.

### ◉ Focus on Evidence _____

Research has shown that it is preferable to perform place-and-hold exercises with the wrist extended and the MCP joints placed in flexion because wrist extension is the position in which the IP joints can be moved by contraction of the FDS and FDP with the *least* amount of contraction force and, therefore, a very low-level load on the repaired tendon.[102]

---

● ***Minimum-tension, short-arc motion.*** Some programs begin active, dynamic finger flexion during the first few days after surgery if the suturing technique and strength of the repair allow.[44,46,47] Active contractions that generate minimum tension, just enough tension to overcome the resistance of the extensors and cause flexor tendon excursion, are performed with the wrist in slight extension and the MCP joints flexed.

### Exercise: Moderate Protection Phase
The moderate protection phase begins at about 4 weeks and continues until 8 weeks postoperatively. The focus during this phase is on safely increasing stresses on the repaired tendon, achieving full active flexion and extension of the wrist and digits, and differential gliding of the tendons. If a tenodesis splint was worn for early active exercises, it is discontinued at the beginning of this phase. However, use of the static dorsal blocking splint continues during the day except for exercise until at least 6 to 8 weeks. Use of a night splint continues for protection or to decrease or prevent a flexion contracture. Exercises include:

● ***Place-and-hold exercises.*** Continuation of place-and-hold exercises but with gradually increasing tension.
● ***Active ROM.*** Continuation or initiation of active composite flexion and extension of the IP joints with the MCP joints flexed, MCP flexion/extension with the IP joints relaxed, and active wrist flexion and extension with the fingers relaxed.
● ***Tendon-gliding and blocking exercises.*** These exercises are initiated at about 5 to 6 weeks (see Fig. 19.17A–E, Fig. 19.18 A–C, and descriptions in the final section of this chapter).

PRECAUTION: Avoid finger extension combined with wrist extension for about 6 to 8 weeks, as this position places extreme tension on the repaired flexor tendon.

### Exercise: Minimum Protection/Return to Function Phase

The minimum protection/return to function phase begins at approximately 8 weeks postoperatively and is characterized by gradual but progressive use of resistance exercises to improve strength and endurance, dexterity exercises, and use of the hand for light (1 to 2 lb) functional activities. (Refer to the final section of this chapter for suggested exercises and activities.)

Protective splinting is discontinued, but intermittent splinting may be necessary if the patient has a persistent extensor lag or flexion contracture. After primary flexor tendon repairs, most patients return to full activity by 12 weeks after surgery.

### Exercise: Delayed Motion Approach

In instances where continuous immobilization of a repaired flexor tendon extends for 3 to 4 weeks (indications already noted in Box 19.14), some degree of tendon healing and adhesion formation already has occurred by the time exercises can be initiated.

PRECAUTION: Despite the extended period of immobilization, at 3 to 4 weeks the tendon repair must still be protected in a dorsal blocking splint, and exercises must be performed in protected positions and progressed gradually.

Exercises such as passive ROM, tendon-blocking and tendon-gliding, and active ROM can be initiated when the cast is removed. Exercises used in early motion approaches are appropriate. The reader also is referred to additional resources that provide detailed exercise programs when delayed mobilization is necessary.[17,89,112]

### Outcomes

*Functional outcomes.* There is a substantial body of evidence on flexor tendon repairs, some of which is based on longitudinal clinical outcome studies.[35,55,105,115,116] One review of the literature[115] indicated that with the advances made in flexor tendon surgery and rehabilitation techniques over the past few decades, recovery of good or excellent function can be expected in 80% or more of patients after flexor tendon injury and repair. Two factors that have contributed considerably to a high rate of favorable outcomes are the use of improved suturing techniques that produce a strong repair site and implementation of early motion in rehabilitation programs.

There are several quantitative assessment tools used in outcome studies of tendon repair.[89] It is helpful to become familiar with the more frequently used assessments in order to understand the findings of studies. With some of these tools, results are reported as excellent, good, fair, and poor. For the most part, these terms are not simply subjective descriptors but, rather, are associated with objective measurement tools. For example, in the Strickland system[43,89] the terms refer to a percentage of "normal" total active motion (total active flexion minus

deficits in active extension) of the PIP and DIP joints achieved after zone I, II, or III repairs and rehabilitation.

Some generalizations can be made about outcomes after flexor tendon repair. Findings in the literature indicate that immediate primary and delayed primary repairs (up to 10 days after injury) yield equally positive outcomes.[105] However, late reconstructions and multistage reconstructions, not surprisingly, result in poorer outcomes (less active and passive ROM, greater functional limitations) than primary repairs.[105] This is consistent with the findings that the greater the severity and number of associated injuries, the less favorable are the outcomes.[116]

Studies dating back to the 1980s have documented that the use of 4 weeks of uninterrupted immobilization leads to a slower return of tensile strength in the repaired tendon and greater adhesion formation than the use of early mobilization.[35] Although extended immobilization continues to be the treatment of choice for children under 7 to 10 years of age, a recent study indicated that the incidence of chronic contractures or diminished hand function is minimal in this age group.[86]

Studies of various approaches to early motion, passive or active, after flexor tendon repair demonstrate superior outcomes when compared with outcomes after extended immobilization.[27,104,128] Although the use of early motion in rehabilitation after flexor tendon repair has been well documented for more than two to three decades, the results of early active motion compared with early passive motion continue to be investigated. In one such study, carried out retrospectively, a "passive flexion–active extension" program of exercises in a dynamic traction splint was compared with a "controlled active motion" program that included therapist-supervised, active contractions of the repaired FDS and FDP muscle-tendon units.[7] The investigators reported that although there were no significant differences in outcomes (total active flexion and active extension deficit) 16 weeks after surgery between groups in patients who had zone I repairs there were substantial differences between groups in patients with zone II repairs. In the "passive flexion– active extension" group, 50% of patients had good or excellent results, whereas 94% of patients in the "controlled active motion" group had good or excellent results. In addition, 39.7% of the passive flexion group had an active extension deficit >15°, but only 10.5% of the active flexion group had an extensor lag 4 months after repair.

A comparable percentage of excellent and good outcomes for total active motion was reported in a 9-year, prospective follow-up study of 130 patients with zone I and II repairs who began supervised active exercises, including minimal-tension IP flexion and extension (detailed in the study), the day after surgery. Patients also performed active extension exercises in a dynamic traction splint regularly during the day. At the conclusion of the study, 92% of the patients had excellent and good results.[62]

*Complications.* The most frequent early complication after surgery is rupture of the repaired tendon, and the most frequent late complication is flexion contracture or a deficit in active extension of the repaired DIP and/or PIP joints, typically associated with tendon adhesions.[35,117] Rupture may occur because of strong gripping activities, but it also may occur while the patient is asleep if the hand is unprotected during the first few months after surgery.

Although there is general agreement that early motion after tendon repair reduces adhesion formation, there are concerns that implementing early active flexion, which places active tension on the newly repaired tendon, may increase the risk of tendon rupture. Overall, however, rupture rates are low and appear to be relatively equal to those seen with early passive flexion/active extension and early active flexion/extension programs.[115] In studies that have used passive flexion/active extension exercise in a dynamic traction splint, rupture rates have ranged from 3.0%[7,67] to 6.8%.[27] In patients using dynamic traction splinting, who also have participated in a variety of early active exercises, including active flexion, rupture rates have been reported at 3.6%,[107] 5.0%,[7] and 5.7%.[62]

## Lacerated Extensor Tendons of the Hand: Surgical and Postoperative Management

### Background and Indications for Surgery
Laceration and traumatic rupture of the extensor tendons of the fingers, thumb, or wrist are more common than in the flexor tendons.[41] Their superficial location makes the extensor tendons vulnerable to damage when trauma occurs to the dorsum of the hand. Furthermore, extensor tendons in the digits are substantially thinner than flexor tendons, making them more prone to traumatic rupture.[41,84,97]

As with the flexor surface, the extensor surface of the hand, wrist, and forearm is divided into zones (Fig. 19.15). The dorsal surface of the fingers and wrist are divided into seven zones, and the thumb is divided into four zones. Each of these zones is identified by specific anatomical landmarks, as noted in Box 19.17.[41,43,53,84,97] The odd-number zones correspond to the location of the DIP, PIP, MCP, and wrist joint regions. Although not depicted in Figure 19.15, the dorsal surface of the distal and middle forearm are often identified as zones VIII and IX, respectively. The area at the CMC joint of the thumb is often identified as zone T-V.[84]

The extensor mechanism of the hand and wrist is complex. The structural characteristics of these mechanisms vary in each zone. Damage in one zone produces compensatory imbalances in adjacent zones. Knowledge of the anatomy and kinesiology of the extensor mechanism is basic to an understanding of how a patient's physical impairments and functional limitations occur according to the structures damaged in each zone. Box 19.18 identifies key structures and characteristic impairments associated with tendon rupture or laceration by zone.[41,43,84,97,114] Of all the extensor zones, injuries in zones III and VII pose the greatest surgical and rehabilitation problems and challenges.

Depending on the type and location of injury to the extensor mechanism and the extent of associated skeletal,

joint, vascular, or nerve damage, surgery may or may not be indicated. The tendons of the extensor system distal to the dorsum of the hand have many soft tissue attachments along various structures, making extensor tendons far less likely to retract when lacerated or ruptured than flexor tendons.[41,84,97] Consequently, with a rupture (closed injury) or a simple laceration in a peripheral zone, the tendon is re-opposed and managed by uninterrupted immobilization in a splint or cast for 6 weeks as it heals.[41,97] For example, this is a common course of treatment for a *mallet finger* (or thumb) deformity, which is a closed rupture of the terminal extensor tendon in zone I usually from forceful hyperflexion.[84]

| BOX 19.17 | Extensor Tendon Zones: Anatomic Landmarks |

**Zones of the Dorsal Surfaces of the Fingers, Hand, Wrist and Forearm**
- I—DIP joint region
- II—middle phalanx
- III—PIP joint region
- IV—proximal phalanx
- V—apex of the MCP joint region
- VI—dorsum of the hand
- VII—wrist region/dorsal retinaculum
- VIII and IX—distal and middle forearm

**Zones of the Thumb**
- T-I—IP joint region
- T-II—proximal phalanx
- T-III—MCP joint region
- T-IV—metacarpal
- T-V—carpometacarpal joint region

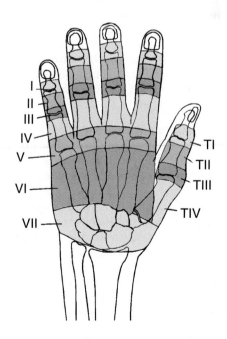

Dorsal

FIGURE 19.15 Extensor tendon zones; dorsal aspect of the hand and wrist.

## BOX 19.18    Consequences of Injury to the Dorsal Structures of the Hand and Wrist

- *Zones I and II.* Damage to the terminal extensor leads to inability to actively extend the DIP joint (extensor lag) and eventual DIP flexion contracture and deformity (mallet finger). A swan-neck deformity secondary to an unopposed central slip and migration of the extensor mechanisms proximally may also develop. Damage in those zones is usually the result of a closed rupture rather than a laceration.
- *Zones III and IV.* Damage to the central slip tendon and possibly the lateral bands results in an inability to actively extend the PIP joint from a 90° flexed position. Flexion contracture of the PIP joint and eventually a boutonnière deformity develops as the lateral bands slip volarward and cause hyperextension of the DIP joint.
- *Zone V.* Damage to the common extensor tendons (EDC), extensor indicis proprius (EIP), and extensor digiti minimi (EDM), and sagittal bands that surround the MCP joints cause inability to actively extend the MCP joints, eventually resulting in MCP flexion contractures.

- *Zones VI and VII.* The juncturae tendium along the dorsum of the hand (VI) and the dorsal retinaculum (VII) under which multiple extensor tendons of the wrist and digits pass in close proximity can be damaged. A bowstring effect occurs in the extensor tendons if the retinaculum, which acts as a pulley, is lacerated. The synovial sheath through which the tendons glide in zone VII can also be damaged, subsequently compromising synovial diffusion and nutrition to the tendons. Injuries in zones VI and VII can result in loss of extension of the digits and wrist.
- *T-I and T-II.* Damage to the EPL and possibly the EPB (if laceration is in the proximal region of the proximal phalanx) leads to loss of hyperextension of the IP joint (mallet thumb deformity) and weakened MCP extension.
- *T-III and T-IV.* Damage to EPB leads to weakened MCP extension and transfers extension forces to IP joint, leading to a flexion deformity of the MCP joint and a hyperextension deformity of the IP joint if the EPL is intact.

Nevertheless, surgical intervention, even for a simple distal tendon injury, usually is necessary to restore active ROM, muscular balance, strength, and function to the hand and prevent contractures and deformity. Although the extensor muscles of the digits are substantially weaker than the flexors, an intact extensor mechanism is essential for functional grasp.

### Procedures

***Types of repairs.*** Surgical options for extensor tendon repair include a direct (end-to-end) repair or a reconstruction. As with flexor tendon repair, surgeries are classified as *primary* (immediate or delayed up to 10 days), *secondary*, *late*, or *staged*.[22,41,84,97] These terms already have been defined in the previous section of this chapter on flexor tendon repair and rehabilitation. Operative procedures, such as tendon transfers, for ruptured, diseased extensor tendons associated with RA also were described earlier in the chapter.

***Overview of operative procedures.*** Although similarities of definition exist for extensor and flexor tendon procedures, there are substantial differences in operative techniques used to repair extensor versus flexor tendons. These differences are based largely on the fact that extensor tendons are morphologically thinner than flexor tendons. This fact led to the belief that extensor tendon repairs are more prone to gapping, have less tensile strength, and are more likely to rupture than flexor tendons after repairs. However, stronger suturing techniques, specifically designed for extensor tendon repair and reconstruction, are used more frequently today, allowing early postoperative mobilization of the repaired tendon while lessening concerns of gapping and rupture.[41,43,111]

Operative procedures for repair of lacerated or ruptured extensor tendons vary significantly in the distal versus the proximal zones. In this overview only repair of a zone III/IV laceration (the most common cause of injury in these zones) is described, simply as an example. Detailed descriptions of operative techniques for primary repair and late reconstruction of extensor tendons in all zones of the hand, wrist, and forearm can be found in several sources.[9,22,41,53,84,97]

With an acute laceration of the PIP joint and middle phalanx, the wound often enters the joint space. Therefore, the area must be débrided, cleansed, and treated with antibiotics. The central slip, which refers to the extensor mechanism in zones III and IV, then can be managed with a direct repair.[41,53,84] The severed tendon is repaired and then sutured into the fibrocartilaginous dorsal plate of the middle phalanx, which is thicker and holds sutures better than the central slip, thereby producing a stronger repair.[41]

NOTE: The suturing and repair technique in zones III/IV may decrease the overall length of the tendon by 2 to 3 mm, causing a loss of 2° to 5° of PIP flexion.[84]

If damaged, the lateral bands are repaired. If a boutonnière deformity is evident or likely to develop, a K-wire may be inserted to immobilize the PIP joint in extension for about 3 weeks and then be removed. After closure of the area, a bulky compression dressing immobilizes the repaired tissues and controls edema.

### Postoperative Management

***General considerations.*** The overall goal of postoperative rehabilitation after extensor tendon injury and repair is the same as after flexor tendon repair—that is, to restore mobility and strength to the hand and wrist for functional activities. Adhesion formation is a concern in the extensor tendons after repair, just as it is after repair of the flexor tendons. As noted previously, extensor tendons of the fingers are less likely to retract after laceration or rupture because of the extensor mechanism's multiple soft tissue linkages to surrounding structures. However, these attachments make extensor tendons prone to adhesion formation and loss of excursion during the healing process. At the level of the dorsum of the hand, although the extensor tendons are relatively mobile, they also are surrounded by synovial sheaths to which they may adhere if immobilized over a period of time.[41,84,97] As with management after flexor tendon repair, emphasis after extensor tendon repair is placed on preventing adhesions that restrict tendon gliding and limit joint ROM and functional use of the hand. (Refer to Box 19.12 to review factors that contribute to adhesion formation.)

The components and progression of postoperative rehabilitation and eventual outcomes after extensor tendon repair are influenced by many of the same factors that influence rehabilitation and outcomes of flexor tendon repair, including the location (level) and severity of the injury, the specifics of the surgical procedure(s), particularly the type of suturing technique and strength of the repair, and the timing of and the patient's access and commitment to a supervised rehabilitation program with an experienced hand therapist.[26,43,111,114,129]

***Approaches to postoperative management.*** Two general approaches to rehabilitation after surgical repair of extensor tendon injuries are described in the literature: prolonged, uninterrupted immobilization with motion of the injured region(s) delayed for 3 to 6 weeks or, in carefully selected patients, early controlled passive or active motion initiated during the first few postoperative days. The latter is based on the same rationale for early mobilization of flexor tendon repairs (see Box 19.13).

Historically, prolonged immobilization has been used more widely than early motion after extensor tendon repair, perhaps because of concerns that inadvertent but forceful or rapid movements could cause gapping or rupture of the repair if the splint or cast is removed early in the healing process[9] or simply that alternative forms of immobilization, such as dynamic splinting, are cumbersome and more costly for the patient.[92] Given these issues, the use of early motion after extensor tendon repair has evolved more slowly than it has for use after flexor tendon repair.

There are situations when an extended immobilization/delayed motion approach is the only appropriate method of management (see Box 19.14), and current studies continue to show that in many instances this traditional approach yields acceptable reults.[92] However, during the past two decades, some studies have shown that extensor tendon repairs, managed with prolonged immobilization, are more likely to develop adhesions, resulting in only marginal outcomes (increased incidence of extensor lag, joint contracture, boutonnière deformity).[28,85] In addition, these and other studies have demonstrated that early motion programs after *primary* repair of acute extensor tendon injuries in zones III and VII are effective and safe[18,19,34,44,45,56,60,99,124] and produce superior outcomes compared with prolonged immobilization/delayed motion programs.[28,34,44,85,99] Consequently, early motion approaches have become more widely used in recent years.

It should be noted, however, that prolonged immobilization continues to be the most frequently selected method of treating zone I and II extensor tendon injuries.[41,84,97] Late reconstruction, which is more complex and usually involves tendon grafts, also is managed in most cases with continuous, extended immobilization and delayed motion.[22]

The first early motion programs for extensor tendons involved passive mobilization, with dynamic extension splinting, which allows active flexion followed by passive extension (see Fig. 19.11).[28,45,85,99] In these programs, although active flexion is initiated just a few days after surgery, active digital extension at least at the level of the repair typically is delayed for 4 to 5 weeks.[18,19,28,34,56,99] For an explanation of dynamic extension splinting after extensor tendon repair, refer to the earlier section of this chapter on repair of tendon ruptures associated with RA.

Although dynamic extension splinting for early mobility of the extensor tendons continues to be used, there is a growing trend to incorporate controlled active extension into early mobilization programs.[26,43,44,60,124] Following a brief overview of immobilizaion procedures, key elements of early active motion and delayed motion approaches to rehabilitation after extensor tendon repair are presented.

### Immobilization

Immobilization typically is maintained with a volar (palmar) splint after the bulky surgical dressing is removed a few days postoperatively. The duration of immobilization, the type(s) of immobilization selected, the joints immobilized, and the position of immobilization are based on the location (zone) of the injury and repair and the structures involved.

***Duration of immobilization.*** If a patient is a good candidate for an early motion program, the duration of uninterrupted immobilization often is just a few days. If delayed motion is a more appropriate course of action, uninterrupted immobilization ranges from 3 to 6 weeks. In early motion programs, some type of protective splinting is used during exercise for about 6 weeks after surgery.

***Types of immobilization.*** Either static or dynamic splinting or a combination of both is used. Depending on the joints immobilized, a forearm and wrist-based or a hand-base splint is indicated to block excessive flexion at the region of the repair and prevent stretching of the repaired tendon(s). A static splint is considered a low-profile splint, whereas a dynamic splint (see Fig. 19.11) with its outrigger secured to the dorsal surface of the splint for the elastic band and sling attachments is a high-profile splint. The slings and elastic band attachments hold the digits in extension at rest but allow active flexion.

For a delayed motion program, a static volar or bivalved circumferential splint is fabricated and worn on a continuous basis (other than daily skin care). A dynamic splint, worn during the day for frequent exercise sessions, is an integral aspect of many early motion programs. At night a static splint is worn to protect the repair. However, some early active motion programs use only static splints that allow active motion when the straps are loosened but prevent excessive motion of joints. In some early active motion programs, special static template splints for the digits are fabricated and used only during exercises to limit the range of allowable motion (see Fig. 19.16).

The joints are immobilized in an extended position or a position that places only minimal tension on the tendon to protect the repair from excessive stretch and potential gapping. As examples, for a zone III/IV repair, the PIP and sometimes the DIP joints are placed in extension, but for a zone V/VI repair, the wrist is held in 30° of extension and the MCP joints in 30° to 45° of flexion. Recommended positions of the joints proximal or distal to the injured zone vary considerably. Several resources provide detailed information on immobilization and splinting procedures after extensor tendon repairs.[26,43,111]

### Exercise: Early Controlled Active Motion Approach

As interest in the application of early active motion after tendon repair has grown, so have the number of studies describing details of exercise programs and outcomes. In addition to one example of an early active motion program for zone III/IV repairs presented in this section, guidelines for early mobilization of zones V, VI, and VII also have been proposed and detailed in the literature.[26,43,60,111,124] The distinguishing feature common to all early active motion programs following extensor tendon repair is that low-intensity and controlled active contractions of the repaired muscle-tendon units are initiated during the first few postoperative days, albeit in the confines of some type of static volar splint.

As noted previously, extensor tendon repairs in zones III and IV are especially prone to adhesion formation because of multiple soft tissue attachments of the extensor mechanism to surrounding structures and the broad bone–tendon interface of the proximal phalanx along which the extensor mechanism must glide.[41,43,53,84,97] Evans[43,44] proposed an early motion program of splinting and exercise for repairs of the central slip that involves minimal active tension of the repaired extensors for controlled, short-arc motion of the PIP and DIP joints.

 **Focus on Evidence** _____

Evans[44] compared the results of a prolonged immobilization/delayed motion program and an early short-arc motion (SAM) program in 55 patients who had undergone primary repair of 64 fingers for injury of the central slip. Patients in one group (36 digits) were managed with 3 to 6 weeks (mean 32.9 days) of continuous immobilization, whereas patients in the early motion group (28 digits) began active motion in a protected range at 2 to 11 days (mean 4.59 days) after surgery. After 6 weeks of treatment, patients in the delayed motion group had significantly less PIP flexion (44°) than the early motion group (88°). At discharge, the delayed motion group continued to have significantly less PIP flexion (72° after 76 days) than the early motion group (88° at 51 days). In addition, at discharge the delayed motion group had significantly less DIP flexion than the early motion group (37.6° and 45.0°, respectively). It also is interesting to note that at discharge the delayed motion group compared to the early motion group had significantly greater PIP extensor lag (8.1° and 2.9° respectively). However, at the initiation of treatment, the delayed motion group had a 13° PIP extensor lag, whereas the early motion group had only a 3° lag.

Key elements of the early short-arc, active motion program for central slip repairs include the following splinting and exercise procedures.[26,43,44]

***Use of customized static volar splints.*** A static, hand-based volar splint is fabricated and applied as soon as the surgical dressing is removed. It holds only the PIP and DIP joints in 0° extension; the wrist and MCP joints are free. This splint is removed for exercise on an hourly basis during the day but replaced between exercise sessions. A forearm-based resting splint is worn at night for protection for at least 6 weeks postoperatively.

Two static, volar, finger-based, template splints are fabricated and worn only during exercise to limit joint motion extensor tendon excursion, and the level of stress on the repaired central slip. One splint (Fig. 19.16) is

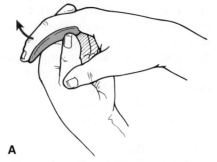
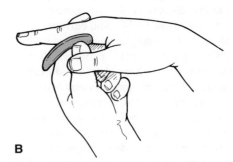

**A**    **B**

FIGURE 19.16 One of two static volar template splints used during early short-arc exercises of the PIP and DIP joints after repair of the extensor mechanism in zones III/IV. During exercise the patient actively holds the wrist in approximately 30° of flexion and manually holds the MCP joint in neutral to slight flexion. (*A*) Using minimal active tension during combined active PIP and DIP flexion, the splint initially limits PIP and DIP flexion to 30° and 20° to 25°, respectively, to prevent excessive stretch of the repair site. (*B*) The patient actively and slowly extends the PIP and DIP joints to full extension and briefly holds the extended position.

molded to limit PIP flexion to 30° and DIP flexion to 20° or 25° during exercise. A second template splint is fabricated to hold the PIP joint in full extension during isolated DIP flexion limited to 30° to 35°.

The PIP exercise splint is revised during the second week of exercise to allow 40° of flexion if no extensor lag is present. The PIP flexion allowed by the splint is increased incrementally by 10° each week thereafter.

***Exercise progression.*** The patient is taught the concept of minimum active tension (MAT) to protect healing tissues during tendon excursion. MAT is just enough tension generated during an active muscle contraction to overcome the elastic resistance of an antagonist.[44] Exercises are initiated within the first few postoperative days and performed hourly during the day. While actively holding the wrist in 30° of flexion and manually stabilizing the MCP joint in neutral to slight flexion, the patient performs active PIP and DIP flexion within the limits allowed by the PIP exercise splint (see Fig. 19.16A), followed by full active extension held for several seconds (see Fig. 19.16B). The patient also performs active, isolated DIP flexion/extension in the second volar template splint that stabilizes the PIP joint in full extension.

Exercises continue regularly during the day for several weeks using revised exercise splints. Ideally, by the end of 4 weeks the patient achieves 70° to 80° of active flexion and full extension of the PIP joint. Composite MCP, PIP, and DIP flexion (full fist) is postponed for at least 4 weeks or when the exercise splints have been discontinued. By 6 to 8 weeks, low-intensity resisted exercises are initiated along with gradual use of the hand for functional activities.

### Exercise: Delayed Mobilization Approach

If a traditional approach to postoperative management of extensor tendon repairs is used, exercises are delayed for at least several weeks after surgery. Special considerations and precautions for exercise using a delayed motion approach are summarized by zones in Box 19.19.[17,26,43,48,92,111,129]

Guidelines for resistance exercises to strengthen the hand and continuation or modification of splinting for protection are not addressed in this summary. In general, splinting is continued during the day if an extensor lag persists and at night for protection for about 12 weeks. If grasp is limited because of insufficient finger flexion, passive stretching is initiated, or dynamic flexor splinting may be incorporated into the program by alternating flexion and extension splints.

Resistance to the repaired muscle-tendon unit is not initiated until 8 to 12 weeks postoperatively regardless of the site of the repair. First, emphasis is placed on gradually strengthening the extensors to prevent or minimize an extensor lag. After 10 to 12 weeks *low-intensity* resisted grasp and pinch activities are initiated to gradually strengthen the flexors if no extensor lag is present.

### Outcomes

Outcomes, including complications, after extensor tendon repair and postoperative rehabilitation are well documented in the literature. Early and late complications are similar to those occurring after flexor tendon repair, including rupture, adhesion formation, and limited motion. Outcomes typically measured and reported after extensor tendon repair are ROM of the wrist and/or digits and grip strength with only limited information reported on use of the hand for functional activities.

Digital motion often is expressed in terms of "pad-to-palm" distances or total active motion (active flexion minus extensor lag). These figures are then compared to the contralateral hand or to the "normal" population and are typically expressed as excellent, good, fair, or poor. For example, if ROM is only 75% of that found in normal individuals or if there is < 15° of extensor lag in a digit and sufficient digital flexion to touch the pad of the distal phalanx to the mid-palm, the result is described as "good." To understand the results of studies on tendon repair, it is necessary to have some understanding of the various assessment tools.

Some generalizations about outcomes can be drawn from the literature regarding the severity and location of the injury. As with flexor tendon injuries, the greater the extent of associated skeletal, joint, vascular, or nerve injuries, the poorer are the results of the repair with respect to extensor lag and digital flexion for grasp. For example, in a study of outcomes after extended immobilization following extensor tendon repair, 64% of patients with simple tendon injuries had good results, whereas only 47% of patients with associated skeletal or joint injuries had a good result.[85] In the same study, investigators found that repairs of distal injuries (zones I to IV) have less favorable results than repairs of more proximal injuries (zones V to VIII).

Outcomes of the various approaches to postoperative management of extensor tendon injuries are reported in the literature on an ongoing basis. With regard to the timing of the surgical intervention, for example, primary repairs of acute injuries (rupture or laceration), whether repaired immediately or delayed for up to 10 days, yield equally good results.[41,84] As noted throughout this section on extensor tendon injury and repair, numerous studies have been published describing outcomes of the various approaches to postoperative management. Although some current studies support the use and effectiveness of prolonged immobilization of extensor tendon repairs,[92] there is growing use and ongoing modification and refinement of early controlled motion approaches to help patients achieve the best possible outcomes.

For example, dynamic extension splinting, a mainstay of early passive mobilization protocols for more than 20 years, now is being re-evaluated. Although some recent studies[19,34] have demonstrated that high-profile, dynamic splinting continues to be used and is effective,

## BOX 19.19   Special Considerations for Exercise After Extensor Tendon Repair and Extended Immobilization

### Zones I and II
- Tendon injuries in these zones are typically managed non-operatively.
- PIP and MCP AROM while the DIP is continuously immobilized in extension for at least 4 weeks but more often 6 to 8 weeks.
- When splint can be removed for exercise, perform active DIP extension and very gentle active flexion with the MCP and PIP joints stabilized in neutral. Briefly hold the extended position with each repetition.
- Emphasize active extension more than flexion to avoid an extensor lag.
- After initiating exercises, splint between exercise sessions an additional 2 weeks or longer if an extensor lag develops.

PRECAUTION: Increase active flexion of the DIP joint *very gradually,* initially limiting flexion to 20° to 25° during the first week of exercise. The strong FDP can easily place excessive stress on the terminal extensor tendon and cause gapping or rupture of the repair. Progress active flexion by about 10° per week. Do not attempt full DIP flexion for about 3 months.

### Zones III and IV
- If the lateral bands were intact, begin DIP AROM 1 week postoperatively while the PIP joint is immobilized in extension in a volar splint or cylinder cast. Early DIP motion prevents adherence and loss of extensibility of the lateral bands and oblique retinacular ligaments and loss of mobility of the DIP joint.
- If the lateral bands were damaged and repaired, postpone DIP ROM until 4 to 6 weeks postoperatively.
- At a minimum of 3 to 4 weeks but more often at 6 weeks, the volar splint is removed for active ROM of the PIP joints with the MCP joints stabilized. Emphasize active extension more than flexion.

PRECAUTIONS: Progress PIP flexion in *very gradual* increments; limit PIP flexion to 30° the first week of PIP ROM exercises. Increase an additional 10° per week if no extensor lag.

- If the wrist and MCP joints have been immobilized postoperatively, include active ROM of the wrist with the MCP and PIP joints stabilized and active MCP ROM with the wrist and PIP joints stabilized in extension.

### Zones V and VI
- When the volar splint can be removed for exercise (between 3 and 4 weeks or as late as 6 weeks postoperatively), begin active or assisted MCP extension and passive flexion with the wrist and IP joints stabilized in neutral and the forearm *pronated.* Actively hold the extended position for a few seconds with each repetition. Let the extensors relax to flex the MCP joints.
- Add carefully controlled active MCP flexion within a protected range with the wrist stabilized in extension.
- Emphasize active MCP extension more than flexion to prevent an extensor lag.

PRECAUTION: Initially limit active MCP flexion to 30° in the index and middle fingers and 35° to 40° in the ring and small fingers.
- During active IP flexion and extension exercises, stabilize the MCP joints in neutral and the wrist in slight extension. Encourage full-range DIP motion.
- Combine active MCP extension with active PIP flexion (hook fist position) and PIP extension (straight hand position).
- Incrementally progress to full fist position over several weeks if no extensor lag develops.

### Zone VII
- If the wrist extensors are intact and only extrinsic finger extensors have been repaired, follow the guidelines for zone V/VI repairs.
- If the wrist extensors were repaired, begin active wrist extension from neutral to full extension in a gravity-eliminated position (forearm in mid-position) at 3 to 4 weeks.
- Incrementally increase wrist flexion beyond neutral between 5 and 8 weeks postoperatively.
- Perform radial and ulnar deviation with the wrist in neutral.

other studies reflect a return to the use of low-profile, static splinting if coupled with early active motion.[44,60,124]

In a prospective, randomized study, Khandawala et al.[60] compared the effectiveness of two early mobilization programs for patients with zone V/VI extensor tendon repairs—a dynamic splinting program and a static splinting program combined with early active exercise. One group of 50 patients performed exercises in a volar, wrist-based dynamic extension splint that allowed free movement of IP joints and active MCP flexion to the level of the splint. The elastic bands and slings passively extended the MCP joints to a neutral position as the flexors relaxed. A second group of 50 patients wore a static volar blocking splint that positioned the wrist in 30° of extension and the MCP joints in 45° of flexion. The IP

joints were free. With the stabilization straps loosened, this group performed active MCP flexion to 45° (further motion was blocked by the splint) and MCP extension to neutral. In both groups IP motion was unrestricted. After 6 weeks of exercise, splinting was discontinued and outcomes were measured by two assessment tools. As reflected by scores on the two assessment instruments, a high percentage of patients in both groups had good and excellent results, specifically 95% and 98% of the dynamic splinting group and 93% and 95% of the static splinting/active exercise group. These results, when analyzed, demonstrated that there were no significant differences in outcomes between the groups. With two splinting and early motion approaches yielding equally favorable results, the investigators concluded that static splinting could be considered a less cumbersome and expensive alternative to dynamic splinting for early motion programs. Additional research is needed to determine if modification of early active motion programs could provide significantly better outcomes over early passive motion programs.

## EXERCISE INTERVENTIONS FOR THE WRIST AND HAND

### TECHNIQUES FOR MUSCULOTENDINOUS MOBILITY

Active muscle contraction and specific motions of the digits and wrist are used to maintain or develop mobility between the multijoint musculotendinous units and other connective tissue structures in the wrist and hand. Because adhesions between the various structures can become restrictive or incapacitating, *tendon-gliding exercises* and *tendon-blocking exercises* are used, whenever possible, to develop or maintain mobility. This is particularly important when there has been immobilization after trauma, surgery, or a fracture, and scar tissue adhesions have developed. If restrictions occur as a result of scar tissue adherence between tendons or between tendons and surrounding tissues, mobilization techniques described in this section may be necessary. General stretching techniques may also be necessary; they are described in the next section. The tendon-gliding and tendon-blocking exercises described here may also be used to develop neuromuscular control and coordinated movement.

### Tendon–Gliding and Tendon–Blocking Exercises

#### Place–and–Hold Exercises
Place-and-hold exercises are a form of gentle muscle setting (static/isometric) exercises that are used during the early postoperative period following tendon repair before active ROM is initiated but when a minimal level of stress on the repaired tendon and passive joint movement are beneficial for maintaining joint mobility and tendon excursion.

- Following flexor tendon repair, the patient usually wears a dorsal blocking splint[46,47,107] or a tenodesis splint.[24,25,115–117] With the MCP joints in flexion, passively place the IP joints in a partially flexed position and have the patient hold the position independently for 5 seconds with a minimum static contraction of the finger flexors.
- If the patient is wearing a tenodesis splint, combine place-and-hold finger flexion with active wrist extension (see Fig 19.14 B&C). Have the patient relax and allow the wrist to passively flex and the digits to passively extend.

- Following extensor tendon repair, when the volar blocking splint may be removed for exercise, passively position the joint in the zone of the repair first in a neutral and later in a slightly extended position. Then, have the patient hold the position. This emphasizes end-range extension to prevent an extensor lag.
- Have the patient practice the exercise with the uninjured hand or use biofeedback to learn how to hold the position with a minimum of force production.

#### Flexor Tendon–Gliding Exercises
Flexor tendon-gliding exercises are designed to maintain or develop free gliding between the flexor digitorum profundus and superficialis tendons and between the tendons and bones in the wrist, hand, and fingers.[101,109,130] There are five positions in which the fingers move during tendon-gliding exercises: straight hand (all the joints are extended), hook (claw) fist (MCP joints are extended, IP joints are flexed), full fist (all the joints are flexed), table-top position, also known as the intrinsic plus hand (MCP joints are flexed, IP joints are extended), and straight fist (MCP and PIP joints are flexed, IP joints are extended) (Fig. 19.17). The following progression is suggested.

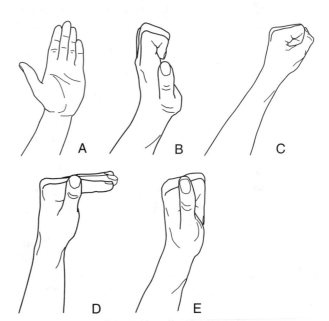

FIGURE 19.17 The five finger positions used for flexor tendon gliding exercises: (*A*) straight hand, (*B*) hook fist (claw fist), (*C*) full fist, (*D*) table top (intrinsic plus), and (*E*) straight fist.

- Initiate the exercises with the wrist in neutral position.
- Once full range of the finger motions is achieved, progress to doing the gliding exercises with the wrist in flexion and in extension to establish combined finger and wrist mobility.
- Full excursion and tendon-gliding of all the extrinsic muscles are accomplished by starting with the wrist and fingers in full extension and moving to full wrist and finger flexion and then reversing the motion.

### Hook (Claw) Fist Position

Have the patient move from the straight hand to the hook fist position by flexing the DIP and PIP joints while maintaining MCP extension (Fig. 19.17 A&B). Maximum gliding occurs between the profundus and superficialis tendons and between the profundus tendon and the bone. (There is also gliding of the extensor digitorum communis tendons; this motion is used with the extensor gliding exercises.)

### Full Fist

Have the patient move to the full fist position by flexing all the MCP and IP joints simultaneously (Fig. 19.17C). Maximum gliding of the profundus tendon with respect to the sheath and bone as well as over the superficialis tendon occurs.

### Straight Fist (Sublimis Fist)

Have the patient move from the table-top position (Fig. 19.17D) to the straight fist position by flexing the PIP joints while maintaining the DIP joints in extension (Fig. 19.17E). Maximum gliding of the superficialis tendon occurs with respect to the flexor sheath and bone.

### Thumb Flexion

Have the patient flex the MCP and IP joints of the thumb full range. This promotes maximum gliding of the flexor pollicis longus.

### Flexor Tendon–Blocking Exercises

Blocking exercises for the flexor tendons (Fig. 19.18) not only develop gliding of the tendons with respect to the sheaths and related bones, they also require neuromuscular control of individual joint motions. Therefore, they use the mobility gained by the flexor tendon-gliding exercises and are a progression of the flexor tendon-gliding exercises. Progress to manual resistance as the tissues heal and can tolerate resistance.

PRECAUTION: These exercises should not be used in the early stages after flexor tendon repair because of the stress placed on the tendons.

*Patient position and stabilization:* Sitting with the forearm supinated and the back of the hand resting on a table. The opposite hand provides stabilization and "blocking" against unwanted movement. Each finger performs the exercise separately.

### Isolated MCP Flexion (Lumbricales and Palmar Interossei)

⊚ Have the patient flex only the MCP joint of one digit (Fig. 19.18A).
⊚ If necessary, the rest of the fingers are stabilized in extension against the table with the other hand.
⊚ With improved control, the hand does not have to be stabilized against the table.

### PIP Flexion (Flexor Digitorum Superficialis)

⊚ Have the patient stabilize the proximal phalanx of one digit with the other hand, and if possible, flex just the PIP joint of the one digit while keeping the DIP joint extended and the rest of fingers on the table (Fig. 19.18B).

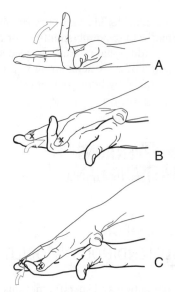

FIGURE 19.18 Flexor tendon blocking exercises: (*A*) isolated MCP flexion of one digit, (*B*) isolated PIP flexion (flexor digitorum superficialis) of one digit, and (*C*) isolated DIP flexion (flexor digitorum profundus) of one digit.

⊚ If the patient has difficulty doing this, the other digits are stabilized in extension with the other hand.

### DIP Flexion (Flexor Digitorum Profundus)

⊚ The middle phalanx of one digit is stabilized with the other hand.
⊚ Have the patient attempt to flex just the distal phalanx (Fig. 19.18C).
⊚ Vary this exercise by increasing the range of MCP and PIP flexion to where the patient just begins to lose DIP motion; stabilize in this position and have the patient attempt DIP flexion.

### Full Fist

When full independent tendon-gliding is available, the patient should be able to make a full fist. Progress the exercises described by adding resistance.

### Exercises to Reduce Extensor Lag

The extrinsic finger extensors (extendor digitorum communis, extensor digitorum indicis, and extensor digiti minimi) are more superficial than the flexor tendons and therefore more easily damaged. Their prime function is to extend the MCP joints. Extension of the IP joints requires active interaction with the intrinsic muscles of the hand via the extensor mechanism. Adhesions within their sheaths at the wrist or between tendon and bone restrict tendon-gliding both proximally (restricting active finger extension) and distally (restricting active and passive finger flexion). When full passive range of extension is available, but the person cannot actively move the joint through the full range of extension, it is called an *extensor lag*. It can occur as the result of weakness but is frequently caused by adhesions that prevent gliding of the tendons when the muscles contract.

One of the purposes of the following exercises is to maintain mobility and thus prevent adhesions. The exercises are also used to regain control of finger extension. Mobilization of adhesions is described immediately following the differential gliding of extensor tendon exercises. Stretching techniques are described in the next section.

### Isolated MCP Extension

- Have the patient move from the full fist position (see Fig. 19.17C) to the hook fist position (see Fig. 19.17B).
- If the patient has difficulty maintaining the IP joints in flexion, have him or her hook the fingers around a pencil while extending the MCP joints.
- Begin with the wrist in neutral and progress to positioning the wrist in flexion and extension while performing MCP extension.

### Isolated PIP and DIP Extension

Extension of the interphalangeal joints requires intrinsic and extrinsic muscle (extensor digitorum communis) control.

- For strongest participation of the lumbricales, stabilize the MCP joint in flexion while the patient attempts IP extension, moving from the full fist position (see Fig. 19.17C) to the table-top position (see Fig. 19.17D).
- Progress to stabilizing the palm of the hand on the edge of a table (or block) with the PIP or DIP joint partially flexed over the edge.
- Have the patient extend the involved phalanx through the ROM.

### Terminal-Range Extension of IP Joints

- Progress to the terminal range by stabilizing the entire hand, palm side down on a flat surface, and have the patient extend the involved phalanx into hyperextension.
- If there is not enough range available, place a pencil or block under the proximal phalanx or middle phalanx so the PIP or DIP joint can go through a greater range (Fig. 19.19).

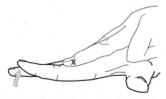

FIGURE 19.19 Terminal extension of the PIP joint. The MCP joint is stabilized in extension, and the patient lifts the middle and distal phalanges off the table.

### Extensor Tendon-Gliding Exercises

*Differential gliding* of the extensor digitorum communis tendons to each of the fingers can be achieved by the following progression.

- Teach the patient to passively flex the MCP and IP joints of one finger with the opposite hand while actively maintaining the other fingers in extension.
- If the patient has difficulty doing this, begin with the involved hand resting on a table with the palm up. Stabilize three of the four fingers against the table while pas-

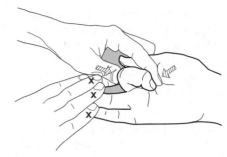

FIGURE 19.20 Differential gliding of the extensor digitorum tendons. Move each digit into flexion while stabilizing the other digits in extension.

sively flexing one of the digits (Fig. 19.20). Then instruct the patient to attempt to actively keep the fingers against the table while one of the digits is passively flexed.

- Progress by having the patient actively maintain the fingers in extension with the fingers spread out and then actively flex each finger in turn while the other fingers remain extended.
- Have the patient flex the middle and ring fingers while maintaining extension of the index and little fingers (long horn sign). This promotes isolated control of the extensor indicis and extensor digiti minimi tendons and promotes their gliding on the extensor digitorum communis tendons.

## Scar Tissue Mobilization for Tendon Adhesions

Ideally, the tendon-gliding exercises described previously in this section maintain or develop mobility between the long tendons and surrounding connective tissues or within their sheaths. However, when there has been inflammation and immobilization during the healing process following trauma or surgery, scar tissue adhesions may form and prevent gliding of the tendons. Contraction of the muscle does not result in movement of the joint or joints distal to the site of the immobile scar.

Techniques to mobilize the adhesive scar tissue include the application of friction massage directly to the adhesion. This is superimposed on active and passive stretching techniques (described in the next section), and the tendon-gliding techniques already described. To apply friction massage, hold the tendon in its lengthened position; apply pressure with your thumb, index, or middle finger and massage perpendicular to the tendon and longitudinally in proximal and distal directions. A sustained force against the adhesion allows for creep and eventual movement of the scar. Techniques to mobilize the flexor and extensor tendons follow.

### To Mobilize the Long Finger Flexor Tendons

Adhesions between the flexor tendons and their sheaths or between tendons and underlying bones restrict tendon-gliding in both a proximal and distal direction so the joints distal to the scar do not flex when the muscle contracts. Passive movement into flexion of the joints distal to the adhered scar is possible if there are no capsular restrictions. Full range of extension of the joints distal to the scar is not possible actively or passively owing to the inability of the tendon to glide distally.

The following is a suggested progression in intensity of scar tissue mobilization.

- ◉ Begin the stretching routine by passively moving the tendon in a distal direction by extending the finger joints as far as possible and apply a sustained hold to allow for creep. Follow this with active contraction of the flexor muscle to create a stretch force against the adhesion in a proximal direction[109] using the patterns of movement described for tendon-gliding exercises (see Fig. 19.17).
- ◉ If active and passive stretching, described in the above technique, does not release the adhesion, extend the MCP and IP joints as far as allowed, stabilize them, then apply friction massage with your thumb or finger at the site of the adhesion while the tendon is held in its stretched position.[36] As indicated above, apply the massaging stretch force across the tendon and in a longitudinal direction, both proximally and distally. When applying friction massage in a proximal direction, ask the patient to simultaneously contract the flexor muscle in order to superimpose an active stretch force.
- ◉ After friction massage, have the patient repeat the flexor tendon-gliding exercises to utilize any gained mobility.

### To Mobilize the Extensor Tendons and the Extensor Mechanism

As with the flexor tendons, if the extensor tendons or extensor mechanism has restricted mobility because of adhesions, muscle action is not transmitted through the mechanism to extend the joint or joints distal to the restriction. Without free gliding, an extensor lag may result. As defined earlier, an extensor lag is the loss of active extension when there is full passive extension. The following is a progression in intensity of scar tissue mobilization.

- ◉ Stretch the adhesion in a distal direction by passively flexing the joint distal to the site. Follow this by having the patient attempt to actively extend the joint and put tension on the scar in a proximal direction.

PRECAUTION: If the extensor lag increases (i.e., flexion increases, but there is no active extension through the increased range), the tendon distal to the adhesion may be stretching, not the adhesion. Do not continue with passive stretching into flexion but, rather, emphasize friction massage applied to the scar tissue.

- ◉ Apply friction massage at the site of the adhesion with the tendon kept taut by holding the joint at the end of its range of flexion. Apply friction massage across the fibers and in a distal and proximal direction. When applying friction massage in a proximal direction, have the patient actively contract the extensors to assist with the mobilization effort.
- ◉ Follow these mobilization techniques with extensor tendon-gliding exercises, as described in the previous section.

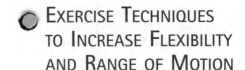

# EXERCISE TECHNIQUES TO INCREASE FLEXIBILITY AND RANGE OF MOTION

Stretching the muscles and connective tissue structures of the wrist and hand requires knowledge of the unique anatomical relationships of the multijoint musculotendinous units and the extensor mechanism of the digits. These are described in the first section of this chapter. The principles and techniques of stretching are presented in Chapter 4, and special note is made of the importance of stabilization when stretching the multijoint muscles of the hand and fingers. This is re-emphasized here. In addition, because scarring and adhesions can restrict tendon-gliding and therefore motion of the digits, it is important to recognize these restrictions and utilize specific techniques that address the adhesions as presented in the previous section (see Scar Tissue Mobilization for Tendon Adhesions). Before stretching muscle or connective tissue, there also should be normal gliding of the joint surfaces to avoid joint damage. Use joint mobilization techniques to stretch the joint capsule and restore gliding (see Chapter 5).

NOTE: Patient position for most wrist and hand exercises is sitting with the forearm supported on a treatment table unless otherwise noted.

## General Stretching Techniques

When stretching to increase wrist flexion or extension, it is important that the fingers are free to move so the extrinsic finger flexor and extensor musculotendinous units do not restrict motion at the wrist. Similarly, when stretching ligaments and other periarticular connective tissues across individual finger joints, it is important that there is no tension on the multijoint tendons. The following techniques are initially applied by the therapist and then are taught to the patient as self-stretching techniques for a home exercise program when he or she understands how to safely apply the stretch force and stabilization.

### To Increase Wrist Extension

- ◉ Have the patient place the palm of the hand on a table with the fingers flexed over the edge. The other hand stabilizes the dorsal surface of the hand to maintain the palm against the table. Then have the patient move the forearm up over the stabilized hand (similar to Fig. 19.22 except the fingers are over the edge of the table so they are free to flex and the stretch occurs only at the wrist).
- ◉ Have the patient place the palms of the hands together at right angles to each other and allow the fingers to intertwine and flex. Instruct the patient to press the restricted hand in a dorsal direction with the palm of the other hand and sustain the stretch.

### To Increase Wrist Flexion

- ◉ Have the patient place the dorsal surface of the hand on a table. The other hand provides stabilization against the palm of the hand. Have the patient move the forearm up over the stabilized hand.

● Have the patient sit with the forearm pronated and resting on a table and the wrist at the edge of the table. The patient then presses the hand toward flexion with the opposite hand.

● Have the patient place the dorsum of both hands together. Then, with the fingers relaxed, move the forearms so the wrists flex toward 90°.

### To Increase Flexion or Extension of Individual Joints of the Fingers or Thumb

To increase extension at any one joint, the patient's forearm is supinated; to increase flexion, the forearm is pronated, and the phalanx to be stretched is at the edge of the table. Show the patient how to apply the force against the distal bone while stabilizing the proximal bone against the table.

## Stretching Techniques for the Intrinsic and Multijoint Muscles

### Self-Stretching the Lumbricales and Interossei Muscles

Have the patient actively extend the MCP joints and flex the IP joints and apply a passive stretch force at the end of the range with the opposite hand (Fig. 19.21A).

### Self-Stretching the Interossei Muscles

Have the patient place the hand flat on a table with the palm down and the MCP joints extended. Instruct the patient to abduct or adduct the appropriate digit and apply the stretch force to the distal end of the proximal phalanx. Stabilization is provided by holding the adjacent digit.

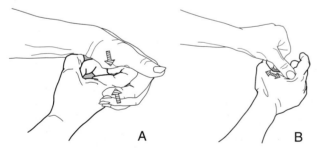

FIGURE 19.21 Self-stretching (A) the lumbricales with MCP extension and IP flexion; and (B) the adductor pollicis with CMC abduction of the thumb. To increase thumb abduction, it is critical that the stretch force is applied against the metacarpal head not the proximal or distal phalanges.

### Self-Stretching the Adductor Pollicis

Have the patient rest the ulnar border of the hand on the table and abduct the thumb perpendicular to the palm of the hand. Instruct the patient to apply the stretch force with the crossed thumb and index or long finger of the other hand against the metacarpal head of the thumb and index finger and attempt to increase the web space (Fig. 19.21B).

PRECAUTION: It is critical that the patient does not apply the stretch force against the proximal or distal pha-

lanx. This places stress on the ulnar collateral ligament of the MCP joint of the thumb and leads to instability at that joint with poor functional usage of the thumb. Abduction occurs at the CMC joint at the articulation between the metacarpal and the trapezium.

### Manual Stretching of the Extrinsic Muscles

Because they are multijoint muscles, the final step is to elongate each tendon of the extrinsic muscles over all the joints simultaneously but *do not* initiate stretching procedures in this manner because joint compression and damage can occur to the smaller or less stable joints. Begin by allowing the wrist and more proximal finger joints to relax; stretch the tendon unit over the most distal joint first. Stabilize the distal joint at the end of the range and then stretch the tendon unit over the next joint. Next, stabilize the two joints, and stretch the tendon over the next joint. Progress in this manner until the desired length is reached.

PRECAUTION: Do not let the PIP and MCP joints hyperextend as the tendons are stretched over the wrist.

### Self-Stretching the Flexor Digitorum Profundus and Superficialis

Have the patient begin by resting the palm of the involved hand on a table and first extend the DIP joint, using the other hand to straighten the joint; keeping it extended, then have the patient straighten the PIP and MCP joints in succession. If the patient can actively extend the finger joints to this point, the motion should be performed unassisted. With the hand stabilized on the table, have the patient then begin to extend the wrist by bringing the arm up over the hand. The patient goes just to the point of feeling discomfort, holds the position, then progresses as the length improves (Fig. 19.22).

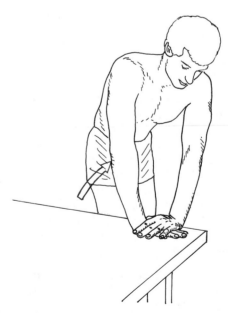

FIGURE 19.22 Self-stretching of the extrinsic finger flexor muscles, showing stabilization of the small distal joints. To isolate stretch to the wrist flexors, allow the fingers to flex over the edge of the table.

### Self-Stretching the Extensor Digitorum Communis

The fingers are flexed to the maximum range, beginning with the distalmost joint first and progressing until the wrist is simultaneously flexed. The opposite hand applies the stretch force.

# Exercises to Develop and Improve Muscle Performance, Neuromuscular Control, and Coordinated Movement

Exercises described in this section are for use during the controlled motion and return to function phases of rehabilitation when the tissues are in the subacute and chronic stages of healing and require only moderate or minimum protection. In addition to the conditions already described in this chapter, imbalances in the length and strength of the wrist and hand muscles can occur as the result of a variety of causes, such as nerve injury, trauma, disuse, or immobilization. Appropriate exercises to develop fine finger dexterity or strength and muscular endurance for strong or repetitive gripping can be selected from the following exercises or their adaptations. The flexor tendon blocking exercises and extensor tendon-gliding exercises described previously in this section may also be used to strengthen the musculature by adding resistance manually or mechanically. Exercises for shoulder, elbow, and forearm strength and muscular endurance should also be included to restore proper function in the upper extremity.

## Techniques to Strengthen Muscles of the Wrist and Hand

If the musculature is weak, use progressive strengthening exercises, beginning at the level of the patient's ability. Use active-assistive, active, or manual resistance exercises as described in Chapters 3 and 6 of this text. Progress to mechanical resistance.

### To Strengthen Wrist Musculature

Allow the fingers to relax. Exercise the wrist muscles in groups if their strength is similar. If one muscle is weaker, the wrist should be guided through the range desired to minimize the action of the stronger muscles. For example, with wrist flexion, if the flexor carpi radialis is stronger than the flexor carpi ulnaris, have the patient attempt to flex the wrist toward the ulnar side as you guide the wrist into flexion and ulnar deviation. If the muscle is strong enough to tolerate resistance, apply manual resistance over the fourth and fifth metacarpals.

### Wrist Flexion (Flexor Carpi Ulnaris and Radialis) and Extension (Extensor Carpi Radialis Longus and Brevis and Extensor Carpi Ulnaris)

The patient sits with the forearm supported on a table, grasping a weight or elastic resistance that is secured on

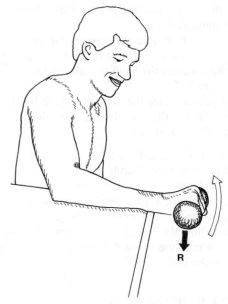

FIGURE 19.23 Mechanical resistance to strengthen wrist extension. Note that the forearm is pronated. To resist wrist flexion, the forearm is supinated.

the floor. The forearm is supinated to resist flexion or pronated to resist extension (Fig. 19.23).

### Wrist Radial Deviation (Flexor and Extensor Carpi Radialis Muscles and Abductor Pollicis Longus) and Ulnar Deviation (Flexor and Extensor Carpi Ulnaris Muscles)

The patient stands and holds a bar with a weight on one end. To resist radial deviation the weight is on the radial side of the wrist (Fig. 19.24A); to resist ulnar deviation the weight is on ulnar side of the wrist (Fig. 19.24B).

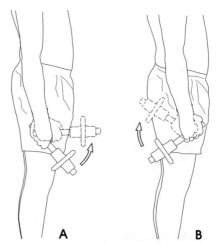

FIGURE 19.24 Mechanical resistance to strengthen (A) radial deviation and (B) ulnar deviation of the wrist using a weighted bar.

### Functional Progressions

Progress to controlled patterns of motion requiring stabilization of the wrist for functional hand activities such as repetitive gripping, picking up and releasing objects of various sizes and weights, and opening and closing the screw lid on a jar. Develop endurance and progress to the desired functional pattern by loading the upper extremity to the tolerance of the wrist stabilizers. When the stabilizers begin to fatigue, stop the activity.

### To Strengthen Weak Intrinsic Musculature

N O T E : Imbalance from weak intrinsic muscles leads to a claw hand.

### MCP Joint Flexion with IP Joint Extension (Lumbricales)

- Begin with the MCP joints stabilized in flexion. Have the patient actively extend the PIP joint against resistance along the middle phalanx. Increase the resistance by resisting the distal phalanx. Resistance may be applied manually or with rubber bands.
- Have the patient start with the MCP joints extended and the PIP joints flexed; then actively push the fingertips outward, performing the desired combined motion (Fig. 19.25 A&B). For resistance, have the patient push the fingers into the palm of the other hand (Fig. 19.25C), or push the fingers into exercise putty with the desired motion.

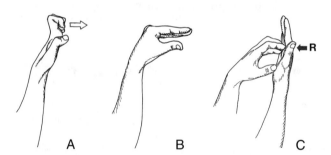

FIGURE 19.25 To strengthen intrinsic muscle function for combined MCP flexion and IP extension, the patient begins with (A) MCP extension and IP flexion and (B) pushes his fingertips outward. The same motion is resisted by (C) pushing the fingertips against the palm of the other hand.

- Begin with all the finger joints extended. Have the patient maintain the IP joints in extension and flex the MCP joints to the table-top position. Apply resistance against the proximal phalanx.

### Isolated or Combined Abduction/Adduction of Each Finger (Dorsal and Volar Interossei)

- Have the patient rest the palm of the hand on a table. Apply resistance at the distal end of the proximal phalanx, one finger at a time, for either abduction or adduction.
- To resist adduction, have the patient interlace the fingers of both hands (or with your hand) and squeeze the fingers together or squeeze exercise putty between two adjacent fingers.
- To resist abduction, place a rubber band around two digits and have the patient spread them apart.

### Abduction of the Thumb (Abductor Pollicis Brevis and Longus)

- The patient rests the dorsum of the hand on a table. Apply resistance at the base of the first phalanx of the thumb as the patient lifts the thumb away from the palm of the hand.
- Place a rubber band or band of exercise putty around the thumb and base of the index finger and have the patient abduct the thumb against the resistance.

### Opposition of the Thumb (Opponens Pollicis)

- Have the patient use various prehension patterns such as tip-to-tip and tip-to-pad, with the thumb opposing each digit in succession, and pad-to-side, with the thumb approximating the lateral side of the index finger.
- Use elastic resistance or have the patient pinch exercise putty, a pliable ball, or a spring-loaded clothespin.

### To Strengthen Weak Extrinsic Musculature of the Fingers

N O T E : The wrist must be stabilized for the action of the extrinsic hand musculature to be effective. If wrist strength is inadequate for stabilization, manually stabilize it during exercises and splint it for functional usage.

### Metacarpophalangeal Extension (Extensor Digitorum Communis, Indicis, and Digiti Minimi)

Have the hand resting on a table with the palm down and digits over the edge. Place a small strap over the distal end of the proximal phalanx with a small weight hanging down from it or secure. Elastic band or tubing around the proximal phalanx and have the patient extend the MCP joint.

### Interphalangeal Flexion (Flexor Digitorum Profundus and Superficialis)

Teach the patient to apply self-resistance by starting with the hands pointing in opposite directions and placing the pads of each finger of one hand against the pads of each finger of the other hand (or against your hand), and then curl the fingers against the resistance provided by the other hand (Fig. 19.6). The same technique is used to resist thumb flexion.

### Mechanical Resistance Techniques for Combined Intrinsic and Extrinsic Muscle Function

N O T E : Proper stabilization is important; either the patient's stabilizing muscles must be strong enough or

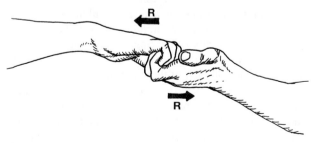

FIGURE 19.26 Self-resistance to strengthen extrinsic finger flexor muscles.

the weakened areas must be supported manually. If a weight causes stress because the patient cannot control it, the exercise is detrimental rather than beneficial.

### Towel or Newspaper Crumple
Spread a towel out on a table. Have the patient place the palm of the hand down at one end of the towel and crumple the towel into the hand while maintaining contact with the heel of the hand. The same exercise can be carried out by placing a stack of newspapers under the hand. The patient crumples the top sheet into a ball (and tosses it into a basket for coordination and skill practice), then repeats it with each sheet in succession.

### Disk Weight
Have the patient grasp a disk weight in the manner described in each of the following exercises.

- With the forearm pronated (palm down), pick up the disk with the tips of all five digits spread around the outer edge. Have the patient hold the position for isometric resistance. To increase the effect of the resistance to the flexors, have the patient extend one digit at a time.
- Pick up the side of the disk with either tip-to-tip or pad-to-pad prehension of thumb and fingers.
- With the hand palm down on a table, place the disk on the dorsum of the fingers and then hyperextend the fingers by lifting the disk.

### Other Resistance Aids
Resistive devices such as putty, spring-loaded hand exercisers, and various grades and sizes of soft balls can be used for specific muscles or general strengthening. Observe the pattern used by the patient and be sure he or she does not substitute or develop damaging forces.

### Fine-Finger Dexterity
Functional use of the hand for manipulating small objects or skillfully controlling delicate devices requires use of the thumb in opposition to the index and middle fingers. Have the patient perform activities such as picking up small objects of various sizes, twisting nuts on and off bolts, drawing, writing, tying, opening, and closing small bottles or boxes, and typing on a keyboard.

## Functional Activities

Progress to specific patterns needed for ADL, job activities, hobbies, or recreational function. For the patient to return to independent function using the hand, he or she must not only have neuromuscular control and strength but must have muscular endurance, coordination, and fine finger dexterity for the desired activity. This requires careful questioning and analysis of the patient's desired outcomes. Each of the power grips and prehension patterns should be considered. Exercises should be adapted to meet the goals.

## INDEPENDENT LEARNING ACTIVITIES

### ● Critical Thinking and Discussion

1. Falling on an outstretched hand can cause several injuries, including posterior shoulder dislocation, radial head subluxation (pushed elbow), Colles' fracture, and scaphoid fracture. Complications can develop including complex regional pain syndrome (reflex sympathetic dystrophy) and carpal tunnel syndrome. Describe the mechanism and typical clinical signs and symptoms for each of these injuries and identify how to recognize the development of complications.
2. Review all the power grips and prehension patterns and identify the primary muscles that function when performing each action.
3. Summarize the sensory and motor impairments, deformities, and functional limitations that occur in the wrist and hand as the result of a lesion of: (1) the median nerve, (2) the radial nerve, and (3) the ulnar nerve.
4. Differentiate between a boutonnière deformity and a swan-neck deformity of the fingers. What are the underlying factors that contribute to these deformities? After surgical repair of each of these deformities, how should an exercise program be designed to increase hand function but prevent recurrence of these deformities?
5. Identify key structures by the zone in the hand and wrist that could be damaged as the result of a laceration at

each zone of the dorsal and volar aspects of the hand and wrist. What functional impairments occur as the result of damage in each zone?
6. Make a case for the use of early controlled motion after surgical repair of a flexor or extensor tendon injury. Explain the key features of different approaches to the use of early motion in an exercise program. Also identify circumstances in which the use of early controlled motion would be inadvisable or not possible.
7. Analyze and summarize the similarities and differences in the components and progression of exercise programs after flexor or extensor tendon repairs using early controlled mobilization versus delayed mobilization approaches.

### ● Laboratory Practice

1. Mobilize each forearm, wrist, and finger joint with joint mobilization and passive stretching techniques.
2. Practice each tendon-gliding exercise and identify the purpose for each one.
3. Teach your partner strengthening exercises for each muscle or muscle group in the hand using resistance putty.
4. Identify three alternative resistance devices that can be used to strengthen each muscle and patterns of motion in the hand.

5. Observe someone tying laces on a shoe, identify the muscles functioning, and design an exercise program that could be used to develop neuromuscular control or strengthen each of the muscles.

## ● Case Studies

1. A patient is referred to you early in the development of symptoms that stem from RA. He currently is in remission after his first serious flare of the disease and desires a home exercise program to safely improve the use of his hands. He is a salesman who travels frequently. He keeps his records on a computer. His grip strength is reduced 50%; he has 25% loss of joint ROM and decreased joint play in the wrist, MCP, and IP joints. Detectable synovial hypertrophy is minimal, and there are no joint subluxations. Consider what precautions should be followed with this disease to prevent the deforming forces of improperly applied exercises and daily forces. Establish a program of intervention for this patient.

2. A patient is referred to you 2 months after a Colles' fracture. Her hand is swollen and sensitive to touch, and she currently is developing contractures and weakness in the hand related to reflex sympathetic dystrophy (see Chapter 13). Joint contractures exist in the forearm, wrist, and hand. You determine that the patient is in the second stage of the disease. Establish a plan for intervention.

3. A patient with RA who has just undergone MCP implant arthroplasties of the ring and small fingers has been referred to you for an exercise program. The patient has been wearing a dynamic extension splint for the past 4 weeks that allows active MCP flexion and assists MCP extension. The patient is now allowed to remove the splint for active ROM of the wrist and hand. Your examination reveals that the patient has an extensor lag and also has restricted flexion of the fingers. Design and progress an exercise program for this patient. What precautions should be incorporated into each phase of the program?

4. A patient has been referred to you who underwent a ligament reconstruction tendon interposition arthroplasty for post-traumatic arthritis of the CMC joint of the thumb 4 weeks ago. The thumb spica cast was removed at $3^1/_2$ weeks postoperatively, and the patient is now wearing a thumb spica splint that may be removed for exercise. Develop and progress an exercise program for the patient. The patient has already returned to his or her position in an office. The patient would like to be able to resume golf on a recreational basis.

5. An 8-year-old child who sustained a zone III laceration of the volar aspect of the index and middle fingers of the nondominant hand while carving a pumpkin has been referred to you after surgical repair of the FDP and FDS tendons. The child's hand has been immobilized in a cast for 3 weeks after the repair in a position of wrist and finger flexion. The child is now wearing a dorsal blocking splint that may be removed for exercise. The child's active and passive extension is significantly limited. Design and progress an exercise program for this child. Identify activities that the child must do under direct supervision and those that he or she may do independently.

## REFERENCES

1. Amadio, PC, Murray, PM, Linscheid, RL: Arthroplasty of the proximal interphalangeal joint. In Morrey, BF (ed) Joint Replacement Arthroplasty, ed 3. Churchill Livingstone, Philadelphia, 2003, pp 163–174.

2. American Physical Therapy Association: Guide to Physical Therapist Practice, ed 2. Phys Ther 81:9–744, 2001.

3. Anderson, RJ: Rheumatoid arthritis: clinical and laboratory features. In Klippel, JF (ed) Primer on Rheumatic Diseases, ed 11. Arthritis Foundation, Atlanta, 1997, p 161.

4. Angst, F, John, M, Goldhahn, J, et al: Comprehensive assessment of clinical outcome and quality of life after resection interposition arthroplasty of the thumb saddle joint. Arthritis Rheum 53(2):205–213, 2005.

5. Austin, NM: The Wrist and Hand Complex. In Levange, PK, Norkin, CC (eds) Joint Structure and Function: A Comprehensive Analysis. FA Davis, Philadelphia, 2005, p 305.

6. Backstrom, KM: Mobilization with movement as an adjunct intervention in a patient with complicated de Quervain's tenosynovitis: a case report. J Orthop Sports Phys Ther 32(3):86–97, 2002.

7. Baimbridge, LC, Bobertson, C, Gillies, D, Elliot, D: A comparison of postoperative mobilization of flexor tendon repairs with "passive flexion-active extension" and "controlled active motion" techniques. J Hand Surg [Br] 19:517–521, 1994.

8. Baxter-Petralia, P, Penney, V: Cumulative trauma. In Stanley, BG, Tribuzi SM (eds): Concepts in Hand Rehabilitation. FA Davis, Philadelphia, 1992, p 419.

9. Beasley, RW: Surgery of the Hand. Thieme, New York, 2003.

10. Beckenbaugh, RD: Arthroplasty of the wrist. In Morrey, BF (ed) Joint Replacement Arthroplasty, ed 3. Churchill Livingstone, Philadelphia, 2003, pp 244–265.

11. Beckenbaugh, RD: Total wrist arthroplasty. In Cooney, WP, Linschied, RL, Dobyns, JH (eds) The Wrist: Diagnosis and Operative Treatment, Vol 2. CV Mosby, St. Louis, 1998, p 924.

12. Berger, RA, Beckenbaugh, RD, Linschied, RL: Arthroplasty of the hand and wrist. In Green, DP, Hotchkiss, RN, Pederson, WC (eds) Green's Operative Hand Surgery, Vol 1, ed 4. Churchill Livingstone, New York, 1999, p 147.

13. Bielefeld, T, Neumann, DA: The unstable metacarpophalangeal joint in rheumatoid arthritis: anatomy, pathomechanics, and physical rehabilitation considerations. J Orthop Sports Phys Ther 35(8):502–520, 2005.

14. Biese, J, Goudzward, P: Postoperative management of metacarpophalangeal implant resection arthroplasty. Orthop Phys Ther Clin North Am 10(4):595–616, 2001.

15. Blair, WF, Schurr, DG, Buckwalter, JA: Metacarpophalangeal joint arthroplasty with a silastic spacer. J Bone Joint Surg Am 66:365–370, 1984.

16. Bodell, LS, Leonard, L: Wrist arthroplasty. In Berger, RA, Weiss, A (eds) Hand Surgery, Vol II. Lippincott Williams & Wilkins, Philadelphia, 2004, pp 1340–1394.

17. Brotzman, SB, Calandruccio, JH, Jobe, JT, Jupiter, JB: Hand and wrist injuries. In Brotzman, SB, Wilk, KE (eds) Clinical Orthopedic Rehabilitation, ed 2. Mosby, Philadelphia, 2003, pp 1–83.

18. Browne, EZ Jr, Ribick, CA: Early dynamic splinting for extensor tendon injuries. J Hand Surg [Am] 14:72, 1989.
19. Brüner, S, Wittemann, M, Jester, A, et al: Dynamic splinting after extensor tendon repair in zones V to VII. J Hand Surg [Br] 28(3): 224–227, 2003.
20. Buckwalter, JA, Ballard, WT: Operative treatment of arthritis. In Klippel, JH (ed) Primer of the Rheumatic Diseases, ed 12. Arthritis Foundation, Atlanta, 2001, pp 613–623.
21. Burr, N, Pratt, AL, Smith, PJ: An alternative splinting and rehabilitation protocol for metacarpophalangeal arthroplasty in patients with rheumatoid arthritis. J Hand Ther 15(1):41–47, 2002.
22. Burton, RI, Melchior, JA: Extensor tendons—late reconstruction. In Green, DP, Hotchkiss, RN, Pederson, WC (eds) Green's Operative Hand Surgery, Vol 2, ed 4. Churchill Livingstone, New York, 1999, p 1988.
23. Burton, RI, Pellegrini, VD: Surgical management of basal joint arthritis of the thumb. Part II. Ligament reconstruction with tendon interposition arthroplasty. J Hand Surg [Am] 11:324–332, 1986.
24. Cannon, N: Post flexor tendon repair protocol. Indiana Hand Center Newslett 1:13, 1993.
25. Cannon, NM: Diagnosis and Treatment Manual for Physicians and Therapists, ed 4. Hand Rehabilitation Center of Indiana, Indianapolis, 2001.
26. Carney, KL, Griffin-Reed, N: Rehabilitation after extensor injury and repair. In Berger, RA, Weiss, APC (eds) Hand Surgery, Vol I. Lippincott Williams & Wilkins, Philadelphia, 2004, pp 767–778.
27. Chow, JA, et al: A combined regimen of controlled motion following flexor tendon repair in "no man's land." Plast Reconstr Surg 79(3): 447–453, 1987.
28. Chow, JA, Dovelle, S, Thomes, LJ, et al: A comparison of results of extensor tendon repair followed by early controlled mobilization versus static immobilization. J Hand Surg [Br] 14(1):18–20, 1989.
29. Cook, SD, Beckenbaugh, RD, Redondo, J, et al: Long-term follow-up of pyrolytic carbon metacarpophalangeal implants. J Bone Joint Surg Am 81:635–648, 1999.
30. Cooney, WP III, Linscheid, RL, Beckenbaugh, RD: Arthroplasty of the metacarpophalangeal joint. In Morrey, BF (ed) Joint Replacement Arthroplasty, ed 3. Churchill Livingstone, Philadelphia, 2003, pp 175–203.
31. Cooney, WP III: Arthroplasty of the thumb axis. In Morrey, BF (ed) Joint Replacement Arthroplasty, ed 3. Churchill Livingstone, Philadelphia, 2003, pp 204–225.
32. Cooney, WP, III, Leddy, TP, Larson, DR: Revision of thumb trapeziometacarpal arthroplasty. J Hand Surg [Am] 31(2):219–227, 2006.
33. Creighton, JJ, Steichen, JB, Strickland, JW: Long-term evaluation of silastic trapezial arthroplasty in patients with osteoarthritis. J Hand Surg [Am] 16:510, 1991.
34. Crosby, CA, Wehbe, MA: Early protected motion after extensor tendon repair. J Hand Surg [Am] 24:1061–1070, 1999.
35. Culp, RW, Taras, JS: Primary care of flexor tendon injuries. In Mackin, EJ, Callahan, AD, Skirven, TM, et al (eds) Rehabilitation of the Hand and Upper Extremity, ed 5. Mosby, St. Louis, 2002, pp 415–427.
36. Cyriax, J: Textbook of Orthopaedic Medicine, ed 8. Vol 1. Diagnosis of Soft Tissue Lesions. Bailliere Tindall, London, 1982.
37. Degnan, GG, Lichtman, DM: Soft tissue arthroplasty about the wrist. In Lichtman, DM, Alexander, AH (eds) The Wrist and Its Disorders, ed 2. WB Saunders, Philadelphia, 1997, p 609.
38. Delaney, R, Stanley, J: A postoperative study of the range of movement following metacarpophalangeal joint replacement: optimum time of recovery. Br J Hand Ther 5(3):85–87, 2000.
39. Delaney, R, Trail, IA, Nutall, D: A comparative study of outcome between the Neuflex and Swanson Silastic metacarpophalangeal joint replacements. J Hand Surg [Br] 30(1):3–7, 2005.
40. Divelbiss, BJ, Sollerman, C, Adams, BD: Early results of the Universal total wrist arthroplasty in rheumatoid arthritis. J Hand Surg [Am] 27:195–204, 2002.
41. Doyle, JR: Extensor tendons—acute injuries. In Green, DP, Hotchkiss, RN, Pederson, WC (eds) Green's Operative Hand Surgery, Vol 2, ed 4. Churchill Livingstone, New York, 1999, p 1950.
42. Duran, RJ, Houser, RC: Controlled passive motion following flexor tendon repair in zones II and III. In AAOS Symposium on Tendon Surgery in the Hand. CV Mosby, St. Louis, 1975.
43. Evans, RB: Clinical management of extensor tendon injuries. In Mackin, EJ, Callahan, AD, Skirven, TM, et al (eds) Rehabilitation of the Hand and Upper Extremity, ed 5. Mosby, St Louis, 2002, pp 542–579.
44. Evans, RB: Early active short arc motion for the repaired central slip. J Hand Surg [Am] 19:991, 1994.
45. Evans, RB, Burkhalter, WE: A study of the dynamic anatomy of extensor tendons and implications for treatment. J Hand Surg [Am] 11:774, 1986.
46. Evans, RB, Thompson, DE: The application of force to the healing tendon. J Hand Ther 6(4):266–284, 1993.
47. Evans, RB, Early active motion after flexor tendon repairs. In Berger, RA, Weiss, APC (eds) Hand Surgery, Vol I. Lippincott Williams & Wilkins, Philadelphia, 2004, pp 709–735.
48. Falkenstein, N, Weiss-Lessard, S: Hand Rehabilitation: A Quick Reference Guide and Review. CV Mosby, St. Louis, 1999.
49. Feldon, PG, Nalebuff, EA, Terrono, AL: Partial wrist fusions: intercarpal and radiocarpal. In Lichtman, DM, Alexander, AH (eds) The Wrist and Its Disorders, ed 2. WB Saunders, Philadelphia, 1997, p 652.
50. Feldon, PG, Terrono, AL, et al: Rheumatoid arthritis and other connective tissue diseases. In Green, DP, Hotchkiss, RN, Pederson, WC (eds) Green's Operative Hand Surgery, Vol 2, ed 4. Churchill Livingstone, New York, 1999, p 1651.
51. Ferlic, DC: Repair of ruptured finger extensors in rheumatoid arthritis. In Strickland, JW, Graham, TJ (eds) The Hand, ed 2. Lippincott Williams & Wilkins, Philadelphia, 2005, pp 457–462.
52. Gellman, H, Stetson, W, Brumfield, RH, et al: Silastic metacarpophalangeal joint arthroplasty in patients with rheumatoid arthritis. Clin Orthop 342:16–21, 1997.
53. Germann, G, Sherman, R, Levin, LS: Decision Making in Reconstructive Surgery: Upper Extremity. Springer-Verlag, Berlin, 2000.
54. Groth, GN: Pyramid of progressive force exercises to the injured flexor-tenson. J Hand Ther 17(1):31–42, 2004.
55. Hunter, JM, Mackin, EJ: Staged flexor tendon reconstruction. In Mackin, EJ, Callahan, AD, Skirven, TM, et al (eds) Rehabilitation of the Hand and Upper Extremity, ed 5. Mosby, St. Louis, 2002, pp 469–497.
56. Ip, WY, Crow, SP: Results of dynamic splintage following extensor tendon repair. J Hand Surg [Br] 22(2):283–287, 1997.
57. Jeter, E, Degnan, GG, Lichtman, DM: Postoperative wrist rehabilitation. In Lichtman, DM, Alexander, AH (eds) The Wrist and Its Disorders. CV Mosby, St. Louis, 1997, p 709.
58. Jolly, SL, et al: Swanson silicone arthroplasty of the wrist in rheumatoid arthritis: a long-term follow-up. J Hand Surg [Am] 17:142, 1992.
59. Kapandji, IA, Kandel, MJ: The Physiology of the Joints, Vol I, ed 5. Churchill-Livingstone, Edinburgh, 1997.
60. Khandawala, AR, Webb, J, Harris, SB, et al: A comparison of dynamic extension splinting and controlled active mobilization of complete divisions of extensor tendons in zones 5 and 6. J Hand Surg [Br] 25(2):140–146, 2000.
61. Kistler, U, Weiss, APC, Simmen, BR, Herren, DB: Long-term results of silicone wrist arthroplasty in patients with rheumatoid arthritis. J Hand Surg [Am] 30(6):1282–1287, 2005.
62. Kitsis, CK, Wade, PJF, Krikler, NK, et al: Controlled active motion following primary flexor tendon repair: a prospective study over a year. J Hand Surg [Br] 23(3):344–349, 1998.
63. Kleinert, HE, Kutz, JE, Cohen, MJ: Primary repair of zone 2 flexor tendon lacerations. In AAOS Symposium on Tendon Surgery in the Hand. CV Mosby, St. Louis, 1975.
64. Kleinman, WB, Eckenrode, JF: Tendon suspension sling arthroplasty for thumb trapeziometacarpal arthritis. J Hand Surg [Am] 16:983, 1991.
65. Kriegs-AU, G, Petje, G, Fojti, E, et al: Ligament reconstruction with or without tendon interposition to treat primary thumb carpometacarpal osteoarthritis: a prospective randomized study. J Bone Joint Surg Am 86(2):209–218, 2004.
66. Linschied, RL, et al: Development of a surface replacement arthroplasty for proximal interphalangeal joints. J Hand Surg [Am] 22:286, 1997.
67. Lister, GD, Kleinert, HE, et al: Primary flexor tendon repair followed by immediate controlled mobilization. J Hand Surg 2:441, 1977.

68. Long, R, et al: Intrinsic-extrinsic muscle control of the hand in power grip and precision handling. J Bone Joint Surg Am 52:853, 1970.

69. Long, C: Normal and Abnormal Motor Control in the Upper Extremities. Final Report. Case Western Reserve University, Cleveland, 1970.

70. Lubahn, JD, Wolfe, TL: Joint replacement in the rheumatoid hand: surgery and therapy. In Mackin, EJ, Callahan, AD, Skirven, TM, et al (eds) Rehabilitation of the Hand and Upper Extremity, ed 5. Mosby, St. Louis, 2002, pp 1583–1597.

71. Lubahn, JD, Wolfe, TL: Surgical treatment and rehabilitation of tendon ruptures in the rheumatoid hand. In Mackin, EJ, Callahan, AD, Skirven, TM, et al (eds) Rehabilitation of the Hand and Upper Extremity, ed 5. Mosby, St. Louis, 2002, pp 1598–1607.

72. Magee, DJ: Orthopedic Physical Assessment, ed 4. WB Saunders, Philadelphia, 2002.

73. Manuel, JL, Weiss, AC: Silicone metacarpal phalangeal joint arthroplasty. In Strickland, JW, Graham, TJ (eds) Master Techniques in Orthopedic Surgery: The Hand, ed 2. Lippincott Williams and Wilkins, Philadelphia, 2005, pp 391–403.

74. Marx, H: Rheumatoid arthritis. In Stanley, BG, Tribuzi, SM (eds) Concepts in Hand Rehabilitation. FA Davis, Philadelphia, 1992, p 395.

75. Mass, DP: Early repairs of flexor tendon injuries. In Berger, RA, Weiss, APC (eds) Hand Surgery, Vol 1. Lippincott Williams & Wilkins, Philadelphia, 2004, pp 679–698.

76. Meuli, HC, Fernandez, DL: Uncemented total arthroplasties. J Hand Surg [Am] 20:115–122, 1995.

77. Morgan, RL, Lindner, MM: Common wrist injuries. Am Family Physician 55(3):857, 1997.

78. Mulligan, BR: Manual Therapy "NAGS," "SNAGS," MWM'S: etc., ed 4. Plane View Press, Wellington, 1999.

79. Murphy, MS, Astifidis, R, Saunders, R: Current management of tendon injuries in the hand. Orthop Phys Ther Clin North Am 10(4): 567–593, 2001.

80. Nalebuff, EA, Terrono, AL, Feldon, PG: Arthrodesis of the wrist: Indications and surgical technique. In Lichtman, DM, Alexander, AH (eds) The Wrist and Its Disorders, ed 2. WB Saunders, Philadelphia, 1997, p 671.

81. Nalebuff, EA: Silicone arthroplasty of the metacarpophalangeal joint. In Blair, WF, Steyers, CM (eds) Techniques in Hand Surgery. Williams & Wilkins, Baltimore, 1996, p 936.

82. Napier, JR: The prehensile movements of the human hand. J Bone Joint Surg Br 38:902, 1956.

83. Neuman, DA, Bielefeld, T: The carpometacarpal joint of the thumb: stability, deformity, and therapeutic intervention. J Orthop Sports Phys Ther 33(7):386–399, 2003.

84. Newport, ML: Early repair of extensor tendon injuries. In Berger, RA, Weiss, APC (eds) Hand Surgery, Vol I. Lippincott Williams & Wilkins, Philadelphia, 2004, pp 737–752.

85. Newport, ML, Blair, WF, Steyers, CM Jr.: Long term results of extensor tendon repair J Hand Surg [Am] 15:961, 1990.

86. O'Connell, SJ, et al: Results of zone I and zone II flexor tendon repairs in children. J Hand Surg [Am] 19:48, 1994.

87. Ottawa Panel: Ottawa Panel evidence-based clinical practice guidelines for therapeutic exercises in the management of rheumatoid arthritis in adults: Phys Ther 84(10):934–972, 2004.

88. Palmer, AK, Werner, FW, Murphy, D, Grissom, R: Functional wrist motion: a biomechanical study. J Hand Surg [Am] 10:39–46, 1985.

89. Pettengill, KM Stewart, van Strien, G: Postoperative management of flexor tendon injuries. In Mackin, EJ, Callahan, AD, Skirven, TM, et al (eds) Rehabilitation of the Hand and Upper Extremity, ed 5. Mosby, St. Louis, 2002, pp 431–456.

90. Phillips, CA: Rehabilitation of the patient with rheumatoid hand involvement. Phys Ther 69:1091, 1989.

91. Phillips, CA: Therapist's management of patients with rheumatoid arthritis. In Hunter, JM, Mackin, EJ, Callahan, AD (eds) Rehabilitation of the Hand: Surgery and Therapy, Vol II, ed 4. CV Mosby, St. Louis, 1995, p 1345.

92. Purcell, T, Eadie, PA, Murugan, S, et al: Static splinting of extensor tendon repairs. J Hand Surg [Br] 25(2):180–182, 2000.

93. Randall, T, Portney, L, Harris, BA: Effects of joint mobilization on joint stiffness and active motion of the metacarpal-phalangeal joint. J Orthop Sports Phys Ther 16:30, 1992.

94. Rettig, LA, Luca, L, Murphy, MS: Silicone implant arthroplasty in patients with idiopathic osteoarthritis of the metacarpophalangeal joint. J Hand Surg [Am] 30:667–672, 2005.

95. Richterman, I, Keenan, MA: Surgical interventions. In Walker, JM, Helewa, A (eds) Physical Therapy in Arthritis. WB Saunders, Philadelphia, 1996, p 95.

96. Rizzo, M, Beckenbaugh, RD: Results of biaxial total wrist arthroplasty with a modified (long) metacarpal stem. J Hand Surg [Am] 28:577–584, 2003.

97. Rosenthal, EA: The extensor tendons: anatomy and management. In Mackin, EJ, Callahan, AD, Skirven, TM, et al (eds) Rehabilitation of the Hand and Upper Extremity, ed 5. Mosby, St. Louis, 2002, pp 498–541.

98. Ryu, JY, Cooney, WP 3rd, Askew, LJ, et al: Functional ranges of motion of the wrist joint. J Hand Surg [Am] 16:409–419, 1991.

99. Saldama, MJ, et al: Results of acute zone III extensor tendon injuries treated with dynamic extension splinting. J Hand Surg [Am] 16: 1145, 1991.

100. Saunders, RJ: Thumb carpometacarpal joint arthroplasty. In Clark, GL, et al (eds) Hand Rehabilitation: A Practical Guide. Churchill Livingstone, New York, 1998, p 363.

101. Saunders, SR: Physical therapy management of hand fractures. Phys Ther 69:1065, 1989.

102. Savage, R: The influence of wrist position on the minimum force required for active movement of the interphalangeal joints. J Hand Surg [Br] 13:262, 1988.

103. Savage, R, Risitano, G: Flexor tendon repair using a "six strand" method of repair and early active motion. J Hand Surg [Br] 14:396, 1989.

104. Schenk, RR, Lenhart, DE: Results of zone II flexor tendon lacerations in civilians treated by the Washington regimen. J Hand Surg [Am] 21:984, 1996.

105. Schneider, LH: Flexor tendons—late reconstruction. In Green, DP, Hotchkiss, RN, Pederson, WC (eds) Green's Operative Hand Surgery, Vol 2, ed 4. Churchill Livingstone, New York, 1999, p 1898.

106. Silfverskiöld, KL, May, EJ, Thornvall, AH: Flexor digitorum profundis excursions during controlled motion after flexor tendon repair in zone II: a prospective clinical study. J Hand Surg [Am] 17:122, 1992.

107. Silfverskiöld, KL, May, EJ: Flexor tendon repair in zone II with a new suture technique and an early mobilization program combining passive and active flexion. J Hand Surg [Am] 19:53–62, 1994.

108. Smith, LK, Weiss, EL, Lehmkuhl, LD: Brunnstrom's Clinical Kinesiology, ed 5. FA Davis, Philadelphia, 1996.

109. Stanley, B: Therapeutic exercise: maintaining and restoring mobility in the hand. In Stanley, BG, Tribuzi, SM (eds) Concepts in Hand Rehabilitation. FA Davis, Philadelphia, 1992, p 178.

110. Stanley, JK, Tolat, AR: Long-term results of Swanson Silastic arthroplasty in the rheumatoid wrist. J Hand Surg [Br] 18:381, 1993.

111. Steinberg, B: Extensor tendon repair. In Clark, GL, et al (eds) Hand Rehabilitation: A Practical Guide, ed 2. Churchill Livingstone, New York, 1998, p 93.

112. Steinberg, B: Flexor tendon repair. In Clark, GL, et al (eds) Hand Rehabilitation: A Practical Guide, ed 2. Churchill Livingstone, New York, 1998, p 103.

113. Steinberg, DR: Osteoarthritis of the hand and digits: metacarpophalangeal and carpometacarpal joints. In Berger, RA, Weiss, APC (eds) Hand Surgery, Vol II. Lippincott Williams & Wilkins, Philadelphia, 2004, pp 1269–1278.

114. Stewart, KM: Review and comparisons in the postoperative management of tendon repair. Hand Clin 7(3):447–460, 1991.

115. Strickland, JW: Development of flexor tendon surgery: twenty-five years of progress. J Hand Surg [Am] 25(2):214–235, 2000.

116. Strickland, JW: Flexor tendons—acute injuries. In Green, DP, Hotchkiss, RN, Pederson, WC (eds) Green's Operative Hand Surgery, Vol 2, ed 4. Churchill Livingstone, New York, 1999, p 1851.

117. Strickland, JW: Flexor tendon injuries. In Strickland, JW, Graham, TJ (eds) Master Techniques in Orthopedic Surgery: The Hand, ed 2. Lippincott Williams & Wilkins, Philadelphia, 2005, pp 251–266.

118. Strickland, JW, Dellacqua, D: Rheumatoid arthritis in the hand and digits. In Berger, RA, Weiss, APC (eds) Hand Surgery, Vol II. Lippincott Williams & Wilkins, Philadelphia, 2004, pp 1179–-211.

119. Swanson, AB, deGroot Swanson, G: Implant arthroplasty in the carpal and radiocarpal joints. In Lichtman, DM, Alexander, AH (eds)

The Wrist and Its Disorders, ed 2. WB Saunders, Philadelphia, 1997, p 616.

120. Swanson, AB, deGroot Swanson, G: Flexible implant resection arthroplasty of the proximal interphalangeal joint. Hand Clin 10:261, 1994.

121. Swanson, AB, deGroot Swanson, G, Leonard JB: Postoperative rehabilitation programs in flexible implant arthroplasty of the digits. In Hunter, JM, Mackin, EJ, Callahan, AD (eds) Rehabilitation of the Hand: Surgery and Therapy, Vol 2, ed 4. CV Mosby, St. Louis, 1995, p 1351.

122. Swanson, AB, Swanson, GD, Maupin, BK: Flexible implant arthroplasty of the radiocarpal joint: surgical techniques and long-term study. Clin Orthop 187:94, 1984.

123. Swanson, AB: Pathogenesis of arthritic lesions. In Hunter, JM, Mackin, EJ, Callahan, AD (eds) Rehabilitation of the Hand: Surgery and Therapy, Vol 2, ed 4. CV Mosby, St. Louis, 1995, p 1307.

124. Sylaidis, M, Youatt, M, Logan, A: Early active mobilization for extensor tendon injuries: the Norwich regime. J Hand Surg [Br] 22(5):594–596, 1997.

125. Terrono, AL, Nalebuff, EA, Phillips, CA: The rheumatoid thumb. In Mackin, EJ, Callahan, AD, Skirven, TM, et al (eds) Rehabilitation of

the Hand and Upper Extremity, ed 5. Mosby, St. Louis, 2002, pp 1555–1568.

126. Theisen, L: Metacarpophalangeal joint arthroplasty. In Clark, GL, et al (eds) Hand Rehabilitation: A Practical Guide, ed 2. Churchill Livingstone, New York, 1998, p 349.

127. Theisen, L: Proximal interphalangeal and distal interphalangeal joint arthroplasty. In Clark, GL, et al (eds) Hand Rehabilitation: A Practical Guide, ed 2. Churchill Livingstone, New York, 1998, p 355.

128. Tottenham, VM, Wilton-Bennet, K, Jeffrey, J: Effects of delayed therapeutic intervention following zone II flexor tendon repair. J Hand Ther 8:23–26, 1995.

129. Waite, J: Physical therapy management of patients with wrist and hand disorders. Orthop Phys Ther Clin North Am 8:135, 1999.

130. Wehbé, MA, Hunter, JM: Flexor tendon gliding in the hand. Part II. Differential gliding. J Hand Surg [Am] 10:575–579, 1985.

131. Weiss, APC, Wiedeman, G Jr, Quenzer, D, et al: Upper extremity function after wrist arthodesis. J Hand Surg [Am] 20:813–817, 1995.

132. Wood, MB: Soft tissue reconstruction. In Cooney, WP, Linscheid, RL, Dobyns, JH (eds) The Wrist: Diagnosis and Operative Treatment, Vol 2. CV Mosby, St. Louis, 1998, p 887.

133. Wynn Parry, CB, Stanley, JK: Synovectomy of the hand. Br J Rheumotol 32:1089, 1993.

# The Hip

The hip is often compared with the shoulder in that it is a triaxial joint, able to function in all three planes, and that it is also the proximal link to its extremity. In contrast to the shoulder, which is designed for mobility, the hip is a stable joint, constructed for weight bearing. However, to carry out activities of daily living (ADL) in what is considered a "normal" manner, at least 120° of hip flexion and at least 20° each of abduction and external rotation are necessary.[97] Forces from the lower extremities are transmitted upward through the hips to the pelvis and trunk during gait and other lower extremity activities. The hips also support the weight of the head, trunk, and upper extremities.

This chapter is divided into three major sections. The first section briefly reviews highlights of the anatomy and function of the hip and its relation to the pelvis and lumbar spine. The second section then describes common disorders of the hip and guidelines for conservative and postoperative management, expanding on the information and principles of management presented in Chapters 10 through 13. The reader should be familiar with that material as well as the components of a comprehensive examination of the hip and pelvis before determining a diagnosis and proceeding to establish a therapeutic exercise program. The last section describes exercise interventions commonly used to meet the goals of treatment for the hip region.

## STRUCTURE AND FUNCTION OF THE HIP

The pelvic girdle links the lower extremity to the trunk and plays a significant role in the function of the hip as well as the spinal joints. The bones of the hip joint consist of the proximal femur and the pelvis (Fig. 20.1). The unique characteristics of the pelvis and femur that affect hip function are reviewed in this section. The function of the pelvis with respect to spinal mechanics is described in greater detail in Chapter 14.

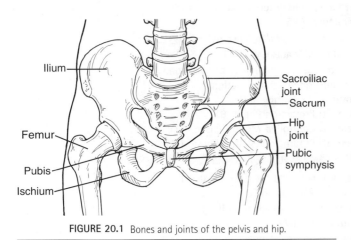

FIGURE 20.1  Bones and joints of the pelvis and hip.

## ⬤ ANATOMICAL CHARACTERISTICS OF THE HIP REGION

### Bony Structures

The structure of the pelvis and femur are designed for weight bearing and transmitting forces through the hip joint.

### The Pelvis
Each innominate bone of the pelvis is formed by the union of the ilium, ischium and pubis bones and therefore is a structural unit. The right and left innominate bones articulate anteriorly with each other at the pubic symphysis and posteriorly with the sacrum at the sacroiliac joints.[69] Slight motion occurs at these three joints to attenuate forces as they are transmitted through the pelvic region, but the pelvis basically functions as a unit in a closed chain.

### The Femur
The shape of the femur is designed to bear body weight and to transmit ground reaction forces through the long bone, neck, and head to the acetabulum of the pelvis. In the frontal plane there is an angle of inclination (normally 125°) between the axis of the femoral neck and the shaft of the femur. The angle of torsion formed by the transverse axis of the femoral condyles and the axis of the neck of the femur ranges from 8° to 25°, with an average angle of 12°. There is also slight bowing of the shaft in the sagittal plane.[69]

## Hip Joint Characteristics and Arthrokinematics

### Characteristics
The hip is a ball-and-socket (spheroidal) triaxial joint made up of the head of the femur and acetabulum of the pelvis. It is supported by a strong articular capsule that is reinforced by the iliofemoral, pubofemoral, and ischiofemoral ligaments. The two hip joints are linked to each other through the bony pelvis and to the vertebral column through the sacroiliac and lumbosacral joints.[69,123]

**Articular Surfaces**
The concave bony partner of the hip joint, the acetabulum, is located in the lateral aspect of the pelvis and faces laterally, anteriorly, and inferiorly (see Fig. 20.1). The acetabulum is deepened by a ring of fibrocartilage, the acetabular labrum. The articular cartilage is horseshoe-shaped, being thicker in the lateral region where the major weight-bearing forces are transmitted. The central portion of the acetabular surface is nonarticular.

The convex bony partner is the spherical head of the femur, which is attached to the femoral neck. It projects anteriorly, medially, and superiorly.

The shapes of the articulating surfaces of the hip joint and the reinforcing properties of the capsule and ligaments, as well as the hip musculature, lend mobility coupled with stability for functional tasks that require wide ranges of combined movements, such as squatting, tying shoes while seated, standing up from a chair or walking.

**Ligaments**
Of the three ligaments that reinforce the joint capsule, the iliofemoral and pubofemoral ligaments are situated anteriorly (Fig. 20.2A), whereas the ischiofemoral ligament is located posteriorly (Fig. 20.2B).[69,94,98]

There is general agreement in the literature that these three capsular ligaments limit excessive extension of the hip and that the iliofemoral ligament, also known as the Y ligament of Bigelow, is the strongest of the hip ligaments.[53,69,94,98] However, there is some dispute as to the functions of each of these ligaments on an individual basis. The iliofemoral ligament, which reinforces the anterior portion of the capsule, also is thought to limit external rotation of the hip[94,98]; and the pubofemoral ligament, lending support to the inferior as well as anterior portion of the

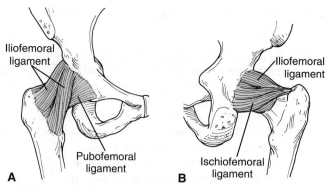

FIGURE 20.2 Ligaments supporting the hip joint. (*A*) Anterior view. (*B*) Posterior view.

capsule, is believed to limit abduction.[94,98] Lastly, the ischiofemoral ligament, although reinforcing the posterior aspect of the capsule, may also limit internal rotation and, when the hip is flexed, adduction.[53,94,98]

### Arthrokinematics of the Hip Joint

During many activities, such as squatting, walking, or doing leg-press exercises, both the pelvis and femur are moving. Therefore, joint mechanics can be described by the movement of the femur in the acetabulum or as the pelvis moving on the femur.

***Motions of the femur.*** The convex femoral head slides in the direction opposite the physiological motion of the femur. Thus, with hip flexion and internal rotation the articulating surface slides posteriorly; with extension and external rotation it slides anteriorly; with abduction it slides inferiorly; and with adduction it slides superiorly (Box 20.1).

***Motions of the pelvis.*** When the lower extremity is stabilized (fixated) distally, as when standing or during the stance phase of gait, the concave acetabulum moves on the convex femoral head, so the acetabulum slides in the same direction as the pelvis. The pelvis is a link in a closed chain; therefore, when the pelvis moves, there is motion at both hip joints as well as the lumbar spine.

| BOX 20.1 | Summary of Arthrokinematics of the Femoral Head in the Hip Joint | |
|---|---|---|
| **Physiological Motions of the Femur** | **Roll** | **Slide** |
| Flexion | Anterior | Posterior |
| Extension | Posterior | Anterior |
| Abduction | Lateral | Inferior |
| Adduction | Medial | Superior |
| Internal rotation | Medial | Posterior |
| External rotation | Lateral | Anterior |

## Influence of the Hip Joint on Balance and Posture Control

The joint capsule is richly supplied with mechanoreceptors that respond to variations in position, stress, and movement for control of posture, balance, and movement. Reflex muscle contractions of the entire kinematic chain, known as balance strategies, occur in a predictable sequence when standing balance is disturbed and regained. Joint pathologies, restricted motion, or muscle weakness can impair balance and postural control.[33,48] Refer to Chapter 8 for an in-depth discussion of these concepts.

# FUNCTIONAL RELATIONSHIPS OF THE HIPS AND PELVIS

## Pelvic Motions and Muscle Function

The pelvis is the connecting link between the spine and lower extremities (Fig. 20.3A). Movement of the pelvis causes motion at the hip joints and lumbar spine articulations. The hip musculature causes pelvic motion through reverse action. Hip flexors cause an anterior pelvic tilt; hip extensors, a posterior pelvic tilt; and abductors and adductors, a lateral pelvic tilt. Rotators cause pelvic rotation. To prevent excessive pelvic motion when moving the femur at the hip joint, the pelvis must be stabilized by the abdominals, erector spinae, multifidus, and quadratus lumborum muscles.

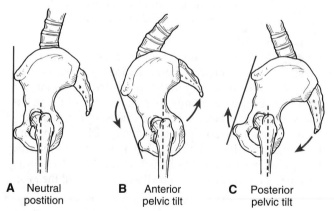

**A** Neutral position    **B** Anterior pelvic tilt    **C** Posterior pelvic tilt

FIGURE 20.3 (*A*) Neutral position of the pelvis. (*B*) Anterior pelvic tilt. (*C*) Posterior pelvic tilt. With anterior pelvic tilt the decreased angle between the pelvis and femur results in hip flexion, and with posterior pelvic tilt the increased angle results in hip extension.

### Anterior Pelvic Tilt

The anterior superior iliac spines of the pelvis move anteriorly and inferiorly and thus closer to the anterior aspect of the femur as the pelvis rotates forward around the transverse axis of the hip joints (Fig. 20.3B). This results in hip flexion and increased lumbar spine extension.[69]

- Muscles causing this motion are the hip flexors and back extensors.
- During standing, the line of gravity of the trunk falls anterior to the axis of the hip joints; the effect is an anterior pelvic tilt moment. Stability is provided by the abdominal muscles and hip extensor muscles.

## Posterior Pelvic Tilt

The posterior superior iliac spines of the pelvis move posteriorly and inferiorly, thus closer to the posterior aspect of the femur as the pelvis rotates backward around the axis of the hip joints (Fig. 20.3C). This results in hip extension and lumbar spine flexion.[69]

- Muscles causing this motion are the hip extensors and trunk flexors.
- During standing when the line of gravity of the trunk falls posterior to the axis of the hip joints, the effect is a posterior pelvic tilt moment. Dynamic stability is provided by the hip flexors and back extensors and passive stability by the iliofemoral ligament.

## Pelvic Shifting

During standing, a forward translatory shifting of the pelvis results in extension of the hip and extension of the lower lumbar spinal segments. There is a compensatory posterior shifting of the thorax on the upper lumbar spine with increased flexion of these spinal segments. This is often seen with slouched or relaxed postures (see Fig. 14.12B in Chapter 14). Little muscle action is required; the posture is maintained by the iliofemoral ligaments at the hip, anterior longitudinal ligament of the lower lumbar spine, and posterior ligaments of the upper lumbar and thoracic spine.

## Lateral Pelvic Tilt

Frontal plane pelvic motion results in opposite motions at each hip joint. Pelvic motion is defined by what is occurring to the iliac crest of the pelvis that is opposite the weight-bearing extremity (that is, the side of the pelvis that is moving). When the pelvis elevates, it is called hip hiking; when it lowers, it is called hip or pelvic drop. On the side that is elevated, there is hip adduction; on the side that is lowered, there is hip abduction (Fig. 20.4A). During standing, the lumbar spine laterally flexes toward the side of the elevated pelvis (convexity of the lateral curve is toward the lowered side).[69]

- Muscles causing lateral pelvic tilting include the quadratus lumborum on the side of the elevated pelvis and reverse muscle pull of the gluteus medius on the side of the lowered pelvis.
- With an asymmetrical slouched posture, the person shifts the trunk weight onto one lower extremity and allows the pelvis to drop on the other side. Passive support comes from the iliofemoral ligament and iliotibial band on the elevated side (stance leg).
- When standing on one leg, there is an adduction moment at the hip, tending to cause the pelvis to drop on the unsupported side (hip or pelvic drop). This is prevented by the gluteus medius stabilizing the pelvis on the stance side.

## Pelvic Rotation

Rotation occurs around one lower extremity that is fixed on the ground. The unsupported lower extremity swings forward or backward along with the pelvis. When the unsupported side of the pelvis moves forward, it is called *forward rotation* of the pelvis.[69] The trunk concurrently rotates in the opposite direction, and the femur on the stabilized side concurrently rotates internally. When the unsupported side of the pelvis moves backward, it is called *posterior rotation*; the femur on the stabilized side concurrently rotates externally, and the trunk rotates opposite (Fig. 20.4B).

## Lumbopelvic Rhythm

A coordinated movement between the lumbar spine and pelvis occurs during maximum forward bending of the trunk[25] as when reaching toward the floor or the toes. As the head and upper trunk initiate flexion, the pelvis shifts posteriorly to maintain the center of gravity over the base of support. The trunk continues to forward-bend, being controlled by the extensor muscles of the spine, until at approximately 45°. At this point for an individual with relatively normal flexibility, the posterior ligaments become taut, and the facets of the zygapophyseal joints approximate. Both of these factors provide stability for the intervertebral joints, and the muscles relax.[126] Once all of the

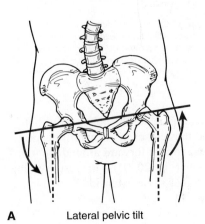

**A**    Lateral pelvic tilt

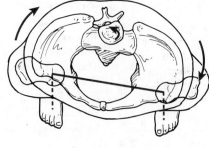

**B**    Pelvic rotation

**FIGURE 20.4** (*A*) Lateral pelvic tilt. Elevation of the iliac crest (hip liking) causes relative adduction of the hip on the elevated side; and lowering of the iliac crest (hip drop) causes relative abduction of the hip on the lower side. (*B*) Pelvic rotation. Forward motion (forward rotation) of the pelvis causes relative external rotation of the hip; and backward motion (posterior rotation) of the pelvis causes relative internal rotation of the hip.

vertebral segments are at the end of the range and stabilized by the posterior ligaments and facets, the pelvis begins to rotate forward (anterior pelvic tilt), being controlled by the gluteus maximus and hamstring muscles. The pelvis continues to rotate forward until the full length of the muscles is reached. Final range of motion (ROM) in forward bending is dictated by the flexibility of the various back extensor muscles and fasciae as well as hip extensor muscles.

The return to the upright position begins with the hip extensor muscles rotating the pelvis posteriorly through reverse muscle action (posterior pelvic tilt) then the back extensor muscles extending the spine from the lumbar region upward. Variations in the normal synchronization of this activity occur because of training (as with dancers and gymnasts), faulty habits, restricted muscle or fascia length, or injury and faulty proprioception.

## Pathomechanics in the Hip Region

Abnormal structure or impaired function of the hip—such as a leg-length discrepancy, decreased flexibility, or muscle imbalances—can contribute to stress in the spine or other joints of the lower extremities.

### Decreased Flexibility
Decreased flexibility in the structures around the hip joint cause weight-bearing forces and movement to be transmitted to the spine rather than absorbed in the pelvis. Tight hip extensors cause increased lumbar flexion when the thigh flexes. Tight hip flexors cause increased lumbar extension as the thigh extends. Hip flexion contractures with incomplete hip extension during weight bearing also place added stresses on the knee because the knee cannot lock while the hip is in flexion unless the trunk is bent forward. During weight bearing tight adductors cause lateral pelvic tilt opposite the side of tightness and side bending of the trunk toward the side of tightness. The opposite occurs with tight abductors.

### Asymmetrical Leg Length
Functional as well as structural asymmetries of the lower extremities affect the posture of the pelvis.

*Unilateral short leg.* A unilateral short *leg* causes lateral pelvic tilting (drop on the short side) and side-bending of the trunk away from the short side (convexity of lateral lumbar curve toward side of short leg). This may lead to a functional or eventually a structural scoliosis. Causes of a short leg could be unilateral lower extremity asymmetries such as flat foot, genu valgum, coxa vara, tight hip muscles, anteriorly rotated innominate bone, poor standing posture, or asymmetry in bone growth.

*Coxa valga and coxa vara.* A pathologically large angle of inclination between the femoral neck and shaft of the femur is called *coxa valga*, and a pathologically smaller angle is called *coxa vara*. Unilateral coxa valga results in a relatively longer leg on that side and associated genu varum. Unilateral coxa vara leads to a relatively shorter leg with associated genu valgum.

*Anteversion and retroversion.* An increase in the torsion of the femoral neck is called *anteversion* and causes the shaft of the femur to be rotated medially; a decrease in the torsion is called *retroversion* and causes the shaft of the femur to be rotated laterally. Anteversion often results in genu valgum and pes planus. Unilateral anteversion results in a relatively shorter leg on that side; retroversion causes the opposite effects.

### Hip Muscle Imbalances and Their Effects
Muscles function through habit. Faulty mechanics from inadequate or excessive length and an imbalance in strength cause hip, knee, or back pain.[116] Overuse syndromes, soft tissue stress, and joint pain develop in response to continued abnormal stresses. The related muscle imbalances due to postural impairments are summarized in Box 20.2. Common muscle length-strength imbalances include the following.

- *Shortened iliotibial (IT) band with shortened tensor fasciae latae (TFL) or gluteus maximus.* Postural impairments often associated with a shortened TFL or gluteus maximus include an anterior pelvic tilt posture, slouched posture, or flat back posture (see Chapter 14).
- *Dominance of the two-joint hip flexor muscles (TFL, rectus femoris, sartorius) over the iliopsoas.* This imbalance may cause faulty hip mechanics or knee pain from overuse of these muscles as they cross the knee.

---

**BOX 20.2 Hip Muscle Imbalances Related to Postural Impairments**

**Anterior Pelvic Tilt Posture**
- Short TFL and IT band
- General limitation of hip external rotation
- Weak, stretched posterior portion of the gluteus medius and piriformis
- Excessive medial rotation of the femur during the first half of stance phase of gait with increased stresses on the medial structures of the knee
- Associated lower extremity compensations including medial rotation of the femur, genu valgum, lateral tibial torsion, pes planus, and hallux valgus

**Slouched Posture**
- Shortened rectus femoris and hamstrings
- General limitation of hip rotators
- Weak, stretched iliopsoas
- Weak and shortened posterior portion of the gluteus medius
- Weak, poorly developed gluteus maximus
- Associated lower extremity compensations including hip extension, sometimes medial rotation of the femur, genu recurvatum, genu varum, and pes valgus

**Flat Back Posture**
- A shortened rectus femoris, IT band, and gluteus maximus
- Variations of the above two postures

- *Dominance of the TFL over the gluteus medius.* This imbalance leads to lateral knee pain from IT band tension or medial rotation of the femur with medial knee stresses from an increased bowstring effect.
- *Dominance of hamstring muscles over the gluteus maximus.* The gluteus maximus becomes short and the range of hip flexion decreases; compensation occurs with excessive lumbar spine flexion whenever the thigh is flexed. Limited mobility in the gluteus maximus also causes increased tension on the IT band with associated trochanteric or lateral knee pain. Overuse of the hamstring muscles causes decreased flexibility as well as muscle imbalances with the quadriceps femoris muscle at the knee. The hamstrings dominate the stabilizing function by pulling posteriorly on the tibia to extend the knee in closed-chain activities. This alters the mechanics at the knee and may lead to overuse syndromes in the hamstring tendons or anterior knee pain from imbalances in quadriceps pull.
- *Use of lateral trunk muscles for hip abductors.* This results in excessive trunk motion and increased stress in the lumbar spine.

# THE HIP AND GAIT

During the normal gait cycle, the hip goes through a ROM of 40° of flexion and extension (10° extension at terminal stance to 30° flexion at midswing and initial contact). There is also some lateral pelvic tilt and hip abduction/adduction of 15° (10° adduction at initial contact, 5° abduction at initial swing); and hip internal/external rotation along with pelvic rotation totaling 15° transverse plane motion (peak internal rotation at the end of loading, peak external rotation at the end of pre-swing). Loss of any of these motions affects the smoothness of the gait pattern.[105]

## Hip Muscle Function During Gait

### Hip Flexors
The hip flexors control hip extension at the end of stance, then contract concentrically to initiate swing.[105] With loss of flexor function, a posterior lurch of the trunk to initiate swing is seen. Contractures in the hip flexors prevent complete extension during the second half of stance; the stride is shortened. To compensate, a person increases the lumbar lordosis or walks with the trunk bent forward.

### Hip Extensors
The hip extensors control the flexor moment at initial foot contact, and the gluteus maximus initiates hip extension.[105] With loss of extensor function, a posterior lurch of the trunk occurs at foot contact to shift the center of gravity of the trunk posterior to the hip. With contractures in the gluteus maximus, some decreased range occurs in the terminal swing as the femur comes forward, or the person

may compensate by rotating the pelvis more forward. The lower extremity may rotate outward because of the external rotation component of the muscle, or the gluteus maximus may place greater tension on the iliotibial band through its attachment, leading to irritation along the lateral aspect of the knee with excessive activity.

### Hip Abductors
The hip abductors control the lateral pelvic tilt during swinging of the opposite leg.[105] With loss of function of the gluteus medius, lateral shifting of the trunk occurs over the weak side during stance when the opposite leg swings. This lateral shifting also occurs with a painful hip because it minimizes the torque at the hip joint during weight bearing. The tensor fasciae latae also functions as an abductor and may become tight and affect gait with faulty use.

## Effect of Musculoskeletal Impairments on Gait

Bony and joint deformities change alignment of the lower extremity and therefore the mechanics of gait. Painful conditions cause antalgic gait patterns, which are characterized by minimum stance on the painful side to avoid the stress of weight bearing.

# REFERRED PAIN AND NERVE INJURY

The hip is innervated primarily from the L3 spinal level; hip joint irritation is usually felt along the L3 dermatome reference from the groin, down the front of the thigh to the knee.[35,72] For a detailed description of referred pain patterns and peripheral nerve injuries in the hip and buttock region, see Chapter 13.

## Major Nerves Subject to Injury or Entrapment

*Sciatic nerve.* Entrapment may occur when the sciatic nerve passes deep to the piriformis muscle (occasionally it passes over or through the piriformis).

*Obturator nerve.* Isolated injury is rare, although uterine pressure and damage during labor may occur.

*Femoral nerve.* Injury may result from fractures of the upper femur or pelvis, during reduction of congenital dislocation of the hip, or from pressure during a forceps labor and delivery.

## Common Sources of Referred Pain in the Hip and Buttock Region

If painful symptoms are referred to the hip and buttock region from other sources, primary treatment must be directed to the source of the irritation. Common sources of referred pain into the hip and buttock region include:

- Nerve roots or tissues derived from spinal segments L1, L2, L3, S1, and S2
- Lumbar intervertebral and sacroiliac joints

## MANAGEMENT OF HIP DISORDERS AND SURGERIES

To make sound clinical decisions when treating patients with hip disorders, it is necessary to understand the various pathologies, surgical procedures, and associated precautions and identify presenting impairments, functional limitations, and possible disabilities. In this section common pathologies and surgeries are presented and related to corresponding preferred practice patterns (groupings of impairments) described in the *Guide to Physical Therapist Practice*[1] (Table 20.1). Conservative and postoperative management of these conditions is also described in this section.

## JOINT HYPOMOBILITY: NONOPERATIVE MANAGEMENT

### Related Pathologies and Etiology of Symptoms

#### Osteoarthritis (Degenerative Joint Disease)
Osteoarthritis is the most common arthritic disease of the hip joint. The etiology may be the aging process, joint trauma, repetitive abnormal stresses, obesity, or disease. The degenerative changes include articular cartilage breakdown and loss, capsular fibrosis, and osteophyte formation at the joint margins.[40] These effects usually occur in regions undergoing the greatest loading forces, such as along the superior weight-bearing surface of the acetabulum (see Fig. 11.6).

#### Other Joint Pathologies
Rheumatoid arthritis, aseptic necrosis, slipped epiphyses, dislocations, and congenital deformities can also lead to degenerative changes in the hip joint (see Fig. 11.2).

---

**TABLE 20.1  Hip Pathologies and Related Preferred Practice Patterns**

| PATHOLOGY/SURGICAL PROCEDURE | PREFERRED PRACTICE PATTERNS AND ASSOCIATED IMPAIRMENTS[1] |
|---|---|
| • Abnormal posture (anterior pelvic tilt posture, posterior pelvic tilt posture, rotated or shifted pelvis related to spinal and lower extremity flexibility and strength imbalances or structural malalignment) | Pattern 4B—Impaired posture |
| • Arthritis (osteoarthritis, rheumatoid arthritis, traumatic arthritis)<br>• Aseptic necrosis<br>• Slipped epiphyses<br>• Dislocation<br>• Postimmobilization arthritis (stiffness) | Pattern 4D—Impaired joint mobility, motor function, muscle performance, and ROM associated with connective tissue dysfunction |
| • Acute arthritis<br>• Acute tendonitis, bursitis, muscle pull | Pattern 4E—Impaired joint mobility, motor function, muscle performance, and ROM associated with localized inflammation |
| • Fracture (femoral or pelvic) | Pattern 4G—Impaired joint mobility, muscle performance, and ROM associated with fracture |
| • Total hip arthroplasty<br>• Surface replacement arthroplasty<br>• Hemiarthroplasty | Pattern 4H—Impaired joint mobility, motor function, muscle performance, and ROM associated with joint arthroplasty |
| • Labral tear<br>• Osteotomy<br>• Open reduction and internal fixation of femoral fracture or fracture-dislocation | Pattern 4I—Impaired joint mobility, motor function, muscle performance, and ROM associated with bony or soft tissue surgery |
| • Sciatic, obturator, or femoral nerve injury or entrapment in the pelvis and hip region | Pattern 5F—Impaired peripheral nerve integrity and muscle performance associated with peripheral nerve injury |

## Postimmobilization Hypomobility

A restriction in the capsular tissues leading to joint hypo-mobilities as well as tightness in the surrounding periarticular tissues may occur anytime the joint is immobilized after a fracture or surgery.

## Common Impairments

● Pain experienced in the groin and referred along the anterior thigh and knee in the L3 dermatome.
● Stiffness after rest.
● Limited motion with a firm capsular end-feel. Initially, limitation is only in internal rotation; in advanced stages the hip is fixed in adduction, has no internal rotation or extension past neutral, and is limited to 90° flexion.[35]
● Antalgic gait usually with a compensated gluteus medius (abductor) limp.
● Limited hip extension leading to increased extension forces on the lumbar spine and possible back pain.
● Limited hip extension preventing full knee extension when standing or during gait leading to increased knee stresses.
● Impaired balance and postural control.[48]

## Common Functional Limitations/Disabilities

Hip joint impairments interfere with many weight-bearing activities and ADL.[30,49]

*Early stages.* There is progressive pain with continued weight bearing and gait or at the end of the day after repetitive lower extremity activities. The pain may interfere with work (job-specific) or routine household activities that involve weight bearing, such as meal preparation, cleaning, and shopping.

*Progressive degeneration.* The individual experiences increased difficulty arising from a chair, climbing stairs, squatting, and other weight-bearing activities, as well as restricted routine ADL such as bathing, toileting, and dressing (putting on pants, hose, socks).

## Management: Protection Phase

Chapter 11 describes the general principles and plan of care in the treatment of osteoarthritis and rheumatoid arthritis, and Chapter 10 describes general management of joints during acute, subacute, and chronic stages of tissue injury and repair. In conjunction with medical management of the disease for inflammation and pain, correction of faulty mechanics is an integral part of decreasing pain in the hip. Faulty hip mechanics may be caused by conditions such as obesity, leg-length differences, muscle length and strength imbalances, sacroiliac dysfunction,[30] poor posture, or injury to other joints in the chain.[23] The following goals and interventions are emphasized during the acute stage of tissue healing and the protection phase of nonoperative management.

### Decrease Pain at Rest

● Apply grade I or II oscillation techniques with the joint in the resting position.
● Have the patient rock in a rocking chair to provide gentle oscillations to the lower extremity joints as well as a stimulus to the mechanoreceptors in the joints.[138]

### Decrease Pain During Weight-Bearing Activities

● Provide assistive devices for ambulation to help reduce stress on the hip joint. If the pain is unilateral, teach the patient to walk with a single cane or crutch on the side opposite the painful joint.
● If leg-length asymmetry is causing hip joint stress, gradually elevate the short leg with lifts in the shoe.
● Modify chairs to provide an elevated and firm surface, and adapt commodes with an elevated seat to make sitting down and standing up easier.

### Decrease Effects of Stiffness and Maintain Available Motion

● Teach the patient the importance of frequently moving the hips through their ROM throughout the day. When the acute symptoms are medically controlled, have the patient perform active ROM if he or she can control the motion or with assistance if necessary.
● If a pool is available, have the patient perform ROM in the buoyant environment.
● Initiate nonimpact activities such as swimming, gentle water aerobics, or stationary cycling.

## Management: Controlled Motion and Return to Function Phases

As healing progresses and symptoms subside, the emphasis of management includes the following goals and interventions.

### Progressively Increase Joint Play and Soft Tissue Mobility

*Joint mobilization techniques.* Progress joint mobilization to stretch grades (grade III sustained or grade III and IV oscillation) using the glides that stretch restricting capsular tissue at the end of the available ROM (see Box 20.1 and Figs. 5.45 through 5.47 in Chapter 5). Vigorous stretching should not be undertaken until the chronic stage of healing.

*Passive stretching, neuromuscular inhibition, and self-stretching techniques.* Stretch any range-limiting tissues. Suggested techniques are described in Chapter 4 and in the exercise section later in this chapter.

### Improve Joint Tracking and Pain-Free Motion
Mobilization with movement (MWM) techniques[87] may be applied through the use of a mobilization belt to produce a pain-free inferolateral glide and then superimposing motion to the end of the available range. As with all MWM techniques, no pain should be experienced during application of the technique. Principles of MWM are described in Chapter 5; specific hip MWM techniques are described here.

## Increase Internal Rotation

*Patient position:* Supine with the involved hip flexed and a mobilization belt secured around the proximal thigh and your pelvis.

*Procedure:* Stabilize the patient's pelvis with the palm of the hand closest to the patient's head. Use the mobilization belt to produce a pain-free inferolateral glide while the caudal hand grips around the flexed thigh and shin to create pain-free end-range internal rotation (Fig. 20.5A).

## Increase Flexion

*Patient position:* Supine with the involved hip flexed and a mobilization belt secured around the proximal thigh and the pelvis.

*Procedure:* Stabilize the patient's pelvis with the palm of the hand closest to the patient's head. Use the mobilization belt to produce a pain-free inferolateral glide while the caudal hand grips around the flexed thigh and shin to create pain-free end-range flexion (Fig. 20.5B).

## Increase Extension

*Patient position:* Supine with the pelvis near the end of the treatment table in the Thomas test position (opposite thigh held against the chest) and a mobilization belt secured around the proximal thigh and your pelvis.

*Procedure:* Stabilize the patient's pelvis with the palm of the hand closest to the patient's head. Use the mobilization belt to produce a pain-free inferolateral glide while the caudal hand presses against the extended thigh to create pain-free end-range extension (Fig. 20.5C).

### Increase Extension During Weight Bearing

*Patient position:* Standing with the unaffected foot up on a stool and a mobilization belt secured around the proximal thigh and your pelvis.

*Procedure:* Stabilize the pelvis with both hands and apply a pain-free lateral glide with the mobilization belt while the patient lunges forward to produce painless extension of the affected hip (Fig. 20.5D).

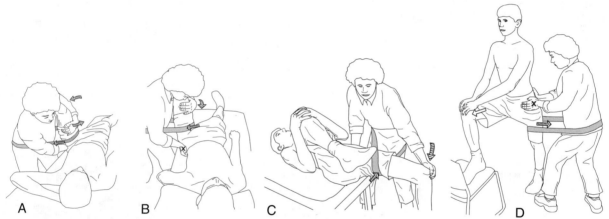

**FIGURE 20.5** Mobilization with movement using an inferolateral glide increasing (*A*) pain-free internal rotation, (*B*) pain-free flexion, (*C*) pain-free extension, and (*D*) extension during weight bearing.

## Improve Muscle Performance in Supporting Muscles

- Initiate exercises that develop strength and control of the hip musculature (especially the gluteus maximus, gluteus medius, and rotators) and that improve stability and balance when performing weight-bearing activities. Begin with submaximal isometric resistance; progress to dynamic resistance as the patient tolerates movement. If any exercises exacerbate the joint symptoms, reduce the intensity. Also reassess the patient's functional activities and adapt them to reduce the stress.
- Progress to functional exercises as tolerated using closed-chain and weight-bearing activities. The patient may require assistive devices while weight bearing. Use a pool or tank to reduce the effects of gravity to allow partial weight-bearing exercises without stress.
- Develop postural awareness and balance.
- Progress the low-impact aerobic exercise program (swimming, cycling, or walking within tolerance).

## Patient Education

Help the patient establish a balance between activity and rest and learn the importance of minimizing stressful deforming forces by maintaining muscle strength and flexibility in the hip region.

###  Focus on Evidence

Two systematic reviews of studies designed to examine evidence of the effects of exercise in the management of hip and knee OA describe support for aerobic exercise and strengthening exercises to reduce pain and disability.[112,113] The consensus of expert opinion cited by Roddy et al.[112] is that there are few contraindications and that exercise is relatively safe in patients with OA; however, exercise should be individualized and patient-centered with consideration for age, co-morbidity, and general mobility.

An outcome review[36] summarized that moderate- or high-intensity exercises in patients with rheumatoid arthritis (RA) have minimal effect on the disease activity, but there is insufficient radiological evidence on the effect in large joints. Long-term moderate- or high-intensity exercises that are individualized to protect radiologically damaged joints improve aerobic capacity, muscle strength, functional ability, and psychological well-being in patients with RA.

## JOINT SURGERY AND POSTOPERATIVE MANAGEMENT

Many joint surgeries are available to treat early- and late-stage joint disease of the hip and some fractures that compromise the vascular supply to the head of the femur. As a result of advances in arthroscopy of the hip over the past decade, small to medium-size full-thickness lesions of the articular cartilage of the acetabulum and head of the femur, as well as other joint pathologies such as acetabular labral tears and capsular laxity, now can be managed arthroscopically.[38] One such procedure, *microfracture*, involves creating small fractures of subchondral bone in the area of the chondral lesion to stimulate growth of fibrocartilage to replace the damaged hyaline cartilage.[38]

Surgical procedures to manage late-stage deterioration of the hip joint include *osteotomy* (which is actually an extra-articular procedure) and arthroplasty, specifically *resurfacing arthroplasty (surface replacement)*,[47] *hemiarthroplasty*,[79] and *total joint replacement arthroplasty*.[31,61,75] *Arthrodesis* and *resection arthroplasty* of the hip are considered salvage procedures after failure of arthroplasty and when revision arthroplasty is contraindicated or not feasible.[75]

The goals of joint surgery and postoperative management are to provide a patient with (1) a pain-free hip, (2) a stable joint for lower extremity weight bearing and functional ambulation, and (3) adequate ROM and strength of the lower extremity for functional activities.

It is important for the therapist to have a basic understanding of the more common surgical procedures for management of joint disease and deformity and a thorough knowledge of appropriate therapeutic exercise interventions and their progression for an effective, safe postoperative rehabilitation program. An overview of two of the more common procedures, total hip arthroplasty and hemiarthroplasty, and guidelines for postoperative management are described in the following sections.

### Total Hip Arthroplasty

One of the most widely performed surgical interventions for advanced arthritis of the hip joint is total hip arthroplasty (Fig. 20.6). Osteoarthritis is the underlying pathology that accounts for most primary total hip procedures.[31]

#### Indications for Surgery
The following are common indications for total hip arthroplasty (THA), also referred to as total hip replacement (THR).[26,31,39,44,75,81]

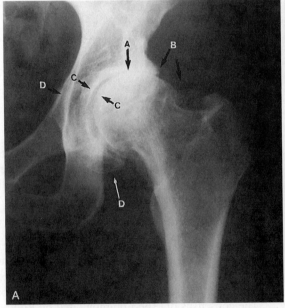
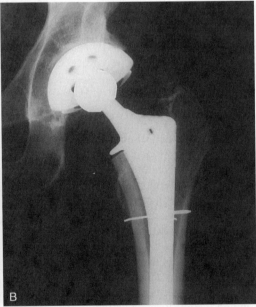

**FIGURE 20.6** Total hip arthroplasty. (*A*) The preoperative film of a severely degenerative hip joint demonstrates the classic signs of degenerative joint disease. A, N; B arrowed, joint space with superior migration of the femoral head; B, osteophyte formation at the joint margins of both the acetabulum and femoral head; C, sclerosis of subchondral bone on both sides of the joint surface; D, acetabular protrusion (a bony outpouching of the acetabular cup in response to the progressive superior and medial migration of the femoral head). (*B*) Postoperative film shows a total hip arthroplasty. Both the acetabular and femoral portions of the joint have been resected and replaced with prosthetic components. (*From McKinnis,*[78] *p. 312, with permission.*)

● Severe hip pain with motion and weight bearing and marked limitation of motion as the result of joint deterioration and loss of articular cartilage associated with osteoarthritis, rheumatoid or traumatic arthritis, ankylosing spondylitis, or osteonecrosis (avascular necrosis) leading to impaired function and health-related quality of life

● Nonunion fracture, instability or deformity of the hip

● Bone tumors

● Failure of conservative management or previous joint reconstruction procedures (osteotomy, resurfacing arthroplasty, femoral stem hemiarthroplasty, total hip replacement)

Historically, primary THA was reserved for patients older than 60 to 65 years of age or the very inactive younger patient with multiple joint involvement because the projected life span of primary THA procedures is less than 20 years.[31,44] For the younger patient with significant hip joint deterioration, surface replacement (resurfacing) arthroplasty, a more bone-conserving surgery than THA, is an alternative that may be considered.[47] However, with advances in designs, materials, and particularly cementless fixation and subsequent broadening of patient selection criteria, THA also is considered an option for some younger, moderately active patients after evaluation on a case-by-case basis.[5] These individuals are counseled by the surgeon to anticipate the need for revision arthroplasty later in life.

There are a number of instances in which THA is contraindicated. Absolute and relative contraindications are noted in Box 20.3.[5,14,31]

## Preoperative Management

Preoperative patient education has been advocated as an important aspect of the overall rehabilitation plan for many years.[8,12] Patient-related instruction in past years took place the day before surgery when patients were often admitted to the hospital for preoperative tests. In the current health care environment, hospital stays have been shortened dramatically. Preoperative contact with a patient prior to elective surgery now occurs on an outpatient basis individually or in a group several days before surgery. Preoperative management typically includes assessment and documentation of a patient's status as well as patient education about the procedure and what to expect during the early postoperative period.[13,55,75,89,114] Patient information sessions are often coordinated and conducted by a team of professionals from multiple disciplines who are likely to be involved with a patient's postoperative care. Box 20.4 summarizes possible components of preoperative management.[13,55,75,89,114]

## Procedures

### Background

***Prosthetic designs and materials.*** Total hip arthroplasty has been successfully performed since the early 1960s.[28,31,41,44,86] Sir John Charnley,[28] a surgeon from England, is credited with the initial research and clinical application of THA, which subsequently has evolved into contemporary hip arthroplasty. A variety of implant designs, materials, and surgical approaches have been developed and modified over the years since the early replacements.[31,41,44] Today total hip implant systems typically are composed of an inert metal (cobalt-chrome and titanium) modular femoral component and a high-density polyethylene acetabular component. Other designs in use are metal-on-metal systems[122] and systems that utilize ceramic surfaces in the design.[31]

***Cemented versus cementless fixation.*** The revolutionary aspect of the early THA procedures was the use of acrylic cement, methylmethacrylate, for prosthetic fixation. Cement fixation allowed very early postoperative weight bearing and shortened the period of rehabilitation, whereas

---

**BOX 20.3 Contraindications to Total Hip Arthroplasty**

**Absolute**
• Active joint infection
• Systemic infection or sepsis
• Chronic osteomyelitis
• Significant loss of bone after resection of a malignant tumor or inadequate bone stock that prevents sufficient implant fixation
• Neuropathic hip joint
• Severe paralysis of the muscles surrounding the joint

**Relative**
• Localized infection, such as bladder or skin
• Insufficient function of the gluteus medius muscle
• Progressive neurological disorder
• Highly compromised/insufficient femoral or acetabular bone stock associated with progressive bone disease
• Patients requiring extensive dental work—dental surgery should be completed before arthroplasty
• Young patients who must or are most likely to participate in high-demand (high-load, high-impact) activities

---

**BOX 20.4 Components of Therapy-Related Preoperative Management: Preparation for Total Hip Arthroplasty**

• Examination and evaluation of pain, ROM, muscle strength, balance, ambulatory status, leg lengths, gait characteristics, use of assistive devices, general level of function, perceived level of disability
• Information for patients and their families about joint disease and the operative procedure in nonmedical terms
• Postoperative precautions and their rationale including positioning and weight bearing
• Functional training for early postoperative days including bed mobility, transfers, gait training with assistive devices
• Early postoperative exercises
• Criteria for discharge from the hospital

prior to the use of cement fixation patients were subjected to months of restricted weight bearing and limited mobility.[31] Cement fixation continues to be used today but has been noted to have its drawbacks.[15,73,100,109]

A significant postoperative complication, identified a number of years after the first THA procedures were performed, was aseptic (biomechanical) loosening of the prosthetic components at the bone–cement interface. It was shown that loosening subsequently led to a gradual recurrence of hip pain and the need for surgical revision.[31,44,75,109] Patients who most often developed loosening were identified as the younger, physically active patients. In contrast, loosening was not shown to be a particularly prevalent problem in elderly patients or in young patients with multiple joint involvement who typically have a limited degree of physical activity.[44,109]

The long-term problem of mechanical loosening of some cemented implants, most often the acetabular component, gave rise to the development and use of cementless (biological) fixation.[31,44,75] Cementless fixation is achieved either by use of porous-coated prostheses that allow osseous ingrowth into the beaded or mesh-like surfaces of an implant or by a cementless press-fit technique.[16,70,106,131] Smooth (nonporous) femoral components also are being used with cementless arthroplasty. Some components are manufactured with a coating of a bioactive compound called hydroxyapatite designed to promote initial osseous ingrowth.[27] Ingrowth of bony tissue occurs over a 3- to 6-month period with continued bone remodeling beyond that time period.

Improvements in cemented fixation[15,73,100,109,110] as well as noncemented fixation[16,70,106,131] have continued, as has debate over the benefits, indications, and disadvantages of both forms of fixation. Cement fixation is routinely used for patients with osteoporosis and poor bone stock and typically with elderly patients.[15,73,100,109] In contrast, cementless fixation is more often the choice for the patient under 60 years of age who is physically active and has good bone quality.[16,21,70,106,131]

In response to a low rate of loosening of cemented femoral implants but continued problems of loosening of cemented acetabular components, the use of a hybrid procedure with a noncemented acetabular component and a cemented femoral prosthesis is a current alternative.[90]

During the first few postoperative weeks, the method of component fixation may influence a patient's weight-bearing status during ambulation and functional activities.

## Overview of Operative Procedures

The operative approaches used to gain access to the involved joint and to implant the prosthetic components during THA can be divided into two broad categories: *standard* and *minimally invasive* approaches. For decades hip arthroplasty procedures have involved the use of rather long surgical incisions (15 to 25 cm) to expose the joint. Although long-term outcomes have been successful, standard surgical approaches impose substantial trauma to soft tissues and contribute to a lengthy postoperative recovery period.

A recent advance in primary hip arthroplasty—the use of minimally invasive approaches through "mini-incisions"— allows adequate exposure of the joint for insertion of the prosthetic components but reportedly lessens the trauma of soft tissues. Brief overviews of the various types of standard and minimally invasive surgical approaches follow, focusing on which muscles are incised or left intact during the procedure because the integrity of these muscles and other soft tissues that surround the prosthetic hip influences its postoperative stability and the extent of restrictions placed on the patient, most notably during the early phase of postoperative recovery.[2,51,75]

***Standard surgical approaches.*** There are several standard (conventional) approaches that may be used during traditional THA procedures: posterior (or posterolateral), lateral, and anterior (or anterolateral). Each has its advantages and disadvantages.[2,51]

- *Posterolateral approach.* This is the most frequently used approach for primary THA. To access the joint, the gluteus maximus is split in line with the muscle fibers. The short external rotator tendons are transected near their insertion. Consequently, this approach preserves the integrity of the gluteus medius and vastus lateralis muscles. Trochanteric osteotomy is not necessary. The capsule is incised posteriorly in preparation for posterior dislocation of the hip. The primary disadvantage of this approach is that it is associated with the highest incidence of postoperative joint instability and resulting subluxation or dislocation of the hip.[66,83,84] To reduce the risk of postoperative dislocation, repair of the posterior capsule (posterior capsulorrhaphy) is advocated to provide maximal soft tissue constraint to the posterior aspect of the capsule.[29]

- *Direct lateral approach.* This approach requires longitudinal division of the tensor fasciae latae, release of up to one-half of the proximal insertion of the gluteus medius, and longitudinal splitting of the vastus lateralis.[2,51] The gluteus minimus also is partially detached from the trochanter. A lateral approach may, but typically does not, involve a trochanteric osteotomy. Disruption of the abductor mechanism is associated with postoperative weakness and gait abnormalities (positive Trendelenburg sign).

- *Anterolateral approach.* This approach and an anterior approach were frequently used for primary THA during the early years of this procedure.[28,31,51] Today, however, it is most often reserved for revision arthroplasty or arthroplasty that involves complex reconstruction. It is also indicated for patients with muscle imbalances associated with stroke or cerebral palsy whose standing posture is characterized by hip flexion and internal rotation.[2,51] Patients exhibiting this posturing are at high risk of dislocation with a posterolateral approach. The anterolateral approach provides excellent stability of the hip postoperatively but involves detachment and subsequent repair of the gluteus medius muscle, or it may necessitate an osteotomy of the greater trochanter for adequate exposure of the hip joint. In addition to the gluteus medius, soft tissues disturbed in an anterolateral approach include the gluteus minimus, tensor fasciae latae, iliopsoas, rectus femoris, and vastus lateralis muscles as well as the anterior capsule.

If a trochanteric osteotomy is performed, the trochanter must be reattached and wired in place to stabilize the osteotomy site until bone healing occurs. The trochanter is often reattached in a position to improve the mechanical efficiency of the gluteus medius muscle.[2,51] Complications associated with trochanteric osteotomy include nonunion, abductor muscle weakness, and greater than usual soft tissue irritation and pain from a considerable amount of internal fixation.

***Minimally invasive approaches.*** As with traditional THA, minimally invasive THA is an open procedure. However, with minimally invasive procedures, the joint is approached through one or two small incisions, usually defined as ≤ 10 cm in length.[14] The characteristics of minimally invasive approaches for THA are summarized in Box 20.5.

The rationale for minimally invasive THA is that, compared with traditional THA, the use of smaller incisions potentially lessens soft tissue trauma during surgery and therefore should improve and accelerate a patient's postoperative recovery.[6,14] Benefits cited by advocates of

---

**BOX 20.5    Features of Minimally Invasive Total Hip Arthroplasty**

- Length of incison: ≤ 10 cm, depending on the location of the approach and the size of the patient[14]
- Most if not all muscles and tendons left intact
- Single-incision or two-incision approach
  - *Single incision*: usually posterior[45] or anterior,[76] or occasionally lateral.[7,57]
  - *Two-incision*: approach: two 4- to 5-cm incisions, one anterior for insertion of acetabular component and one posterior for placement of femoral component.[4,13,115,125]
- Incision location and muscles disturbed
  - *Posterior approach* a 7- to 10-cm posterior incision extending mostly distal to the greater trochanter between the gluteus medius and piriformis muscles; short external rotators may or may not be incised (later repaired), but the abductor mechanism consistently is left intact.[45,137]
  - *Anterior approach*: approximately a 10 cm incision beginning just lateral and distal of the anterior superior iliac spine extending in a distal and slightly posterior direction along the belly of the tensor fasciae latae (TFL); sartorius and rectus femoris retracted medially and the TFL laterally leaves all muscles intact; no postopertive precautions.[13,76]
  - *Lateral approach*: least commonly used; splits the middle-third of the gluteus medius; anterolateral incision into the capsule leaves the posterior capsule intact, eliminating the need to postoperative precautions.[7,57]

---

minimally invasive THA are reduced blood loss, reduced postoperative pain, shorter length of hospital stay and lower cost of hospitalization, more rapid recovery of functional mobility, and a better cosmetic appearance of the surgical scar.[3,6,13,14,115] However, proponents also note that minimally invasive THA procedures are more technically challenging, specifically with regard to insertion and alignment of the prosthetic components, and that there is likely to be a higher rate of complications depending on the surgeon's experience with the new approach and selection of patients.[3,7]

Although most investigators have indicated that minimally invasive THA procedures hold promise and many reports have provided data about a variety of positive outcomes associated with minimally invasive approaches,[13,14,76] these reports have been limited to descriptions of practitioner or institutional experiences with selected patient populations and did not include a comparison group. Only recently have studies become available that call into question some of the reported benefits and document the rate of surgery-related complications or that directly compare minimally invasive THA procedures with traditional THA.[99,137]

 **Focus on Evidence**

Woolson et al.[137] conducted a retrospective comparative study of 135 patients who had undergone primary, unilateral THA with either a standard posterior approach (85 patients, mean age 63 years) or a minimally invasive posterior approach (50 patients, mean age 60 years). Several surgery-related, in-hospital variables and discharge outcomes were evaluated. The participating surgeons determined which patients met the criteria for the minimally invasive procedure with regard to health history and body mass index. Consequently, the minimally invasive group was thinner and healthier than the conventional THA group. Despite these demographic differences, there were no significant differences found between the groups with respect to the surgery itself (operating time, blood loss, need for transfusion), nor were there significant differences in length of hospital stay or the percentage of patients discharged diectly home. However, an independent investigator, who was blind to the type of approach used, identified a higher rate of complications in the minimally invasive group, including wound complications, component malpositioning, and leg-length discrepancy.

Ogonda and colleagues[99] reported the first randomized controlled trial comparing minimally invasive and traditional THA in 219 patients who underwent primary, unilateral, hybrid THA performed by the same surgeon. In both groups a single incision, posterior approach was used, with the only differences being the length of the skin incision (the minimally invasive incision ≤ 10 cm and the standard incision 16 cm) and the extent of tensor fasciae latae disturbance during the approach (less in the mini-incision group). All patients and evaluators were blinded to the length of the incision, and all participated in exercise and functional training after surgery. No significant differences were found between groups at the conclusion of the study with respect to the variables evaluated, including postoperative pain and use of pain medication, ability to transfer and ambulate with an assistive device, length of hospital stay, and discharge to home or to a transitional facility. At 6 weeks after surgery there continued to be no significant differences between groups related to function or complications.

The investigators in both studies concluded that there was no objective evidence to support that there are short-term benefits of minimally invasive THA compared with traditional THA. Both indicated that long-term, follow-up studies must be conducted.

***Implantation of components and closure.*** After dislocation of the joint, an osteotomy is performed at the femoral neck, and the head is removed. Another option used by some surgeons for minimally invasive procedures is to cut the femoral neck in situ without dislocating the hip.[13,76,125] The acetabulum is reamed and remodeled, and a high-density polyethylene cup is inserted into the prepared acetabulum.[100,110] A patient with developmental dysplasia of the hip may require acetabular bone grafting to improve the stability of the prosthetic joint. The intramedullary canal of the femur may be broadened, primarily when cement fixation is to be used; and a stemmed, metal prosthesis is inserted into the shaft of the femur.[15,109] It is important to note that trial components are inserted and checked radiographically to verify alignment of the components, and the hip is moved through a full ROM to assess its stability before the permanet implants are inserted.

After the prosthetic hip is reduced, the capsule usually is repaired. The remaining layers of soft tissues that were incised or detached are securely repaired and appropriately balanced prior to closure.

### Complications

The incidence of intraoperative and postoperative complications after primary, traditional THA is relatively low. However, there may be a higher incidence of complications after minimally invasive procedures due to decreased exposure of the hip joint and the more technically demanding nature of minimally invasive approaches.[3,7] Although only a small percentage of complications require revision arthroplasty, any complication can hamper rehabilitation and restoration of functional mobility.

Intraoperative complications associated with THA include malpositioning of the prosthetic components, femoral fracture, and nerve injury. In addition to medical complications, such as infection, deep vein thrombosis (DVT), or pneumonia that can occur after any surgery, postoperative complications that may occur during the early period of recovery (before 6 weeks or up to 2 to 3 months) include wound healing problems, dislocation of the prosthetic joint, disruption of a bone graft site before sufficient bone healing has occurred, and leg-length discrepancy.[83] Late complications include dislocation, mechanical loosening of either implant at the bone–cement or bone–implant interface, polyethylene wear, and in rare instances heterotopic ossification.

Dislocation of the operated hip is a complication that occurs most frequently during the first 2 to 3 months postoperatively when soft tissues around the hip joint are healing. The frequency of early dislocation after current-day primary THA is reported to be < 1% to slightly more than 10%, with a mean of just less than 2%.[80] However, this rate increases to 5% at 5 years.[80] Most dislocations are nontraumatic and occur in a posterior direction.[66,84] Posterior dislocations are often but not always associated with a posterior surgical approach.[2,51] However, dislocation also occurs after anterior/anterolateral and direct lateral approaches.[66,75,83,84,104,139] Patient-related and surgery/prothesis-related risk factors that may contribute to dislocation are noted in Table 20.2.[80] Precautions to reduce the risk of dislocation after THA are addressed in the following section on postoperative management (see Box 20.7). Recurrent dislocation after THA usually must be managed surgically.

Inequality of leg lengths is a complaint of some patients during the early period of recovery after THA.[103] Although asymmetry of the pelvis and trunk may be evident

| TABLE 20.2 Risk Factors Contributing to Joint Dislocation after Total Hip Arthroplasty | |
|---|---|
| **Patient-Related Factors** | **Surgery/Prosthesis-Related Factors** |
| • Age > 80 to 85 years[80,84]<br>• THA for femoral neck fracture<br>• Medical diagnosis: higher risk in patients with inflammatory arthritis (mostly RA) than patients with OA[139]<br>• Poor quality soft tissue from chronic inflammatory disease<br>• History of prior hip surgery<br>• Preoperative and postoperative muscle weakness and contractures<br>• Cognitive dysfunction, dementia | • Surgical approach: higher risk with posterior than anterior or lateral approaches<br>• Malpositioning of the acetabular component<br>• Inadequate soft tissue balancing during surgery or poor quality soft tissue repair<br>• Experience of the surgeon |

during standing and walking, in most instances this is the result of muscle spasm, muscle weakness (particularly the gluteus medius), and residual contracture of hip muscles, which can be managed conservatively. However, a true leg-length discrepancy, associated with low back and hip pain or hip dislocation, may be the result of malpositioning of the prosthetic implants (usually the acetabular component). If significant, it may necessitate revision arthroplasty.[103]

## Postoperative Management

### Immobilization

After THA there is no need for immobilization of the operated hip. To the contrary, postoperative rehabilitation emphasizes early movement. Depending on the type of surgical approach used and the stability of the prosthetic hip, the operated limb may need to remain in a position of slight abduction and neutral rotation when the patient is lying in bed in the supine position. An abduction pillow or wedge typically is sufficient to maintain the position.[75]

### Weight-Bearing Considerations

After cemented THA, typically patients are permitted to bear as much weight as tolerated almost immediately after surgery.[15,73,100,109] In contrast, with cementless or hybrid THA, it is often necessary to limit weight bearing on the operated limb for the first few weeks or up to 3 months. A number of factors affect the extent and duration of postoperative weight-bearing restrictions and the need for an ambulation aid during transfers, walking, and ascending and descending stairs. Box 20.6 summarizes these factors.

---

**BOX 20.6  Early Postoperative Weight–Bearing Restrictions After Total Hip Arthroplasty**

**Method of Fixation**
- *Cemented.* Immediate postoperative weight bearing as tolerated.[15,73,75,100]
- *Cementless and hybrid.* Recommendations vary from partial weight bearing (toe-touch or touch-down) for at least 6 weeks[16,70,75,90] to weight bearing as tolerated (no restrictions) immediately after surgery.[13,19,21]

**Surgical Approach**
- *Standard versus minimally invasive.* Weight-bearing usually more restricted after standard (traditional) approach because of more extensive surgical disturbance and repair than minimally invasive approach.[14] Weight bearing as tolerated may be permissible immediately after minimally invasive procedure.[13]
- *Trochanteric osteotomy.* Although used infrequently, restricted weight bearing at least 6 to 8 weeks or possibly 12 to 16 weeks for bone healing

**Other Factors**
- *Use of bone grafts.* Non-weight-bearing or restricted weight bearing during bone healing.
- *Poor quality of patient's bone.* Extended restrictions so as not to jeopardize the stability of the prosthetic implants.

---

Although it is customary to limit weight bearing on the operated lower extremity after cementless and hybrid THA,[16,59,131] this practice deserves a closer look. The rationale for restricting weight bearing is based on the assumption that early, excesssive loading of the operated limb could cause micromovement at the bone–implant interface, thereby jeopardizing the initial stability of the implant(s), interfering with osseous ingrowth, and contributing to eventual loosening of the prosthetic implants.

Nonetheless, there are also potential benefits of safe levels of early weight bearing after THA, specifically the reduction of bone demineralization from decreased weight bearing and the earlier recovery of functional mobility.[19,21] It has been established that many patients have difficulty learning and integrating prescribed weight-bearing limitations into daily functional activities and consequently place greater loads than recommended on the operated extremity, particularly once postoperative pain has subsided.[133] It is also known that in the supine position resisted movements of the lower extremity impose loads on the hip considerably greater than body weight.[97]

In light of these considerations, the need for weight-bearing restrictions after cementles THA currently is being re-examined.

 **Focus on Evidence**_____

In two recent randomized, controlled investigations,[19,21] the effects of immediate weight bearing as tolerated during ambulation and other functional activities after cementless or hybrid arthroplasty were compared with the effects of restricted weight bearing. No short-term or long-term adverse effects of immediate weight bearing were identified in either study. It is important to note that patients in both studies were relatively young compared with most patients undergoing hip arthroplasty, and their bone quality was described as excellent. In addition, all patients in both studies participated in a comprehensive, supervised postoperative rehabilitation program.

In one study,[21] patients assigned to the immediate weight-bearing group were placed on no weight-bearing restrictions. These patients were also encouraged to discontinue use of ambulation aids as soon as possible. In contrast, those in the restricted weight-bearing group were required to ambulate with two crutches and were limited to toe-touch weight bearing for 6 weeks. After 6 weeks these patients were permitted to bear weight as tolerated.

In the other study,[19] patients in the immediate weight-bearing group initially used one crutch but were encouraged to place as much weight as tolerated on the operated lower extremity. Patients in the delayed weight-bearing group ambulated with two crutches and were allowed to place only 10% of body weight on the operated leg for 3 months.

There were no significant differences found between the two groups in either study on several follow-up evaluations. Authors of both studies suggested that early weight bearing as tolerated after cementless or hybrid primary THA can be safe in a young patient population ($< 60$ to 65 years of age) with excellent bone quality. However, in the clinical setting, the responsibility of determining the need for protected weight bearing during the early phase of postoperative rehabilitation after THA remains with the surgeon.

## Exercise and Functional Training

The use of therapeutic exercise interventions for patients after THA has been reported in the literature for several decades.[12,24,34,54,111] Although the time frame for and extent of patient-therapist contact have decreased substantially since these early descriptive reports were published, the ultimate goal of rehabilitation remains the same: to optimize a patient's postoperative level of function. However, specific components, frequency, and progression of rehabilitation programs have not been consistent or standardized.[37] More often than not rehabilitation programming has centered on protocols developed by and based on the opinions or assumptions of individual surgeons or therapy departments rather than on evidence-based research on the effects of specific exercises or weight-bearing activities on the hip joint or on functional outcomes. In addition, exercise protocols often must be adjusted to meet the needs and abilities of individual patients. Consequently, the effectiveness of postoperative exercise has not been clearly supported.

A report from the National Institutes of Health (NIH) has identified the need for consistently applied and evaluated long- and short-term intervention strategies for rehabilitation after THA.[95] A consensus survey on physical therapy-related intervention for early inpatient total hip (and knee) rehabilitation is a step forward in the development of consistent guidelines for postoperative management.[37] The exercises and functional activities identified in the consensus document were elements common to most postoperative programs and only those agreed upon by the participating physical therapists.

The goals, guidelines, and precautions for exercise and functional activities after THA discussed in this section represent not only those interventions identified in the aforementioned consensus survey but also exercises selected from other resources in the current literature,[22,26,56,75,89,134] including those for an accelerated rehabilitation program after minimally invasive THA.[13] The suggested exercises, functional activities, and precautions are also based on the results of the available, albeit limited, research on the impact of specific exercises and functional activities on the hip joint.

 **Focus on Evidence**_____

Several related, single-subject studies have measured in vivo forces acting on the hip and acetabular contact pressures during exercise and gait.[46,64,65,124] Although these studies involved only two patients after insertion of a femoral endoprosthesis, not a total joint replacement, the results raise questions about assumptions made by clinicians with regard to the selection and progression of common exercises and functional activities during rehabilitation after hip arthroplasty. The results of these studies suggest that active or resistive exercises, per-

formed statically or dynamically, should be initiated and progressed cautiously. During the acute or postacute phases of rehabilitation some exercises, such as maximal effort gluteal setting or unassisted heel slides typically used during the acute phase of rehabilitation and manually resisted isometric abduction during the postacute stage in preparation for gait and other weight-bearing activities, may actually generate greater acetabular contact pressures than the weight-bearing activities themselves.[46,124]

## Exercise: Maximum Protection Phase After Traditional THA

Common impairments exhibited by patients during the acute and subacute stages of soft tissue healing and the initial phase of postoperative rehabilitation after THA are pain secondary to the surgical procedure, decreased ROM, muscle guarding and weakness, impaired postural stability and balance, and diminished functional mobility (transfers and ambulation activities). Depending on the type of THA procedure and the surgeon's preference, weight-bearing restrictions initially may interfere with functional activities.

The emphasis of this phase rehabilitation after a standard surgical approach is on patient education to reduce the risk of early postoperative complications, in particular dislocation of the operated hip. (Risk factors for dislocation after THA are noted in Table 20.2.) Precautions during functional activities are determined by the surgical approach used and input from the surgeon about the stability of the hip replacement (Box 20.7).[66,75,83,84,104] (Also refer to Box 20.6 for weight-bearing restrictions.)

Although a posterior surgical approach is associated with the highest risk of dislocation, all patients routinely are asked to limit flexion of the hip to < 90° and rotation to < 45° for about 6 weeks regardless of the approach used.[104]

Selected exercises and functional training begin the day of or after surgery. The frequency of treatment by a therapist is often twice a day until the patient is discharged from the hospital,[37] typically by 3 to 4 days postoperatively. Ideally, the prescribed exercises are performed hourly by the patient.

*Goals and interventions.* The following goals and interventions apply to the initial postoperative days while the patient is hospitalized, continuing through the first few weeks after surgery when the patient is at home or in another health care facility.

◎ *Prevent vascular and pulmonary complications.*
  • Ankle pumping exercise to prevent venous stasis, thrombus formation, and the potential for pulmonary embolism.
  • Deep breathing exercise and bronchial hygiene to prevent postoperative atelectasis or pneumonia continued until the patient is up and about on a regular basis.
◎ *Prevent postoperative dislocation or subluxation of the operated hip.*
  • Patient and caregiver education about motion restrictions, safe bed mobility, transfers, and precautions during other ADL (see Box 20.7).

## BOX 20.7   Early Postoperative Motion Precautions After Total Hip Arthroplasty*

**Posterior/Posterolateral Approaches**

**ROM**
- Avoid hip flexion > 80° to 90° and adduction and internal rotation beyond neutral.

**ADL**
- Transfer to the sound side from bed to chair or chair to bed.
- Do not cross the legs.
- Keep the knees slightly lower than the hips when sitting.
- Avoid sitting in low, soft chairs.
- If the bed at home is low, raise it on blocks.
- Use a raised toilet seat.
- Avoid bending the trunk over the legs when rising from or sitting down in a chair or dressing or undressing.
- For bathing, take showers or use a shower chair in the bathtub.
- When ascending stairs, lead with the sound leg. When descending, lead with the operated leg.
- Pivot on the sound lower extremity.
- Avoid standing activities that involve rotating the body toward the operated extremity.

- Sleep in supine position with an abduction pillow; avoid sleeping or resting in a side-lying position.

**Anterior/Anterolateral and Direct Lateral Approaches With or Without Trochanteric Osteotomy**

**ROM**
- Avoid flexion > 90°.
- Avoid hip extension, adduction, and external rotation past neutral.
- Avoid the combined motion of flexion, abduction, and external rotation.
- If the gluteus medius was incised and repaired or a trochanteric osteotomy was done, do not perform active, antigravity hip abduction for at least 6 to 8 weeks or until approved by the surgeon.

**ADL**
- Do not cross the legs.
- During early ambulation, step to, rather than past, the operated hip to avoid hyperextension.
- Avoid activities that involve standing on the operated extremity and rotating away from the involved side.

*Note: These precautions apply to traditional total hip arthroplasty and may or may not be necessary after minimally invasive procedures, depending on the surgeon's guidelines.

---

- Monitor the patient for signs and symptoms of dislocation, such as shortening of the operated lower extremity not previously present.

◉ *Achieve independent functional mobility prior to discharge.*
- Bed mobility and transfer training, integrating weight-bearing and motion restrictions.
- Ambulation with an assistive device (usually a walker or two crutches) immediately after surgery, adhering to weight-bearing restrictions and gait-related ADL precautions.

N O T E : Arising from a low chair imposes particularly high loads across the hip joint, producing loads approximately eight times body weight.[97] If the posterior capsule was incised during surgery, this places the involved hip at a high risk of posterior dislocation until soft tissues around the hip joint have healed sufficiently (at least 6 weeks) or until the surgeon indicates that unrestricted functional activities are permissible.

◉ *Maintain a functional level of strength and muscular endurance in the upper extremities and unoperated lower extremity.*
- Active-resistive exercises in functional movement patterns, targeting muscle groups used during transfers and ambulation with assistive devices.

◉ *Prevent reflex inhibition and atrophy of musculature in the operated limb.*
- *Submaximal* muscle-setting exercises of the quadriceps, hip extensor, and hip abductor muscles—just enough to elicit a muscle contraction.

P R E C A U T I O N : If a trochanteric osteotomy was performed, avoid even low-intensity isometric contractions of the hip abductors during the early postoperative phase unless initially approved by the surgeon and performed strictly at a minimum intensity. (See Box 20.7 for additional precautions after trochanteric osteotomy.)

◉ *Regain active mobility and control of the operated extremity.*
- While in bed, active-assistive (A-AROM) exercises of the hip within protected ranges.
- Active knee flexion and extension exercises while seated in a chair, emphasizing terminal extension progressing to active hip and knee flexion (heel slides), gravity-eliminated hip abduction (if permissible) by sliding the leg on a low-friction surface, and active rotation between external rotation or internal rotation to neutral depending on the surgical approach. Do these exercises while lying supine in bed.
- Active hip exercises in the standing position with the knee flexed and extended with hands on a stable surface to maintain balance.
- Closed-chain hip flexion and extension, placing only the allowable amount of weight on the operated extremity.

◉ *Prevent a flexion contracture of the operated hip.*
- Avoid use of a pillow under the knee of the operated extremity.

**Exercise: Moderate and Minimum Protection Phases**
After traditional THA the intermediate and late phases of rehabilitation begin about 4 to 6 weeks postoperatively.

The degree of protection of the operated hip required varies substantially from patient to patient. Some degree of moderate protection may be necessary for 12 weeks postoperatively. However, full healing of soft tissue and bone continues for up to a year after surgery.

The exercises described for these phases usually are a part of a home program that a patient has learned during home-based therapy, on an outpatient basis, or in an extended care facility. Exercises and functional training focus on restoration of strength, postural stability and balance, muscular and cardiopulmonary endurance, and ROM to functional levels and gradual resumption and necessary modification of functional activities. Postoperative precautions during ADL are continued for at least 12 weeks and often considerably longer.[75,89] Patient education continues throughout these phases of rehabilitation in preparation for a return to anticipated activities in the home, workplace, or recreational setting. Return to a full level of functional activities may take 6 to 8 months.

To prolong the life of the prosthesis, particularly in patients under 50 to 60 years of age, patients are routinely advised to refrain from high-impact sports and recreational activities.[77] If a patient's employment involves heavy labor, vocational retraining or an adjustment in work-related activities is advised.

***Goals and interventions.*** The following are the goals and interventions during the intermediate and advanced phases of rehabilitation.

 ***Regain strength and muscular endurance.***
- Open-chain exercises within the permissible ranges in the operated leg against light resistance. Emphasize increasing the number of repetitions rather than the resistance to improve muscular endurance.
- Bilateral closed-chain exercises such as mini-squats against light-grade elastic resistance or while holding light weights in both hands when unsupported standing is permitted.
- Unilateral closed-chain exercises such as forward and lateral step-ups (to a low step) and partial lunges with the involved foot forward when full weight bearing is permitted on the operated lower extremity.
- Resistive exercises to other involved areas in order to improve function.

 ***Improve cardiopulmonary endurance.***
- Nonimpact aerobic conditioning program, such as progressive stationary cycling, swimming, or water aerobics.

 ***Reduce contractures while adhering to motion precautions.***
- Gravity-assisted supine stretch to neutral in the Thomas test position. Pull the uninvolved knee to the chest while relaxing the operated hip. (At least 10° of hip extension beyond neutral is needed for a normal gait pattern.)
- Resting in a prone position for a prolonged passive stretch of the hip flexor muscles when rolling to prone-lying is permissible and is also tolerable.
- Integrate gained ROM into functional activities.

PRECAUTION: Check with the surgeon before initiating a stretch of the hip flexors to neutral or into hyperextension if the patient has undergone an anterolateral approach.

 ***Improve postural stability, balance, and gait.***
- Emphasize use of a cane (in the hand *contralateral* to the operated hip) and progressive weight bearing on the operated limb.
- While using a cane, walk over uneven and soft surfaces to challenge the balance system.
- Integrate posture training during ambulation, emphasizing an erect trunk, vertical alignment, equal step lengths, and a neutral symmetrical position of the legs.
- Continue cane use until weight-bearing restrictions are discontinued or if the patient exhibits gait deviations, such as a positive Trendelenburg sign on the operated lower extremity, indicating gluteus medius weakness. Cane use is also recommended during extended periods of ambulation to decrease muscle fatigue.

### ◉ Focus on Evidence_____

Use of a cane in the contralateral hand by patients after a hip replacement has been shown to decrease electromyographic (EMG) activity in the hip abductor muscles to a significant degree regardless of whether moderate or near-maximum force is applied on the cane.[93] In the same study, ipsilateral cane use produced no significant decrease in EMG activity in the hip abductor muscles. The degree to which the decreases in EMG activity reflected a reduction in forces imposed on the prosthetic hip joint was not determined in this study. However, in single-subject studies of two patients with femoral endoprotheses, acetabular contact pressures were reduced by using a cane in the contralateral hand.[46,64,65]

 ***Prepare for a full level of functional activities.***
- Integrate strength, endurance, and balance exercises into functional activities but continue to avoid applying high loads during exercise. When weight-bearing restrictions have been discontinued, strengthen hip and knee musculature with functional activities such as ascending and descending stairs step over step.
- Progressively increase the length of time and distance of a low-intensity walking program 2 to 4 days a week.
- When walking and carrying a heavy object in one hand, suggest that the patient hold it on the same side as the operated hip. Theoretically, this reduces the amount of stress imposed over time on the prosthetic hip replacement.
- Through patient education reinforce the importance of selecting activities that reduce or minimize the forces and demands placed on the prosthetic hip.

### ◉ Focus on Evidence_____

The results of research suggest that the forces imposed on the abductor muscles of the prosthetic hip, as measured by EMG, are significantly lower when a load is carried in the arm on the same side as the prosthetic hip compared to when the load is carried in the contralateral arm. This was found to hold true with and without cane usage.[91,92] As the patient's activity level increases, have the patient avoid high-impact activities or activities that impose heavy rotational forces on the operated limb. Both factors can contribute to long-term loosening and wear of the prosthetic implants and eventual failure of the hip replacement.

## Accelerated Rehabilitation After Minimally Invasive THA

For carefully selected patients who have undergone minimally invasive primary THA, an accelerated rehabilitation program may be feasible to achieve optimal outcomes as rapidly as possible. However, few guidelines have been published to date.

Berger and colleagues[13] developed and implemented a program specifically designed for patients undergoing primary cementless THA with a two-incision approach. Patients eligible for the minimally invasive surgery and accelerated rehabilitation program had to be between the ages of 40 to 75 years with a body mass index of $< 35$, no previous hip surgery, and no history of cardiac, vascular, or pulmonary disorders. The following are key elements of the accelerated program described by Berger et al.[13]

*Preoperative activities.* Prior to surgery, educate the patient about the surgical procedure and postoperative rehabilitation program, wound care, and the home exercise program. Initiate gait training (weight bearing as tolerated) using crutches and a cane.

*Immediate postoperative therapy.* Approximately 5 to 6 hours after surgery, if the patient is medically stable, begin the following activities.

- Postoperative bed and chair transfers (weight bearing as tolerated)
- Ambulation with crutches, progressing to a cane as tolerated
- Ascending and descending stairs, one step at a time

*Criteria for hospital discharge.* The patient is discharged from the hospital to home when able to perform the following tasks independently while using an ambulation aid.

- Transfer in and out of bed
- Stand up from and sit down in a standard, firm chair
- Walk 100 feet
- Ascend and descend a flight of stairs

Berger et al.[13] reported that 97 of the 100 participants in the study met the crteria for same-day discharge. The three remaining patients, who delayed therapy because of nausea or orthostatic hypotension, were discharged the day after surgery.

*Home-based and outpatient therapy.* Patients participate in a home-based therapy program followed by outpatient therapy once able to drive. There are no specific positioning or ROM precautions or weight-bearing restrictions.

- Progress to ambulation with a cane as soon as possible. Continue cane use until able to ambulate with a symmetrical gait pattern and no noticable limp.

- Have patient maintain an activity log to document functional outcomes.

Some of the short-term outcomes of this accelerated rehabilitation program reported by Berger et al.[13] were that patients discontinued use of narcotic pain medication, transitioned to a cane, and started driving after an average of 6 days. Patients who worked returned to work at an average of 8 days. Patients walked without an assistive device at an average of 9 days. At 3 months there were no serious complications identified.[13]

PRECAUTION: These highlights are presented as an example of a rapid rehabilitation program after minimally invasive primary THA performed by the same surgeon and carried out at one institution with a carefully selected group of patients. Such a program is not appropriate for many patients undergoing minimally invasive THA and should be implemented only with necessary planning and ongoing communication between the surgeon, therapist, and patient.

## Outcomes

The assessment of outcomes of THA has focused on numerous variables, ranging from patient satisfaction and the impact of THA on function and quality of life to the assessment of prosthetic designs, materials, methods of fixation, and rates of complications. The number of follow-up studies on any one of these areas is extensive. A 1990s NIH report pointed out that THA and subsequent rehabilitation have resulted in a high degree of success related to pain reduction, improvement in physical function, and health-related quality of life.[68,95] The report went on to say that THA results in good to excellent long-term results for 90% to 95% of patients.[95] However, the findings of numerous follow-up studies reflect considerable variability of outcomes.

*Pain relief, patient satisfaction, and quality of life.* Patient satisfaction after THA as well as the assessment of pain and perceived level of function and quality of life as judged by the patient and/or the surgeon generally reflect a marked decrease in pain and improvement in function.[107] Historically, patient-related outcomes were assessed by the surgeon rather than the patient. During the past decade or two, assessing outcomes from a patient's perspective has become increasingly evident in the literature. One outcomes study, in particular, pointed out why there is a need for evaluations by both the patient and the surgeon to fully assess the long-term outcomes of THA. During postoperative follow-up when patients reported little or no pain, patients' and physicians' assessments of pain and level of satisfaction were similar. However, as a patient's report of continuing pain increased, the disparity increased between the patient's and the physician's assessment of the level of patient satisfaction.[71]

Two recent studies have identified several factors that contribute to unsatisfactory outcomes. Fortin and colleagues[42] investigated the timing of THA and outcomes. Although intuitively known by experienced practitioners, this study confmed that patients who had the worst physical function and pain before surgery had the poorest outcomes 2 years after surgery. The findings of a long-term (mean 3.6 years), prospective study by Nils-dotter et al.[96] of patients who had undergone unilateral THA for OA also confirmed that a higher preoperative level of pain predicted poorer outcomes. In addition, their study revealed that an older age at the time of surgery and postoperative low back pain were predictors of poor self-assessed outcomes.

***Improvements in physical function.*** Improvements in ROM, postural stability, strength, and functional mobility are significant but occur gradually after THA. Patients typically achieve 90% of their expected level of overall functional improvement by the end of the first year. During the next 1 to 2 years, patients have self-reported additional gains in strength, with improvement in function reaching a plateau at approximately 2 to 3 years.[107]

Several studies have documented deficits in physical function that persist at 1 year and beyond after THA. Trudelle-Jackson and co-investigators,[132] compared ROM, static muscle strength, and postural stability (balance during one-leg stance) in a group of 15 patients with a mean age 62 years (range 51–77 years) 1 year after unilateral THA. They found no significant differences in ROM for the operated and uninvolved hips and small but not statistically significant differences in the strength of hip and knee musculature. However, they did find substantial differences between the operated leg and the uninvolved leg for all parameters of postural stability measured during one-leg stance. In addition, patients' self-assessed level of physical function was moderately associated with muscle strength but only weakly with postural stability.

In another study, Shih and colleagues[120] identified muscle weakness in the operated lower extremity compared with the uninvolved side in all patients 2 years after THA, with strength in the hip flexors showing the slowest rate of recovery. The investigator suggested that persistent muscle weakness and muscle fatigue during activities that require endurance may increase the stresses placed on the prosthetic implants and contribute to biomechanical loosening of the implant over time.[120] The findings of both of these studies suggest that some patients benefit from a long-term program of strength and balance training, even after returning to a full level of functional activity.

***Implant design, fixation, and surgical approach.*** Two to three decades of studies indicate that both cemented and cementless THA have yielded equally positive postoperative outcomes in all areas of assessment, with the most consistent being reduction of pain.[70,109] Despite the success of both cemented and uncemented THA, debate continues as to the benefits and limitations of both types of fixation. What can be said is that as surgical technique, prosthetic designs, and materials continue to improve the rate of failure because of wear and loosening continues to decrease. A higher rate of loosening continues to occur in the acetabular component.[109,110]

Results of a study of 92 cementless THA procedures revealed a 100% survival rate of the femoral component after 10 years and a 96.4% rate for the acetabular component.[3] In-depth analyses and current information on outcomes of specific prosthetic designs[41] as well as outcome assessments of cemented,[15,73,100,109] uncemented,[16,70,106,131] and hybrid[90] procedures can be found in the references noted.

Outcomes of minimally invasive THA compared with traditional THA are just beginning to be investigated.[99,137] Significantly more short- and long-term studies are needed before the value of minimally invasive approaches can be determined.

***Impact of rehabilitation.*** Despite the number of sources in the literature that emphasize the importance of rehabilitation programs or, more specifically, a postoperative exercise and ambulation program after THA, the impact of these postoperative interventions has not been clearly established. The NIH reported that there is currently insufficient evidence to determine what constitutes an appropriate level of physical therapy utilization after THA. The report went on to say that there does appear to be a role for these interventions but that the efficacy of these postoperative programs has not yet been determined.[95] Studies have demonstrated that access to inpatient physical therapy services does[43,88] and does not[67] decrease a patient's length of stay in an acute care facility after THA. The use of physical therapy services after THA also has been shown to increase the probability of discharge to the home setting rather than to another health-care facility.[43]

Studies with control groups that have evaluated the impact of exercise on functional outcomes in patients who have undergone THA are few in number. Most of these studies have looked at the effect of exercise several months or even a year or two after surgery, not during the first 6 to 12 weeks. However, Wang and colleagues[134] conducted a randomized, controlled investigation to determine if a customized exercise program initiated before scheduled THA had an efffect on the ambulatory abilities of patients after surgery. Gait velocity was measured by the 25-meter walk test, and walking endurance was measured by the 6-minute walk test. Participants in the exercise group ($n = 15$) took part in two facility-based and two home-based exercise sessions of stationary bicycling and resistance training two times per week for 8 weeks prior to surgery. At 3 weeks postoperatively, these patients resumed their individualized exercise regimens, modified to incorporate postoperative precautions, and continued until 12 weeks. Patients in the control goup ($n = 13$) underwent no preoperative intervention and received routine post-THA functional training. At 3 weeks postoperatively the exercise group demonstrated significantly greater gait velocity and stride length and at 12 weeks significantly greater 6-minute walking distance than the control group. The investigators concluded that a customized strength and endurance training program prior to and after THA improved the rate of recovery of ambulatory function.

In a nonrandomized study of the effectiveness of a 6-week home exercise program with patients who were 6 to 48 months post-THA, the two exercise groups (one performing ROM and isometric exercises of the hip and the other performing ROM, isometric, and eccentric exercises) increased their walking speed, whereas a control group (no exercise program) did not. Interestingly, strength improvements were noted in all three groups.[117] The results of these two studies provide useful information, but a great deal more research needs to be done on the effects of exercise on function after THA.

## Hemiarthroplasty of the Hip

### Indications for Surgery
The following are possible indications for prosthetic replacement of the proximal femur.[61,63,73]

- Acute, displaced intracapsular (subcapital, transcervical) fractures of the proximal femur in an elderly patient with poor bone stock and an anticipated low-demand level of activity after surgery[61,81,101,102,127]
- Failed internal fixation of intracapsular fractures associated with osteonecrosis of the head of the femur[61,81,101]
- Severe degeneration of the head of the femur (but an intact acetabulum) associated with long-standing hip disease or deformity resulting in disabling pain and loss of function that cannot be managed with nonoperative procedures[61,81,102]

NOTE: Patients with preexisting degenerative hip disease who sustain a femoral fracture are candidates for primary THA rather than hemiarthroplasty.[39,81] Acute, severely comminuted intertrochanteric fractures are *infrequently* managed by primary hemiarthroplasty.[81,128]

### Procedures

***Background.*** Historically, acute displaced fractures of the proximal femur in the elderly were treated with unipolar (fixed head), uncemented metal-stemmed endoprostheses with marginal results. With the introduction of cement fixation during the 1960s, these results improved.[81] The primary complication associated with the single-component unipolar implants, regardless of design or fixation, was progressive erosion of the acetabular cartilage and subsequent pain.

To decrease the problem of acetabular wear, the bipolar hemiarthroplasty was developed. The bipolar design is composed of multiple components: a metal ball-and-stem femoral prosthesis (may be modular) that moves within a free-riding polyethylene shell, which in turn inserts into a metal cup that moves within the acetabulum. The purpose of the multiple-surface, load-bearing design is to displace forces incurred by the acetabulum through the interposed components rather than directly to the acetabulum to lessen erosion of the acetabular cartilage.[58,81,101] Both current-day modular unipolar and bipolar prostheses are in use today.

Considerable differences of opinion exist among surgeons regarding the advantages and disadvantages of one design versus the other.[58,81,101]

***Operative procedure.*** As with THA, a posterolateral approach is most commonly used. After removing the head of the femur, the metal-stemmed prosthesis is inserted into the shaft of the proximal femur. The femoral stem is usually cemented in place, although bioingrowth fixation has also been used. Procedures for closure are consistent with THA.

### Postoperative Management
There are no studies in the literature that have examined the effects of comprehensive postoperative exercise programs exclusively for patients who have undergone current-day hemiarthroplasty. This is because, for the most part, considerations and precautions for positioning and ADL, as well as the components and progression of the exercise and ambulation program, are similar to those for postoperative management of THA. These guidelines are detailed in the previous section of this chapter. As with postoperative management after THA, selection and progression of exercises and functional activities after hemiarthroplasty also tend to be based on the opinions of surgeons and therapists as to the potential of specific exercises to remediate impairments and improve functional performance. Consequently, the effectiveness of exercise after hemiarthroplasty also remains unclear. Only limited information on the impact of specific exercises and gait-related activities on the hip joint per se after hemiarthroplasty is available in the literature. Some findings from several single-subject studies of two patients with femoral endoprostheses have already been discussed in the previous section of this chapter on THA.[46,64,65,124]

PRECAUTION: Given the significant concerns for long-term erosion of acetabular cartilage after hemiarthroplasty, it may be even more critical to avoid exercises that impose the greatest compressive or shearing forces across the hip joint and therefore pose the greatest potential for eroding the cartilaginous surface of the acetabulum. Exercises should be performed initially at a submaximal level and then progressed gradually. *Unassisted* heel slides and *maximum* effort gluteal setting exercises may need to be avoided during the acute phase of postoperative rehabilitation.[124] During the postacute period of rehabilitation exercises, such as maximum-effort manually resisted hip abduction may actually generate greater forces across the hip than protected weight-bearing activities.[46]

### Outcomes
Present-day modular unipolar and bipolar hemiarthroplasty procedures appear to yield similar results in pain relief, functional outcomes, and type and rate of complications.[61,81,101] Although acetabular wear was identified as the primary concern after the unipolar replacement used during the 1960s and 1970s, the mechanical effectiveness of the bipolar prosthesis in preventing acetabular erosion has yet to be firmly established.[61] In a study of community-dwelling patients age 65 years or older

(mean age 80 years) who had undergone hemiarthroplasty with either a bipolar implant or a modular unipolar implant, there were no significant differences between the two groups at 1 year and 4 to 5 years of follow-up with regard to functioning in daily activities or rates of dislocation, infection, or mortality.[135] Another study has suggested that joint ROM may decrease over time after bipolar hemiarthroplasty possibly due to the design of the implants. This decreased range was not associated with diminished functional abilities.[58]

# FRACTURES OF THE HIP—SURGICAL AND POSTOPERATIVE MANAGEMENT

## Hip Fracture—Incidence and Risk Factors

One of the more common musculoskeletal problems in the elderly is fracture of the hip or, more correctly, fracture of the most proximal portion of the femur in the hip joint area. The acute signs and symptoms of hip fracture are pain in the groin or hip region, pain with active or passive motion of the hip, or pain with lower extremity weight bearing. The lower extremity appears to be shorter by several centimeters and assumes a position of external rotation.[61,102]

More than 70% of hip fractures occur in individuals who are more than 70 years of age, and they occur in women significantly more often than in men.[18,61] In the United States, for example, women sustain 84.6% of all hip fractures.[108] Worldwide, the incidence of hip fracture has stabilized; but the total number of hip fractures per year is increasing, in part because of the aging of the population.[18,61,74,102] Fewer than 2% to 3% of fractures are sustained by persons who are less than 50 years of age.[61,102] These fractures or fracture-dislocations are usually associated with high-force, high-impact trauma but may also be seen with repetitive microtrauma.[61,102]

Multiple factors contribute to the increasing incidence of hip fracture with age. Osteoporosis, a condition associated with age-related loss of bone density and strength, typically occurs in the proximal femur and the distal radius and spine.[61,102] A sudden twisting motion of the lower extremity or the impact from a fall can cause pathological fracture of a fragile proximal femur. Although 90% of all hip fractures in the elderly are associated with a fall,[61] there is always the question of whether trauma from the fall caused the hip fracture or a pathological fracture of the hip caused the fall. Despite the increasing incidence of osteoporosis with age, the cause of most hip fractures appears to be impaired functional mobility rather than osteoporosis.[10]

Balance, protective reactions, and muscle power deteriorate with age, thus increasing the likelihood of a fall. These changes, combined with decreasing ability to absorb the impact of a fall, contribute to the risk of sustaining a fracture.[102] Characteristics of falling change with age, which may also increase the risk of hip fracture in the elderly. As walking speed decreases with age, particularly past 70 to 80 years, when a loss of balance and fall occurs

an older person usually drops and falls to the side, rather than falling forward on outstretched hands as occurs with faster walking speeds.[61,102]

Hip fracture in the elderly is associated with a high rate of disability because of a loss of independence in mobility.[32] Many patients require long-term nursing care and often are permanently institutionalized in extended care or assisted living facilities. For example, among women who sustain a hip fracture, approximately 15% to 25% lose the ability to live independently within the first year.[18] Although postoperative mortality rates remain high (approximately 20%),[32] improved surgical techniques over the past few decades have decreased the need for prolonged immobilization or restricted weight bearing, thus decreasing postoperative complications such as pneumonia and thromboemboli.

## Sites and Types of Hip Fracture

Fractures of the proximal femur are broadly classified as intracapsular or extracapsular and then further subdivided by specific location. Sites and specific types of hip fracture are noted in Box 20.8.[61,78,81,102,127-129] Of these sites, fractures in the intertrochanteric region are most common, accounting for approximately 50% of all fractures of the proximal femur.[78] Intracapsular fractures can potentially compromise the vascular supply to the head of the femur, which in turn increases the risk of delayed healing, nonunion, or osteonecrosis (avascular necrosis) of the head of the femur. These complications occur far more frequently with displaced versus nondisplaced intracapsular fractures.[61,81] Intracapsular fractures are most often sustained by elderly women.[61,81]

In contrast, fracture-dislocation and acetabular trauma are most common in the young, active individual.[61] Most fracture-dislocations occur in a posterior direction. This

---

**BOX 20.8    Common Sites and Types of Hip Fracture**

Intracapsular
- Fracture site proximal to the attachment of the hip joint capsule
- Further subdivided into *femoral head*, *subcapital* and *femoral neck* (*transcervical* or *basicervical* fractures)
- May be displaced, nondisplaced, or impacted
- May disturb the blood supply to the head of the femur resulting in avascular necrosis or nonunion

Extracapsular
- Fracture site distal to the capsule to a line 5 cm distal to the lesser trochanter
- Further subdivided into *intertrochanteric* (between the greater and lesser trochanters) or *subtrochanteric* and *stable* or *unstable* (comminuted)
- Does not disturb the blood supply to the head of the femur, but nonunion may occur as the result of fixation failure

type of fracture often causes traumatic disruption of the vascular supply to the head of the femur and damage to joint cartilage, resulting in osteonecrosis and post-traumatic arthritis, eventually necessitating prosthetic replacement of the hip joint. However, this need may not arise for many years.

## Open Reduction and Internal Fixation of Hip Fracture

### Indications for Surgery

Surgical intervention by means of open (or possibly closed) reduction followed by stabilization with internal fixation (Figs. 20.7 and 20.8) is indicated for the following types of fractures of the proximal femur.[61,102,127-129]

- Displaced or nondisplaced intracapsular femoral neck fractures
- Fracture-dislocations of the head of the femur
- Stable or unstable intertrochanteric fractures
- Subtrochanteric fractures

In the elderly patient, displaced intracapsular fractures are typically managed with prosthetic replacement of the femoral head to avoid a relatively high incidence of nonunion.[101] Some severely comminuted (unstable) intertrochanteric fractures also may be managed in this manner.[61,81,128]

In a few situations, nonoperative management is the only option for treatment after hip fracture. Traction is an appropriate alternative for nonambulatory individuals or for medically unstable patients who cannot undergo a sur-

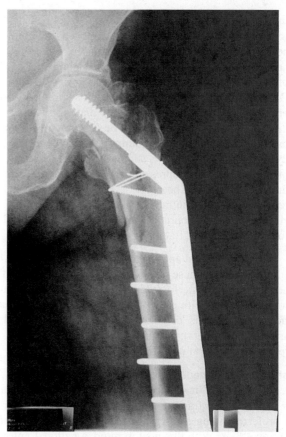

FIGURE 20.8 Intertrochanteric fracture of the hip. This postoperative image shows fracture fixation via a side plate and screw combination device. The fracture line is evident, extending through the intertrochanteric region to the proximal femoral shaft. Some comminution is evident, and a large fragment on the medial shaft is noted. The imposed added densities of swelling of the soft tissues is seen. *(From McKinnis,[78] p. 310, with permission.)*

gical procedure.[61,102] The patient remains in bed in traction just long enough for early healing to occur. Bed to chair mobilization follows. If weight bearing or ambulation is feasible, it is delayed until bone healing is sufficient, usually 10 to 12 weeks or as long as 16 weeks postoperatively.

### Procedures

The goal of surgery is to achieve maximum stability and restore alignment of bony structures of the hip. Surgery is indicated during the first 24 to 48 hours after injury, particularly with femoral neck fractures where the risk of disruption of the vascular supply to the head of the femur is high. A variety of internal fixation devices are used after open or closed reduction to stabilize the many types of fracture of the proximal femur. The type and severity of the fracture and the associated injuries as well as the patient's age and physical and cognitive status all influence the surgeon's choice of procedure.[61,102] The type of procedure performed, in turn, affects the progression of postoperative rehabilitation.

*Types of fixation and surgical approach.* The most common current-day internal fixation devices used, based on the type of fracture, include the following.[61,102,127-129]

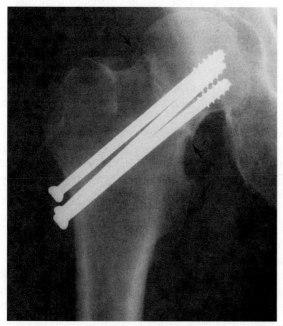

FIGURE 20.7 Reduction and internal fixation of a complete fracture of the femoral neck. Restoration of alignment and good compression is obtained via fixation with three compression screws. The black arrows mark the extent of the fracture line. *(From McKinnis,[78] p. 309, with permission.)*

- In situ fixation with multiple parallel cancellous lag screws or pins for nondisplaced or impacted femoral neck fractures and possibly for displaced femoral neck fractures in active patients less than 65 years of age.
- Dynamic extramedullary fixation with a sliding (compression) hip screw and lateral side plate for stable intertrochanteric fractures; may be combined with an osteotomy for unstable (comminuted) fractures. The dynamic hip screw allows sliding between the screw and plate and creates compression across the fracture site during early weight bearing.
- Static interlocking intramedullary nail fixation or a sliding hip screw coupled with an intramedullary nail for subtrochanteric fractures.

An open surgical approach along the lateral aspect of the hip is used for these procedures. Aspects of some of the procedures may be performed percutaneously. Soft tissue disruption differs with each procedure. The tensor fasciae latae, vastus lateralis, or gluteus medius may be incised (parallel to the fibers); a capsulotomy is generally performed with femoral neck fractures.

## Postoperative Management

The ultimate goal of surgical intervention and postoperative care after hip fracture is to return a patient to his or her preferred living environment[85] at a preinjury level of function.[54,61,102] With this goal in mind, a national, interdisciplinary consensus conference of health professionals met and developed recommendations for optimal care. Among the recommendations was the need for rehabilitation services during recovery, including postoperative exercise and functional training across the continuum of care.[85]

During the initial phase of postoperative rehabilitation, which begins in the acute care setting, the focus is to get the patient up and moving as quickly as possible to prevent or minimize the adverse effects of prolonged bed rest, including thromboemboli and pulmonary complications, while protecting the surgically stabilized fracture site. In addition to helping the patient learn to move safely in bed, transfer, and ambulate independently with an assistive device, early postoperative rehabilitation typically includes patient or caregiver education for wound care, deep breathing and coughing exercises, edema control (use of compressive stockings), proper positioning in bed to avoid contractures, and an exercise program.

After discharge from the hospital, postoperative functional training and exercise typically continue in a transitional, subacute rehabilitation or skilled nursing facility or at home. Despite consensus that rehabilitation after hospital discharge is an essential aspect of postoperative care,[85] according to the results of a recent systematic review of the literature[11] there is little evidence derived from randomized controlled investigations of patients' functional outcomes to support that one setting for rehabilitation is superior to another; nor is there sufficient evidence to identify the optimal timing for or components of subacute rehabilitation.

What is known, however, is that most patients are discharged from rehabilitation services after achieving independence in ambulation using an assistive device and necessary daily living activities, parameters typically set by health care plans. Often services must be discontinued despite persistent deficits in muscle performance (strength and endurance impairments) and well before patients have attained a preinjury level of function, which in turn increases the risk of future injury.[17]

## Weight-Bearing Considerations

The amount of weight bearing permissible during early ambulation and transfers is always determined by the surgeon for each patient on an individual basis. Factors that influence the decision are the patient's age and bone quality, the fracture location and pattern, the type of fixation used to stabilize the fracture site, and the degree of intraoperative stability achieved.[54,61,63,102] Recommendations range from non-weight-bearing, toe-touch, or touch-down weight bearing (<10 lb) to weight bearing as tolerated. Current methods of internal fixation of the fracture site have decreased the need for an extended non-weight-bearing status after surgery.

Many fixation procedures used today make early weight bearing possible. Some examples of fractures and fixation procedures in which weight bearing as tolerated is permissible immediately after surgery are:

- Undisplaced, rigidly fixed, or impacted femoral neck fractures managed with in situ fixation[61,63,102,127]
- Stable (noncomminuted) intertrochanteric fractures managed with a dynamic (sliding) hip screw and lateral side plate fixation[61,102,128]
- Stable subtrochanteric fractures managed with interlocking intramedullary nailing and bone-to-bone fixation[61,102,129]

Even when weight bearing is curtailed during ambulation and transfers, the fracture site is still subjected to significant forces. For example, moving in bed, getting up to the side of the bed, and active and resisted ROM exercises all generate forces across the hip that approach or even exceed those incurred during unsupported (full weight bearing) ambulation.[97] Considering this, studies have been implemented to investigate the risks associated with early weight bearing after open reduction and internal fixation of hip fractures.

### ● Focus on Evidence

In one such study, elderly patients with stable as well as comminuted intertrochanteric fractures treated with dynamic hip screw and plate fixation were all allowed to bear weight as tolerated during ambulation with an assistive device immediately after surgery. One year postoperatively there was no significant difference between the rate of implant failure and revision surgery in the patients with stable fractures and those with comminuted fractures. The investigators concluded that at least in elderly patients with comminuted and noncomminuted intertrochanteric fractures that could be stabilized intraoperatively there was little biomechanical justification for non-weight-bearing restrictions postoperatively.[63]

Excluded from this generalization were patients with complex fractures in whom satisfactory intraoperative stabilization could not be achieved, young patients with displaced femoral neck fractures with in situ fixation, and patients with severe bone disease (e.g., as the result of malignancy).

Despite the finding of this study and the recognized benefits of early ambulation and exercise, there is always risk, albeit small, of failure of an internal fixation device in some patients. Therefore, it is important to recognize the signs of possible displacement or loosening of the fracture stabilization device as summarized in Box 20.9. The presence of any of these signs or symptoms should be reported immediately to the surgeon.[54,61,102]

### Exercise

Impaired joint mobility, ROM, muscle performance, and balance are the most common impairments after open reduction and internal fixation of hip fracture. Exercise is one of the interventions routinely included in postoperative rehabilitation to reduce these impairments.

Hip and even knee motions are quite painful during the initial postoperative period, affecting ROM and strength of the operated lower extremity. In addition, some degree of protection is necessary over the course of soft tissue healing (approximately 6 weeks) and bone healing (10 to 16 weeks).[127-129] All of these factors affect the progression of exercise, as do the location and stability of the fracture site, type of internal fixation used, and which soft tissues were traumatized at the time of the injury and during surgery. Special considerations for exercise and ambulation after various types of hip fracture and with specific surgeries are noted in Box 20.10.[61,102,127-129]

The following sections outline a progression of exercises after open reduction and internal fixation of hip fractures.

### Exercise: Maximum Protection Phase

Exercises begin on the first postoperative day to prevent postoperative complications and to restore a patient's con-

---

**BOX 20.9**  **Signs and Symptoms of Possible Failure of the Internal Fixation Mechanism**

- Severe, persistent groin, thigh, or knee pain that increases with limb movement or weight bearing
- Progressive limb length inequality (shortening of the involved lower extremity) that was not present immediately after surgery
- Persistent external rotation of the operated limb
- A positive Trendelenburg sign during weight bearing on the involved limb that does not resolve with strengthening exercises

---

**BOX 20.10**  **Special Considerations for Exercise and Gait After Internal Fixation of Fractures of the Proximal Femur**

- Multiple hip muscles are traumatized by fracture of the hip leading to postoperative pain, reflex inhibition, and weakness. Fractures that involve the following sites cause damage to the following muscles.
  - Greater trochanter: gluteus medius
  - Lesser trochanter: iliopsoas
  - Subtrochanteric region: gluteus maximus
- The tensor fasciae latae (TFL) and vastus lateralis (VL) are usually incised during surgery, causing postoperative pain, inhibition, and weakness during hip abduction and knee flexion.
- Adhesion formation may develop between the incised TFL and VL and restrict motion. Hip adduction and internal rotation and knee flexion place a stretch on the TFL and VL, respectively, during ROM exercises and therefore are often painful.
- If there is shortening of the involved limb after fracture and internal fixation, the distance between the distal insertion of the gluteus medius on the greater trochanter and the center of axis of hip motion is often decreased, thus diminishing the mechanical advantage of the muscle and causing weakness and a positive Trendelenburg sign during ambulation.
- Intracapsular fractures typically traumatize the capsule, and internal fixation requires an incision into the capsule (capsulotomy). Both predispose the capsule to postoperative restriction.

---

trol of the operated hip during functional activities. All exercises are performed within a patient's level of comfort. Initially, exercises are directed toward restoring ROM of the operated hip and developing strength in the upper extremities and unoperated lower extremity to facilitate ambulation with an assistive device. It is reasonable to expect to achieve 80° to 90° of active hip flexion (with the knee flexed) by 2 to 4 weeks postoperatively.[54,61]

There is lack of consensus about the appropriate time to begin resistance exercises to strengthen the operated lower extremity. Low-intensity resistance exercises of the operated hip often are delayed until 4 to 6 weeks postoperatively to allow time for the hip muscles incised during surgery to heal. However, resistance exercises of knee and ankle musculature may be initiated sooner.

 **Focus on Evidence** _____

Mitchell and colleagues[82] conducted a randomized controlled trial to determine the effects of 6 weeks of quadriceps resistance exercises during the early phase of postoperative rehabilitation after hip fracture. All of the 80 patients in the study, described as "frail elderly" (all ≥ 65 years of age, mean 80 years), began a program of ROM exercises and functional training (described as "standard" therapy) after surgery. In addition, at 16 days postoperatively half of the patients (intervention group) performed three sets of 12 repetitions of resisted knee extension of the operated and unoperated lower extremities initially at the 50% 1-RM intensity twice a week, progressing to 80% intensity by the fifth week. Of the 80 patients in the study, 75% completed the 6-week study.

After 6 weeks of resistance training the quadriceps strength of the intervention group increased bilaterally to a significantly greater extent than that of the control group. The intervention group also demonstrated significantly greater improvement and, as such, a greater reduction in disability than the control group on a functional mobility test measuring locomotion, balance, and transfers. However, there were no significant differences in improvement between groups regarding gait velocity or on a test that measures independence in ADL. There were no training-related adverse events during the study.

The authors concluded that moderate- to high-intensity postoperative quadriceps resistance training during early recovery after hip fracture was functionally beneficial and well tolerated by the participants despite their age and fraility.

---

The following are goals and exercise-related interventions for the initial phase of postoperative rehabilitation.

◉ *Prevent vascular and pulmonary complications.*
  • Active ankle exercises (pumping exercises) performed regularly throughout the day to maintain circulation and reduce the risk of DVTs and thromboemboli.
  • Deep breathing exercises and airway clearance to prevent pulmonary complications.
◉ *Improve strength in the upper and sound lower extremities.*
  • Exercises against progressive levels of resistance targeting key muscle groups used to lift body weight during bed mobility, standing transfers, and ambulation with assistive devices.
  • Emphasis on closed-chain training to simulate the movement patterns used during these activities.
◉ *Prevent postoperative reflex inhibition of hip and knee musculature.*
  • Low-intensity isometric (setting) exercises of the hip and knee musculature of the operated extremity. Depending on the fracture site and its stability, perform submaximal gluteal, abductor, adductor, and quadriceps and hamstring setting exercises.
◉ *Restore active mobility and dynamic control of the involved hip and adjacent joints.*
  • Assisted, progressing to active ROM of the involved hip and knee in progressively more challenging positions as pain and fracture healing permit. For example, in the supine position, perform heel slides before straight leg raises (SLRs) in the supine position. The shorter moment arm when the knee is flexed places lower rotational loads on the fracture site than a long moment arm.

  • Unassisted SLRs (flexion, abduction, extension) *while standing* on the sound leg and holding onto a stable surface for balance before progressing to SLRs in a horizontal position.
  • Pelvic tilts and knee-to-chest movements with the *uninvolved* leg to prevent stiffness in the low back region.
  • Low-intensity dynamic resistance exercises in weight-bearing and non-weight-bearing positions as the stability of the fracture site allows.

PRECAUTION: When initiating setting and dynamic exercises of the operated hip after comminuted subtrochanteric fractures that required medial cortex reconstruction, postpone contractions of the abductor and adductor muscles for 4 to 6 weeks to avoid stresses across the fracture site.[129]

**Exercise: Moderate and Minimum Protection Phases**
By 6 weeks soft tissues are healed; and by 8 to 12 weeks, depending on the age and health of the patient, some degree of bone healing has occurred. By the sixth week of rehabilitation, except in unusual situations, at least partial weight bearing or full weight bearing as tolerated, if not initiated previously, now is permissible. By 8 to 12 weeks, although a patient gradually can be weaned from use of an assistive device during ambulation, most continue to use at least a cane well beyond this time frame.

The emphasis during the intermediate and final phases of rehabilitation focuses on increasing strength and functional control of the involved lower extremity and gradually increasing the patient's level of functional activities. Patients typically are discharged from therapy no later than 8 to 12 weeks postoperatively and often earlier.

*Extended exercise programs after hip fracture.* For many years there was lack of agreement about the value of an extended exercise program or if it was appropriate to include moderate-intensity resistance exercises of the operated extremity in an elderly patient's rehabilitation program before and even after the fracture site was fully healed.[54] (Bone healing typically takes 8 to 16 weeks and up to 6 months in some patients.) However, during the past few years the findings of several studies have demonstrated that after a standard course of postoperative rehabilitation and with clearance from the patient's surgeon, an extended program of properly supervised, carefully progressed resistance exercises for strength training, begun 6 to 19 weeks postoperatively, is safe and effective.[17,52,74,118,119]

The intensity, frequency, and duration of the extended exercise program varied in these studies, and the equipment used for resistance training ranged from elastic resistance products to weight machines. Features of the exercise programs implemented in three of the studies are summarized in Table 20.3. Additional details and outcomes of these studies are addressed at the conclusion of this section on postoperative management after hip fracture.

The following goals and exercises are appropriate during the intermediate and advanced phases of rehabilitation.

| TABLE 20.3 | Summary of Studies of Extended Exercise Programs Following Surgery for Hip Fracture | | | |
|---|---|---|---|---|
| First Author and Type of Study | Subjects: (n) and Mean Age | Setting, Format, and Timing of Intervention | Frequency, Duration, and Types of Exercise | Features of PRE Training |
| Binder[17] RCT with two groups | n = 90 Intervention group: n = 46; 80 years Control group: n = 44; 81 years | Facility-based; group format for intervention group and home-based program for control group Begun no more than 16 weeks postsurgery | *Intervention group*: Two 3-month phases, three weekly sessions Phase 1: total of 22 exercises (flexibility, balance, aerobic training, low-intensity resistance exercises) Phase 2: Moderate- to high-intensity PRE added to shortened phase 1 program *Control group*: A portion of phase 1 exercises, no PRE | One or two sets, six to eight reps at 65% of initial 1-RM progressing to three sets, 8 to 12 reps at 85–100% initial 1-RM Weight machines Exercises: bilateral knee flexion and extension, leg press, seated bench press, biceps curl, seated rowing |
| Hauer[52] RCT with two groups | n = 28; all at least 75 years Intervention group: n = 15; 81.7 years Control group: n = 13; 80.8 years | Facility-based; group format; begun 6–8 weeks postfracture | *Intervention group*: Three weekly sessions for 3 months; PRE, balance, and functional training *Control group*: Stretching, seated calisthenics, memory tasks. | Two sets at 70–90% of 1-RM intensity Weight machines and body weight resistance Exercises: leg press, hip/knee extension, plantarflexion |
| Mangione[74] RCT with three groups | n = 33 Resistance group: n = 11; 77.9 years Aerobic group: n = 12; 79.8 years Control group: n = 10; 77.8 years | Home-based; individual format; begun 19.4, 19.7, and 12.6 weeks after surgery, respectively, for resistance, aerobic, and control groups | Total of 3 months: two sessions weekly for 2 months, followed by 1 session weekly for 1 month | Three sets of eight reps at the 8-RM intensity Portable resistance unit or body weight resistance Exercises: supine hip and knee extension, hip abduction, standing hip extension; standing plantarflexion (heel raises) |

PRE, progressive resistance exercise; RCT, randomized controlled trial; RM, repetition maximum.

● *Increase flexibility of any chronically shortened muscles.* Muscles typically involved include the ankle plantarflexors, hip flexors and hamstrings. Suggested stretching techniques include:
- Heel cord stretching with a towel while sitting on a bed with the knee straight or the assistance of a caregiver and later while standing.
- Hip flexor stretching in the supine/Thomas test position.
- Hamstring stretching by sitting on the edge of a table with one leg supported in hip flexion and knee extension and the other in extension over the side of the support surface (see Fig. 20.15).

● *Improve strength and muscular endurance in the lower extremities for functional activities.* Refer to the section on exercise interventions later in the chapter for descriptions of the following exercises.
- Bilateral closed-chain active exercises, such as mini-squats and heel raises using a table or walker for support and balance and body weight as the source of resistance as soon as partial-weight bearing on the operated lower extremity is permissible.
- Lunges and forward and lateral step-ups when weight bearing to tolerance is allowable.

- Open-chain hip and knee exercises initially against light to moderate resistance (up to 5 lb) with elastic resistance or cuff weights. Emphasize hip extension and abduction for a positive impact on ambulation.
- Task-specific training, such as stair-climbing or carrying small loads while ambulating.

◉ *Improve postural stability and standing balance.*
- A progression of balance activities appropriate for the patient's age and desired activity level.
- Progressive ambulation on various surfaces.

◉ *Increase aerobic capacity/cardiopulmonary endurance.*
- Stationary bicycling, upper body ergometry, or treadmill walking.
- Aerobic conditioining activities, possibly in an age-appropriate, community-based exercise class, to increase walking distance and velocity.

### Outcomes

*General outcomes.* The true measure of success of surgical intervention and postoperative rehabilitation after hip fracture is the extent to which a patient can return to his or her prefracture level of function. The level of preinjury functional mobility in patients with femoral neck fractures has been shown to be a critical factor in postoperative survival.[55] In one follow-up study of patients after hip fracture, only 33% had regained their preinjury level of function in basic ADL and IADL 1 year postoperatively.[59] Given the advanced age and health status of the "average" patient who sustains a hip fracture, it is not surprising that mortality rates 1 year postoperatively are high, ranging from 12% to 36% depending on the mean age, general health status, and severity of the fracture.[61] After 1 year mortality rates are equal to age-matched subjects who have not sustained a hip fracture.[61]

Among patients who survive 1 year postoperatively, the ability to ambulate independently (50 feet on an uncarpeted surface) was seen in 83% in one study.[9] In a more recent study 92% of patients returned to independent ambulation, but only 41% regained their prefracture level of ambulation.[62] In a follow-up study[121] of 90 community-dwelling older adults (mean age 83.4 years) 6 months after discharge from the hospital following a fall-related hip fracture, 53.3% (48/90) had experienced one or more falls. The need for an assistive device during ambulation after hip fracture and the patient's prefracture fall history were predictors of a fall after hospital discharge.

*Impact of rehabilitation.* According to a report of the National Center for Medical Rehabilitation Research (NCMRR), the use of therapeutic exercise is one of the least examined factors affecting outcomes after hip fracture.[136] However, there are at least a few studies, some of which are randomized controlled trials, available that have addressed the impact of exercise and functional training on outcomes. For example, the number of visits to physical therapy has been positively associated with the ability to ambulate independently.[9] The results of

another study indicated that the frequency of physical therapy visits increased the likelihood of regaining functional independence and going directly home from an acute care setting after hip fracture surgery.[50]

As noted previously, the benefits and risks of resistance training have been investigated. In an early randomized, controlled study, subjects (most of whom were living in the community and were an average of 7 months postfracture surgery) who participated in a 1-month home exercise program increased the strength of the knee extensors and increased their walking velocity to a greater extent than the control group.[118] Another study compared the effects of a 2-week program of weight-bearing versus non-weight-bearing exercises initiated during inpatient rehabilitation. It found that both groups demonstrated substantial improvements in lower extremity muscle strength, balance, gait, and other functional tasks. However, there were no significant differences between groups.[119] This study lends support to the value of both types of exercise during early rehabilitation.

Recently, studies of the effects of extended, comprehensive exercise programs after hip fracture have included moderate- to high-intensity resistance training of multiple muscle groups (see Table 20.2). In the three studies described in Table 20.2, muscle strength and performance on a variety of functional mobility and ADL tests improved to a significantly greater extent in the groups who participated in resistance training than in the groups who participated in low-intensity or no resistance training.[17,52,74] The resistance training group in the study by Binder and colleagues[17] also reported a significant decrease in the perceived levels of disability, whereas the control group, who performed only low-intensity exercises, did not. The resistance training group in the investigation by Hauer et al.[52] noted improved perception of walking steadiness but no change in fear of falling.

Moderate- to high-intensity resistance training after discharge from a "standard" postoperative program of exercise and functional training appears to be not only feasible but safe. Other than reports of mild muscle soreness during the early weeks of resistance exercise programs, training-related adverse events were reported in only one study (3 of 46 participants in the resistance training group).[17] One individual fell during exercise and sustained a rib fracture; another incurred a metatarsal fracture that was discovered a few days after an exercise session; and a third developed ecchymosis at the ankle after an exercise session. All three participants chose to complete the program.

Not all types of extended rehabilitation after hip fracture have been shown to be effective. The results of a study of individuals in a long-term, home-based, multifaceted rehabilitation program (including extensive ADL and IADL training) for 6 months postoperatively in comparison to a traditional postoperative exercise and ambulation program for an equal period of time demonstrated no significant differences.[130]

# PAINFUL HIP SYNDROMES/ OVERUSE SYNDROMES: NONOPERATIVE MANAGEMENT

## Related Pathologies and Etiology of Symptoms

### Tendinitis or Muscle Pull

Overuse or trauma to any of the muscles in the hip region can result from excessive strain while the muscle is contracting (often in a stretched position) or from repetitive use and not allowing the injured tissue to heal between activities. Common problems include hip flexor, adductor, and hamstring strains. Poor flexibility and fatigue may predispose an individual to strain and injury during an activity or sporting event; and sudden falls, such as slipping on ice, may cause a strain.

### Trochanteric Bursitis

Pain is experienced over the lateral hip and possibly down the lateral thigh to the knee when the iliotibial band rubs over the trochanter. Discomfort may be experienced after standing asymmetrically for long periods with the affected hip elevated and adducted and the pelvis dropped on the opposite side. Ambulation and climbing stairs aggravate the condition. Muscle flexibility and strength imbalances and the resulting faulty posture of the pelvis may be the predisposing factors leading to bursal irritation (see Box 20.2).

### Psoas Bursitis

Pain is experienced in the groin or anterior thigh and possibly into the patellar area. It is aggravated during activities requiring excessive hip flexion.

### Ischiogluteal Bursitis (Tailor's or Weaver's Bottom)

Pain is experienced around the ischial tuberosities, especially when sitting. If the adjacent sciatic nerve is irritated from the swelling, symptoms of sciatica may occur.

## Common Impairments and Functional Limitations/Disabilities

*Pain.* Symptoms occur when the involved muscle contracts, when it is stretched, or when the provoking activity is repeated.

*Gait deviations.* Slightly shorter stance occurs on the painful side. There may be a slight lurch when the involved muscle contracts to protect the muscle resulting in impaired gait.

*Imbalance in muscle flexibility and strength.* Muscle flexibility or dominance in use may be the precipitating factor in many painful hip syndromes. Common imbalances are described in the introductory section of this chapter; and imbalances from postural impairments are summarized in Box 20.2. Overuse syndromes are associated with (1) dom-inance of the tensor fasciae latae and rectus femoris as hip flexors and abductors, with weak gluteus medius and min-imus muscles; (2) dominance of the hamstrings over the gluteus maximus; and (3) shortened lateral rotators. Because of the relationship of these muscles with the pelvis and knee, patients may present with low back or knee symptoms.

*Decreased muscular endurance.* Muscle fatigue may lead to faulty postures, stress, and flexibility imbalances as described above.

## Management: Protection Phase

### Control Inflammation and Promote Healing

When there is chronic irritation or inflammation from an acute injury, follow the guidelines as described in Chapter 10, with emphasis on resting the involved tissue by not stressing or putting pressure on it. Have the patient avoid the provoking activity; and if necessary, decrease the amount and time walking or use an assistive device.

### Develop Support in Related Areas

Initiate exercises to develop neuromuscular control for alignment of the pelvis and hip. Avoid stressing the inflamed tissue. Patient education and cooperation are necessary to reduce repetitive trauma.

## Management: Controlled Motion Phase

N O T E : When the acute symptoms have decreased, initiate a progressive exercise program within the tolerance of the involved tissues to improve muscle performance. The program should emphasize regaining a balance in length, neuromuscular control, strength, and endurance in the muscles of the hip and the rest of the lower extremity.

### Develop a Strong Mobile Scar and Regain Flexibility

Remodel the scar in muscle or tendon by applying cross-fiber massage to the site of the lesion followed by multiple-angle submaximal isometrics in pain-free positions.

### Develop a Balance in Length and Strength of the Hip Muscles

Specific exercises are described in the exercise sections of this chapter.

- Stretch any muscles that are restricting motion with gentle, progressive neuromuscular inhibition techniques. Instruct the patient to do self-stretching with proper stabilization to ensure that the stretches are performed safely and effectively.
- Begin developing neuromuscular control to train the involved muscles to contract and control alignment of the femur. Initially, the emphasis is on control, not strengthening.
- Once the patient is aware of proper muscle control and is able to maintain alignment, progress to strengthening the weakened muscles through the range.

● Muscles not directly injured should be stretched and strengthened if they are contributing to asymmetrical forces. The patient may not have sufficient trunk coordination or strength, which may be contributing to the overuse because of compensations in the hip. See Chapter 16 for suggestions on developing control and stabilizing function in the trunk muscles.

### Develop Stability and Closed–Chain Function

● Initiate controlled weight-bearing exercises when tolerated. Because the individual is probably standing and walking, he or she may not tolerate much more closed-chain activities than those previously initiated early during the healing stage, so proceed with caution. Carefully observe the exercises so proper movement patterns are used.

● Use exercises such as biking or partial weight-bearing and weight-shifting activities in the parallel bars. Observe coordination between trunk, hip, knee, and ankle motions; and exercise only to the point of fatigue, substitute motions, or pain in the weakest segment in the chain.

### Develop Muscle and Cardiopulmonary Endurance

● For muscle endurance, teach the patient how to perform each exercise safely for 1 to 3 minutes before progressing to the next level of difficulty.

● Determine aerobic activities that do not exacerbate the patient's symptoms. It may be that the patient just needs to modify the intensity or the techniques used in his or her current program.

### Patient Education

Initiate a home exercise program as soon as the patient has learned neuromuscular control techniques and correct stretching, strengthening, and aerobic activities. Provide follow-up instruction for modification and progression of the program.

## Management: Return to Function Phase

### Progress Strength and Functional Control

● Progress closed-chain and functional training to include balance and muscular endurance for each activity.

● Use specificity principles; increase eccentric resistance and demand for controlled speed if necessary for return-to-work activity or sporting events.

● Progress to patterns of motion consistent with the desired outcome. Use acceleration/deceleration drills and plyometric training; assess the total body functioning while doing the desired activity. Practice timing and sequencing of events.

### Return to Function

Prior to returning to the desired function have the patient practice the activity in a controlled environment and for a limited period. As tolerated, introduce variability in the environment and increase the intensity of the endurance activities.

## EXERCISE INTERVENTIONS FOR THE HIP REGION

No matter what the cause, muscle strength or flexibility imbalance in the hip can lead to abnormal lumbopelvic and hip mechanics, which predisposes a patient to or perpetuates low back, sacroiliac, or hip pain. (See Chapters 14 through 16 for discussion of impaired posture, common spinal diagnoses, plans of care, and exercise interventions for the spinal regions.) Poor hip mechanics from muscle flexibility and strength imbalances can also affect the knee and ankle during weight-bearing activities, causing overuse syndromes or stress to these regions.

## ◐ EXERCISE TECHNIQUES TO INCREASE FLEXIBILITY AND RANGE OF MOTION

The exercise techniques in this section are suggestions for correcting limited flexibility of the musculature and periarticular tissues crossing the hip. Principles and techniques of passive stretching and neuromuscular inhibition are presented in Chapter 4 and those of joint mobilization in Chapter 5. Specific manual and self-stretching techniques are described in this section.

Flexibility (self-stretching) exercises, chosen according to the degree of limitation and ability of the patient to participate, can be valuable for reinforcing therapeutic interventions performed by the therapist. Not all of the following exercises are appropriate for every patient; the therapist should select each exercise and intensity appropriate for each patient's level of function and progress each exercise as indicated. Whenever the patient is able to contract the muscle opposite the range-limiting muscle, there are the added benefits of reciprocal inhibition of the shortened muscles as well as training the agonist (the muscle opposite the tight muscle) to function for effective control in the gained ROM.

### Techniques to Stretch Range-Limiting Hip Structures

NOTE: Two-joint muscles can restrict full ROM at the hip. This first section describes stretches to increase just hip motions, so the two-joint muscles are kept on a slack across the knee during these stretches. Techniques to stretch the specific two-joint muscles are described in the second section.

### To Increase Hip Extension

**Prone Press-Ups**

*Patient position and procedure:* Prone with hands on a table at shoulder level. Have the patient press the thorax upward and allow the pelvis to sag (see Fig. 15.7).

PRECAUTION: This exercise also moves the lumbar spine into extension; if it causes radiating pain down the patient's leg, rather than just a stretch sensation in the anterior trunk, hip, and thigh, it must not be performed.

### "Thomas Test" Stretch

*Patient position and procedure:* Supine with the hips near the end of the treatment table, both hips and knees flexed, and the thigh on the side opposite the tight hip held against the chest. Have the patient slowly lower the thigh to be stretched toward the table in a controlled manner and allow the knee to extend so the two-joint rectus femoris does not limit the range. Do not allow the thigh to externally rotate or abduct. Direct the patient to let the weight of the leg cause the stretch force and to relax the tight muscles at the end of the range (Fig. 20.9). A passive stretch force may be applied manually, or a hold-relax technique may be used by applying a force to the distal thigh (see Fig. 4.26).

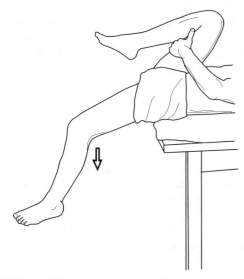

FIGURE 20.9 Self-stretching to increase hip extension. The pelvis is stabilized by holding the opposite hip in flexion. The weight of the thigh provides a stretch force as the patient relaxes. Allowing the knee to extend emphasizes the one-joint hip flexors (iliopsoas), whereas maintaining the knee in flexion and hip neutral to rotation as the thigh is lowered emphasizes the two joint rectus femoris and tensor fasciae latae muscles.

### Modified Fencer Stretch

*Patient position and procedure:* Standing in a fencer's lunge-like posture, with the back leg in the same plane as the front leg and the foot pointing forward. Have the patient first do a posterior pelvic tilt and then shift the body weight onto the anterior leg until a stretch sensation is felt in the anterior hip region of the back leg (Fig. 20.10). If the heel of the back foot is kept on the floor, this exercise may also stretch the gastrocnemius muscle.

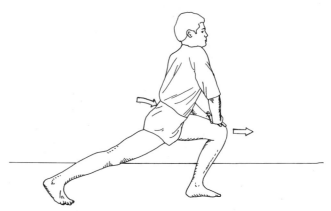

FIGURE 20.10 Self-stretching of hip flexor muscles and soft tissue anterior to the hip using a modified fencer's squat posture.

### To Increase Hip Flexion

#### Bilateral Knee to Chest

*Patient position and procedure:* Supine. Have the patient bring both knees toward the chest and grasp the thighs firmly until a stretch sensation is felt in the posterior hip region. Monitor the position carefully because if the pelvis lifts up off the mat the lumbar spine flexes and the stretch force is transmitted there instead of to the hips.

#### Unilateral Knee to Chest

*Patient position and procedure:* Supine. Have the patient bring one knee to the chest and grasp the thigh firmly against the chest while keeping the other lower extremity extended on the mat. This position isolates the stretch force to the hip being flexed and helps stabilize the pelvis. To emphasize a stretch of the gluteus maximus, have the patient pull the knee toward the opposite shoulder.

#### Quadruped (All Fours) Stretch

*Patient position and procedure:* On hands and knees. Have the patient rock the pelvis into an anterior tilt, causing lumbar extension (Fig. 20.11A); then maintain the lumbar extension and shift the buttocks back in an attempt to sit on the heels. The hands remain forward (Fig. 20.11B). It is important not to let the lumbar spine flex while holding the stretch position so the stretch affects the hip.

#### Chair Stretch

*Patient position and procedure:* Sitting in a chair with the pelvis rotated anteriorly and the low back extended to stabilize the spine. Have the patient grasp the front of the chair seat and lean or pull the trunk forward, keeping the back arched so the motion occurs only at the hips.

### To Increase Hip Abduction

*Patient position and procedure:* Supine with both hips flexed 90°, knees extended, and legs and buttocks against the wall. Have the patient abduct both hips as far as possible with gravity causing the stretch force (Fig. 20.12).

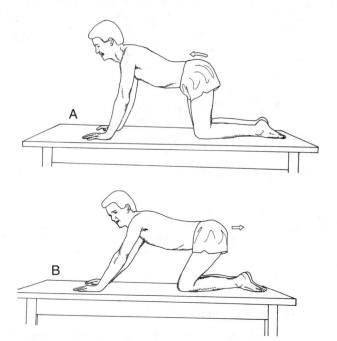

FIGURE 20.11  Gluteus maximus self-stretch with lumbar spine stabilization. (A) The patient on all fours rocks into an anterior pelvic tilt, causing lumbar extension. (B) While maintaining lumbar extension, the patient shifts the buttocks back, attempting to sit on the heels. When lordosis can no longer be maintained, the end-range of hip flexion is reached; this position is held for the stretch.

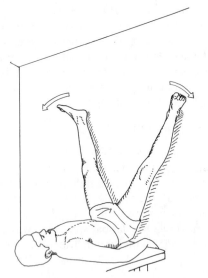

FIGURE 20.12  Self-stretching of the adductor muscles with the hips at 90° of flexion.

### To Increase Hip Abduction and External Rotation Simultaneously

*Patient position and procedure:* Sitting or supine with soles of feet together and hands on the inner surface of the knees. Have the patient push the knees down toward the floor with a sustained stretch. The stretch can be increased by pulling the feet closer to the trunk.

PRECAUTION: When this stretch is performed supine, teach the patient to stabilize the pelvis and lumbar spine by actively contracting the abdominal muscles and maintaining a neutral spinal position.

*Patient position and procedure:* Standing in a fencer's position but with the hind leg externally rotated. Have the patient shift the weight onto the front leg until a stretch sensation is felt along the medial thigh in the hind leg.

## Techniques to Stretch Range-Limiting Two-Joint Muscles

### Rectus Femoris Stretches

#### "Thomas Test" Stretch

*Patient position and procedure:* Supine with the hips near the end of the treatment table, both hips and knees flexed, and the thigh on the side opposite the tight hip held against the chest with the arms. While keeping the knee flexed, have the patient lower the thigh to be stretched toward the table in a controlled manner. Do not allow the thigh to externally rotate or abduct. Direct the patient to let the weight of the leg cause the stretch force and to relax the tight muscles at the end of the range. The patient can attempt to further extend the hip by contracting the extensor muscles. (See Figure 20.10 but with the knee flexed.)

NOTE: This is the same stretch used to increase hip extension—except to stretch the rectus femoris the knee is kept flexed so the range for hip extension is less.

#### Prone Stretch

*Patient position and procedure:* Prone with the knee flexed on the side to be stretched. Have the patient grasp the ankle on that side (or place a towel or strap around the ankle to pull on) and flex the knee. As the muscle increases in flexibility, place a small folded towel under the distal thigh to further extend the hip.

NOTE: Do not let the hip abduct or laterally rotate or let the spine hyperextend.

#### Standing Stretch

*Patient position and procedure:* Standing with the hip extended and knee flexed and grasping the ankle. Instruct the patient to maintain a posterior pelvic tilt and not let the back arch or the side bend during this stretch (Fig. 20.13).

NOTE: If the rectus femoris is too tight to stretch safely in this manner, the patient may place his or her foot on a chair or bench located behind the body rather than grasping the ankle.

### Hamstring Stretches

#### Straight Leg Raising

NOTE: Straight leg raising (SLR) exercises elongate the hamstrings by stretching them across the hip using hip flexion while maintaining the knee in extension.

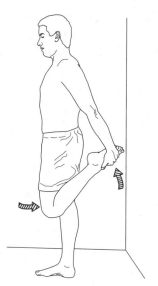

FIGURE 20.13 Self-stretch of the rectus femoris while standing. The femur is kept in line with the trunk. Care must be taken to maintain a posterior PT and not arch or twist the back.

*Patient position and procedure:* Supine with a towel under the thigh. Have the patient perform SLR with one extremity and apply the stretch force by pulling on the towel to move the hip into more flexion.

### Doorway Stretch

*Patient position and procedure:* Supine, on the floor, with one leg through a doorway and the other leg (the one to be stretched) propped up against the door frame. For an effective stretch, the pelvis and opposite leg must remain on the floor with the knee extended.

- To increase the stretch when the patient is able, have the patient move the buttock closer to the doorframe, keeping the knee extended (Fig. 20.14A).
- Teach the patient to perform the hold–relax/agonist contraction technique by pressing the heel of the leg being stretched against the doorframe, causing an isometric contraction, relaxing it, then lifting the leg away from the frame (Fig. 20.14B).

### Chair Stretch

*Patient position and procedure:* Sitting with the leg to be stretched extended across to another chair, or sitting at the edge of a treatment table, with the leg to be stretched on the table and the opposite foot on the floor. Have the patient lean the trunk forward toward the thigh, keeping the back extended so there is motion only at the hip joint (Fig. 20.15).

### Bilateral Toe Touching

NOTE: Bilateral toe touching exercises are often used to stretch the hamstring muscles in exercise classes. It is important to recognize that having the patient reach for the toes does not selectively stretch the hamstrings but stretches the low back and mid-back as well. Toe touching

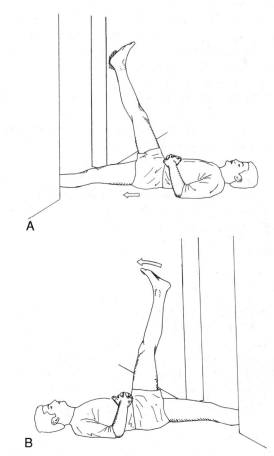

A

B

FIGURE 20.14 Self-stretching of the hamstring muscles. Additional stretch can occur if the person either (*A*) moves the buttock closer to the door frame or (*B*) lifts the leg away from the doorframe.

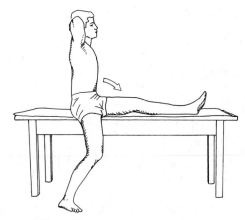

FIGURE 20.15 Self-stretching the hamstring muscles by leaning the trunk toward the extended knee, flexing at the hips.

is considered a general flexibility exercise and tends to mask shortening of soft tissues in one region and overstretch areas already flexible. Whether a person can touch the toes depends on many factors (e.g., body type; arm, trunk, and leg length; flexibility in the thoracic and lumbar regions; hamstring and gastrocnemius length).[60]

*Patient position and procedure:* Standing. To discourage the "toe touch" idea, teach the patient to place the hands on the hips when bending forward. To specifically stretch the hamstrings using the standing forward-bend method, teach the patient to first do an anterior pelvic tilt to extend the spine; then keep the back stable and bend only at the hips ("hinge at the hips") and go only through the range of forward bending where the spine can be maintained in extension. The stretch sensation should be felt in the hamstring region.

P R E C A U T I O N : This stretching technique should not be used when the patient has low back impairments because forward bending greatly increases mechanical stress to the tissues of the low back.

## To Stretch the Tensor Fasciae Latae

### Standing Stretch

*Patient position and procedure:* Standing with the side to be stretched toward a wall and the hand on that side placed on the wall. Have the patient extend, adduct, and externally rotate the extremity to be stretched and cross it behind the other extremity. With both feet on the floor, have the patient shift his or her pelvis toward the wall and allow the normal knee to bend slightly (Fig. 20.16). There is a slight side-bending of the trunk away from the side being stretched.

### Side-Lying Stretch

*Patient position and procedure:* Side-lying, with the leg to be stretched uppermost. The bottom extremity is flexed for support and the pelvis tilted laterally so the waist is against the mat or floor. Abduct the top leg and align it in the

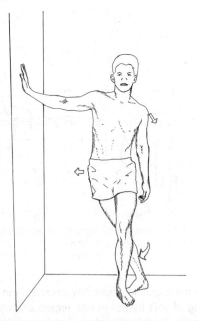

**FIGURE 20.16** Self-stretching the tensor fasciae latae occurs as the trunk bends away from and the pelvis shifts toward the tight side. Increased stretch occurs when the extremity is positioned in external rotation prior to the stretch.

plane of the body (in extension). While maintaining this position, have the patient externally rotate the hip and then gradually lower (adduct) the thigh to the point of stretch (Fig. 20.17). Flex the knee to obtain additional stretch.

N O T E : It is critical to keep the trunk aligned and not allow it to roll backward because the hip would then flex and the iliotibial tract would slip in front of the greater trochanter, and an effective stretch would not take place.

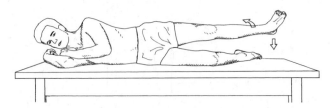

**FIGURE 20.17** Tensor fasciae latae self-stretching: side-lying position. The thigh is abducted in the plane of the body; then it is extended and externally rotated, then slowly lowered. Additional stretch can occur by flexing the knee.

## EXERCISES TO DEVELOP AND IMPROVE MUSCLE PERFORMANCE AND FUNCTIONAL CONTROL

During the controlled motion and return to function phases of intervention when only moderate or minimum protection of healing tissues is necessary, it is important that the patient learns to develop control of hip movement while using good trunk stability. For a muscle that has not been properly used or that has been dominated by another muscle, exercises begin with developing patient awareness of muscle contractions and movements through controlled ROM exercises. If muscle shortening has prevented full ROM, development of muscle control in any new range must immediately follow stretching activities. Principles for improving muscle performance as well as techniques for manual resistance exercise and methods of mechanical resistance are described in Chapter 6. Manually applied resistance should be used when muscles are weak or when helping the patient focus on specific muscles. Exercises described in the following sections may be adapted for home exercise programs. Choose exercises that challenge the patient to progress toward the functional goals established in the plan of care.

### Non-Weight-Bearing Exercises

Even though weight-bearing activities dominate lower extremity function, when a patient is weak or has poor control of specific muscles or patterns of motion, it is advantageous to begin exercises in non-weight-bearing positions so the individual can learn to isolate muscle activity and control specific motions. In addition, many functional activities have a non-weight-bearing component, such as the swing phase in gait, lifting the leg up to a step when going upstairs, and lifting the lower extremity into a car or onto a bed.

### To Develop Control of and Strengthen Hip Abduction (Gluteus Medius and Tensor Fasciae Latae)

N O T E : Muscle imbalances in the hip that contribute to hip and/or low back pain may be seen if abduction is dominated by the tensor fasciae latae and the stabilizing forces from the gluteus medius are poorly controlled.[116] This is seen if the patient flexes and internally rotates the thigh when abducting the hip. The posterior fibers of the gluteus medius must be trained to contract while the tensor relaxes. Techniques to do this are described below. If the patient has good control of rotation, abduction utilizing the synergy between these muscles is used.

#### Supine Abduction

Supine abduction is the easiest position in which to initiate motion because the effects of gravity on the abductors are eliminated. Have the patient concentrate on isolated hip abduction while keeping the trunk still. Do not let the femur roll outward into external rotation.

- For very weak patients, provide assistance or place a skate or towel under the leg to minimize the effects of friction.
- If the patient is not strong enough to progress to the side-lying position, place a weight, such as a sandbag, along the outside of the thigh or ankle and have the patient push the weight outward.

#### Side-Lying Abduction

Have the patient flex the bottom leg for balance, and then lift the top leg into abduction, keeping the hip neutral to rotation and in slight extension. Do not allow the hip to flex or the trunk to roll backward. Add ankle weights to provide resistance as the patient's strength improves.

If the patient has difficulty controlling hip abduction in the side lying position, use the following training sequence.

- First have the patient practice externally rotating the thigh. This may be done with the hip and knee in slight flexion while the patient lifts the uppermost knee off the mat or with the hip and knee extended while the patient rolls the uppermost extremity outward.
- Once the patient can control external rotation, have him or her extend the hip (without arching the spine) and then abduct the top leg (it should be aligned in the plane of the body). The patient then slowly adducts and abducts the thigh against gravity.

N O T E : If the tensor fasciae latae is tight, the range into extension or adduction may be limited. Stretching of this muscle should be done prior to this exercise (see Fig. 20.17). It is important that the patient does not let the hip flex or internally rotate during this exercise to minimize action of the tensor fasciae latae.

#### Standing Abduction

Have the patient, while standing on one leg, bring the other lower extremity out to the side. Instruct the patient to maintain the trunk upright, in neutral alignment, and not let the abducting hip flex or rotate.

- Add resistance by applying an ankle weight on the moving leg or by using pulleys or elastic resistance applied at right angles to the moving extremity.
- The abductors on the stationary lower extremity experience closed-chain resistance while stabilizing the pelvis, and the abductors on the moving extremity experience open-chain resistance.

### To Develop Control of and Strengthen Hip Extension (Gluteus Maximus)

#### Gluteal Muscle Setting

Use gluteal setting exercises to increase awareness of the contracting muscle. Position the patient prone or supine and teach the patient to "squeeze" (contract) the buttocks.

#### Forward-Bending Leg Lifts

With the patient standing at the edge of the treatment table and the trunk flexed and supported on the table, have the patient alternately extend one hip, then the other. This is done with the knee flexed to train the gluteus maximus while relaxing the hamstrings. If the hamstrings cramp from active insufficiency, the patient is attempting to use them and should practice relaxing them before progressing with this exercise. Progress by adding weights or elastic resistance to the distal thigh.

#### Quadruped Leg Lifts

Have the patient alternately extend each hip while keeping the knee flexed (Fig. 20.18). Combine this exercise with trunk stabilization by first having the patient find the neutral pelvic position, drawing in the abdominal muscles, then extending the hip (see Chapter 16).

P R E C A U T I O N : Care is taken not to extend the hip beyond the available range of hip extension; otherwise, the motion causes stress in the sacroiliac joint or lumbar spine.

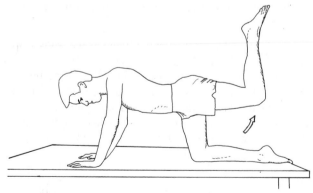

FIGURE 20.18 Isolated training and strengthening of the gluteus maximus. Starting in the quadruped position, extend the hip while keeping the knee flexed to rule out use of the hamstring muscles. Do not to extend the hip beyond the available ROM to avoid causing stress to the sacroiliac or lumbar spinal joints.

## To Develop Control of and Strengthen Hip External Rotation

### Prone

The patient's knees are flexed and about 10 inches apart. Have the patient press the heels together, causing an isometric contraction of the external rotators.

### Side-Lying

With both lower extremities partially flexed at the hips and knees and the heel of the top leg resting on the heel of the bottom leg, have the patient lift the knee of the top leg, keeping the heels together.

*Progression.* Have the patient extend the top hip and knee, aligning the lower extremity with the trunk, then rolling the leg outward. Progress this to lifting the entire lower extremity into abduction once the hip is externally rotated.

N O T E : Do not allow the patient to roll the trunk backward, as this exercise is done to minimize substitution with the hip flexor muscles.

### Standing

With feet parallel and about 4 inches apart, have the patient flex the knees slightly, then externally rotate the thighs (so the knees are pointing laterally) while keeping the feet stationary on the floor. Tell the patient to maintain external rotation while extending the knees, then relax the rotation slightly until the patellae point forward.

### Sitting

With knees flexed over the edge of the treatment table, secure elastic material around the patient's ankle and the table leg on the same side. Have the patient move the foot toward the opposite side, pulling against the resistance, causing external rotation of the hip.

N O T E : Do not allow substitution with knee flexion or extension or hip abduction.

## To Develop Control of and Strengthen Hip Adduction

### Side-Lying

With the bottom leg aligned in the plane of the trunk (hip extension) and the top leg flexed forward with the foot on the floor or with the thigh resting on a pillow, have the patient lift the bottom leg upward into adduction. Weights can be added to the ankle to progress strengthening (Fig. 20.19A). A more difficult position is to have the patient hold the top leg in abduction and adduct the bottom leg up to meet it (Fig. 20.19B).

### Standing

Have the patient adduct the leg across the front of the weight-bearing leg. Add ankle weights to provide resistance, or fasten elastic resistance or a pulley at right angles to the moving leg.

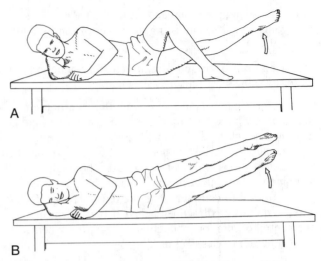

FIGURE 20.19 Training and strengthening the hip adductors. (*A*) The top leg is stabilized by flexing the hip and resting the foot on the mat while the bottom leg is adducted against gravity. (*B*) The top leg is isometrically held in abduction while the bottom leg is adducted against gravity.

## Closed-Chain Weight-Bearing Exercises

Weight-bearing exercises in the lower extremity involve all of the joints in the closed chain and are therefore not limited to hip muscles. Most activities bring into play antagonistic two-joint muscles in which each muscle is being lengthened across one joint while it is shortening across another, thus maintaining an optimal length–tension relationship. In addition to causing motion, a prime function of the muscles in weight bearing is to control against the forces of gravity and momentum for balance and stability. Therefore, the exercises described in this section include balance and stabilization training as well as strengthening and functional exercises.

### Closed-Chain Strengthening and Functional Training

Strengthening and balance activities in weight-bearing postures described in the following section are closely related and are progressed concurrently as the patient is able.

### Hip Hiking/Pelvic Drop

Position the patient with one leg on a 2- to 4-inch block and alternately lower and elevate the pelvis on the side of the unsupported leg (Fig. 20.20). This develops control in the abductors of the stance leg and hip hikers on the unsupported side.

 **Focus on Evidence** _____

In an EMG study by Bolglia and Uhl,[20] a series of 16 healthy subjects performing six different abductor exercises using a constant weight. The authors documented significantly greater maximum voluntary contraction of the gluteus medius in the stance leg (weight-bearing leg) during the pelvic drop exercise than during other hip abduction exercises. In addition, standing hip abduction showed significantly greater hip abductor activity on the

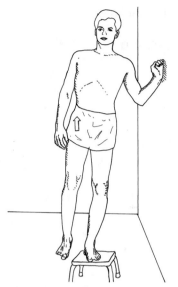

FIGURE 20.20 Training the hip abductor and hiker muscles for frontal plane strenthening and stability.

weight-bearing side than on the moving (open-chain) side; the activity on the weight-bearing side had a comparable maximum voluntary contraction as side-lying hip abduction.

### Bridging

Beginning in the hook-lying position, have the patient press the upper back and feet into the mat, elevate the pelvis, and extend the hips (Fig. 20.21).

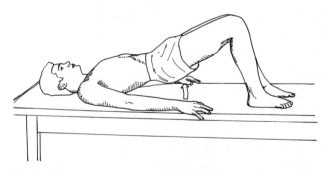

FIGURE 20.21 Training and strengthening the hip extensor muscles using bridging exercises. Resistance can be added against the pelvis.

*Progressions.* Apply resistance against the anterior pelvis manually or by strapping a weighted belt around the pelvis. To challenge proprioception and balance, have the patient perform bridging exercises using a large gym ball positioned either under the back with feet on the floor or under the feet while lying on the floor.

### Single-Leg Stance Against Resistance

Have the patient stand on the involved leg. Place elastic resistance around the thigh of the other extremity and

secure it to a stable upright structure. If the knee is stable, the resistance can be applied around the ankle. Fatigue is determined when the patient can no longer hold the weight-bearing extremity or pelvis stable.

- To resist *hip flexion*, the patient faces away from where the resistance is secured.
- To resist *extension*, the patient faces toward where the resistance is secured (Fig. 20.22A).
- To resist *abduction* and *adduction* the patient faces so the band is directed toward one side and then the other (Fig. 20.22B).

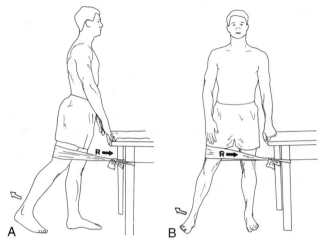

FIGURE 20.22 Closed-chain exercise with elastic resistance around the opposite leg. (*A*) Resisting extension on the right requires stabilization of anterior muscles of the left side. (*B*) Resisting abduction on the right requires stabilization of the left frontal plane muscles. To increase difficulty, the resistance is moved distally onto the leg.

N O T E : This activity is open-chain on the side of the moving extremity and closed-chain on the weight-bearing side.

### Step-Ups

Begin with a low step, 2 to 3 inches in height; progress the height as the patient is able. Have the patient step up sideways, forward, or backward. Be sure that the entire foot is planted on the step and that the body is lifted and then lowered with smooth motion, with no lurching of the trunk or pushing off with the trailing extremity.

*Progressions:* In addition to increasing the step height, resistance can be added with a weight belt, with weights in the hands or around the ankle of the non-weight-bearing leg.

### Lunges

Have the patient stride forward and flex the hip and knee of the forward extremity and then return upright. Repeat, or alternate legs. Begin with flexing the knee a small range and progressing to 90° knee flexion.

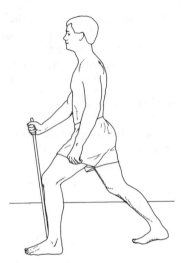

FIGURE 20.23 Lunge with cane assistance to develop balance and control for lowering body weight.

● If the patient has difficulty with balance or control, have him or her use a cane or rod for balance, or begin the activity holding on in the parallel bars or beside a treatment table (Fig. 20.23).

● It is important to instruct the patient to keep the toes pointing forward, bend the knee in the same plane as the feet, and keep the back upright.

*Progressions:* Progressions include using weights in the hands for resistance, taking a longer stride, or lunging forward onto a small step. This exercise is progressed to a functional activity by having the patient lunge and pick up objects from the floor.

N O T E : A patient with an anterior cruciate ligament (ACL) deficiency or a surgically repaired ACL should not flex the knee forward of the toes when performing lunges because this increases the shear force and stress to the ACL. Individuals with patellofemoral compression syndrome experience increased pain under these circumstances because the compressive force from the body weight is greater when it is kept posterior to the knee. Adapt the position of the knee based on the patient's symptoms and presenting pathology.

### Wall Slides

Have the patient rest the back against a wall with feet forward and shoulder-width apart. Instruct the patient to slide the back down the wall by flexing the hips and knees and dorsiflexing the ankle; then slide up the wall by extending hips and knees and plantarflexing the ankles (Fig. 20.24A). If sliding the back directly against the wall causes excessive friction, place a towel behind the patient's back.

*Progressions:* A large exercise ball (Swiss ball) placed behind the back requires additional control because it is less stable (Fig. 20.24B). Add arm motions and weights to develop coordination or add resistance. To develop isometric strength, have the patient hold the flexed position and superimpose arm motions with weights.

### Partial Squats/Mini-Squats

Have the patient lower the trunk by flexing the hips and knees as if sitting on a chair. Add resistance by having the patient hold weights in the hands or use elastic resistance secured under the feet (see Fig. 21.20). Progress to safe lifting techniques that involve squatting.

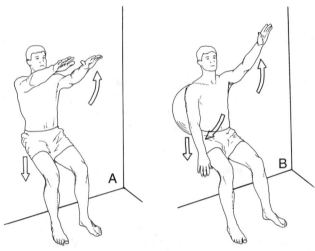

FIGURE 20.24 Wall slides/partial squats to develop eccentric control of body weight. (*A*) The back sliding down a wall, superimposing bilateral arm motion for added resistance. (*B*) The back rolling a gym ball down the wall, superimposing antagonistic arm motion to develop coordination.

N O T E : To protect the ACL, knee flexion range is limited to 0° to 60°, and the patient is instructed to lower the hips as if preparing to sit on a chair so the knees stay behind the toes. To protect a patellofemoral compression problem, instruct the patient to squat only through pain-free ranges and avoid deep knee bends.

### Equipment

Mechanical equipment such as a leg press, Total Gym® treadmill, bicycle, slide board, or Profitter™ may be used for strengthening, balance, coordination, and endurance.

### Postural Control and Balance Activities

As noted earlier, weight-bearing control and balance training begin as soon as the patient tolerates partial weight bearing. For a detailed discussion on balance, see Chapter 8.

### Weight Shifting

● If the patient cannot bear full weight, begin in the parallel bars with part of the weight borne by the hands. An overhead harnessing system can also be used to unweight the lower extremities.

● Have the patient shift anterior to posterior, side to side, and obliquely.

● Add manual resistance to the motion by applying pressure against the patient's pelvis.

### Balance Activities with Arm Movements

- Begin with bilateral weight bearing and progress to unilateral weight bearing. First have the patient move his or her arms in the sagittal and frontal planes, then progress to the transverse and diagonal planes.
- As the patient demonstrates the ability to balance with simple arm movements, progress to moving the arms and following the movement with the eyes and head. Then progress to moving the entire trunk through planes of motion following the arm motions.

### Marching and Resisted Walking

- Once the patient can shift weight and maintain balance with arm movements, have him or her alternately pick up each foot and march in place.
- Progress to moving each leg forward and backward and learning to accept weight on the moving leg.
- Once the patient can step and walk, progress to resisted walking by applying resistance at the pelvis or have the patient walk against an elastic or pulley resistance secured around the pelvis (Fig. 20.25).

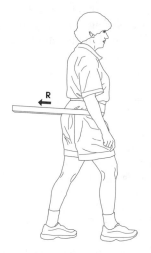

FIGURE 20.25 Resisted walking using a large elastic resistance band secured around the pelvis.

### Alternating Isometrics and Rhythmic Stabilization
Alternating isometrics and rhythmic stabilization develop postural adjustments to applied forces.

- Apply manual resistance against the pelvis in alternating directions and ask the patient to hold (with isometric contractions). There should be little or no movement.
- Vary the force and direction of resistance; also vary where the force is applied by shifting the resistance from the pelvis to the shoulders and eventually against outstretched arms (see Fig. 22.15).
- At first, use verbal cueing. Then, as the patient learns control, apply the varying forces without warning. Progress the patient to unilateral standing.

- Teach the patient a self-applied stabilization technique using elastic resistance secured around the thigh or leg of one extremity and then rapidly move the extremity forward and backward against the elastic force (see Fig. 20.22 for the setup). The rapid motion requires stabilization on the weight-bearing side.

### Balance Training on Unstable Surfaces

- Have the patient stand with bilateral support on foam, a rocker board, wobble board, or BAPS board and begin with single-plane weight shifting forward/backward and side to side.
- Progress by placing the extremities in a diagonal plane and have the patient shift the weight from one extremity to the other.
- When able, have the patient progress to single-leg activities on an unstable surface.

### Advanced Stability and Balance Activities

- Have the patient stand on an unstable surface, such as a rocker or wobble board, and maintain balance without the edges of the board touching the ground while a partner tosses a weighted ball to the patient from various angles.
- Have the patient hold onto the two ends of an elastic resistance band while someone pulls against it in various directions and with varying speeds.

## Functional Training

The level of challenge of the exercise program depends on the activities the patient is required to perform in his or her ADL, IADL, work, or sport-related tasks; and the challenge level therefore affects the desired outcomes. An outcome may be simply learning how to ambulate forward, backward, and around obstacles safely, or it may involve developing a high level of coordination, balance, and skill to climb, perform complicated dance maneuvers, engage in gymnastics, or run and jump. Analyze the patient's exercise techniques and adapt them whenever necessary to avoid unsafe stresses.

Suggestions for progressive functional training include:

- Increase challenges for ambulation, such as having the patient walk on uneven surfaces, turn, maneuver backward, and walk up and down ramps first under supervision and then unassisted. As soon as the patient is able, have him or her practice rising up and sitting down from chairs of various heights and climbing and descending flights of stairs.
- Incorporate exercises that prepare the musculature for safe body mechanics such as repetitive squats and lunges. Progress the exercises by having the patient lift and carry or push and pull various loads as part of the exercise routine. Utilize safe patterns of motion that replicate functional requirements.

- Use agility drills such as maneuvering around and stepping over obstacles. Incorporate running, jumping, hopping, skipping, and side-shuffle drills.
- If the patient is returning to activities that require strength and power, incorporate plyometric drills. For example, have the patient jump from a box or step; flex the hips, knees, and ankles to absorb the impact of landing; and immediately jump back up to the box or step.
- Use maximum eccentric loading. Any of the previously described exercises can be adapted, but it is critical to assist the patient through the concentric phase of the exercise and guard him or her through the eccentric phase as the resistance is great. These are not exercises the patient can do alone.

# INDEPENDENT LEARNING ACTIVITIES

## ● Critical Thinking and Discussion

1. Describe the function of the primary muscle groups of the hip joint in open- and closed-chain situations. Include their role in stabilizing the pelvis during single leg stance and the effects on the spine when the pelvis is moved by the hip musculature.
2. Describe the role of the hip during the gait cycle. Include muscle activity, motion needed, and pathological gait patterns when there is muscle weakness or restricted motion.
3. Analyze the type of gait deviations a patient might exhibit after internal fixation of a fracture of the proximal femur, total hip arthroplasty, or hemiarthroplasty of the hip.
4. After total hip arthroplasty or internal fixation of a hip fracture, what are the signs that dislocation of the hip or loss of fracture stabilization has occurred?

## ● Laboratory Practice

1. Identify and practice the techniques you would use to treat a mobility impairment if the results of your examination included decreased joint play versus restricted flexibility in the hip musculature. Include exercises that could be used in a home exercise program.
2. Demonstrate a progression of exercises to develop control and strength in the gluteus medius muscle after total hip replacement.
3. Develop an exercise routine and progression for an individual with hip muscle weakness who wants to return to work that requires walking, lifting objects that weigh up to 45 lb, and climbing ladders with 45-lb weights.

## ● Case Studies

1. Mr. C., 57 years of age, is a mail carrier; he has walked his mail route for 32 years and is proud "that he has no heart problems." Over the past year he has noticed that his hip hurts after sitting for more than 1 hour and that there is a marked increase in pain when first getting up out of a chair and walking. He also has noticed that there is increased discomfort in his hip and knees near the end of each workday. The medical diagnosis is osteoarthritis. Strength testing reveals generally 4/5 on manual muscle tests except the gluteus medius, which is 3+/5. There is mild tightness in the hip flexors, including the rectus femoris and tensor fasciae lata. He wants to avoid being a "candidate for total hip replacement surgery."
   - Explain why the patient's job would perpetuate these symptoms.
   - Outline a plan to manage the symptoms; identify measurable goals and interventions you would use to reach the goals.
   - What can the patient do to protect his hip joints?
2. Ms. J., a 31-year-old mother, recreational tennis player, and bowler, is recovering from multiple femoral fractures that she sustained in an automobile accident 3 months ago. There is radiological healing of all the fracture sites, and she is now allowed full weight bearing and no restrictions in activities. She has significant hip mobility impairments from joint restrictions and muscle weakness.
   - What joint ranges and muscle strength levels are needed for her to return to her functional activities?
   - Outline a plan to manage the symptoms; identify measurable goals and interventions you would use to reach the goals. Using the taxonomy or motor skills described in Chapter 1, develop a series of progressively more challenging motor tasks under varying environmental conditions.
3. Mr. C. is a 32-year-old firefighter who strained his hamstrings at the ischial tuberosity while pulling a 250-lb individual out of a burning building. It happened 4 days ago. Currently, he is experiencing considerable pain, is unable to sit on hard surfaces (because of pressure as well as flexing the hip), and has pain when arising from or lowering himself into a chair and climbing or descending stairs. Hip flexion is limited to 90° and straight-leg raising to 45°. He tolerates minimal resistance to hip extension or knee flexion. This individual must be able to climb a ladder while wearing his gear (40 lb) and air pack (40 lb) and carrying a 20-lb hand tool; in addition, he must be able to carry a 175-lb individual across his shoulder, drag a heavy body across the floor, climb five flights of stairs wearing full gear, and run $1/2$ mile in 5 minutes to be able to return to work.
   - Explain why this patient has impaired function in biomechanical terms.

- Establish goals that reflect treatment of the impairments and desired functional outcomes.
- Design a program of intervention at each stage of tissue healing.
- Design a series of exercises that can be used to prepare Mr. C. for return to function once the muscle has healed.

4. A 78-year-old woman who lives at home with her husband has been referred to you for home-based physical therapy. Ten days ago she underwent cemented THA with a posterolateral approach for late-stage post-traumatic arthritis associated with injuries sustained in a horseback riding accident 30 years ago. She has been home from the hospital for 5 days. She is ambulating with a walker on level surfaces, and weight bearing is tolerated. The patient's long-term goals

are to be able to participate in a community-based fitness program for older adults and resume travel vacations with her husband.

- Continue progressing her exercise program that was initiated in the hospital.
- Review the precautions she must take for the next 6 to 12 weeks during ADL.
- Make suggestions on how she or her husband might adapt the home environment to help her adhere to the precautions.
- To help her meet her long-term goals, design a sequence of progressively more demanding functional activities, integrating the taxonomy of motor tasks (addressed in Chapter 1) and the principles of aerobic conditioning (discussed in Chapter 5).

## REFERENCES

1. American Physical Therapy Association: Guide to Physical Therapist Practice, ed 2. Phys Ther 81:9–744, 2001.
2. Antoniou, J, Greidanus, NV, Proprosky, WG: Surgical approaches and anatomic considerations. In Pellicci, PM, Tria, AJ, Garvin, KL (eds) Orthopedic Knowledge Update. 2. Hip and Knee Reconstruction. American Academy of Orthopedic Surgeons, Rosemont, IL, 2000, p 91.
3. Archibeck, MJ, Berger, RA, Jacobs, JJ, et al: Second-generation cementless total hip arthroplasty: eight to eleven year results. J Bone Joint Surg Am 83:1666–1673, 2001.
4. Archibeck, MJ, White, RE: Learning curve for the two-incision total hip replacement. Clin Orthop 429:232–238, 2004.
5. Babis, GC, Morrey, BF, Berry, DJ: The young patient indications and results. In Morrey, BF (ed) Total Joint Replacement Arthroplasty, ed 3. Churchill Livingstone, Philadelphia, 2003, pp 696–707.
6. Baerga-Varela, L, Malanga, GA: Rehabilitation and minimally invasive surgery. In Hozack, WJ, Krismer, M, Nogler, M, et al (eds) Minimally Invasive Total Joint Arthroplasty. Springer Verlag, Heidelberg, 2004, pp 2–5.
7. Bal, BS, Halton, G, Aleto, T, Barrett, M: Early complications of primary total hip replacement performed with a two-incision minimally invasive technique. J Bone Joint Surg Am 87(11):2432–2438, 2005.
8. Ball, PB, Wroe, MC, MacLeod, L: Survey of physical therapy preoperative care in total hip replacement. Phys Ther Health Care 1:83, 1986.
9. Barnes, B, Dunovan, K: Functional outcomes after hip fracture. Phys Ther 67:1675, 1987.
10. Barrick, EF: Orthopedic trauma. In Kauffman, TL (ed) Geriatric Rehabilitation Manual. Churchill Livingstone, New York, 1999, p 125.
11. Beaupre, LA, Jones, A, Saunders, LD, et al: Best practices for elderly hip fracture patients: a systematic overview of the evidence. J Gen Intern Med 20(11):1019–1025, 2005.
12. Beber, C, Convery, R: Management of patients with total hip replacement. Phys Ther 52:823, 1972.
13. Berger, RA, Jacobs, JJ, Meneghini, RM, et al: Rapid rehabilitation and recovery with minimally invasive total hip arthroplasty. Clin Orthop 429:239–247, 2004.
14. Berry, DJ, Berger, RA, Callaghan, JJ, et al: Minimally invasive total hip arthroplasty: development, early results, and critical analysis. J Bone Joint Surg Am 85:2235–2246, 2003.
15. Berry, DJ, Duffy, GP: Cemented femoral components. In Morrey, BF (ed) Joint Replacement Arthroplasty, ed 3. Churchill Livingstone, Philadelphia, 2003, pp 617–636.
16. Berry, DJ, Morrey, BF, Cabanela, MG: Uncemented femoral components. In Morrey, BF (ed) Joint Replacement Arthroplasty, ed 3. Churchill Livingstone, Philadelphia, 2003, pp 637–656.

17. Binder, EF, Brown, M, Sinacore, DR, et al: Effects of extended outpatient rehabilitation after hip fracture: a randomized controlled trial. JAMA 292(7):837–846, 2004.
18. Birage, SJ, Morrow-Howell, N, Proctor, EK: Hip fracture. Clin Geriatr Med 10:589, 1994.
19. Bodén, H, Adolphson, P: No adverse effects of early weight bearing after uncemented total hip arthroplasty. Acta Orthop Scand 75(1):21–29, 2004.
20. Bolgla, LA, Uhl, TL: Electromyographic analysis of hip rehabilitation exercises in a group of healthy subjects. J Orthop Sports Phys Ther 35(8):487–494, 2005.
21. Bottner, F, Zawadsky, M, Su, EP, et al: Implant migration after early weightbearing in cementless hip replacement. Clin Orthop 436:132–137, 2005.
22. Bukowski, EL: Practice guidelines: acute care management following total hip arthroplasty (postoperative days 1-4). Orthop Phys Ther Pract 17(3):10–14, 2005.
23. Bullock-Saxton, JE: Local sensation changes and altered hip muscle function following severe ankle sprain. Phys Ther 74:17,1994.
24. Burton, D, Imrie, S: Total hip arthroplasty and postoperative rehabilitation. Phys Ther 53:132, 1973.
25. Cailliet, R: Low Back Pain Syndrome, ed 4. FA Davis, Philadelphia, 1988.
26. Cameron, H, Brotzman, SB: The arthritic lower extremity. In Brotzman, SB, Wilk, KE (eds) Clinical Orthopedic Rehabilitation, ed 2. Mosby, Philadelphia, 2003, p 441.
27. Capello, WN, D'Antonio, JA, Manley, MT, Feinberg, JR: Arc-deposited hydroxyapatite-coated cups. Clin Orthop 441:305–312, 2005.
28. Charnley, J: Total hip replacement by low friction arthroplasty. Clin Orthop 72:721, 1974.
29. Chu, FY, Chen, CM, Ghung, TY, et al: The effect of posterior capsulorrhaphy in primary total hip arthroplasty. J Arthroplasty 15:194, 2000.
30. Cibulka, MT, Delitto, A: A comparison of two different methods to treat hip pain in runners. J Orthop Sports Phys Ther 17:173, 1993.
31. Coventry, MB, Morrey, BF: Historical perspective of hip arthroplasty. In Morrey, BF (ed) Joint Replacement Arthroplasty, ed 3. Churchill Livingstone, Philadelphia, 2003, pp 557–565.
32. Craik, RL: Disability following hip fracture. Phys Ther 74:388, 1994.
33. Crutchfield, CA, et al: Balance and coordination training. In Scully, RM, Barnes, MR (eds) Physical Therapy. JB Lippincott, Philadelphia, 1989.
34. Cullen, S: Physical therapy program for patients with total hip replacement. Phys Ther 53:1293, 1973.
35. Cyriax, J: Textbook of Orthopaedic Medicine, ed 8, Vol 1. Diagnosis of Soft Tissue Lesions. Bailliere Tindall, London, 1982.
36. De Jong, Z, Vlieland, TP: Safety of exercise in patients with rheumatoid arthritis. Curr Opin Rheumatol 17(2):177–182, 2005.

37. Enloe, J, et al: Total hip and knee replacement treatment: a report using consensus. J Orthop Sports Phys Ther 23:3, 1996.
38. Enseki, KR, Martin, RL, Draovitch, P, et al: The hip joint: arthoscopic procedures and postoperative rehabilitation. J Orthop Sports Phys Ther 336(7):516–525, 2006.
39. Fehring, TK, Rosenberg, AG: Primary total hip arthroplasty: indications and contraindications. In Callaghan, JJ, Rosenberg, AG, Rubash, HE (eds) The Adult Hip, Vol II. Lippincott-Raven, Philadelphia, 1998, p 893.
40. Fife, RS: Osteoarthritis, epidemiology, pathology, and pathogensis. In Klippel, JF (ed) Primer on Rheumatic Diseases, ed 11. Arthritis Foundation, Atlanta, 1997, p 216.
41. Finerman, GA, et al: Commentary. In Finerman, GA, et al (eds) Total Hip Arthroplasty Outcomes. Churchill Livingstone, New York, 1998, p 3.
42. Fortin, PR, Penrod, JR, Clarke, AE, et al: Timing of total joint replacement affects clinical outcomes among patient with osteoarthritis of the hip or knee. Arthritis Rheum 46(12):3327–3330, 2002.
43. Freburger, JK: An analysis of the relationship between utilization of physical therapy services and outcomes of care for patients after total hip arthroplasty. Phys Ther 80:448, 2000.
44. Galante, JO: An overview of total joint arthroplasty. In Callaghan, JJ, Rosenberg, AG, Rubash, HE (eds) The Adult Hip, Vol II. Lippincott-Raven, Philadelphia, 1998, p 829.
45. Gerlinger, TL, Ghate, RS, Paprosky, WG: Posterior approach: backdoor in. Orthopedics 28(9):931–933, 2005.
46. Givens-Heiss, DL, et al: In vivo acetabular contact pressures during rehabilitation. Part II. Post acute phase. Phys Ther 72:700, 1992.
47. Goldberg, VM: Surface replacement solutions for the arthritic hip. Orthopedics 28(9):943–944, 2005.
48. Goldstein, TS: Determining the cause of disability. In Functional Rehabilitation in Orthopedics. Aspen, Gaithersburg, MD, 1995.
49. Gucione, AA: Arthritis and the process of disablement. Phys Ther 74:408, 1994.
50. Gucione, AA, Fogerson, TL, Anderson, JJ: Regaining functional independence in the acute care setting following hip fracture. Phys Ther 76:818, 1996.
51. Hanssen, AD: Anatomy and surgical approaches. In Morrey, BF (ed) Joint Replacement Arthroplasty, ed 3. Churchill Livingstone, Philadelphia, 2003, pp 566–593.
52. Hauer, K, Specht, N, Schuler, M, et al: Intensive physical training in geriatric patients after severe falls and hip surgery. Age Aging 31:49–57, 2002.
53. Hewitt, J, Glisson, R, Guilak, F, Vail, T: The mechanical properties of the human hip capsule ligaments. J Arthroplasty 17:82–89, 2002.
54. Hielema, F, Summerfore, R: Physical therapy for patients with hip fracture or joint replacement. Phys Ther Health Care 1:89, 1986.
55. Holt, EM, et al: 1000 Femoral neck fractures: the effect of pre-injury mobility and surgical experience on outcome. Injury 25:91, 1994.
56. Howe, JG, Lambert, B: Critical pathways in total hip arthroplasty. In Callaghan, JJ, Rosenberg, AG, Rubash, HE (eds) The Adult Hip, Vol II. Lippincott-Raven, Philadelphia, p 865, 1998.
57. Hozack, WJ: Direct lateral approach: splitting the difference. Orthopedics 28(9):937–938, 2005.
58. Izumi, H, et al: Joint motion of bipolar femoral prostheses. J Arthroplasty 10:237, 1995.
59. Jette, AM, Harris, BA, Clearly, PD: Functional recovery after hip fracture. Arch Phys Med Rehabil 68:735, 1987.
60. Kendall, F: Criticism of current tests and exercises for physical fitness. Phys Ther 45:187, 1965.
61. Koval, KJ, Zuckerman, JD Hip Fractures: A Practical Guide to Management. Springer-Verlag, New York, 2000.
62. Koval, KJ, et al: Ambulatory ability after hip fracture: a prospective study in geriatric patients. Clin Orthop 310:150, 1995.
63. Koval, K, et al: Weight bearing after hip fracture: a prospective series of 596 geriatric hip fracture patients. J Orthop Trauma 10:526, 1996.
64. Krebs, DE, et al: Exercise and gait effects on in vivo hip contact pressures. Phys Ther 71:301, 1991.
65. Krebs, DE, et al: Hip biomechanics during gait. J Orthop Sports Phys Ther 28: 51, 1998.
66. Lachiewicz, PF: Dislocation. In Pellicci, PM, Tria, AJ, Garvin, KL (eds) Orthopedic Knowledge Update, 2. Hip and Knee Reconstruction. American Academy of Orthopedic Surgeons, Rosemont, IL, 2000, p 149.
67. Lang, KE: Comparison of 6- and 7-day physical therapy coverage on length of stay and discharge outcome for individuals with total hip and knee arthroplasty. J Orthop Sports Phys Ther 28:15, 1998.
68. Laupacis, A, et al: The effect of elective total hip replacement on health-related quality of life. J Bone Joint Surg Am 75:1619, 1993.
69. Levangie, PK: The hip comples. In Levangie, PK, Norkin, CC (eds) Joint Structure and Function: A Comprehensive Analysis, ed 4. FA Davis, Philadelphia, 2005, pp 355–391.
70. Lewallen, DG: Cementless primary total hip arthroplasty. In Pellicci, PM, Tria, AJ, Garvin, KL (eds) Orthopedic Knowledge Update, 2. Hip and Knee Reconstruction. American Academy of Orthopedic Surgeons, Rosemont, IL, 2000, p 195.
71. Lieberman, JR, et al: Differences between patients' and physicians' evaluation of outcome after total hip arthroplasty. J Bone Joint Surg Am 78:835, 1996.
72. Magee, DJ: Orthopedic Physical Assessment, ed 4. WB Saunders, Philadelphia, 2002.
73. Maloney, WJ, Hartford, JM: The cemented femoral component. In Callaghan, JJ, Rosenberg, AG, Rubash, HE (eds) The Adult Hip, Vol II. Lippincott-Raven, Philadelphia, p 959, 1998.
74. Mangione, KK, Craik, RL, Tomlinson, SS, Palombaro, KM: Can elderly patients who have had a hip fracture perform moderate- to high-intensity exercise at home? Phys Ther 85(8):727–739, 2005.
75. Martin, SD, et al: Hip surgery and rehabilitation. In Melvin, JL, Gall, V (eds) Rheumatologic Rehabilitation Series. Vol 5. Surgical Rehabilitation. American Occupational Therapy Association, Bethesda, 1999, p 81.
76. Matta, JM, Ferguson, TA: The anterior approach for hip replacement. Orthopedics 28(9):927–928, 2005.
77. McGrorey, BJ, Stewart, MJ, Sim, FH: Participation in sports after total hip and knee arthroplasty: a review of the literature and survey of surgical preferences. Mayo Clin Proc 70B:202, 1995.
78. McKinnis, LN: Fundamentals of Musculoskeletal Imaging, ed 2. FA Davis, Philadelphia, 2005.
79. McMinn, DJW: Avascular necrosis in the young patient: a triology of arthroplasty options. Orthopedics 28(9):945–947, 2005.
80. Meek, RMD, Allan, DB, McPhillips, G, et al: Epidemiology of dislocation after total hip arthroplasty. Clin Orthop 447:9–18, 2006.
81. Meere, PA, DiCesare, PE, Zuckerman, JD: Hip fractures treated by hip arthroplasty. In Callaghan, JJ, Rosenberg, AG, Rubash, HE (eds) The Adult Hip, Vol II. Lippincott-Raven, Philadelphia, 1998, p 1221.
82. Mitchell, SL, Stott, DJ, Martin, BJ, Grant, SJ: Randomized controlled trial of quadriceps training after proximal femoral fracture. Clin Rehabil 15(3):282–290, 2001.
83. Mohler, CG, Collis, DK: Early complications and their management. In Callaghan, JJ, Rosenberg, AG, Rubash, HE (eds) The Adult Hip, Vol II. Lippincott-Raven, Philadelphia, 1998, p 1125.
84. Morrey, BF: Dislocation. In Morrey, BF (ed) Joint Replacement Arthroplasty, ed 3. Churchill Livingstone, Philadelphia, 2003, pp 875–890.
85. Morris, AH, Zuckerman, JD: National consensus conference on improving the continuum of care for patients with hip fracture. J Bone Joint Surg Am 84:670–674, 2002.
86. Muller, WE: Total hip prosthesis. Clin Orthop 72:460, 1970.
87. Mulligan, BR: Manual Therapy "NAGS", "SNAGS", MWM'S: etc., ed 4. Plane View Press, Wellington, 1999.
88. Munin, ME, et al: Early inpatient rehabilitation after elective hip and knee arthroplasty. JAMA 279:847, 1998.
89. Munin, MC, et al: Rehabilitation. In Callaghan, JJ, Rosenberg, AG, Rubash, HE (eds) The Adult Hip, Vol II. Lippincott-Raven, Philadelphia, 1998, p 1571.
90. Nelson, C, Lombardi, PM, Pellicci, PM: Hybrid total hip replacement. In Pellicci, PM, Tria, AJ, Garvin, KL (eds) Orthopedic Knowledge Update. 2. Hip and Knee Reconstruction. American Academy of Orthopedic Surgeons, Rosemont, IL, 2000, p 207.
91. Neumann, DA: An electromyographic study of the hip abductor muscles as subjects with hip prostheses walked with different methods of using a cane and carrying a load. Phys Ther 79:1163, 1999.
92. Neumann, DA: Hip abductor muscle activity in patients with a hip prosthesis while carrying loads in one hand. Phys Ther 76:1320, 1996.
93. Neumann, DA: Hip abductor muscle activity as subjects with hip prostheses walk with different methods of using a cane. Phys Ther 78:490, 1998.

94. Neumann, DA: Hip. In Neuman, DA: Kinesiology of the Musculoskeletal System. Mosby, St. Louis, 2002, pp 387–433.

95. NIH Consensus Development Panel on Total Hip Replacement. JAMA 273:1950, 1995.

96. Nilsdotter, A-K, Peterson, IF, Roos, RM, Lohmander, LS: Predictors of patient relevant outcomes after total hip replacement for osteoarthritis: a prospective study. Ann Rheum Dis 62(10):923–930, 2003.

97. Nordin, M, Frankel, VH: Biomechanics of the Hip. In Nordin, M, Frankel, VH (eds) Basic Biomechanics of the Musculoskeletal System, ed 3. Lippincott Williams & Wilkins, Philadelphia, 2001, p 202.

98. Oatis, CA: Kinesiology—The Mechanics and Pathomechanics of Human Movement. Lippincott Williams & Wilkins, Philadelphia, 2004.

99. Ogonda, L, Wilson, R, Archbold, P, et al: A minimal-incision technique in total hip arthroplasty does not improve early postoperative outcomes: a prospective, randomized, controlled trial. J Bone Joint Surg Am 87(4):701–710, 2005.

100. Papagelopoulos, PJ, Morrey, BF: Cemented acetabular components. In Morrey, BF (ed) Joint Replacement Arthroplasty, ed 3. Churchill Livingstone, Philadelphia, 2003, pp 602–608.

101. Papagelopoulos, PJ, Sim, FH: Proximal femoral fracture: femoral neck fracture. In Morrey, BF (ed) Joint Replacement Arthroplasty, ed 3. Churchill Livingstone, Philadelphia, 2003, pp 722–732.

102. Parker, MJ, Pryor, GA, Thorngren, K: Handbook of Hip Fracture Surgery. Butterworth-Heinemann, Oxford, 1997.

103. Parvizi, J, Sharkey, PF, Bissett, GA, et al: Surgical treatment of limb-length discrepancy following total hip arthroplasty. J Bone Joint Surg Am 85(12):2310–2317, 2003.

104. Peak, EL, Parvizi, J, Ciminiello, M, et al: The role of patient restrictions in reducing the prevalence of early dislocation following total hip arthroplasty. J Bone Joint Surg Am 87(2):247–253, 2005.

105. Perry, J: Gait Analysis: Normal and Pathological Function. Slack, Thorofare, NJ, 1992.

106. Peters, CL, Dunn, HK: The cementless acetabular component. In Callaghan, JJ, Rosenberg, AG, Rubash, HE (eds) The Adult Hip, Vol II. Lippincott-Raven, Philadelphia, 1998, p 993.

107. Poss, R: Total joint replacement: optimizing patient expectations. J Am Acad Orthop Surg 1:18, 1993.

108. Praemer, A, Furner, S, Rice, DP: Musculoskeletal Conditions in the United States. American Academy of Orthopedic Surgeons, Chicago, 1992.

109. Ranawat, CS, Rasquinna, VJ, Rodriguez, JA: Results of cemented total hip replacement. In Pellicci, PM, Tria, AJ, Garvin, KL (eds) Orthopedic Knowledge Update, 2. Hip and Knee Reconstruction. American Academy of Orthopedic Surgeons, Rosemont, IL, 2000, p 181.

110. Ranawat, CS, Rodriguez, JA: The cemented acetabular component. In Callaghan, JJ, Rosenberg, AG, Rubash, HE (eds) The Adult Hip, Vol II. Lippincott-Raven, 1998, p 981.

111. Richardson, R: Physical therapy management of patients undergoing total hip replacement. Phys Ther 55:984, 1975.

112. Roddy, E, Zhang, W, Doherty, M, et al: Evidence-based recommendations for the role of exercise in the management of osteoarthritis of the hip or knee—the MOVE consensus. Rheumatology 44(1):67–73, 2005.

113. Roddy, E, Zhang, W, Doherty, M: Aerobic walking or strengthening exercise for osteoarthritis of the knee? A systematic review. Ann Rheum Dis 64(4):544–548, 2005.

114. Roach, JA, Tremblay, LM, Bowers, DL: A preoperative assessment and education program: implementation and outcomes. Patient Educ Couns 25:83, 1995.

115. Rosenberg, AG: A two-incision approach: promises and pitfalls. Orthopedics 28(9):935–937, 2005.

116. Sahrmann, SA: Diagnosis and Treatment of Movement Impairment Syndromes. CV Mosby, St. Louis, 2002.

117. Shashika, H, Matsuba, Y, Watanabe, Y: Home program of physical therapy: effect on disabilities of patients with total hip arthroplasty. Arch Phys Med Rehabil 77:273, 1996.

118. Sherrington, C, Lord, SR: Home exercise to improve strength and walking velocity after hip fracture: a randomized, controlled trial. Arch Phys Med Rehabil 78:208–212, 1997.

119. Sherrington, C, Lord, SR, Herbert, RD: A randomised trial of weight-bearing versus non-weight-bearing exercise for improving physical abilities in inpatients after hip fracture. Aust J Physiother 49:15–22, 2003.

120. Shih, CH, Du, YK, Lu, YH, Wu, CC: Muscular recovery around the the hip joint after total hip arthroplasty. Clin Orthop 302:115–120, 1994.

121. Shumway-Cook, A, Ciol, MA, Gruber, W, Robinson, C: Incidence of and risk factors for falls following hip fracture in community-dwelling older adults. Phys Ther 85(7):648–655, 2005.

122. Silva, M, Heisel, C, Schmalzied, TP: Metal-on-metal total hip replacement. Clin Orthop 430:53–61, 2005.

123. Smith, LK, Weiss, EL, Lehmkuhl, LD: Brunnstrom's Clinical Kinesiology, ed 5. FA Davis, Philadelphia, 1996.

124. Strickland, EM, et al: In vivo acetabular contact pressures during rehabilitation. Part I. Acute phase. Phys Ther 72:691, 1992.

125. Tanzer, M: Two-incision total hip arthroplasty. Clin Orthop 441:71–79, 2005.

126. Taylor, JR, Twomey, LT: Age changes in lumbar zygapophyseal joint. Spine 11(7):739, 1986.

127. Taylor, KW, Murphy, VL: Femoral neck fractures. In Hoppenfeld, S, Murthy, VL (eds) Treatment and Rehabilitation of Fractures. Lippincott Williams & Wilkins, Philadelphia, 2000, p 258.

128. Taylor, KW, Hoppenfeld, S: Intertrochanteric fractures. In Hoppenfeld, S, Murthy, VL (eds) Treatment and Rehabilitation of Fractures. Lippincott Williams & Wilkins, Philadelphia, 2000, p 274.

129. Taylor, KW, Murphy, VL: Subtrochanteric femur fractures. In Hoppenfeld, S, Murthy, VL (eds) Treatment and Rehabilitation of Fractures. Lippincott Williams & Wilkins, Philadelphia, 2000, p 288.

130. Tinetti, ME, Baker, DI, Gottschalk, M, et al: Home-based multicomponent rehabilitation program for older persons after hip fracture: a randomized trial. Arch Phys Med Rehabil 80:916–922, 1999.

131. Trousdale, TR, Cabahela, ME: Uncemented acetabular components. In Morrey, BF (ed) Joint Replacement Arthroplasty, ed 3. Churchill Livingstone, Philadelphia, 2003, pp 609–616.

132. Trudelle-Jackson, E, Emerson, R, Smith, S: Outcomes of total hip arthroplasty: a study of patients one year postsurgery. J Orthop Sports Phys Ther 32(6):260–267, 2002.

133. Tveit, M, Kärrholm, J: Low effectiveness of partial weight bearing: continuous recording of vertical loads using a new pressure-sensitive insole. J Rehabil Med 33:42–46, 2001.

134. Wang, AW, Gilbey, HJ, Ackland, TR: Perioperative exercise programs improve early return of ambulation function after total hip arthroplasty: a randomized, controlled trial. Am J Phys Med Rehabil 81(11):801–806, 2002.

135. Wathe, RA, Koval, KJ, et al: Modular unipolar versus bipolar prosthesis: a prospective evaluation of functional outcomes after femoral neck fracture. J Orthop Trauma 9:298, 1995.

136. Weinrich, M, Good, DC, Reding, M, et al: Timing, intensity, and duration of rehabilitation for hip fracture and stroke: report of a workshop at the National Center for Medical Rehabilitation Research. Neurorehabil Neural Repair 18(1):12–28, 2004.

137. Woolson, ST, Mow, CS, Syquia, JF, et al: Comparison of primary total hip replacement performed with a standard incision or a mini-incision. J Bone Joint Surg Am 86:1353–1358, 2004.

138. Wyke, B: Neurological aspects of pain for the physical therapy clinician. Physical Therapy Forum, Ohio Chapter APTA Conference, Columbus, OH, 1982.

139. Zwartelé, RE, Brand, R, Doets, HC: Increased risk of dislocation after primary total hip arthroplasty in inflammatory arthritis. Acta Orthop Scand 75(6):684–690, 2004.

# The Knee

The knee joint is designed for mobility and stability; it functionally lengthens and shortens the lower extremity to raise and lower the body or to move the foot in space. Along with the hip and ankle, it supports the body when standing, and it is a primary functional unit in walking, climbing, and sitting activities.

As in the other chapters in this section of the text, this chapter is divided into three primary sections. Highlights of the anatomy and function of the knee complex are reviewed in the first section of this chapter, followed by material on the management of disorders and surgeries. The third section includes exercise interventions for the knee region. Chapters 10 through 13 present general information on principles of management. The reader should be familiar with the material in these chapters as well as have a background in examination and evaluation in order to effectively design a therapeutic exercise program to improve knee function in patients with impairments due to injury or pathology or following surgery.

## STRUCTURE AND FUNCTION OF THE KNEE

The bones of the knee joint consist of the distal femur with its two condyles, the proximal tibia with its two tibial plateaus, and the large sesamoid bone in the quadriceps tendon, the patella. It is a complex joint both anatomically and biomechanically (Fig. 21.1).[223] The proximal tibiofibular joint is anatomically close to the knee but is enclosed in a separate joint capsule and functions with the ankle. Therefore, the proximal tibiofibular joint is discussed in Chapter 22.

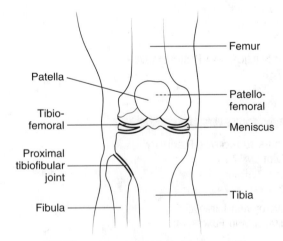

FIGURE 21.1  Bones and joints of the knee and leg.

## JOINTS OF THE KNEE COMPLEX

A lax joint capsule encloses two articulations: the tibiofemoral and the patellofemoral joints. Recesses from the capsule form the suprapatellar, subpopliteal, and gastrocnemius bursae. Folds or thickenings in the synovium persist from embryologic tissue in up to 60% of individuals and may become symptomatic with microtrauma or macrotrauma.[19,107]

### Tibiofemoral Joint

***Characteristics.*** The knee joint is a biaxial, modified hinge joint with two interposed menisci supported by ligaments and muscles. Anteroposterior stability is provided by the cruciate ligaments; mediolateral stability is provided by the medial (tibial) and lateral (fibular) collateral ligaments, respectively (Fig. 21.2).[31,221,223]

- The convex bony partner is composed of two asymmetrical condyles on the distal end of the femur. The medial condyle is longer than the lateral condyle, which contributes to the locking mechanism at the knee.
- The concave bony partner is composed of two tibial plateaus on the proximal tibia with their respective

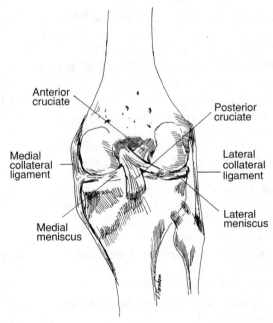

FIGURE 21.2  The medial meniscus is attached to the medial collateral, anterior cruciate, and posterior cruciate ligaments. The lateral meniscus is also attached to the posterior cruciate ligament (the joint capsule has been removed for visualization). *(From Snyder-Mackler.[223] In: Levangie and Norkin, p. 398, with permission.)*

fibrocartilaginous menisci. The medial plateau is larger than the lateral plateau.

● The menisci improve the congruency of the articulating surfaces. They are connected to the tibial condyles and capsule by the coronary ligaments, to each other by the transverse ligament, and to the patella via the patellomeniscal ligaments.[223] The medial meniscus is firmly attached to the joint capsule as well as to the medial collateral ligament, anterior and posterior cruciate ligaments, and semimembranosus muscle. The lateral meniscus attaches to the posterior cruciate ligament and the tendon of the popliteus muscle through capsular connections.[223] Because of the relatively secure attachment of the medial meniscus compared to the lateral meniscus (see Fig. 21.2), it has a greater chance of sustaining a tear when there is a lateral blow to the knee.

***Arthrokinematics.*** Joint mechanics are affected by open- and closed-chain positions of the extremity and are summarized in Box 21.1. Rotation occurs as the knee flexes and extends.

● With motions of the tibia (open kinematic chain), the concave plateaus slide in the same direction as the bone motion. Terminal extension results in the tibia rotating externally on the femur; with flexion, the tibia rotates internally.

● With motions of the femur on a fixated tibia (closed kinematic chain), the convex condyles slide in the direction opposite to the bone motion.

***Screw-home mechanism.*** The rotation that occurs between the femoral condyles and the tibia during the final degrees of extension is called the locking, or screw-home, mechanism. When the tibia is fixed with the foot on the ground (closed kinematic chain), terminal extension results in the femur rotating internally (the medial condyle slides farther posteriorly than the lateral condyle). Concurrently, the hip moves into extension. Tautness in the iliofemoral ligament, which occurs with hip extension, reinforces the medial rotation of the femur. As the knee is unlocked, the femur rotates laterally. Unlocking of the knee occurs indirectly with hip flexion and directly from action of the popliteus muscle. An individual who lacks full hip extension (hip flexion contracture) cannot stand upright and lock the knee, thus lacking this passive stabilizing function.

## Patellofemoral Joint

***Characteristics.*** The patella is a sesamoid bone in the quadriceps tendon. It articulates with the intercondylar (trochlear) groove on the anterior aspect of the distal portion of the femur. Its articulating surface is covered with smooth hyaline cartilage. The patella is embedded in the anterior portion of the joint capsule and is connected to the tibia by the ligamentum patellae. Many bursae surround the patella.[223]

***Mechanics.*** As the knee flexes, the patella enters the intercondylar groove with its inferior margin making first contact and then slides caudally along the groove. With extension, the patella slides superiorly. If patellar movement is restricted, it interferes with the range of knee flexion and may contribute to an extensor lag with active knee extension.[235]

##  PATELLAR FUNCTION

The primary function of the patella is to increase the moment arm of the quadriceps muscle in its function to extend the knee. It also redirects the forces exerted by the quadriceps.

### Patellar Alignment

The alignment of the patella in the frontal plane is influenced by the line of pull of the quadriceps muscle group and by its attachment to the tubial tubercle via the patellar tendon. The result of these two forces is a bowstring effect on the patella, causing it to track laterally. One method of describing the bowstring effect is to measure the Q-angle. The *Q-angle* is the angle formed by two intersecting lines: one from the anterior superior iliac spine to the mid-patella, the other from the tibial tubercle through the mid-patella (Fig. 21.3).[141,223] A normal Q-angle, which tends to be greater in women than men, is 10° to 15°.

---

**BOX 21.1**

Summary of Arthrokinematics of the Knee Joint

| Physiological Motion | Roll | Slide |
|---|---|---|
| *Tibial motion—open chain* | | |
| Flexion | Posterior and medial rotation | Posterior |
| Extension | Anterior and lateral rotation | Anterior |
| *Femoral motion—closed chain* | | |
| Flexion | Posterior and lateral rotation | Anterior |
| Extension | Anterior and medial rotation | Posterior |

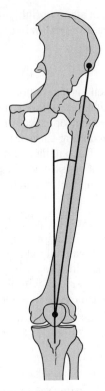

FIGURE 21.3 The *Q-angle* is the angle formed by the intersection of a line drawn from the center of the patella to the anterosuperior iliac spine and a line drawn from the center of the patella to the tibial tuberosity. These two lines represent the bowstring effect on the patella from the pull of the quadriceps femoris muscle and the patellar tendon. An increased Q-angle is a factor contributing to excessive lateral tracking of the patella. *(From McKinnis,[141] p. 332, with permission.)*

## Forces Maintaining Alignment

In addition to the bony restraints of the trochlear groove (femoral sulcus), the patella is stabilized by passive and dynamic (muscular) restraints. The superficial portion of the extensor retinaculum, to which the vastus medialis and vastus lateralis muscles have an attachment, provides dynamic stability in the transverse plane. The medial and lateral patellofemoral ligaments, which attach to the adductor tubercle medially and iliotibial band laterally provide passive restraints to the patella in the transverse plane.[223] Longitudinally, the medial and lateral patellotibial ligaments and patellar tendon fixate the patella inferiorly against the active pull of the quadriceps muscle superiorly (Fig. 21.4).

### Patellar Malalignment and Tracking Problems

Malalignment and tracking problems of the patella may be caused by several factors that may or may not be interrelated.[81,135]

***Increased Q-angle.*** With an increased Q-angle there may be increased pressure of the lateral facet against the lateral femoral condyle when the knee flexes during weight bearing. Structurally, an increased Q-angle occurs with a wide pelvis, femoral anteversion, coxa vara, genu valgum, and laterally displaced tibial tuberosity. Lower extremity motions in the transverse plane that may increase the Q-angle are external tibial rotation, internal femoral rotation, and a pronated subtalar joint. Functional knee valgus that occurs during dynamic activities also increases the Q-angle.[189]

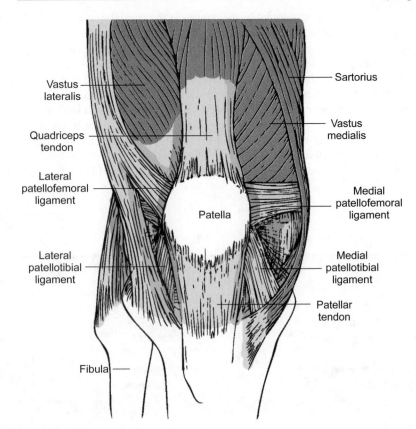

Vastus lateralis

Quadriceps tendon

Lateral patellofemoral ligament

Patella

Lateral patellotibial ligament

Fibula

Sartorius

Vastus medialis

Medial patellofemoral ligament

Medial patellotibial ligament

Patellar tendon

FIGURE 21.4 The extensor retinaculum is reinforced medially by the transversely oriented medial patellofemoral ligament and the longitudinally oriented medial patellotibial ligament. Laterally, the lateral patellofemoral ligament and lateral patellotibial ligament help resist an excessive medial glide of the patella. *(From Snyder-Mackler.[223] In: Levangie and Norkin, p. 401, with permission.)*

***Muscle and fascial tightness.*** A tight iliotibial (IT) band and lateral retinaculum prevent medial gliding of the patella. Tight ankle plantarflexors result in pronation of the foot when the ankle dorsiflexes, causing medial torsion of the tibia and functional lateral displacement of the tibial tuberosity in relationship to the patella. Tight rectus femoris and hamstring muscles may affect the mechanics of the knee, leading to compensations.[135]

***Lax medial capsular retinaculum or an insufficient VMO muscle.*** The vastus medialis obliquus (VMO) muscle may be weak from disuse or inhibited because of joint swelling or pain, leading to poor medial stability.[225] Poor timing of its contraction, which alters the ratio of firing between the VMO and vastus lateralis (VL) muscle, may lead to an imbalance of forces.[201,242] Weakness or poor timing of VMO contractions increase the lateral drifting of the patella.

***Hip muscle weakness.*** Weakness of the hip abductors and external rotators may result in adduction of the femur and valgus at the knee under loaded weight bearing.[100,189]

## Patellar Compression

***Patellar contact.*** The posterior surface of the patella has several facets. It is not completely congruent as it articulates with the trochlear groove on the femur. When the knee is in complete extension (0°), the patella is superior to the trochlear groove. By 15° of flexion the inferior border of the patella begins to articulate with the superior aspect of the groove. As the knee flexes, the patella slides distally in the groove, and more surface area comes in contact. Beyond 60° there is controversy as to whether the contact area continues to increase, level off, or decrease.[80,81] In addition, as the knee flexes past 90°, the quadriceps tendon comes in contact with the trochlear groove as the patella slides inferiorly.

***Compression forces.*** In full extension, because there is minimal to no contact of the patella with the trochlear groove, there is no compression of the articular surfaces. Furthermore, because the femur and tibia are almost parallel, the line of pull of the quadriceps muscle and patellar tendon causes a very small resultant compressive load. The resultant force of the quadriceps and patellar tendon forces rises as the knee flexes, but there is also greater surface area of the patella in contact with the groove to dissipate this force. The joint reaction force on the articular surface rises rapidly between 30° and 60°. There is controversy as to the extent of joint reaction forces in greater degrees of flexion.

- During squatting, the joint reaction force continues to rise until 90° and then levels off or decreases because the quadriceps tendon begins making contact with the trochlear groove and therefore dissipates some of the force.[80]
- In an open-chain exercise with a free weight on the distal leg, the greatest joint reaction force occurs at around 30°

of flexion.[80] This is because of the changing moment arm of the resistive force more than the line of pull of the quadriceps and patellar tendons. In an open-chain with variable resistance, the peak stress is at 60° and peak compression at 75°.[56]

- An increased Q-angle causes increased lateral facet pressure as the knee flexes.[189]

 ## MUSCLE FUNCTION

### Knee Extensor Muscle Function

The quadriceps femoris muscle group is the only muscle crossing anterior to the axis of the knee and is the prime mover for knee extension. Other muscles that can act to extend the knee require the foot to be fixated, creating a closed chain. In this situation, the hamstrings and the soleus muscles can cause or control knee extension by pulling the tibia posteriorly.

***Closed-chain function.*** During standing and the stance phase of gait, the knee is an intermediate joint in a closed chain. The quadriceps muscle controls the amount of flexion at the knee and also causes knee extension through reverse muscle pull on the femur. In the erect posture, when the knee is locked, the quadriceps need not function when the gravity line falls anterior to the axis of motion. In this case, tension in the hamstring and gastrocnemius tendons supports the posterior capsule.

***Patella.*** The patella improves the moment arm of the extensor force by increasing the distance of the quadriceps tendon from the knee joint axis. Its greatest effect on the leverage of the quadriceps is during extension of the knee from 60° to 30° and rapidly diminishes from 15° to 0° of extension.[83,223]

***Torque.*** The peak torque of the quadriceps muscle occurs between 70° and 50°.[28] The physiological advantage of the quadriceps rapidly decreases during the last 15° of knee extension because of its shortened length. This, combined with its decreased moment arm in the last 15°, requires the muscle to significantly increase its contractile force when large demands are placed on the muscle during terminal extension.[83]

- During standing, assistance for extension comes from the hamstring and soleus muscles as well as from the mechanical locking mechanism of the knee. In addition, the anterior cruciate ligament and the pull of the hamstring muscle group counter the anterior translation force of the quadriceps muscle.[63,134]
- During open-chain knee extension exercises in the sitting or supine position, when the resistive force is maximum in terminal extension because of the moment arm of the resistance a relatively strong contraction of the quadriceps muscle is required to overcome the physiological and mechanical disadvantages of the muscle to complete the final 15° of motion.[83] However, it is worth mention-

ing that the compressive loads on the patella also decrease in terminal extension because of its superior location with respect to the trochlear groove and the resultant force of the line of pull of the quadriceps and patellar tendon.

● The therapist needs to be aware of the effect of the resistance and where in the range of motion the muscle is being challenged. During open-chain exercises with fixed resistance, when the resistance torque challenges the quadriceps in terminal extension there is little challenge mid-range where the muscle is capable of generating greater tension.

## Knee Flexor Muscle Function

The hamstring muscles are the primary knee flexors and also influence rotation of the tibia on the femur. Because they are two-joint muscles, they contract more efficiently when they are simultaneously lengthened over the hip (during hip flexion) as they flex the knee. During closed-chain activities, the hamstring muscles can assist with knee extension by pulling on the tibia.

● The gastrocnemius muscle can also function as a knee flexor, but its prime function at the knee during weight bearing is to support the posterior capsule against hyperextension forces.

● The popliteus muscle supports the posterior capsule and acts to unlock the knee.

● The pes anserinus muscle group (sartorius, gracilis, semitendinosus) provides medial stability to the knee and affects rotation of the tibia in a closed chain.

## Dynamic Stability of the Knee

Because of the incongruity of the femoral condyles and tibial plateaus, there is little stability from the bony architecture. The cruciate and collateral ligaments provide significant passive stability in the various ranges of joint motion. Dynamic stability involves motor control of the neuromuscular system to coordinate muscle activity around the joint. The complex feedforward and feedback responses mediated by the central nervous system modulate muscle stiffness and are important for providing dynamic knee stability under varying loads and stresses imposed on the joint structures.[254] As summarized in a clinical commentary by Williams,[254] clinical and scientific evidence is accumulating to substantiate exercise programs that have the purpose of training dynamic knee stability; that is, to improve control of the knee via neuromuscular responses in order to reduce knee ligament stress and injury during high-intensity activities.

## ● THE KNEE AND GAIT

During the normal gait cycle, the knee goes through a range of 60° (0° extension at initial contact or heel strike to 60° at the end of initial swing). There is some medial rotation of the femur as the knee extends at initial contact and just prior to heel-off.[185,223]

## Muscle Control of the Knee During Gait

Stability during the gait cycle is efficiently controlled by the normal function of the muscles that attach at the knee.[172,185]

*Quadriceps.* The quadriceps muscle controls the amount of knee flexion during initial contact (loading response) and then extends the knee toward mid-stance. It again controls the amount of flexion during pre-swing (heel-off to toe-off) and prevents excessive heel rise during initial swing. With loss of quadriceps function, the patient lurches the trunk anteriorly during initial contact to move the center of gravity anterior to the knee so it is stable or rotates the extremity outward to lock the knee.[228] With fast walking, there may be excessive heel rise during initial swing.

*Hamstrings.* The hamstring muscles primarily control the forward swing of the leg during terminal swing. Loss of function may result in the knee snapping into extension during this period. The hamstrings also provide posterior support to the knee capsule when the knee is extended during stance. Loss of function results in progressive genu recurvatum.[228]

*Soleus.* The unijoint ankle plantarflexor muscles (primarily the soleus) help control the amount of knee flexion during pre-swing by controlling the forward movement of the tibia. Loss of function results in hyperextension of the knee during pre-swing (also loss of heel rise at the ankle and thus a lag or slight dropping of the pelvis on that side during the pre-swing phase).

*Gastrocnemius.* The gastrocnemius muscle provides tension posterior to the knee when it is in extension (end of loading response or foot flat and just prior to pre-swing or heel-off). Loss of function results in hyperextension of the knee during these periods as well as loss of plantarflexion during pre-swing or push-off.

## Hip and Ankle Impairments

Because the knee is the intermediate joint between the hip and foot, problems in these two areas can interfere with knee function during gait. Examples:

*Hip flexion contractures.* Inability to extend the hip prevents the knee from extending just before terminal stance (heel-off).

*Length/strength imbalances.* Most of the muscles functioning to control the hip are two-joint muscles that also cross the knee. With asymmetry of length and strength, unbalanced forces may stress various structures in the knee, giving rise to pain during walking or running. For example, a tight tensor fasciae latae or gluteus maximus muscle increases stress on the IT band, which could lead to lateral knee pain; or it could affect tracking of the patella and lead to anterior knee pain. Overuse of the hamstring muscle group increases posterior translation forces on the tibia, requiring compensation in the quadriceps femoris muscle and resulting in anterior knee pain (see Chapter 20).

*Foot impairments.* The position and function of the foot and ankle affect the stresses transmitted to the knee. For example, with pes planus or pes valgus, there is medial rotation of the tibia and an increased bowstring effect on the patella, increasing the lateral tracking forces.

# REFERRED PAIN AND NERVE INJURIES

For a detailed description of referred pain patterns and peripheral nerve injuries in the knee region see Chapter 13.

## Major Nerves Subject to Injury at the Knee

The sciatic nerve divides into the tibial and common peroneal nerves just proximal to the popliteal fossa. These nerves are relatively well protected deep in the fossa.

- The *common peroneal nerve* (L2-4) becomes superficial where it winds around the fibula just below the fibular head, a common site for injury. Symptoms of sensory loss and muscle weakness are distal to that site.
- The *saphenous nerve* (L2-4) is a sensory nerve that innervates the skin along the medial side of the knee and leg. It may be injured with trauma or surgery in that region.

## Common Sources of Referred Pain

Nerve roots and tissues derived from spinal segments L3 refer to the anterior aspect, and those from S1 and S2 refer to the posterior aspect of the knee.[38] The hip joint, which is primarily innervated by L3, may refer symptoms to the anterior thigh and knee. Therapeutic exercise for the knee is beneficial only for preventing disuse of the part. Primary treatment must be directed to the source of the irritation.

## MANAGEMENT OF KNEE DISORDERS AND SURGERIES

To make sound clinical decisions when treating patients with knee disorders, it is necessary to understand the various pathologies, surgical procedures, and associated precautions and to identify presenting impairments, functional limitations, and possible disabilities. In this section common pathologies and surgical procedures are presented and related to corresponding preferred practice patterns (group-

ings of impairments) described in the *Guide to Physical Therapist Practice*[2] (Table 21.1). Conservative and postoperative management of these conditions is described in this section.

# JOINT HYPOMOBILITY: NONOPERATIVE MANAGEMENT

## Common Joint Pathologies and Associated Impairments

Osteoarthritis (OA) and rheumatoid arthritis (RA) as well as acute joint trauma can affect knee articulations at the tibiofemoral joint. Decreased flexibility and adhesions develop in the joints and surrounding tissues any time the joint is immobilized for a period of time. Reflex inhibition and resulting weakness of the quadriceps femoris muscle occurs because of joint distention.[225] The etiology of these arthritic and joint symptoms and general management guidelines are described in Chapter 11.

### Osteoarthritis (Degenerative Joint Disease)

Osteoarthritis, often referred to as degenerative joint disease (DJD), is the most common disease affecting weight-bearing joints (Fig. 21.5). One-third of individuals over the age of 65 have radiographic evidence of OA.[12] Pain, muscle weakness, and joint limitations affect function and lead to disability. Deformity such as genu varum commonly develops. Factors such as excess weight, joint trauma, developmental deformities, weakness in the quadriceps muscle and abnormal tibial rotation are identified as risk factors for developing OA.[12]

*Post-traumatic arthritis* in the knee occurs in response to any injury that affects the joint structures but particularly

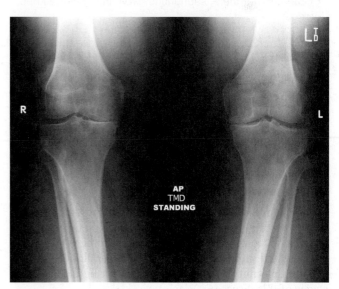

FIGURE 21.5 Advanced bilateral, medial compartment degenerative joint disease in the knees of a 52-year-old computer programmer/analyst who subsequently underwent right total knee arthroplasty.

**TABLE 21.1    Knee Pathologies/Surgical Procedures and Preferred Practice Patterns**

| PATHOLOGY/SURGICAL PROCEDURE | PREFERRED PRACTICE PATTERN AND ASSOCIATED IMPAIRMENTS[2] |
|---|---|
| • Abnormal knee posture (related to hip and foot alignment) | • Pattern 4B—Impaired posture |
| • Arthritis (osteoarthritis, rheumatoid arthritis, traumatic arthritis)<br>• Synovitis<br>• Postimmobilization arthritis (stiff knee)<br>• Joint instability, ligament tears<br>• Meniscus lesions<br>• Patellofemoral syndromes (patellar instability, malalignment, plica syndrome, fat pad syndrome, patellar tendonitis, bursitis, chondromalacia)<br>• Apophysitis (Osgood-Schlatter's disease) | • Pattern 4D—Impaired joint mobility, motor function, muscle performance, and ROM associated with connective tissue dysfunction |
| • Acute arthritis<br>• Acute tendinitis, bursitis<br>• Acute capsulitis<br>• Acute patellofemoral pain | • Pattern 4E—Impaired joint mobility, motor function, muscle performance, and ROM associated with localized inflammation |
| • Arthroscopic débridement<br>• Articular cartilage repair: microfracture, osteochondral autograft transfer, autologous chrondrocyte implantation<br>• Arthroscopic synovectomy<br>• Total knee arthroplasty | • Pattern 4H—Impaired joint mobility, motor function, muscle performance, and ROM associated with joint arthroplasty |
| • Lateral retinacular release<br>• Extensor mechanism realignment<br>• Arthroscopic or open ligament repair/reconstruction<br>• Meniscectomy or meniscal repair<br>• Repair of ruptured patellar tendon<br>• Osteotomy<br>• Patellectomy | • Pattern 4I—Impaired joint mobility, motor function, muscle performance, and ROM associated with bony or soft tissue surgery |
| • Common peroneal, saphenous nerve injury in the knee region | • Pattern 5F—Impaired peripheral nerve integrity and muscle performance associated with peripheral nerve injury |

following acute ligament and meniscal tears. Joint swelling (effusion) may be immediate, indicating bleeding within the joint, or progressive (more than 4 hours to develop), indicating serous effusion. Acute symptoms include pain, limited motion, and muscle guarding. Trauma, including repetitive microtrauma, is a common cause of degenerative changes in the knee joint.

### Rheumatoid Arthritis

Early-stage RA usually manifests in the hands and feet first. With progression of the disease process, the knees also may become involved. The joints become warm and swollen, and limited motion develops. In addition, a genu valgum deformity commonly develops during the advanced stages of this disease.

### Postimmobilization Hypomobility

When the knee has been immobilized for several weeks or longer, such as after healing of a fracture or after surgery,

the capsule, muscles, and soft tissue develop contractures, and motion becomes restricted. Adhesions may restrict caudal gliding of the patella, which limits knee flexion, and may cause pain as the patella is compressed against the femur. An extensor lag may occur with active knee extension if the patella does not glide proximally when the quadriceps muscle contracts.[183] This usually occurs after operative repairs of some knee ligaments, when the knee is immobilized in flexion for a prolonged period.

### Common Impairments

◉ With joint involvement, the pattern of restriction at the knee is usually more loss of flexion than extension.
◉ When there is effusion (swelling within the joint), the joint assumes a position near 25° of flexion, at which there is the greatest capsular distensibility. Little motion is possible because of the swelling.

● Symptoms of joint involvement, such as distention, stiffness, pain, and reflex quadriceps inhibition, may cause extensor (quadriceps) lag in which the active range of knee extension is less than the passive range available.[226]

● Disturbed balance responses also have been reported in patients with arthritis.[245]

## Common Functional Limitations/Disabilities

● With acute symptoms and in advanced stages of degeneration, there is pain during motion, weight bearing, and gait that may interfere with work or routine household and community activities.

● There is limitation of, or difficulty controlling, weight-bearing activities that involve knee flexion, such as sitting down and rising from a chair or a commode, descending or ascending stairs, stooping, or squatting.[62]

● With end-stage OA, physical activity is markedly curtailed with less participation in leisure activities (e.g., walking, gardening, swimming, athletic activities) and household activities (e.g., dusting, washing floors, cleaning, shopping).[237]

## Joint Hypomobility: Management— Protection Phase

See Chapter 11 for general guidelines for the management of acute joint lesions and specific guidelines for RA and DJD.

### Control Pain and Protect the Joint

***Patient education.*** It is important to teach the patient methods to protect the joint including bed positioning or use of splints in order to avoid deforming contractures, range of motion (ROM) and muscle setting exercises to maintain mobility, and safe functional activities that reduce stresses on the knee.

***Functional adaptations.*** To reduce the amount of knee flexion and patellar compression instruct the patient to minimize stair climbing, use elevated seats on commodes, and avoid deep-seated or low chairs. If necessary during an acute flare of arthritis have the patient use crutches, canes, or a walker to distribute forces through the upper extremities while walking.

### Maintain Soft Tissue and Joint Mobility

***Passive, active-assistive or active ROM.*** Use ROM techniques within the limits of pain and available motion. The patient may be able to perform active ROM in the gravity-eliminated, side-lying position, or self-assisted ROM.

***Grade I or II tractions or glides.*** Apply gentle techniques, if tolerated, with the joint in resting position (25° flexion). These techniques are used to inhibit pain as well as maintain joint mobility. Stretching is contraindicated at this stage.

### Maintain Muscle Function and Prevent Patellar Adhesions

***Setting exercises.*** Have the patient perform pain-free quadriceps ("quad sets") and hamstring muscle-setting exercises with the knee in various pain-free positions, quad sets with leg raising, and submaximal closed-chain muscle setting exercises. Muscle setting exercises are described in detail in the last section of this chapter. Quad sets may help maintain mobility of the patella when the tibiofemoral joint is immobilized and therefore are routinely taught following surgery or when the joint is immobilized in a cast.

## Joint Hypomobility: Management—Controlled Motion and Return to Function Phases

As the inflammation decreases and the joint tissues are able to tolerate increased stresses, the goals of treatment change to deal with the impairments that interfere with functional activities. The patient is progressed through controlled motion exercises and activities that focus on safely returning to the desired functional outcome.

### Educate the Patient

● Inform the patient about his or her condition, what to expect regarding recovery, and how to protect the joints.

● Teach the patient safe exercises to do at home, how to progress them, and how to modify them if symptoms are exacerbated by the disease or from overuse. Exercises that include specifically designed strengthening, stretching, ROM, and use of a stationary bicycle have been shown to improve funtional outcomes in patients with OA in a home exercise program.[43] It is important to emphasize that maintaining strength in the supporting muscles helps protect and stabilize the joint and that balance exercises help reduce the incidence of falls.

● Instruct the patient to perform active ROM and muscle-setting techniques frequently during the day, especially prior to bearing weight in order to reduce the painful symptoms that occur with initial weight bearing.[62]

● The patient with OA or RA should be cautioned to alternate activity with rest.

 **Focus on Evidence** _____

There have been no studies comparing outcomes from home exercise programs versus physical therapy-directed interventions in a clinic setting until recently. In a randomized controlled study of 134 patients with OA of the knees, a clinic treatment group ($n = 66$) underwent supervised exercise, manual therapy, and home exercises for 4 weeks; and a home exercise group ($n = 68$) underwent home exercises only (instructions and a follow-up examination were provided for the same exercises as the clinic group). Outcomes that were measured consisted of the distance walked in 6 minutes and the Western Ontario and McMaster Universities Osteoarthritis Index (WOMAC). Both groups improved in the outcome measures at 4 weeks; the clinic treatment group improved 52% on the WOMAC, whereas the home exercise group improved 26%. Both groups improved 10% on the 6-minute walk distances. At 1 year there was no difference between the groups, and both groups demonstrated improvement over baseline measurements, although it was noted that the clinic treatment group was less likely to be taking medication for the arthritis and were more satisfied with the outcome of their rehabilitation.[43]

### Decrease Pain from Mechanical Stress

Continue use of assistive devices for ambulation, if necessary. The patient may progress to using less assistance or may ambulate for periods without assistance. Continue use of elevated seats on commodes and chairs, if needed, to reduce the mechanical stresses imposed when attempting to stand up.[62]

### Increase Joint Play and Range of Motion

PRECAUTION: Do not increase ROM unless the patient has sufficient strength to control the motion already available. A mobile weight-bearing joint with inadequate muscle control causes impaired stability and makes lower extremity weight-bearing function difficult.

*Joint mobilization.* When there is loss of joint play and decreased mobility, joint mobilization techniques should be used. Apply grade III sustained or grade IV oscillation techniques to the tibiofemoral and patellofemoral articulations with the joint positioned at the end of its available range before applying the mobilization technique. See Figures 5.49 through 5.54 and their descriptions in Chapter 5. As ROM increases, it is important to emphasize the rotational accessory motions that accompany flexion and extension.[105]

● To increase *flexion*, position the tibia in medial rotation and apply the posterior glide against the anterior aspect of the medial tibial plateau.
● To increase *extension*, position the tibia in lateral rotation and apply the anterior glide against the posterior aspect of the lateral tibial plateau.
● Medial and lateral gliding of the tibia on the femur may also be done to regain mobility for flexion and extension.

*Stretching techniques.* Passive and muscle inhibition stretching techniques are used to increase flexibility in the muscles and extracapsular noncontractile soft tissues that restrict knee motion. Specific techniques are described in the last section of this chapter.

PRECAUTIONS: Techniques that force the knee into flexion by using the tibia as a lever or by using strong quadriceps contractions (during hold-relax maneuver) may exacerbate joint symptoms.

Incorporate the following to minimize joint trauma from stretching.

● Mobilize the patellofemoral and tibiofemoral joints before stretching in order to improve gliding of the joint surfaces during the stretch maneuvers.

● Apply soft tissue or friction massage to loosen adhesions or contractures prior to stretching. Include deep massage around the border of the patella.
● Modify the intensity of contraction when applying muscle inhibition techniques to restricting muscles in order to decrease the effects of joint compression. If hold–relax aggravates anterior knee pain when attempting to increase knee flexion, use agonist contraction to the hamstring muscles to minimize compression from a strong quadriceps muscle contraction.
● Use low intensity, long-duration stretches within the patient's tolerance.

*Mobilization with Movement.* Mobilization with movement (MWM) may be applied to increase ROM and/or decrease the pain associated with movement by improving joint tracking. Mulligan[154] stated that MWM is more effective with loss of flexion than extension. The principles of MWM are described in Chapter 5.

### Lateral or Medial Glides

*Patient position and procedure*: Supine for extension or prone for flexion. Apply a pain-free medial or lateral glide to the tibial plateau by hand or through the use of a mobilization belt. The direction of glide is often in the direction of the pain (i.e., lateral knee pain responds best to a lateral glide of the tibia and medial knee pain to a medial glide).[154]

● While sustaining the mobilization, ask the patient to move to the end of the available pain-free range of flexion or extension.
● Add pain-free overpressure to achieve the benefit of end-range loading.

### Internal Tibial Rotation for Flexion—Manual Technique

*Patient position and procedure*: Supine with the knee flexed to the end of its available pain-free range. Apply internal rotation mobilization to the tibia with manual pressure from one hand on the anteromedial tibial plateau simultaneously with pressure from the other hand on the posterolateral tibial plateau, posterior to the fibular head.

● Sustain the internal rotation mobilization and ask the patient to flex the knee through the use of a mobilization belt looped around the foot. Hold the position at the end of the available pain-free range for several seconds (Fig. 21.6).

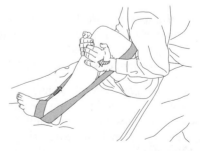

FIGURE 21.6 MWM with internal tibial rotation to increase knee flexion.

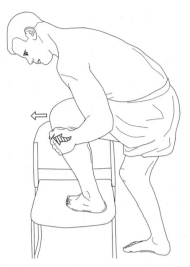

FIGURE 21.7 Self-treatment using MWM with internal tibial rotation to increase knee flexion.

### Internal Rotation for Flexion—Self-Treatment

*Patient position and procedure*: Standing with the foot of the involved leg on a chair and knee flexed. Position the foot such that the tibia is internally rotated. Have the patient apply internal rotation pressure against the anteromedial and posterolateral tibial plateaus and shift the weight forward to flex the knee to the end of the available pain-free range (Fig. 21.7).

### Improve Muscle Performance in Supporting Muscles

Exercises identified in this section are described in detail in the last section of this chapter.

***Progressive strengthening.*** Begin with multiple-angle isometrics to both knee flexion and extension, short-arc terminal extension exercises in open- and closed-chain positions, and a moderate progression of repetitions and resistance in wider arcs of motion so long as the motion is pain-free. Exercises intensity should be within the tolerance of the joint and not exacerbate symptoms.

● When doing open-chain exercises, patients experience less pain with faster speeds and lighter resistance than when doing the exercises slowly with heavy resistance.

● Resistance through the mid-range (45° to 90°) tends to exacerbate patellofemoral pain because of the compressive forces on the patella. Apply resistance in arcs of motion that are pain-free on either side of the symptomatic range. This could be done using manual or mechanical resistance in the pain-free ranges.

● Strengthen both hip and ankle musculature using open- and closed-chain activities in order to balance forces throughout the lower extremities and progress the patient toward functional independence. (See Chapters 20 and 22 for hip and ankle exercises.)

***Muscular endurance.*** For muscular endurance, increase repetitions at each resistance level before progressing with greater resistance.

***Functional training.*** Climbing steps, sitting down and rising up from chairs and commodes, and using safe body mechanics to lift objects from the floor are often compromised in individuals with knee arthritis. It is imperative to strengthen the knee musculature using modifications of functional activities, progressing the difficulty as strength improves.

● ***Step-up and step-down exercises (forward, backward, lateral).*** Begin with blocks or steps 4 to 6 inches in height and progress to the step height the patient requires for home and community mobility. Progress to functional activities such as climbing stairs or ladders, depending on the desired outcome.

● ***Wall slides and mini-squats to 90° if tolerated.*** Stay within a range that does not exacerbate symptoms or cause crepitation. Practice sitting and sit-to-stand with arm assistance in various chair heights. Determine if chair adaptation is needed for safe function.

● ***Partial lunges.*** This activity is progressed to include lunging to pick up small objects from the floor. Lunges are an effective way to teach body mechanics for an individual with unilateral knee impairment. Concentrate on trunk control during the motion. Have the patient contract the abdominals to stabilize the pelvis during the lunge activity.

● ***Balance activities.*** Balance activities are initiated at the level the patient can control. Detailed suggestions are outlined in Chapters 8 and 20.

● ***Ambulation.*** Decrease use of assistive devices as quadriceps strength improves to a manual muscle test level of 4/5. Practice on a variety of terrains, up and down ramps, and reversing directions, first with assistance and then independently.

### Improve Cardiopulmonary Endurance

Develop and improve cardiopulmonary fitness for the individual with joint symptoms by adapting activities to minimize irritating stresses.

● ***Swimming, water aerobics, and aquatic exercises*** provide an environment for improving muscular and cardiopulmonary function with less joint trauma.

● ***Bicycling*** is a low-impact form of exercise. Adjust the seat height so the knee goes into complete extension (but not hyperextension) when the pedal is down. On a stationary bike, use low resistance.

● ***High impact—with caution.*** For some patients, progression to running or jumping rope and other high-impact, faster paced, or more intense activities can be undertaken so long as the joint remains asymptomatic. If joint deformity is present and proper biomechanics cannot be restored, the patient probably cannot progress to these activities.

 **Focus on Evidence** _____

Two systematic reviews of studies designed to examine evidence of the effects of exercise in the management of hip and knee OA describe support for aerobic exercise and strengthening exercises to reduce pain and disability.[196,197]

The consensus of expert opinion cited by Roddy[196] is that (1) there are few contraindications and (2) exercise is relatively safe in patients with OA but it should be individualized and patient-centered with consideration for age, co-morbidity, and general mobility. Similarly the Cochrane Database of Systematic Reviews[66] and the Philadelphia Panel Evidence-Based Clinical Practice Guidelines[186] indicated that there is evidence to support strengthening, stretching, and functional exercises as interventions for the management of knee pain as the result of OA and to improve physical function.

In another study that followed 285 patients with knee OA for 3 years, investigators found that factors that protected the individuals from poor functional outcomes included strength and activity level as well as factors such as mental health, self-efficacy, and social support.[210]

An outcome review[44] summarized that moderate- or high-intensity exercises for patients with RA have minimal effect on the disease activity but that there is insufficient radiological evidence on the effect in large joints. Long-term moderate- or high-intensity exercises that are individualized to protect radiologically damaged joints improve aerobic capacity, muscle strength, functional ability, and psychological well-being of patients with RA.[44]

# ⬤ JOINT SURGERY AND POSTOPERATIVE MANAGEMENT

A range of surgical options for management of arthritis of the knee is available when joint pain and synovitis cannot be controlled with conservative therapy and appropriate medical management or when destruction of articular surfaces, deformity, or restriction of motion have progressed to the point that functional abilities are significantly impaired.

The surgical procedure selected depends on the patient's signs and symptoms, activity level and age, type of disease, severity of articular damage or joint deformity, and involvement of other joints. *Arthroscopic débridement* and *lavage* are used to remove loose bodies that may be causing swelling and intermittent locking of the knee.[14,205] A number of procedures to repair damaged articular cartilage have been developed. *Abrasion arthroplasty*, a procedure designed to smooth worn articular surfaces and stimulate growth of replacement cartilage has met with only limited success.[14,205] More recently developed procedures used to repair small, localized articular cartilage defects of the knee, such as *microfracture*,[76,207] *osteochondral autograft transplantation/mosaicplasty*,[8,20,86,110] and *autologous chondrocyte implantation*[36,77,248] appear to hold promise.

*Synovectomy* may be the procedure of choice for a young patient with unremitting joint effusion, synovial proliferation, and pain as the result of RA or juvenile RA (JRA) but with minimal destruction of articular surfaces.[29,87,182,205] *Osteotomy* of the distal femur or proximal tibia (an extra-articular procedure) redistributes weight-bearing forces between the tibia and femur in an attempt to reduce joint pain during weight-bearing activities and delays the need for arthroplasty of the knee for up to 10 years.[14,29,193,205] In the past, high tibial osteotomy was considered a surgical option for the active patient under 50 to 55 years of age without active systemic disease and significant limitation of motion or joint deformity.[193] However, because arthroplasty now is being performed in younger patients than was the case a decade or two ago, osteotomy is an infrequently selected surgical option.[33]

When erosion of articular surfaces becomes severe and pain is unremitting, *total knee replacement arthroplasty* is the surgical procedure of choice to reduce pain, correct deformity, and improve functional movement.[98,131,203] Only in highly selective situations is *arthrodesis* (fusion) of the knee used as a salvage procedure to provide a patient with a stable and pain-free knee.

Regardless of the type of surgery selected, the goals of surgery and postoperative management are to (1) reduce pain, (2) correct deformity or instability, and (3) restore lower extremity function. Carefully progressed postoperative rehabilitation is essential for optimal functional outcomes.

## Repair of Articular Cartilage Defects

Injuries of the ligaments or menisci of the knee and acute or chronic patellofemoral dysfunction often are associated with damage to an articular surface of the knee. Surgical management of chondral defects has proven challenging because of the limited capacity of articular cartilage to heal.[36] However, several surgical procedures introduced during the 1990s are available for repairing small lesions in the symptomatic knee when nonoperative management or arthroscopic débridement and lavage have been unsuccessful.

Procedures include microfracture,[76,118,207,227] osteochondral autograft transplantation/mosaicplasty,[8,13,20,86,110] and autologous chondrocyte implantation.[77,114,118,248] These procedures are designed to stimulate growth of hyaline cartilage for repair of focal defects of articular cartilage and for preventing progressive deterioration of joint cartilage leading to osteoarthritis.[36,118]

Descriptions of procedures specific to the knee are presented in this section. Regardless of the cartilage procedure selected, each requires the patient's ability and willingness to adhere to a lengthy rehabilitation process.

### Indications for Surgery

The primary indication for repair of an articular cartilage defect is a symptomatic knee caused by a small to relatively large focal lesion of the tibiofemoral or patellofemoral joint. Sites typically involved are the weight-bearing portions of the medial or lateral femoral condyles, the trochlear groove, and the articulating facets of the patella.

Selection criteria when choosing the procedure include the size of the chondral lesion (in general, defects greater than 1 to 2 cm² but no more than 4 cm² are considered suitable for repair), the depth of the lesion, the location of the lesion, the elapsed time since the occurrence of the defect, and the patient's age and intended activity level. Most patients, who undergo articular cartilage repair are young and active.[36,118]

### Procedures

*Microfracture.* Microfracture is indicated for repair of very small defects usually of the medial or lateral femoral condyle or the posterior aspect of the patella. The procedure is performed arthroscopically and involves the use of a nonmotorized awl to systematically penetrate the subchondral bone and expose the bone marrow. The procedure is designed to stimulate a marrow-based repair response leading to local ingrowth of cartilagenous repair tissue (fibrocartilage) to repair the lesion.[36,76,118,207,227]

*Osteochondral autograft transplantation/mosaicplasty.* For focal lesions involving chondral or subchondral tissue of the weight-bearing surfaces of the knee, osteochondral graft transplantation may be selected. It is an arthroscopic or mini open procedure involving transplantation of *intact* articular cartilage along with some underlying bone, resulting in a bone-to-bone graft.[8,13,20,86,110] Rather than using a single piece of tissue and creating a similar size osteochondral defect at the donor site, mosaicplasty is used in which multiple, small-diameter osteochondral plugs are harvested and press-fit into the chondral defect.[8,13,86,110]

Donor sites typically are non-weight-bearing, non-articulating portions of the supracondylar ridge of the lateral femoral articulating surfaces or elsewhere in the knee.[8]

*Autologous chondrocyte implantation.* This procedure, also referred to as chondrocyte transplantation, is used for for full-thickness chondral and osteochondral defects (2 to 4 cm²) of the femoral condyles or patella.[36,77,114,248] The procedure occurs in two stages. First, healthy articular cartilage is harvested arthroscopically from the patient. Then chondrocytes are extracted from the articular cartilage, cultured for several weeks, and processed in a laboratory to increase the volume of healthy tissue. The second phase is the implantation phase, which currently requires an arthrotomy (open procedure). After the chondral defect sites have been débrided, they are covered with a periosteal patch, typically harvested from the proximal medial tibia. Then millions of autologous chondrocytes are injected under the patch and into the articular defect.

Patient positioning during the first 4 hours after surgery is critical. Patients are positioned so the effect of gravity distributes the chondrocytes evenly along the base of the defect.[192] For example, after a patellofemoral repair, the patient is placed in the prone position.

Maturation of the implanted chondrocytes is a lengthy process. It may take up to 6 months for the graft site to become firm and as long as 9 months for the graft to become as durable as the healthy tissue surrounding the graft.[77]

*Osteochondral allograft transplantation.* For defects larger than 4 cm², the only option for repair, although used infrequently, is an osteochondral allograft of intact articular cartilage from a cadaveric donor. However, only fresh, intact grafts, which are in limited supply and can be stored for only a few days, can be used. A frozen allograft cannot be used because freezing the graft material kills the articular chondrocytes, leading to graft failure.[36,118]

*Other procedures.* If coexisting ligament or meniscus pathology or tibiofemoral or patellofemoral malalignment are identified prior to or concomitant with surgical repair, reconstruction or realignment must be carried out for the articular cartilage repair to be successful. The most common procedures are ACL reconstruction and meniscus repair for tibiofemoral articular defects and lateral retinacular release for patellar defects.[8,77]

### Postoperative Management

A cautiously progressed and closely monitored rehabilitation program after articular cartilage repair procedures is critical for a successful outcome. The components and progression of a rehabilitation program, including exercise, ambulation, and functional activities, must be graded to protect the repair or graft and prevent further articular damage while applying controlled stresses to stimulate the healing process.

The progression of postoperative exercises and functional activities after microfracture, osteochondral autologous transplantation, and autologous chondrocyte implantation has many common elements, yet they vary to some degree. Detailed postoperative protocols for each of these procedures have been published in the literature.[8,77,110,192] In addition to the type of repair employed, the rehabilitation progression is based on the size, depth, and location of the articular defect, the need for concomitant surgical procedures, and patient-related factors such as age, body mass index, health history, and preoperative activity level.

The goals during rehabilitation after articular cartilage repair are similar to those found for most knee rehabilitation programs presented in this chapter. Protected weight bearing over an extended period of time and early motion are essential after articular cartilage repair to promote maturation and maintain the health of the repaired or implanted cartilage. Special considerations for exercise and weight bearing associated with the various articular cartilage procedures are summarized in Box 21.2.[8,77,110,192,248]

## Synovectomy

Hypertrophic synovitis develops most frequently in patients with RA or JRA.[29,87,182,205] Resection of proliferated synovium in patients without significant cartilage erosion alleviates pain and stiffness of the knee for a period of time. Although it is unclear if synovectomy alters the course of the underlying disease, it delays the need for arthroplasty in the young patient.

| BOX 21.2 | Special Considerations and Precautions for Rehabilitation after Articular Cartilage Repair* |
|---|---|

- The larger the lesion, the slower/more cautious the progression of rehabilitation.
- Early, but controlled, ROM is advocated to facilitate the healing process and begins immediately or within a day or two after surgery (CPM, passive or assisted exercise).
- Controlled (protected) weight bearing initiated as early as possible is beneficial to the healing process, but adherence to weight-bearing restrictions is critical.
- Duration and degree of weight-bearing restrictions vary with the size of the defect and type and location of the repair.*
  - Longer period of protected weight bearing for osteochondral transplantation/mosaicplasty and autologous chondrocyte implantation than after microfracture.
  - Longer period of protected weight bearing for a femoral condyle repair (up to 8 to 12 weeks) than for a patellar defect (up to 4 weeks).
  - Full weight bearing is delayed for as long as 8 to 12 weeks.
- Protective bracing may be used postoperatively.
  - Typically locked in extension, except during exercise.
  - Worn during weight bearing activities 4 to 6 weeks.
  - Worn during sleep for up to 4 weeks.
  - An unloading brace may be used after repair of a femoral condyle defect to shift the weight away from the repair during the period of protected weight bearing.

*Considerations and precautions vary with the size, depth, and location of the articular defect, type of surgical repair and concomitant procedures, and patient-related factors (age, body mass index, health history, preoperative activity level).

## Indications for Surgery

The following are frequently cited indications for synovectomy of the knee.[29,87,182,205]

- Chronic, proliferative synovitis, joint pain, restricted joint mobility lasting 6 months or longer secondary to unremitting but early-stage RA or JRA that cannot be controlled by medical management
- Synovial hypertrophy and joint pain secondary to recurrent hemarthrosis as the result of hemophilia
- Intact or minimally eroded articular surfaces

## Procedures

*Arthroscopic synovectomy* involves the use of multiple portals for access to and endoscopic removal of as much synovium as possible from all compartments of the knee.[87,182,205] A partial meniscectomy often is performed during synovectomy because chronically inflamed synovium can invade a portion of a meniscus leading to a tear.[193]

An arthroscopic approach to synovectomy is routinely preferred over an open approach. *Open synovectomy* necessitates arthrotomy of the knee through a longitudinal medial and/or lateral parapatellar incision(s) of the capsule and,

therefore, causes greater postoperative morbidity and a lengthier recovery. It is also more difficult to preserve the menisci with an open approach than an arthroscopic approach.[87] However, an open approach may be selected by the surgeon if synovectomy is performed in conjunction with other open procedures.

## Postoperative Management

Postoperative management after arthroscopic synovectomy, summarized in Table 21.2, is progressed based on the patient's signs and symptoms rather than strict adherence to timelines.[167] Exercises and weight-bearing activities are progressed relatively rapidly after arthroscopic synovectomy. A patient often achieves nearly full ROM of the operated knee and is able to ambulate without assistive devices as early as 10 to 14 days postoperatively depending on involvement of unoperated joints. Nevertheless, return to a full level of functional activity should occur gradually with some degree of protection continuing until joint swelling, limitation of active and passive knee ROM, and muscle weakness are resolved.

### Immobilization and Weight Bearing

The knee is immobilized for 24 to 48 hours in a compression dressing and a posterior splint that holds the knee in extension. During that time the leg is elevated to control postoperative edema. Ambulation with crutches begins the day of surgery, with weight bearing as tolerated. The patient should wear the posterior splint during ambulation until full, active knee extension has been achieved.

### Exercise

The choices and progression of exercises are based not only on the status of the operated knee but also on the extent of involvement of other joints of the upper or lower extremities affected by chronic arthritis. The goals and exercise interventions commonly included in successive phases of postoperative rehabilitation are described in the following sections.

### Exercise: Maximum Protection Phase

Immediately after surgery and for the next 2 to 3 weeks, early movement must be balanced with protection of the operated knee. Attention to wound care is particularly important because of the systemic nature of inflammatory arthritis. Regaining full, active knee extension is essential for ambulation without crutches or a cane. The goals and interventions implemented during the first phase of rehabilitation include the following.[87,205]

- ***Control pain and peripheral edema and decrease the risk of deep vein thrombosis.***
  - Elevation of the lower extremity and application of cold to the operated knee.
  - Active ankle pumping exercises.
- ***Regain or maintain neuromuscular control of hip and knee musculature on the operated side.***
  - Quadriceps and hamstring setting exercises performed frequently during the day
  - Straight-leg raising exercises (SLRs) in the supine, prone, and side-lying positions.

| TABLE 21.2 | Arthroscopic Synovectomy—Interventions for Each Phase of Rehabilitation | | |
|---|---|---|---|
| **Phase and General Time Frame** | **Maximum Protection Phase: Weeks 1–2** | **Moderate to Minimum Protection Phases: Weeks 3–6** | **Return to Activity Phase: Week 6** |
| Patient presentation | • Patient enters rehabilitation within 2 days<br>• Postoperative compression dressing<br>• Minimal postoperative pain<br>• ROM minimally limited<br>• Weight bearing as tolerated | • Minimum gain<br>• Full weight bearing<br>• Nearly full ROM<br>• Joint effusion controlled | • Muscle function: 70% of noninvolved side<br>• No symptoms of pain or swelling during the previous phase |
| Key examination procedures | • Pain assessment: 1–10 scale<br>• Monitor for hemarthrosis<br>• ROM<br>• Patellar mobility<br>• Muscle control<br>• Soft tissue palpitation | • Pain assessment<br>• Joint effusion—girth<br>• ROM<br>• Patellar mobility<br>• Muscle strength<br>• Gait analysis | • Pain assessment<br>• Muscle strength<br>• Patellar alignment/stability<br>• Functional strength |
| Goals | • Control postoperative swelling<br>• Minimize pain<br>• ROM: 0°–115°<br>• 3/5 to 4/5 muscle strength<br>• Ambulate without assistance unless weight bearing is delayed<br>• Establish home exercise program | • Control swelling<br>• Full ROM<br>• Full weight bearing<br>• 4/5 to 5/5 strength<br>• Improve cardiopulmonary fitness<br>• Improve balance<br>• Unrestricted ADL<br>• Adherence to home program | • Transition to maintenance program for self-management and prevention<br>• Reinforce lifelong joint protection |
| Interventions | • Compressive wrap to control effusion<br>• Pain modulation modalities (cryotherapy)<br>• Ankle pumps to prevent peripheral edema<br>• A-AROM and AROM<br>• Patellar mobilization<br>• Muscle setting: quadriceps, hamstrings and adductors (may augment with E-stim)<br>• SLRs—four positions (assisted to unassisted)<br>• Flexibility program: hamstrings, plantarflexors, IT band<br>• Trunk/pelvis strengthening | • LE flexibility program<br>• Closed-chain strengthening<br>• Limited-range PRE<br>• Tibiofemoral joint and patellar mobilization, if needed<br>• Proprioceptive training<br>• Stabilization exercises<br>• Gait training<br>• Protected aerobic exercise: swimming or walking program | • Continue previous phase activities and advance as appropriate<br>• Implement exercise specific to functional tasks |

◉ *Regain ROM of the knee.*
- Active-assistive knee flexion and extension exercises within the pain-free ROM.
- Gentle superior and inferior patellar mobilization techniques as swelling decreases.
- Gravity-assisted knee extension with a rolled towel under the ankle and the posterior aspect of the knee unsupported.
- Continuous passive motion (CPM), if requested by the surgeon.

**Exercise: Moderate, Minimum Protection and Return to Function Phases**

As joint swelling and postoperative pain subside, emphasis is placed on re-establishing functional control of the operated knee necessary for independence during daily living activities. Goals and interventions for the intermediate and final phases of rehabilitation after arthroscopic synovectomy, noted in Table 21.2, are consistent with those for nonoperative management of joint dysfunction described in the previous section of this chapter.

## Outcomes

Synovectomy has been shown to be of benefit in alleviating chronic synovitis and joint pain and, in most cases, improving ROM and postponing deterioration of the involved joint.[205] After recovery from surgery, joint pain and swelling are reduced in approximately 90% to 95% of patients.[87] Long-term results of arthroscopic and open approaches are reported to be comparable. A review of several studies indicated that at 2.0 to 2.5 years after arthroscopic synovectomy 78% to 90% of patients continued to report a reduction of symptoms and general satisfaction with the procedure. However, by 4 to 5 years, positive outcomes after both arthroscopic and open procedures tended to deteriorate to approximately 60% to 70% in the presence of recurrent synovitis.[87] Progression of inflammatory joint disease, as reflected by radiographic changes, is common several years after synovectomy. Therefore, there is little evidence to support the claim that synovectomy can reverse the disease process.[29,87,205]

## Total Knee Arthroplasty

Total knee arthroplasty (TKA), also called total knee replacement, is a widely performed procedure for advanced arthritis of the knee, primarily in older patients (≥ 70 years of age) with osteoarthritis. However, during the decade between 1990 and 2000, the proportion of younger patients undergoing TKA increased significantly. During this period the proportion of knee replacements performed in the 40- to 49-year-old age group increased by 95.2% and in the 50- to 59-year-old age group by 53.7%. This indicates the criteria for TKA, traditionally reserved for the patient over 65 years of age, are broadening.[101]

The primary goals of TKA are to relieve pain and improve a patient's physical function and quality of life.[149,203]

### Indications for Surgery

The following are common indications for TKA.[98,131,203,205]

- Severe joint pain with weight bearing or motion that compromises functional abilities
- Extensive destruction of articular cartilage of the knee secondary to advanced arthritis
- Marked deformity of the knee such as genu varum or valgum
- Gross instability or limitation of motion
- Failure of nonoperative management or a previous surgical procedure

### Procedure

**Background**
Prosthetic replacement of one or more surfaces of the knee joint began to develop during the 1960s. Initially, only the tibial plateau was replaced (hemiarthroplasty). This was followed by the first generation of TKA, which involved a noncemented, double-stemmed, hinged, metal prosthesis that replaced the articulating surfaces of the distal femur and proximal tibia. This early design had a high failure rate

because of progressive component loosening.[98,131,203] The next major step was the development of an unconstrained, metal-to-plastic system that replaced the entire articular surfaces of the tibia and femur or just the medial or lateral compartment of the knee. The implants were held in place with acrylic cement. Completely unconstrained TKA also was associated with early failure because of a high incidence of instability or dislocation.[98,131,203] To address these problems, semiconstrained, two-component designs evolved. For the patient with severe anterior knee pain resulting from advanced patellofemoral deterioration, a three-component, total condylar design that included resurfacing the patellofemoral joint was developed.

These early designs were forerunners of current-day designs of TKA and unicompartmental knee arthroplasty (UKA).[98,131,156,203,236] A therapist's knowledge of the different types of TKA and UKA used today enhances communication between the therapist and surgeon and provides a foundation for decisions made during rehabilitation.

***Types of knee arthroplasty.*** Contemporary knee replacement procedures can be divided into several categories based on component design, surgical approach, and type of fixation (Box 21.3).[99,131,153,203] One category is based on

---

| BOX 21.3 | Total Knee Arthroplasty—Design, Surgical Approach, Fixation |
|---|---|

**Number of Compartments Replaced**
- *Unicompartmental*: only medial or lateral joint surfaces replaced
- *Bicompartmental*: entire femoral and tibial surfaces replaced
- *Tricompartmental*: femoral, tibial, and patellar surfaces replaced

**Implant Design**
- Degree of constraint
  - *Unconstrained:* no inherent stability in the implant design; used primarily with unicompartmental arthroplasty
  - *Semiconstrained*: provides some degree of stability with little compromise of mobility; most common design used for total knee arthroplasty
  - *Fully constrained*: significant congruency of components; most inherent stability but considerable limitation of motion
- Fixed-bearing or mobile-bearing design
- Cruciate-retaining or cruciate-excising/substituting

**Surgical Approach**
- Standard/traditional or minimally invasive
- Quadriceps-splitting or quadriceps-sparing

**Implant Fixation**
- Cemented
- Uncemented
- Hybrid

the number of components implanted or articulating sur-faces replaced. Another is based on the degree of con-straint (i.e., the amount of inherent congruency/stability in the design). Most TKA procedures today involve a two-component (bicompartmental), semiconstrained prosthetic system to replace the proximal tibia and distal femur (Fig. 21.8). These systems typically are composed of a modular or nonmodular femoral component with a metal articulat-ing surface and a single all-polyethylene or metal-backed modular or nonmodular tibial component with a polyethyl-ene articulating surface.[99,131,203]

Occasionally, a tricompartmental design, which also resurfaces the posterior aspect of the patella with a poly-ethylene component, is selected if the patellofemoral joint is symptomatic.[98,131,203] For the younger patient (< 55 years of age) with advanced disease of only the medial or lateral aspect of the knee joint, a unicompartmental design often is selected to replace just one tibial and one femoral condyle.[156,177,203,236]

Intact medial and lateral collateral ligaments are nec-essary prerequisites for semiconstrained and unconstrained TKA.[98,131,203] Fully constrained designs, now used infre-quently, are reserved for the low-demand patient who has marked instability of the knee, extensive bone loss, or severe deformity or who has had previous TKA revi-sions.[98,131] Contemporary fully constrained designs are not hinged but have inherent medial-lateral (ML) and anterior-posterior (AP) stability and some degree of rotation of the tibia on the femur to lessen the problem of progressive loosening of the prosthetic components over time.[98,131]

TKA designs also are classified as mobile-bearing or fixed-bearing. The most recent development in the evolu-tion of TKA is introduction of the mobile-bearing, bicom-partmental prosthetic knee. A mobile-bearing knee has a rotating platform inserted between the femoral and tibial components whose top surface is congruent with the femoral implant (round-on-round articulation) but whose undersurface is flat for rotation and sliding of the tibial component (flat-on-flat articulation).[32,153,203] A fixed-bearing knee does not have such an insert.[46,203] The purpose of the mobile-bearing insert is to decrease long-term wear of the polyethylene tibial component. A mobile-bearing knee design is recommended most often for the active patient, under 55 to 65 years of age.[203]

Another way to classify TKA design is based on the status of the posterior cruciate ligament (PCL). Designs are described as cruciate-retaining or cruciate-excising/substituting.[98,131,173,176,203] Although the ACL is routinely excised during knee replacement, except with UKA, the PCL can be preserved or excised. If the PCL is intact to provide posterior stability to the knee, one of several cru-ciate-retaining designs that require less congruency and allow some degree of AP glide can be used. If the PCL is irreparably deficient, a cruciate-substituting prosthesis is selected. This type of design has inherent posterior sta-bility from the congruency of the components, a posterior prominence in the tibial component, or a cam-post mecha-nism built into the design. Cruciate-retaining and cruciate-

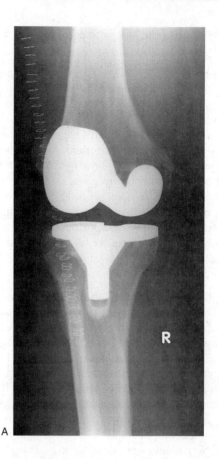

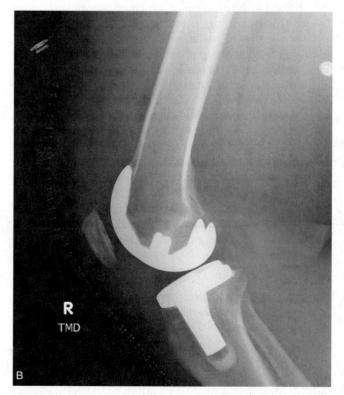

FIGURE 21.8 Posterior cruciate-retaining total knee arthroplasty of the right knee with cemented fixation. (A) Anteroposterior view. (B) Lateral view. Preop-erative ROM is 0° to 125°; ROM 1 month after surgery is 0° to 120°.

substituting designs can have a fixed-bearing or mobile-bearing design.[203]

***Surgical approach.*** TKA and UKA procedures are also described in terms of the surgical approach employed.[21,34,156,203] Since the inception of knee arthroplasty, an open approach requiring a relatively long anterior incision traditionally has been employed to provide sufficient exposure of the knee joint during the procedure. A recent advance is the development of *minimally invasive* knee arthroplasty.[21,156] Although minimally invasive, as with traditional joint arthroplasty it is an open procedure. However, minimally invasive TKA involves a smaller incision and less soft tissue disruption to reduce postoperative pain and increase the rate of postoperative recovery. Standard (traditional) and minimally invasive surgical approaches are described later in this section.

***Fixation.*** The method of fixation—cemented, uncemented, or "hybrid"—is another way to classify TKA procedures. That is, implants are held in place with acrylic cement, bone ingrowth (uncemented), or a combination of these two methods.[131,175,191,247] Initially, almost all total knee replacements relied on cemented fixation. In fact, cemented fixation revolutionized knee arthroplasty.[98,191] However, a long-term complication associated with early designs of cemented prostheses was biomechanical loosening, primarily of the tibial component at the bone-cement interface. Young, active patients were believed to be at highest risk for component loosening.[247]

To address the problem of loosening, cementless (biological) fixation relying on rapid growth of bone into the surfaces of a porous-coated or beaded prosthesis was introduced and recommended primarily for the young, active patient.[98,131,175,203,247] In addition, the use of a hydroxyapatite coating on the prosthesis has been advocated to enhance the ingrowth of bone.[205] However, long-term follow-up demonstrated that although the femoral component reliably achieved fixation to bone tibial component loosening occurred at an even higher rate with all-cementless fixation compared with cemented fixation.[175,247] This finding gave rise to the "hybrid" TKA, which combines

cemented fixation of the tibial component and cementless fixation of the femoral component.

Currently, all-cemented fixation is used most often and all-cementless used least often. A surgeon's decision whether to employ hybrid fixation is based on the patient's age, bone quality, expected activity level, and the tightness of fit of the femoral component achieved during surgery.[203] Design modifications to augment fixation of the tibial component (e.g., with pegs or screws) continue, although the long-term value of these design changes has yet to be determined.[98,257]

In summary, research continues on the biomechanics of knee arthroplasty, modifications of designs, development of better methods of fixation and new materials with better wear qualities, as well as improved surgical techniques and use of sophisticated instrumentation for alignment and placement of prosthetic components. Ongoing developments in all of these areas will continue to contribute to the success of current-day and improvement of future TKA procedures.[203,257]

### Operative Overview

One of several variations of standard or minimally invasive approaches along the anteromedial aspect of the knee can be used. Key features of these two types of approaches are compared in Table 21.3.[21,34,156,203] A quadriceps-splitting or a quadriceps-sparing approach is used to reach the capsule for an arthrotomy. The knee is flexed; and osteophytes, menisci, and the ACL are resected. If a posterior cruciate-substituting prosthesis is to be implanted, the PCL is also excised.

A series of surgical techniques are performed prior to inserting the implants.[99,203] Small portions of the distal femur and proximal tibia are removed and prepared for the implants. If a patellar implant is indicated, the patellar surface also is prepared and the prosthesis inserted. After trial components are inserted, soft tissue tension, collateral ligament balance, ROM, and patellar tracking are checked. The lateral retinaculum may be released to improve patellar tracking.[111,203] Permanent components are inserted, and the capsule and other soft tissues are repaired. The area

| TABLE 21.3 | Features of Standard and Minimally Invasive Surgical Approaches for Total Knee Arthroplasty |
|---|---|
| **Standard Approach** | **Minimally Invasive Approach** |
| • Anteromedial parapatellar vertical or curved incision from the distal aspect of the femoral shaft, running medial of the patella to just medial of the tibial tubercle, ranging from 8 to 12 cm[21] or 13 to 15 cm[204] in length<br>• Necessary soft tissue releases prior to eversion of the patella<br>• Anterior capsule release<br>• Dislocation of the tibiofemoral joint prior to bone cuts and implantation of components | • Reduced length of anteromedial skin incision 6–9 cm in length[21]<br>• No patellar eversion<br>• Anterior capsule release<br>• No tibiofemoral dislocation<br>• In situ bone cuts<br>• In situ implantation of components |

is thoroughly irrigated, and the wound is closed with the knee extended or in 90° of flexion[96] and with a small suction drain in place. A sterile dressing is placed over the incision, and the area is covered from foot to thigh with a compression wrap.

## Complications

Overall, the incidence of complications after TKA is low. Intraoperative complications during knee arthroplasty, such as intercondylar fracture or damage to a peripheral nerve (e.g., the peroneal nerve), are uncommon. Because minimally invasive TKA is considered more technically challenging than traditional TKA, early reports suggest that the rate of intraoperative complications, such as fracture or malpositioning of an implant, is higher with a minimally invasive than a standard approach.[21]

Early and late postoperative complications include infection, joint instability, polyethylene wear, and component loosening. As with arthroplasty of other joints, there is a risk of wound-healing problems and deep vein thrombosis (DVT) during the first few months after surgery. Although the incidence of deep periprosthetic infection is low, it is the most common reason for early failure and the need for revision arthroplasty. In contrast, polyethylene wear of the patellar and tibial components is the most common late complication requiring revision.[40,155] The incidence of biomechanical loosening has been reduced significantly with the newer prosthetic designs and improved surgical techniques.[155,204] If mechanical loosening develops over time, it occurs most often at the tibial component and more often with cementless or hybrid TKAs than fully cemented replacements.[175,205]

Other postoperative complications that can compromise a patient's functional recovery include limited knee flexion, joint instability leading to subluxation,[40,203] and patellar instability or tracking problems leading to impaired function of the extensor mechanism (most often an extensor lag).[111,203]

## Postoperative Management

Goals and interventions during progressive phases of postoperative rehabilitation after TKA are summarized in Table 21.4. Guidelines are similar for management after UKA. Interventions also may include preoperative patient education on an individual or group basis.[205] After surgery, patients routinely receive gait training and exercise instruction while hospitalized and in a subacute rehabilitation facility. Many patients also receive home-based or outpatient therapy after discharge from inpatient care.

A patient is advanced from one phase of rehabilitation to the next based on an evaluation of their signs and symptoms and responses to selected interventions rather than at designated time periods.[167] Accordingly, the timelines noted in Table 21.4 and described in the following sections are intended to serve only as general guidelines.

NOTE: The postoperative guidelines in Table 21.4 and the following sctions reflect recommendations for patients who have undergone *primary* TKA in which a *standard* surgical

approach was used. The suggested timelines for the progression of exercises and weight bearing tend to be more rapid after UKA than TKA and minimally invasive compared with traditional arthroplasty but slower after complex revision arthroplasty versus primary arthroplasty.

## Immobilization and Early Motion

Typically, after primary TKA the knee is immobilized in a bulky compression dressing for a day, or sometimes continuous passive motion (CPM) is initiated in the recovery room or within a day after surgery. After complicated revision arthroplasty, an extended period of immobilization may be required. The position of immobilization after primary TKA usually is extension.[203] Although atypical, an alternative approach is to immobilize the knee in a 90° flexion splint immediately after surgery and for brief intervals during the next day or two to achieve knee flexion as soon as possible while maintaining knee extension with exercises.[93]

During the initial postoperative period, it is advisable to have a patient wear a posterior extension splint during ambulation until quadriceps control is re-established. A extension splint also is indicated at night for a patient who is having difficulty achieving full knee extension after surgery or who had a significant preoperative knee flexion contracture.[33,203]

During the 1980s and 1990s CPM was used routinely during a patient's hospital stay after TKA.[51,79] At that time a number of studies describing the benefits of CPM, such as decreased need for postoperative pain medication, decreased incidence of deep vein thrombosis, and increased or more rapid recovery of ROM, were reported in the literature.[103,120,140] However, in some of the investigations that reported greater ROM with CPM, the knees of patients in the control groups, who did not undergo CPM, were immobilized for several days to a week after surgery.[103,140]

Customary practice for the past decade or more has been to initiate early postoperative exercise except in some instances of complex revision arthroplasty.[55] To evaluate postoperative CPM in the context of current practice, several randomized, controlled studies have been conducted comparing the effects of early postoperative exercise with and without the use of CPM after TKA.[9,35,42,112,122] The results of these studies have demonstrated that although the addition of CPM in the recovery room or within a day after surgery increased the rate of return of knee flexion during the early postoperative period in one study[35] it provided no significant long-term benefits as to gains in ROM and functional mobility.[9,35,42,112,122]

Although CPM continues to be used at the surgeon's discretion, the literature currently reflects that it is either no longer recommended after primary TKA[42,112,175] or, if used, is recommended as an adjunct to, not a replacement for, a postoperative exercise program.[9,35,42,122,203]

## Weight-Bearing Considerations

The extent to which weight bearing is allowable after primary TKA depends on the type of prosthesis implanted,

**TABLE 21.4    Total Knee Arthroplasty—Interventions for Each Phase of Rehabilitation**

| Phase and General Time Frame | Maximum Protection Phase: Weeks 1–4 | Moderate Protection Phases: Weeks 4–8 | Minimum Protection/Return to Function Phases: Beyond Week 8 |
|---|---|---|---|
| Patient presentation | • Patient enters rehabilitation 1–2 days postoperatively<br>• Postoperative compression dressing<br>• Postop pain controlled<br>• ROM 10°–60°<br>• Weight bearing as tolerated with cemented prosthesis, delayed with uncemented or hybrid | • Minimum pain<br>• Full weight bearing except with uncemented or hybrid<br>• ROM 0°–90°<br>• Joint effusion controlled | • Muscle function: 70% of noninvolved extremity<br>• No symptoms of pain or swelling during previous phase |
| Key examination procedures | • Pain (0–10 scale)<br>• Monitor for hemarthosis<br>• ROM<br>• Patellar mobility<br>• Muscle control<br>• Soft tissue palpation | • Pain assessment<br>• Joint effusion—girth<br>• ROM<br>• Patellar mobility<br>• Gait analysis | • Pain assessment<br>• Muscular strength<br>• Patellar alignment/stability<br>• Functional status |
| Goals | • Control postoperative swelling<br>• Minimize pain<br>• ROM 0°–90°<br>• 3/5 to 4/5 muscle strength<br>• Ambulate with or without assistive device<br>• Establish home exercise program | • Reduce swelling<br>• ROM 0°–110° or more<br>• Full weight bearing<br>• 4/5 to 5/5 strength<br>• Unrestricted ADL function<br>• Adherence to home exercise program | • Develop maintenance program and educate patient on importance of adherence including methods of joint protection<br>• Improve cardiopulmonary endurance/aerobic fitness |
| Interventions | • Pain modulation modalities<br>• Compression wrap to control effusion<br>• Ankle pumps to minimize risk of DVT<br>• A-AROM and AROM<br>• Muscle setting quadriceps, hamstrings, and adductors (may augment with E-stim)<br>• Patellar mobilization (grades I and II)<br>• Flexibility program hamstrings, calf, IT band<br>• Trunk/pelvis strengthening<br>• Gait training | • Patellar mobilization<br>• LE stretching program<br>• Closed-chain strengthening<br>• Limited range PRE<br>• Tibiofemoral joint mobilization, if appropriate and needed<br>• Proprioceptive training<br>• Stabilization exercises<br>• Gait training<br>• Protected aerobic exercise—swimming, cycling or walking | • Continue as previous phase; advance as appropriate<br>• Implement exercise specific to functional tasks |

the type of fixation used, the patient's age, size, and bone quality, and whether a knee immobilizer is worn during ambulation or transfers. With *cemented fixation*, weight bearing typically is permitted as tolerated immediately after surgery using crutches or a walker. During the first few days after surgery, use of a knee immobilizer may be required. The patient progresses to full weight bearing over 6 weeks.[191]

With *biological/cementless fixation*, recommendations for weight bearing vary from permitting only touch-down weight bearing for 4 to 8 weeks while using crutches or a walker[175] to weight bearing as tolerated within a few days after surgery while using crutches or a walker.[33,203,205]

Cane use is indicated as a patient progresses from partial to full weight bearing. Ambulation without an assistive device, particularly during outdoor walking, is not advisable until the patient has attained full or nearly full active knee extension and adequate strength of the quadriceps and hip musculature to control the operated lower extremity.[33,131,175,205]

## BOX 21.4    Exercise Precautions Following TKA

- Postpone straight-leg raises (SLRs) in side-lying positions for 2 weeks after cemented arthroplasty and for 4 to 6 weeks after cementless/hybrid arthroplasty to avoid varus and valgus stresses to the operated knee.
- Monitor the integrity of the surgical incision during knee flexion exercises. Watch for signs of excessive tension on the wound, such as drainage or skin blanching.
- Check with the surgeon to determine when it is permissible to initiate exercises against low-intensity resistance. It may be as early as 2 weeks or as late as 3 months postoperatively.[20]
- Tibiofemoral joint mobilization techniques to increase knee flexion or extension may or may not be appropriate, depending on the design of the prosthetic components. It is advisable to discuss the use of these techniques with the surgeon before initiating them.
- Postpone unsupported or unassisted weight-bearing activities until strength in the quadriceps and hamstrings is sufficient to stabilize the knee.

### Exercise

Guidelines for exercise after TKA have been reported in the literature since the mid-1970s.[130,244] Goals and exercises for progressive phases of postoperative rehabilitation after current-day TKA, noted in Table 21.4, are discussed in the following sections.[33,51,55,205] Precautions for exercise during rehabilitation are summarized in Box 21.4.

Many of the exercises described for the early phase of rehabilitation were reported in a consensus document developed by physical therapists on the management of patients during the period of hospitalization after TKA.[55] Prior to discharge from inpatient rehabilitation, a home exercise program serves as the foundation for the remainder of the rehabilitation process, with some patients also undergoing home-based or outpatient rehabilitation for a limited number of visits.

### Exercise: Maximum Protection Phase

The focus of management during the first phase of rehabilitation, which extends for about 4 weeks, is to control pain and swelling (with cold and compression), achieve independent ambulation and transfers while using a walker or crutches, prevent early postoperative medical complications, such as pneumonia and deep vein thrombosis, and minimize the adverse effects of postoperative immobilization. The goal is to attain 90° of knee flexion and full knee extension by the end of this first phase of rehabilitation. However, full knee extension may not be possible until joint swelling subsides.

It is well established that pain and joint swelling limit the function of the quadriceps.[45] In addition, there is a high correlation between quadriceps muscle weakness and impaired functional abilities during the initial period of recovery after TKA.[147] Regaining quadriceps muscle strength, particularly in terminal extension, as

early as possible after TKA is essential for functional control of the knee during ambulation and negotiating stairs. In addition to early postoperative exercise, neuromuscular electrical stimulation or biofeedback is recommended.

 **Focus on Evidence** _____

A study by Mizner and co-investigators[148] measured the voluntary activation and force-producing capacity of the quadriceps femoris muscle group in 52 patients (mean age 64.9 years, range 49 to 78 years) 3 to 4 weeks after unilateral, cemented primary TKA for OA and in 52 healthy individuals (mean age 72.2 years, range 64 to 85 years) without knee pathology. All patients in the TKA group had participated in a standard exercise program following surgery. Force production (maximum voluntary isometric contraction) and volitional activation of the quadriceps muscle group of the operated limb were, respectively, 64% and 26% less in the TKA group than in the healthy group. There was a weak relationship ($r^2 = 0.17$) between these results and postoperative knee pain. There were no significant differences in quadriceps muscle force production and volitional activation of the noninvolved knees in the TKA group compared with the healthy group. Based on the results of their study, the investigators recommended the use of neuromuscular electrical muscle stimulation or biofeedback as an adjunct to an individualized postoperative exercise program to augment quadriceps muscle force production after TKA.

Results of a prospective, randomized, controlled study conducted by Avramidis and colleagues[6] support the use of neuromuscular electrical stimulation in addition to a postoperative exercise program after TKA. Thirty patients scheduled to undergo primary TKA were randomly assigned to two groups (15 patients per group). Postoperatively, patients in both groups underwent an individualized program of exercise and gait training. In addition, the treatment group received electrical stimulation to the vastus medialis muscle 4 hours a day for 6 weeks beginning on postoperative day 2. Patients in the electrical stimulation group demonstrated a significantly faster walking speed than those in the control group at 6 weeks and 12 weeks postoperatively.

_____

The following goals and exercise interventions are included in the first phase of rehabilitation after TKA.[33,51,55,102,205]

- ◉ *Prevent vascular and pulmonary complications.*
  - Ankle pumping exercises with the leg elevated immediately after surgery to prevent a DVT or pulmonary embolism
  - Deep breathing exercises
- ◉ *Prevent reflex inhibition or loss of strength of knee and hip musculature.*
  - Muscle-setting exercises of the quadriceps (preferably coupled with neuromuscular electrical stimulation), hamstrings, and hip extensors and adductors.

- Assisted progression to active SLRs in supine and prone positions the first day or two after surgery, postponing SLRs in side-lying positions for 2 weeks after cemented TKA and for 4 to 6 weeks after cementless/hybrid replacement to avoid varus or valgus stresses to the operated knee.
- Active assisted ROM (A-AROM) progressing to assisted ROM (AROM) of the knee while seated and standing for gravity-resisted knee extension and flexion, respectively.
- As weight bearing on the operated lower extremity permits, wall slides in a standing position, mini-squats, and partial lunges to develop control of the knee extensors and reduce the risk of an extensor lag.

◐ *Regain knee ROM.*
- Heel-slides in a supine position or while seated with the foot on the floor to increase knee flexion.
- Neuromuscular facilitation and inhibition technique, such as the agonist-contraction technique (described in Chapter 4), to decrease muscle guarding, particularly in the quadriceps, and increase knee flexion.
- Gravity-assisted knee flexion by having the patient sit and dangle the lower leg over the side of a bed.
- Gravity-assisted knee extension in the supine position by periodically placing a rolled towel under the ankle and leaving the knee unsupported or in a seated position with the heel on the floor and pressing downward just above the knee with both hands.
- Gentle inferior and superior patellar gliding techniques to prevent restricted mobility.

P R E C A U T I O N : Avoid placing a pillow under the knee while lying supine or while seated with the operated leg elevated to reduce the risk of developing a knee flexion contracture.

### Exercise: Moderate Protection Phase

The emphasis of the moderate protection phase of rehabilitation, which begins at about 4 weeks and extends to 8 to 12 weeks postoperatively, is to achieve approximately 110° knee flexion and active knee extension to 0° and gradually to regain lower extremity strength, muscular endurance, and balance. By 4 to 6 weeks postoperatively if nearly full knee extension has been achieved and the strength of the quadriceps is sufficient, most patients transition to using a cane during ambulation activities. This makes it possible to focus on improving the patient's gait pattern and the speed and duration of walking.

The goals and exercise interventions for this phase of rehabilitation are the following.[33,51,55,102,147,205]

◐ *Increase strength and muscular endurance of knee and hip.*
- Multiple-angle isometrics and low-intensity dynamic resistance exercises of the quadriceps and hamstrings against a light grade of elastic resistance or a cuff weight around the ankle. Perform in a variety of positions to strengthen knee and hip musculature.

- Resisted SLRs in various positions to increase the strength of hip musculature, with emphasis on the hip extensors and abductors.
- As weight bearing allows, continue or begin closed-chain exercises including wall slides, mini-squats, and partial lunges. Add forward and backward, progressing to lateral step-ups and step-downs (initially using a low block or stool and progressing the height of the block) and scooting forward and backward on a wheeled stool to improve functional control of the knee.
- Stationary cycling with the seat positioned as high as possible to emphasize knee extension.

◐ *Continue to increase knee ROM.*
- Low-intensity self-stretching using a prolonged stretch or hold–relax exercises to increase knee flexion and extension if limitation persists. Flexibility of the hip flexors, hamstrings, and calf muscles also may need to be increased for standing and ambulation activities.
- Stationary cycling with seat lowered to increase knee flexion.
- Grade III inferior or superior patellar mobilization techniques to increase knee flexion or extension, respectively, if insufficient patellar mobility is restricting ROM.

◐ *Improve standing balance.*
- Proprioceptive and balance training progressing from bilateral to unilateral stance on stable surface, then to balance activities on an unstable surface.
- Functional reaching activities while standing, stooping.
- Heel-toe walking; ambulation on a variety of surfaces and inclines.
- Stepping over small objects.

### Exercise: Minimum Protection and Return to Function Phases

From the 8th to 12th week and beyond after surgery, the emphasis of rehabilitation is on task-specific strengthening exercises, proprioceptive training, and cardiopulmonary conditioning so the patient develops the strength, balance, and endurance needed to return to a full level of functional activities. However, patients often are discharged from supervised therapy 2 to 3 months postoperatively after attaining functional ROM of the knee and the ability to ambulate independently with an assistive device despite persistent strength deficits and functional limitations. These deficits have been shown to persist for a year or more after surgery.[247]

It is likely that some patients, especially those living in the community, could benefit from an intensive exercise program during the late phases of rehabilitation to perform demanding physical activities more efficiently, such as ascending and descending stairs and returning to selected recreational activities.

⬤ **Focus on Evidence** _____

Moffet et al.[149] conducted a single-blind, randomized controlled study to determine the effectiveness of an intensive, supervised functional training program initiated 2 months after primary TKA for OA. Patients in the experimental group (n = 38) participated in facility-based, twice weekly, 60- to 90-minute exercise sessions consisting of hip and knee strengthening exercises, task-specific functional exercises, and aerobic conditioning exercises. These exercises were preceded by a warm-up and followed by a cool-down period. The full cohort of exercises was phased in gradually during the first 2 weeks of the program. Patients also received a home program to be followed on the days they did not participate in the supervised program. Patients in the control group (n = 39) participated in a home exercise program for 6 weeks with periodic home visits by a therapist. No exercise-related adverse events occurred during the study.

Patients were evaluated by means of the 6-minute walk test and two functional outcome and quality-of-life (QOL) measures prior to beginning the exercise program (baseline measurement at 2 months after surgery), at the conclusion of the 6-week exercise program, and at 6 and 12 months postoperatively. The two groups were comparable at baseline. At the conclusion of the intervention and at the 6- and 12-month follow-ups, patients in the intensive exercise group walked significantly longer distances during the 6-minute walk test than did those in the control group. Functional abilities and QOL measures also were significantly better for the intensive exercise group than the control group immediately after the 6-week program and at 6 months postoperatively. At 1 year after surgery there were no significant differences in function or QOL measures between the two groups.

The investigators concluded that an intensive, functionally oriented exercise program initiated 2 months after primary TKA was safe and effective for improving physical function and quality of life.

---

With the trend toward an increasing number of young (< 60 years of age) and active patients undergoing TKA,[101] patient education is essential to help patients understand the detrimental effects of repetitive, high-impact activities (work-related, fitness-related, recreational) on the prosthetic implants and learn how to select activities that promote fitness but are least likely to reduce the longevity of the prosthetic knee.[88,113,138] Accordingly, patients are advised to participate in low-impact physical activities after TKA to reduce the risk of component wear and mechanical loosening over time and the premature need for revision arthroplasty.

For the patient who wishes to participate in athletic activities after TKA, there are a number of considerations. Factors that influence participation include the level of demand (intensity and load) of an athletic activity, a patient's body weight, overall level of fitness, and preoperative experience with the activity, and the technical quality of the knee replacement and related soft tissue balancing or reconstruction.[88,113]

Physical activities for fitness and recreation that are highly recommended, recommended with caution, or not recommended after TKA are noted in Box 21.5.[88,113,138]

---

**BOX 21.5 Recommendations for Participation in Physical Activities Following TKA**

**Highly Recommended***
- Stationary cycling
- Swimming, water aerobics
- Walking
- Golf (preferably with golf cart)
- Ballroom or square dancing
- Table tennis

**Recommended If Experienced Before TKA****
- Road cycling
- Speed/power walking
- Low-impact aerobics
- Cross-country skiing (machine or outdoor)
- Table tennis
- Doubles tennis
- Rowing
- Bowling, canoeing

**Not Recommended*****
- Jogging, running
- Basketball
- Volleyball
- Singles tennis
- Baseball, softball
- High-impact aerobics
- Stair-climbing machine
- Handball, racquetball, squash
- Football, soccer
- Gymnastics, tumbling
- Water-skiing

*Low impact, low load; appropriate at moderate- or high-intensity on a regular basis for aerobic fitness.

**Moderate impact; appropriate on a recreational basis if performed at low or moderate intensity.

***High impact, high load; peak load occurs during knee flexion.

---

**Outcomes**

Extensive research has been published in the orthopedic literature on patient-related outcomes after knee arthroplasty and the survivorship associated with a wide variety of prosthetic designs, surgical techniques, methods of fixation, and types of materials that have evolved over the past three to four decades.[98,99,203,257] Because of this variability, it is difficult to draw general conclusions.[204] What can be said, however, is that knee arthroplasty is a successful procedure for patients with advanced joint disease, although the ideal total knee replacement that replicates the normal biomechanics of the knee has yet to be developed. The effects of minimally invasive TKA and UKA on long-term patient-related outcomes and the longevity of implants have yet to be determined.

Patient-related outcomes after knee arthroplasty that have the most influence on patient satisfaction are relief of pain and an improved ability to perform necessary and desired functional activities for an extended number of years. Approximately 90% of patients who undergo primary TKA can expect 10 to 20 years of satisfactory function before revision arthroplasty may need to be considered.[203] For example, Dixon and colleagues[46] reported a 92.6% survival rate of modular, fixed-bearing TKA in patients followed for a minimum of 15 years.

Parameters typically measured to determine the success of knee replacement surgery are the level of pain, overall QOL, knee ROM, strength of the knee musculature, and a patient's ability to perform functional activities safely and with ease.

***Pain relief.*** Almost all patients who undergo knee arthroplasty report a significant reduction of pain during knee motion and weight bearing, with most patients reporting good to excellent pain relief.[59,203,204,220,243]

***ROM.*** Improvements in knee ROM are not as predictable as relief of pain. Stiffness often persists after the initial recovery from surgery has occurred.[59] However, it also has been reported that ROM may continue to improve up to 12 to 24 months postoperatively.[220] Factors that influence postoperative ROM include preoperative ROM, the underlying disease, postoperative pain, and whether a primary or a revison arthroplasty was performed. Complications such as component malpositioning, inadequate soft tissue balancing or reconstruction, infection, and mechanical loosening of an implant can adversely affect postoperative ROM.[179,217]

Patients with restricted ROM preoperatively usually continue to have limited knee flexion, extension, or both postoperatively despite an aggressive postoperative exercise program.[217,220] In fact, the most important predictor of long-term postoperative knee ROM is preoperative ROM.[119,202,217] For example, in a study of 358 patients who underwent primary TKA for OA, total ROM of the knee was 110° preoperatively and 113° postoperatively due to a reduction in the average knee flexion contracture from 12° to 9°.[202] The results of two other studies found that despite patients' participation in a outpatient or home-based postoperative rehabilitation program, there was no significant change in preoperative or postoperative knee ROM at 6 months[147] or at 12 months after surgery.[190]

Differences in prosthetic design, such as mobile-bearing versus fixed-bearing[32,133,203] or PCL-retaining versus PCL-substituting designs,[173,176,203] and the method of fixation[175,203] do not appear to affect ROM outcomes after primary TKA. A comparison of five designs of posterior cruciate-substituting implants, for example, showed no significant differences in the extent of improvement of knee ROM among designs.[202]

Limited knee ROM has a substantial impact on postoperative function, particularly if knee flexion is less than 90° and knee extension is limited by more than 10° to 15°.[203] With less than 90° to 100° of knee flexion, it is difficult to negotiate stairs; and having less than 105° makes it difficult to stand up from a standard height chair without using arm support.[203] In contrast, lack of full knee extension because of contracture or an extensor lag is thought to be a source of a patient's perception of knee pain or instability during ambulation activities particularly when ascending and descending stairs.[111,203]

***Strength and endurance.*** It takes a minimum of 3 to 6 months after surgery for a patient to regain strength in the quadriceps and hamstrings to a preoperative level.[111,147,220] Quadriceps weakness tends to persist longer after knee arthroplasty than does knee flexor weakness.[220]

Studies of patients after unilateral TKA with a conventional surgical approach have demonstrated that quadriceps strength in the operated leg correlates highly with performance on tests of functional abilities during the first 6 months after surgery.[147] Quadriceps strength also is significantly less than in similarly aged healthy individuals 6 months to a year after surgery[59,147,243] and the noninvolved leg 1 to 2 years postoperatively.[199,218] It has been suggested that eversion of the patella during a conventional surgical approach may contribute to impaired function of the quadriceps mechanism after surgery.[124,218] Given the number of studies that identified significant quadriceps weakness after TKA and the high correlation between quadriceps strength and functional performance, there is substantial evidence to support the importance of quadriceps strengthening exercises in postoperative rehabilitation programs to optimize function after TKA.

***Physical function and activity level.*** Relief of pain as the result of TKA significantly improves a patient's QOL and ability to perform functional activities. In general, when comparing preoperative with postoperative function, patients with high preoperative scores on functional measures achieved a higher level of function postoperatively than patients with low preoperative functional scores.[65] An insufficient number of studies have been conducted directly comparing the effects of various prosthetic designs (e.g., cruciate-retaining versus cruciate-substituting and mobile-bearing versus fixed-bearing designs) on knee control during functional activities (e.g., walking or negotiating stairs) to draw conclusions.

A systematic review of the literature by Ethgen and colleagues[57] revealed that a patient's postoperative level of function and QOL, as measured by self-report questionnaires, typically begins to surpass the preoperative level at approximately 3 months, with most improvement in function occurring by 6 months, although additional improvements may occur for a year or more postoperatively.[220,243]

A survey by Weiss et al.[246] of 176 patients (mean age 70.5 years) 1 year or more after TKA identified patients' level of participation in activities of graduated difficulty and determined which activities were most important to patients. The survey also identified activities that were difficult after TKA. The results of the survey indicated that in addition to basic activities of daily living (ADL)—walking, stair-climbing, personal care—patients performed a wide range of therapeutic and recreational activities after TKA. The activities in which the highest percentage of patients participated were stretching exercises (73%), leg-strengthening exercises (70%), gardening (57%), and stationary cycling (51%). These same activities were rated as important by patients. Functions that were the most difficult and most often caused knee pain were squatting (75%) and kneeling (70%).

Bradbury and colleagues[23] studied the pre- and postoperative sports participation of 160 patients who had undergone TKA 5 years earlier. Preoperatively, there were no significant differences in knee ROM, walking abilities, and radiographs in the patients who did and did not participate in sports activities. Postoperatively, the investigators found that 51 (65%) of the 79 patients (mean age 73 at the 5-year follow-up) who had regularly (at least twice a week) participated in sports activities during the year prior to surgery were participating in some type of sport at the 5-year follow-up. Patients were more likely to return to low-impact rather than high-impact activities. Of the patients who did not regularly participate in a sport before surgery, none took up a sport postoperatively.

Despite an overall positive impact of TKA on physical function, long-term studies indicate that functional abilities typically remain below norms for age-matched populations.[59,65] A follow-up study of 276 community-dwelling patients 6 months after primary TKA revealed that overall physical function improved significantly for all patients, although 60% reported moderate to extreme difficulty descending stairs and 64% continued to have a similar degree of difficulty with heavy household tasks.[104]

Results of another study indicated that 1 year after TKA, despite a relative absence of pain and some improvement in functional abilities, significant deficits in strength and function were apparent when compared with the abilities of age-matched, healthy individuals.[243] The post-TKA patients had less strength of the knee musculature, slower walking and stair-climbing speeds, and a higher perceived level of exertion during activities than healthy individuals. The authors pointed out that the post-TKA patients as a group were heavier than the control group and suggested that general physical deconditioning may have contributed to the postoperative group's functional limitations. This study emphasizes the need for inclusion of a low-impact aerobic conditioning program during rehabilitation after TKA.

## PATELLOFEMORAL DYSFUNCTION: NONOPERATIVE MANAGEMENT

### Related Patellofemoral Pathologies

Historically, the differential diagnosis of patellofemoral pathologies has been plagued with confusion, largely related to the use of broadly inclusive terminology such as chondromalacia patellae and patellofemoral pain syndrome. In an attempt to more clearly identify the anatomical structures involved and the biomechanical changes leading to dysfunction, several classification systems have been proposed. These classifications include guidelines for intervention based on impairments and functional limitations.[96,252]

### Patellofemoral Instability

Instability includes subluxation or dislocation of a single or recurrent episode. There may be an abnormal Q-angle, dysplastic trochlea (shallow groove or flat lateral femoral condyle), patella alta, tight lateral retinaculum, and inadequate medial stabilizers (VMO). There may be associated fractures. Usually the instability is in a lateral direction. The dislocation may derive from direct trauma to the patella or from a forceful quadriceps contraction while the foot is planted and the femur is externally rotating while the knee is flexed. Recurrent dislocation is usually an indication for surgery to redirect the forces through the patella.

### Patellofemoral Pain with Malalignment or Biomechanical Dysfunction

Patellofemoral pain due to malalignment or a biomechanical dysfunction includes impairments that cause an increased functional Q-angle such as femoral anteversion, external tibial torsion, genu valgum, or foot hyperpronation. There may be a tight lateral retinaculum, weak VMO, patella alta, patella baja, or dysplastic femoral trochlea. There is usually abnormal patellar tracking, and there may be discordant firing of the quadriceps muscle.[96]

### Patellofemoral Pain Without Malalignment

Patellofemoral pain without malalignment includes many subcategories of lesions that cause anterior knee pain.

***Soft tissue lesions.*** Soft tissue lesions include plica syndrome, fat pad syndrome, tendinitis, iliotibial band friction syndrome, and bursitis.

- *Plica syndrome* describes a condition related to irritation of remnants of embryological synovial tissue around the patella. With chronic irritation, the tissue becomes an inelastic, fibrotic band that is tender during palpation. When acute, the tissue is painful during palpation. The band is usually palpable medial to the patella, although there are variations in its location.[19,107]
- *Fat pad syndrome* involves irritation of the infrapatellar fat pad from trauma or overuse.
- *Tendinitis* of the patellar or quadriceps tendons often occurs from overuse as the result of repetitive jumping. Tenderness occurs along the attachment of the tendon to the patella.
- *Iliotibial (IT) band friction syndrome* is irritation of the IT band as it passes over the lateral femoral condyle. Contributing factors could be tight tensor fasciae latae or tight gluteus maximus (see discussion in Chapter 20). Because the IT band attaches to the patella and lateral retinaculum, it may cause anterior knee pain.
- *Prepatellar bursitis,* also known as housemaid's knee results from prolonged kneeling or recurrent minor trauma to the anterior knee. When inflamed there may be restricted motion due to the swelling and pain caused by direct pressure or pressure from the patellar tendon.

***Tight medial and lateral retinacula or patellar pressure syndrome.*** There is increased contact pressure of the patella in the trochlear groove.

***Osteochondritis dissecans of the patella or femoral trochlea.*** Osteochondral lesions result in pain on the retro surface of the patella that is worse during squatting, stooping, ambulation, and descending steps. The knee may give way or may lock. There may be loose bodies within the joint.

***Traumatic patellar chondromalacia.*** With chondromalacia there is softening and fissuring of the cartilaginous surface of the patella, which is diagnosed with arthroscopy or arthrography.[96] It may eventually predispose the joint to degenerative arthritis or basal degeneration of the middle and deep zones of the cartilage.[78] Causes of the degeneration may include trauma, surgery, prolonged or repeated stress, or lack of normal stress such as during periods of immobilization.[174]

***Patellofemoral osteoarthritis.*** Osteoarthritis may be idiopathic or posttraumatic and is diagnosed by radiographic changes consistent with degeneration.

***Apophysitis.*** Osgood-Schlatter's disease (traction apophysitis of the tibial tuberosity) and Sinding-Larsen-Johansson syndrome (traction apophysitis on the inferior pole of the patella) occur during adolescence owing to overuse during rapid growth. They are self-limiting conditions.

***Symptomatic bipartite patella.*** Most bipartite patellae (due to patellar ossification variants) are asymptomatic, but trauma may disrupt the chondro-osseous junction leading to symptoms.[96]

***Trauma.*** Trauma includes *tendon rupture, fracture, contusion,* and *articular cartilage damage* that results in inflammation, swelling, limited motion, and pain with dysfunction whenever contracting the quadriceps, such as during stair climbing, squatting, and resisted knee extension.

## Etiology of Symptoms

The cause of anterior knee pain may be direct trauma, overuse, faulty patellar tracking from malalignment due to anatomical variations or soft tissue length and strength imbalances, degeneration, or a combination of these factors.[27,47,135,189,201,215,242,256] An attempt should be made to determine the causative factors based on the patient's history and a comprehensive and sequential examination.

## Common Impairments and Functional Limitations/Disabilities

Impairments that may be associated with patellofemoral dysfunction include the following.[27,47,100,116,135,189,201,215,242,256]

- Weakness, inhibition, or poor recruitment or timing of firing of the VMO
- Overstretched medial retinaculum

- Restricted lateral retinaculum, IT band, or fascial structures around the patella
- Decreased medial gliding or medial tipping of the patella
- Pronated foot
- Pain in the retropatellar region
- Tight gastrocnemius soleus, hamstring, or rectus femoris muscles
- Irritated patellar tendon or subpatellar fat pads
- Patellar crepitus, swelling, or locking
- Weakness in the hip abductor or external rotator musculature

Limitations associated with the impairments include the following.

- Pain or poor knee control when descending or ascending stairs
- Pain with walking, jumping, or running interfering during ADL, instrumental ADL (IADL), work, and community, recreational, or sport activities
- Pain and stiffness with prolonged flexed knee postures, such as sitting or squatting

## Patellofemoral Symptoms: Management—Protection Phase

When symptoms are acute, treat them as any acute joint problem—with modalities, rest, gentle motion, and muscle-setting exercises in pain-free positions. Pain and joint effusion inhibit the quadriceps,[231] so it is imperative to reduce irritating forces. Splinting the patella with a brace or tape may unload the joint and relieve the irritating stress.[107]

## Patellofemoral Symptoms: Management—Controlled Motion and Return to Function Phases

When signs of inflammation are no longer present, management is directed toward correcting or modifying the biomechanical forces that may be contributing to the impairment. Because no one factor or combination of factors has been identified as the direct cause or effect of patellofemoral pain symptoms, it is imperative to develop interventions that address the patient's specific impairments.[189]

### Educate the Patient

***Patient advice.*** Because end-range stress and prolonged postures tend to exacerbate symptoms, the following information should be provided.
- Until the knee is symptom-free, avoid positions and activities that provoke the symptoms.
- Minimize or avoid stair climbing and descending until the hip and knee muscles are strengthened to a level at which they can control knee function without symptoms.
- Do not sit with the knees flexed excessively for prolonged periods. During sitting, periodically perform ROM to the knee to relieve stasis.

***Home exercise program.*** Use a home exercise program to reinforce training. Prior to discharge provide instructions for safe progression of the exercises.

## Increase Flexibility of Restricting Tissues

Identify any structures that could be contributing to faulty mechanics and establish a stretching program. The gastrocnemius, soleus, quadriceps, and hamstring muscles have been identified as specific muscles with decreased flexibility in individuals with patellofemoral dysfunction.[187] In addition to self-stretching techniques described in the exercise section of this chapter, techniques to stretch the two-joint muscles that cross the hip and knee are described in Chapter 20, and those that cross the knee and ankle are described in Chapter 22.

Because restrictions related to insertion of the IT band and the lateral retinaculum may contribute to decreased patellar mobility and faulty patellar tracking in some patients with patellofemoral pain syndrome, specific techniques to address these impairments are described in this section.

***Patellar mobilization—medial glide.*** Position the patient side-lying. Stabilize the femoral condyles with one hand under the femur and glide the patella medially with the base of the other hand (Fig. 21.9).[81,136] There is usually greater mobility with the knee near extension; progress by positioning the knee in greater flexion prior to performing the medial glide.

***Medial tipping of the patella.*** Position the patient supine. Place the thenar eminence at the base of the hand over the medial aspect of the patella. Direct posterior force tips the patella medially. While the patella is held in this position, friction massage can be applied with the other hand along the lateral border (Fig. 21.10). Teach the patient to self-stretch in this manner.

***Patellar taping.*** Use tape to realign the patella and apply a prolonged stretch as well as maintain alignment of the patella for nonstressful training.[81,135,136]

***Self-stretching— insertion of IT band.*** Position the patient side-lying with a belt or sheet strapped around the ankle and the other end placed over the shoulder and held in the hand. The hip is positioned in extension,

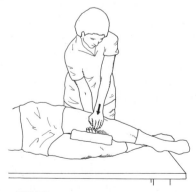

FIGURE 21.9 Medial glide of the patella.

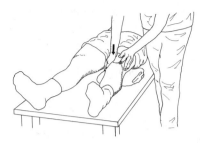

FIGURE 21.10 Medial tipping of the patella with friction massage along the lateral border.

adduction, and slight lateral rotation and the knee in flexion.

- Instruct the patient to first flex the knee and abduct the hip; then extend the hip (this ensures that the IT band is over the greater trochanter).
- The femur is then adducted with slight lateral rotation until tension is felt in the IT band along the lateral knee.
- The patient stabilizes himself/herself in this position by holding onto the strap. If tolerated, a 2- to 5-lb weight is placed distally over the lateral thigh for added stretch, and the position is maintained for 20 to 30 minutes (Fig. 21.11).

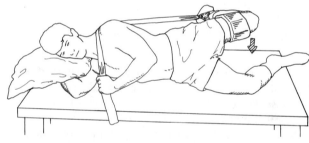

FIGURE 21.11 Self-stretch to the insertion of IT band.

## Improve Muscle Performance for Functional Control

Because many possible diagnoses fall under the category of patellofemoral pain syndromes, various biomechanical influences may be the precipitating or perpetuating cause of the symptoms. Not all patients benefit from the same exercises. Research studies have not identified interventions that have led to consistent results.[189] It is imperative that the therapist design an exercise program that addresses the specific impairments of each patient, considering factors such as trunk, hip, and foot strength and alignment.[100,132,189] Exercises for impairments in these regions are described in Chapters 16, 20, and 22, respectively.

### Non-Weight-Bearing (Open-Chain) Exercises

N O T E : There is controversy regarding compressive forces and stress in the patellofemoral joint with open-chain exercises.[56,80] The type of resistance (constant, variable, or isokinetic) places different demands on the quadriceps muscle in terms of maximum effort at various ranges. The resultant force from the quadriceps tendon and patellar tendon and the patellar contact area also vary through the ROM. Therefore, the stress to the articulating surface of the patella varies. There is little or no contact of the patella with the trochlear groove from 0° to 15° of flexion,[56] so pain felt in that range could derive from irritation of the patellar fat pads or synovial tissue. Greatest patellar stress is at 60° and compression loads at 75°, so pain may be provoked in these ranges when maximum torque from the resistance force is applied in these ranges.[56] Where the pathology is located affects where in the range the patient feels pain.[80] It is recommended that when examining the patient the range where pain is felt is noted and resistance loads that cause pain in that range be avoided.

***Vastus medialis obliquus emphasis.*** Although it is not possible to isolate contraction of the VMO, it is accepted that the line of pull of this component of the quadriceps muscle influences the tracking of the patella, and thus effort is directed toward developing awareness of the VMO contraction during quadriceps muscle activity. Use tactile cues over the muscle belly, electrical stimulation, or biofeedback to reinforce the VMO contraction during open- and closed-chain extension exercises.

***Quadriceps setting (quad sets) in pain-free positions.*** Have the patient set the quads with the knee in various positions while focusing on tension development in the VMO. Because the site of irritation varies among patients, identify pain-free positions for each patient to ensure nondestructive loading.[56,80]

***Quad sets with straight-leg raising.*** Because many fibers of the VMO originate on the adductor tendons and medial intramuscular septum, some popular exercise programs suggest that by laterally rotating the femur while performing SLR exercises the adductors contract and provide a firm base for the VMO.[4,47,135] However, electromyography (EMG) studies do not support the claim of increased activity in the VMO.[106]

***Progression of resisted isometrics.*** When the patient tolerates it, isometric resistance to knee extension may be utilized in pain-free positions.

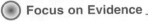 **Focus on Evidence** _____

To determine if there is preferential recruitment of the VMO over the VL, five knee extension exercises in symptomatic and control subjects were studied during various combinations of adduction and medial rotation of the tibia.[116] Investigators found that the VMO/VL ratio was greatest when there was simultaneous resistance to medial tibial rotation and knee extension. The test was conducted with the knee at 70° of flexion and the tibia laterally rotated. The ratio with resisted adduction in extension was less than with resisted extension alone. This study did not evaluate the effects of exercise on pain or improved function.

***Short-arc terminal extension.*** Begin with the patient supine and knee flexed around 20° (see Fig. 21.17). If tolerated and the motion is not painful, light resistance is added at the ankle. Strengthening in terminal extension trains the muscle to function where it is least efficient because of its shortened position and where there is minimal patellar compression because it is superior to the femoral groove. This action is needed when lifting the leg into bed and moving the covers, as well as when lifting the leg into a car.

PRECAUTION: If there is irritation of the synovial lining of the suprapatellar pouch or bursa, terminal knee extension may be painful and should be avoided until the pain subsides.

### Weight-Bearing (Closed-Chain) Exercises
See the last section of this chapter for detailed descriptions of various weight-bearing exercises.

- If weight bearing is painful, begin with partial weight-bearing exercises. Progress to standing exercises as tolerated.
- To improve strength and muscular endurance, the patient should perform the repetitions of the appropriate exercise until symptoms or loss of control just begins. It is important to not push beyond that point in order to avoid faulty mechanics or loss of control.
- Mini-squats, which may be useful for improving patellar tracking, are introduced early in the exercise program when weight bearing and partial squatting are tolerated and do not provoke symptoms.

NOTE: A recent study suggests that mini-squats are effective in causing a greater VMO/VL ratio than a maximum voluntary isometric quadriceps contraction.[97]

- Observe the lower extremity positioning as the patient squats or descends steps; it is important for the knee to maintain alignment over the foot and not go into increased valgus.[189] Valgus alignment may be indicitative of weak hip abductor musculature, which should be addressed with strengthening exercises to develop dynamic control.

PRECAUTION: Because there are higher patellar compressive loads when the knee is flexed beyond 60° during weight bearing, exercises and activities with the knee flexed beyond this angle may provoke symptoms. Use caution when the patient is ready to progress beyond 60°. Have the patient carefully monitor symptoms and stop the exercise if symptoms develop.

### Functional Activities
Exercises are progressed as described in the exercise section of this chapter so long as the patient is able to maintain control and not exacerbate the symptoms. Use activity-specific drills to prepare the patient to return to the desired activity.

## Modify Biomechanical Stresses

If the patient has foot pronation, a foot orthosis may relieve the stresses at the knee.[53,84] Assess lower extremity mechanics, and modify any faulty patterns.

 **Focus on Evidence** _____

A systematic review of the literature focusing on quality randomized controlled studies for patellofemoral pain syndrome revealed that interventions most effective for reducing pain and improving function were acupuncture, quadriceps strengthening, and combinations of interventions that include quadriceps strengthening with patellar taping and use of biofeedback.[18] The effectiveness of a patellar brace was not refuted or supported, nor was the use of manual therapy techniques such as stretching and manipulation. No particular exercise approach was superior to another for improving pain and function, although exercise interventions in general have been shown to improve symptoms sooner than in control groups. The authors emphasized the importance of developing effective methods for classifying patients and gearing interventions to each patient's impairments.[18]

---

 ## PATELLOFEMORAL AND EXTENSOR MECHANISM DYSFUNCTION: SURGICAL AND POSTOPERATIVE MANAGEMENT

Any number of factors, noted in the previous section, can contribute to chronic patellofemoral pain and crepitation, degeneration of the articular surface of the patella, or recurrent instability of the patella. When conservative (nonoperative) management of patellofemoral dysfunction fails, surgery may be indicated.

Surgical intervention can be used to alter the alignment of the patellofemoral joint, correct imbalances of static stabilizers (see Fig. 21.4) of the patella and knee, decrease an abnormal Q-angle (see Fig. 21.3 for depiction of Q-angle measurement), improve tracking of the patella, and débride or repair the articular surface of the patella. However, before a surgical procedure is selected, the etiology of symptoms and identification of contributing factors must be determined by a thorough physical examination and radiographic and arthroscopic evaluation.

Categories of surgical options for patellofemoral dysfunction are noted in Box 21.6.[72,73,95,144,145,180,188] Numerous variations of procedures fall under each of these categories. Often a combination of procedures is necessary.[73,158] Of the procedures noted, lateral retinacular release is the procedure performed most often for patellofemoral pain. In contrast, only in rare instances is a patellofemoral joint replacement (as an alternative to TKA) or patellectomy performed for chronic patellofemoral pain and dysfunction. If used, these

---

**BOX 21.6    Surgical Options for Patellofemoral Dysfunction**

- Lateral retinacular release, including release of the lateral patellofemoral and patellotibial ligaments
- Repair, imbrication, or reconstruction of the medial patellofemoral ligament
- Proximal realignment of the extensor mechanism (medialization or advancement and medialization of the VMO)
- Distal realignment of the extensor mechanism (anteromedialization of the tibial tubercle and insertion of the patellar tendon)
- Arthroscopic débridement
- Repair of patellofemoral articular cartilage lesions (microfracture, osteochondral autograft transfer/mosaicplasty, autologous chondrocyte implantation)
- Abrasion arthroplasty/chondroplasty of the posterior surface of the patella (used less frequently with the advent of surgeries to repair articular cartilage)
- Interposition trochleoplasty for trochlear dysplasia
- Replacement arthroplasty of the posterior surface of the patella or patellectomy (salvage procedures for advanced degeneration of the articular surface)

---

procedures are reserved as salvage procedures for patients with end-stage articular degeneration and collapse of the joint space.[73,145,180]

The goals and interventions for rehabilitation after surgeries for patellofemoral and extensor mechanism dysfunction are directed toward restoring and improving the function of the entire lower extremity and trunk, not just the knee, and are derived from resources dealing with postoperative and nonoperative management.[10,67,126,132,189] Depending on the phase of rehabilitation, the goals and interventions discussed in the previous section on nonoperative management of patellofemoral dysfunction are applicable to postoperative management.

The goals of postoperative rehabilitation are to: (1) control pain and swelling; (2) prevent or reduce the adverse effects of immobilization (3) restore postoperative knee ROM quickly and safely; (4) maximize the function of the extensor mechanism, especially the VMO, to restore full active knee extension and prevent an extensor lag; (5) remediate deficits in the length and strength of the hip and ankle to develop stability and flexibility proximal and distal to the knee; and (6) educate the patient and possibly alter the lifestyle to prevent recurrence of patellofemoral pain or instability.

A number of factors influence the rate of progression of postoperative rehabilitation. These factors include the patient's age, general health, and severity of symptoms prior to the surgical procedure, the presence of other pathology, the desired functional outcomes, and the patient's adherence to the prescribed home exercise program and motivation to return to functional activities.

## Lateral Retinacular Release

Depending on the underlying pathologies, lateral retinacular release (LRR) may be performed in isolation or in conjunction with other procedures, such as proximal or distal realignment of the extensor mechanism, imbrication of the medial structures, joint débridement, articular cartilage repair, chondroplasty, or synovectomy.

### Indications for Surgery

Although opinion varies, the following are often cited as indications for LRR.[67,70,73,75,145,188] Chronic patellofemoral pain and functional limitations without improvement in symptoms after 6 months of conservative (nonoperative) management including exercise, taping, bracing, anti-inflammatory medication, and modification of daily activities.

- Restricting and often tender lateral retinaculum with documented rotational malalignment of the patella, specifically a lateral patellar tilt (without subluxation), and resulting lateral compression syndrome.[70,73,145,188]
- Minimal or no evidence of patellofemoral chondrosis or abnormal Q-angle.
- In conjunction with other surgical procedures performed to correct instability (subluxation or dislocation) of the patella, inadequate dynamic medial stabilizers, increased Q-angle, and inadequate size/shape of the trochlear groove.

### Procedures

#### Background and Operative Overview

The LRR is designed to reduce an identified lateral tilt of the patella, alleviate excessive compressive forces on the lateral facet of the patella, and consequently reduce pain and the risk of lateral subluxation of the patella.[73,188] Typically, LRR is perfomed arthroscopically through several parapatellar portals, but it also may be performed through an open approach that involves a longitudinal parapatellar incision immediately lateral to the patella when done concomitantly with other open procedures.[67,70,73,75,145,180,188]

The procedure "releases" the lateral structures supporting the patellofemoral joint, specifically the superficial and deep portions of the lateral retinaculum and the lateral patellofemoral and patellotibial ligaments by means of an incision extending from the superior lateral pole of the patella to just lateral and inferior to the patellar tendon. Any loose chondral flaps are removed.[145] The location of the incision is such that the superior lateral and inferior lateral geniculate arteries are cut and must be cauterized immediately and tied. However, the release leaves the tendinous portion of the vastus lateralis (VL) muscle intact so as not to compromise the function of the quadriceps.

Electrocautery[158] and, most recently, radiofrequency ablation[75] are alternatives to surgically incising the retinaculum. The advantages of these methods for releasing the lateral structures is less bleeding and subsequent hemarthrosis.

After the release has been completed, patellar tracking is assessed. The wounds are closed and covered with a sterile dressing, and a compression dressing is placed around the knee.

### Complications

Several complications may occur with LRR.[75,126,188] The most common complication associated with LRR is hemarthrosis if the geniculate artery is not adequately cauterized during surgery. Thermal injury to overlying skin can occur with radiofrequency ablation or electrocautery.[75] As with any surgery, there is always the risk of the patient developing a DVT. A superficial infection also can occur, but intra-articular infection is rare.

Other complications include postoperative arthrofibrosis or medial patellar subluxation as the result of the release extending too far proximally, causing weakness of the VL muscle. In rare instances rupture of the quadriceps tendon or complex regional pain syndrome (reflex sympathetic dystrophy) may occur.[37] Any of these complications can affect postoperative rehabilitation and compromise the outcome.

### Postoperative Management

Postoperative management of LRR is a fairly straightforward intervention process that progresses quite rapidly, especially after arthroscopic LRR because of less postoperative tissue morbidity.[10,70,75,126] The patient is progressed through the phases of rehabilitation based on signs and symptoms and the attainment of phase-specific goals.[167] Management of each phase of rehabilitation following arthroscopic LRR is summarized in Table 21.5.

#### Immobilization and Weight-Bearing Considerations

The knee is immobilized postoperatively in full extension with a compression dressing and patella-stabilizing orthosis or posterior splint.[10,75,126] A Cryo-Cuff®, which combines cold and compression, or another form of cryotherapy is applied to minimize the postoperative joint effusion often associated with hemarthrosis. The patient is permitted to ambulate, weight bearing as tolerated with crutches, immediately after surgery. When control of the quadriceps is sufficient to hold the knee in full extension, use of the knee immobilizer and assistive devices for ambulation may be discontinued.

#### Exercise: Maximum Protection Phase

Emphasis during the maximum protection phase after arthroscopic LRR, which extends approximately 2 weeks postoperatively, is prevention of complications, such as a DVT, control of pain and joint swelling, restoration of quadriceps function, and regaining ROM. Maintaining adequate patellar mobility to prevent formation of adhesions that could position the patella in the same alignment that was evident preoperatively or even in a more lateral position is also a priority. By the end of this first phase of rehabilitation, as swelling subsides and tissues heal, the goal is to achieve 115° of knee flexion to full extension.

**TABLE 21.5** Lateral Retinacular Release—Interventions for Each Phase of Rehabilitation

| Phase and General Time Frame | Maximum Protection Phase: Weeks 1–2 | Moderate Protection Phase: Weeks 3–4 | Minimum Protection Phase: Weeks 5–6 | Return to Function Phase: Beyond Week 6 |
|---|---|---|---|---|
| Patient presentation | • Patient enters rehabilitation within 1–2 days after surgery<br>• Minimum postoperative pain<br>• ROM minimally limited<br>• Weight bearing as tolerated | • Minimum pain<br>• Full weight bearing<br>• Nearly full ROM<br>• Joint effusion controlled | • No swelling or tenderness<br>• Good to normal strength<br>• Unrestricted ADL function | • Muscle function 75% of noninvolved extremity<br>• No signs or symptoms of patellar subluxation, pain, or swelling during the previous phase |
| Key examination procedures | • Pain (0–10 scale)<br>• Monitor for hemarthosis<br>• ROM<br>• Patellar mobility<br>• Muscle control<br>• Soft tissue palpation | • Pain assessment<br>• Joint effusion—girth<br>• ROM<br>• Patellar mobility<br>• Muscle strength<br>• Gait analysis | • Pain assessment<br>• Muscle strength<br>• Patellar alignment and stability<br>• Functional status | • Pain assessment<br>• Muscle strength<br>• Patellar alignment and stability<br>• Functional status |
| Goals | • Control postoperative swelling<br>• Minimize pain<br>• ROM 0°–115°<br>• 3/5 to 4/5 muscle strength<br>• Ambulate without assistive device<br>• Establish home exercise program | • Control swelling<br>• Full ROM<br>• 4/5 to 5/5 strength<br>• Gradual return to ADL<br>• Adherence to home program | • 70% Muscle strength<br>• Educate patient on resuming activity slowly monitoring signs and symptoms | • Develop maintenance program and educate patient on importance of adherence |
| Interventions | • A-AROM and AROM<br>• Patellar mobilization (grade I and II)<br>• Muscle setting quadriceps, hamstrings, and adductors (may augment with E-stim)<br>• SLRs—four positions<br>• Flexibility program hamstring, calf, IT band<br>• Ankle pumps<br>• Trunk/pelvis strengthening<br>• Pain modulation modalities<br>• Lateral felt pad to apply medial glide to patella<br>• Compression wrap to control effusion | • LE flexibility program<br>• Continued open- and closed-chain strengthening<br>• Limited-range PREs<br>• Tibiofemoral joint mobilization if needed<br>• Proprioceptive training<br>• Stabilization exercises<br>• Gait training<br>• Aerobic conditioning program: swimming or walking program as incision healing permits | • Continue LE flexibility<br>• Advance PRE strengthening<br>• Advance closed-chain exercise<br>• Advance endurance training<br>• Task specific training. Simulated functional tasks based on signs and symptoms | • Continue stretching and strengthening; advance as appropriate<br>• Advance agility drills<br>• Advance running drills<br>• Implement drills specific to sport or occupation<br>• Consider bracing for high-demand activity |

Adapted from: Mangine et al.,[126] page 327, with permission.

Exercises are initiated the day of surgery, even after an open release, and include setting exercises of the knee and hip musculature and assisted ROM. These exercises, summarized in Table 21.5, are similar to those for nonoperative management of patellofemoral dysfunction during the acute stage of tissue healing (detailed in the previous section of this chapter). All exercises are progressed within the patient's comfort level. Exercises to develop control of the quadriceps can be performed in non-weight-bearing and protected weight-bearing positions. As noted in Table 21.5, the use of a felt pad wedge placed under the compression dressing along the lateral border of the patella,[126] which applies a slight medial glide, or the use of McConnell taping[81,135] to maintain patellar alignment and unload the lateral soft tissue structures may enable the patient to perform knee exercises more comfortably.

Although grades I and II patellar mobilization procedures should be initiated during the early postoperative period to maintain patellar gliding and to prevent patellofemoral adhesions, these glides should be performed within the patient's pain parameters.[126] With proper instruction the patient can be taught to carry out patellar mobilization techniques at home and should do so regularly throughout the day.

### Exercise: Moderate Protection Phase
The moderate protection phase after arthroscopic LRR, which begins by the third postoperative week, places emphasis on attaining full active ROM of the knee as well as the hip and ankle. Interventions are aimed at developing muscular strength and endurance of the entire lower extremity and the trunk, as well as re-establishing balance as pain and joint effusion reach a minimal level. Closed-chain and open-chain exercises, performed while maintaining appropriate alignment, are progressed for knee, hip, and ankle musculature at levels of intensity and positions in the ROM that do not evoke pain. In addition to quadriceps training, emphasis is placed on improving the function of the hip abductors, extensors, and external rotators.[132] If the patient is having difficulty re-establishing active control of the quadriceps, electrical stimulation or biofeedback is beneficial. Aerobic conditioning on a stationary bicycle to re-establish cardiopulmonary fitness also is begun during this phase.

Flexibility exercises for the lower extremity should continue, with particular emphasis placed on stretching the gastrocnemius, soleus, and hamstring muscles, which have been shown to be tight in patients with patellofemoral dysfunction.[187] Stretching the IT band also may be necessary. If restricted, the IT band can contribute to excessive compression over the lateral femoral condyle and lateral border of the patella during knee motion.

Available motion and strength are incorporated into progressive functional activities. Any number of exercises (described in the final section of this chapter) and individually designed exercises can be incorporated and progressed in a patient's rehabilitation program so long as the selected exercises do not cause a recurrence of patellofemoral symptoms.

### Exercise: Minimum Protection and Return to Function Phases
The advanced phases of rehabilitation, which begin about 5 weeks after surgery, are characterized by the progression of interventions initiated during the moderate protection phase, and activity-specific training for return to work or sport function. The aim is to educate the patient to resume full activity slowly while monitoring signs and symptoms. The return to function phase focuses on advanced training for sport or occupational demands.

NOTE: Continued use of patellar taping or a patellar tracking orthosis during exercise may be useful during the progression of exercises and transition to functional activities.

During this phase a self-managed maintenance program and plan for adherence should be developed. Patients usually can return to a full level of activity by 6 to 8 weeks postoperatively.

### Outcomes
As an independent procedure, LRR can be useful for alleviating or reducing patellofemoral pain if the cause of the pain stems from compression of lateral structures of the knee as the result of an excessive lateral tilt of the patella.[70,73,180,188] Comparably favorable outcomes have been reported for arthroscopic and open procedures.[70] Good to excellent short-term reduction of pain and associated patellofemoral symptoms have been reported for 65% to 75% of patients, although it may take 3 to 6 months after surgery to achieve maximum function.[75] Long-term effectiveness of LRR is questionable, especially in patients with a history of patellar instability.[188]

## Proximal Realignment of the Extensor Mechanism

Proximal realignment of the extensor mechanism usually is reserved for the patient with a history of recurrent lateral instability (dislocation/subluxation) of the patella who continues to be symptomatic despite a course of nonoperative management. It is often performed in the skeletally immature patient with patellar instability or in conjunction with distal realignment involving an osteotomy in the skeletally mature patient.[73,95] If performed in isolation, it is not appropriate solely for the management of patellofemoral pain.[73]

### Indications for Surgery
Proximal realignment of the extensor mechanism is indicated for a combination of the following findings.[73,74,95,158,180,188]

- Deficiency (acute injury, chronic laxity) of the medial patellar support structures, in particular the medial patellofemoral ligament, leading to extensor mechanism malalignment and recurrent instability of the patella
- Excessive (or abnormal) lateral tracking of the patella and insufficiency of the VMO

⊙ Painful, lateral compressive forces at the patello-femoral joint and persistent lateral tilt of the patella despite an LRR

⊙ Appropriate realignment option for the skeletally immature patient with patellar instability

CONTRAINDICATIONS: Proximal realignment is not appropriate for patients with articular degeneration of the medial patella, patella alta, or trochlear dysplasia as it may exacerbate or have no impact on symptoms.[73,95]

## Procedures

### Background and Operative Overview

A proximal realignment procedure, which is performed as an open procedure through a medial parapatellar incision after arthroscopic examination of the knee and removal of loose osteochondral fragments, is characterized by a repair or reconstruction (tightening/imbrication) of the medial patellofemoral ligament, often coupled with advancement of the VMO muscle to a more central and distal location to improve its resting length-tension relationship.[73,158,180,188] For the patient with an acute dislocation who does not respond to nonoperative management, direct repair of the medial patellofemoral ligament, rather than reconstruction, often is sufficient.[95]

The medial patellofemoral ligament is repaired or imbricated with nonabsorbable sutures at its patellar or medial epicondylar attachment, depending on the location of damage. Use of an autogenous hamstring or fascia lata graft also has been advocated to reinforce the reconstruction of the medial patellofemoral ligament damaged in an acute dislocation.[49] Sometimes the medial patellotibial and medial patellomeniscal ligaments also must be tightened or repaired.[73,74]

If a lateral release is indicated to restore or maintain the balance of the patella in the trochlea, it is performed arthroscopically. The use of a concomitant soft tissue or bony distal realignment procedure has been advocated in the presence of an abnormally increased Q-angle.[74,158]

### Complications

In addition to complications that can occur with other patellofemoral surgeries, such as hemarthrosis, adhesions, infection, or a DVT, there are complications seen in proximal realignment procedures.[73,126] For example, significant scarring or overtightening of the medial patellofemoral ligament and/or VMO can exacerbate pain caused by increased loads on a medial articular lesion that may have occurred as the result of an acute dislocation. Scarring or overtightening also can cause increased patellar rotation and excessive medial tracking leading to retropatellar erosion or increased risk of *medial* instability of the patella. However, inadequate transfer of the VMO may result in no change in patellar position, tracking, or a patient's symptoms.

Entrapment, irritation, or a neuroma of the saphenous nerve as it passes the adductor tubercle and splits at the pes anserine tendon can occur with procedures involving structures on the medial side of the knee. Reflex sympathetic dystrophy, also referred to as complex regional pain syndrome, occasionally develops (see Chapter 13).[37]

Complications are more likely to occur with an open rather than an arthroscopic realignment procedure.[126] Surgical advances in proximal realignment procedures by arthroscopic intervention have decreased the morbidity of this surgery.

### Postoperative Management

Postoperative rehabilitation after proximal realignment follows a course similar to that seen after LRR (see Table 21.5) with the exception of a longer maximum protection phase and more gradual progression of exercise and weight bearing to allow adequate time for the reconstructed soft tissues to heal (about 5 to 6 weeks).[10,126]

As with postoperative management after LRR and nonoperative management of patellofemoral dysfunction, many of the exercises selected for a patient's rehabilitation traditionally have focused on regaining pain-free ROM, maintaining patellar mobility, and recruiting the quadriceps mechanism as a unit and the VMO in particular. These interventions are designed to prevent or remediate patellar restrictions and an extensor lag (quadriceps lag).[4,10,47,106,126,226,235] Equally important to the success of rehabilitation following repair of the extensor mechanism is remediating deficits in strength, endurance, and flexibility of the trunk, hip and ankle musculature.[100,132,187,189]

### Immobilization and Weight-Bearing Considerations

The knee is immobilized in a range-limiting, hinged orthosis or a posterior splint in full or nearly full extension to protect the reconstructed soft tissues. Some surgeons allow removal of the immobilizer for early ROM in a protected range within a few days after surgery or while wearing the hinged orthosis,[126] whereas others advocate continuous immobilization for a week postoperatively.[10,95,126,188]

During ambulation with crutches, the knee immobilizer should be locked in extension. Either no weight or touch-down/toe-touch weight bearing is permitted on the operated extremity for the first 10 to 14 days postoperatively, followed by gradual progression to 75% weight bearing by 4 weeks. Full weight bearing without assistive devices should be achieved by weeks 8 to 10 but only in the absence of an extensor lag.[126,188]

### Exercise Progression

Refer to goals and interventions for LRR (see Table 21.5), but progress exercises to increase the range of knee flexion and to improve strength and muscular endurance more gradually than after LRR. Too rapid progression after extensor mechanism realignment may cause suture failure in the approximated soft tissues leading to an inability to control patellar position.[126]

Goals, a progression of exercise interventions, and criteria to advance from one phase of rehabilitation to the next after proximal realignment procedures are summarized in the following sections.[74,126] Exercise precautions after proximal and distal extensor realignment procedures are noted in Box 21.7.[10,95,126]

---

**BOX 21.7    Exercise Precautions after Proximal or Distal Realignment of the Extensor Mechanism**

- Initiate A-AROM and AROM exercises in a hinged, range-limiting orthosis to prevent excessive knee flexion or a valgus stress to the knee.
- Progress knee flexion gradually so as not to disrupt sutures after advancement of the VMO or medial transfer of the patellar tendon and tibial tubercle.
- When assisting with supine-lying hip and knee flexion/extension ROM, stand on the contralateral side of the operated extremity to avoid placing a valgus stress on the knee and stretching repaired medial structures.
- To protect the medial structures during the initial phase of healing after a proximal repair, use patellar taping to maintain the patella in a central or slightly medial position during quadriceps training.
- Postpone unilateral closed-chain exercises that involve full weight bearing on the operated side for at least 4 to 6 weeks after soft tissue reconstruction and for at least 8 weeks or until radiographic healing has occcured after a distal realignment involving a bony procedure.
- Do not perform a maximum voluntary contraction (MVC) of the quadriceps for at least 12 weeks after proximal or distal realignment procedures.

---

### Exercise: Maximum Protection Phase

**Goals.** During the first 4 weeks after surgery, goals are to control pain and swelling, prevent adhesions, regain mobility and muscle control, and establish a home exercise program while protecting the reconstructed soft tissues.

**Interventions.** While symptoms are acute, apply cold intermittently. Limit weight bearing and the range of knee motion permissible and include the following interventions while the reconstructed extensor mechanism is most vulnerable to excessive stresses.

- **ROM.** Perform knee flexion/extension exercises (A-AROM and AROM) in the range-limiting orthosis from 0° to 60° during the first 2 weeks, to 90° by end of week 3, and to 110° to 120° by end of week 4.[74,126] Stretch hip and ankle musculature, if restricted.
- **Joint mobility.** Use gentle (grade I and II) joint mobilizations of the patellofemoral and tibiofemoral joints to decrease pain and prevent adhesions.
- **Muscle performance.** Begin isometrics for quadriceps control and active superior patellar gliding with emphasis on VMO activation augmented with neuromuscular electrical muscle stimulation or biofeedback. While wearing the knee immobilizer, initiate SLRs in supine, prone, and side-lying positions for hip control. Also, begin partial-range heel-slides in the supine position.

**Criteria to advance to next phase.** Criteria include minimal pain, full active knee extension, and 110° to 120° of knee flexion.

### Exercise: Moderate Protection Phase: 4 to 8 Weeks

**Goals.** During the second phase of rehabilitation, goals are to attain unassisted, pain-free ambulation, full active knee flexion/extension, increase flexibility of hip and ankle structures if restricted, increase strength and endurance of lower extremity and trunk musculature, improve balance, and progress and reinforce the home exercise program.

**Interventions.** As symptoms subside, and the patient gradually places full weight on the operated extremity, the following interventions are appropriate.

- **ROM and joint mobility.** Begin low-intensity, prolonged stretching and grade III joint mobilization to increase ROM of restricted areas.
- **Muscle performace and balance.** Initiate pain-free, closed-chain and open-chain resistance training to increase strength and endurance in the entire lower extremity and proprioceptive training to improve balance control. Perform resisted exercises only in pain-free ranges and in positions consistent with weight-bearing precautions.

**Criteria to advance to next phase.** No swelling or extensor lag, pain-free functional ROM of the knee (0° to 135°), 4/5 strength of knee musculature.[126]

### Exercise: Minimum Protection/Return to Function Phases: Beyond 8 to 10 Weeks

**Goals.** The goals of the final phases of rehabilitation are to participate in gradually more demanding activities without recurrence of pain, patellar instability, or joint effusion and to return to a full level of activity without symptoms by 14 to 20 weeks postoperatively with modification of some activities, as necessary.

**Interventions.** Emphasize activity-specific training. Efforts should be made to modify the patient's lifestyle to avoid symptom-provoking activities at least on a temporary basis.

Refer to the exercise progression previously discussed for advanced nonoperative management and the selected exercises described in the final sections of this chapter.

---

**Outcomes**

Outcomes for proximal realignment of the extensor mechanism vary considerably among studies with most involving a combination of lateral release or distal realignment with proximal realignment. However, in a retrospective case series Drez and co-investigators[49] reported the use of medial patellofemoral ligament reconstruction with a soft tissue graft (and no distal realignment) in 15 patients with recurrent lateral instability after patellar dislocation. At a mean follow-up of 31.5 months (minimum of 2 years), 93% of patients had excellent results (10 patients) or good results (3 patients) on an objective functional outcome and patient satisfaction scale. Only 1 of the 15 patients reported one episode of subluxation during the follow-up period.

Poor results reported in the literature appear to be due more to retropatellar pain than to recurrent instability.[95] Patients with generalized joint hypomobility or uncorrected trochlear dysplasia tend to have a high rate of redislocation.[74]

## Distal Realignment of the Extensor Mechanism

For a patient with recurrent subluxation/dislocation of the patella with or without degeneration of the lateral and distal articular surfaces of the patella, distal realignment of the extensor mechanism may be the surgical intervention of choice. A medial transfer and possibly anteriorization of the tibial tubercle decreases laterally directed forces on the patella to improve patellar tracking and shifts contact stresses in a medial and proximal direction away from chondral lesions of the distal and lateral articular surface of the patella.[72] Distal realignment procedures often are coupled with an LRR and sometimes with advancement of the VMO and repair of medial structures.[74,158]

### Indications for Surgery
The following are indications for distal realignment procedures.[72,73,145,158,180,188]

- Recurrent episodes of patellar instability (dislocation/subluxation) and a sense of the knee "giving way" because of patellar malalignment due to lateralization of the tibial tubercle and patellar tendon insertion that cannot be corrected with LRR and proximal realignment procedures.
- Abnormally increased Q-angle.
- Patellofemoral arthrosis (chondral or osteochondral defects) on the lateral and distal retropatellar surfaces

C O N T R A I N D I C A T I O N : Bony procedures are not recommended for the skeletally immature patient whose tibial tubercle growth plate is open. Recurvatum of the knee can develop with premature closure of this epiphyseal plate.[72,95,158]

### Procedures

**Background and Operative Overview**
The purpose of distal realignment procedures is to transfer the patellar tendon medially to reduce the Q-angle and improve patellar tracking by decreasing the laterally directed moment.[72,73,180,188] Distal realignment procedures are performed using an open surgical approach. However, examination of the knee joint and débridement of the articular surface of the patella typically precede the distal realignment procedure.

Several techniques of distal realignment have been reported. An osteotomy of the tibial tubercle is performed; the bony prominence is then transferred medially and secured with single-screw or double-screw fixation.[72,74] Anteriorization (elevation) of the tibial tubercle serves to reduce shear forces and articular stresses on the patella.[72,188] The procedure involves anteriorly displacing the tibial tubercle by means of a bone graft.[188] For the skeletally immature patient, a distal medialization procedure involves only a soft tissues transfer. When the patellar tendon and tibial tubercle are reattached, often the knee is flexed 30° to prevent overtightening the quadriceps mechanism.[158]

### Complications
Uncommon but serious complications associated with distal realignment procedures include tibial fracture during placement of fixation screws, neurovascular injury during surgery, inadequate skin closure or sloughing over the osteotomy site, soft tissue infection or osteomyelitis, and nonunion of the transposed bone.[72,188] Redislocation can occur laterally because of undercorrection or medially with overcorrection, particularly in patients who return to high-demand activities.[72,158]

Pain at the anterior tibial tubercle from the fixation screws is not unusual. Therefore, screws are removed routinely 6 to 12 months after surgery.[72] As with all patellofemoral surgeries, patellar adhesions can occur, restricting knee motion. Because distal realignment shifts retropatellar loads medially and proximally, arthrosis in these areas also can develop over time, causing knee pain.

### Postoperative Management
Depending on the type of fixation used, rehabilitation after distal realignment involving bony procedures may progress even more gradually than rehabilitation following LRR and proximal realignment of soft tissues to allow time for bony healing. Ambulation with crutches while wearing a knee immobilizer locked in extension is permissible the day after surgery. Weight bearing is limited to touch-down/toe-touch for the first 4 weeks or until radiographic verification of bone callus formation at the osteotomy site has occurred.[10,72,126] Weight bearing is progressed gradually, with full weight bearing permissible without the immobilizer at 8 weeks if quadriceps control is sufficient.[126]

ROM also is progressed more gradually than after soft tissue procedures. (Refer to exercise precautions noted in Box 21.7.) A range-limiting orthosis is worn that allows motion from only 0° to 30°[126] or 0° to 60°[74] of flexion during the first week, to 90° of flexion by the end of week 4, and 135° (full knee flexion) by the end of week 8.[126] Otherwise, exercises are similar to those for nonoperative management, LRR, and proximal realignment procedures. The return to full activity generally takes about 5 to 6 months and is based on bone healing and lower extremity strength.

### Outcomes
Successful outcomes after distal realignment surgeries for patellar instability, possibly associated with chronic knee pain from chondral lesions, are contingent on correctly determining the underlying causes of the patient's symptoms. Patients without degeneration of the retropatellar surface or those with lateral and distal lesions tend to have better results than those with medial articular lesions.[145]

Often distal realignment procedures are coupled with a proximal repair and/or lateral release to correct malalignment and relieve symptoms. Results of studies of combined procedures reflect good to excellent outcomes for most patients measured by one or more objective assessment tools. For example, Garth and colleagues[74] studied a group of young adults (mean age 18 years) with recurrent patellar instability despite a course of conservative management after sustaining an acute, traumatic, lateral dislocation of the patella. After undergoing distal realignment coupled with repair of the medial patellofemoral ligament and advancement of the patellomeniscal ligament, 90% (18/20) patients reported good to excellent results in knee function and patient satisfaction and no recurrence of symptoms at a minimum follow-up of 24 months. The results of another study in which three procedures were performed (lateral release, repair of medial supporting structures, and distal realignment) revealed that 32 of 42 knees (76%) in 37 patients had good or excellent outcomes at follow-up a mean of 44 months (minimum follow-up 25 months, range 25 to 85 months). At the time of follow-up, redislocation had occurred in four knees (9.5%).

 # LIGAMENT INJURIES: NONOPERATIVE MANAGEMENT

## Mechanisms of Injury

Ligament injuries occur most frequently in individuals between 20 and 40 years of age as the result of sport injuries (e.g., skiing, soccer, football) but can occur in individuals of all ages. The anterior cruciate ligament (ACL) is the most commonly injured ligament. Often more than one ligament is damaged as the result of a single injury.

### Anterior Cruciate Ligament

Anterior cruciate ligament (ACL) injuries occur from both contact and noncontact mechanisms. The most common contact mechanism is a blow to the lateral side of the knee resulting in a valgus force to the knee. This mechanism can result in injury not only to the ACL but to the medial collateral ligament (MCL) and the medial meniscus as well. This injury is termed the "unholy triad" injury because of the frequency of these three structures being injured from a common blow. The most common noncontact mechanism is a rotational mechanism in which the tibia is externally rotated on the planted foot. Literature supports that this mechanism can account for up to 78% of all ACL injuries.[165] The second most common noncontact mechanism is forceful hyperextension of the knee.

With prolonged ambulation on a knee that has a deficient ACL, the secondary restraints (lateral collateral ligament and posterolateral joint capsule) are stressed and become lax, and the individual may develop a "quadriceps avoidance gait."[92] The quadriceps avoidance gait in ACL-deficient knees was originally documented and described by Berchuck and collegues[11] as a reduction in the magnitude of the flexion moment about the knee during the limb loading phase of gait due to the patient's effort to reduce contraction of the quadriceps.

### Posterior Cruciate Ligament

The posterior cruciate ligament (PCL) is most commonly injured by a forceful blow to the anterior tibia while the knee is flexed, such as a blow to the dashboard or falling onto a flexed knee.

### Medial Collateral Ligament

Isolated injuries to the medial collateral ligament (MCL) can occur from valgus forces being placed across the medial joint line of the knee. Whereas most injuries to the ACL and PCL are complete tears of the ligament, injuries to the MCL can be partial or incomplete and are graded utilizing a I, II, III grading classification of ligament injuries described in Chapter 10.

### Lateral Collateral Ligament

Injuries to the lateral collateral ligament (LCL) are infrequent and usually result from a traumatic varus force across the knee. It is not uncommon that more than one ligament, joint capsule, and sometimes the menisci are damaged as the result of a single injury.

## Ligament Injuries in the Female Athlete

With an increase in the number of female athletes since the passage of Title IX in 1972, a concurrent increase in the number of injuries to female athletes has been seen, most significantly an increase in the number of knee injuries. What is interesting is that when injury to the ACL is sustained in a noncontact manner, a woman is three times more likely to tear the ACL than a man.[5] With the increased number of noncontact ACL injuries in female athletes being reported, the American Academy of Orthopaedic Surgeons published a consensus paper examining the risk factors and prevention strategies of noncontact ACL injuries.[82] In addition, results from a research retreat on "ACL Injuries—The Gender Bias" were published in the *Journal of Orthopaedic and Sports Physical Therapy*.[41] Risk factors fall into four major categories: environmental, anatomical, hormonal, and biomechanical.

- *Environmental factors* center on the use of prophylactic knee braces to prevent knee injuries and a shoe-to-surface interface that may improve performance but may also increase the risk of injury.
- *Anatomical risk factors* include femoral notch size, ACL size, and lower extremity alignment. Insufficient data relating to each of these factors have resulted in an incomplete understanding of the influence of these factors at this time.
- *Hormonal differences* between males and females have also been postulated to be one possible factor related to the increased incidence of female ACL injuries. In 1996, hormone receptor sites for estrogen and progesterone were found in the ACL of humans. Since that time, research has been conducted to study the effects of such hormones on the mechanical properties of the ACL and other musculoskeletal tissues. To date, however, results of multiple studies differ in their conclusions.

- *Biomechanical risk factors* summarized by the consensus panel[82] included the effect of the total chain (trunk, hip, knee, and ankle) on ACL injuries, awkward or improper dynamic body movements, deceleration and change of direction, and neuromuscular control of the joint.

## Common Impairments and Functional Limitations/Disabilities

- Following trauma, the joint usually does not swell for several hours. If blood vessels are torn, swelling is usually immediate.
- If tested when the joint is not swollen, the patient feels pain when the injured ligament is stressed.
- If there is a complete tear, instability is detected when the torn ligament is tested.
- When swollen, motion is restricted, the joint assumes a position of minimum stress (usually flexed 25°), and inhibition (shut down) of the quadriceps muscle occurs.[225]
- When acute, the knee cannot bear weight, and the person cannot ambulate without an assistive device.
- With a complete tear, there is instability, and the knee may give way during weight bearing.

## Ligament Injuries: Nonoperative Management

Acute sprains and partial ligament tears of the knee can be treated conservatively with rest, joint protection, and exercise. After the acute stage of healing, exercises should be geared toward regaining normal ROM, balance control, normalization of gait, and strengthening of muscles that support and stabilize the joint during functional activities. The degree of instability with ligament tears affects the demands the patient can place on the knee when returning to full activity. An intensive rehabilitation program, including balance/perturbation training to stimulate neuromuscular control, has been shown to be effective in selected athletes after ACL injury.[63,64] With extensive damage and in general for those desiring to return to high-level work or sports, surgical repair often is necessary for return to a desired level of function.

If the collateral or coronary ligaments are involved, because of their superficial location cross-fiber massage to the structure helps align the healing fibers and maintain their mobility. Because of the structural characteristics of the MCL (a broad, flat ligament with deep and superficial portions, parallel alignment of collagen fibers, and fan-shaped attachments both proximally and distally), injuries to the MCL are typically managed with a conservative (nonsurgical) approach.[251] Conservative management of MCL injuries is described in Table 21.6; progression is based on presenting signs and symptoms.[167] A similar rehabilitation program for ACL injuries is followed with appropriate precautions (as noted below) regarding stress to the the ligament.

### Nonoperative Management: Maximum Protection Phase
Follow the principles described for an acute joint lesion.

- If possible, examine before effusion sets in.
- Utilize cold and compression with rest and elevation.
- Protect the joint during ambulation with use of crutches; partial weight bearing as tolerated. Teach safe transfer activities to avoid pivoting on the involved extremity.
- Initiate quadriceps-setting exercises. The knee may not fully extend for end-range muscle-setting exercises, so begin the exercises in the range most comfortable for the patient. As the swelling decreases, initiate ROM within tolerance.

### Nonoperative Management: Moderate Protection (Controlled Motion) Through Return to Activity
As the swelling decreases, examine the patient for impairments and functional losses. Initiate joint movement and exercises to improve muscle performance, functional status, and cardiopulmonary conditioning.

**Improve Joint Mobility and Protection**

*Joint mobility.* Use supine wall slides (see Fig. 21.14), patellar mobilizations, and stationary cycling; encourage as much movement as possible. Unless there has been an extended period of immobilization, there should be minimal need to stretch contractures.

*Protective bracing.* Bracing may be necessary for weight-bearing activities to decrease stress to the healing ligament or to provide stability where ligament integrity has been compromised. Bracing can be one of two types: range-limiting postoperative type braces that are used to protect healing tissues and discarded during later phases of rehabilitation or functional braces that are used during rehabilitation and also when returning to functional activities. The patient must be advised to modify activities until appropriate stability is obtained.

**Improve Muscle Performance and Function**

*Strength and endurance.* Initiate isometric quadriceps and hamstring exercises and progress to dynamic strength and muscular endurance training. Neuromuscular control is compromised when stabilizing muscles fatigue.[94]

- Utilize both open-chain and closed-chain resistance. Reinforce quadriceps contractions with high-intensity electrical stimulation if there is an extensor lag.[222] Progress muscular endurance and strengthening exercises using partial squats, step-ups, leg press, and heel-raises
- Emphasize neuromuscular control with stabilization and perturbation training in weight-bearing positions.

PRECAUTIONS: Open-chain terminal knee extension exercises (from 40° to 0°) with resistance applied to the distal leg and squatting between 60° and 90° cause increased anterior translation of the tibia and stress to the ACL. Exercises using either of these activities in the designated ranges should not be attempted with ACL injuries.[82,250,253] Teach the patient closed-chain strengthening activities from 60° to 0° and open-chain strengthening from 90° to 40°.[253] Isolated open-chain knee flexion exercises (hamstring curls)

**TABLE 21.6  Nonoperative Management of MCL Injuries—Intervention for Each Phase of Rehabilitation***

| Phase and General Time Frame | Maximum Protection Phase: Weeks 1–3 | Moderate Protection Phase: Weeks 3–6 | Minimum Protection Phase: Weeks 5–8 | Return to Activity Phase: Weeks 6–10 |
|---|---|---|---|---|
| Patient presentation | • Joint effusion<br>• Pinpoint tenderness<br>• Decreased ROM | • Minimal tenderness<br>• Joint effusion controlled<br>• No increased instability<br>• Full of nearly full ROM | • No instability<br>• No effusion of tenderness<br>• 4/5 to 5/5 strength (MMT)<br>• Unrestricted ADL function | • No instability<br>• Muscle function 70% of noninvolved extremity<br>• No symptoms of instability, pain, or swelling during the previous phase |
| Key examination procedures | • Pain scale<br>• Joint effusion<br>• Ligament stability<br>• ROM<br>• Muscle control<br>• Functional status<br>• Patellar mobility | • Pain scale<br>• Joint effusion<br>• Ligament stability<br>• ROM<br>• Muscle control/strength<br>• Functional status | • Ligament stability<br>• Muscle control<br>• Functional status | • Full clinical examination<br>• Ligament stability<br>• Muscle strength<br>• Functional status |
| Goals | • Protect healing tissues<br>• Prevent reflex inhibition of muscle<br>• Decrease joint effusion<br>• Decrease pain<br>• Establish home exercise program | • Full pain-free ROM<br>• Restore muscular strength<br>• Normalize gait without assistive device<br>• Normalize ADL function<br>• Adherence to home program | • Increase strength<br>• Increase power<br>• Increase endurance<br>• Improve neuromuscular control<br>• Improve dynamic stability | • Increase strength<br>• Increase power<br>• Increase endurance<br>• Regain ability to function at highest desired level<br>• Transition to maintenance program |
| Interventions | • PRICE (ice, compression, elevation, and protective bracing)<br>• Ambulation training with crutches; weight bearing as tolerated<br>• PROM/A-AROM<br>• Patellar mobilization (grades I and II)<br>• Muscle setting quadriceps, hamstrings, and adductors (may augment with E-stim)<br>• SLRs<br>• Aerobic conditioning | • Continue multiple-angle isometrics<br>• Initiate PRE<br>• Closed-chain strengthening<br>• LE flexibility exercises<br>• Endurance training (e.g., bike, pool, ski machine)<br>• Perturbation/balance training<br>• Stabilization exercises<br>• Initiate a walk/jog program at the end of this phase<br>• Initiate skill specific drills at the end of this phase | • Continue LE flexibility<br>• Advance PRE strengthening<br>• Advance closed-chain exercises<br>• Advance perturbation training<br>• Advance endurance training<br>• Isokinetic training (if available)<br>• Progress running program; full speed jog, sprints, figure-eight running and cutting | • Continue flexibility and strengthening; advance as appropriate<br>• Advance agility drills<br>• Advance running drills<br>• Advance perturbation drills<br>• Implement drills specific to sport or occupation<br>• Determine need for protective bracing prior to return to sport or work |

*Note: this is based on grade II ligament injury but may be accelerated for grade I or decelerated for grade III injuries

Adapted from Wilk and Clancy,[251] with permission.

increase posterior translation of the tibia and should not be done with PCL injuries.

***Cardiopulmonary conditioning.*** Utilize a program that is consistent with the patient's goals such as biking (begin with a stationary bike), jogging (begin with walking on a treadmill), ski machine, or swimming.

***Functional training.*** Progress neuromuscular training. Develop activity-specific drills that replicate the demands of the individual's outcome goals.[240] Suggestions for functional training are described in the exercise section of this chapter.

 **Focus on Evidence** _____

In a randomized controlled study, 26 level I or level II athletes with an acute ACL injury or rupture of ACL grafts participated in a standard rehabilitation program or a standard rehabilitation program with perturbation training.[63] Of those in the perturbation group (*n* = 12), only one had unsuccessful rehabilitation, with the knee giving way while playing football prior to completing the program. In the control group (no perturbation training; *n* = 14) one-half of the subjects had unsuccessful outcomes and were considered at high risk for reinjury at the 6-month follow-up examination. The authors stated that although both groups returned to high-level physical activities those in the perturbation training group demonstrated greater long-term success.[63]

 ## LIGAMENT INJURIES: SURGICAL AND POSTOPERATIVE MANAGEMENT

### Background

Ligaments of the knee provide the key stabilizing forces for accessory motions of the knee (see Fig. 21.2). Specifically, these accessory motions are anterior and posterior translation and medial/lateral pivots (valgus/varus/rotation). Strong ligamentous support is necessary, in part, because of the shallow design of the concave tibial articulating surface that allows significant translatory motions if unrestrained. Acute traumatic disruption or chronic laxity of the ligaments results in excessive accessory motions of the joint, which can impair functional abilities.[26,68,146] Although injuries to each of the four primary knee ligaments (ACL, PCL, MCL, LCL) are discussed extensively in the literature, the ACL is, by far, the most frequently injured and surgically repaired.[15,165]

Factors influencing the decision for surgical reconstruction of a knee ligament include the ligament injured (differences in healing capacities among ligaments), the location and size of the lesion, the degree of instability experienced by the patient, the presence of other pathology such as a meniscal or articular damage, the desired level of function to which the patient wishes to return, and the risk of reinjury.[12,60,108,146,233] Prevention of future impairment is

also a consideration because acute ligament injury can lead to chronic instability and degeneration of joint structures over time if not managed and monitored adequately.[15]

***General indications for ligament surgery.*** Surgical intervention for ligament injury is indicated if the patient has failed to meet functional goals established in a conservative rehabilitation program or early degenerative changes of the joint are apparent. Many authors[15,26,69,146,213,233] recommend surgical intervention for acute, isolated ACL and LCL injuries after a brief period of acute symptom management in recreationally active individuals. Surgical management of chronic ligament injuries is advocated when the patient's function has become limited or when secondary pathology (e.g., meniscus damage, other ligament involvement, articular surface degeneration) has developed.

***Types of ligament surgery.*** Ligament surgeries are classified as *intra-articular*, *extra-articular*, or combined procedures and can be performed using an open, arthroscopically assisted, or endoscopic approach.[26,115,146] Prior to the development and refinement of arthroscopy, an open approach involving a large incision and arthrotomy was the only option available for surgically managing a ligament injury.

The first type of intra-articular procedure was a *direct repair* through an open approach. The repair was accomplished by reopposing and suturing the torn ligament. Postoperatively, a long period of immobilization and restricted weight bearing were required because of extensive tissue disruption associated with the open approach and the poor healing qualities of ligamentous tissue.[115] Results of this procedure were unacceptable due to postimmobilization contractures, patellofemoral dysfunction, weakness, and an unacceptably high incidence of rerupture. Consequently, use of direct repair was abandoned as procedures involving intra-articular or extra-articular *reconstruction* were developed.

Intra-articular reconstruction of ligament injuries, which has evolved over the past four decades, has become the primary means by which ACL and PCL injuries are managed surgically. In general terms, reconstruction involves the use of a tissue graft to replicate the function of the damaged ligament and act as an inert restraint of the knee.[16,26,115,129,146,162,233] Early reconstruction procedures were performed through an open approach. Although open reconstruction restored knee stability, the need for lengthy postoperative immobilization continued.[115] Today, intra-articular ligament reconstruction is performed through an arthroscopically assisted or an endoscopic approach, causing far less tissue morbidity and resulting in a faster postoperative recovery.

N O T E : Overviews of intra-articular ACL and PCL reconstruction procedures are described in this chapter.

Extra-articular reconstruction procedures, which involve the transposition of dynamic musculotendinous stabilizers or inert restraints around the knee, such as the IT band, were designed to provide external stability to the knee joint. Extra-articular procedures, in common use in the past, particularly for MCL and LCL injuries, are used rarely today as primary procedures because they do not restore normal kinematics to the knee as effectively as intra-articular procedures. Use of extra-articular procedures to augment intra-articular reconstruction in difficult cases also has been shown to have little benefit.[115]

***Grafts: types, healing characteristics, and fixation.*** Intra-articular reconstruction is achieved through the use of tissue grafts, most often an *autograft* (the patient's own tissue) or occasionally an *allograft* (donor tissue) or a *synthetic graft*.[109,115,143,162] An allograft or synthetic graft is used only when a suitable autogenous graft is not available, for example when a patient's own tissue is not suitable for graft harvesting.[115,162] However, there is concern that remodeling and incorporation of the graft after implantation may be slower with an allograft (possibly due to sterilization to prevent disease transmission) or a synthetic graft than with an autograft.[143] (Refer to Chapter 12 and Box 12.7 for additional information about tissue grafts.)

Although a variety of tissues have been used for knee ligament reconstruction,[109,117,129,143,150,162] a bone–patellar tendon–bone autograft has been used reliably and has been considered the gold standard for ACL reconstruction for several decades.[117,166] It remains the most frequently selected graft material for this procedure.[16,26,60,68,109,117,129,146] A frequently selected alternative to a patellar tendon graft for ACL reconstruction is a semitendinosus–gracilis tendon graft.[115,117,150,209,234] Research has shown that the strength and stiffness of a bone–patellar tendon–bone graft and a quadrupled (four-strand) hamstring tendon graft are actually greater than that of the ACL ligament.[209]

An extensive body of knowledge exists on graft healing, placement, and fixation as well as the strength and stiffness of various tissues selected as grafts and their responses to imposed loads. Most research has focused on grafts for ACL reconstruction.[16,24,68,91,108,117,219] Because the characteristics of grafts and graft fixation affect the rehabilitation process and the outcome of surgery, it is important to understand that a graft undergoes a series of changes after implantation as it heals. Initially, there is a period of avascular necrosis during which the graft loses substantial strength. This period is followed by a period of revascularization, then remodeling, and finally maturation, which typically takes at least 1 year. During the first 6 to 8 weeks postoperatively the graft is most vulnerable to excessive loads because the strength of the graft is derived solely from the fixation device, not the graft itself.[16,24,108,109]

The need for a long postoperative period of immobilization and protected weight bearing after ligament reconstruction has been eliminated following primary ACL reconstruction for some time because of advances in graft selection, preparation, placement and fixation, and the evolution of arthroscopic techniques.[16,24,219] Nevertheless, there is still a need to select and progress the stresses imposed on the healing graft carefully during early rehabilitation.

***Goals of ligament surgery and rehabilitation.*** The goals of surgery and postoperative rehabilitation after ligament reconstruction are (1) restoration of joint stability and motion, (2) pain-free and stable weight bearing, (3) sufficient postoperative strength and endurance to meet functional demands, and (4) the ability to return to preinjury activities.

To meet these goals, successful postoperative outcomes start whenever possible with a *preoperative* program that includes edema control, exercise to minimize atrophy and maintain as much ROM as possible, protected ambulation, and patient education.[45,183,211,253] Preoperative intervention is often possible because ligament reconstruction typically is delayed until acute symptoms subside. Exercises are similar to those used for the acute phase of nonoperative management of ligament injuries already discussed. Preoperative exercises should not further irritate the injured tissues or cause additional swelling or pain.

The *rate* and *progression* of postoperative rehabilitation programs vary; and no one program has been shown to be most effective or most efficient. Emphasis is placed on restoring a patient's functional abilities while protecting the healing graft and preventing postoperative complications and reinjury. Early controlled motion and weight bearing, hallmarks of current-day rehabilitation, have been shown to decrease the incidence of postoperative complications, such as contracture, patellofemoral pain, and muscle atrophy,[183,211,214,253] and to allow patients to return to activity more quickly without compromising the integrity of the reconstructed ligament.[214]

For more than a decade there has been a move away from adherence to strict time-based rehabilitation protocols toward guidelines that are progressed based on the attainment of specific criteria and measurable goals or performance on functional tests.[45,52,90,125,127,157,167,253] For example, an exercise program is progressed only after full active knee extension has been achieved or arthrometer testing indicates that a particular level of joint stability is present. Open communication with the surgeon enables the therapist to discuss any precautions or concerns specific to individual patients and procedures.

## Anterior Cruciate Ligament Reconstruction

Unlike the MCL, which heals readily with nonoperative management, the healing capacity of a torn ACL is poor, giving rise to the frequent need for surgical reconstruction to restore knee stability, particularly in the young, active individual.[108] The incidence of reinjury of the knee is lower after ACL reconstruction than with nonoperative management, particularly in patients younger than 25 years of age.[50]

### Indications for Surgery
Although there are no rigid criteria for patient selection, the most frequently cited indications for reconstruction of the anterior cruciate ligament include the following.[15,26,129,146,150,162]

- Disabling instability of the knee due to ACL deficiency caused by a complete or partial acute tear or chronic laxity
- Frequent episodes of the knee giving way (buckling) during routine ADLs despite a course of nonoperative management
- A positive pivot-shift test because an ACL deficit is often associated with a lesion of other structures of the knee, such as the MCL, resulting in rotatory instability of the joint
- Injury of the MCL at the time of ACL injury to prevent lax healing of the MCL
- High risk of reinjury because of participation in high-demand, high-joint-load activities related to work, sports, or recreational activities

NOTE: Increased anterior translation of the tibia on the femur compared with the contralateral, noninvolved knee, as measured by an arthrometer, is considered a questionable indication because a strong correlation between these measurements of stability and a patient's symptoms of instability has not been established.[15]

CONTRAINDICATIONS: Relative, not absolute, contraindications for ACL reconstruction are noted im Box 21.8.[15,26,129,150]

## Procedures

### Operative Overview

***Surgical approach, graft selection, and harvesting.*** Over the past 20 years, surgical management of the deficient ACL has evolved and continues to be refined with a move away from entirely open reconstruction to most procedures now using arthroscopically assisted or endoscopic techniques to reduce tissue morbidity and reduce recovery time.[15,16,58,115] In an arthroscopically assisted approach only the intra-articular portions of the procedure, such as meniscus débridement or repair, enlargement of the intra-condylar notch of the femur, or drilling the femoral and tibial bone tunnels, are performed arthroscopically.[115]

The most common ACL reconstruction procedure today is an arthroscopically assisted or endoscopic procedure using an autograft. If a bone–patellar tendon–bone

graft is selected, it is harvested through a small, longitudinal incision over the patellar tendon from the patient's involved knee[17,26,60,129,146] or occasionally from the contralateral knee.[213] The central one-third portion of the tendon is dissected along with small bone plugs attached to the tendon. If a semitendinosus–gracilis tendon autograft (hamstring tendon graft) is selected, it is harvested through an incision centered over the tibial insertion of the semitendinosus and gracilis tendons.[58,150,209,216,219,234]

There are a number of advantages, disadvantages, and potential complications associated with bone–patellar tendon–bone and hamstring tendon autografts. For example, transition from mechanical fixation to biological fixation is thought to occur more rapidly with a patellar tendon graft, which involves bone-to-bone healing, than a hamstring tendon graft, which requires tendon-to-bone healing (6 to 8 weeks versus 12 weeks, respectively).[219] Other reported advantages and disadvantages of these two types of autografts are summarized in Boxes 21.9 and 21.10.[1,58,115,117,198,209,216,234] It should be noted, however, that recently the use of a bone–hamstring tendon–bone autograft for ACL reconstruction was reported, allowing bone-to-bone healing and affording some of the same advantages associated with a bone–patellar tendon–bone autograft.[133]

***Graft placement and fixation.*** After the graft is harvested and prepared for implantation, the arthroscopic instrumentation is reinserted to drill femoral and tibial bone tunnels.[16,69,115,129] Graft placement is achieved by passing the graft through the tunnels to its final position in the tibia and femur. Precise, anatomical graft placement is crucial for restoration of joint stability and mobility.[91] Improper graft placement can lead to loss of ROM postoperatively.[1] A graft placed too far posteriorly may result in failure to

---

### BOX 21.8 Relative Contraindications to ACL Reconstruction

- Relatively inactive individual with little to no exposure to work, sport, and recreational activities that place high demands on the knee
- Ability to make lifestyle modifications to eliminate high-risk activities
- Ability to cope with infrequent episodes of instability
- Advanced arthritis of the knee
- Poor likelihood of complying with postoperative restrictions and adhering to a rehabilitation program

---

### BOX 21.9 Advantages and Disadvantages/Complications of the Bone–Patellar Tendon–Bone Autograft

**Advantages**
- High tensile strength/stiffness, similar or greater than the ACL
- Secure and reliable bone-to-bone graft fixation with interference screws
- Rapid revascularization/biological fixation (6 weeks) at the bone-to-bone interface permitting safe, accelerated rehabilitation
- Ability to return to preinjury, high-demand activities safely

**Disadvantages/Potential Complications**
- Anterior knee pain in area of graft harvest site
- Pain during kneeling
- Extensor mechanism/patellofemoral dysfunction
- Long-term quadriceps muscle weakness
- Patellar fracture during graft harvest (rare, but significant adverse effects)
- Patellar tendon rupture (rare)

**Advantages and Disadvantages/ Complications of the Semitendinosus– Gracilis Autograft**

**Advantages**
- High tensile strength/stiffness greater than ACL with quadrupled graft
- No disturbance of epiphyseal plate in skeletally immature patient
- Evidence of hamstring tendon regeneration at donor site
- Loss of knee flexor muscle strength remediated by 2 years postoperatively

**Disadvantages/Potential Complications**
- Tendon-to-bone fixation devices (particularly tibial fixation) not as reliable as bone-to-bone fixation
- Longer healing time (12 weeks) at tendon-bone interface
- Hamstring muscle strain during early rehabilitation
- Short- and long-term knee flexor muscle weakness (not associated with functional limitation)
- Possible increased anterior knee translation (not associated with functional limitations)

regain full flexion, and a graft placed too far anteriorly may limit extension.[24]

N O T E : Limited ROM into extension also may be caused by graft impingement due to an inadequate femoral notch size or buildup of scar tissue in the notch.[1] A *femoral notchplasty* (enlargement of the intercondylar notch) is performed to ensure adequate clearance of the graft as the knee extends.

Graft fixation is vital to the success of ACL reconstruction. With a bone–patellar tendon–bone graft, the bone plugs are secured at each end in the prepared tunnels (bone-to-bone fixation) by means of screw fixation (metal or bioabsorbale interference screws).[24,26,69,117,129,219] Several types of soft tissue fixation device have been used to secure a hamstring tendon graft, including endobuttons, washers, and staples. Recently, several types of soft tissue screw (interference and transfixation) have been introduced.[24,58,115,150,209] Despite these advances, strong tendon–bone fixation, particularly tibial fixation, remains a challenge.

An advantage of current-day fixation devices is that they can withstand early, but controlled, tensile forces placed across the graft with a low risk of compromising the security of the graft itself provided proper placement and fit of the fixation devices are achieved.[16,24,58] This, in turn, permits early initiation of weight bearing and ROM of the knee, both typical elements of today's accelerated rehabilitation programs.[90,127,209,214,253]

After graft fixation and prior to closure, the knee is moved through the ROM to check the graft's integrity and the tension on the graft during knee movement. As with graft placement, proper graft tension at the time of fixation has a direct effect on postoperative joint mobility and stability. Too little tension can result in excessive knee laxity and potential instability, and too much tension can limit knee ROM.[16] After the incision is closed, a small compression dressing is immediately placed on the knee, and often the leg is placed in a knee immobilizer for protecion.

**Complications**
There are a number of operative and postoperative complications that can compromise outcomes after ACL reconstruction. Some of these complications were noted in Boxes 21.9 and 21.10. Even minor technical errors during reconstruction can affect function adversely. As discussed in the previous section, inappropriate placement of the graft or bone tunnels, problems with graft harvesting such as inadequate graft length, and improper graft tension can adversely affect joint stability and mobility.[1,206,232] Insufficient graft length occurs more frequently during hamstring than patellar tendon graft harvesting. If graft fixation is insufficient, graft slippage and early failure can occur.[206,209] With a bone–patellar tendon–bone graft, a bone plug can fracture during harvesting or implantation, necessitating an alternative autograft or an allograft.[206]

Postoperatively, potential complications are knee pain, loss of motion, persistent strength deficits, and inadequate joint stability.[1,150,206,232] Anterior knee pain at the donor site of a patellar tendon graft or at the patellofemoral joint may affect functional activities. A neuroma of the infrapatellar branch of the saphenous nerve can cause significant knee pain during kneeling. Loss of full knee extension and quadriceps weakness are recognized as significant complications after ACL reconstruction. There may be permanent damage to the extensor mechanism after patellar tendon graft harvesting, leading to quadriceps weakness or even patellar tendon rupture in rare instances. Limited ROM of the knee may have been present prior to surgery or may develop after surgery. One possible cause is a buildup of scar tissue in the intracondylar notch, necessitating arthroscopic notchplasty. Loss of patellar mobility also may be a source of limited knee ROM. It has been suggested that a patient's preoperative strength and ROM also may have an impact on postoperative knee motion and strength.

🔘 **Focus on Evidence** _____

McHugh et al.[139] evaluated 102 patients (age 31 ± 1 year) within 2 weeks of primary ACL reconstruction and 6 months after surgery to determine preoperative indicators of postoperative motion loss (lack of full knee extension) and quadriceps weakness. They found that patients with loss of knee extension preoperatively (in comparison to the noninvolved contralateral knee) were more likely to have limited knee extension postoperatively. However, a preoperative deficit of quadriceps muscle strength (≥ 20% compared with contralateral quadriceps strength) was not an indicator of postoperative quadriceps weakness 6 months after surgery.

_____

Finally, graft failure and the need for revision reconstruction may occur even in the absence of risk factors related to surgical technique. It has been shown that graft failure is most likely to occur during the early months after surgery.[71] It has also been suggested that the most common cause of graft failure is poor adherence to postoperative rehabilitation, in particular returning to high-risk, high-joint-load activities prematurely.[1,71,206]

## Postoperative Management

Just over two decades ago, rehabilitation after ACL reconstruction involved long periods of continuous immobilization of the knee in a position of flexion and an extended period (often 6 to 8 weeks) of restricted weight bearing. Return to full activity often took a full year.[25,125,171,212] With advances in surgical techniques and a better understanding of graft healing and the impact of stress on the healing graft, early postoperative motion and weight bearing—often referred to as "accelerated rehabilitation"—has become the standard of care after primary ACL reconstruction with an autogenous graft for the active, typically young patient.[52,90,127,181,183,211,212,214,253]

Accelerated rehabilitation is based on the premise that a precisely placed and appropriately tensioned graft not only is strong enough to withstand the stresses of early motion and weight bearing, but that the graft responds favorably to these stresses during the healing process.[16,211,212,214,253] Table 21.7 outlines a contemporary, accelerated program for postoperative management after primary ACL reconstruction.

NOTE: It is important to recognize that although the descriptor "accelerated" is used frequently in the literature to characterize current-day rehabilitation after primary ACL reconstruction, there is no consensus on the components, progression, or duration of postoperative exercise, weight bearing, and other interventions. Therefore, the sequence of goals and interventions described in Table 21.6 reflects guidelines common to a number of programs published in the literature.[30,52,90,127,157,181,183,195,211,214,253]

| TABLE 21.7 | ACL Reconstruction—Intervention for Accelerated Rehabilitation | | | |
|---|---|---|---|---|
| Phase and General Time Frame | Maximum Protection Phase: Day 1 to Week 4 | Moderate Protection Phase: Weeks 4–10 | Minimum Protection Phase: Weeks 11–24 | Return-to-Activity Phase: ≥ 6 Months |
| Patient presentation | • Postoperative hemarthrosis, pain<br>• Postoperative pain<br>• Decreased ROM<br>• Diminished voluntary quadriceps activation<br>• Ambulation with crutches<br>• Protective bracing (may or may not be worn) | • Pain controlled<br>• Joint effusion controlled<br>• Full or near full ROM<br>• Fair plus to good muscle strength (3+/5 to 4/5)<br>• Muscular control of joint<br>• Independent ambulation | • No instability<br>• No swelling<br>• No pain<br>• Good to normal muscle strength (4/5 to 5/5 on MMT)<br>• Unrestricted ADL function<br>• Possible use of functional brace | • No instability<br>• Muscle function 70% of noninvolved extremity<br>• No symptoms of instability, pain or swelling during the previous phase<br>• Possible use of functional brace or sleeve during high-demand work or sports |
| Key examination procedures | • Pain scale<br>• Joint effusion—girth<br>• Ligament stability—joint arthrometer (days 7–14)<br>• ROM<br>• Patellar mobility<br>• Muscle control<br>• Functional status | • Pain scale<br>• Effusion—girth<br>• Ligament stability—joint arthrometer<br>• ROM<br>• Patellar mobility<br>• Muscle strength<br>• Functional status | • Ligament stability—joint arthrometer<br>• Muscle strength<br>• Functional status | • Full clinical examination<br>• Ligament stability<br>• Muscle strength<br>• Functional testing |
| Goals | • Protect healing tissues<br>• Prevent reflex inhibition of muscle<br>• Decrease joint effusion<br>• ROM 0°–110°<br>• Active control of ROM<br>• Weight bearing 75% to WBAT<br>• Establish home exercise program | • Full pain-free ROM<br>• 4/5 Muscular strength (MMT)<br>• Dynamic control of knee<br>• Improved kinesthetic awareness<br>• Normalize gait pattern and ADL function<br>• Adherence to home program | • Increase strength<br>• Increase power<br>• Increase muscular endurance<br>• Improve neuromuscular control, dynamic stability, balance<br>• Improve cardiopulmonary fitness | • Increase strength<br>• Increase power<br>• Increase endurance<br>• Regain ability to function at highest desired level<br>• Transition to maintenance program<br>• Reduce risk of re-injury |

(table continued on page 730)

| TABLE 21.7 | ACL Reconstruction—Intervention for Accelerated Rehabilitation (continued) | | | |
|---|---|---|---|---|
| Phase and General Time Frame | Maximum Protection Phase: Day 1 to Week 4 | Moderate Protection Phase: Weeks 4–10 | Minimum Protection Phase: Weeks 11–24 | Return-to-Activity Phase: ≥ 6 Months |
| Intervention | Early: days 1–14<br>• PRICE: protective bracing, ice, compression, elevation<br>• Gait training: crutches, partial weight bearing to WBAT<br>• PROM/A-AROM (range-limiting braces may or may not be used)<br>• Patellar mobilization (grades I and II)<br>• Muscle setting, isometrics: quadriceps, hamstrings, adductors at multiple angles (may augment with E-stim)<br>• Assisted SLRs—supine<br>• Ankle pumps<br>Late: weeks 2–4<br>• Continue as above<br>• Progress to full weight-bearing; begin closed chain squats; heel/toe raises<br>• SLRs in four planes cont'd<br>• Low-load PRE: hamstrings<br>• Initiate open-chain knee extension (range 90°–40°)<br>• Trunk/pelvis stabilization<br>• Aerobic conditioning: stationary cycle | Early: weeks 5–6<br>• Multiple-angle isometrics<br>• Advance closed-chain strengthening and PRE<br>• LE stretching program<br>• Endurance training (e.g., bike, pool, ski machine)<br>• Proprioceptive training: single-leg stance, tilt board, BAPS board<br>• Stabilization exercises, elastic bands, band walking<br>Late: weeks 7–10<br>• Continue as above; advance strengthening (include PNF patterns), endurance and flexibility<br>• Advance proprioceptive training to high speed stepping drills, unstable surface challenge drills, and balance beam<br>• Initiate a walk/jog program at the end of this phase<br>• Initiate plyometric drills: bounding, jumping | • Continue LE stretching program<br>• Advance PRE/initiate isokinetic training (if desired)<br>• Advanced closed-chain exercise, ply-ometric drills (bouncing, jumping rope, box jumps: double-/single-leg)<br>• Advanced proprioceptive training<br>• Progressive agility drills (figure-8, skill-specific patterns)<br>• Simulated work or sport-specific endurance training<br>• Progress running program: full-speed jogging, sprints, running and cutting | • Continue to progress PRE and flexibility exercises<br>• Advance agility drills<br>• Advance running drills<br>• Implement drills specific to sport or occupation<br>• Determine the need for protective bracing prior to return to sport or work |

**Immobilization and Protective Bracing**

The rationale for bracing after ACL reconstruction is protection of the graft and prevention of a knee flexion contracture during early rehabilitation.[16] However, with advances in graft fixation, the need for and benefits of protective bracing during rehabilitation has become a point of debate—recommended by some but not by others.[16,181,211,253]

The decision about whether postoperative bracing is prescribed is based on many factors, including the surgeon's philosophy, the type of graft used, intraoperative observations about the quality of fixation, co-morbidities and concomitant surgical procedures (e.g., meniscus or collateral ligament repair), and an assessment of the patient's expected level of adherence to a postoperative rehabilitation program.[90,183]

***Position and duration of immobilization.*** If bracing is prescribed during early recovery, it usually is a hinged and possibly range-limiting orthosis. The following are commonly recommended guidelines for the position and duration of immobilization. When the brace is locked, it holds the knee in full extension to prevent a knee flexion contracture or excessive hyperextension.[26,45,52,90,150,181,183,211,214,253] In addition, the hinged orthosis initially may be set to limit full knee flexion during exercise (e.g., allowing movement from 0° to 90° or more the first week after surgery). Even though the greatest stress on the graft occurs between 20° of flexion and full knee extension, precise graft placement and tension allow full knee extension without disrupting the graft's integrity.

Typically, the brace is worn throughout the day for anywhere from a few weeks to 6 weeks[16] and sometimes is also worn during sleep for the first week postoperatively.[183] During the first week or two the protective brace is locked in full extension during ambulation with crutches in the event of a fall.[90,183,211,253] By the beginning of week 3 the brace is unlocked, allowing motion between full extension to 125° of flexion during ambulation and other weight-bearing activities. Depending on the stability of the knee, sometimes the protective brace may need to be worn for 2 to 3 months or possibly longer. These timelines are progressed more slowly when ACL reconstruction is combined with another procedure, such as a collateral ligament, meniscus, or articular cartilage repair.[181] Some patients are advised to wear a functional brace during the advanced phases of rehabilitation and during high-demand sports or heavy manual labor after completing their rehabilitation program.

The literature provides some insight into the effectiveness of protective bracing during early rehabilitation.

 **Focus on Evidence** _____

A review of the literature by Beynnon and colleagues[16] identified only three randomized, controlled studies of the effects of brace use after primary ACL reconstruction. After analyzing the studies, the reviewers concluded that there was general consensus among investigators that use of a hinged brace during early recovery after surgery was associated with less joint swelling, wound drainage, and pain. However, at follow-up 1 and 2 years after surgery, no significant differences were identified in anterior-posterior knee stability, ROM, functional testing (hop test), thigh muscle strength, or patients' activity level and subjective assessment of outcomes in groups who did and did not use bracing during early rehabilitation.

### Weight-Bearing Considerations

As with ROM, early weight bearing is possible after primary ACL reconstruction with a bone–patellar tendon–bone or hamstring tendon autograft because of advances in graft fixation. However, recommendations for a period of protected weight bearing immediately after surgery vary, ranging from some degree of restricted weight bearing the first 2 weeks to weight bearing as tolerated with use of two crutches immediately after surgery.[17,58,139,181,198,211,240,253] Weight bearing is increased during the next 2 to 3 weeks based on the patient's symptoms. Protected weight bearing continues for a longer period of time if other structures in the knee have been injured and/or repaired (e.g., after repair of an articular cartilage defect of a femoral or tibial condyle).[253]

Full weight bearing and ambulation without crutches while wearing an unlocked protective brace usually is permitted by 3 to 4 weeks if weight bearing is pain-free and the patient has achieved full, _active_ knee extension and sufficient strength of the quadriceps to control the knee.[90,150,183]

Weight-bearing recommendations do not appear to be based on the type of graft or graft fixation used or whether protective bracing is worn but, rather, are determined on an empirical basis. The few randomized studies in the literature indicate that immediate and delayed weight bearing during the first few weeks after surgery produce similar outcomes.[16]

 **Focus on Evidence** _____

Tyler and colleagues[241] conducted a prospective, randomized, controlled study with 49 patients comparing the effects of immediate versus delayed weight bearing during the first 2 weeks after ACL reconstruction with bone–patellar tendon–bone fixation. The immediate weight-bearing group was advised to bear weight as tolerated and discontinue crutch use as soon as they felt comfortable doing so. The delayed weight-bearing group was advised not to wear a shoe on the operated side and remain non-weight bearing during ambulation with crutches for the first 2 weeks. After that, there were no restrictions placed on the progression of weight bearing. Neither group wore protective bracing. With the exception of weight-bearing status, the rehabilitation program for all patients was the same.

At a mean of 7.3 months, there were no significant differences between groups with respect to knee ROM, knee stability (measured by clinical examination and arthrometer), VMO activation (measured by EMG activity), or overall function. However, patients in the immediate weight-bearing group had a lower incidence of anterior knee pain than patients in the delayed weight-bearing group (8% and 35%, respectively). The investigators concluded that immediate weight bearing did not compromise knee joint stability or function and was beneficial in that it resulted in a lower incidence of postoperative anterior knee pain.

### Exercise Progression

A progression of carefully selected exercises and functional activities coupled with patient education is a foundation of rehabilitation following ACL injury and reconstruction. Because surgery typically is delayed after injury until acute symptoms have subsided, there is ample time to implement a _preoperative_ exercise program to restore full knee ROM, particularly extension, prevent atrophy and weakness of thigh musculature, and improve the strength and flexibility of hip and ankle musculature.[45,183,211,253]

After reconstruction of the ACL, exercise begins immediately on the first postoperative day. Use of strong grafts, such as bone–patellar tendon–bone and quadrupled hamstring autografts, and reliable graft fixation make early motion possible.[90,127,181,183,211,253]

Sometimes CPM is used while a patient is hospitalized or at home after discharge. Although a valid mechanism for controlling postoperative pain and initiating early motion,[48,134,169,211] it is used less frequently today than in the recent past.[90] It has been suggested that the CPM unit should be used without a calf band to minimize anterior translation of the tibia and prevent excessive stress to the graft site.[48]

It is important to remember that a tendon graft goes through a necrotizing process the first 2 to 3 weeks postoperatively before revascularization commences and maturation gradually occurs.[16,68,108,109] Therefore, exercises are progressed cautiously during each phase of rehabilitation, even during an accelerated program. If protective bracing has been prescribed, exercises are carried out while wearing the brace.

The rate of progression of exercise and functional training after ACL reconstruction depends on many factors. For example, patient-related facts, such as age and preinjury health status, affect the healing process, enabling younger, healthier patients to progress exercises more rapidly. The type of graft and graft fixation also may influence the progression of exercise. Some resources advocate more rapid progression of exercise for bone-to-bone fixation with a patellar tendon graft than for tendon-to-bone fixation with a quadrupled hamstring graft, suggesting that bone-to-bone healing may be faster than soft tissue-to-bone healing.[90,183,253] In contrast, others advocate the same accelerated program for both procedures.[58,198,209]

If, in addition to an ACL reconstruction, concomitant injuries are present or were managed surgically, the progression of exercises, as with weight bearing, typically is more gradual than after isolated ACL injury and reconstruction.[203]

Exercises for progressive phases of rehabilitation after ACL reconstruction, summarized in Table 21.6, are described in the following sections. Exercise precautions are noted in Box 21.11.[90,139,211,222,249,253]

### Exercise: Maximum Protection Phase

During the early postoperative period, a delicate balance exists between adequate protection of the healing graft and donor site and prevention of adhesions, contractures, articular degeneration, and muscle weakness and atrophy associated with immobilization. Early motion places beneficial stresses that strengthen the graft but must be carefully controlled to avoid stretching the graft while in a weakened state, particularly during the first 6 to 8 weeks after implantation.

The following goals and exercise interventions are emphasized during the first 4 weeks after surgery when considerable protection of knee structures is required.[90,127,139,181,183,211,253]

***Goals.*** Immediately after surgery through the first few postoperative weeks, in addition to controlling pain and

---

| BOX 21.11 | Exercise Precautions after ACL Reconstruction |

**Resistance Training—General Precautions**
- Progress exercises more gradually for reconstruction with hamstring tendon graft than bone-patellar tendon-bone graft.
- Progress knee flexor strengthening exercises cautiously if a hamstring tendon graft was harvested and knee extensor strengthening if a patellar tendon graft was harvested.

**Closed-Chain Training**
- When squatting in an upright position be sure that the knees do not move anterior to the toes as the hips descend because this increases shear forces on the tibia and could potentially place excess stress on the autograft.
- Avoid closed-chain strengthening of the quadriceps between 60° to 90° of knee flexion.*

**Open-Chain Training**
- During PRE to strengthen hip musculature, initially place the resistance above the knee until knee control is established.
- Avoid resisted, open-chain knee extension between 45° to 15°.*
- Avoid applying resistance to the distal tibia during quadriceps strengthening.*

*Contraction of the quadriceps in these positions and ranges causes the greatest anterior tibial translation and can create potentially excessive stress to the graft during the early stage of healing.[56,83,249,253]

---

swelling and initiating ambulation with crutches, exercise goals are to prevent reflex inhibition of knee musculature, prevent adhesions, restore full knee mobility, regain kinesthetic awareness and neuromuscular control (static and dynamic) of the lower extremity, and improve strength and flexibility of hip and ankle musculature.

The goal for knee ROM is to achieve 90° of flexion and full passive extension by the end of the first week as joint swelling subsides and then 110° to 125° of flexion by 3 to 4 weeks.

***Interventions.*** Pain, swelling, and peripheral edema are controlled in a standard manner. Exercises begin the day of or the day after surgery with an emphasis on (1) preventing vascular complications (DVTs); (2) activating knee musculature, particularly the quadriceps; and (3) establishing knee mobility. Patient education during the first phase of rehabilitation focuses on the home exercise program.

When weight-bearing exercises are initiated, they are performed in a protective brace if one has been prescribed. Low-intensity closed-chain exercises and proprioceptive/neuromuscular control training are initiated as soon as weight bearing is permissible. The value of closed-chain exercises and proprioceptive/neuromuscular control training after ACL reconstruction has been supported by many authors and is discussed in the exercise section of this chapter.[7,30,45,90,127,195,211,253]

 **Focus on Evidence** _____

Bynum and colleagues[30] conducted a prospective, randomized controlled study comparing open-chain and closed-chain rehabilitation after primary ACL reconstruction with a bone–patellar tendon–bone autograft. Immediately after surgery all patients followed the same exercise program, emphasizing early ROM (against no external resistance) and isometric quadriceps control. All patients wore a protective brace and ambulated with crutches, bearing weight as tolerated. When strengthening exercises were initiated, one group followed an open-chain regimen and the other a closed-chain regimen. One year after surgery 66% of patients participated in a follow-up examination that included subjective and objective measurements; it was conducted by someone blind to group assignment. Patients in the closed-chain exercise group compared with the open-chain group had significantly less anterior knee pain, knee stability closer to normal as measured by an arthrometer, earlier return to functional activities, and greater overall satisfaction with the outcome of the surgery.

---

The following exercises are advocated for the maximum protection phase.[90,127,139,183,195,211,249,253]

● *Voluntary activation of knee musculature.* Begin muscle setting of quadriceps, hamstrings, and hip abductors and adductors within the patient's comfort level. Use electrical stimulation or biofeedback to augment quadriceps activation. Perform four-position SLRs, first with assistance, then progressing to active hip motions with the knee maintained in extension. Add external resistance when the patient is able to maintain knee control during hip movements. Initiate low-intensity, multiple-angle isometrics of the knee musculature with emphasis on quadriceps control. To activate the hamstrings dynamically include supine heel-slides to a comfortable level of hip and knee flexion, active knee flexion in a standing position (hamstring curls without resistance added), and scooting *forward* while seated on a rolling stool (see Fig. 21.22).

● *ROM and patellar mobility.* Begin ROM in a protected range. Include therapist-controlled PROM or A-AROM within the patient's comfort level. Include patellar mobilization to prevent adhesions. To increase passive knee extension, assume a supine or long-sitting position and prop the heel on a rolled towel or bolster with the knee unsupported. To increase knee flexion, include supine, gravity-assisted wall slides. Stretch hip and ankle musculature if flexibility is limited.

● *Neuromuscular control, proprioception, and dynamic stability of the operated lower extremity.* While wearing a protecitve brace, if prescribed, begin trunk and lower extremity stabilization exercises in a standing position with weight distributed equally on both lower extremities and some weight on the hands for support, progressing

to bilateral mini-squats in the 0° to 30° range and weight-shifting, stepping, and marching movements. Gradually decrease upper extremity support. When the knee is pain-free and full weight bearing is possible, begin unilateral activities. Add stationary cycling and exercise on a seated leg press machine or in a semi-reclining position on a Total Gym® unit at 3 to 4 weeks and exercises in a pool as incision healing allows.

N O T E : A quadriceps contraction with the knee in full extension generates little to no anterior translation of the tibia on the femur because the knee is in a closed-pack position.

*Criteria to advance to next phase.* Criteria include minimal pain and swelling, full *active* knee extension (no extensor lag), 50% to 60% quadriceps strength (measured isometrically at 60°), greater than 110° of knee flexion, and no evidence of excessive joint laxity (determined by arthrometry measurements).

**Exercise: Moderate Protection Phase**
The moderate protection phase, which begins about 4 to 5 weeks postoperatively or at a point when identified criteria have been met, extends to about 10 to 12 weeks postoperatively. The emphasis of this phase is to achieve full knee ROM and increase strength, endurance, and balance in preparation for a transition to functional activities without compromising the stability of the knee. The hinged, protective brace is worn for gait and most exercises.

N O T E : By 8 to 10 weeks revascularization of the graft is becoming well established, and therefore exercises can be performed more vigorously.[68,108,109]

*Goals.* Rehabilitation goals during the intermediate phase are to attain full ROM (full knee extension and 125° to 135° flexion), improve lower extremity strength and muscular endurance, ambulate without assistive device and protective brace using a normal gait pattern, continue to improve neuromuscular control, proprioception, and balance, and regain cardiopulmonary fitness.

*Interventions.* Include and progress the following interventions during the moderate protection phase.[90,127,139,183,195,211,253]

● *ROM and joint mobility.* Continue low-intensity, end-range self-stretching to gain full knee ROM. Use grade III joint mobilization techniques to restore full knee flexion. Contine flexibility exercises for hip and ankle musculature, especially the hamstrings, IT band, and plantarflexors.

● *Strength and muscle endurance.* Initiate closed-chain and open-chain PRE in appropriate portions of knee ROM (see Box 21.11). Emphasize progressive closed-chain quadriceps training.

● *Neuromuscular control, proprioceptive training, and balance activities.* Progress closed-chain training, adding standing wall-slides, unilateral squats or lunges on the Total Gym®, lateral and diagonal step-ups, step-downs, partial lunges, and use of a stair-stepping machine. Perform balance activities bilaterally, progressing to unilateral balance activities on stable and then unstable surfaces. Initiate beginning-level plyometric training during the later weeks of this phase.

◉ *Gait training.* Practice ambulation in a controlled environment with the protective brace unlocked and without crutches. Emphasize symmetrical alignment, step length, and timing. Gradually discontinue protective bracing; use a functional brace or sleeve if necessary.

◉ *Aerobic conditioning.* Begin a swimming or pool walking/running program or ski machine or treadmill training; or continue stationary cycling, increasing the duration and speed.

◉ *Activity-specific training.* Integrate simulated functional activities or components of activities into the exercise program.

*Criteria to advance to next phase.* Criteria to progress to the advanced phases of rehabilitation include absence of pain, full active knee ROM, 75% strength of knee musculature compared to the contralateral side, no evidence of knee instability on arthrometer readings or clinical examination.

### Exercise: Minimum Protection and Return-to-Activity Phases

The advanced phases of rehabilitation and preparation for a return to a preinjury level of activity begin at about 10 to 12 weeks postoperatively or at a point when the patient has met specified criteria. Most post-ACL reconstruction rehabilitation programs described in the literature continue until about 6 months postoperatively.[16,90,181,183,253] The intensity and duration of training typically are based on the patient's goals and the level of activity to which the patient wishes to return. Individuals involved in high-joint-loading, work-related activities or competitive sports are advised to participate in a maintenance exercise program.

*Goals.* From 12 to 24 weeks postoperatively the aim is to further increase strength, endurance, and power; further enhance neuromuscular control and agility; and participate in progressively more demanding functional activities. A functional knee brace often is worn to reduce the risk of reinjury during high-demand activities, particularly those that involve turning, twisting, cutting, or jumping motions.

*Interventions.* Exercise interventions during the final phases of rehabilitation include PRE with an emphasis on eccentric training, advanced neuromuscular and balance training, plyometrics, agility drills, and activity-specific training coupled with a gradual return to high-demand activities. Patient education, emphasizing prevention of reinjury, continues throughout the advanced phases of rehabilitation and as the patient returns to full activity.

*Return to activity.* Recommended timelines for returning to vigorous activities, including competitive sports, vary considerably, ranging from as early as 4 to 6 months[198,209,214] to a year after surgery. Criteria to return to a preinjury level

---

| **BOX 21.12** | **Criteria to Return to High-Demand Activities after ACL Reconstruction** |
|---|---|

- No knee pain or joint effusion
- Full active knee ROM
- Quadriceps strength $\geq$ 85% of contralateral side *or* peak torque/body mass 40% and 60% for men and 30% and 50% for women (tested at 300°/sec and 180°/sec, respectively).
- Hamstring strength 100% of contralateral side
- No postoperative history of knee instability/giving way
- Negative pivot shift test
- Knee stability measured by arthrometer: < 3 mm difference between reconstructed and uninjured side
- Proprioceptive testing: 100%
- Functional testing (hop, jump, and squat tests): $\geq$ 85% of contralateral side or normative values
- Acceptable patient-reported score on comprehensive, quantitative knee function measurement tool, such as the International Knee Documentation Committee Subjective Knee Form

---

of activity must be individualized for each patient and are contingent on clinical examination findings, particularly the stability of the knee, and the expected work-related, recreational, or sports-related demands. Box 21.12 identifies criteria, suggested by several sources,[114,157,214,249,253] that should be met prior to a return to high-risk, high-joint-loading activities.

### Outcomes

Reconstruction of the ACL followed by a carefully progressed postoperative rehabilitation program is a reliable means of re-establishing knee stability. Consequently, ACL reconstruction results in a high rate (> 90%) of patient satisfaction.[219] However, outcomes are predicated on numerous factors, including the patient's age, sex, and overall health status, the presence or absence of injuries associated with the ACL injury, various aspects of the surgical procedure, postoperative complications, and the patient's adherence to the rehabilitation program. The effects of several of these variables are addressed in this section.

*Graft selection and outcomes.* Numerous prospective and retrospective studies have been conducted comparing the effects of graft selection on outcomes. Bone–patellar tendon–bone and hamstring tendon autografts are studied most often. An extensive review and analysis of the literature revealed that although both types of grafts have their merits and limitations (summarized in Boxes 21.9 and 21.10) long-term (2 years or more) functional outcomes are essentially the same.[216]

*Functional bracing.* The effect of functional bracing during the intermediate and advanced phases of rehabilitation and its use during high-risk sports after completion of rehabilitation is unclear. Risberg et al.[194] carried out a prospective investigation in which 60 patients were randomly assigned to a braced or a nonbraced group. After ACL reconstruction with a patellar tendon autograft, patients in the braced group wore a protective brace for 2 weeks and then wore a functional brace most of the time for an additional 10 weeks. At the conclusion of rehabilitation the braced group was advised to wear the functional brace for all high-joint-loading activities. The nonbraced group had no brace at any time during or after rehabilitation. Otherwise, both groups underwent the same rehabilitation program and patient education. At a 2-year follow-up there were no significant differences between groups for knee ROM, knee joint laxity, muscle strength, functional testing, or incidence of reinjury to the ACL. The results of this study are similar to the findings of a more recent randomized, controlled multicenter study by McDevitt et al.,[137] who found that use of an "off the shelf" functional brace for 1 year after ACL reconstruction during all high-demand activities (jumping, pivoting, cutting) had no significant impact on knee function or reinjury.

Sterett et al.[229] also investigated the role of functional bracing in preventing reinjury in patients returning to an advanced, high-demand activity after ACL reconstruction, specifically snow skiing. Over several consecutive ski seasons at a large ski resort, the investigators conducted a prospective, nonrandomized cohort study of 820 skiers who were employees of the ski resort and had undergone ACL reconstruction with a patellar tendon autograft at least 2 years previously. Of the 820 post-ACL reconstruction skier/employees, 257 were considered at significant risk for reinjury of the ACL based on the results of preseason screening. These individuals were given and advised to wear a functional knee brace during skiing. The remaining 563 skier/employees were not determined to be at significant risk for reinjury and were not issued a functional brace.

Analysis of data during the course of the study over several years indicated that 61 ACL reinjuries occurred: 51 in the nonbraced skiers and 10 in the braced skiers. The nonbraced group was 2.74 times more likely to sustain reinjury to the ACL than the braced group. Based on the results of their study, the authors recommended functional knee bracing after recovery from ACL reconstruction for patients returning to the high-demand sport of skiing regardless of their assessed risk of reinjury. The authors, although noting the limitations of this nonrandomized study, suggested that the findings of this study were of interest because of the large number of participants in the study.

*Approaches to rehabilitation.* There is limited evidence in the literature to determine the effects of variables in a postoperative exercise program, such as the degree of supervison or the duration of the program, on outcomes. Beynnon and co-investigators[17] conducted a prospective, randomized, double-blind study comparing the results of an accelerated (19 weeks) and nonaccelerated (32 weeks) rehabilitation program following ACL reconstruction with bone–patellar tendon–bone autografts. The two programs contained the same components but were implemented over two different timelines. A total of 25 patients entered the study, and 22 patients (10 in the accelerated/19-week program and 12 in the nonaccelerated/32-week program) completed the program and were available for final follow-up. At 24 months postoperatively there were no significant differences in knee laxity, functional testing, or patient satisfaction and activity level.

The effect of supervision during rehabilitation has also been studied. Specifically, home-based rehabilitation with limited therapist supervision has been compared with clinic-based rehabilitation with therapist supervision throughout the program. A review of the literature revealed that, for the most part, these two approaches produced similar outcomes.[16] However, the reviewers pointed out that all patients who participated in the various studies had some instruction and supervision from a therapist. The reviewers emphasized the importance of therapist-directed assessments and initial instruction in an exercise program but recommended periodic, rather than continuous, supervision over the course of rehabilitation.

## Posterior Cruciate Ligament Reconstruction

In contrast to injury of the ACL, injury of the posterior cruciate ligament (PCL) is relatively infrequent.[255] When an injury does occur, it usually is accompanied by damage to other structures of the knee. There is general agreement that a PCL injury, combined with an injury to another ligament or other structures of the knee, usually warrants early surgical intervention.[61,168,170]

When an isolated PCL injury occurs, most patients respond well to nonoperative management and are able to return to a preinjury level of activity without surgical intervention. However, after a severe PCL injury an increased incidence of OA in the medial compartment of the knee over time has been observed.[225] Recently, motion analysis of the PCL-deficient knee, as the result of an isolated rupture, has demonstrated altered kinematics of the medial compartment of the knee, specifically anterior subluxation of the medial femoral condyle (posterior subluxation of the medial tibial plateau).[121] These findings provide a possible explanation for the degenerative changes observed in the PCL-deficient knee and lend support for surgical intervention.

### Indications for Surgery
Although there is limited consensus, the most frequently cited indications for surgical reconstruction of the PCL include the following.[3,61,159,170,233,255]

- Complete tear or avulsion of the PCL with posterolateral, posteromedial, or rotary instability of the knee combined with damage to another ligament and often the menisci or articular cartilage.
- Isolated, symptomatic, grade 3 PCL tear with more than 10 to 15 mm posterior displacement resulting in instability during functional activities.

● Chronic PCL insufficiency associated with posterolateral instability, pain, limitations in functional activities, and deterioration of articular surfaces of the knee.

## Procedures

### Operative Overview

There are a number of arthroscopic, arthroscopically assisted, or open procedures available for management of a torn or ruptured PCL. Although an acute bony avulsion occasionally is managed with primary repair, reconstruction is by far the more frequently selected option.[61] As with the ACL, PCL reconstruction involves implantation of a graft to replace the damaged ligament. Graft options using single-bundle or double-bundle reconstruction include a bone–patellar tendon–bone autograft, a hamstring (semitendinosus–gracilis) or quadriceps tendon autograft, an Achilles tendon allograft, or occasionally a synthetic graft.[3,61,159,170,233,255] Of these choices, the patellar tendon graft reconstruction is the most common.

The operative procedure begins with diagnostic arthroscopy followed by graft harvest if an autograft is to be used for reconstruction. After femoral and tibial tunnels are drilled and prepared, the grafts are drawn through and secured in the tunnels with bony or soft tissue fixation devices, such as interference screws and washers or staples. Graft placement must be precise to mimic the function of the PCL. Prior to closure, the knee is flexed and extended to be certain that graft placement and tension allow full ROM. After wound closure, a sterile compression dressing is applied, and the knee is immobilized in full extension.

### Complications

Because PCL reconstruction involves the posterior aspect of the knee, there is risk of damage to the popliteal neurovascular bundle. Risk is highest during drilling of the tibial bone tunnel. Postoperatively, bleeding can lead to compartment syndrome. If a patellar tendon autograft was harvested, the patient may experience anterior knee pain and pain during kneeling. If motion is lost postoperatively, usually knee flexion becomes limited. As with any ligament reconstruction, graft failure can occur, leading to loss of joint stability and the need for revision reconstruction.[61]

### Postoperative Management

#### Immobilization, Protective Bracing, and Weight Bearing

Initially, the knee is immobilized in a hinged, range-limiting brace locked in full extension. The immobilizer is worn during the day and even during sleep for the first 4 weeks to prevent posterior displacement of the tibia as the result of gravity or sudden knee flexion. It is unlocked or removed for exercise 1 day to a week after surgery.[3,61,168,170,255] The protective brace remains locked in extension during weight bearing for an extended period of time.

In contrast to weight bearing after ACL reconstruction, weight bearing is progressed more gradually after PCL surgery.[54,61,168,170,255] The time frame for initiating

and progressing weight bearing varies considerably in the literature. Recommendations range from partial weight bearing immediately after surgery using two crutches and wearing the protective brace locked in extension[39,168,170] to non-weight bearing for a week to 5 weeks postoperatively.[61,255] Weight bearing is increased over several weeks while keeping the brace locked in extension. As quadriceps control improves, enabling the patient to fully extend the knee, and pain and joint effusion are well controlled, the brace is unlocked, allowing movement in a protected range during ambulation with crutches and weight-bearing exercises. Crutches are discontinued and full weight bearing with the brace unlocked is permitted when the patient has minimal to no pain or joint effusion, approximately 70% quadriceps strength, and active knee motion from 0° to 120°, which typically is possible at approximately 8 to 10 weeks.[39,168,170] Brace use is then discontinued gradually.

### Exercise

After PCL reconstruction many of the postoperative exercises performed during progressive phases of rehabilitation are similar to those following ACL reconstruction (see Table 21.7).[39,54,61,168,170] The key differences are that exercises are progressed more slowly and those that place posterior shear forces on the tibia are postponed during the early phase of rehabilitation when the graft is most vulnerable. When resistance exercises for hamstring strengthening are initiated during advanced rehabilitation, they are adjusted based on the stability of the knee. Box 21.13 summarizes precautions for exercise and functional activities after PCL reconstruction.[39,168,170]

#### Exercise: Maximum Protection Phase

The emphasis during the first, maximum protection phase of rehabilitation, which extends for 4 to 6 weeks, is to protect the integrity of the graft while simultaneously regaining a functional degree of mobility and developing quadriceps control.[39,54,61,168,170]

*Goals.* During this phase of rehabilitation goals are to control or reduce acute symptoms (pain, swelling), prevent vascular complications (DVTs), re-establish control of the quadriceps mechanism, maintain patellar mobility, regain approximately 90° of knee flexion by 2 to 4 weeks after initiating knee motion, begin to re-establish proprioception, neuromuscular control, and balance, improve the strength and flexibility of the hip and ankle musculature if limited, and improve cardiopulmonary fitness.[39,168,170]

*Interventions.* Control pain and swelling in a standard manner. Immediately after surgery begin ankle pumping exercises, patellar gliding techniques, quadriceps-setting exercises (augmented by neuromuscular electrical stimulation), and multiplanar SLRs while wearing the protective brace locked in full extension. Use an upper extremity ergometer for aerobic conditioning.

When knee motion is permitted, follow the exercise precautions for early rehabilitation described in Box 21.13. Begin multiple-angle isometrics of the quadriceps from full extension to 25° to 30° of flexion. Perform assisted knee

**Exercise Precautions After PCL Reconstruction**

*General Precaution:* Avoid exercises and activities that place excessive posterior shear forces and cause posterior displacement of the tibia on the femur, thus disrupting the healing graft.

### Early and Intermediate Rehabilitation

- Begin exercise to restore knee flexion while in a seated position, allowing gravity to passively flex the knee and the hamstrings to remain essentially inactive.
- Postpone open-chain, active knee flexion against the resistance of gravity (prone or standing) for 6 to 12 weeks.
- During squatting exercises to increase quadriceps strength, avoid excessive trunk flexion as it causes increased activity in the hamstrings.

### Advanced Rehabilitation

- Postpone resistance training for the knee flexors, such as use of a hamstring curl machine, for 5 to 6 months.
- When performing resisted hamstring curls, use low loads.
- Avoid downhill inclines during walking, jogging, or hiking.
- Avoid activities that involve knee flexion combined with rapid deceleration when one or both feet are planted.
- Postpone returning to vigorous functional activities for at least 9 to 12 months. Consider wearing a functional knee brace during high-demand activities.

extension, progressing to active knee extension while seated. To regain knee flexion, begin with gravity-assisted flexion. Hold the patient's leg in full knee extension and have the patient control leg lowering as gravity flexes the knee.

To the extent that weight-bearing restrictions allow and while wearing the locked brace, begin trunk and lower extremity stabilization exercises in a supported standing position (in the parallel bars or with crutches). Begin bilateral closed-chain quadriceps strengthening while holding on to a stable surface for support when it is permissible to unlock the protective brace. Stretch the hip and ankle musculature, in particular the hamstrings, IT band, and plantarflexors.

***Criteria to advance to next phase.*** If there is minimal joint swelling and the patient has minimal pain and has achieved full active knee extension (no extensor lag) and at least 100° of knee flexion, it is appropriate to progress to the next phase of rehabilitation.[39,168,170]

### Exercise: Moderate and Minimum Protection Phases

***Goals and interventions.*** As with early rehabilitation, the goals and interventions during the intermediate and advanced phases of rehabilitation following PCL reconstruction are similar to those following ACL reconstruction (see Table 21.7), although the suggested timelines continue to be more extended. The exercises and activities during

the intermediate phase of rehabilitation are essentially an extension of those initiated during the first phase. By 9 to 12 weeks postoperatively the patient should have achieved full knee ROM (0° to 135°), making it possible to discontinue use of the protective brace if quadriceps control is sufficient.[39,168,170]

During the intermediate and advanced phases of rehabilitation, precautions to prevent excessive posterior shear forces on the tibia during exercises and functional activities continue (see Box 21.13). Strengthening focuses on the quadriceps to re-establish full active knee extension and sufficient strength in the quadriceps, hip, and ankle musculature for functional weight-bearing activities. Resistance training to improve strength and muscular endurance of the hamstrings (hamstring curls) is based on the posterior stability of the knee. Strengthening of the knee flexors typically is delayed until 2 to 3 months postoperatively and, when initiated, is progressed cautiously.

Advanced neuromuscular training with plyometrics, balance activities, and agility drills, progressive aerobic conditioning, and activity-specific training are critical for a safe transition to a full level of functional activities. A full return to vigorous activities after PCL reconstruction often takes 9 months to a year.[39,61,168,170]

 ## MENISCAL TEARS: NONOPERATIVE MANAGEMENT

### Mechanisms of Injury

The medial meniscus is injured more frequently than the lateral meniscus. Insult may occur when the foot is fixed on the ground and the femur is rotated internally, as when pivoting, getting out of a car, or receiving a clipping injury. An ACL injury often accompanies a medial meniscus tear. Lateral rotation of the femur on a fixed tibia may tear the lateral meniscus. Simple squatting or trauma may also cause a tear.

### Common Impairments and Functional Limitations/Disabilities

Meniscal tears can cause acute locking of the knee or chronic symptoms with intermittent locking. Pain occurs along the joint line (due to stress to the coronary ligament) along with joint swelling and some degree of quadriceps atrophy. When there is joint locking, the knee does not fully extend, and there is a springy end-feel when passive extension is attempted. If the joint is swollen, there is usually slight limitation of flexion or extension. The McMurray or Apley grinding tests may be positive.[123]

When the meniscus tear is acute, the patient may be unable to bear weight on the involved side. Unexpected locking or giving way during ambulation often occurs, causing safety problems.

## Management

- Often the patient can actively move the leg to "unlock" the knee, or the unlocking happens spontaneously.
- Passive manipulative reduction of the medial meniscus may unlock the knee (Fig. 21.12). *Patient position and procedure*: Supine. Passively flex the involved knee and hip and simultaneously rotate the tibia internally and externally. When the knee is fully flexed, externally rotate the tibia and apply a valgus stress at the knee. Hold the tibia in this position and extend the knee. The meniscus may click into place. Once reduced, the knee may react as an acute joint lesion. If this occurs, treat as described earlier in the chapter in the section on nonoperative management of joint hypomobility.
- After acute symptoms have subsided, exercises should be performed in open-chain and closed-chain positions to improve strength and endurance in isolated muscle groups and to prepare the patient for functional activities.

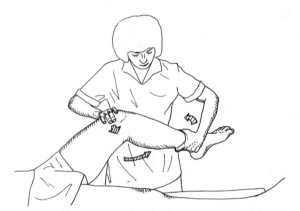

FIGURE 21.12 Manipulative reduction of a medial meniscus. Internally and externally rotate the tibia as you flex the hip and knee (not shown); then laterally rotate the tibia and apply a valgus stress at the knee as you extend it. The meniscus may click into place.

## ● MENISCAL TEARS: SURGICAL AND POSTOPERATIVE MANAGEMENT

When a significant tear or rupture of the medial or lateral meniscus occurs or if nonoperative management of a partial tear has been unsuccessful, surgical intervention often is necessary. Current-day surgical procedures are designed to retain as much of the meniscus as possible as a means of preserving the load transmission and shock-absorbing functions of the menisci and to reduce stress on the tibiofemoral articular surfaces.

Primary surgical options are *partial meniscectomy* and *meniscal repair*, both of which are considered preferable to total meniscectomy.[230,238] The location and nature of the tear influences the selection of a procedure, as does the patient's age and level of activity. Tears of the outer area of a meniscus, which has a rich vascular supply, heal well, whereas tears extending into the central portion, where the vascular supply is considerably less, have marginal healing

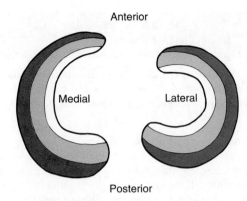

FIGURE 21.13 Vascularity of the medial and lateral menisci. The peripheral zone (outer one-third) is highly vascular; the central one-third is relatively avascular; and the inner one-third is avascular.

properties (Fig. 21.13).[239] Age and the patient's activity level factor into the decision-making process because it has been shown that loss of even a portion of a meniscus increases the long-term risk of articular degeneration.[239]

Traditionally, partial meniscectomy has been performed to manage complex, fragmented tears and tears involving the central (middle third), relatively avascular zone of a meniscus.[238] In contrast, peripheral tears involving the highly vascular portion of a meniscus have been shown to lend themselves well to repair rather than excision of the torn portion.[239] However, if a patient with a central zone tear is young or physically active but older, some surgeons now advocate repair of the torn meniscus.[89,142,160,161] If there is extensive damage to a major portion of the meniscus and it is determined to be unsalvagable, total meniscectomy remains the only surgical option.[238]

For the relatively young and/or active patient, who previously underwent total meniscectomy and now is symptomatic as the result of early osteoarthritic changes in the tibiofemoral joint, a recently developed option, *meniscal transplantation*, using human allograft tissue has become available.[89,163,184]

The progression of postoperative rehabilitation and the time required to return to full activity after each of these procedures depends on the extent and location of the tear and the type of surgical approach and procedure performed. Rehabilitation proceeds more conservatively after repair or implantation of a meniscus or total meniscectomy than after partial meniscectomy. Damage and repair or reconstruction of other soft tissues of the knee, such as the ACL, also affect the course and progression of rehabilitation after surgery.

### Meniscus Repair

#### Indications for Surgery
Repair of a torn meniscus is indicated in the following situations.[89,160,230,238]

- A lesion in the vascular outer third of the medial or lateral meniscus

● A tear extending into the central, relatively avascular third of the meniscus of a young (under age 40 to 50) or physcially active older (over age 50) individal

CONTRAINDICATIONS: Contraindications include the presence of a tear localized to the inner, avascular third of the meniscus; a tear in which there is considerable tissue fragmentation; or a tear that cannot be completely reopposed during surgery.[89]

## Procedure

### Operative Overview

Prior to the operative procedure, a comprehensive arthroscopic examination of the joint is performed to determine if a meniscus tear is suitable for repair and to identify any concomitant injuries, such as ACL damage. The repair itself typically is performed using an arthroscopically assisted open approach or a fully arthroscopic approach.[89,151,152,160] The determination of which approach is selected generally is based on the location and nature of the tear.[238]

There are several surgical procedures—referred to as inside-out, outside-in, or all-inside techniques—for meniscus repair. The inside-out and outside-in techniques are arthroscopically assisted, with a portion of the procedure being performed through an incision at the posteromedial or posterolateral aspect of the knee.[151,160] The all-inside technique is fully arthroscopic.[152,239]

There are also various suturing techniques with nonabsorable or bioabsorbable sutures that can be used during the repair. Use of other fixation devices, such as darts or staples, also has been reported. Of the many variations of meniscus repair, the arthroscopically assisted, inside-out suture repair is most common and considered by some in the orthopedic community to be the "gold standard."[89,151,160,239]

At the beginning of the procedure small incisions are made at the knee for portals, and saline is arthroscopically introduced into the joint to distend the capsule. After the joint has been examined, arthroscopic débridement is performed to remove all unstable tissue fragments and prepare the torn meniscus for repair. During the repair itself (performed endoscopically or through a posteromedial or posterolateral incision), the edges of the tear are closely approximated, and sutures are placed every 3 to 4 mm to ensure complete closure (no gapping) along the tear line. All sutures are tied with the knee fully extended or in 10° of flexion to allow full extension postoperatively without causing undue stress on the repaired meniscus.

After closure, a compression dressing, extending above and below the knee, is applied to control postoperative joint effusion, and the knee is placed in an immobilizer.

NOTE: Detailed descriptions of medial and lateral meniscal allograft transplantation techniques are published in several resources.[89,163,164,184]

### Complications

Complications specific to meniscus surgery include intraoperative damage to the neurovascular bundle at the posterior aspect of the knee during the suturing process. With a medial meniscus repair there is a risk of damage to the saphenous nerve; and with a lateral meniscus repair there is risk of damage to the peroneal nerve. Postoperatively, these same nerves can become entrapped by adherent scar tissue.[151,238,239]

A flexion contracture or an extensor lag postoperatively compromises knee alignment and stability during gait and functional activities. The risk of failure of the repair is greatest during activities that involve joint loading and knee flexion beyond 45°. This risk is greatest during the first few postoperative months.[142,230]

### Postoperative Management

Factors that influence the components and progression of postoperative rehabilitation after meniscus repair are noted in Box 21.14.[39,89,142,160] Some variables permit relatively rapid rehabilitation, whereas others necessitate a more cautious progression. For example, exercise and weight bearing are progressed more rapidly after repair of a peripheral zone tear than a central tear and after a single tear than after a complex pattern tear.

Another factor, malalignment of the knee, affects forces placed on a repaired meniscus and thus influences the progression of weight bearing during ambulation and exercise. With varus alignment, a repaired medial meniscus is subjected to increased stress and increased risk of displacement during healing. Therefore, weight bearing must be progressed more slowly in this situation than is necessary when there is normal alignment of the knee.[39]

NOTE: Although timelines vary somewhat in published protocols, the progression of exercises presented in the following sections are appropriate after *isolated* meniscus repair in a cruciate-stable knee. These same guidelines are appropriate after meniscal transplantation, although the duration of rehabilitation and protection of the transplanted meniscus is longer.[89,184] If a concomitant procedure, such as ligament reconstruction, is performed, adjustments also are made.

### Immobilization, Protective Bracing, and Weight Bearing

***Immobilization and protective bracing.*** The knee is held in full extension, first in the postoperative immobilizer and then in a long-leg brace when the bulky compression dressing is removed a few days after surgery.[39,89,238] Occasional-

---

| BOX 21.14 | Factors Influencing the Progression of Rehabilitation After Meniscus Repair |
|---|---|

- Location and size of the tear [i.e., the zone(s) affected and their vascularity]
- Type of tear (tear pattern and complexity)
- Security of the suture fixation observed intraoperatively
- Alignment of the knee joint (normal, varus, valgus)
- Concomitant injuries (ligament, chondral defect) *with or without* reconstruction or repair

ly, for carefully selected patients with a peripheral zone repair, no protective bracing is used after the postoperative dressing is removed.[151] The patient continues to wear a thigh-high compression stocking to control swelling.

To protect the repaired meniscus during the first few postoperative weeks, the range-limiting brace is worn continuously (day and night) and locked in full extension, except during ROM exercises. Depending on the site of the lesion and repair, the protective brace is set to allow 0° to no more than 90° of flexion for the first 2 weeks or longer. Each week the range allowed by the brace is increased by about 10° until full flexion has been achieved.[89] The brace is unlocked during daily activities as early as 2 weeks if the patient has achieved full knee extension.

After a central zone repair, the patient typically wears the brace for about 6 weeks or until adequate quadriceps control has been established. After a meniscal transplant, the brace may be worn a few weeks longer.

*Weight bearing.* Partial weight bearing (ranging from 25% to 50%) during ambulation with crutches and the brace locked in full extension is allowed during the immediate postoperative period. The percent of body weight permitted during weight bearing is progressed more cautiously after a central zone or transplant than after a peripheral zone repair. Regardless of the type of procedure, however, weight bearing is progressed gradually and always is based on the patient's signs and symptoms.

If quadriceps control is sufficient, full weight bearing may be permitted by 4 to 6 weeks after a peripheral repair[89] and by 6 to 8 weeks after a central repair or transplant.[39,89,142,163,184]

### Exercise: Maximum Protection Phase

Exercises and gait training with crutches are begun the first postoperative day. A standard approach (cold, compression, elevation) to control pain, joint effusion, and vascular complications (ankle pumping exercises) is used. Patient education focuses on establishing a home exercise program and reinforcing weight-bearing precautions. Exercise precautions are noted in Box 21.15.[39,89,142,238,239]

*Goals.* During the first 4 weeks after surgery, exercise goals are to regain functional ROM, prevent patellar restrictions, re-establish control of knee musculature, restore postural stability, improve strength and flexibility of the hip and ankle, and maintain cardiopulmonary fitness. By 4 weeks the patient should achieve full, active knee extension. Recommendations for maximum flexion during the first 2 weeks vary from 60° to 90°.[22,39,89,142,208,230,238] After 4 weeks the patient should attain 120° of knee flexion.[89]

*Interventions.* During the first 4 weeks after meniscus repair, the following interventions are included.[22,39,89,102,142,208]

- ◐ *ROM of the knee.* CPM is prescribed at the surgeon's discretion. Begin A-AROM and AROM exercises of the knee the day after surgery. Knee flexion is restricted by

---

| BOX 21.15 | Exercise Precautions After Meniscus Repair* |

**General Precautions**
- Progress exercises and weight bearing more gradually after a central zone meniscus repair or meniscus transplantations than after a peripheral zone repair.
- If the patient experiences a clicking sensation in the knee during exercise or weight-bearing activities, report it immediately to the surgeon.

**Early and Intermediate Rehabilitation**
- Increase knee flexion gradually, especially after a central zone repair.
- If a stationary bicycle is used for cardiopulmonary conditioning, set the seat height as high as possible to limit the range of knee flexion.
- During weight-bearing exercises, such as lunges and squatting, do not perform knee flexion beyond 45° for 4 weeks or beyond 60° to 70° for 8 weeks. Flexion beyond 60° to 70° places posterior translation forces on a repaired meniscus, increasing the risk of displacement during early healing.
- Postpone use of a leg press machine until about 8 weeks. Limit motion from 0° to 60°.
- Avoid twisting motions during weight-bearing activities.
- Postpone hamstring curls until about 8 weeks.

**Advanced Rehabilitation**
- Do not perform exercises that involve deep squatting, deep lunges, twisting, or pivoting for at least 4 to 6 months. (The greater the flexion angle, the greater is the stress on the meniscus.)
- Do not begin jogging or running program until 5 to 6 months.

**Return to Activity**
- Refrain from recreational and sports activities that involve repetitive, high joint compressions and shear forces.
- Avoid prolonged squatting in full flexion.

*These precautions also are applicable after meniscus transplantation, but time frames for the precautions are longer.

---

a hinged, controlled-motion brace. Include exercises such as gravity-assisted knee flexion in a sitting position and assisted progressing to active heel slides in a supine position.
- ◐ *Patellar mobility.* Teach the patient grade I and II patellar gliding exercises.
- ◐ *Activation of knee musculature.* Emphasize quadriceps control in full extension with quadriceps setting exercises, assisted SLRs in the supine position, and assisted progressing to active open-chain knee extension/flexion in a sitting position for concentric/eccentric quadriceps control. Augment quadriceps activation with electrical muscle stimulation or biofeedback. Also, perform hamstring-setting exercises and multiple-angle isometrics.

- *Neuromuscular control, proprioception, and balance.* Begin balance activities in a standing position within the limits of weight-bearing restrictions and with the brace locked. Emphasize trunk and lower extremity stabilization exercises. When it is permissible to unlock the brace during carefully controlled weight bearing, initiate bilateral closed-chain exercises, such as mini-squats and standing wall-slides, initially limiting flexion to no more than 45°.
- *Flexibility and strength of the hip and ankle musculature.* Stretch the hamstrings and plantarflexors, if restricted. Begin gluteal and adductor setting exercises the first postoperataive day. Perform four-position SLRs with the brace locked or when the patient can perform an SLR in supine position without an extensor lag. Perform bilateral heel raises when 50% weight bearing is permitted.
- *Cardiopulmonary function.* Use an upper body ergometer for aerobic conditioning exercises.

*Criteria to advance to next phase.* Joint effusion and pain should be minimal, and the patient should have evidence of superior gliding of the patella with quadriceps setting, full active knee extension, and approximately 120° of knee flexion.

### Exercise: Moderate Protection Phase
The moderate protection phase extends from 4 to 6 weeks to about 12 weeks postoperatively. The knee brace is discontinued at about 6 to 8 weeks if there is adequate control of the knee and no extensor lag. Use of a cane or single crutch is advisable to provide some degree of protection during ambulation.

*Goals.* Restoring full knee ROM, improving lower extremity flexibility, strength, and muscular endurance, continuing to re-establish neuromuscular control and balance, and improving overall aerobic fitness are emphasized during the moderate protection phase of rehabilitation.

*Interventions.* Include and progress the following exercises and activities during the intermediate phase of rehabilitation.[22,39,89,102,142,208]

- *ROM.* Progress low-load, long-duration stretching exercises if the patient is having difficulty achieving full knee ROM.
- *Muscle performance (strength and muscular endurance).* Initiate stationary cycling against light resistance. Use elastic resistance for low-intensity, open-chain and closed-chain exercises. Progress hip and ankle strengthening exercises
- *Neuromuscular control, proprioception, and balance.* Continue or, if not initiated previously, begin closed-chain exercises. Add disturbed balance activities (perturbation training) standing on an unstable surface, such as a mini-trampoline or wobble board. When full weight bearing is permissible, begin unilateral balance activities, partial lunges, step-ups, and step-downs. Practice walking on an unstable surface, such as high-density foam rubber. Initiate low-intensity agility drills.

- *Flexibility of the hip and ankle.* Stretch the IT band and rectus femoris after the patient has achieved full knee flexion with hip flexion.
- *Cardiopulmonary fitness.* Begin stationary cycling or a pool-walking program at the beginning of this phase. Initiate treadmill training, land walking, or use of a cross-country ski machine at around 9 to 12 weeks.
- *Functional activities.* Gradually resume light functional activities during this phase.

*Criteria to advance to next phase.* By 12 to 16 weeks postoperatively, there should be no pain or joint effusion and full active knee ROM. Lower extremity strength (maximum isometric contraction) should be at the 60% to 80% level.

### Exercise: Minimum Protection/ Return-to-Activity Phase
Some degree of protection still is warranted at the beginning of the final phase of rehabilitation, which typically begins at around 12 to 16 weeks and may continue until 6 to 9 months. The return to a high level of physical activity depends on achieving adequate strength, full, nonpainful ROM, and an acceptable clinical examination.[39,89,142]

*Goals.* The primary goal of this phase is to prepare the patient to resume a full level of functional activities while continuing patient education to reinforce the importance of selecting activities that do not overstress the repaired meniscus (see Box 21.15).

*Interventions.* During resistance training incorporate movement patterns that simulate functional activities. Begin and gradually progress drills to improve power, such as plyometric training. Increase the duration or intensity of the aerobic conditioning program. Transition from a walking program to a jogging/running program, if desired, at about 5 to 6 months. A detailed progression of aerobic conditioning activities after meniscus repair is available in the literature.[89,142]

---

### Outcomes
Repair of a torn medial or lateral meniscus using any one of several surgical techniques is a well tested procedure designed to preserve these important structures and results in predictably successful outcomes. This is particularly true for suture repair of a peripheral zone tear.[89,151,239] Although the results of repair of tears extending into the central zone are not as predictable, there is increasing evidence that repairs in this zone heal well and provide long-term relief of symptoms.[160,161]

Although the use of various surgical techniques and the frequency of concomitant pathologies and surgeries make it difficult to compare outcomes of studies, several generalizations can be made. One of the most important factors influencing outcomes of meniscus repair is the status of the ACL. When an ACL injury occurs in combination with a menicus tear, patients who undergo ACL reconstruction have better outcomes than patients with ACL deficiency. A recurrent tear of a repaired meniscus occurs more frequently in an ACL-deficient knee than an ACL-stable knee.[161,239]

Although the age of a patient typically is cited as a factor influencing the decision of whether to repair a torn meniscus, particularly a tear in the central zone, and although most repairs are performed in patients under age 40, a study by Noyes and colleagues[160] demonstrated a high success rate in a group of patients 40 years of age or older who had central zone tears.

With regard to postoperative rehabilitation, no single protocol has been shown to result in superior outcomes.[239]

Lastly, short-term results of meniscus transplantation with an allograft are promising, but the long-term effectiveness of this procedure remains unclear.[163,184]

## Partial Meniscectomy

### Indications for Surgery
The following are indications for partial menisectomy as a surgical option for a tear of the medial or lateral meniscus.[238]

- A symptomatic (pain and locking), displaced tear of the meniscus sustained by an older, inactive individual associated with pain and locking of the knee
- A tear extending into the central, less vascular third of the meniscus if not determined repairable when arthroscopically visualized and probed
- A tear localized to the inner, avascular third of the meniscus

### Procedure
Arthroscopic meniscectomy typically is performed on an outpatient basis under local anesthesia. Small incisions are made at the knee for portals (usually three); and saline solution is injected through one of the portals, distending the knee. The torn portion of the meniscus is identified, grasped, and divided endoscopically by knife or scissors and removed by vacuum. Intra-articular debris or loose bodies also are removed. After the knee is irrigated and drained, skin incisions at the portal sites are closed, and a compression dressing is applied to the knee.[230,238]

### Postoperative Management
The overall goal of rehabilitation after partial meniscectomy is to restore ROM of the knee and develop strength in the lower extremity to reduce stresses on the knee and protect its articular surfaces.

### Immobilization and Weight Bearing
A compression dressing is placed on the knee, but it is not necessary to immobilize the knee postoperatively with a splint or motion-controlling orthosis. For the first few postoperative days, cryotherapy, compression, and elevation of the operated leg are used to control edema and pain. Weight bearing is progressed as tolerated.[39,208,238]

### Exercise: Maximum and Moderate Protection Phases
Although the ideal situation is to begin exercise instruction on the day of or after surgery, most patients do not see a therapist for supervised exercise immediately after an outpatient procedure. When a patient is referred for supervised therapy, the emphasis typically is placed on establishing a home exercise program. Under these circumstances it is preferable to teach the patient initial exercises to reduce atrophy and prevent contracture *preoperatively* so he or she can initiate the exercises at home immediately after surgery.

After arthroscopic partial meniscectomy there is no need for an extended period of maximum protection postoperatively as there is little soft tissue trauma during surgery. However, moderate protection is warranted for approximately 3 to 4 weeks. All exercises and weight-bearing activities should be pain-free and progressed gradually during the first few postoperative weeks.[22,208]

*Goals and interventions.* Immediately after surgery, begin muscle-setting exercises, SLRs, active knee ROM, and weight bearing as tolerated. Full weight bearing usually is achieved by 4 to 7 days, and at least 90° of knee flexion and full extension are attained by 10 days. Initiate closed-chain exercises and stationary cycling a few days after surgery or as pain and weight bearing status allow, with the goal of regaining dynamic strength and endurance of the knee.

PRECAUTION: Patients who have undergone partial meniscectomy must be cautioned not to push themselves too quickly. Too rapid progression of exercise can cause recurrent joint effusion and possible damage to articular cartilage.

### Exercise: Minimum Protection and Return-to-Activity Phases
By 3 or 4 weeks postoperatively, minimum protection of the knee is necessary, but full active knee ROM should be achieved before progressing to high-demand exercises. Resistance training, endurance activities, bilateral and unilateral closed-chain exercises, and proprioceptive/balance training to develop neuromuscular control all can be progressed rapidly. Advanced activities such as plyometrics, maximum effort isokinetic training, and simulated high-demand functional activities can be initiated as early as 4 to 6 weeks or 6 to 8 weeks postoperatively.

PRECAUTION: High-impact weight-bearing activities such as jogging or jumping, if included in the program, should be added and progressed cautiously to prevent future or additional articular damage to the knee.

## EXERCISE INTERVENTIONS FOR THE KNEE

Strength and flexibility imbalances between muscle groups can result from a variety of causes, some of which are disuse, faulty joint mechanics, joint swelling, immobilization (due to fracture, surgery, or trauma), and nerve injury. In addition to the hamstrings and rectus femoris, most of the two-joint muscles crossing the knee function primarily at the hip or the ankle, yet they also have an effect on the knee. If there is an imbalance in length or strength in the hip or ankle muscles, altered mechanics usually occur throughout the lower extremity. Refer to the chapters on the hip and the ankle and the foot for a complete picture of these interrelationships.

##  EXERCISE TECHNIQUES TO INCREASE FLEXIBILITY AND RANGE OF MOTION

When attempting to increase ROM, the mechanics of the tibiofemoral and patellofemoral joints and their importance in lower extremity function must be respected. Because the knee is a weight-bearing joint, the need for stability takes precedence over the need for mobility, although mobility coupled with adequate strength is also necessary for normal function.

Principles of neuromuscular inhibition and passive stretching were presented in Chapter 4, joint mobilization in Chapter 5, and techniques directed toward specific joint restrictions at the knee and patella earlier in the chapter. Additional manual and self-stretching techniques to increase knee ROM are described in this section.

### To Increase Knee Extension

Decreased flexibility in the hamstring musculature and periarticular tissue posterior to the knee can restrict full knee extension. Increasing knee extension is a two-step process. First, full extension of the knee is obtained without placing tension on the hamstrings at the hip (the hip is maintained at or near 0° extension). After full knee extension has been attained, a stretch is applied to the two-joint hamstring muscle group by progressively flexing the hip while maintaining the knee in extension (SLR position). Techniques to stretch the hamstrings using SLRs are described in Chapter 4 and the exercise section of Chapter 20.

#### Neuromuscular Inhibition Techniques

- *Patient position and procedure:* Supine, with the hip and knee extended as much as possible. Resist knee flexion with an isometric hold using your hand proximal to the ankle; have the patient relax and then passively (or have the patient actively) extend the knee into the end of the range (hold–relax and hold–relax/agonist-contraction techniques, respectively).
- *Patient position and procedure:* Prone, with the hip and knee extended as much as possible. Place a small pad or folded hand towel under the femur proximal to the patella to protect the patella from compressive forces. Stabilize the pelvis to prevent hip flexion and then apply the hold–relax technique to increase knee extension.

#### Passive Stretching Techniques
Use a low-intensity, long-duration stretch to ensure that the patient stays as relaxed as possible.

- *Patient position and procedure:* Prone, hips extended with the patient's foot off the edge of the treatment table. Place a rolled towel under the patient's femur just proximal to the patella and a cuff weight around the ankle. As the muscle relaxes, the weight places a sustained passive stretch on the hamstrings, which increases knee extension.
- *Patient position and procedure:* Supine, with the knee extended as far as possible. Place a rolled towel or padding under the distal leg to elevate the calf and knee off the table. Secure a cuff weight across the distal femur for a sustained stretch.
  N O T E : This position is not effective for severe knee flexion contractures. Use it only for restrictions that are near the end of the range of knee extension.

#### Self-Stretching Technique
*Patient position and procedure*: Long sitting, with the distal leg supported on a rolled towel. Have the patient press down with the hands against the femur just above (not on) the patella to cause a sustained force to increase knee extension.

### To Increase Knee Flexion

Before stretching to increase knee flexion, be sure the patella is mobile and is able to glide distally in the trochlear groove as the knee flexes; otherwise, it restricts knee flexion. Patellar mobilization techniques to increase patellar gliding are described in Chapter 5 (see Figs. 5.53 and 5.54). Once full range of knee flexion is reached, the two-joint rectus femoris and tensor fasciae latae muscles should be stretched across the hip joint while maintaining the knee in flexion. These techniques are described in Chapter 20.

#### Neuromuscular Inhibition Techniques
*Patient position and procedure*: Sitting, with the knee at the edge of the treatment table and flexed as far as possible. Manually resist an isometric contraction of the knee extensors proximal to the ankle. Have the patient relax and then passively (or have the patient actively) flex the knee to the end of the range.

#### Passive Stretching Technique
*Patient position and procedure*: Sitting with knee flexed to the end of its available range. Instruct the patient to relax the muscles and let the weight of the leg cause a low-intensity, long-duration stretch. Apply a manual stretch force, or strap a light weight around the distal leg to increase the stretch force.

#### Self-Stretching Techniques

**Gravity-Assisted Supine Wall Slides**
*Patient position and procedure*: Supine, with buttocks close to the wall and lower extremities resting vertically against

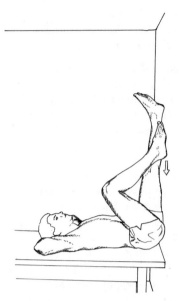

FIGURE 21.14 Gravity-assisted supine wall slide. The patient flexes the knee to the limit of its range and holds it there for a sustained stretch to the quadriceps femoris muscle.

the wall (hips flexed, knees extended). Instruct the patient to slowly flex the involved knee by sliding the foot down the wall until a gentle stretch sensation is felt, hold in a comfortable position, then slide the foot back up the wall (Fig. 21.14).

### Rocking Forward on a Step

*Patient position and procedure*: Standing, with the foot of the involved knee on a step. Have the patient rock forward over the stabilized foot, flexing the knee to the limit of its range, then rock back and forth in a slow, rhythmic manner or hold the stretched position (Fig. 21.15). Begin with a low step or stool; increase the height as more range is obtained.

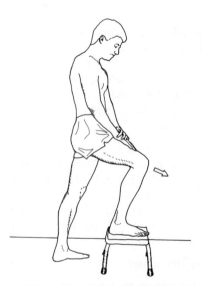

FIGURE 21.15 Self-stretching rock on step. The patient places the foot of the involved side on a step, then rocks forward over the stabilized foot to the limit of knee flexion to stretch the quadriceps femoris muscle. Use a higher step for greater flexion.

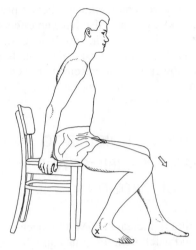

FIGURE 21.16 Self-stretching in a chair. The patient fixates the foot of the involved leg on the floor, then moves forward in the chair over the stabilized foot to place a sustained stretch on the quadriceps femoris muscle and increase knee flexion.

### Sitting

*Patient position and procedure*: Sitting in a chair, with the involved knee flexed to the end of its available range and the foot firmly planted on the floor. Have the patient move forward in the chair, not allowing the foot to slide, then hold the position for a comfortable, sustained stretch of the knee extensors (Fig. 21.16).

## EXERCISES TO DEVELOP AND IMPROVE MUSCLE PERFORMANCE AND FUNCTIONAL CONTROL

When strengthening exercises for knee musculature are selected, implemented, and progressed in a rehabilitation program, the stability of the knee (which involves co-contraction of the quadriceps and hamstrings muscles) and safe patellofemoral and extensor mechanism biomechanics (which allow appropriate patellar tracking) are primary concerns. After stability and patellar mechanics are well established, coordination and timing of muscle contractions as well as endurance are emphasized. *Closed-chain exercises* with an emphasis on low-intensity (low resistance)/high-repetition activities are more effective than open-chain exercises for improving stability and muscular endurance of the knee for dynamic control during weight-bearing activities.

Although closed-chain control of the knee is essential, remember that the knee functions in both an open- and closed-chain fashion during most ADLs. The quadriceps and hamstrings must contract simultaneously (co-contraction) as well as contract concentrically and eccentrically during functional activities. Therefore, exercises under all of these varying conditions should be incorporated into a comprehensive knee rehabilitation program. It is also important to change the position of the hip during quadriceps- and hamstring-strengthening exercises to affect the length–tension relationship of the rectus femoris and hamstrings.[62] Only after a thorough examination and understanding of a patient's pathology, impairments, and functional limitations can a therapist select and design an exercise plan to meet an individual patient's needs.

Considerable research has been done comparing joint reaction forces and muscle function during open-chain and closed-chain exercises. Comparisons of outcomes are difficult because of differing research designs and exercise variables.[56] Table 21.8 summarizes results from a recent study comparing two dynamic exercises, with recommendations for exercise modification with specific knee impairments. Special adaptations also have been highlighted in the conservative management and surgical management sections of this chapter.

In the exercises that follow, open-chain exercises are described before closed-chain exercises simply because weight bearing after knee injury or surgery is often restricted for a time. Isolated activation of knee musculature also is necessary for ADLs that involve open-chain movements, such as lifting the leg to get in and out of bed or a car or flexing and extending the knee during dressing. Closed-chain exercises during partial weight bearing and later during full weight bearing should be initiated as soon as healing allows progressing to balance and proprioceptive training and functional weight-bearing activities.

## Nonweight-Bearing Exercises

### To Develop Control of Knee Extension and Progress Strength (Quadriceps Femoris)

A wide variety of static and dynamic exercises can be used to improve the function of the quadriceps femoris muscles in open-chain positions. Because of variations in muscle fiber orientation and attachments of the knee extensor muscles, individual components of the quadriceps femoris muscle group place different biomechanical stresses on the patella. Even though it is not possible to isolate contraction of the different parts of the quadriceps femoris muscle because of the common innervation, emphasis is often placed on activation of the vastus medialis obliquus (VMO) and vastus medialis (VM) muscles to develop appropriate patellar tracking. Tactile cues, biofeedback, and electrical muscle stimulation over the VMO can reinforce awareness of the muscle contracting for patellar control. In this section, the effectiveness of various quadriceps exercises with regard to training and strengthening the VMO are discussed.

### Quadriceps Setting (Quad Sets)

N O T E : Of the many variations of static and dynamic exercises that have been proposed to selectively train the VMO, quadriceps setting coupled with electrical stimulation or biofeedback has been shown to be most effective.[224]

*Patient position and procedure*: Supine, sitting in a chair (with the heel on the floor) or long-sitting with the knee extended (or flexed a few degrees) but not hyperextended. Have the patient contract the quadriceps isometrically, causing the patella to glide proximally; then hold for a count of 10 and repeat.

- Use verbal cues such as, "Try to push your knee back and tighten your thigh muscle" or "Try to tighten your thigh muscle and pull your kneecap up." When the patient sets the muscle properly, offer verbal reinforcement immediately and then have the patient repeat the activity.
- Have the patient dorsiflex the ankle and then hold an isometric contraction of the quadriceps.[4]

### Straight-Leg Raise

N O T E : An SLR in supine combines dynamic hip flexion with an isometric contraction of the quadriceps. The effec-

## TABLE 21.8 Comparison of Forces and Muscle Action at the Knee During Dynamic Open-Chain and Closed-Chain Exercises[56,249]

| Parameter | Open-Chain Exercise—Variable Resistance: Sitting, Knee Extension Machine | Closed-Chain Exercise—Variable Resistance: Squatting, Leg-Press Machine (Body Moves Away from Fixed Feet) |
|---|---|---|
| Rectus femoris development | More effective | Less effective |
| VMO development | Less effective | More effective for VMO (and VL) |
| Other muscle development | None | Effective for hamstrings |
| ACL tensile forces* | ACL under tension <25° | |
| PCL tensile forces* | PCL under tension of 25°– 95° (peak at 1.0 × body weight) | PCL under tension throughout range (1.5–2.0 × body weight) |
| Patellofemoral compression | Peak stress at 60°, peak compression at 75°‡ | Compression increases with knee flexion, peaking at 90°† |
| Tibiofemoral compression | Higher compression (more stability) < 30° | Higher compression (more stability) >70° |

*The 0–25° range should be excluded in open-chain exercises following ACL injury, but may be included after PCL injury.
†Squat exercises: exercise only from 0° to 50° with patellofemoral dysfunctions.
‡Open-chain exercise from 0° to 30° and 75° to 90° with patellofemoral dysfunctions. (Note: there is controversy in the literature regarding compressive forces in the patellofemoral joint from 0° to 30°.)

tive resistance of gravity (or any additional weight added at the ankle) decreases as the lower extremity elevates because of the decreasing moment arm of the resistance force. The rectus femoris is the primary muscle in the quadriceps group that is active during SLR exercise.[224]

*Patient position and procedure*: Supine, with the knee extended. To stabilize the pelvis and low back, the opposite hip and knee are flexed, and the foot is placed flat on the exercise table. First, instruct the patient to set the quadriceps muscle; then lift the leg to about 45° of hip flexion while keeping the knee extended; hold the leg in that position for a count of 10 and then lower it.

- As the patient progresses, have the patient lift to only 30° of hip flexion and hold the position. Later, have the patient flex the hip to only 15°. The most significant resistance to the quadriceps is during the first few degrees of SLR.
- To increase resistance, place a cuff weight around the patient's ankle.

 **Focus on Evidence** _____

It has been proposed that if an SLR in the supine position is coupled with external rotation or isometric adduction of the hip, the VMO or VM muscles are preferentially activated and strengthened.[4,10,28,47,135] The rationale for advocating these exercises is that many fibers of the VMO muscle originate from the adductor magnus tendon.[4,106] Although a number of authors[4,10] have advocated these adaptations to SLRs to increase the medially directed forces on the patella, there is lack of evidence to substantiate the effect. In two quantitative studies comparing quadriceps muscle activity during quad sets and variations of SLRs, quad sets were found to be associated with significantly more VMO or VM activity than several variations of SLRs.[106,224]

_____

### Straight-Leg Lowering

*Patient position and procedure*: Supine. If the patient cannot perform an SLR because of a quadriceps lag or weakness, begin by passively placing the leg in a 90° of SLR position (or as far as the flexibility of the hamstrings allows) and have the patient gradually lower the extremity while keeping the knee fully extended.

- Be prepared to control the descent of the leg with your hand under the heel as the torque created by gravity increases.
- If the knee begins to flex as the extremity is lowered, have the patient stop at that point, then raise the extremity upward to 90°.
- Have the patient repeat the motion and attempt to lower the extremity a little farther each time while keeping the knee extended.
- Once the patient can keep the knee extended while lowering the leg through the full ROM, SLRs can be initiated.

### Multiple-Angle Isometric Exercises

- *Patient position and procedure*: Supine or long-sitting. Have the patient perform bent leg raises with the knee in multiple angles of flexion.
- *Patient position and procedure*: Seated at the edge of a treatment table. When tolerated, resistance is applied at the ankle manually or mechanically to strengthen the quadriceps isometrically in varying degrees of knee flexion. An effective co-contraction with the hamstrings can be activated (except in the last 10° to 15° of knee extension) by having the patient push the thigh downward into the table while holding the knee in extension against maximum resistance.[85]

### Short-Arc Terminal Extension

N O T E : Although in the past it was thought that the VMO was responsible for the terminal phase of knee extension, it is now well documented that all components of the quadriceps femoris muscle group are active throughout active knee extension and that the VMO primarily affects patellar alignment.[224]

*Patient position and procedure*: Supine or long-sitting. Place a rolled towel or bolster under the knee to support it in flexion (Fig. 21.17). The patient can also assume a short-sitting position at the edge of a table with the seat of a chair or a stool placed under the heel to stop knee flexion at the desired angle. Begin with the knee in a few degrees of flexion. Increase the degrees of flexion as tolerated by the patient or dictated by the condition.

- Initially have the patient extend the knee only against the resistance of gravity. Later, add cuff weights around the ankle to increase the resistance if the patient does not experience pain or crepitation.
- Combine short-arc terminal extension with an isometric hold and/or SLR when the knee is in full extension.
- To prevent lateral shear forces at the knee, have the patient invert the foot as he or she extends the knee.[4,83]

P R E C A U T I O N : When adding resistance to the distal leg, the amount of torque generated by the quadriceps muscle increases significantly in the terminal ranges of knee

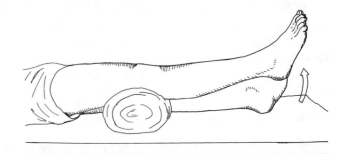

**FIGURE 21.17** Short-arc terminal extension exercise to strengthen the quadriceps femoris muscle. When tolerated, resistance is added proximal to the ankle.

extension. In this portion of the range, the quadriceps has a poor mechanical advantage and poor physiological length while having to contract against an external resistance force that has a long lever arm. The amount of muscle force generated causes an anterior translation force on the tibia, which is restrained by the ACL. This exercise is not appropriate for a person with an unstable knee after an ACL injury or during postoperative rehabilitation before the ligament has healed.

### Full-Arc Extension

*Patient position and procedure*: Sitting or supine. Have the patient extend the knee from 90° to full extension. Apply resistance to the motion as tolerated.

N O T E : Resistance from 90° to 60° causes less anterior tibial translation than closed-chain squatting in this range. Resistance applied in open-chain extension from 30° to 0°, however, increases anterior translation more than does performing mini-squats in the same range.[249]

- Apply resistance through the full arc of motion only during the later stages of rehabilitation if the knee is pain-free, stable, and asymptomatic. If there is pain, resistance should be applied only through those parts of the range with no symptoms.
- Various forms of mechanical resistance equipment discussed in Chapter 6 can be used to strengthen the knee extensors. Emphasize high-repetition, low-resistance training with weight-training equipment and medium- to high-speed training with isokinetic equipment to minimize compressive and shear forces to knee joint structures during exercise. When using equipment, the tibial pad against which the patient pushes while extending the knee can be placed more proximally than distally on the lower leg to minimize excessive stress to supporting structures of the knee.
- If a cuff weight is applied to the tibia to provide resistance, it causes a distraction to the joint and stress on the ligaments when the patient sits or lies supine with the knee flexed to 90° and the tibia over the edge of the treatment table. To avoid this stress to ligaments, place a stool under the foot so it can be supported when the leg is in the dependent position.[31]

### To Strengthen Knee Flexion (Hamstrings)

### Hamstring-Setting (Hamstring Sets)

*Patient position and procedure*: Supine or long-sitting, with the knee in extension or slight flexion with a towel roll under the knee. Have the patient isometrically contract the knee flexors just enough to feel tension developing in the muscle group by gently pushing the heel into the treatment table and holding the contraction. Have the patient relax and then repeat the contraction.

### Multiple-Angle Isometric Exercises

*Patient position and procedure*: Supine or long-sitting. Apply either manual or mechanical resistance to a static hamstring muscle contraction with the knee flexed to several positions in the ROM.

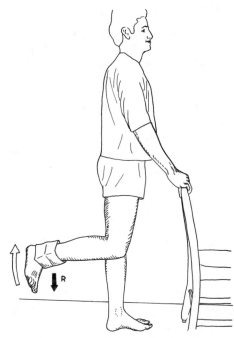

FIGURE 21.18 Hamstring curls; resistance exercises to the knee flexors with the patient standing. Maximal resistance occurs when the knee is at 90°.

- Place the tibia in internal or external rotation prior to resisting knee flexion to emphasize the medial or lateral hamstring muscles, respectively.
- Teach the patient to apply self-resistance at multiple points in the ROM by placing the opposite foot behind the ankle of the leg to be resisted.

### Hamstring Curls (Open-Chain Knee Flexion)

- *Patient position and procedure:* Standing, holding onto a solid object for balance. Have the patient pick up the foot and flex the knee (Fig. 21.18). Maximum resistance from gravity occurs when the knee is at 90° flexion. Add resistance with ankle weights or a weighted boot. If the patient flexes the hip, stabilize it by having the patient place the anterior thigh against a wall or solid object.
- *Patient position and procedure:* Prone. Place a small towel roll or foam rubber under the femur just proximal to the patella to avoid compression of the patella between the treatment table and the femur. With a cuff weight around the ankle, have the patient flex the knee to only 90°. Maximum resistance from gravity occurs when the knee first starts to flex at 0°. If hamstring curls are performed in the prone position using manual resistance, a weight-pulley system or isokinetic equipment resistance to the knee flexors can be applied throughout the range of knee flexion.

P R E C A U T I O N : Open-chain hamstring curls performed against resistance placed on the distal tibia cause posterior tibial translation. A patient with a PCL injury or reconstruction should avoid this exercise during the early stages of rehabilitation.

## Closed-Chain Exercises

Progressive closed-chain exercises are beneficial for activating and training the musculature of the lower extremity to respond to specific functional demands. As the quadriceps contract eccentrically to control knee flexion or contract concentrically to extend the knee, the hamstrings and soleus function to stabilize the tibia against the anterior translating force of the quadriceps at the knee joint. This synergy along with the compressive loading on the joints provides support to the cruciate ligaments.[56,178] In addition, because the hip extends and the ankle plantarflexes as the knee extends (and vice versa) during closed-chain activities, the two-joint hamstrings and gastrocnemius and the one-joint soleus are maintaining favorable length–tension relationships through action at the hip and ankle, respectively.

In a rehabilitation program, closed-chain exercises can be incorporated in an exercise regimen as soon as partial or full weight bearing is safe. Closed-chain strengthening exercises generate less shear force on knee ligaments, particularly anterior tibial translation, than open-chain quadriceps-strengthening activities.[52] Therefore, resistance can be added to closed-chain activities sooner after injury or surgery than to open-chain exercises while still protecting healing structures such as the ACL. Clinically, closed-chain exercises enable a patient to develop strength, endurance, and stability of the lower extremity in functional patterns sooner after knee injury or surgery than do open-chain exercises. The progression of closed-chain exercises described in Chapter 20 also are appropriate for knee rehabilitation programs.

If the patient does not tolerate or is not permitted to be full weight bearing, begin exercises in the parallel bars or in a pool to partially unload body weight. During the healing phase after surgical procedures or with anterior knee pain problems, the knee should be taped or supported in a hinged brace during exercise. Begin exercises at a level tolerated by the patient and at which there is complete control and no exacerbation of symptoms.

Because the knee is the intermediate link in the lower extremity chain, it is influenced by hip and trunk as well as foot and ankle function during weight bearing. Proximal stability of the hip and the trunk may influence the kinematics of the knee,[189] and therefore exercises for these regions should be included in the rehabilitation of the knee if any impairments are detected during the examination.

### Closed-Chain Isometric Exercises

Closed-chain isometric exercises are done to facilitate co-contraction of the quadriceps and hamstrings.

### Setting Exercises

*Patient position and procedure*: Sitting on a chair, with the knee extended or slightly flexed and the heel on the floor. Have the patient press the heel against the floor and the thigh against the seat of the chair and concentrate on contracting the quadriceps and hamstrings simultaneously to facilitate co-contraction around the knee joint. Hold the muscle contraction, relax, and repeat. Use biofeedback to enhance learning of the co-contraction.

### Stabilization Exercises

*Patient position and procedure*: Standing, with weight equally distributed through both lower extremities. Apply manual resistance to the pelvis in alternating directions as the patient holds the position. This facilitates isometric contractions of muscles in the ankles, knees, and hips.
- Increase the speed of application of the resistive forces to train the muscles to respond to sudden shifts in forces.
- Progress the stabilization activity by applying the alternating resistance against the shoulders to develop trunk stabilization and then by having the patient bear weight only on the involved lower extremity while resistance is applied.

### Closed-Chain Isometrics Against Elastic Resistance

*Patient position and procedure*: Standing on the involved extremity, with elastic resistance looped around the thigh of the opposite extremity and secured to a stable object (see Fig. 20.22). Have the patient flex and extend the hip of the non-weight-bearing lower extremity to facilitate co-contraction of muscles and stability of the weight-bearing leg. This closed-chain exercise also facilitates proprioceptive input and balance on the weight-bearing (involved) lower extremity.

### Closed-Chain Dynamic Exercises

Patient position is standing in all of the following exercises.

### Unilateral Closed-Chain Terminal Knee Extension

Loop elastic resistance around the distal thigh and secure it to a stationary structure (Fig. 21.19). Have the patient actively perform terminal knee extension while bearing partial to full weight on the involved extremity.

### Partial Squats, Mini-Squats, and Short-Arc Training

Begin by having the patient flex both knees up to 30° to 45° and then extend them. Progress by using elastic resistance placed under both feet (Fig. 21.20) or by holding

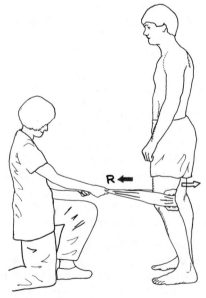

FIGURE 21.19 Unilateral closed-chain extension.

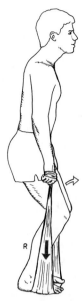

FIGURE 21.20 Resisted mini-squats; closed-chain short-arc training. Elastic resistance to knee extension is provided for short-arc motion. It is important to use the quadriceps femoris muscles rather than substitute with the hamstring muscles for proper strengthening.

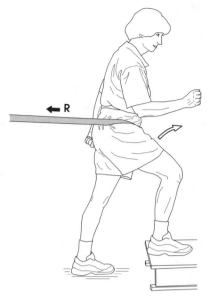

FIGURE 21.21 Resisted step-ups against elastic resistance or a pulley to strengthen knee extension.

weights in the hands. The patient should maintain the trunk upright and concentrate on the sensation of the quadriceps muscle contracting, not pulling back on the femur with the hip extensors.

● Progress squats to greater ranges of knee flexion during the advanced phases of treatment if necessary.
● Increase the difficulty of the exercise by performing unilateral resisted mini-squats.
● It has been suggested but not documented through research that if partial squats are performed with the legs slightly externally rotated the VMO muscle is in an optimal line of pull and may be more readily activated.[10]

N O T E : Squatting can be accomplished in one of two ways, each with positive and negative effects. When the knees move anterior to the toes, as the hips descend there is increased shear forces on the tibia and strain on the ACL. This can be dangerous if the patient squats while carrying considerable weight or after ACL surgery. Yet this is a more normal method for squatting and maintaining balance over the base of support. Squatting, as if sitting on a chair, during which the tibia remains relatively vertical, requires greater trunk flexion to maintain balance and a stronger quadriceps contraction to support the load of the pelvis posterior to the knee axis at an angle where patellar compressive loads are great. Yet this method reduces stress on the ACL. Positioning should be based on the patient's symptoms and pathological condition.

### Forward, Backward, and Lateral Step-Ups and Step-Downs

● Begin with a low step, 2 to 3 inches in height, and increase the height as the patient is able. Make sure the patient keeps the trunk upright.

● Emphasize control of body weight during concentric (step-up) and eccentric (step-down) quadriceps activity. To emphasize the quadriceps and minimize pushing off with the plantarflexors of the trailing extremity, instruct the patient that the heel is to be the last to leave the floor and the first to return or to "keep the toes up."
● Add resistance with a weight belt, handheld weights, or ankle weights around the non-weight-bearing leg if there is good ligamentous integrity, or place elastic resistance or a belt attached to a pulley system around the patient's hips and have the patient step up against the resistance force (Fig. 21.21).

### Standing Wall Slides
*Patient position and procedure*: Standing, with back against the wall (see Fig. 20.24A); flex the hips and knees and slide the back down and then up the wall, lowering and lifting the body weight.

● As control improves, have the patient move into greater knee flexion, up to a maximum of 60°. Knee flexion beyond 60° is not advocated to avoid excessive shear forces on ligamentous structures of the knee and compressive forces on the patellofemoral joint.
● Add isometric training by having the patient stay in the partial-squat position. If the patient is able, he or she maintains the partial squat and alternately extends one leg and then the other.
● Wall slides performed with a gym ball behind the back decrease stability and require more control (see Fig. 20.24B).
● Unpublished data suggest that doing wall slides with a small ball between the knees activates a stronger contraction in the VMO.[128]

### Partial and Full Lunges

- Have the patient assume a step-forward stance position and rock his or her body weight forward, allowing the knee to flex slightly, and then rock backward and control knee extension.
- Progress the activity with full lunges (see Fig. 20.23). The patient begins with the feet together and then lunges forward with the involved extremity, beginning with a small stride and a small amount of knee flexion. He or she then returns upright by extending the knee and then bringing the foot back beside the other foot. Instruct the patient to keep the flexing knee in alignment with the toes and not to flex beyond a vertical line coming up from the toes. As the patient gains control, the stride length is increased and knee flexion is increased accordingly. Weights can be added to the trunk or be placed in the patient's hands for progressive strengthening. The speed of the activity is also increased as control improves.
- Progress by having the patient lunge diagonally forward, then out to the side, then diagonally backward, and then backward. This is facilitated by placing four intersecting lines on the floor (like spokes on a wheel) and having the patient stand in the middle of the intersecting lines. The patient then steps out onto one of the lines and returns. This same motion can be repeated multiple times before progressing to the next line, or the patient can step out onto each line in succession.

### Chair Scooting

*Patient position and procedure*: Sitting, on a rolling stool or chair. Have the patient "walk" forward to use the hamstrings or "walk" backward to use the quadriceps. Increase the challenge of the exercise by having the patient steer around an obstacle course, roll the stool across carpeting, or pull against a resistance (such as pulling another person who is also on a rolling stool) (Fig. 21.22).

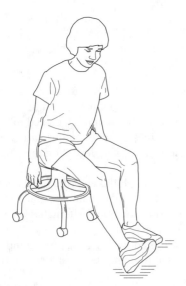

FIGURE 21.22 Forward chair scooting to strengthen knee flexion and backward scooting to strengthen knee extension.

## Techniques to Simulate Functional Activities

To prepare for functional activities, it is important to develop muscular endurance, control of balance, and ability to respond to expected or unexpected perturbations. The principle of specificity of training is used to progress the patient's activities toward the desired outcome. Activities previously described are progressed for endurance by increasing the number of repetitions or time element at each resistance level. Once control has developed, emphasis is placed on balance, coordination, timing, and skill acquisition specific to the desired activity of the patient. Also refer to the exercises described in the hip chapter for balance stability and training.

### Strength and Muscle Endurance Training

Mechanical equipment such as a leg press, Total Gym® unit, isokinetic dynamometer, treadmill, stationary bicycle, and stair-stepping units is useful for strengthening and endurance training and provides motivational feedback to the patient. When implementing isokinetic training for the quadriceps and hamstrings, use velocity-spectrum rehabilitation at medium to fast velocities.[200] Place the tibia pad in a relatively proximal position on the knee to decrease anterior shear forces[250] and program in range-limiting parameters whenever necessary.

### Conditioning Activities

Activities such as swimming, progressive walking, running, cross-country ski machine training, and biking are designed for general cardiovascular/pulmonary conditioning and are graded to the patient's tolerance. If the patient is planning on returning to a sport activity, choose a conditioning activity that best replicates the muscle activity used in the sport

### Proprioceptive and Balance Activities (Perturbation Training)

Begin as early as weight bearing is allowed with balance activities. Suggestions include:

- Partial weight bearing in parallel bars and shifting weight; progress to full weight bearing.
- Stabilization exercises against alternating resistive forces.
- Stepping and marching in place.
- Balancing with arm movements in sagittal, frontal, and transverse planes; then progressing to diagonal planes.
- Walking; progress to walking in different directions, walking against resistance, and walking on uneven surfaces.
- Bilateral then unilateral stance on a balance (rocker) board, roller board, or BAPS board. Increase the challenge by adding destabilizing forces while the patient is balancing, such as tossing a weighted ball to the patient or pulling against elastic resistance that the patient is holding.
- If the patient is returning to a sport activity, replicate the stresses that will be placed on the knee in a controlled and then progressively uncontrolled manner.[63,64,240,254]

## Plyometric Training

High-speed, stretch-shortening exercises, which are designed to improve power, are appropriate for selected patients intending to return to high-demand functional or recreational activities. Jumping on and off surfaces of varying heights (Fig. 21.23) and incorporating directional changes in the movements are appropriate during the later stages of knee rehabilitation.

## Drills

To improve coordination and agility, have the patient begin by stepping over and around objects that are placed on the ground as obstacles. Progress the training by increasing the speed of moving around the obstacles, or jump or hop over the obstacles. Initiate running, sprinting, pivoting, cutting, and sport-specific drills, monitoring for appropriate progression and correct mechanics.

## Simulated Work–Related Activities

A patient returning to a repetitive lifting job requires strength in the trunk stabilizers as well as hip and knee extensors for safe body mechanics. A progression of lifting tasks, including squats and lunges, should also include use of proper body mechanics during lifting tasks. This progression is described in detail in Chapter 16.

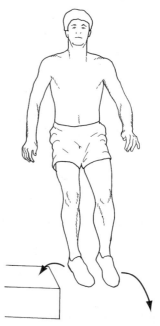

FIGURE 21.23 Plyometric training using lateral jumps from a step. When the patient lands on the ground the hips and knees flex, then quickly extend to jump back up on the step. This plies a quick lengthening prior to shortening of the quadriceps muscle.

# INDEPENDENT LEARNING ACTIVITIES

## ● Critical Thinking and Discussion

1. Observe a functional activity, such as putting on a pair of socks, rising from a chair, or climbing on to a city bus.
   • What ROM is needed in the knee joint? Also include hip and ankle in the analysis.
   • If motion is restricted, what muscles would have decreased mobility? What joint glides would have decreased mobility?
   • What muscles are functioning, and what level of strength is needed?
   • Assume there is 50% loss of range and strength. Design an exercise program to progress functional recovery.
2. Describe the function of all the two-joint muscles that cross the knee; include the function of each muscle at its "other joint" and how each muscle can function most efficiently at the knee in terms of its length–tension relationship.
3. Describe the role of the knee musculature during the gait cycle.
   • What ROM is needed, and when during the gait cycle does the maximum degree of flexion and extension occur?
   • During the gait cycle, when is each of the muscles active at the knee, and what is their function?
   • What gait deviations occur when there is muscle shortening, muscle weakness, and joint pain? Explain why each deviation occurs.

4. Two patients, both in their seventies, who underwent TKA 10 days ago because of joint degeneration from OA of the right knee have been referred to you in your home health practice. One patient had a cemented TKA and the other had a "hybrid" TKA. How does their postoperative management differ or how is it similar?
5. Differentiate among structures involved with a lateral retinacular release, a proximal realignment of the extensor mechanism, and a distal realignment procedure. How would these differences have an impact on postoperative rehabilitation?

## ● Laboratory Practice

1. Design, set up, and then perform a circuit training course for hamstring and quadriceps activation and strengthening and balance exercises. Sequence the activities from basic to advanced. Observe the accuracy and safety with each exercise and note the stresses involved.
2. Using mechanical resistance (pulleys, elastic resistance, and free weights), set up exercises to meet each of the following situations.
   • Strengthen the quadriceps with the greatest mechanical torque occurring when the knee is at 90°, at 45°, and at 25°.
   • Strengthen the hamstrings with the greatest mechanical torque occurring when the knee is at 90°, at 45°, and at 0°.

3. Review all the joint mobilization techniques for the knee; include basic glides, accessory motions, patellar mobilizations, and mobilization with movement techniques.
   - Identify and practice techniques that increase knee extension, beginning with the knee at 45° and progressing by 15° increments until full extension is reached.
   - Do the same for knee flexion, beginning at 25° and progressing at 15° increments until full range is achieved. What accessory motions are necessary?
   - What motions are restricted if the patella does not glide distally?
   - What function is lost if the patella does not glide proximally?
4. Review and practice soft tissue and patellar mobilization techniques that can be used to increase the mobility of the lateral retinaculum around the patella. How does mobilizing this tissue improve patellar tracking?
5. Identify all the two-joint muscles that cross the knee. Review and practice self-stretching techniques with and without equipment for each of these muscles.

## ● Case Studies

1. Mrs. J. is a 49-year-old mother of three children. She is in good health but recently has experienced considerable right knee pain, especially after sitting for prolonged periods and then standing up, when descending stairs, and when shopping at the mall for longer than 2 hours. She has a history of a proximal tibial fracture 15 years ago. She reports that it took about a year before relatively normal mobility returned. On examination, you note no obvious deformities or joint swelling. Knee flexion is 125° with firm end-feel and pain on overpressure; extension is 0° with firm end-feel and pain on overpressure. There is a slight decrease in posterior glide accessory motion of the tibia and decreased mobility of the patella

on the right compared to the left. Strength of the knee flexors and extensors is 4/5 bilaterally. She complains of pain in the right knee when squatting; pain begins at 45° flexion. She stops when the knees are at 75°, saying it hurts too much. She bends forward from the waist to pick up objects from the floor. She has difficulty lowering herself down to a low chair in a controlled manner.
   - List her impairments and functional limitations, and state appropriate goals.
   - Develop an exercise program to meet the goals. How do you begin the exercises; how do you progress each exercise and the program?
   - Describe a rationale for each manual technique you would use and for each exercise you would teach the patient.
2. Mr. R., 25 years of age, was in a serious automobile accident and sustained multiple femoral and patellar fractures on the left side. His leg was immobilized in a long-leg cast for 3 months followed by a short leg cast for an additional month. He was allowed to perform partial weight bearing when in the short-leg cast. The cast was removed this morning, and now he is to begin his rehabilitation, although he will not be allowed to perform full weight bearing for an additional month. He describes significant stiffness and discomfort when attempting to flex his knee. Observation reveals significant atrophy in the thigh and leg. There are no open sores or joint swelling. Range is minimal: flexion to 25°, extension to 20°, and no joint play in the tibiofemoral or patellofemoral joints. He demonstrated the ability to do quad and hamstring sets, but strength could not be tested.
   - Answer the same questions as in the previous case.
   - Even though patients in this and the previous case have restricted motion and demonstrate weakness, what are the differences in your intervention strategies? Are there different precautions that you will follow during treatment? If so, what are they?

---

## REFERENCES

1. Allum, R: Aspects of current management: complications of arthroscopic reconstruction of the anterior cruciate ligament. J Bone Joint Surg Br 85:12–16, 2003.
2. American Physical Therapy Association: Guide to Physical Therapist Practice, ed 2. Phys Ther 81:9–744, 2001.
3. Anderson, JK, Noyes, FR: Principles of posterior cruciate ligament reconstruction. Orthopedics 18:493, 1995.
4. Antich, TJ, Brewster, CE: Modification of quadriceps femoris muscle exercises during knee rehabilitation. Phys Ther 66:1246, 1986.
5. Arendt, E, Dick, R: Knee injury patterns among men and women in collegiate basketball and soccer. Am J Sports Med 23:694, 1995.
6. Avramidis, K, Strike, PW, Taylor, PN, Swain, ID: Effectiveness of electrical stimulation of the vastus medialis muscle in the rehabilitation of patients after total knee arthroplasty. Arch Phys Med Rehabil 84(12):1850–1853, 2003.
7. Barber-Westin, SD, Noyes, FR, et al: The effect of exercise and rehabilitation on anterior posterior knee displacements after anterior cruciate ligament autograft reconstruction. Am J Sports Med 27:2, 1999.
8. Bartha, L, Vajada, A, Duska, Z, et al: Autologous osteochondral mosaicplasty grafting. J Orthop Sports Phys Ther 36(10):739–750, 2006.

9. Beaupré, LA, Davies, DM, Jones, CA, Cinarts, JG: Exercise combined with continuous passive motion or slider board therapy compared with exercise only: a randomized controlled trial of patients following total knee arthroplasty. Phys Ther 81:1029–1037, 2001.
10. Bennett, JG: Rehabilitation of patellofemoral joint dysfunction. In Greenfield, BH (ed) Rehabilitation of the Knee: A Problem-Solving Approach. FA Davis, Philadelphia, 1993, p 177.
11. Berchuck, M, Andriacchi, TP, Bach, BR, et al: Gait adaptations by patients who have a deficient anterior cruciate ligament. J Bone Joint Surg Am 72(6):871–877, 1990.
12. Berenbaum, F: Osteoarthritis, epidemiology, pathology, and pathogenesis. In Primer on the Rheumatic Diseases, ed 12. Arthritis Foundation, Atlanta, 2001.
13. Bertlet, GC, Mascia, A, Miniaci, A: Treatment of unstable osteochondritis dessicans lesions of the knee using autogenous osteochondral grafts (mosaicplasty). Arthroscopy 15:312–316, 1999.
14. Bert, JM: Arthroscopic treatment of degenerative arthritis of the knee. In Insall, JN, Scott, WN (eds) Surgery of the Knee, Vol 1, ed 3. Churchill Livingstone, New York, 2001, p 381.
15. Beynnon, BD, Johnson, RJ, Abate, JA, et al: Treatment of anterior cruciate ligament injuries. Part 1. Am J Sports Med 33(10):1579–1602, 2005.

16. Beynnon, BD, Johnson, RJ, Abate, JA, et al: Treatment of anterior cruciate ligament injuries. Part 2. Am J Sports Med 33(11): 1751–1767, 2005.

17. Beynnon, BD, Uh, BS, Johnson, RJ, et al: Rehabilitation after anterior cruciate ligament reconstruction: a prospective, randomized, double-blind comparison of programs administered over 2 different time intervals. Am J Sports Med 33(3):347–355, 2005.

18. Bizzini, M, Childs, JD, et al: Systematic review of the quality of randomized controlled trials for patellofemoral pain syndrome. J Orthop Sports Phys Ther 33(1):4–20, 2003.

19. Blackburn, TA, Eiland, WG, Bandy, WG: An introduction to the plica. J Orthop Sports Phys Ther 3:171, 1982.

20. Bobic, V: Autologous osteo-chondral grafts in the management of articular cartilage lesions. Orthopaedics 28:19, 1999.

21. Bonutti, PM: Minimally invasive total knee arthroplasty—midvastus approach. In Hozack, WJ, Krismer, M, Nogler, M, et al (eds) Minimally Invasive Total Joint Arthroplasty. Springer, Heidelberg, 2004, pp 139–145.

22. Boyce, DA, Hanley, ST: Functional based rehabilitation of the knee after partial meniscectomy or meniscal repair. Orthop Phys Ther Clin North Am 3:555, 1994.

23. Bradbury, N, Borton, D, Spoo, G, Cross, MJ: Participation in sports after total knee replacement. Am J Sports Med 26(4):530–535, 1998.

24. Brand, J, Jr, Weiler, A, Caborn, DN, et al: Graft fixation in cruciate ligament reconstruction. Am J Sports Med 28:761–774, 2000.

25. Brewster, CE, Moynes, DR, Jobe, FW: Rehabilitation for anterior cruciate reconstruction. J Orthop Sports Phys Ther 5:121, 1983.

26. Brodersen, MP: Anterior cruciate ligament reconstruction. In Morrey, BF (ed) Reconstructive Surgery of the Joints, ed 2. Churchill Livingstone, New York, 1996, p 1639.

27. Brody, LT, Thein, JM: Nonoperative treatment for patello-femoral pain. J Orthop Sports Phys Ther 28:336, 1988.

28. Brownstein, BA, Lamb, RL, Mangine, RE: Quadriceps, torque and integrated electromyography. J Orthop Sports Phys Ther 6:309, 1985.

29. Buckwalter, JA, Ballard, WT: Operative treatment of arthritis. In Klippel, JH (ed) Primer on the Rheumatic Diseases, ed 12. Arthritis Foundation, Atlanta, 2001, pp 613–623.

30. Bynum, EB, Barrick, RL, Alexander, AH: Open versus closed kinetic chain exercises after anterior cruciate ligament reconstruction: a prospective study. Am J Sports Med 23:401, 1995.

31. Cailliet, R: Knee Pain and Disability, ed 3. FA Davis, Philadelphia, 1992.

32. Callaghan, JJ, Insall, JN, Greenwald, AS, et al: Mobile-bearing knee replacement. J Bone Joint Surg Am 82:1020–1041, 2000.

33. Cameron, H, Brotzman, SB: The arthritic lower extremity. In Brotzman, SB, Wilk, KE (eds) Clinical Orthopedic Rehabilitation, ed 2. Mosby, Philadelphia, 2003, pp 441–474.

34. Carrey, CT, Tria, AJ: Surgical principles of total knee replacement: Incisions, extensor mechanism, ligament balancing. In Pellicci, PM, Tria, AJ, Garvin, KL (eds) Orthopedic Knowledge Update, 2. Hip and Knee Reconstruction. American Academy of Orthopedic Surgeons, Rosemont, IL, 2000, p 281.

35. Chiarello, CM, Gunderson, L, O'Halloran, T: The effect of continuous passive motion duration and increment on range of motion in total knee arthroplasty patients. J Orthop Sports Phys Ther 25(2):119–127, 1997.

36. Chu, C: Cartilage therapies: chondrocyte transplantation, osteochondral allografts, and autographs. In Pedowitz, RA, O'Conor, JJ, Akeson, WH (eds) Daniel's Knee Injuries: Ligament and Cartilage Structure, Function, Injury and Repair, ed 2. Lippincott Williams & Wilkins, Philadelphia, 2003, pp 227–237.

37. Cooper, DE, DeLee, MD, Ramamurthy, S: Reflex sympathetic dystrophy of the knee. J Bone Joint Surg Am 71:365, 1989.

38. Cyriax, J: Textbook of Orthopaedic Medicine. Vol. 1. Diagnosis of Soft Tissue Lesions, ed 8. Bailliere Tindall, London, 1982.

39. D'Amato, M, Bach, BR: Knee injuries. In Brotzman, SB, Wilk, KE (eds) Clinical Orthopedic Rehabilitation, ed 2. Mosby, Philadelphia, 2003, pp 251–370.

40. D'Antonio, JA: Complications of total hip and knee arthroplasty: lessons learned. In Hozack, WJ, Krismer, M, Nogler, M, et al (eds) Minimally Invasive Total Joint Arthroplasty. Springer, Heidelberg, 2004, pp 304–308.

41. Davis, IM, Ireland, ML: ACL injuries—the gender bias. J Orthop Sports Phys Ther 33(8):A2–A8, 2003.

42. Denis, M, Moffet, H, Caron, F, et al: Effectiveness of continuous passive motion and conventional physical therapy after total knee arthroplasty: a randomized clinical trial. Phys Ther 86:174–185, 2006.

43. Deyle, GD, Allison, SC, Matekel, RL, et al: Physical therapy treatment effectiveness for osteoarthritis of the knee: a randomized comparison of supervised clinical exercise and manual therapy procedures versus a home exercise program. Phys Ther 85:1301–1317, 2005.

44. De Jong, Z, Vlieland, TP: Safety of exercise in patients with rheumatoid arthritis. Curr Opin Rheumatol 17(2):177–182, 2005.

45. Dietrichson, J, Souryal, TO: Preoperative and postoperative rehabilitation of anterior cruciate ligament tears. Orthop Phys Ther Clin North Am 3:539, 1994.

46. Dixon, MC, Brown, RR, Parsch, D, Scott, RD: Modular fixed-bearing total knee arthroplasty with retention of the posterior cruciate ligament: a study of patients followed for a minimum of fifteen years. J Bone Joint Surg Am 87(3):598–603, 2005.

47. Doucette, SA, Goble, EM: The effect of exercise on patellar tracking in lateral patellar compression syndrome. Am J Sports Med 20:434, 1992.

48. Drez, D, et al: In vivo measurement of anterior tibial translation using continuous passive motion devices. Am J Sports Med 19:381, 1991.

49. Drez, D, Edwards, TB, Williams, CS: Results of medial patellofemoral ligament reconstruction in the treatment of patellar dislocations. Arthroscopy 17(3):298–306, 2001.

50. Dunn, WR, Lyman, S, Lincoln, AE, et al: The effect of anterior cruciate ligament reconstruction on the risk of knee re-injury. Am J Sports Med 32(8):1906–1914, 2004.

51. Ecker, ML, Lotke, PA: Postoperative care of the total knee patient. Orthop Phys Ther Clin North Am 20:55, 1989.

52. Einhorn, AR, Sawyer, M, Tovin B: Rehabilitation of intra-articular reconstructions. In Greenfield, BH (ed) Rehabilitation of the Knee: A Problem-Solving Approach. FA Davis, Philadelphia. 1993, p 245.

53. Eng, JJ, Peirrynowsk, MR: Evaluation of soft foot orthotics in the treatment of patellofemoral pain syndrome. Phys Ther 73:840, 1993.

54. Engle, RP, Meade, TD, Canner, GC: Rehabilitation of posterior cruciate ligament injuries. In Greenfield, BH (ed) Rehabilitation of the Knee: A Problem-Solving Approach. FA Davis Philadelphia, 1993, p 304.

55. Enloe, J, et al: Total hip and knee replacement programs: a report using consensus. J Orthop Sports Phys Ther 23:3, 1996.

56. Escamilla, RF, et al: Biomechanics of the knee during closed kinetic chain and open kinetic chain exercises. Med Sci Sports Exerc 30:556, 1998.

57. Ethgen, O, Bruyere, O, Richy, F, et al: Health-related quality of life in total hip and total knee arthroplasty: a qualitative and systematic review of the literature. J Bone Joint Surg Am 86:963–974, 2004.

58. Feller, JA, Webster, KE: A randomized comparison of patellar tendon and hamstring tendon anterior cruciate ligament reconstruction. Am J Sports Med 31(4):564–573, 2003.

59. Finch, E, Walsh, M, Thomas, SC, Woodhouse, LJ: Functional ability perceived by individuals following total knee arthroplasty compared to age-matched individuals without knee disability. J Orthop Sports Phys Ther 27:255–263, 1998.

60. Fineberg, MS, Zarins, B, Sherman, OH: Practical considerations in anterior cruciate ligament replacement surgery. Arthroscopy 16:715, 2000.

61. Finger, S, Paulos, LE: Arthroscopic-assisted posterior cruciate ligament repair/reconstruction. In Jackson, DW (ed) Master Techniques in Orthopedic Surgery: Reconstructive Knee Surgery, ed 2. Lippincott Williams & Wilkins, Philadelphia, 2003, pp 159–177.

62. Fisher, NM, et al: Quantitative effects of physical therapy on muscular and functional performance in subjects with osteoarthritis of the knees. Arch Phys Med Rehabil 74:840, 1993.

63. Fitzgerald, GK, et al: The efficacy of perturbation training in nonoperative anterior cruciate ligament rehabilitation programs for physically active individuals. Phys Ther 80:128, 2000.

64. Fitzgerald, GK, et al: Proposed practice guidelines for nonoperative anterior cruciate ligament rehabilitation of physically active individuals. J Orthop Sports Phys Ther 30:194, 2000.

65. Fortin, PR, Clarke, AE, Joseph, L, et al: Outcomes of total hip and knee replacement: preoperative functional status predicts outcomes at six months after surgery. Arthritis Rheum 42:1722–1728, 1999.

66. Fransen, M, McConnell, S, Bell, M: Exercise for osteoarthritis of the hip or knee. The Cochrane Database of Systematic Reviews 2001, Issue 2. Art. No.: CD004376.DOI: 10.1002/14561858.CD004376.

67. Ford, DH, Post, WR: Open or arthroscopic lateral release: Indications, techniques and rehabilitation. Clin Sports Med 16:29, 1997.

68. Fu, FH, et al: Current trends in anterior cruciate ligament reconstruction. Part I. Biology and biomechanics of reconstruction. Am J Sports Med 27:821, 1999.

69. Fu, FH, et al: Current trends in anterior cruciate ligament reconstruction. Part II. Operative procedures and clinical correlations. Am J Sports Med 28:124:2000.

70. Fu, FH, Maday, M: Arthroscopic lateral release and the patellar compression syndrome. Orthop Clin North Am 23:601, 1992.

71. Fujimoto, E, Sumen, Y, Urabe, Y, et al: An early return to vigorous activity may destabilize anterior cruciate ligaments reconstructed with hamstring grafts. Arch Phys Med Rehabil 85:298–302, 2004

72. Fulkerson, JP: Anteromedial tibial tubercle transfer. In Jackson, DW (ed) Master Techniques in Orthopedic Surgery: Reconstructive Knee Surgery, ed 2. Lippincott Williams & Wilkins, Philadelphia, 2006, pp 13–25.

73. Fulkerson, JP: Diagnosis and treatment of patients with patellofemoral pain (review). Am J Sports Med 30:447–456, 2002.

74. Garth, WP, DiChristina, DG, Holt, G: Delayed proximal repair and distal realignment after patellar dislocation. Clin Orthop 377:132–144, 2000.

75. Gasser, SI, Jackson, DW: Arthroscopic lateral release of the patella with radiofrequency ablation. In Jackson, DW (ed) Master Techniques in Orthopedic Surgery: Reconstructive Knee Surgery, ed 2. Lippincott Williams & Wilkins, Philadelphia, 2006, pp 3–13.

76. Gill, TJ, Asnis, PD, Berkson, EM: The treatment of articular cartilage defects using the microfracture technique. J Orthop Sports Phys Ther 36(10):728–738, 2006.

77. Gillogly, SD, Myers, TH, Reinold, MM: Treatment of full-thickness chondral defects in the knee with autologous chondrocyte implantation. J Orthop Sports Phys Ther 36(10):751–764, 2006.

78. Goodfellow, J, Hungerford, D, Woods, C: Patello-femoral joint mechanics and pathology of chondromalacia patellae. J Bone Joint Surg Br 58:291, 1976.

79. Gose, JC: CPM in the postoperative treatment of patients with total knee replacements. Phys Ther 67:39, 1987.

80. Grelsamer, RP, Klein, JR: The biomechanics of the patellofemoral joint. J Orthop Sports Phys Ther 28:286, 1998.

81. Grelsamer, RP, McConnell, J: The Patella: A Team Approach. Aspen, Gaithersburg, MD, 1998.

82. Griffin, LY, et al: Non-contact anterior cruciate ligament injuries: risk factors and prevention strategies. J Am Acad Orthop Surg 8:141, 2000.

83. Grood, ES, et al: Biomechanics of the knee: extension exercise. J Bone Joint Surg Am 66:725, 1984.

84. Gross, MT, Foxworth, JL: The role of foot orthoses as an intervention for patellofemoral pain. J Orthop Sports Phys Ther 33(11):661–670, 2003.

85. Gryzlo, SM, et al: Electromyographic analysis of knee rehabilitation exercises. J Orthop Sports Phys Ther 20:36, 1994.

86. Hangood, L: Mosaicplasty. In Insall, JN, Scott, WN (eds) Surgery of the Knee, Vol 1, ed 3. Churchill Livingstone, New York, 2001, p 357.

87. Hattrup, SJ: Synovectomy. In Morrey, BF (ed) Reconstructive Surgery of the Joints, ed 2. Churchill Livingstone, New York, 1996, p 1599.

88. Healy, WL, Iorio, R, Lemos, MJ: Athletic activity after total knee arthroplasty. Clin Orthop 390:65–71, 2000.

89. Heckman, TP, Barber-Westin, SD, Noyes, FR: Meniscal repair and transplantation: indications, techniques, rehabilitation, and clinical outcomes. J Orthop Sports Phys Ther 36(10):795–815, 2006.

90. Heckman, TP, Noyes, FR, Barber-Westin, SD: Autogenic and allogenic anterior cruciate ligament rehabilitation. In Ellenbecker, TS (ed) Knee Ligament Rehabilitation. Churchill Livingstone, New York, 2000, p 132.

91. Hefzy, MS, Grood, ES, Noyes, FR: Factors effecting the region of most isometric femoral attachments. Part II. The anterior cruciate ligament. Am J Sports Med 17:208, 1989.

92. Hewett, TE, Blum, KR, Noyes, FR: Gait characteristics of the anterior cruciate ligament-deficient varus knee. Am J Knee Surg 10:246, 1997.

93. Hewitt, B, Shakespeare, D: Flexion versus extension: a comparison of postoperative total knee arthroplasty mobilization regimes. Knee 8:305–309, 2001.

94. Hiemstra, LA, Lo, I, Fowler, PJ: Effect of fatigue on knee proprioception: implications for dynamic stabilization. J Orthop Sports Phys Ther 31(10):598–605, 2001.

95. Hinton, RY, Sharma, KM: Acute and recurrent patellar instability in the young athlete. Orthop Clin North Am 34:385–396, 2003.

96. Holmes, SW, Clancy, WG: Clinical classification of patellofemoral pain and dysfunction. J Orthop Sports Phys Ther 28:299, 1998.

97. Hung, V, Gross, MST: Effect of foot position on electromyographic activity of the vastus medialis oblique and vastus lateralis during lower-extremity weight-bearing activities. J Orthop Sports Phys Ther 29:91, 1999.

98. Insall, JN, Clark, HD: Historic development, classification and characteristics of total knee protheses. In Insall, JN, Scott, WN (eds) Surgery of the Knee, Vol 2, ed 3. Churchill-Livingstone, New York, 2001, p 1516.

99. Insall, JN, Easley, ME: Surgical techniques and instrumentation in total knee arthroplasty. In Insall, JN, Scott, WN (eds) Surgery of the Knee, Vol 2, ed 3. Churchill Livingstone, New York, 2001, p 1553.

100. Ireland, ML, Willson, JD, et al: Hip strength in females with and without patellofemoral pain. J Orthop Sports Phys Ther 33(11): 671–676, 2003.

101. Jain, NB, Higgins, LD, Ozumba, D, et al: Trends in epidemiology of knee arthroplasty in the United States 1990-2000. Arthritis Rheum 52(12):3928–3933, 2005.

102. Jaramillo, J, Worrell, TW, Ingersoll, CD: Hip isometric strength following knee surgery. J Ortho Sports Phys Ther 20:160, 1993.

103. Johnson, DP: The effect of continuous passive motion on wound healing and joint mobility after knee arthroplasty. J Bone Joint Surg Am 72(3):421–426, 1990.

104. Jones, CA, Voaklander, DL, Suarez-Almazor, ME: Determinents of function after total knee arthroplasty. Phys Ther 83(8):696–706, 2003.

105. Kaltenborn, FM: The Kaltenborn Method of Joint Examination and Treatment. Vol I. The Extremities, ed 5. Olaf Norlis Bokhandle, Oslo, 1999.

106. Karst, GM, Jewett, PD: Electromyographic analysis of exercises proposed for differential activation of medial and lateral quadriceps femoris muscle components. Phys Ther 73:286, 1993.

107. Kegerreis, S, Malone, T, Ohnson, F: The diagonal medical plica: an underestimated clinical entity. J Orthop Sports Phys Ther 9:305, 1988.

108. Khatod, M, Akeson, WH: Ligament injury and repair. In Pedowitz, RA, O'Connor, JJ, Akeson, WH (eds) Daniel's Knee Injuries: Ligament and Cartilage Structure, Function, Injury and Repair, ed 2. Lippincott Williams & Wilkins, Philadelphia, 2003, pp 185–201.

109. Kim, CW, Pedowitz, RA: Principles of surgery. Part A. Graft choice and the biology of graft healing. In Pedowitz, RA, O'Connor, JJ, Akeson, WH (eds) Daniel's Knee Injuries: Ligament and Cartilage Structure, Function, Injury and Repair, ed 2. Lippincott Williams & Wilkins, Philadelphia, 2003, pp 435–455.

110. Koh, JL, Hangody, L, Rathonyi, GK: Osteochondral autograft transfer (OATS/mosaicplasty). In Mirzayan, R (ed) Cartilage Injury in the Athlete, Thieme Medical Publishing, New York, 2006, pp 124–140.

111. Kolessar, DJ, Rand, JA: Extensor mechanism problems following total knee arthroplasty. In Morrey, BF (ed) Reconstructive Surgery of the Joints, ed 2. Churchill Livingstone, New York, 1996, p 1533.

112. Kumar, PJ, McPherson, EJ, Dorr, LD, et al: Rehabilitation after total knee arthroplasty: a comparison of 2 rehabilitation techniques. Clin Orthop 331:93–101, 1996.

113. Kuster, MS: Exercise recommendations after total joint replacement: a review of the current literature and proposal of scientifically based guidelines. Sports Med 32(7):433–445, 2002.

114. Kvist, J: Rehabilitation following anterior cruciate ligament injury: current recommendations for sports participation. Sports Med 34:269–280, 2004.

115. Laimins, PD, Powell, SE: Principles of surgery. Part C. Anterior cruciate ligament reconstruction: techniques past and present. In Pedowitz, RA, O'Connor, JJ, Akeson, WH (eds) Daniel's Knee Injuries: Ligament and Cartilage Structure, Function, Injury, and Repair, ed 2. Lippincott Williams & Wilkins, Philadelphia, 2003, pp 472–491.

116. Laprade, J, et al: Comparison of five isometric exercises in the recruitment of the vastus medialis oblique in persons with and

without patellofemoral pain syndrome. J Orthop Sports Phys Ther 27:197, 1998.

117. Lee, S, Seong, SC, Jo, H, et al: Outcome of anterior cruciate ligament reconstruction using quadriceps tendon autograft. Arthroplasty 20:795–802, 2004.

118. Lewis, PB, McCarthy, LP III, Kang, RW, et al: Basic science and treatment options for articular cartilage injuries. J Orthop Sports Phys Ther 36(10):717–728, 2006.

119. Lizaur, A, Marco, L, Cebrian, R: Preoperative factors influencing the range of movement after total knee arthroplasty for severe osteoarthritis. J Bone Joint Surg Br 79(4):626–629, 1997.

120. Lynch, PA, et al: Deep venous thrombosis and continued passive motion after total knee arthroplasty. J Bone Joint Surg Am 70:11, 1988.

121. Logan, M, Williams, A, Lavelle, J, et al: The effect of posterior cruciate ligament deficiency on knee kinematics. Am J Sports Med 32(8):1915–1922, 2004.

122. MacDonald, SJ, Bourne, RB, Rorabeck, CH, et al: Postoperative randomized clinical trial of continuous passive motion after total knee arthroplasty. Clin Orthop 380:30–35, 2000.

123. Magee, DJ: Orthopedic Physical Assessment, ed 4. Saunders (Elsevier), Philadelphia, 2002.

124. Mahoney, OM, McClung, CD, de la Rosa, MA, Schmalzried, TP: The effect of total knee arthroplasty design on extensor mechanism function. J Arthroplasty 17:416–421, 2002.

125. Malone, TR, Garrett, WE: Commentary and historical perspective of anterior cruciate ligament rehabilitation. J Orthop Sports Phys Ther 15:265, 1992.

126. Mangine, RE, Eifert-Mangine, M, et al: Postoperative management of the patellofemoral patient. J Ortho Sports Phys Ther 28:323, 1998.

127. Mangine, RE, Kremchek, ET: Evaluation-based protocol of the anterior cruciate ligament. J Sport Rehabil 6:157, 1997.

128. Mangine, RE, Quillen, WS: EMG analysis of closed-chain squat with and without hip adduction. Presented at Combined Sections Meeting, American Physical Therapy Association, Seattle, 1999.

129. Manifold, SG, Cushner, FD, Scott, WN: Anterior cruciate ligament reconstruction with bone-patellar tendon-bone autograft: indications, technique, complications, and management. In Insall, JN, Scott, WN (eds) Surgery of the Knee, Vol 1, ed 3. Churchill Livingstone, New York, 2001, p 665.

130. Manske, PR, Gleason, P: Rehabilitation program following polycentric total knee arthroplasty. Phys Ther 57:915–918, 1977.

131. Martin, SD, Scott, RD, Thornhill, TS: Current concepts of total knee arthroplasty. J Orthop Sports Phys Ther 28:252, 1998.

132. Mascal, CL, Landel, R, Powers, C: Management of patellofemoral pain targeting hip, pelvis, and trunk muscle function: 2 case reports. J Orthop Sports Phys Ther 33(11):642–660, 2003.

133. Matsumoto, A, Yoshiya, S, Muratsu, H, et al: A comparison of bone-patellar tendon-bone and bone-hamstring tendon-bone autografts for anterior cruciate ligament reconstruction. Am J Sports Med 34(2):213–219, 2006.

134. McCarthy, MR, et al: The effects of immediate continuous passive motion on pain during the inflammatory phase of soft tissue healing following anterior cruciate ligament reconstruction. J Orthop Sports Phys Ther 17:96, 1993.

135. McConnell, J: The management of chondromalacia patellae: a long term solution. Aust J Physiother 32:215, 1986.

136. McConnell, J: McConnell Institute Workshop on Management of Patellofemoral Pain. Columbus, OH, 1994.

137. McDevitt, ER, Taylor, DC, Miller, MD, et al: Functional bracing after anterior cruciate ligament reconstruction: a prospective, randomized, multicenter study. Am J Sports Med 32(8):1887–1892, 2004.

138. McGrory, BJ, Stuart, MJ, Sim, FH: Participation in sports after hip and knee arthroplasty: review of literature and survey of surgeon preferences. Mayo Clin Proc 70:342–348, 1995.

139. McHugh, MP, Tyler, TF, Gleim, GW, Nicholas, SJ: Preoperative indicators of motion loss and weakness following anterior cruciate ligament reconstruction. J Orthop Sports Phys Ther 27(6):407–411, 1998.

140. McInnes, J, Larson, M, Daltroy, LH, et al: A controlled evaluation of continuous passive motion in patients undergoing total knee arthroplasty. JAMA 268(11):1423–1428, 1992.

141. McKinnis, LN: Fundamentals of Musculoskeletal Imaging, ed 2. FA Davis, Philadelphia, 2005.

142. McLaughlin, J, et al: Rehabilitation after meniscus repair. Orthopedics 17:463, 1994.

143. Miller, SL, Gladstone, JN: Graft selection in anterior cruciate ligament reconstruction. Orthop Clin North Am 33:675–638, 2002.

144. Minas, T, Bryant, T: The role of autologous chondrocyte implantation in the patellofemoral joint. Clin Orthop 436:30–39, 2005.

145. Minas, T: Surgical management of patellofemoral disease. In Mizrayan, R (ed) Cartilage Injury in the Athlete. Thieme, New York, 2006, pp 273–285.

146. Mirza, F, et al: Management of injuries to the anterior cruciate ligament: results of a survey of orthopaedic surgeons in Canada. Clin J Sport Med 10:85, 2000.

147. Mizner, RL, Petterson, SC, Snyder-Mackler, L: Quadriceps strength and time course of functional recovery after total knee arthroplasty. J Orthop Sports Phys Ther 35(7):424–436, 2005.

148. Mizner, RL, Stevens, JE, Snyder-Mackler, L: Voluntary activation and decreased force production of the quadriceps femoris muscle after total knee arthroplasty. Phys Ther 83(4):359–365, 2003.

149. Moffet, H, Collet, JP, Shapiro, SH, et al: Effectiveness of intensive rehabilitation on functional ability and quality of life after first total knee arthroplasty: a single-blind randomized trial. Arch Phys Med Rehabil 85:546–555, 2004.

150. Mologne, TS, Friedman, MJ: Arthroscopic anterior cruciate reconstruction with hamstring tendons: indications, surgical technique, complications and their treatment. In Insall, JN, Scott, WN (eds) Surgery of the Knee, Vol 1, ed 3. Churchill Livingstone, New York, 2001, p 681.

151. Mooney, Mf, Rosenberg, TD: Meniscus repair: the inside-out technique. In Jackson, DW (ed) Master Techniques in Orthopedic Surgery: Reconstructive Knee Surgery, ed 2. Lippincott Williams & Wilkins, Philadelphia, 2003, pp 57–71.

152. Morgan, CD, Leitman, EH: Meniscus repair: the all-inside arthroscopic technique. In Jackson, DW (ed) Master Techniques in Orthopedic Surgery: Reconstructive Knee Surgery, ed 2. Lippincott Williams & Wilkins, Philadelphia, 2003, pp 73–91.

153. Morrey, BF, Pagnano, MW: Mobile-bearing knee. In Morrey, BF (ed) Joint Replacement Arthroplasty, ed 3. Churchill Livingstone, Philadelphia, 2003, pp 1013–1022.

154. Mulligan, BR: Manual Therapy "NAGS", "SNAGS", "MWM's": etc, ed 4. Plane View Press, Wellington, 1999.

155. Mulvey, TJ, et al: Complications associated with total knee arthroplasty. In Pellicci, PM, Tria, AJ, Garvin, KL (eds) Orthopedic Knowledge Update 2. Hip and Knee Reconstruction. American Academy of Orthopedic Surgeons, Rosemont, IL, 2000, p 323.

156. Murray, DW: Mobile bearing unicompartmental knee replacement. Orthopedics 28(9):985–987, 2005.

157. Myer, GD, Paterno, MV, Ford, KR, et al: Rehabilitation after anterior cruciate ligament reconstruction: criterion-based progression through the return-to-sport phase. J Orthop Sports Phys Ther 26(6):385–399, 2006.

158. Myers, P, Williams, A, Dodds, R, Bulow, J: The three-in-one proximal and distal soft tissue patellar realignment procedure: results and its place in the management of patellofemoral instability. Am J Sports Med 27:575–579, 1999.

159. Noyes, FR, Barber-Westin, SD: Surgical restoration to treat chronic deficiency of the posterolateral complex and cruciate ligaments of the knee. Am J Sports Med 24:415, 1996.

160. Noyes, FR, Barber-Westin, SD: Arthroscopic repairs of meniscus tears extending into the avascular zone with or without anterior cruciate ligament reconstruction in patients 40 years of age and older. Arthroscopy 16(8):882–829, 2000.

161. Noyes, FR, Barber-Westin, SD: Arthroscopic repairs of meniscal tears extending into the avascular zone in patients younger than twenty years of age. Am J Sports Med 30(4):589–600, 2002.

162. Noyes, FR, Barber, SD, Mangine, RE: Bone-patellar ligament-bone and fascia lata allografts for reconstruction of the anterior cruciate ligament. J Bone Joint Surg Am 72:125, 1990.

163. Noyes, FR, Barber-Westin, SD, Rankin, M: Meniscal transplantation in symptomatic patients less than fifty years old. J Bone Joint Surg Am 86(7):1392–1404, 2004.

164. Noyes, FR, Barber-Westin, SD, Rankin, M: Meniscal transplantation in symptomatic patients less than fifty years old: surgical technique. J Bone Joint Surg Am 87(Suppl 1, Pt 2):149–165, 2005.

165. Noyes, FR, et al: Arthroscopy in acute traumatic hemarthrosis of the knee: incidence of anterior cruciate tears and other injuries. J Bone Joint Surg Am 62:687, 1980.

166. Noyes, FR, Butler, DL, Grood, ES, et al: Biomechanical analysis of human ligament grafts used in knee ligament repairs and reconstructions. J Bone Joint Surg Am 66:334, 1984.

167. Noyes, FR, DeMaio, M, Mangine, RE: Evaluation-based protocol: a new approach to rehabilitation. J Orthop Phys Ther 14:1383, 1991.

168. Noyes, FR, Heckman, TP, Barber-Westin, SD: Posterior cruciate ligament and posterolateral reconstruction. In Ellenbecker, TS (ed) Knee Ligament Rehabilitation. Churchill Livingstone, New York, 2000, pp 167–185.

169. Noyes, FR, Mangine, RE: Early knee motion after open and arthroscopic anterior cruciate ligament reconstruction. Am J Sports Med 15:149, 1987.

170. Noyes, FR, Barber-Westin, SD, Grood, ES: New concepts in the treatment of posterior cruciate ligament ruptures. In Insall, JN, Scott, WN (eds) Surgery of the Knee, Vol 1, ed 3. Churchill Livingstone, New York, 2001, p 841.

171. O'Donoghue, DH: Surgical treatment of fresh injuries to the major ligaments of the knee. J Bone Joint Surg Am 32:721, 1950.

172. Olney, SJ: Gait. In Levangie, PK, Norkin, CC (eds) Joint Structure & Function: A comprehensive Analysis, ed 4. FA Davis, Philadelphia, 2005.

173. Ortiguera, CJ, Hanssen, AD, Stuart, MJ: Posterior cruciate-substituting and -sacrificing total knee arthroplasty. In Morrey, BF (ed) Joint Replacement Arthroplasty, ed 3. Churchill Livingstone, Philadelphia, 2003, pp 982–992.

174. Outerbridge, RE, Dunlop, J: The problem of chondromalacia patellae. Clin Orthrop 110:177, 1975.

175. Pagnano, MW, Papagelopoulas, PJ, Rand, JA: Uncemented total knee arthroplasty. In Morrey, BF (ed) Joint Replacement Arthroplasty, ed 3. Churchill Livingstone, Philadelphia, 2003, pp 993–1001.

176. Pagnano, MW, Rand, JA: Posterior cruciate ligament retaining total knee arthroplasty. In Morrey, BF (ed) Joint Replacement Arthroplasty, ed 3. Churchill Livingstone, Philadelphia, 2003, pp 976–981.

177. Pagnano, MW, Rand, JA: Unicompartmental total knee arthroplasty. In Morrey, BF (ed) Joint Replacement Arthroplasty, ed 3. Churchill Livingstone, Philadelphia, 2003, pp 1002–1012.

178. Palmitier, RA, et al: Kinetic chain exercises in knee rehabilitation. Sports Med 11:402, 1991.

179. Papagelopoulos, PJ, Sim, FH: Limited range of motion after total knee arthroplasty: etiology, treatment and prognosis. Orthopedics 20:1061–1065, 1997.

180. Papagelopoulos, PJ, Sim, FH, Morrey, BF: Patellectomy and reconstructive surgery for disorders of the patellofemoral joint. In Morrey, BF (ed) Reconstructive Surgery of the Joints, ed 2. Churchill Livingstone, New York, 1996, p 1671.

181. Paris, MJ, Wilcon, RB, III, Millett, PJ: Anterior cruciate ligament reconstruction: surgical management and postoperative rehabilitation considerations. Orthop Phys Ther Pract 17(4):14–24, 2005.

182. Patel, D: Arthroscopic synovectomy. In Jackson, DW (ed) Master Techniques in Orthopedic Surgery: Knee Surgery, ed 2. Lippincott Williams & Wilkins, Philadelphia, 2003, pp 417–425.

183. Paulos, LE, Walther, CE, Walker, JA: Rehabilitation of the surgically reconstructed and nonsurgical anterior cruciate ligament. In Insall, JN, Scott, WN (eds) Surgery of the Knee, Vol 1, ed 3. Churchill Livingstone, New York, 2001, p 789.

184. Pepe, MD, Giffin, JR, Haner, CD: Meniscal transplantation. In Jackson, DW (ed) Master Techniques in Orthopedic Surgery: Reconstructive Knee Surgery, ed 2. Lippincott Williams & Wilkins, Philadelphia, 2003, pp 93–101.

185. Perry, J: Gait Analysis: Normal and Pathological Function. Slack, Thorofare, NJ, 1992.

186. Philadelphia Panel Evidence-Based Clinical Practice Guidelines on Selected Rehabilitation Interventions for Knee Pain. Phys Ther 81(10):1675–1700, 2001.

187. Piva, SR, Coodnight, EA, Childs, JD: Strength around the hip and flexibility of soft tissues in individuals with and without patellofemoral pain syndrome. J Orthop Sports Phys Ther 35(12):793–801, 2005.

188. Post, WR, Fulkerson, JP: Surgery of the patellofemoral joint: indications, effects, results and recommendations. In Insall, JN, Scott, WN (eds) Surgery of the Knee, Vol 1, ed 3. Churchill Livingstone, New York, 2001, p 1045.

189. Powers, CM: The influence of altered lower-extremity kinematics on patellofemoral joint dysfunction: a theoretical perspective. J Orthop Sports Phys Ther 33(11):639–646, 2003.

190. Rajan, RA, Pack, Y, Jackson, H, et al: No need for outpatient physiotherapy following total knee arthroplasty. Acta Orthop Scand 75(1):71–73, 2004.

191. Rand, JA: Cemented total knee arthroplasty: techniques. In Morrey, BF (ed) Reconstructive Surgery of the Joints, ed 2. Churchill Livingstone, New York, 1996, p 1389.

192. Reinold, MM, Wilk, KE, Macrina, LC, et al: Current concepts in rehabilitation following articular cartilage repair procedures in the knee. J Orthop Sports Phys Ther 38(10):774–795, 2006.

193. Richterman, I, Keenan, MA: Surgical interventions. In Walker, JM, Helenwa, A (eds) Physical Therapy in Arthritis. WB Saunders, Philadelphia, 1996, pp 95–112.

194. Risberg, MA, Holm, I, Steen, H, et al: The effect of knee bracing after anterior cruciate ligament reconstruction: a prospective, randomized study with two years' follow-up. Am J Sports Med 27:76–83, 1999.

195. Risberg, MA, Mork, M, Jensen, HK, et al: Design and implementation of a neuromuscular training program following anterior cruciate ligament reconstruction. J Orthop Sports Phys Ther 31(11):620–631, 2001.

196. Roddy, E, Zhang, W, Doherty, M, et al: Evidence-based recommendations for the role of exercise in the management of osteoarthritis of the hip or knee—the MOVE consensus. Rheumatology 44(1):67–73, 2005.

197. Roddy, E, Zhang, W, Doherty, M: Aerobic walking or strengthening exercise for osteoarthritis of the knee? A systematic review. Ann Rheum Dis 64(4):544–548, 2005.

198. Roe, J, Pinczewski, LA, Russell, VJ, et al: A 7-year follow-up of patellar tendon and hamstring grafts for arthroscopic anterior cruciate ligament reconstruction: differences and similarities. Am J Sports Med 33(9):1337–1345, 2005.

199. Rossi, MD, Hassan, S: Lower-limb force production in individuals after unilateral total knee arthroplasty. Arch Phys Med Rehabil 85:1279–1284, 2003.

200. Sandor, SM, Hart, JAL, Oakes, BW: Case study: rehabilitation of a surgically repaired medial collateral knee ligament using a limited motion cast and isokinetic exercise. J Orthop Sports Phys Ther 7:154, 1986.

201. Scaepanski, TL, et al: Effect of contraction type, angular velocity, and arc of motion on VMO:VL EMG ratio. J Orthop Sports Phys Ther 14:256, 1991.

202. Schurman, DJ, Rojer, DE: Total knee arthroplasty: range of motion across five systems. Clin Orthop 430:132–137, 2005.

203. Scott, RD: Total Knee Arthroplasty. Saunders, Philadelphia, 2006.

204. Scott, RD, et al: Long-term results of total knee replacement. In Pellicci, JM, Tria, AJ, Garvin, KL (eds) Orthopedic Knowledge Update, 2. Hip and Knee Reconstruction. American Academy of Orthopedic Surgeons, Rosemont, IL, 2000, p 301.

205. Sculco, T, et al: Knee surgery and rehabilitation. In Melvin, JL, Gall, V (eds) Rheumatologic Rehabilitation Series. Vol 5. Surgical Rehabilitation. American Occupational Therapy Association, Bethesda, 1999, p 121.

206. Sekiya, JK, Ong, BC, Bradley, JP: Complications in anterior cruciate ligament surgery. Orthop Clin North Am 34:99–105, 2003.

207. Sethi, P, Mirzayan, R, Kharrazi, D: Microfracture technique. In Mirzayan, R (ed) Cartilage Injury in the Athlete. Thieme Medical Publishers, New York, 2006, pp 116–123.

208. Seto, JL, Brewster, CE: Rehabilitation of meniscal injuries. In Greenfield, BH (ed) Rehabilitation of the Knee: A Problem-Solving Approach. FA Davis, Philadelphia, 1993, pp 381–409.

209. Shaieb, MD, Kan, DM, Chang, SK, et al: A prospective randomized comparison of patellar tendon versus semitendinosus and gracilis tendon autografts for anterior cruciate ligament reconstruction. Am J Sports Med 30(2):214–220, 2002.

210. Sharma, L, Cahue, S, Song, J, et al: Physical functioning over three years in knee osteoarthritis: role of psychosocial, local mechanical, and neuromuscular factors. Arthritis Rheum 48(12):3359–3370, 2003.

211. Shelbourne, KD, Kloutwyk, TE: Rehabilitation after anterior cruciate ligament reconstruction. In Pedowitz, RA, O'Connor, JJ, Akeson, WH (eds) Daniel's Knee Injuries: Ligament and Cartilage Structure, Function, Injury and Repair, ed 2. Lippincott Williams & Wilkins, Philadelphia, 2003, pp 493–500.

212. Shelbourne, KD, Trumper, RV: Anterior cruciate ligament reconstruction: evolution of rehabilitation. In Ellenbecker, TS: Knee Ligament Rehabilitation. Churchill Livingstone. New York, 2000, pp 106–117.

213. Shelbourne, KD, Urch, SE: Primary anterior cruciate ligament reconstruction using the contralateral autogenous patellar tendon. Am J Sports Med 18:651, 2000.

214. Shelbourne, KD, Nitz, P: Accelerated rehabilitation after anterior cruciate ligament reconstruction. J Orthop Sports Phys Ther 15:256, 1992.

215. Shelton, GL, Thigpen, LK: Rehabilitation of patellofemoral dysfunction: a review of literature. J Orthop Sports Phys Ther 14:143, 1991.

216. Sherman, OH, Banffy, MB: Anterior cruciate ligament reconstruction: which graft is best? Arthroscopy 20(9):974–980, 2004.

217. Shoji, H, Solomonov, M: Factors affecting postoperative flexion in total knee arthroplasty. Clin Orthop 13:643, 1990.

218. Silva, M, Schmalzried, T: Knee strength after total knee arthroplasty. J Arthroplasty 18:605–611, 2003.

219. Singhal, MC, Fites, BS, Johnson, DL: Fixation devices in ACL surgery: what do I need to know? Orthopedics 28(9):920–924, 2005.

220. Smidt, GL, Albright, JP, Deusinger, RH: Pre- and postoperative functional changes in total knee patients. J Orthop Sports Phys Ther 6:25, 1984.

221. Smith, LK, Weiss, EL, Lehmkuhl, LD: Brunnstrom's Clinical Kinesiology, ed 5. FA Davis, Philadelphia, 1996.

222. Snyder-Mackler, L, et al: Strength of the quadriceps femoris muscle and functional recovery after reconstruction of the anterior cruciate ligament. J Bone Joint Surg Am 77:1166, 1995.

223. Snyder-Mackler, L: The knee. In Levangie, PK, Norkin, CC (eds) Joint Structure & Function: A Comprehensive Analysis, ed 5. FA Davis, Philadelphia, 2005, p 393.

224. Sodeberg, GL, Cook, TM: An electromyographic analysis of quadriceps femoris muscle setting and straight leg raising. Phys Ther 63:1434–1438, 1983.

225. Spencer, JD, Hayes, KC, Alexander, IJ: Knee joint effusion and quadriceps reflex inhibition in man. Arch Phys Med Rehabil 65: 171, 1984.

226. Sprague, R: Factors related to extension lag at the knee joint. J Orthop Sports Phys Ther 3:178, 1982.

227. Steadman, JR, Briggs, KK, Rodrigo, JJ, et al: Outcomes of microfracture for traumatic chondral defects of the knee: average 11-year follow-up. Arthroscopy 19:477–484, 2003.

228. Steindler, A: Kinesiology of the Human Body Under Normal and Pathological Conditions. Charles C Thomas, Springfield, IL, 1955.

229. Sterret, WI, Briggs, KK, Farley, T, Steadman, JR: Effect of functional bracing on knee injury in skiers with anterior cruciate ligament reconstruction: a prospective cohort study. Am J Sports Med 34(10):1581–1585, 2006.

230. Stone, RC, Frewin, PR, Gonzales, S: Long term assessment of arthroscopic meniscus repair: a two to six year follow-up study. Arthroscopy 6:73, 1990.

231. Stratford, P: Electromyography of the quadriceps femoris muscles in subjects with normal and acutely effused knees. Phys Ther 62:279, 1982.

232. Strum, GM, et al: Acute anterior cruciate ligament reconstruction: analysis of complications, Clin Orthop 253:184, 1990.

233. Stuart, MJ: Posterior cruciate ligament reconstruction. In Morrey, BF (ed) Reconstructive Surgery of the Joints, ed 2. Churchill Livingstone, New York, 1996, p 1651.

234. Tadokoro, K, Matsui, N, Yagi, M, et al: Evaluation of hamstring strength and tendon regrowth after harvesting for anterior cruciate ligament reconstruction. Am J Sports Med 32(7):1644–1650, 2004.

235. Tamburello, T, et al: Patella hypomobility as a cause of extensor lag. Research presentation. Overland Park, KS, May 1985.

236. Tanavalee, A, Choi, YJ, Tria, AJ: Unicondylar knee arthroplasty: past and present. Orthopedics 28(12):1423–1433, 2005.

237. Thomas, SG, Pagura, SM, Kennedy, D: Physical activity and its relationship to physical performance in patients with end stage knee osteoarthritis. J Orthop Sports Phys Ther 33(12):745–754, 2003.

238. Torchia, ME: Meniscal tears. In Morrey, BF (ed) Reconstructive Surgery of the Joints, ed 2. Churchill Livingstone, New York, 1996, p 1607.

239. Tsai, AMH, Pedowitz, RA: Meniscus injury and repair. In Pedowitz, RA, O'Connor, JJ, Akeson, WH (eds) Daniel's Knee Injuries: Ligament and Cartilage Structure, Function, Injury and Repair, ed 2. Lippincott Williams & Wilkins, Philadelphia, 2003, pp 239–251.

240. Tyler, TF, McHugh, MP: Neuromuscular rehabilitation of a female Olympic ice hockey player following anterior cruciate ligament reconstruction. J Orthop Sports Phys Ther 31(10):577–587, 2001.

241. Tyler, TF, McHugh, MP, Gleim, GW, Nicholas, SJ: The effect of immediate weightbearing after anterior cruciate ligament reconstruction. Clin Orthop 357:141–148, 1998.

242. Voight, ML, Wieder, DL: Comparative reflex response times of vastus medialis obliquis and vastus lateralis in normal subjects and subjects with extensor mechanism dysfunction. Am J Sports Med 19:131, 1991.

243. Walsh, M, Woodhoude, LU, Thomas, SG, Finch, E: Physical impairments and functional limitations: a comparison of individuals 1 year after total knee arthroplasty with control subjects. Phys Ther 78: 248–258, 1998.

244. Waters, EA: Physical therapy management of patients with total knee replacement. Phys Ther 54:936–944, 1974.

245. Wegener, L, Kisner, C, Nichols, D: Static and dynamic balance responses in persons with bilateral knee osteoarthritis. J Orthop Sports Phys Ther 25:13, 1997.

246. Weiss, JM, Noble, PC, Condit, MA, et al: What functional activities are important to patients with knee replacements? Clin Orthop 404:172–188, 2002.

247. Whiteside, LA: Fixation in total knee replacement: bone ingrowth. In Pellicci, PM, Tria, AJ, Garvin, KL (eds) Orthopedic Knowledge Update, 2. Hip and Knee Reconstruction. American Academy of Orthopedic Surgeons, Rosemont, IL, 2000, p 275.

248. Wiley, JW, Bryant, T, Minas, T: Autologous chondrocyte implantation. In Mirzayan, R (ed) Cartilage Injury in the Athlete. Thieme Medical Publishers, New York, 2006, pp 141–157.

249. Wilk, KE, Andrews, JR: Current concepts in the treatment of anterior cruciate ligament disruption. J Orthop Sports Phys Ther 15:279, 1992.

250. Wilk, KE, Andrews, JR: The effects of pad placement and angular velocity on tibial displacement during isokinetic exercise. J Orthop Sports Phys Ther 17:24, 1993.

251. Wilk, KE, Clancy, WG: Medial collateral ligament injuries: diagnosis, treatment, and rehabilitation in knee ligament injuries. In Engle, RP (ed): Knee Ligament Rehabilitation. Churchill Livingstone, New York, 1991, p 71.

252. Wilk, KE, et al: Patellofemoral disorders: a classification system and clinical guidelines for nonoperative rehabilitation. J Orthop Sports Phys Ther 28:307, 1998.

253. Wilk, KE, Reinold, MM, Hooks, TR: Recent advances in the rehabilitation of isolated and combined anterior cruciate ligament injuries. Orthop Clin North Am 34:107–137, 2003.

254. Williams, GN, Chmielewski, T, Rudolph, KS, et al: Dynamic knee stability: current theory and implications for clinicians and scientists. J Orthop Sports Phys Ther 31(10):546–566, 2001.

255. Wind, WM, Bergfeld, JA, Parker, RD: Evaluation and treatment of posterior cruciate ligament injuries: revisited. Am J Sports Med 32(7):1765–1775, 2004.

256. Woodall, W, Welsh, J: A biomechanical basis for rehabilitation programs involving the patellofemoral joint. J Orthop Sports Phys Ther 11:535, 1990.

257. Wright, TM: Biomechanics of total knee design. In Pellicci, PM, Tria, AJ, Garvin, KL (eds) Orthopedic Knowledge Update, 2. Hip and Knee Reconstruction. American Academy of Orthopedic Surgeons, Rosemont, IL, 2000, p 265.

# The Ankle and Foot

The joints, ligaments, and muscles of the ankle and foot are designed to provide stability and mobility in the terminal structures of the lower extremity. During standing, the foot must bear the body weight with a minimum of muscle energy expenditure. In addition, the foot must be capable of being either pliable or relatively rigid depending on various functional demands such as adapting to absorb forces and accommodate to uneven surfaces, or becoming a structural lever to propel the body forward during walking and running.

The anatomy and kinesiology of the ankle and foot are complex, but it is important to understand and be able to apply this knowledge to treat impairments in this region of the body effectively. The first section of this chapter reviews highlights of these areas that the reader should know and understand. The second section contains guidelines for the management of disorders and surgeries in the foot and ankle region, and the third section describes exercise interventions for this region. Chapters 10 through 13 present general information on principles of management; the reader should be familiar with the material in these chapters, and have a background in examination and evaluation in order to effectively design a therapeutic exercise program to improve ankle and foot function in patients with impairments from injury, pathology, or following surgery.

## STRUCTURE AND FUNCTION OF THE ANKLE AND FOOT

The bones of the ankle and foot consist of the distal tibia and fibula, 7 tarsals, 5 metatarsals, and 14 phalanges (Fig. 22.1).

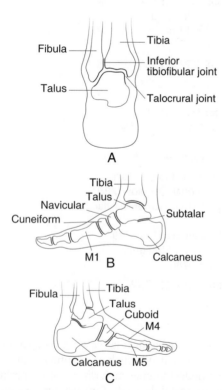

FIGURE 22.1 Bones of the ankle and foot. (*A*) Anterior view of the lower leg and ankle, (*B*) medial view, and (*C*) lateral view of the ankle and foot.

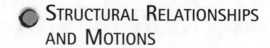

# STRUCTURAL RELATIONSHIPS AND MOTIONS

## Anatomical Characteristics

The leg is structurally designed to transmit the ground reaction forces from the foot upward to the knee joint and femur, and adapt as needed to provide stability to or allow motion of the ankle. The resulting motions in the ankle and foot are defined using primary plane descriptors and triplanar descriptors.

### Leg
The tibia and fibula make up the leg. These two bones are bound together by an interosseous membrane along the shafts of the bones, by strong anterior and posterior inferior tibiofibular ligaments that hold the distal tibiofibular articulation together, and by a strong capsule that encloses the proximal tibiofibular articulation. Unlike the radius and ulna in the upper extremity, the tibia and fibula do not rotate around each other, but there is slight movement between the two bones that allows greater movement of the ankle joints.

### Foot
The foot is divided into three segments: the hindfoot, midfoot, and forefoot.

***Hindfoot.*** The talus and calcaneus make up the posterior segment.

***Midfoot.*** The navicular, cuboid, and three cuneiforms make up the middle segment.

***Forefoot.*** Five metatarsals and 14 phalanges make up the anterior segment. Each toe has three phalanges except for the large toe, which has two.

## Motions of the Foot and Ankle Defined

### Primary Plane Motions
Although motions in the foot and ankle do not occur purely in the cardinal planes, they are still defined as follows.[19,20,70,88]

***Sagittal plane motion around a frontal (coronal axis).*** *Dorsiflexion* is movement in a dorsal direction which decreases the angle between the leg and dorsum of the foot, and *plantarflexion* is movement in a plantar direction. Motion occurring at the toes may also be called dorsiflexion or extension, and plantarflexion or flexion.

***Frontal plane motion around a sagittal (anteroposterior) axis.*** *Inversion* is inward turning of the foot and *eversion* is outward turning. Normally, an inward and outward motion is described by the terms abduction and adduction, but because the foot is at a right angle to the leg, the terms abduction and adduction are not used here.

***Transverse plane motion around a vertical axis.*** *Abduction* is movement away from the midline, and *adduction* is movement toward the midline.

## Triplanar Motions

Triplanar motion occurs around an oblique axis at each articulation of the ankle and foot. The definitions are descriptive of the movement of the distal bone on the proximal bone. When the proximal bone moves on the stabilized distal bone, as occurs in weight bearing, the motion of the proximal bone is opposite, although the relative joint motion is the same as defined.

***Pronation.*** Pronation is a combination of dorsiflexion, eversion, and abduction. During weight bearing, pronation of the subtalar and transverse tarsal joints causes the arch of the foot to lower, and there is a relative supination of the forefoot with dorsiflexion of the first and plantarflexion of the fifth metatarsals. This is the loose-packed or mobile position of the foot and is assumed when the foot absorbs the impact of weight bearing and rotational forces of the rest of the lower extremity and when the foot conforms to the ground.[20]

***Supination.*** Supination is a combination of plantarflexion, inversion, and adduction. In the closed-chain, weight-bearing foot, supination of the subtalar and transverse tarsal joints with a pronation twist of the forefoot (plantarflexion of the first and dorsiflexion of the fifth metatarsals) increases the arch of the foot and is the close-packed or stable position of the joints of the foot. This is the position the foot assumes when a rigid lever is needed to propel the body forward during the push-off phase of ambulation.[70,88]

N O T E : The terms inversion and supination, as well as eversion and pronation, are often interchanged.[76] This text uses the terms as defined above.

## Leg, Ankle, and Foot Joint Characteristics and Arthrokinematics

The characteristics of each joint in the leg, ankle, and foot dictate how they contribute to the function of the foot.[70,75,88,94]

## Tibiofibular Joints

Anatomically, the superior and inferior tibiofibular joints are separate from the ankle but provide accessory motions that allow greater movement at the ankle. Fusion or immobility in these joints impairs ankle function. The strong mortise formed by the distal ends of the tibia and fibula forms the proximal surface of the ankle (talocrural) joint.

***Superior tibiofibular joint characteristics.*** The superior tibiofibular joint is a plane synovial joint made up of the fibular head and a facet on the posterolateral aspect of the rim of the tibial condyle. The facet faces posteriorly, inferiorly, and laterally. Although near the knee joint, it has its own capsule which is reinforced by the anterior and posterior tibiofibular ligaments.

***Inferior tibiofibular joint characteristics.*** The inferior tibiofibular joint is a syndesmosis with fibroadipose tissue between the two bony surfaces. This strong articulation is supported by the crural tibiofibular interosseous ligament and the anterior and posterior tibiofibular ligaments.

***Accessory motions.*** With dorsiflexion and plantarflexion of the ankle, there are slight accessory movements of the fibula. The direction of movement is variable depending on facet orientation of the proximal tibiofibular joint and elasticity in the tibiofibular ligaments. However, movement is necessary to allow full range of the talus in the mortise during ankle dorsiflexion.

### Ankle (Talocrural) Joint

***Characteristics.*** The ankle (talocrural) joint is a synovial hinge joint formed by the mortise (distal end of the tibia and tibial and fibular malleoli) and trochlea (dome) of the talus, and is enclosed by a relatively thin and weak capsule. It, along with the subtalar joint, is supported medially by the medial collateral (deltoid) ligament and laterally by the lateral collateral (anterior and posterior talofibular and calcaneofibular) ligaments (Fig. 22.2).

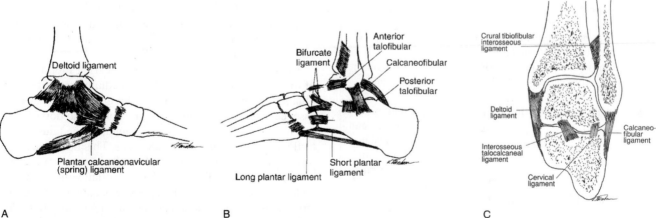

FIGURE 22.2 Ligaments of the ankle and foot. (*A*) Medial view, (*B*) lateral view, and (*C*) posterior (cross-sectional) view. (From Mueller in Levangie and Norkin,[70] A and B, p 442; C p 447, with permission.)

The fibular malleolus extends farther distally and posteriorly than the tibial malleolus so that the mortise angles outward and downward. This causes the axis of motion to be rotated laterally 20° to 30° and inclined downward 10°. The surface of the mortise is congruent with the articulating surface of the body of the talus.

The surface of the talus is wedge-shaped, being wider anteriorly, and is also cone-shaped, with the apex pointing medially. As a result of the orientation of the axis and shape of the talus when the foot dorsiflexes, the talus also abducts and slightly everts (pronation). When the foot plantarflexes, the talus also adducts and slightly inverts (supination). Dorsiflexion is the close-packed, stable position of the talocrural joint. Plantarflexion is the loose-packed position. The ankle joint is more vulnerable to injury when an individual is walking in high heels because of the less stable plantarflexed position at the same time that the subtalar and transverse tarsal joints are in their close-packed (rigid) position.

*Arthrokinematics.* The concave articulating surface is the mortise; the convex articulating surface is the body of the talus. With physiological motions of the foot, the articulating surface of the talus slides in the opposite direction (Box 22.1).

## Subtalar (Talocalcaneal) Joint

*Characteristics.* The subtalar (talocalcaneal) joint is a complex joint with three articulations between the talus and calcaneus. It has an oblique axis of motion lying approximately 42° from the transverse plane and 16° from the sagittal plane, which allows the calcaneus to pronate and supinate in a triplanar motion on the talus. Frontal plane inversion (turning heel inward) and eversion (turning heel outward) can be isolated only with passive motion. The subtalar joint is supported by the medial and lateral collateral ligaments, which also support the talocrural joint; by the interosseous talocalcaneal ligament in the tarsal canal; and by the posterior and lateral talocalcaneal ligaments. In closed-chain activities, the joint attenuates the rotatory forces between the leg and foot so that, normally, excessive inward or outward turning of the foot does not occur as the foot maintains contact with the supporting surface.

Of the three articulations between the talus and calcaneus, the posterior is separated from the anterior and middle by the tarsal canal. The canal divides the subtalar joint into two joint cavities. The posterior articulation has its own capsule. The anterior articulations are enclosed in the same capsule as the talonavicular articulation, forming the talocalcaneonavicular joint. Functionally, these articulations work together.

*Arthrokinematics.* The facet on the bottom of the talus in the posterior compartment is concave and the opposing facet on the calcaneus is convex. The facets of the anterior and middle articulations on the talus are convex, whereas the opposing facets on the calcaneus are concave. With open-chain physiological motions of the subtalar joint, the convex posterior portion of the calcaneus slides opposite to the motion; the concave anterior and middle facets on the calcaneus slide in the same direction, similar to turning a doorknob. Therefore, with the component motion of eversion, as the calcaneus swings laterally, the posterior articulating surface slides medially, and with inversion, the posterior articulating surface slides laterally (see Box 22.1).

## Talonavicular Joint

*Characteristics.* The talonavicular joint is anatomically and functionally part of a complex articulation between the talus and navicular as well as anterior and medial facets of the subtalar joint. It is supported by the spring, the deltoid, the bifurcate, and the dorsal talonavicular ligaments. The triplanar motions of the navicular on the talus function with the subtalar joint, resulting in pronation and supination.

During pronation, in the weight-bearing foot, the head of the talus drops plantarward and medially, resulting in a pliable foot and decreased medial longitudinal arch. In essence, as the calcaneus everts, it cannot also dorsiflex and abduct with the foot on the ground, so the talus plantarflexes and inverts on the calcaneus. This downward and inward motion of the talar head results in an upward and outward motion of the navicular and a flattening of the arch. During supination, the opposite occurs, resulting in a structurally stable foot and an increased medial longitudinal arch. The calcaneus inverts, and the talus dorsiflexes and everts, resulting in the navicular plantarflexing, inverting, and adducting.

| BOX 22.1 | Arthrokinematics of the Ankle and Foot Joints | |
|---|---|---|
| **Physiologic motion** | **Roll** | **Slide** |
| **Talocrural joint: motion of talus** | | |
| Dorsiflexion | Anterior | Posterior |
| Plantarflexion | Posterior | Anterior |
| **Subtalar joint: motion of calcaneus (posterior articulating surface)** | | |
| Supination with inversion | Medial | Lateral |
| Pronation with eversion | Lateral | Medial |
| **Talonavicular joint: motion of navicular (open-chain)** | | |
| Supination | Plantar and medial | Plantar and medial |
| Pronation | Dorsal and lateral | Dorsal and lateral |
| **Metatarsophalangeal and interphalangeal joints: motion of the phalanges** | | |
| Flexion | Plantar | Plantar |
| Extension | Dorsal | Dorsal |

*Arthrokinematics.* The head of the talus is convex; the proximal articulating surface of the navicular is concave. With physiological motions of the foot, the navicular slides in the same direction as the motion of the forefoot. In the open-chain motion of pronation, the navicular slides dorsally and laterally (abduction and eversion), resulting in a flattening of the medial longitudinal arch. With supination, the navicular slides volarly and medially (adduction and inversion) (see Box 22.1).

### Transverse Tarsal Joint

*Characteristics.* This functionally compound joint between the hind- and midfoot includes the anatomically separate talonavicular and calcaneocuboid joints. The *talonavicular joint* was described in the previous section. The *calcaneocuboid joint* is saddle-shaped. The transverse tarsal joint participates in the triplanar pronation/supination motions of the foot and makes compensatory movements to accommodate variations in the ground. Passive accessory motions include abduction/adduction, inversion/eversion, and dorsal/plantar gliding.

*Arthrokinematics.* The articulating surface of the calcaneus is convex in a dorsal-to-plantar direction and concave in a medial-to-lateral direction. The articulating surface of the cuboid is reciprocally concave and convex.

### Remaining Intertarsal and Tarsometatarsal Joints

The remaining intertarsal and tarsometatarsal joints are plane joints that reinforce the function of transverse tarsal joints, and during weight bearing, help regulate the position of the forefoot on the ground.

### Metatarsophalangeal and Interphalangeal Joints of the Toes

The metatarsophalangeal and interphalangeal joints of the toes are the same as the metacarpophalangeal and interphalangeal joints of the hand except that, in the toes, extension range of motion (ROM) is more important than is flexion (the opposite is true in the hand). Extension of the metatarsophalangeal (MTP) joints is necessary for normal walking. Also, unlike the thumb, the large toe does not function separately.

## ● FUNCTION OF THE ANKLE AND FOOT

### Structural Relationships

*Interdependence of leg and foot motions.* In the weight-bearing foot, subtalar motion and tibial rotation are interdependent. Supination of the subtalar joint results in or is caused by lateral rotation of the tibia, and conversely, pronation of the subtalar joint results in or is caused by medial rotation of the tibia.[70,88]

*Arches.* The arches of the foot are visualized as a twisted osteoligamentous plate, with the metatarsal heads being the horizontally placed anterior edge of the plate, and the cal-

caneus being the vertically placed posterior edge. The twist causes the longitudinal and transverse arches. When the foot is bearing weight, the plate tends to untwist and flatten the arches slightly.[70]

- Primary support of the arches comes from the spring ligament, with additional support from the long plantar ligament, the plantar aponeurosis, and short plantar ligament. During push-off in gait, as the foot plantarflexes and supinates and the metatarsal phalangeal joints go into extension, increased tension is placed on the plantar aponeurosis, which helps increase the arch. This is called the windlass effect.
- In the normal static foot, muscles do little to support the arches, yet without muscle tension the passive support stretches, and foot pronation increases under weight-bearing loads. Muscles contribute to support during ambulation.

*Effect on posture.* During standing with weight equally distributed through both lower extremities, if one foot/ankle complex is more pronated than the other, the overall effect is a frontal plane asymmetry with a "short leg" on that side. All typical landmarks (crest of the ilium, greater trochanter, popliteal crease, head of the fibula, and medial malleolus) on the side of the pronated foot are slightly lower.

*Abnormal foot postures.* A person with a varus deformity of the calcaneus (observed nonweight-bearing) may compensate by standing with a pronated (or everted) calcaneus posture.[19,21] The terms pes planus, pronated foot, and flat foot are often interchanged to mean a pronated posture of the hindfoot and decreased medial longitudinal arch. Pes cavus and supinated foot describe a high-arched foot.[76]

### Muscle Function in the Ankle and Foot

*Plantarflexors.* Plantarflexion is caused primarily by the two-joint gastrocnemius muscle and the one-joint soleus muscle, these muscles attach to the calcaneus via the Achilles tendon.

*Secondary plantarflexors.* Other muscles passing posteriorly to the axis of motion of plantarflexion contribute little to that motion, but they do have other functions.

- Tibialis posterior is a strong *supinator* and *invertor* that helps to control and reverse pronation during midstance of gait.
- The flexor hallucis longus and flexor digitorum longus muscles flex the toes and help support the medial longitudinal arch. To prevent clawing of the toes (MTP extension with IP flexion), intrinsic muscles must also function at the MTP joints.
- The peroneus longus and brevis muscles primarily *pronate* the foot at the subtalar joint, and the longus gives support to the transverse and lateral longitudinal arches during weight-bearing activities.[71]

*Dorsiflexors.* Dorsiflexion of the ankle is caused by the tibialis anterior muscle (which also inverts the ankle), the extensor hallucis longus and extensor digitorum longus (which also extend the toes), and the peroneus tertius muscles.

*Intrinsic muscles.* Intrinsic muscles of the foot function similar to those of the hand (except there is no thumb-like function in the foot). In addition, they provide support to the arches during gait.

*Stability in standing.* During normal standing, the gravitational line is anterior to the axis of the ankle joint, creating a dorsiflexion moment. The soleus muscle contracts to counter the gravitational moment through its pull on the tibia. Other extrinsic foot muscles help stabilize the foot during postural sway.

# ● THE ANKLE/FOOT COMPLEX AND GAIT

During the normal gait cycle, the ankle goes through a ROM of 32° to 35°. Approximately 7° of dorsiflexion occurs at the end of midstance as the heel begins to rise, and 25° of plantarflexion occurs at the end of stance (toe off).[78]

## Function of the Ankle and Foot Joints During Gait

The shock-absorbing, terrain-conforming, and propulsion functions of the ankle and foot include the following.[70,78,80]

● During the *loading response* (heel strike to foot flat), the heel strikes the ground in neutral or slight supination. As the foot lowers to the ground, it begins to pronate to its loose-packed position. The entire lower extremity rotates inward, which reinforces the loose-packed position of the foot. With the foot in a lax position, it can conform to variations in the ground contour and absorb some of the impact forces as the foot is lowered.
● Once the foot is fixed on the ground, dorsiflexion begins as the tibia comes up over the foot. The tibia continues to rotate internally, which reinforces pronation of the subtalar joint and loose-packed position of the foot.
● During *midstance* and continuing through *terminal stance*, the tibia begins to rotate externally, which initiates supination of the hindfoot and locking of the transverse tarsal joint. This brings the foot into its close-packed position, which is reinforced as the heel rises and the foot rocks up onto the toes, causing toe extension and tightening of the plantar aponeurosis (windlass effect). This stable position converts the foot into a rigid lever, ready to propel the body forward as the ankle plantarflexes from the pull of the gastrocnemius–soleus muscle group.

## Muscle Control of the Ankle and Foot During Gait[70,78,80]

*Ankle dorsiflexors.* The ankle dorsiflexors function during the initial foot contact and loading response (heel strike to foot flat) to counter the plantarflexion torque and to control the lowering of the foot to the ground. They also function during the swing phase to keep the foot from plantarflexing and dragging on the ground. With loss of the dorsiflexors, foot slap occurs at initial foot contact, and the hip and knee flex excessively during swing (otherwise the toe drags on the ground).

*Ankle plantarflexors.* The ankle plantarflexors function eccentrically early in stance to control the rate of forward movement of the tibia. Then at around 40% of the cycle (midstance) there is a burst of concentric activity to initiate plantarflexion of the ankle for push off. Loss of function results in a slight lag of the lower extremity during terminal stance with no push-off.

*Ankle evertors.* Contraction of the peroneus longus muscle late in the stance phase facilitates transfer of weight from the lateral to the medial side of the foot. It also stabilizes the first ray and facilitates the pronation twist of the tarsometatarsal joints as increased supination occurs in the hindfoot.

*Ankle inverters.* The tibialis anterior helps control the pronation force on the hindfoot during the loading response of gait.

*Intrinsic muscles.* The intrinsic muscles support the transverse and longitudinal arches during gait.

# ● REFERRED PAIN AND NERVE INJURY

Several major nerves terminate in the foot. Injury or entrapment of the nerves may occur anywhere along their course, from the lumbosacral spine to near their termination. For treatment to be effective, it must be directed to the source of the problem. Therefore, a thorough history is obtained, and an examination is performed when the patient reports referred pain patterns, sensory changes, or muscle weakness. For a detailed description of referred pain patterns and peripheral nerve injuries in the foot and ankle region see Chapter 13.

## Major Nerves Subject to Pressure and Trauma

*Common peroneal nerve.* Pressure on the common peroneal nerve may occur as it courses laterally around the fibular neck and passes through an opening in the peroneus longus muscle.

*Posterior tibial nerve.* Entrapment in the tarsal tunnel, causing tarsal tunnel syndrome, may occur from a space-occupying lesion posterior to the medial malleolus.

*Plantar and calcaneal nerves.* These branches of the posterior tibial nerve may become entrapped as they turn under the medial aspect of the foot and pass through openings in the abductor hallucis muscle. Overpronation presses the nerves against these openings. Irritation of the nerves may elicit symptoms similar to those of acute foot strain (tenderness at the posteromedial plantar aspect of the foot), painful heel (inflamed calcaneal nerve), and pain in a pes cavus foot.

## Common Sources of Segmental Sensory Reference in the Foot

The foot is the terminal point for the L4, L5, and S1 nerve roots coursing through the terminal branches of the peroneal and tibial nerves. Referred pain may occur with irritation to tissues derived from the same spinal segments, or sensory changes from irritation or damage to these nerve roots (see Fig. 13.2 in Chapter 13).

# MANAGEMENT OF FOOT AND ANKLE DISORDERS AND SURGERIES

To make sound clinical decisions when managing patients with foot and ankle disorders, it is necessary to understand the various pathologies, surgical procedures, and associated precautions and identify presenting impairments, functional limitations, and possible disabilities. In this section common pathologies and surgeries are presented and related to corresponding preferred practice patterns (groupings of impairments) described in the *Guide to Physical Therapist Practice*[2] (Table 22.1). Conservative and postoperative management of the conditions described in this section are based on principles of tissue healing and exercise intervention.

## TABLE 22.1 Foot and Ankle Pathologies/Surgical Procedures and Preferred Practice Patterns

| PATHOLOGY/SURGICAL PROCEDURE | PREFERRED PRACTICE PATTERNS AND ASSOCIATED IMPAIRMENTS[2] |
|---|---|
| • Abnormal posture (pronated or supinated foot, tibial torsion) | Pattern 4B—Impaired posture |
| • Arthritis (osteoarthritis, rheumatoid arthritis, traumatic arthritis, gout)<br>• Post-immobilization stiffness<br>• Synovitis<br>• Joint instability, subluxation, dislocation (nontraumatic/recurrent)<br>• Overuse syndromes/repetitive trauma syndromes (tendonitis, plantar fasciitis, shin splints) | Pattern 4D—Impaired joint mobility, motor function, muscle performance, and range of motion associated with connective tissue dysfunction |
| • Arthritis—acute stage<br>• Acute capsulitis<br>• Acute plantar fasciitis, tendonitis, shin splints<br>• Acute ankle sprains<br>• Acute muscle tears | Pattern 4E—Impaired joint mobility, motor function, muscle performance, and range of motion associated with localized inflammation |
| • Fractures | Pattern 4G—Impaired joint mobility, muscle performance, and range of motion associated with fracture |
| • Arthroscopic débridement<br>• Osteochondral drilling, mosaicplasty, osteochondral autologous transplantation<br>• Excision arthroplasty with or without implant of the MTP or IP joints<br>• Total joint arthroplasty | Pattern 4H—Impaired joint mobility, motor function, muscle performance and range of motion associated with joint arthroplasty |
| • Fracture stabilization with internal fixation<br>• Tendon and ligament repairs<br>• Capsulorrhaphy<br>• Synovectomy<br>• Arthrodesis | Pattern 4I—Impaired joint mobility, motor function, muscle performance and range of motion associated with bony or soft tissue surgery |
| • Peripheral nerve injury (common peroneal, posterior tibial, tarsal tunnel syndrome) | Pattern 5F—Impaired peripheral nerve integrity and muscle performance associated with peripheral nerve injury |

# ● JOINT HYPOMOBILITY: NONOPERATIVE MANAGEMENT

## Common Joint Pathologies and Etiology of Symptoms

Pathologies such as rheumatoid arthritis (RA); juvenile rheumatoid arthritis (JRA); degenerative joint disease (DJD); and acute joint reactions after trauma, dislocations, or fractures affect the foot and ankle complex. Post-immobilization contractures and adhesions develop in the joint capsules and surrounding tissues any time a joint is immobilized in a cast or splint, typically after dislocations and fractures. The reader is referred to Chapter 11 for background information on arthritis, post-immobilization stiffness, and etiology of symptoms. The following is specific to joint conditions in the ankle and foot:

*Rheumatoid arthritis.* Joint pathology of the foot and ankle as the result of RA commonly affects the forefoot early in the disease process, later the hindfoot, and least frequently, the ankle.[14,41] Involvement may occur in the MTP, subtalar, talocrural joints of the foot, leading to instabilities and painful deformities, such as hallux valgus and subluxation of the metatarsal heads, that increase with the stress of weight bearing. Tendon rupture of foot and ankle musculature also may occur as the result of chronic inflammation and contribute to deformity.[41]

*Degenerative joint disease (DJD) and joint trauma.* Degenerative symptoms occur in joints that are malaligned or repetitively traumatized, and acute joint symptoms are often seen in conjunction with ankle sprains, chronic instability, or fracture. Post-traumatic arthritis leading to DJD is by far the most common type of arthritis that affects the ankle, accounting for approximately 80% of all ankle arthritis. In contrast, primary osteoarthritis, a common type of arthritis in the hip and knee, is rare in the ankle, even in the older adult population.[105]

*Post-immobilization stiffness.* Contractures and adhesions in the capsular tissues leading to joint hypomobilities as well as in the surrounding periarticular tissues may occur any time the joint is immobilized after a fracture or surgery.

*Gout.* Symptoms commonly affect the MTP joint of the great toe, causing pain during terminal stance so that there is a shorter stance and lack of smooth push-off.

## Common Impairments and Functional Limitations/Disabilities

In RA, many of the following impairments and deformities occur with progression of the disease.[18,92] With DJD and post-immobilization stiffness, only the affected joint or joints are limited.[16] Functional limitations and disabilities occur primarily as a result of loss of weight-bearing abilities.

● *Restricted motion.* When symptoms are acute, the patient experiences swelling and restricted, painful motion, particularly during weight-bearing activities. When symptoms are chronic, there is restricted motion, decreased joint play, and a firm capsular end-feel in the affected joint.

- *Decreased mobility in the proximal and distal tibiofibular joints.* Restricted accessory motion in these joints usually occurs with periods of immobilization and limits ankle and subtalar joint motion.[56]
- *Talocrural joint.* Passive plantarflexion is more limited than dorsiflexion (unless the gastrocnemius–soleus muscle group also is shortened, in which case dorsiflexion is limited accordingly).
- *Subtalar and transverse tarsal joints.* Progressive limitation of supination develops until eventually the joint fixes in pronation with flattening of the medial longitudinal arch. The close-packed position of the tarsals (supination) becomes more and more difficult to assume during the terminal stance (push-off) phase of gait.
- *MTP joint of the large toe.* Gross limitation of extension and some limitation of flexion develop; the rest of the MTP joints are variable. Lack of extension restricts the terminal stance phase of gait with an inability to rock up onto the metatarsal heads. This exacerbates the pronation posture and inability to supinate the foot during push-off in gait.

● *Common deformities.* Deformities occur due to a variety of factors including but not limited to muscle imbalances, faulty footware, trauma, and heredity.

- *Hallux valgus.* This deformity in the great (large) toe develops as the proximal phalanx shifts laterally toward the second toe. Eventually the flexor and extensor muscles of the great toe shift laterally and further accentuate the deformity. The bursa over the medial aspect of the metatarsal head may become inflamed and the bone hypertrophies, causing a painful bunion.
- *Hallux rigidus.* Narrowing and eventual obliteration of the first MTP joint space occur with progressive loss of extension. This affects terminal stance by not allowing the foot to roll over the metatarsal heads and great toe for normal push-off. Instead, the individual turns the foot outward and rolls over the medial aspect of the large toe. This faulty pattern accentuates hallux valgus and foot pronation, and usually the MTP joint is quite painful.
- *Dorsal dislocation of the proximal phalanges on the metatarsal heads.* If this occurs, the fat pad, which is normally under the metatarsal heads, migrates dorsally with the phalanges, and the protective cushion on weight bearing is lost, leading to pain, callus formation, and potential ulceration.
- *Claw toe (MTP hyperextension and IP flexion) and hammer toe (MTP hyperextension, PIP flexion, and DIP hyperextension).* These result from muscle imbalances between the intrinsic and extrinsic muscles of the

toes. Friction from shoes may cause calluses to form where the toes rub.

● *Muscle weakness and decreased muscular endurance.* Inhibition resulting from pain and decreased use of the extremities lead to impaired muscle function.

● *Impaired balance and postural control.* The sensory receptors in the ankle joints and ligaments, as well as in the muscle spindles, provide important information for posture and movement, known as the *ankle strategy.* The ankle strategy is used in balance control during perturbations.[37,84] Faulty feedback and balance deficits occur when there is instability, muscle impairments, or arthritis.

● *Increased frequency of falling.* Impaired balance may lead to frequent falling or fear of falling and thus restrict community outings.

● *Painful weight bearing.* When symptoms are acute, weight-bearing activities are painful, preventing independent ambulation and causing difficulty in rising from a chair and ascending and descending stairs.

● *Gait deviations.* If the patient experiences pain during weight bearing, there is a short stance phase, reduced single limb support, and decreased stride length on the side of involvement. Because of the restricting motion and loss of effective plantarflexion and supination in the arthritic foot, as well as pain in the forefoot area under the metatarsal heads, push-off is ineffective during terminal stance. Little or no heel rise occurs; instead, the person lifts up the involved foot.

● *Decreased ambulation.* Because of decreased ankle and foot mobility and resulting decreased length of stride, distance and speed of ambulation are decreased; the person may require use of assistive devices for ambulation. If pain, balance, or restricted motion is severe the person will be unable to ambulate and, therefore, requires a wheelchair for mobility.

## Joint Hypomobility: Management—Protection Phase

The interventions selected for management depend on the signs and symptoms present. For acute problems, follow the general outline presented in Chapter 10 and summarized in Box 10.1. Suggested interventions for the various goals are described in this section.[45,92,105]

### Educate the Patient and Provide Joint Protection

Teach a home exercise program at the level of the patient's abilities. Teach the patient to be aware of signs of systemic fatigue (especially in RA), local muscle fatigue, and joint stress, and how to modify exercises and activities to remain active within safe levels. Emphasize the importance of daily ROM, endurance activities, and joint protection, including avoidance of faulty foot and ankle postures and protection of the feet from deforming weight-bearing forces and trauma imposed by improperly fitting footwear. If necessary, instruct the patient in safe use of assistive devices to decrease the effects of weight bearing and pain.

### Decrease Pain

In addition to physician-prescribed medication, intra-articular injections of corticosteroids, or nonsteroidal anti-inflammatory medications, and therapeutic use of modalities the following are used to manage painful symptoms.

● *Manual therapy techniques.* Gentle grade I or II distraction and oscillation techniques may inhibit pain and move synovial fluid for nutrition within the involved joints.

● *Orthotic devices.* Orthotics and well-constructed shoes help protect the joints by realigning forces and providing support from faulty foot postures.[45,62,65] Such support has been shown to decrease pain and improve functional mobility. Splinting or bracing may also be used to stabilize an arthritic joint.

 **Focus on Evidence**

Kavlak and colleagues[45] reported the effects of prescribed orthotic devices in 18 patients with RA (no control group) and a variety of bilateral foot deformities, including pes planus, hallux valgus, hammer toe, subluxation of the metatarsal heads, and others. All patients in the study were community walkers with no history of surgery of the foot or ankle. All patients were prescribed custom-made orthotic inserts and shoe modifications, such as a medial longitudinal arch support, metatarsal pad, or heel and forefoot wedge, to meet their individual needs. Pain, temporal-distance characteristics of gait, and energy expenditure during walking were measured before and after the patients had been wearing the custom orthoses for 3 months. There was a significant reduction in pain and energy cost during ambulation and increases in step and stride length after use of the orthotic devices for 3 months. There were no significant changes in foot angle or the width of the base of support. The authors concluded that appropriately prescribed orthoses and shoe modifications were important elements of nonoperative treatment of foot pain and impaired gait in patients with RA.

### Maintain Joint and Soft Tissue Mobility and Muscle Integrity

● *Passive, active-assistive, or active ROM.* It is important to move the joints as tolerated. If active exercises are tolerated, they are preferred because of the benefits of muscle action.

● *Aquatic therapy.* Aquatic therapy is an effective method of combining nonstressful buoyancy-assisted exercises with therapeutic heat.

● *Muscle setting.* Apply gentle multiangle muscle-setting techniques in pain-free positions and at an intensity that does not exacerbate symptoms.

## Joint Hypomobility: Management—Controlled Motion and Return to Function Phases

Examine the patient for signs of decreased muscle flexibility, joint restrictions, muscle weakness, and balance impairments. Initiate exercises and mobilization procedures at a level appropriate for the condition of the patient.

**PRECAUTIONS WITH RA:** Modify the intensity of joint mobilization and stretching techniques used to counter any restrictions because the disease process and use of steroid therapy weaken the tensile quality of the connective tissue. Therefore, it is more easily torn. It may be necessary to continue joint protection with orthotics, proper fitting shoes, and assistive devices for ambulation.[92] Encourage the patient to be active, but also to respect pain and fatigue.

### Increase Joint Play and Accessory Motions

***Joint mobilization techniques.*** Determine which articulations are restricted owing to decreased joint play, and apply grade III sustained or grade III and IV oscillation techniques to stretch the limitations. See Figures 5.55 through 5.64 and their descriptions in Chapter 5 for techniques to mobilize the leg, ankle, and foot articulations. Mobilizing the toes is the same as the fingers (see Figs. 5.42 through 5.43).

**NOTE:** Because weight-bearing forces and joint changes with arthritis accentuate pronation, mobilizing to increase pronation usually should not be undertaken in an arthritic foot. Perform these techniques only in the stiff foot after immobilization when the foot does not pronate sufficiently during the loading response in gait. In addition, extension of the toes at the MTP joints is important during terminal stance for normal push-off and development of the windlass effect in gait. The great toe requires from 40° to 50° extension to function effectively during this phase of gait.[78,80]

### Improve Joint Tracking of the Talocrural Joint
Apply mobilization with movement (MWM) techniques to increase ROM and/or decrease pain associated with movement.[72] The principles of MWM are described in Chapter 5.

### Plantarflexion MWM
*Patient position and procedure*: Supine with hip and knee flexed and heel on the table (Fig. 22.3). Stand at the foot of the table facing the patient and contact the patient's anterior tibia with the palm of your hand (for the right foot use the left hand). Produce a pain-free graded posterior glide of the tibia on the talus. The patient should now be unable to plantarflex. While maintaining the posterior tibial glide grip the talus with your other hand (for the right foot, use the right hand) and create a passive end-range plantarflexion movement, causing the talus to roll anteriorly.

The sustained plantarflexion must be painless. Repeat three to four times in sets of 6 to 10 and reassess to confirm improved range.

### Dorsiflexion MWM
*Patient position and procedure*: The patient is standing with the affected foot placed on a chair or stool (Fig. 22.4). Kneel on the floor facing the patient with a mobilization belt around your buttocks and the patient's Achilles tendon

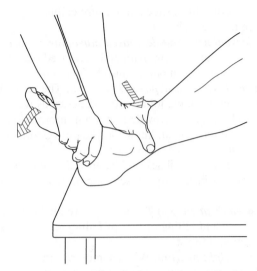

FIGURE 22.3 Mobilization with movement to increase ankle plantarflexion. Maintain a posterior glide of the tibia while moving the talus into planterflexion. This should not cause pain.

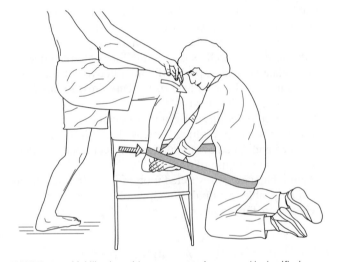

FIGURE 22.4 Mobilization with movement to increase ankle dorsiflexion. Maintain an anterior glide of the tibia with the mobilization belt while the patient lunges forward to move the ankle into dorsiflexion. This should not cause pain.

(padded with a towel). Place the web space of both hands around the neck of the talus with the palms on the dorsum of the foot. Hold the foot down and back and the subtalar joint in neutral pronation/supination. Use the belt to produce a pain-free graded anterior gliding force to the ankle joint. While maintaining this mobilization, have the patient lunge forward, bringing the affected ankle into dorsiflexion and causing painless end-range loading. Repeat in sets of 6 to 10, reassessing for effect.

### Increase Mobility of Soft Tissues and Muscles
Perform passive stretching and inhibition techniques as described in Chapter 4. Self-stretching techniques are described later in this chapter.

### Regain a Balance in Muscle Strength and Prepare for Functional Activities

Initiate resistive exercises at a level appropriate for the weakened muscles. Begin with isometric resistance in pain-free positions, and progress to dynamic resistance exercises through pain-free ranges using open- and closed-chain exercises. Resistive exercises are described later in this chapter. Low-load, weight-bearing exercises may be initiated in a pool or tank and progressed to full weight bearing as tolerated. Develop exercises that prepare the patient to return to functional activities.

### Improve Balance and Proprioception

Initiate protected balance exercises, and progress the intensity as tolerated. Determine the level of stability and safety during ambulation and continue use of assistive devices if necessary to help prevent falls.

### Develop Cardiopulmonary Fitness

Low-impact aerobic exercises should be initiated early in the treatment program and progressed as the patient is able. Repetitive exercises in a pool (water aerobics), swimming, treadmill walking, and bicycling may be within the

patient's tolerance. A person with degenerative or rheumatoid arthritis should not do high-impact (jumping, hopping, and jogging) aerobic exercises.

## JOINT SURGERY AND POSTOPERATIVE MANAGEMENT

Advanced arthritis of the ankle or the joints of the foot can cause severe pain, limitation of motion, gross instability or deformity, and significant loss of function during activities that require weight bearing through the lower extremities (Fig. 22.5). When nonoperative management no longer alleviates symptoms, surgical options for early and advanced joint disease may be necessary (Box 22.2).[6,12,14,41,47,51,105,107,111] The procedure(s) selected depends on the joints involved, the extent of articular damage, the severity of joint instability or deformity, and the postoperative functional goals of the patient.

Arthroscopic débridement of a symptomatic joint is appropriate for management of early joint changes but

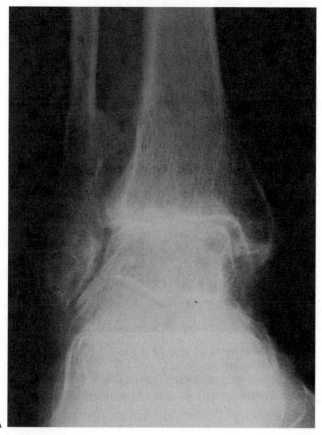 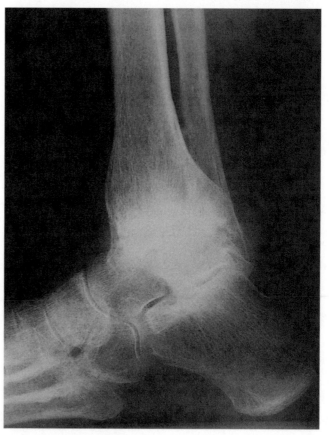

FIGURE 22.5 Late-stage arthritis of the ankle. (*A*) Mortise view of the ankle shows severe loss of the normal joint space and partial erosion of the lateral tibia. (*B*) Lateral view shows tibial erosion with mild joint space loss in the subtalar region and significant osteophyte formation in the anterior ankle. (From Hasselman, CT, Wong, YS, Conti, SF: Total ankle replacement. In Kitaoka, HB (ed): Master Techniques in Orthopedic Surgery: The Foot and Ankle, ed 2. Lippincott Williams & Wilkins, Philadelphia, 2002, figure 39.1, p 583, with permission.)

**Early-Stage Procedures**
- Arthroscopic débridement and cheilectomy (removal of osteophytes)
- Arthroscopic subchondral drilling, mosaicplasty, or osteochondral autologous implantation for small osteochondral lesions of the talus
- Articular distraction (widening of the joint space by means of a temporarily inserted external fixation device)
- Soft tissue reconstruction
- Synovectomy

**Late-Stage Procedures**
- Osteotomy
- Excision arthroplasty with or without implant
- Total joint arthroplasty
- Arthrodesis

offers little if there is significant destruction of articular cartilage.[105] For late-stage arthritis, arthrodesis provides pain-free weight bearing and stability of the involved joint(s) but sacrifices mobility of the operated joints, which, in turn, affects functional movement. Pain-free compensatory movements must be available in adjacent joints to absorb weight-bearing forces during ambulation. Arthrodesis typically is performed in young patients with high functional demands.[6,12,14,47,105] Arthroplasty of the ankle[14,36,51–53,86,105] or toes,[14,107] an option far less frequently selected than arthrodesis, affords pain relief while retaining some degree of joint mobility. It is an alternative to arthrodesis for patients with severe joint symptoms but who are older or relatively inactive.

The anticipated outcomes of joint surgery at the ankle and foot and postoperative rehabilitation are (1) relief of pain with weight bearing and joint motion, (2) correction of deformity, (3) restoration of stability or mobility of the involved joints, and (4) improved strength and muscular endurance of the lower extremities for ambulation and functional activities.[6,14,51,105,107] Rehabilitation includes postoperative exercise; gait training with assistive devices; fabrication of foot orthoses; and patient education including information about shoe selection, fit, and modification and appropriate choices of recreational and activities of daily living (ADLs) as well.

## Total Ankle Arthroplasty

Total ankle arthroplasty (TAA) is an option for carefully selected patients with disabling pain associated with advanced, symptomatic arthritis of the talocrural joint whose only surgical alternative is ankle arthrodesis. This procedure provides pain relief while preserving functional motion of the ankle and therefore reduces stresses on adja-

cent joints more effectively than does arthrodesis. TAA is most appropriate for individuals who are relatively sedentary and do not expect to participate in high-impact recreational activities or heavy labor after surgery.[33,51,86,105]

### Indications for Surgery

Although no consensus exists at this time, the following are frequently cited current-day indications for total ankle arthroplasty.[14,33,41,51,86,105] These indications are far less liberal than those suggested when TAA was first introduced several decades ago.

- Severe, persistent pain, particularly during weight bearing, and compromised functional mobility as the result of advanced degenerative or inflammatory joint disease including post-traumatic arthritis; OA, RA, or JRA; or avascular necrosis of the dome of the talus
- Sufficient integrity of ligaments for ankle stability
- A flexible deformity that can be passively corrected to neutral or no more than 5° or hindfoot valgus
- Appropriate for an older patient with low physical demands
- An option when both ankles are involved and bilateral ankle fusions are impractical and would dramatically restrict functional mobility, such as ascending or descending stairs or rising from a chair.

**Contraindications.** There are numerous contraindications to TAA.[14,33,51,86] Patient-related contraindications include active or chronic infection of the ankle, severe osteoporosis, impaired lower extremity vascular supply, and long-term use of corticosteroids. Young (less than 50 to 60 years of age), physically active patients or obese patients are not good candidates for TAA. Contraindications specific to the ankle include avascular necrosis of a significant portion of the body of the talus, marked ankle instability, a varus or valgus deformity of the hindfoot greater than 20°, less than a 20° total arc of dorsi- and plantarflexion, and peripheral neuropathy leading to decreased sensation, significant weakness, and imbalance of ankle and foot musculature.

### Procedure

**Implant designs, materials, and fixation.** Introduced in the 1970s, the first total ankle arthroplasty designs were two-component, metal-to-polyethylene implants held in place with cement fixation.[108,115] Short-term results of these "first generation" implants, although quite variable, seemed to hold promise. However, the early designs proved to have limited durability because many had highly constrained tibial and talar components and did not replicate the complex biomechanical characteristics of the ankle's articulating surfaces.[108] Functional ROM of the ankle also was difficult to achieve with the more constrained designs. Other early designs were unconstrained, allowing multiplanar movements but providing no ankle stability.[115] Consequently, a high rate of complications occurred, such as loosening at the bone–cement interface and premature component wear with the constrained implants, and ankle dislocation with the unconstrained designs, leading to unsatisfactory long-term results.[33,41,51,86,105]

Advances in prosthetic design, beginning in the late 1980s and early 1990s, based on a more thorough understanding of the biomechanics of the ankle and foot, have incorporated sliding and rotational motions into implant systems. Because contemporary prosthetic designs more closely mimic the characteristics of a normal ankle joint, ROM available in several of these systems now approaches that of a normal ankle.[109] Changes in design combined with improved surgical techniques, such as better soft tissue balancing and ligament reconstruction, and the availability of new implant materials and cementless fixation have led to current-day, "second generation" TAA (Fig. 22.6). These new implant designs, which are minimally constrained or semiconstrained, completely resurface the tibial, fibular, and talar articulating surfaces using either a two- or three-component system. Contemporary TAA also requires far less resection of bone than early replacements and often employs bioingrowth fixation.[4,33,36,51,86,89,91,105] A hydroxyapatite coating on the outer surfaces of the metal implants is used to increase the rate of bone ingrowth.[91] However, cement fixation continues to be used for patients with poor bone stock.[54]

With a two-component system a porous or beaded metal-backed, high-density polyethylene tibial component articulates with a metal talar component that also has a beaded outer surface.[52] A three-component design, sometimes referred to as a mobile bearing design, employs a flat (table-top) tibial component made of metal and a metal talar dome distally with a mobile, polyethylene bearing interposed between the two metal components.[4,36] All of these newer designs allow at least 5° to 10° of dorsiflexion and 20° to 25° of plantarflexion, sufficient for functional activities, and a small degree of rotation of the foot on the tibia to reduce stresses on the implants.[33,51,86,105]

***Operative procedure.*** Although there are numerous variations of operative procedures involved in a TAA, the following represent key components.[4,33,51,91] An anterior longitudinal incision between the tibialis anterior and extensor hallicis longus tendons is the most widely used approach for TAA. The extensor retinaculum and capsule are incised to expose the joint. The joint is débrided and osteophytes are removed. An external distraction device is used to separate the joint surfaces and facilitate bone resection. Small portions of the distal tibia and talar dome are excised, followed by preparation of the joint surfaces. In some cases, the medial and lateral malleolar recesses also are resurfaced. Trial implants are inserted, and ROM is checked to be certain that at least 5° of dorsiflexion is possible. If limited by a contracture of the gastrocnemius–soleus muscle group, a percutaneous lengthening of the Achilles tendon is performed.

Sometimes a second incision is made along the distal fibula for fusion of the tibiofibular syndesmosis with screw fixation to provide a larger surface for fixation of the tibial prosthesis.[51,52] If there is a significant varus or valgus hindfoot deformity, a subtalar arthrodesis may also be performed.[91] After the permanent implants are inserted, soft tissues are balanced and repaired. Ligament reconstruction may be necessary if there is inadequate stability of the ankle and hindfoot. After the wound is closed, a bulky compression dressing and posterior splint are placed on the foot and ankle to control joint swelling and peripheral edema.

## Complications

The incidence of complications after second generation ankle replacements appears to be lower than after first generation prostheses and surgical techniques. However, because few long-term follow-up studies have been reported, the full picture is not yet available. In addition, whether current-day TAA will prove to be as successful as total hip or knee arthroplasty has yet to be determined.[50]

As with all types of joint arthroplasty, postoperative infection and wound healing are always potential complications. Postoperative edema in the ankle and foot also increases the likelihood of delayed wound healing. Wound healing complications, in turn, often prolong the immobilization period, thus delaying early ankle motion and potentially leading to poor ROM outcomes.[33,50,74] Reflex sympathetic dystrophy (complex regional pain syndrome) occasionally develops and causes chronic foot or ankle pain.[4] (Complex regional pain syndromes and interventions are described in Chapter 13.) Intraoperative (perioperative), early postoperative, and long-term complications unique to TAA are noted in Box 22.3.[4,33,50,74] Intraoperative and early

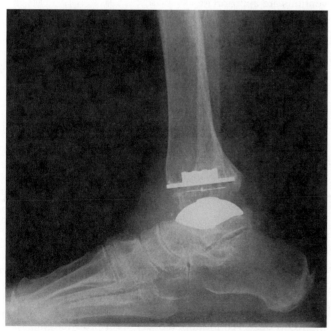

**FIGURE 22.6** Total ankle arthroplasty. Lateral view of a total ankle replacement in a 78-year-old woman 1 year following surgery for post-traumatic arthritis. (From Joint Replacement Arthroplasty, ed 3, Morrey, BF (ed), Chapter 85: Ankle replacement arthroplasty, Kitaoka, HB, Claridge, RJ, page 1148, 2003, with permission from The Mayo Clinic Foundation.)

Complications of Total Ankle Arthroplasty

**Intraoperative Complications**
- Fracture of the medial or lateral malleolus during implant insertion→the necessity for fracture stabilization with internal fixation.
- Malpositioning of an implant→chronic ankle instability, subluxation, dislocation, early mechanical loosening, or premature implant wear.
- Laceration of the posterior tibialis tendon during bone resection due to its close proximity to the medial malleolus→necessity for tendon repair.
- Nerve injury, usually the superficial or deep peroneal→impaired sensory or motor function.
- Insufficient soft tissue balancing or reconstruction→chronic ankle instability or deformity.

**Postoperative: Early and Long-Term Complications**
- Delayed union or nonunion of a tibiofibular syndesmosis fusion→an extended immobilization and nonweight-bearing period.
- Mechanical (aseptic) loosening (most often the talar component)→pain and impaired functional mobility
- Hindfoot arthritis (most often the subtalar joint)→pain and impaired weight-bearing abilities.

postoperative complications can adversely affect rehabilitation and outcomes of ankle replacement and may necessitate revision arthroplasty or arthrodesis.

**Postoperative Management**
There are few guidelines in the literature for postoperative management of patients who have undergone total ankle arthroplasty. Those that are available vary considerably with regard to immobilization, initiation of exercise, and weight bearing. Although opinions often are cited, there is a lack of evidence to support whether ROM exercises should be initiated a few days postoperatively or delayed for several weeks until there is evidence of bone ingrowth into the implants. It also is unclear whether early protected motion has a positive impact on ROM outcomes or if it is detrimental to implant fixation or wound healing.[86]

Therefore, the following guidelines or precautions for postoperative management are a summary of those cited by several authors based on their experience and training.[4,33,51,74,86]

**Immobilization and Weight-Bearing considerations**

*Immobilization.* The ankle is placed in a compression dressing and immobilized in a neutral position in a well-padded, short-leg, posterior splint. The duration of continuous immobilization varies depending on the type of implant fixation used and the types of surgical procedures performed during the arthroplasty. For example, if a tibiofibular syndesmosis or subtalar fusion was performed, no motion is allowed for 6 weeks or until there is evidence of bony union.[51,52] If there was no bony fusion, at least 3

weeks of immobilization after cementless fixation is recommended if the prosthetic implants have a hydroxyapatite coating but approximately 6 weeks for beaded implants without a coating.[86]

*Weight-bearing considerations.* A patient must always wear an ankle immobilizer when initiating weight bearing after TAA. Recommendations for the time at which weight bearing is permissible after cementless fixation range from a maximum of 40 pounds[33] or weight bearing as tolerated[4] immediately after surgery to nonweight bearing for 3 weeks or more.[86] If a tibiofibular syndesmosis fusion was performed, weight bearing is not permitted for at least 6 weeks.[51,52] After a period of restricted weight bearing, patients gradually progress from partial to full weight bearing over several weeks and then gradually discontinue wearing the immobilizer.

**Exercise: Maximum Protection Phase**
The first phase of postoperative rehabilitation, which extends for about 6 weeks, focuses on the patient becoming functionally mobile immediately after surgery with attention to protecting the operated ankle and controlling postoperative edema. *Goals* include maintaining ROM in the joints proximal to the ankle or any other arthritic joints, improving strength in the upper and nonoperated lower extremities, and minimizing atrophy of the ankle and foot muscles of the operated limb. If removal of the immobilization is allowed during the first few weeks after surgery, an additional goal is to prevent stiffness in the operated ankle and loss of extensibility of surrounding soft tissues.

To achieve these goals, the following exercise interventions are appropriate.

- Begin isometric (muscle-setting) exercises of the ankle musculature, gluteal, and quadriceps muscles and active-resistive exercises of hip and knee musculature on the operated side.[93]
- Strengthen the nonoperated lower extremity and upper extremities using resisted exercises in preparation for ambulation.
- Regain active ROM of the operated ankle using gentle, nonforceful motions when it is permissible to remove the immobilization and if wound healing is sufficient. Include dorsiflexion and plantarflexion, inversion, eversion, and circumduction. Perform active ROM of the toes.

**Exercise: Moderate and Minimum Protection Phases**
By 6 weeks it usually is permissible to remove the immobilizer for exercise and gradually discontinue its use during weight-bearing activities except in cases of poor soft tissue healing or delayed bone ingrowth or union. *Goals* during the final phases of rehabilitation are to achieve 100% of the ROM observed intraoperatively[86]; restore strength, muscular endurance, and balance in the lower extremities for unrestricted weight bearing; improve aerobic capacity and cardiopulmonary endurance; and help the patient perform necessary and desired functional activities safely. Patient education is a key to safe participation in recreational and work-related activities.

The following interventions are recommended to meet these goals. Refer to the last section of this chapter for detailed descriptions, progression, and illustrations of exercises. A progression of balance activities is described in Chapter 8.

- Continue or initiate active ROM exercises of the operated ankle and foot.
- Stretch the plantarflexors, if dorsiflexion is restricted, using towel stretches in a long-sitting position, or have the patient stand on a wedge for an extended period of time.
- Perform low-intensity, high-repetition resistance exercises in nonweight-bearing and weight-bearing positions.
- Initiate a stationary cycling program and progress the speed and distance of ambulation to increase cardiopulmonary fitness and lower extremity muscular endurance. The amount of dorsiflexion required during pedaling can be adjusted by raising or lowering the seat height.
- To the extent weight bearing allows, perform a progression of bilateral and unilateral balance activities.
- Through patient education and activity modification, prepare the patient to return to functional activities. Select nonimpact or low-impact activities, and for joint protection avoid activities that involve quick stop-and-go motions.[110]

### Outcomes

As discussed previously, although early total ankle arthroplasty afforded pain relief for a period of time,[89,108,115] there were unacceptably high rates of complications, leading to poor functional outcomes and patient dissatisfaction.[14,51,86,105,108,115] Intermediate and long-term results of second generation systems and surgical techniques used for more judiciously selected surgical candidates are becoming available and are encouraging. However, long-term success is still in question.[33,51,86] The outcomes discussed in this section are reported for contemporary TAA. Ongoing issues leading to complications were addressed in an earlier section. It is important to note that no studies were identified that compared early or late postoperative weight-bearing conditions or exercise programs.

***Pain relief, functional improvement, and patient satisfaction.*** A variety of quantitative assessment instruments are used to measure pain relief, postoperative function, and patient satisfaction. Descriptors of outcomes, from "excellent" to "poor," are based on data from these scales. The Ankle Osteoarthritis Scale and the American Orthopedic Foot and Ankle Society questionnaire are two examples.

There is evidence from prospective studies to suggest that the survival rates of implants are similar for patients with OA (primary or post-traumatic arthritis) and RA at a median follow-up of 14 years[54] and for patients older or younger than 50 years of age at a median follow-up of 6 years.[53] Survival rates (the percentage of protheses not requiring removal) in the former study were 72.7% and 75.5% respectively in the patients with OA and RA and in the latter study were 75% and 80.6% respectively in the younger and older patients.

Outcomes for a frequently used second generation, two-component system and more recently developed three-component (mobile-bearing) designs have been reported but not directly compared. Knecht[52] reported positive outcomes (reduced pain and increased function) in 66 patients who had undergone a two-component ankle replacement a mean of 9 years earlier. The mean total arc of dorsi- and plantarflexion, measured in 33 patients, was 18°.

Buechel and colleagues[4] followed 50 patients (mean age 49 years), who had undergone three-component, mobile-bearing, cementless TAA, and reported 48% excellent and 40% good results at a mean follow-up of 5 years (range 2 to 10 years). Of the 50 patients in the study, 26% reported no pain, 60% reported slight or mild pain, and 14% reported moderate or severe pain that interfered with functional activities. The mean total arc of dorsi- and plantarflexion was 28°. In a short-term follow-up study of 116 patients who had a different mobile-bearing prosthesis implanted in 122 ankles, 84% of patients were satisfied, with 82% reporting good or excellent results at an average of 19.9 months.[36] The mean total arc of ankle dorsi- and plantarflexion was 39°. Although postoperative gains in ROM reported in these studies were small (often as little as 5° to 10°), gains of even a few degrees have been reported to improve functional mobility.[86]

Measurements of pain, ROM, general level of function, patient satisfaction, and postoperative complications are outcomes most often reported in follow-up studies. However, Valderrabano and co-investigators[110] recently reported sport and recreational activities in which 147 patients (mean age 59.6 years, range 28 to 86 years) participated before and after TAA. Of these patients, 89% had a preoperative diagnosis of post-traumatic arthritis or primary OA and only 11% had a diagnosis of RA; 83% reported excellent or good results and 69% were pain-free postoperatively. Prior to surgery, 36% of patients were active in sports/recreational activities, and 56% were active after surgery. This change reflected an increase in the activity level of the patients with post-traumatic arthritis and primary OA, not of the patients with RA. The most frequently reported preoperative activities (in descending order) were cycling, swimming, hiking, and low-impact aerobics. After surgery, hiking was most frequently reported, followed by cycling, swimming, and aerobics. The only significant change before and after surgery was for hiking (from 25.5% to 52.8%). The authors recommended that before initiating any sport activity after ankle replacement, a patient should complete postoperative rehabilitation and be free of complications.

## Arthrodesis at the Ankle and Foot

Arthrodesis is the most frequently used surgery for late-stage arthritis of the ankle or one or more of the joints of the foot and toes. It typically is the procedure of choice for relatively young, active patients with post-traumatic arthritis and gross instability of the ankle and hindfoot.[105] Arthrodesis also is an option for patients with hindfoot or forefoot involvement as the result of RA or JRA.[6,14] Deformities of the forefoot, such as hallux valgus or hallux rigidus, and severe deterioration of the MTP joint of the first toe also are managed with arthrodesis.[1,6,14,17]

## Indications for Surgery

The following are frequent indications for surgical fusion of selected joints of the ankle and foot.[1,6,14,47,95,105]

- Debilitating pain, particularly during weight bearing, and severe articular degeneration secondary to post-traumatic arthritis, OA, RA, infection, or other inflammatory arthropathies
- Marked instability of one or more joints
- Deformity of the toes, foot, or ankle associated with chronic joint malalignment as the result of congenital anomalies, neuromuscular disorders, or arthritis
- Patients with high functional demands and pain-free compensatory movements in adjacent joints
- A salvage procedure after failed total ankle arthroplasty

## Procedures

There are many types of arthrodesis; however, all involve the use of bone grafts coupled with internal fixation devices (see Fig. 12.2) or occasionally external skeletal fixation for bony ankylosis. Internal fixation can be achieved via multiple compression screws, pins, an intramedullary nail, or a plate. The type of fixation selected depends on the joints involved and types of deformity. For correction of severe deformity or tendon rupture, concomitant soft tissue procedures are required.

Arthrodesis at the ankle or foot almost always is performed through an open approach. Over the past decade, however, arthroscopic or arthroscopically assisted arthrodesis of the ankle has become an option for patients with severe pain at the tibiotarsal joint but without significant fixed deformity.[7,77,79,90,102] Specifically, an arthroscopic approach cannot be used if a varus or valgus deformity is greater than 5° to 10°.[102] The most consistently suggested benefit of an arthroscopic approach is a reduced rate of wound healing complications because of less disruption of soft tissues during surgery.[90,105]

There have been reports of a more rapid rate of fusion with an arthroscopic approach compared with an open approach. However, this potential benefit is based largely on data from nonrandomized, retrospective studies and therefore cannot yet be substantiated.[77,79,102,105]

## Common Types of Arthrodesis

**Arthrodesis of the ankle.** When the tibiotalar joint is fused, it is positioned in 0° of dorsiflexion, 5° of hindfoot valgus, and 5° to 10° of external rotation of the foot on the tibia to match the rotation of the opposite lower extremity.[12,47,95,105] Although ankle arthrodesis provides pain relief and ankle stability, dorsiflexion and plantarflexion are lost, conse-

quently altering the biomechanics and speed of gait and increasing energy expenditure during ambulation.[105] Over time the hindfoot and forefoot compensate to a great extent for the loss of motion at the ankle. Nevertheless, an asymmetrical gait pattern is detectable in most patients after ankle arthrodesis.[12]

**NOTE:** For patients with RA involving both ankles, bilateral arthrodesis is rarely performed, because loss of dorsiflexion bilaterally makes it difficult to get up from a chair or to ascend or descend stairs.

**Arthrodesis of the hindfoot.** Severe instability or chronic malalignment and deformity of the hindfoot, such as pes valgus or pes planus, and pain as the result of advanced hindfoot arthritis may require a triple arthrodesis or a single-joint fusion, such as talonavicular or talocalcaneal (subtalar) arthrodesis. A triple arthrodesis, often indicated for a rigid hindfoot deformity, involves fusion of the talocalcaneal, talonavicular, and calcaneocuboid joints.[66] A single-joint fusion, such as a talonavicular arthrodesis, may be sufficient to correct a chronic but flexible hindfoot deformity.[23,49,87] In most instances the hindfoot is positioned in 5° of valgus in each of these fusions.

Talonavicular, subtalar, or triple arthrodesis provides permanent medial–lateral stability and relief of pain in the hindfoot, but pronation and supination of the ankle are eliminated or substantially diminished. It is interesting to note that fusion of the talonavicular joint alone indirectly reduces motion at the subtalar and calcaneocuboid joints, thus providing added frontal plane stability without fusing additional joints.[23,87]

**Arthrodesis of the first toe.** Fusion of the first MTP joint for hallux rigidus and hallux valgus provides relief of pain, most notably during ambulation.[1,17,41] The position of fusion is neutral rotation, 10° to 15° of valgus, 15° to 30° of MTP extension. This allows adequate push-off during ambulation but also enables a patient to wear some types of commercially available shoes.[14,17,41] If the lateral MTP joints also are involved, fusion of the great toe is performed after, not before, excision or implant arthroplasty of the lateral joints.[6,14,107]

**Arthrodesis of the IP joints of the toes.** Fusion of the IP joints of the toes in a neutral position for hammer toes, usually occurring in the second and third toes, provides relief of pain for ambulation and correction of deformities of the toes to improve shoe fit.[41]

## Complications

The overall rate of complications associated with arthrodesis is relatively low but varies with patient population, the joints involved, and surgical techniques.[105] The most common complication is nonunion, occurring in up to 10% of arthrodesis procedures.[87,105] The smaller the area of the bony surfaces and the poorer their vascular supply, the higher the rate of nonunion. Factors that contribute to nonunion include postoperative infection, malalignment of the fused joint, and a patient's use of tobacco before and after surgery.[49,66] Delayed wound healing is a particular problem in patients with poor vascularity of the foot and ankle. Furthermore, nerve damage can occur during surgery or a neuroma can develop postoperatively, causing pain and limiting function. Occasionally a stress fracture of one of the fused bones or adjacent bones occurs.

## Postoperative Management

***Immobilization.*** The method and duration of immobilization of the fused joints are determined by the surgeon based on the site of the fusion, the type of fixation used, the quality of fixation achieved, the patient's bone quality, and the presence of factors that affect bone healing, such as systemic inflammatory disease and preoperative use of corticosteroids.

At the close of surgery, a compression dressing and splint are applied and worn for 48 to 72 hours for edema control. For an ankle or hindfoot arthrodesis, after the compression dressing has been removed, a short-leg cast is applied for an extended period of time, usually 4 to 8 weeks. During the first 6 weeks, frequent cast changes are necessary as swelling subsides. A short-leg walking cast or rigid boot is applied at about 4 to 8 weeks, and immobilization continues for an additional 4 to 6 weeks.[23,49,66,79,87,95] After arthrodesis of the first MTP joint, a short-leg cast or surgical shoe with a flat, rigid sole is worn to protect the joint as it heals.[1,17]

When there is evidence of fusion, the patient is weaned from the immobilizer over several weeks. After splint use is discontinued, the patient should be advised of proper shoe selection, modification, and fit. The use of custom-made foot orthoses may be necessary for support, relief of pressure, or shock absorption.[14]

***Weight-bearing considerations.*** As with postoperative immobilization, published guidelines for the timing and extent of weight bearing permissible after arthrodesis vary considerably. The same considerations that influence decisions about immobilization also influence the progression of postoperative weight bearing on the operated extremity. The most prevalent practice is to substantially restrict weight bearing for many weeks after open or arthroscopic arthrodesis. Typically, patients must ambulate with crutches or a walker and are not allowed to bear weight on the operated side for 4 to 8 weeks.[1,49,66,79,87,95,102] When there is radiographic evidence of bony healing, partial weight bearing is permitted while the patient wears a rigid short-leg boot or shoe. Full weight bearing without wearing an immobilizer usually is permitted by 12 to 16 weeks postoperatively.

In an effort to reduce recovery time and improve a patient's quality of life during recovery, the safety of early weight bearing is being investigated. To date, most studies have assessed the effects of early weight bearing only after arthroscopic ankle arthrodesis. In selected patient populations, early results are encouraging. However, randomized, prospective studies have not been done yet.

 **Focus on Evidence**

Cannon and co-investigators[7] conducted a nonrandomized, retrospective study of two comparable groups of patients who had undergone arthroscopic ankle arthrodesis. One group ($N = 16$; mean age 48) wore a short-leg cast and was not permitted to bear weight on the operated limb for 8 weeks. In contrast, the other group ($N = 23$; mean age 51) was encouraged to bear as much weight as was comfortable on the operated limb within the first few days after surgery while wearing a rigid boot that immobilized the ankle and foot.

At 8 weeks, all patients in both groups had radiographic evidence of bony union, and by 4 months all had achieved ankle fusion. There were no significant differences between groups in the rate of postoperative complications. The investigators concluded that an early weight-bearing regimen is safe after arthroscopic ankle arthrodesis provided the ankle is protected in a rigid splint. However, the investigators pointed out that early weight bearing after arthrodesis is not appropriate for patients with reduced sensation in the foot and ankle.

---

***Postoperative exercises.*** Initially, postoperative exercises focus on ROM of the unoperated joints proximal or distal to the joints that are immobilized. If the patient is wearing a removable splint, ROM exercises of the unoperated joints confined by the immobilizer may be permissible early in the rehabilitation program as well.[7] For example, after ankle or hindfoot arthrodesis, exercises to maintain toe mobility are indicated in addition to knee ROM. For a patient with RA, active ROM is essential in all involved joints not controlled by the immobilization device.

When bony fusion has occurred and use of the immobilizer has been discontinued, often there are signs of post-immobilization muscle weakness, hypomobility of joints adjacent to the arthrodesis, and impaired balance. In such instances, exercises described previously in this chapter for nonoperative management of chronic joint hypomobility are appropriate.

### Outcomes

***Short-term outcomes.*** When healing is complete after arthrodesis, pain relief and joint stability are predictable outcomes, resulting in improved functional mobility. Recent reports indicate that fusion is achieved greater than 90% of the time but varies with the number and location of joint(s) fused, the extent of preoperative deformity, and the underlying pathology.

***Long-term outcomes.*** Although arthrodesis provides pain relief in the fused joint(s), it also imposes increased stresses on contiguous joints. Consequently, there are long-term adverse outcomes after arthrodesis. For example, Coester and colleagues[12] carried out a long-term follow-up study of 23 patients who had undergone isolated ankle arthrodesis for post-traumatic arthritis a mean of 22 years earlier. They found a substantial increase in arthritis in the joints distal but not proximal to the fused tibiotalar joint compared with the same joints of the contralateral lower limb. In addition, ipsilateral foot pain interfered with the functional mobility of almost all patients, based on information from standardized, self-report functional assessment instruments.

# OVERUSE (REPETITIVE TRAUMA) SYNDROMES: NONOPERATIVE MANAGEMENT

An overuse syndrome is a local inflammatory response to stresses from repetitive microtrauma, which may be from faulty alignment in the lower extremity, muscle imbalances or fatigue, changes in exercise or functional routines, training errors, improper footwear for the ground or functional demands placed on the feet, or a combination of several of these factors.[29] The syndrome occurs because continued demand is placed on the tissue before it has adequately healed, so the pain and inflammation continue. A common cause predisposing the foot to overuse syndromes is abnormal pronation of the subtalar joint. The abnormal pronation could be related to a variety of causes including excessive joint mobility, leg-length discrepancy, femoral anteversion, external tibial torsion, genu valgum, or muscle flexibility and strength imbalances.

## Related Pathologies and Etiology of Symptoms

The extrinsic foot musculature may develop symptoms either at or near its proximal attachment in the leg (shin splints), or where coursing around bony prominences in the ankle, or at its distal attachment in the foot (tendinitis/tenosynovitis). Symptoms occur at the site of inflammation when the muscle is stressed. Symptoms may also develop in the intrinsic muscles as well as the plantar fascia (plantar fasciitis). Several common syndromes are described in this section; the principles of management may be used for any overuse syndrome.

### Tendinitis and Tenosynovitis
Any of the tendons of the extrinsic muscles of the foot may become irritated as they approach and cross over the ankle or where they attach in the foot. Pain occurs during or after repetitive activity. When the foot and ankle are tested, pain is experienced at the site of the lesion as resistance is applied to the muscle action and also when the involved tendon is placed on a stretch or palpated.[9,29,73] A common site for symptoms is proximal to the calcaneus in the Achilles tendon or its sheath (*Achilles tendinitis* or *peritendinitis*). Symptoms may develop when the person switches from high-heeled to low-heeled shoes and then does a lot of walking.[29,58,60,83] Symptoms in the anterior or posterior tibialis tendons, or peroneus tendons, are also associated

with athletic activities such as running, tennis, and basketball.[73] Usually there is a hypomobile gastrocnemius–soleus complex and abnormal foot pronation.

### Plantar Fasciitis
Pain is usually experienced along the plantar aspect of the heel where the plantar fascia inserts on the medial tubercle of the calcaneus. The site of the injury is very tender to palpation. Excessive pronation of the subtalar joint, which may be reinforced by hypomobile gastrocnemius–soleus muscles, predisposes the foot to abnormal forces and irritation of the plantar fascia. Conversely, stress forces on the fascia can also occur with an excessively high arch (cavus foot). Pressure transmitted to the irritated site with weight bearing or stretch forces to the fascia, as when extending the toes during push-off, causes pain.

A heel spur may develop at the site of irritation on the calcaneus causing pain whenever the heel is on the ground. The individual usually avoids heel-strike during the loading response of gait.

### Shin Splints
This term is used to describe activity-induced leg pain along the posterior medial or anterior lateral aspects of the proximal two-thirds of the tibia. It may include different pathological conditions such as musculotendinitis, stress fractures of the tibia, periosteitis, increased pressure in a muscular compartment, or irritation of the interosseous membrane.

***Anterior shin splints.*** Most common is overuse of the anterior tibialis muscle. A hypomobile gastrocnemius-soleus complex and a weak anterior tibialis muscle, as well as foot pronation, are associated with anterior shin splints. Pain increases with active dorsiflexion and when the muscle is stretched into plantarflexion.

***Posterior shin splints.*** A tight gastrocnemius–soleus complex and a weak or inflamed posterior tibialis muscle, along with foot pronation, are associated with posterior medial shin splints. Pain is experienced when the foot is passively dorsiflexed with eversion and with active supination. Muscle fatigue with vigorous exercise, such as running or aerobic dancing, may precipitate the problem.

## Common Impairments and Functional Limitations/Disabilities

- Pain with repetitive activity, on palpation of the involved site, when the involved musculotendinous unit is stretched, and with resistance to the involved muscle
- Pain with weight-bearing activities and gait
- Muscle length–strength imbalances, especially tight gastrocnemius–soleus muscle group
- Abnormal foot posture (may be from faulty footwear)
- Functional limitations resulting from the impairments include decreased length of time the individual can stand, decreased distance or speed of ambulation, and restriction of sport or recreational activities

## Overuse Syndromes: Management—Protection Phase

While tissues are inflamed, leg or foot symptoms should be treated as an acute condition, with rest and appropriate modalities (see Chapter 10 for general principles and guidelines). Immobilization in a cast or splint with the foot slightly plantarflexed or a heel lift inside the shoe may be used to relieve stress.[60,83]

- Apply cross-friction massage to the site of the lesion.
- Initiate gentle muscle-setting contractions or electrical stimulation to the involved muscle in pain-free positions.
- Teach active ROM within the pain-free ranges.
- Instruct the patient to avoid the activity that provokes the pain.
- Use supportive taping to provide relief of symptoms.[40]

## Overuse Syndromes: Management—Controlled Motion and Return to Function Phases

When symptoms become subacute, the entire lower extremity as well as the foot should be examined for abnormal alignment or muscle flexibility and strength imbalances. Eliminating or modifying the cause is important to prevent recurrences. Orthotic devices may be necessary to correct alignment.[19,60,62,83] Therapeutic exercises may be helpful to increase flexibility, and, in general, improve muscle performance. Detailed descriptions of stretching and strengthening exercises for the ankle and foot are in the last section of this chapter.

### Educate the Patient and Provide Home Exercises

- Help the patient incorporate home exercises within his or her daily routine.
- With plantar fasciitis the patient experiences the greatest pain when first bearing weight, especially in the morning and after prolonged sitting. Teach the patient to do ROM exercises (especially dorsiflexion) or alphabet writing with the foot for several minutes before standing.
- Teach prevention, including the following principles:
  - Before intense exercise, use gentle repetitive warm-up activities followed by stretching of tight muscles.
  - Use proper foot support for the ground conditions (this cannot be overemphasized).
  - Allow time for recovery from microtrauma after high-intensity workouts

### Stretch Range-Limiting Structures

- The gastrocnemius–soleus muscle complex is frequently hypomobile in cases of foot problems and should be stretched. Restricted mobility causes the foot to pronate when the ankle dorsiflexes.
- With plantar fasciitis and heel spurs, apply deep massage and stretching exercises to the plantar fascia.

### Improve Muscle Performance

- Begin with resistive isometric and progress to resistive dynamic (including isokinetic) exercises to the foot and ankle in open- and closed-chain activities. Develop a balance in strength between the muscle groups, especially the invertors and evertors, for medial and lateral support.
- With plantar fasciitis, the intrinsic muscles need to be strengthened. Include exercises that require toe control such as scrunching tissue paper or a towel and picking up marbles and other small objects with the toes.
- In addition to general strengthening of the extrinsic and intrinsic muscles of the foot, place emphasis on muscular endurance, and train the muscles to respond to eccentric loading.

## LIGAMENTOUS INJURIES: NONOPERATIVE MANAGEMENT

After trauma, the ligaments of the ankle may be stressed or torn. First- and second-degree (grades 1 and 2) sprains are usually treated conservatively. The most common type of ankle sprain is caused by an *inversion stress* and can result in a partial or complete tear of the anterior talofibular (ATF) ligament and often the calcaneofibular (CF) ligament.[38,85] The posterior talofibular (PTF) ligament, the strongest of the lateral ligaments, is torn only with *massive* inversion stresses. If the inferior tibiofibular ligaments are torn after stress to the ankle, the mortise becomes unstable. Rarely do the components of the deltoid ligament become stressed; there is greater likelihood of an avulsion from or fracture of the medial malleolus with an eversion stress. Depending on the severity of injury, the joint capsule may also be involved, and intra-articular pathology, including articular cartilage lesions, may also occur,[55] resulting in symptoms of acute (traumatic) arthritis.

### Common Impairments and Functional Limitations/Disabilities

- Pain when the injured tissue is stressed in mild to moderate injuries
- Excessive motion or instability of the related joint in the case of complete tears
- Proprioceptive deficit manifested as decreased ability to perceive passive motion and development of balance impairments[25]
- Related joint symptoms and reflex muscle inhibition
- Possible decreased ROM in the talocrural joint in recurrent lateral ankle sprains due to anterior subluxation and impaired tracking of the talus in the mortise.[113]
- Functional limitations resulting from the impairments include restricted ambulation (requiring assistance) during the acute and subacute phases. With chronic instability the individual may have difficulty walking or running on uneven surfaces or making quick changes in direc-

tion, may not be able to land safely when jumping, or may fall more frequently.

## Management: Protection Phase

See Chapter 10 for principles of treatment during stages of inflammation and repair.

- If possible, examine the ankle before joint effusion occurs. To minimize the swelling, use compression, elevation, and ice. The ankle should be immobilized in neutral or in slight dorsiflexion and eversion.
- Use gentle joint mobilization techniques to maintain mobility and inhibit pain.
- Educate the patient.
  - Teach the patient the importance of RICE (rest, ice, compression, and elevation) and to apply the ice every 2 hours during the first 24 to 48 hours.
  - Teach partial weight bearing with crutches to decrease the stress of ambulation.[27]
  - Teach muscle-setting techniques and active toe curls to help maintain muscle integrity and assist with circulation.

### Focus on Evidence

Green and associates[28] studied 38 individuals following acute ankle sprain (within 72 hours of injury and requiring partial weight bearing). All subjects received RICE intervention. Those randomly assigned to the experimental group ($N = 19$) also received gentle anterior–posterior (AP) joint mobilization techniques to the talocrural joint with the foot positioned in dorsiflexion. Range of pain-free ankle dorsiflexion, gait speed, step length, and single support time were measured. The majority of those in the experimental group were discharged after fewer treatments (13/19 subjects by the fourth treatment), having gained full range of dorsiflexion, whereas only three subjects in the control group met this criterion and required additional treatment. Also, subjects in the experimental group demonstrated improved stride speed compared to the control group.

## Management: Controlled Motion Phase

- As the acute symptoms subside, continue to provide protection for the involved ligament with a splint during weight bearing. Fabricating a stirrup out of thermoplastic material and holding it in place with an elastic wrap or Velcro straps provides stability to the joint structures while allowing for the stimulus of weight bearing for proprioceptive feedback and proper healing. Commercial splints such as an air splint are also available to provide medial–lateral stability while allowing dorsiflexion and plantarflexion.[30,48]
- Apply cross-fiber massage to the ligaments as tolerated.
- Use grade II joint mobilization techniques to maintain mobility of the joint.
- Teach the patient exercises to be done within tissue tolerance at least three times per day. Suggestions include:

- Nonweight-bearing AROM into dorsiflexion and plantarflexion, inversion and eversion, toe curls and writing the alphabet in the air with the foot.
- Sitting with the heel on floor and scrunching paper or a towel and picking up marbles with the toes.
- If adhesions are developing in the healing ligament, have the patient actively move the foot in the direction opposite the line of pull of the ligament. For the anterior talofibular ligament, the motion is plantarflexion and inversion. Also stretch the gastrocnemius–soleus muscle group for adequate dorsiflexion. Progress to weight-bearing stretches when the patient's recovery allows.
- As swelling decreases and weight-bearing tolerance increases, progress to strengthening, endurance, and stabilization exercises; include isometric resistance to the peroneals, bicycle ergometry, and partial to full weight-bearing balance board exercises. Have the patient wear a brace or splint that restricts end-range motion to control the range and prevent excessive stress on the healing ligament.[27]

## Management: Return to Function Phase

- Progress strengthening exercises by adding elastic resistance to foot movements in long-sitting (open-chain) and sitting with the heel on the floor for partial weight bearing. Use isokinetic resistance if a unit is available.
- Progress stabilization and proprioceptive/balance training for ankle stability, coordination, and reflex response with full weight-bearing activities on a rocker, wobble, or BAPS board.[26,84,116] Depending on the final goals of rehabilitation, train the ankle with weight-bearing activities such as walking, jogging, and running and with agility activities such as controlled twisting, turning, and lateral weight shifting.
- When the patient is involved in sports activities, the ankle should be splinted, taped, or wrapped, and proper shoes should be worn to protect the ligament from reinjury.[17]

###  Focus on Evidence

Twenty-five individuals with post-acute (3 to 4 weeks) lateral ankle sprain (unilateral grade I or II), who exhibited postural sway instability in their sprained ankle (modified Rhomberg Test), were tested under two conditions (with a commercial air splint and nonbraced control) with two dependent variables (shuttle-run and vertical-jump). The tests were repeated after 5 to 7 days of wearing the splint during ADLs to determine if acclimation to the brace affected performance. Results demonstrated immediate performance enhancement while wearing the air splint for the shuttle-run test (mean 9.43 ± 0.72 seconds) compared with the nonbraced condition (mean 9.57 ± 0.75 seconds) in sessions 1 and 2, demonstrating that an acclimation period was not necessary for the stabilizing benefit. The vertical jump did not show improvement when the splint was worn.[30]

# TRAUMATIC SOFT TISSUE INJURIES: SURGICAL AND POSTOPERATIVE MANAGEMENT

## Repair of Complete Lateral Ligament Tears

A third-degree (grade 3) sprain of the lateral ankle, which usually occurs as the result of a severe inversion injury, causes a complete tear or rupture of the anterior talofibular (ATF) ligament, often the calcaneofibular (CF) ligament, and only occasionally the posterior tibiofibular (PTF) ligament (Fig. 22.7).[24,99] When the ATF and CF ligaments are both torn, it leads to combined instability of the tibiotalar and subtalar joints. The ATF ligament is most likely to tear when forceful inversion occurs while the ankle is plantarflexed.[101] Associated injuries that occur include a transverse fracture of the lateral malleolus or an avulsion fracture of the base of the fifth metatarsal.[24,73,85]

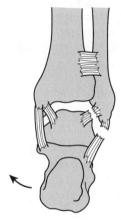

FIGURE 22.7 A complete tear of the lateral collateral ligament complex as the result of a severe (grade 3) inversion injury of the ankle. (From McKinnis, LN: Fundamentals of Musculoskeletal Imaging, ed 2. FA Davis, Philadelphia, 2005, p 389, with permission.)

In addition to significant pain, swelling, and tenderness, a complete tear of one or more lateral ligaments causes marked mechanical instability and functional instability of the ankle during weight-bearing activities. Mechanical instability is defined as ankle mobility beyond the physiological ROM, increased talar tilt, and an anterior drawer sign. Functional instability is characterized by the sensation of the ankle "giving way" experienced by the patient.[103] As many as 20% of patients without evidence of mechanical instability complain of the ankle "giving way" after a severe lateral ankle sprain, thus significantly impairing functional activities.[13]

After an acute, grade 3 inversion injury, nonoperative treatment is successful for most patients. However, some patients sustain recurrent inversion injuries after the acute injury has healed and develop chronic, symptomatic instability. For patients with demonstrated mechanical instability who do not respond to nonoperative management and

for selected patients with acute lateral ankle injuries who regularly engage in high-impact activities, surgical repair or reconstruction may be required to manage the instability and return the patient to a desired level of function.[13,24,81] The goal of surgery and postoperative management is to restore joint stability while retaining pain-free, functional ROM of the ankle and subtalar joints.[13,24,31,32,85,96,99]

### Indications for Surgery

The following are frequently cited indications for surgical repair or reconstruction of the soft tissues of the lateral aspect of the ankle.[24,31,32,81,96,99]

- Chronic mechanical and functional instability of the ankle during activity, which remains unresolved after conservative management.
- Acute, third-degree lateral ankle sprain resulting in a complete tear of the ATF and/or CF ligaments.

### Procedures

#### Types of Procedures

There are numerous surgical procedures that may be used for repair and reconstruction of the lateral ligaments and associated structures of the ankle.[24,39,81,99] Arthroscopy, for the most part, is reserved for preoperative examination to assist the surgeon in identifying pathologies associated with ankle instability that may not be readily evident through physical examination or during surgery.[8] The various repair and reconstruction procedures are performed almost exclusively through an open approach. However, arthroscopic repair of ATF ligament tears by means of staples or bone anchors has been reported.[98]

Open procedures may be classified into two broad categories: those that primarily involve a direct (anatomic) repair of the torn or attenuated (overstretched) ligaments and those that involve tenodesis (tendon graft and transposition) to reconstruct the lateral ankle complex and augment joint stability.[57] Recently an arthroscopic, thermally assisted capsular shift has been introduced as an alternative to open repair for selected patients.[39]

The type of procedure selected depends on the severity and chronicity of the instability, the presence of comorbidities, the age of the patient, and the patient's anticipated postoperative activity level. Some procedures are used predominantly for a primary repair, whereas others are reserved for revision surgery.

*Direct repair.* The surgery used most commonly for a primary repair is an open procedure called the *modified Bröstrom procedure,* also known as the *Bröstrom-Gould procedure.*[31,32,35] This procedure involves an anatomic repair with direct suturing of the torn ATF and CF ligament ends, imbrication (plication) of lax ligaments to tighten the ligament and provide a double layer of reinforcement, or reinsertion of an avulsed ligament to bone. The lateral aspect of the ankle is reinforced by pulling the lateral portion of the extensor retinaculum proximally over the repaired structures and suturing it to the anterior aspect of the distal fibula. The advantages of the modified Bröstrom procedure are that it provides stability (without the need to harvest a soft tissue graft) while retaining full ROM of the tibiotalar and subtalar joints, an outcome particularly important to individuals who wish to return to activities that require full ankle mobility, such as gymnastics and ballet.

***Reconstruction with augmentation.*** The other broad grouping of procedures are those that use a tenodesis, usually a tendon autograft and transposition of the peroneus brevis tendon, to reconstruct the lateral ankle complex with or without ligament repair. Examples include various modifications of the *Evans, Chrisman-Snook,* and *Watson-Jones procedures*.[13,24,35,81,96,99] These procedures all provide additional reinforcement to the joint to augment stability but sacrifice a portion of the ankle evertors and often limit the range of inversion available after surgery.[57] To maintain the integrity of the peroneal tendons, a bone–patellar tendon graft has been proposed as an alternative to a peroneal tendon autograft.[104] These procedures typically are used as revision procedures when previous direct repair has failed to prevent recurrence of lateral instability. Reconstruction with augmentation is used occasionally during a primary repair for large patients, specifically those weighing more than 200 to 250 pounds.[31]

***Arthroscopic thermally assisted capsular shift.*** Similar to its use for glenohumeral joint instability, arthroscopic, thermally assisted capsular shift (capsulorrhaphy) is a relatively new type of repair for the unstable ankle. The procedure shrinks and tightens attenuated lateral ligaments and joint capsule by means of radiofrequency or laser energy for the purpose of improving joint stability. The long-term success of this procedure at the ankle has not yet been determined. (Refer to Chapters 12 and 17 for additional discussions of thermally assisted capsular shift.)

### Operative Overview
Prior to an open repair or reconstruction for lateral ankle instability, arthroscopy is performed to assess the extent of intra-articular pathology, because a high percentage (93%) of patients with complete tears of one or more lateral ligaments also exhibit associated joint pathology, including articular cartilage lesions.[55] After arthroscopy, an oblique or vertical incision is made beginning at the anterior aspect of the distal fibula and extending distally along the lateral aspect of the ankle and foot. Torn or ruptured structures are identified, repaired, and reinforced with the extensor retinaculum.

If a peroneus brevis tendon graft is to be used to reinforce the ankle, the tendon is split longitudinally. One-half of the tendon is harvested by detaching it proximally at its musculotendinous junction and weaving it through drill holes in the fibula, talus, and/or calcaneus. Then it is doubled back and sutured to itself.

Prior to wound closure, the stability and ROM of the ankle are checked. The foot and ankle are placed in a compression dressing and well-padded, short-leg, posterior splint with the ankle in 0° of dorsiflexion and slight eversion. The leg is elevated for control of joint swelling and peripheral edema.

### Postoperative Management
In the past decade there has been a trend to allow early postoperative weight bearing while the ankle is immobilized, and in selected patients, early but protected ROM after lateral ligament reconstruction. The exercise progression after surgery is similar to that used for nonoperative management of lateral ankle sprains. Postoperative management is geared toward not only returning a patient to a pre-injury level of function, but also toward preventing re-injury.

### Immobilization and Weight-Bearing Considerations

***Immobilization.*** After some degree of swelling has subsided, usually within 3 to 5 postoperative days or as late as a week to 10 days, the compression dressing is removed and a short-leg walking cast is applied that immobilizes the ankle in a neutral position. If a short-leg cast is used initially, it may be removed at 4 to 6 weeks and replaced with an air-stirrup type splint,[31] a removable cast-boot, or a controlled active motion (CAM) walking brace, worn for several additional weeks.[24,73,101,103]

By 8 to 12 weeks the patient gradually discontinues use of the immobilizer during ambulation. However, patients returning to athletic activities that involve jumping, running, and quick changes of direction are advised to wear a protective orthotic device or to tape the ankle for at least 3 to 6 months or even indefinitely to prevent re-injury.

***Weight-bearing considerations.*** Immediately after surgery the patient must remain nonweight bearing on the operated extremity while the ankle is in the compression dressing and posterior splint. When the compression dressing is removed and the short-leg walking cast applied, protected weight bearing is initiated and gradually progressed to full weight bearing by 6 weeks.[24,31,101,103]

N O T E : After an arthroscopic thermally assisted capsular shift, the nonweight-bearing period is longer than after an open repair, usually extending for 5 to 6 weeks.[39]

### Exercise: Maximum Protection Phase
The primary goal of the first phase of rehabilitation, which extends for 4 to 6 weeks, is to regain independent mobility for functional activities while protecting the repaired or reconstructed lateral ankle structures. Ambulation with crutches, nonweight bearing on the operated extremity, is initiated directly after surgery. Elevation of the operated foot is essential when the patient is resting to control peripheral edema and reduce pain. ROM of the operated ankle is not permitted during this period. The following treatment goals and exercises are appropriate during the first postoperative phase.

***Maintain strength of nonimmobilized muscle groups.*** Perform active or gentle resisted exercises of the hip and knee of the operated lower extremity and resistance exercises of the upper extremities and sound lower extremity. If the immobilizer, such as a splint or boot, allows a small degree of dorsi- and plantarflexion, perform mini-squats in bilateral stance when partial weight bearing is permissible.

*Prevent reflex inhibition of immobilized muscle groups.*
While the ankle is immobilized, begin gentle, pain-free muscle-setting exercises of the ankle musculature including isometric contractions of the peroneal muscles.

## Exercise: Moderate and Minimum Protection Phases

By 4 to 6 weeks postoperatively only moderate protection of healing structures is necessary as joint symptoms subside. Most patients are allowed to bear full weight on the operated extremity by 6 weeks. The goals of the intermediate and final phases of rehabilitation are to restore full ROM and strength of the operated ankle and to improve balance reactions, and neuromuscular control and reaction times in the operated extremity. All activities are directed toward enabling the patient to return to functional activities safely and preventing recurrence of ankle injuries.[21,73,96,101,103]

With proper precautions a return to functional activities, including selected sports, may be possible by 3 to 4 months postoperatively[31,103] or when peroneal muscle strength is normal (compared to the contralateral ankle) and when multiple, pain-free single-leg hops on the operated lower extremity are possible.[101]

The following exercises and activities are appropriate at this stage to achieve the stated goals.

*Restore ROM.* Begin with pain-free, assisted or active dorsiflexion and plantarflexion of the operated ankle as soon as the immobilizer may be removed for exercise as determined by the surgeon, usually by 4 to 6 weeks postoperatively. Postpone inversion and supination movements until 6 to 8 weeks postoperatively. Progress to multiplanar motions such as figure-of-eight movements.

● If joint restriction limits dorsi- or plantarflexion, perform grade II or III joint mobilization procedures, but avoid stretch mobilization of the subtalar joint.
● If full ankle motion is not achieved with active ROM, add gentle self-stretching exercises to improve flexibility of specific muscle groups, most frequently the gastrocnemius–soleus complex.

P R E C A U T I O N : It is advisable to begin with open-chain stretching, such as a towel stretch or closed-chain stretching in a *seated* position, because closed-chain stretching with the patient standing imposes significant ground reaction forces on the repaired ligaments.

*Increase strength of ankle and foot musculature.* Perform low-intensity resistance exercises of all ankle muscles in open- and closed-chain positions. After surgical repair of the lateral ligaments, improving strength of the evertors is particularly important for dynamic stability of the ankle.

● Isometric strengthening of the evertors can be achieved by having the patient cross the ankles and press the lateral borders of the feet together. Dynamic strengthening of the evertors against elastic resistance is also appropriate (see Fig. 22.12).
● Progress to dynamic exercises using elastic resistance and isokinetic training, if available.

● In the final phase of rehabilitation initiate plyometric training.

N O T E : The extent of strength loss in the ankle musculature has been shown to be associated with the chronicity of the instability.[42]

*Improve neuromuscular control, balance reactions, dynamic stability, and agility.* Initiate proprioceptive/balance training at about 6 weeks postoperatively or when the patient is able to bear full weight on the operated lower extremity without ankle pain. Emphasize a progression of bilateral to unilateral balance activities first on a level, firm surface, then on a soft surface, such as dense foam, and then on a balance board. Progress to jumping, then hopping forward, diagonally, backward, and side-to-side on the floor or a mini-trampoline. Other balance activities are described in the final section of this chapter.

 **Focus on Evidence** _____

For patients with a functionally unstable ankle proprioceptive training, using rocker or wobble boards has been shown to be an effective method of improving joint proprioception (joint position sense) and single-leg standing ability and reducing postural sway and muscle reaction times during balance activities.[22,26,84,116]

In a prospective study by Verhagen and co-investigators,[111] 1127 male and female professional volleyball players from 116 teams were randomly assigned by team to a training group or a control group. Throughout the 36-week volleyball season, the training groups participated in a proprioceptive training program consisting of a variety of balance activities, some on balance boards. The control groups were not given any training program. The training and control groups kept track of injuries sustained during the season. Among players who had a history of a lateral ankle sprain prior to the beginning of the study, those who participated in the balance training program had a significantly lower incidence of acute lateral ankle sprains during the season than those in the control group. Among training and control group players who did not have a history of lateral ankle sprains, there was no significant difference in the incidence of ankle injury during the season. The authors concluded that proprioceptive training was effective in preventing recurrence of lateral ankle injury in adult volleyball players.

Although these studies did not involve patients undergoing rehabilitation after reconstruction of the lateral ankle ligaments, proprioceptive training programs such as these may be beneficial for the postoperative patient.

_____

*Improve muscular endurance and cardiopulmonary fitness.* Begin with swimming, stationary bicycling, treadmill walking, or using a cross-country ski machine. Progress to outdoor walking, jogging or running, being certain the ankle is appropriately supported.

*Safely return to functional activities and prevent re-injury.*
Sport-specific training, beginning with low-intensity simu-

---

**BOX 22.4** **Activity-Related Precautions to Reduce the Risk of Re-injury After Lateral Ligament Reconstruction of the Ankle**

- Modify activities, if possible, by participating in low-impact sports, such as swimming, cycling, low-impact aerobics, or cross country skiing.
- Minimize or avoid participation in activities that involve high-impact (basketball, volleyball), rapid stopping and starting and changes of direction (tennis, soccer), or moving on uneven surfaces
- If involved in activities associated with high risk of ankle injury
  - Participate in a pre-season injury prevention program that includes progressive proprioceptive and plyometric training and continue the program throughout a sport season.[111]
  - Wear a prescribed orthotic device to provide medial-lateral stability of the ankle, such as functional stirrup brace or splint.[101]
  - Tape the ankle or insert a slight lateral lift in the shoe.[65,73]

---

lated movements, usually is permissible by 8 to 12 weeks postoperatively.[31,101,103] Precautions to reduce the risk of re-injury when returning to sports or high-demand activities after reconstruction of lateral ankle ligaments are summarized in Box 22.4.

### Outcomes

A successful postoperative outcome after lateral ankle repair or reconstruction is an ankle that has full mobility but remains stable and pain-free during functional activities. At this time, an open approach for primary repair or reconstruction provides more predictable long-term results than arthroscopic procedures.[13] In some instances, although not an optimal result, a slight loss of ankle motion, possibly 5° to 10° of eversion, occurs most often after tenodesis procedures.[96]

A review of the literature of studies involving patients with chronic lateral ankle instability indicated that 87% to 95% of patients report good to excellent results after surgery.[81] Similar results were reported in a postoperative follow-up study of ballet dancers who had undergone a modified Broström procedure.[32] Several studies have compared the results of an anatomic (direct) repair with reconstruction with a tendon graft (tenodesis). Hennrikus et al.[35] compared two types of lateral ankle reconstruction, one using anatomic repair (modified Broström procedure) and the other involving augmentation with a peroneus brevis tendon graft (Chrisman-Snook procedure). Both procedures yielded good to excellent results in 80% of patients, but the latter was associated with a higher rate of complications.

In a multicenter, retrospective nonrandomized study, Krips and colleagues[57] evaluated two groups of athletes ($N = 77$) who had undergone an anatomic (direct) repair or reconstruction with a tenodesis procedure for chronic lateral ankle instability 2 to 10 (mean 5.4) years earlier. There were no significant differences in preoperative characteristics of the athletes in the two groups. All had participated in a nonoperative treatment program for at least 6 months before surgery. Physical examination at follow-up revealed significantly more patients (15/36) in the tenodesis group had limited ankle ROM than patients (3/41) in the anatomic repair group. Functional abilities reported by patients on a quantitative questionnaire were rated as excellent and good by 21/36 subjects in the tenodesis group and by 36/41 in the anatomic repair group. Those in the tenodesis group reported a noticeably diminished push-off power on the operated side during running. They also reported a lower activity level and a perception of less ankle stability than those in the anatomic repair group. The authors concluded that an anatomic repair was a better choice than tenodesis for primary repair of chronic ankle instability in an athletic population.[57]

## Repair of a Ruptured Achilles Tendon

Acute rupture of the Achilles tendon is a common soft tissue injury, occurring more frequently in men than in women, 30 to 50 years old, who intermittently participate in exercise or athletic activities.[3,46,117] The rupture usually is associated with a forceful concentric or eccentric contraction of the gastrocnemius–soleus muscles (triceps surae) during sudden acceleration or abrupt deceleration, such as jumping or landing.[5] Degenerative and mechanical factors appear to increase the risk of acute rupture, including decreased strength or flexibility of the plantarflexors, excessive body weight, pre-existing tendinosis, corticosteroid injections into the tendon, and decreased vascularity of the tendon.[5]

The tendon often ruptures proximal to the distal insertion of the tendon on the calcaneus.[34] At the time of injury a complete rupture leads to pain, swelling, a palpable defect, and significant weakness in plantarflexion. It also is associated with a positive Thompson test (absence of reflexive plantarflexion when the patient is prone-lying with the foot over the edge of a table and the calf is squeezed).[106]

A complete rupture of the Achilles tendon can be managed conservatively with extended cast immobilization or functional bracing; or it can be managed surgically. There is general agreement in the literature and in clinical practice that surgical intervention is routinely recommended for the young, active patient less than 30 years of age but that nonoperative management is the better option for the sedentary patient older than 50 to 60 years of age.[3,46,117] Furthermore, surgery is considered the only option for the symptomatic patient with a chronic rupture in which the diagnosis or treatment was delayed for 4 weeks or more.[71,114] However, there is lack of agreement in the literature and in practice as to which is the better option for the middle-aged population.

Several recently reported systematic reviews and meta-analyses of the literature that included only prospective, randomized and quasi-randomized studies have revealed there is insufficient evidence to indicate which option is the better treatment strategy or yields better outcomes.[3,46,117] Both options have advantages and disadvantages. With surgical repair there is a lower rate of re-rupture of the tendon than with nonoperative management, but there also is a risk of wound closure problems, infection, and nerve injury with surgery. Nonoperative management requires a longer immobilization and recuperative time and is associated with a higher rate of deep vein thrombosis (DVT).[3,11,46,117] Both patient and surgeon must weigh the different advantages and disadvantages in the decision-making process.

### Indications for Surgery
The following are frequently cited indications for surgical repair or reconstruction of an acute or chronic rupture of the Achilles tendon.

- Acute, complete rupture of the Achilles tendon[5,10,11]
- Chronic, previously undiagnosed or untreated complete rupture in which end-to-end apposition cannot be achieved by conservative means.[72,114]
- Typically indicated for the active individual who wishes to return to high-demand functional activities.[3,11,117]

### Procedures
There are a considerable number of surgical procedures and techniques for repair or reconstruction of a ruptured Achilles tendon.[5,10,11,68,69,114,117] An open or percutaneous approach can be used for a primary repair.[15,61,100]

Primary repair of an acute rupture is performed within a few days to a week after the injury and usually is carried out with a direct, end-to-end repair in which the ends of the torn tendon are reopposed and sutured together.[5] The repair site may or may not be reinforced by some method of tissue augmentation. Delayed repair of a chronic rupture requires reconstruction and augmentation of the tendon most often by an autograft, or tendon transfer, or possibly an allograft.[71,114] Structures that may serve as a donor graft are the flexor hallucis longus, plantaris, or peroneus brevis tendons or a flap of fascia from the gastrocnemius muscle.

In an open primary repair, a posterior incision is made at the distal leg just medial to the Achilles tendon. Placing the incision medial of the tendon avoids possible damage to the sural nerve. The tendon ends are identified, frayed fibers are removed, and the ends reopposed and sutured together while the ankle is maintained in a neutral to slightly plantarflexed position.[5] With a tendon reconstruction a second incision is made to harvest the donor graft. If, for example, the flexor hallucis longus (FHL) tendon is selected, an incision is made along medial aspect of the sole of the foot at the mid-metatarsal level. A sufficient portion of the FHL tendon is left distally so the remaining portion can be sutured to the flexor digitorum longus tendon to retain active flexion of the first toe.[114] The har-

vested portion of the FHL tendon then is woven into and sutured to bridge the gap of the Achilles tendon ends.

Before closure, the ankle is moved through the ROM to assess the stability of the repair or reconstruction. A compression dressing and below-knee posterior splint are applied after closure with the ankle usually positioned in 15° to 20° of plantarflexion.[5,114] If immediate or very early postoperative weight bearing is to be allowed by the surgeon, the ankle is placed in a neutral (0° of dorsiflexion), if possible, and stabilized with a rigid anterior splint.[43]

NOTE: An above-knee cast is applied (and later replaced with a below-knee cast) if the rupture occurred at the myotendinous junction or the quality of the repair is tenuous.[5]

### Postoperative Management
Although guidelines for postoperative rehabilitation after an open repair of an acute Achilles tendon rupture vary considerably in the literature and in clinical practice, these guidelines tend to fall within two categories—use of a conventional (traditional) management strategy or an early remobilization approach. The use of immobilization and the initiation of weight bearing distinguish one approach from the other. Guidelines for management after percutaneous repair are not addressed in the following sections but can be found in other resources.[15,61,100]

#### Immobilization and Weight Bearing Considerations

**Conventional approach.** After an open primary repair of an acute Achilles tendon rupture, conventional postoperative management, a widely used practice for many years, involves approximately 6 weeks of continuous immobilization with the ankle held in plantarflexion at least a portion of that period of time.[3,5,11,63,67] The patient remains nonweight bearing on the operated extremity during this time. After a delayed tendon reconstruction with graft augmentation for a chronic rupture, the time before motion and weight bearing are permissible is longer, usually an additional 2 weeks or more.[114]

Table 22.2 summarizes immobilization and weight-bearing guidelines associated with conventional management after primary Achilles tendon repair.[3,5,11,63,67,68] Although this approach is safe and associated with low risk of rerupture, extended immobilization, traditionally thought to be necessary to protect the healing tendon, has been shown in some studies to lead to deficits in strength, particularly in the plantarflexors, and loss of ROM of the ankle.[9,68,100]

**Early remobilization approach.** For the past two decades or more there has been a trend to decrease the period of continuous postoperative immobilization and to initiate early ankle ROM in a protected range and early weight bearing in a functional orthosis.[9,34,43,63,64,67-69,82,97] This approach, sometimes termed "functional rehabilitation," is an option after primary repair of an acute rupture, not a delayed reconstruction. Early motion and weight bearing are possible because of advances in surgical procedures, such as stronger suturing techniques and sometimes the

**TABLE 22.2    Conventional Postoperative Management After Achilles Tendon Repair or Reconstruction with Graft***

| Postoperative Time Period | Type and Position of Ankle Immobilization | Weight-bearing Guidelines |
|---|---|---|
| At 0–4 weeks | • Compression dressing removed a few days to a week postoperatively<br>• When compression dressing removed, below-knee cast applied; foot in 15° to 30° plantarflexion<br>• At 2–3 weeks new cast applied in less plantar-flexion | • Nonweight bearing<br>• Ambulation with crutches |
| At 4 weeks | • Cast set in equines removed and walking cast applied with ankle positioned in neutral or replaced with a controlled ankle motion (CAM) brace that limits dorsiflexion to 0°; cast or brace worn an additional 2–4 weeks | • Weight bearing initiated while wearing immobilizer<br>• Progressed as tolerated |
| At 6–8 weeks | • If walking cast used; replaced with CAM brace allowing dorsiflexion beyond neutral.<br>• Active ROM exercises initiated | • Full weight bearing wearing functional brace; transition to shoe with 1.0- to 1.5-cm heel lift for an additional 2 to 4 weeks or more |
| Beyond 12 weeks | • Functional brace gradually discontinued** | • Full weight bearing in regular shoes without lift, if ankle is pain-free and 10° dorsiflexion attained |

*All time periods are approximately 2 weeks longer after reconstruction with tendon graft.

   ** Immobilizer may be worn during ambulation for a longer period of time if wound healing is delayed or the quality of the repair is tenuous.

use of soft tissue augmentation to reinforce the primary repair.[10,43,64,68,69,97]

Although published recommendations for early protected motion and weight bearing vary widely, use of a below-knee (boot-like) *dorsal* functional brace or splint is a consistent feature of early remobilization approaches. If bracing is prescribed, it is a hinged, controlled ankle motion (CAM) orthosis that can be locked in various positions.[82] When ankle motion is permissible, the orthosis is adjusted to allow movement but only in a protected range, typically limiting dorsiflexion beyond neutral.[9,34,67] If a rigid splint is used, its dorsal configuration limits dorsiflexion to 0° but allows plantarflexion.[43,63]

Initially, the brace or splint holds the ankle in slight plantarflexion but is adjusted (or refabricated in the case of a splint) to neutral by 2 weeks postoperatively.[13,34,63] During the first 6 weeks of rehabilitation the protective orthosis is worn during ambulation and at all other times except when removed for wound care and selected exercises.

When the patient is able to ambulate on level surfaces without pain while bearing full weight on the operated extremity, the protective boot or splint is discontinued (usually by 8 to 10 weeks postoperatively). As with a conventional approach, after discontinuing the functional brace or splint, many surgeons prescribe a 1.0- or 1.5-cm heel lift for both shoes that are worn for several weeks to decrease ground reaction forces during functional activities.[68]

The guidelines for initiating and progressing weight bearing and ROM exercises recommended in published

programs differ from study to study. A summary of these guidelines is presented in Box 22.5.[43,63,67,82] Common to all early remobilization programs is the use of safe levels of applied stress while protecting the healing tendon. Close communication among the surgeon, therapist, and patient is essential for success with this approach to postoperative management.

 **Focus on Evidence**

Although there have been few randomized studies directly comparing a functional bracing or splinting and early motion program after acute Achilles tendon repair with a program of extended cast immobilization (usually 6 weeks) followed by ROM exercises, a recent meta-analysis of these studies demonstrated that patients managed with an early motion/functional bracing program had a significantly lower rate of adhesion formation and limited ankle ROM. However, the investigators noted that the pooled data from the available studies must be interpreted with caution because of the variety of postoperative regimens used.[46]

**Exercise**

After open, primary repair of an acute Achilles tendon rupture, the types of exercise included in a postoperative program are similar regardless of whether an early motion/early weight-bearing approach or a conventional (extended immobilization/delayed motion and weight bearing)

| BOX 22.5 | Features of Early Remobilization Programs After Repair of Acute Achilles Tendon Rupture* |
|---|---|

**Weight-bearing Guidelines**
- Initiated as tolerated while using crutches immediately after surgery[43,63] or after 2 weeks[67,82] in a below-knee orthosis with the ankle immobilized most often in plantarflexion or possibly neutral
- Progress gradually to full weight-bearing status between 3 to 6 weeks postoperatively[43,82]
- Orthosis worn during all weight-bearing activities for 6 to 8 weeks after surgery[82]
- Full weight bearing without the functional orthosis but wearing regular shoes with bilateral heel lifts when orthosis discontinued beginning at about 6 to 8 weeks postoperatively[43,101]

**ROM Exercises**
- Immediately[43,63,64,97] or by 1 to 2 weeks[67,82,101] after surgery, active plantarflexion and dorsiflexion of the ankle initiated while wearing a dorsal functional brace or splint to prevent dorsiflexion beyond 15° to 30° of equines or to no more than a neutral position while seated or supine
- By 6 to 8 weeks dorsiflexion to 10° permitted in the orthosis and inversion/eversion out of the orthosis[43,67]

*Beyond 6 to 8 weeks postoperatively guidelines are similar for early remobilization and conventional programs.

approach is employed. What is different is the timing and progression of the exercises based on when ROM and weight bearing are permissible.

In the sections that follow a progression of exercises designed to assist a patient achieve a number of treatment goals and ultimately function at the pre-injury level is presented.

**Exercise: Maximum Protection Phase**
Achilles tendon repair frequently is performed on an outpatient basis. Therefore, patient education is essential before surgery or prior to discharge. It focuses on wound care (if the immobilizer is removable), controlling peripheral edema by elevating the operated leg, gait training, and a home exercise program. The following treatment goals and exercises are appropriate during the first 4 to 6 weeks after surgery.

◉ *Maintain ROM of nonimmobilized joints.* Perform active ROM of the hip, knee, and toes of the operated lower extremity while the patient is wearing the immobilizer.
◉ *Prevent reflex inhibition of immobilized muscle groups.* If early ROM is not permitted, begin submaximal, pain-free muscle-setting exercises of the ankle in the immobilizer within the first few days after surgery. Start with setting exercises of the dorsiflexors, invertors, and evertors. At 2 weeks, add setting exercises of the plantarflexors.

◉ *Prevent joint stiffness and soft tissue adhesions in the operated ankle and foot.* If an early motion and weight-bearing approach was planned, begin the ROM exercises described in Box 22.5 within a few days to 2 weeks after surgery. The time frame is determined by the surgeon.
◉ *Maintain cardiopulmonary endurance.* Use an upper extremity ergometry for endurance training, if available.

**Exercise: Moderate Protection Phase**
By 6 weeks postoperatively the patient may be permitted to bear weight as tolerated on the operated extremity regardless of whether an early weight-bearing program or conventional program was implemented. However, a functional CAM orthosis is required during progressive weight-bearing activities for several weeks.

During this phase of rehabilitation, which usually extends from 6 to 12 weeks postoperatively, gradually increasing stress is placed on the operated tendon and surrounding structures. Patients typically begin a supervised exercise program at this time.

**PRECAUTIONS:** Progress all exercises very cautiously that place resistance or a stretch on the gastrocnemius-soleus muscle group. Postpone closed-chain exercises until the patient is able to bear full weight on the operated side without pain. Avoid any high-impact, high-velocity activities to minimize the risk of re-rupture of the Achilles tendon.

◉ *Increase ROM of the operated ankle.* Begin gentle self-stretching exercises in nonweight-bearing and weight-bearing positions. Stretch the gastrocnemius-soleus muscle group with the knee extended and flexed. Examples of stretching activities are:
- Grade III joint mobilization techniques if ankle or foot joints are restricted
- Gentle manual stretching to increase inversion/eversion and dorsiflexion/plantarflexion
- A towel stretch to increase dorsiflexion
- While seated, active ankle ROM with the foot resting on a small rocker or wobble board
- Standing stretch to increase dorsiflexion with the knee flexed and extended
- Descend stairs step over step as ROM improves
◉ *Improve strength of the operated lower extremity.* Initiate open- and closed-chain, low-intensity resistance exercises at 6 to 8 weeks. Examples include.
- Open-chain resistance exercises of the ankle against a light grade of elastic resistance.
- Bilateral, progressing to unilateral closed-chain activities, such as heel and toe raises while seated, mini-squats alternating heel raises and toe raises, and partial lunges using body weight as resistance.
◉ *Re-establish balance reactions.* Initiate proprioceptive training and balance exercises in double-leg stance on a firm surface. Progress to single-leg stance on a soft surface.
◉ *Improve muscular and cardiopulmonary endurance.* Begin and gradually progress level-surface treadmill walking or stationary cycling (recumbent or upright)

while wearing the functional, hinged orthosis, if required, or regular shoes with a heel lift. Raise the seat height of the upright bicycle to accommodate for limited dorsiflexion. Progress to treadmill walking on an incline.

## Exercise: Minimum Protection/ Return to Function Phase

The final phase of rehabilitation, which begins around 12 to 16 weeks postoperatively, is directed toward returning a patient to a pre-injury level of function for expected work-related demands and desired recreational/athletic activities. Stretching exercises continue until full ROM is achieved, and then the patient transitions to a maintenance program. Eccentric resistance exercises of the gastrocnemius–soleus muscle group in weight-bearing positions and eventually plyometric training are added to the strengthening program. More challenging proprioceptive training is added. Jogging, running, agility drills, and sport-specific training usually can be initiated at 16 weeks. Patient education focuses on ways to reduce the risk of rerupture of the repaired tendon, such as warming up before strenuous activity and daily stretching. Most patients are permitted to resume sports gradually at 5 to 6 months if the strength of the operated extremity is relatively comparable to that of the contralateral extremity.[5,63,67]

### Outcomes

The ideal outcome is for a patient to return to a pre-injury level of physical activity without pain or re-rupture of the repaired Achilles tendon. Patients undergoing primary repair of an acute rupture have consistently better outcomes than those who undergo a delayed repair for a chronic rupture. The longer the delay between injury and repair, the poorer the results.[114] The patient population with the highest risk of re-rupture after primary repair of an acute rupture are active individuals 30 years of age or younger.[82]

*Comparison of methods of management.* The results of numerous studies comparing methods of management of acute tendon ruptures have been reported. Methods compared include operative and nonoperative management, open and percutaneous procedures, and conventional and early motion/early weight bearing approaches to postoperative treatment. Outcomes typically reported are rate of rerupture, ROM, strength, functional or sport-related activity level, and patient satisfaction. Some generalizations can be drawn from systematic reviews of the literature and individual studies.

When comparing outcomes of nonoperative (cast immobilization) with operative management of acute ruptures, three systematic reviews and meta-analyses of the literature have revealed that there is a significantly higher rate of re-rupture associated with nonoperative management than with surgical repair.[3,46,117] The authors of one of these reviews of randomized trials concluded that there is a three times higher risk of re-rupture after nonoperative treatment than after surgery. However, excluding re-rupture, operative management is associated with a substantially higher rate of complications than

nonoperative treatment, including infection, adhesions, and nerve injury.[46] The authors of another one of the reviews noted that when patients who sustain a re-rupture are excluded from an analysis of outcomes of nonoperative and operative management, long-term results, including activity level, ROM and strength, are similar.[3]

Comparison of open repair with percutaneous repair indicates no significant difference in the rate of re-rupture between the two techniques, but a higher rate of infection occurs with open repair[61] and a higher rate of sural nerve damage occurs with a percutaneous approach.[117]

Rehabilitation using early motion and weight bearing appears to be as safe as management with prolonged cast immobilization and delayed weight bearing. Early follow-up studies have indicated no increased incidence of tendon rerupture with early postoperative motion.[9,44,64,68] Although early reports are promising, no determination can yet be made on whether early motion and weight bearing enables a patient to return to a full level of functional activity sooner than if managed with a conventional postoperative approach.[44,64,68] However, authors of a systematic review of the available studies concluded that open repair followed by early motion and weight bearing is probably the treatment of choice and leads to better outcomes for active patients.[117]

# EXERCISE INTERVENTIONS FOR THE ANKLE AND FOOT

## EXERCISE TECHNIQUES TO INCREASE FLEXIBILITY AND RANGE OF MOTION

Loss of flexibility in the ankle and foot can result from a variety of causes. Restoration of motion may be necessary to correct alignment or for normal biomechanics during walking and running. Joint mobilization techniques are used to increase accessory motion of the joint surfaces. These techniques are described in detail in Chapter 5. Manual passive stretching and neuromuscular inhibition techniques are described in Chapter 4. Self-stretching techniques to improve flexibility and ROM are the emphasis of this ssection.

### Flexibility Exercises for the Ankle Region

#### Increase Dorsiflexion of the Ankle

The muscles that restrict dorsiflexion of the ankle are the one-joint soleus and the two-joint gastrocnemius. To effectively stretch the gastrocnemius, the knee must be extended while dorsiflexing the ankle. To isolate stretch to the soleus, the knee must be flexed during dorsiflexion to take tension off the gastrocnemius. Most of the following stretching exercises can be adapted with the knee in flexion or extension so that both of the plantarflexor muscles can be stretched.

PRECAUTION: When a patient uses weight-bearing exercises to stretch the plantarflexor muscles, shoes with arch supports should be worn or a folded washcloth can be placed under the medial border of the foot to minimize the stress to the arches of the foot.

● *Patient position and procedure*: Long-sitting (knees extended) or with the knees partially flexed. Have the patient strongly dorsiflex the feet, attempting to keep the toes relaxed.
● *Patient position and procedure*: Long-sitting or with the knee partially flexed and with a towel or belt under the forefoot. Have the patient pull the foot into dorsiflexion.
● *Patient position and procedure*: Sitting with the foot flat on the floor. Have the patient slide the foot backward, keeping the heel on the floor.
● *Patient position and procedure*: Standing. Have the patient stride forward with one foot, keeping the heel of the back foot flat on the floor (the back foot is the one being stretched). If necessary, have the patient brace his or her hands against a wall. To provide stability to the foot, the patient partially rotates the back leg inward so the foot assumes a supinated position and locks the joints. The patient then shifts body weight forward onto the front foot. To stretch the gastrocnemius muscle, the knee of the back leg is kept extended; to stretch the soleus, the knee of the back leg is flexed.
● *Patient position and procedure*: Standing on an inclined board with feet pointing upward and heels downward (Fig. 22.8). Greater stretch occurs if the patient leans forward. Because the body weight is on the heels, there is little stretch on the long arches of the feet. Little effort is required to maintain this position for extended periods.

● *Patient position and procedure*: Standing, with the fore-foot on the edge of a step or stool and heel over the edge. Have the patient slowly lower the heel over the edge (heel drop).

PRECAUTION: This stretch may create muscle soreness because it requires that the patient control an eccentric contraction of the plantarflexors.

### Increase Inversion

● *Patient position and procedure*: Sitting, with the foot to be stretched placed across the opposite knee. Have the patient grasp the mid- and hindfoot with the opposite hand and lift the foot into inversion. Emphasize turning the heel inward, not just twisting the forefoot.
● *Patient position and procedure*: Long-sitting with a towel or belt under the foot. Have the patient pull on the medial side of the towel to cause the heel and foot to turn inward (Fig. 22.9). This technique can also be used to turn the foot outward by pulling on the lateral side of the towel. It is important that the motion includes the heel, not just the forefoot.
● *Patient position and procedure*: Sitting or standing, with feet pointing forward. Have the patient roll to the lateral border of each foot so the soles are turned inward.
● *Patient position and procedure*: Standing or walking, with the involved foot on a slanted board, placing the lateral aspect of the foot to be stretched on the lower side of the board. Bilateral stretching can be accomplished if hinged planks are placed in an inverted-V position and the patient stands or walks on them.

### Increase Ankle Plantarflexion and Eversion

It is not common for plantarflexion and eversion to be restricted because in the supine position gravity plantarflexes the foot and in the standing position the body's weight everts the foot. Eversion, which is a component of pronation, is the loose-packed position of the foot and is perpetuated with weight bearing. The exception for restricted talocrural plantarflexion is when there is a capsular pattern at the joint as a result of arthritis. If the restriction is from joint hypomobility, it is treated with joint mobilization techniques. If there is restriction of

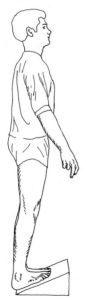

FIGURE 22.8 Self-stretching the ankle into dorsiflexion (stretching the gastrocnemius muscle).

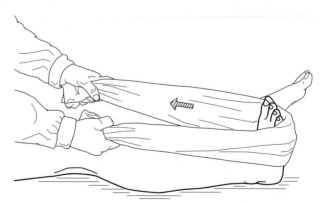

FIGURE 22.9 Self-stretching the foot into inversion using a towel by pulling on the towel on the medial side of the foot.

eversion, a stretching technique was described previously with use of a towel or belt around the foot.

## Flexibility Exercises for Limited Mobility of the Toes

Tight extrinsic muscles of the toes occur with claw toes and hammer toes, causing the MTP joints to extend and IP joints to flex. There is often weakness in the intrinsic muscles. To stretch the intrinsic muscles, emphasize *MTP flexion* and *IP extension.*

### Passive MTP Flexion

*Patient position and procedure*: Sitting with the foot crossed onto the opposite knee. Show the patient how to stabilize the foot under the metatarsal heads (MTP joints) with the thumbs, and passively *flex* the MTP joints by applying pressure against the proximal phalanges. Or have the patient attempt active flexion of the MTP joints, assisting the motion if necessary.

### Passive IP Extension

*Patient position and procedure*: Sitting with the foot crossed onto the opposite knee. Teach the patient to stabilize the proximal phalanx of the involved toe and passively stretch the long flexors across each joint by moving the middle and/or distal phalanx into *extension.*

### Active MTP Flexion

*Patient position and procedure*: Standing with the toes over the edge of a stool or book and the MTP joints at the edge. Have the patient attempt to flex the MTP joints over the edge of the stool. Ideally the patient should try to keep the IP joints of the toes extended, but many individuals cannot do this.

### Great Toe Extension

Extension of the great toe at the MTP joint is critical during the push-off phase of gait. In addition to joint mobilization techniques, passive stretching and self-stretching techniques should be used.

- *Patient position and procedure*: Sitting with the foot resting on the opposite knee. Show the patient how to stabilize the foot around the head of the first metatarsal with one hand, and passively *extend* the MTP joint by applying pressure against the proximal phalanx.
- *Patient position and procedure*: Standing with the involved foot in a backward stride position. The patient may lean his or her hands against a wall for support. Have the patient keep the toes on the ground and rock forward lifting the heel until a stretch is felt under the first toe. A sustained stretch or a gentle rocking stretch can be used.

## Stretching the Plantar Fascia of the Foot

- *Patient position and procedure*: Sitting with the foot placed across the opposite knee. Teach the patient to use his or her thumbs to apply deep massage horizontally and longitudinally across the plantar surface of the foot.

- *Patient position and procedure*: Sitting with a ball or small roller (or bottle) under the foot. Have the patient roll the foot forward and backward across the curved surface, using as much pressure as is comfortable. Pressing down on the knee with one or both hands can exert additional force.

# EXERCISES TO DEVELOP AND IMPROVE MUSCLE PERFORMANCE AND FUNCTIONAL CONTROL

Causes of strength and flexibility imbalances in the ankle and foot include disuse, immobilization, nerve injury, and progressive joint degeneration. In addition, imbalances occur from the weight-bearing stresses that are imposed on the feet. Imbalances can be the cause or the effect of faulty lower extremity mechanics. Because the lower extremities bear weight, realignment by strengthening exercises alone is of limited value. Strengthening exercises undertaken in conjunction with conscious correction, appropriate stretching, balance training, and other necessary measures (such as using orthotic inserts or adaptations for shoes, bracing, splinting, or surgery) improve alignment so that structurally safe weight bearing is possible. In addition, observation of the types of shoes and surfaces that the person uses for walking or sports activities may be a lead to the source of faulty mechanics, which then can be adjusted. (Techniques of orthopedic adaptations for shoes, bracing, and splinting are beyond the scope of this text.)

Most functional demands on the ankle and foot occur in weight-bearing postures. Kinesthetic input from skin, joint, and muscle receptors and the resulting joint and muscle responses are different in open- and closed-chain activities.[25,59] Therefore, whenever possible, use of progressive weight-bearing exercises is important to simulate functional activities. In addition to the exercises described in this section, refer to Chapter 20 for total lower extremity functional exercises performed in the standing position that influence muscle control at the hip, knee, and ankle.

## Activities to Develop Dynamic Neuromuscular Control

- *Patient position and procedure*: Long-sitting or with the knees partially flexed. Have the patient practice contracting each of the major muscles while concentrating on his or her actions, for example, dorsiflexion with inversion (anterior tibialis), plantarflexion with inversion (posterior tibialis), and eversion (peroneus muscles).
- *Patient position and procedure*: Long-sitting or with the knee partially flexed. Instruct the patient to "draw" the alphabet in space leading with the toes but moving at the ankle. For variety have the patient "print" using capital letters, then with lower case letters, or "write" words such as his or her name or address.

● *Patient position and procedure*: Sitting on a chair or low mat table with feet on the floor. Place a number of small objects, such as marbles or dice, to one side of the involved foot. Have the patient pick up one object at a time by curling the toes around it and then placing it in a container on the other side of the foot. This emphasizes the plantar muscles as well as inversion and eversion.

● *Patient position and procedure*: Sitting with feet on the floor or standing. Have the patient curl the toes against the resistance of the floor. Place a towel or tissue paper under the feet, and have the patient attempt to wrinkle it up by keeping the heel on the floor and flexing the toes.

● *Patient position and procedure*: Sitting, with the feet on the floor. Have the patient attempt to raise the medial longitudinal arch while keeping the forefoot and hind-foot on the floor. External rotation of the tibia should occur but not abduction of the hips. The activity is repeated until the patient has consistent control, then it is performed while standing as a progression.

● *Patient position and procedure*: Sitting with a tennis ball placed between the soles of the feet. Instruct the patient to roll the tennis ball back and forth from heel to fore-foot.

● *Patient position and procedure*: Sitting with both feet or just the involved foot on a rocker or balance board. Have patient perform controlled ankle and foot motions (with or without the assistance of the normal foot) into dorsi-flexion and plantarflexion and inversion and eversion (Fig. 22.10). If the equipment permits, the patient also can perform circumduction in each direction. Progress this activity to the standing position to further develop control and to develop balance.

● *Patient position and procedure*: Standing. Have the patient practice walking while concentrating on place-ment of the feet and shifting body weight with each step. The patient begins by accepting body weight on the heel, then shifting the weight along the lateral border of the foot to the fifth metatarsal head and across to the first metatarsal head and great toe for push-off.

## Open-Chain Strengthening Exercises

All of the following exercises in this section are performed without bearing weight through the foot and ankle.

### Plantarflexion

*Patient position and procedure*: Long-sitting with the leg resting on a rolled towel to slightly elevate the heel off the treatment table. Have the patient hold onto the ends of elasticized material that is looped under the forefoot and then plantarflex the foot against the resistance (Fig. 22.11).

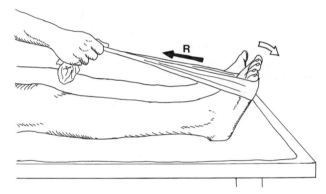

FIGURE 22.11 Resisting the ankle plantarflexor muscles with an elasticized material.

### Isometric Eversion and Inversion

*Patient position and procedure*: Long-sitting or sitting in a chair with knees flexed.

● To resist *eversion*, the ankles are crossed; instruct the patient to press the lateral borders of both feet together against each other.

● To resist *inversion*, the medial borders of the feet are placed beside each other; instruct the patient to press the medial borders of the feet against each other.

### Eversion and Inversion with Elastic Resistance

*Patient position and procedure*: Long-sitting, supine, or sitting with the feet resting on the floor.

● To resist *eversion*, place a loop of elastic tubing around both feet and have the patient evert one or both feet against the resistance (Fig. 22.12). Instruct the patient to keep the knees still and just turn the foot outward, not allowing the thigh and leg to abduct or externally rotate.

● To resist *inversion*, tie the elastic band or tubing to a structure on the lateral side of the foot. Again, have the patient keep the legs stationary and only turn the foot inward without allowing the hip to adduct and internally rotate.

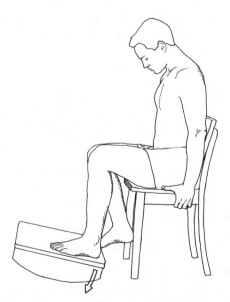

FIGURE 22.10 Using a rocker board to develop control of ankle motions with the patient sitting. When both feet are on the board, the normal foot can assist the involved side. With only the involved foot on the board, the activity is more difficult.

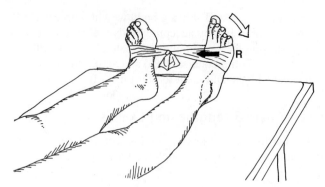

FIGURE 22.12 Resisting the evertor muscles of the foot with an elasticized material.

### Adduction with Inversion and Abduction with Eversion Using Weights

*Patient position and procedure*: Sitting with the foot on the floor. Place a towel under the forefoot and a weight on the end of the towel (Fig. 22.13). Have the patient pull the weighted towel along the floor with the forefoot by keeping the heel fixed on the floor and swinging the foot either inward or outward.

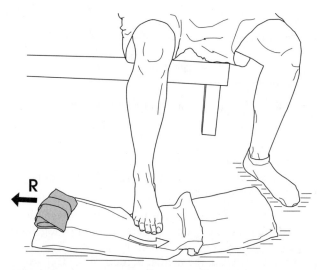

FIGURE 22.13 Resisting adduction and inversion with a weight on the end of the towel. The heel is kept stationary while a windshield wiper motion of the foot is used to pull the towel along the floor. Abduction with eversion is resisted by placing the weight on the towel on the medial side of the foot.

### Dorsiflexion

*Patient position and procedure*: Long-sitting or supine with a rolled towel under the distal leg to elevate the heel slightly. Tie an elastic band or tubing to the foot end of the bed (or other object), and place a loop over the dorsum of the foot. Have the patient dorsiflex against the resistance (Fig. 22.14).

### All Ankle Motions

*Position of patient*: Sitting in a chair or standing with one or both feet in a box filled with sand, foam, dry peas, dry

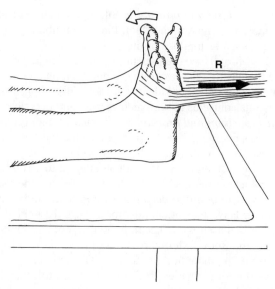

FIGURE 22.14 Resisting the ankle dorsiflexor muscles with an elasticized material.

beans, or other similar type material to offer resistance to various foot motions. Have the patient plantarflex, dorsiflex, invert and evert the foot and ankle, and curl the toes either with the foot on top or with the foot dug into the medium.

## Weight-Bearing Exercises for Strength, Balance, and Function

For these exercises, the patient position is standing. If the patient does not initially tolerate full weight bearing without reproduction of symptoms, begin by standing in the parallel bars or in a pool to reduce weight-bearing forces. Refer to Table 6.8 for general guidelines for progresssion of closed-chain exercises.

### Stabilization Exercises

● Apply resistance to the patient's pelvis in various directions while he or she attempts to maintain control. At first, use verbal cues, then resist without warning, Also increase the speed and intensity of the perturbation forces.
● Have the patient hold onto a wooden dowel rod or cane with both hands. Apply the resistance through the rod in various directions and with varying intensities and speeds as the patient attempts to remain stable (Fig. 22.15).
● Progress to standing only on the involved foot.

### Dynamic Strength Training

Have the patient perform bilateral toe raises, heel raises, and rocking outward to the lateral borders of the feet. Progress to unilateral toe raises, heel raises, and lateral border standing. When tolerated, resistance is added with a weight belt or handheld weights.

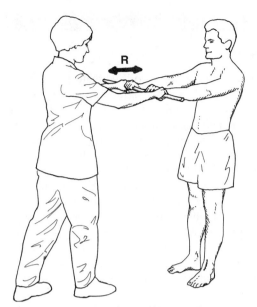

FIGURE 22.15 Stabilization exercises with the patient standing and maintaining balance against the alternating resistance forces from the therapist. The therapist applies force through the rod in backward/forward, side-to-side, and rotation directions.

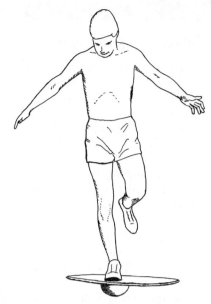

FIGURE 22.16 Advanced training for balance and coordination on a balance board requires that the patient not hold on while balancing with one leg.

### Resisted Walking

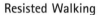 Have the patient walk on heels and on toes against resistance.

⊙ Apply resistance against the patient's pelvis, or have the patient walk against a pulley weight or elastic resistance fixed around the pelvis (see Fig. 20.25).

### Balance Activities

Exercises and functional activities to improve balance are described in detail in Chapter 8. Additional balance activities are described in Chapter 20. Begin with partial weight-bearing activities in the parallel bars if necessary; progress to full, bilateral weight bearing, then unilateral weight bearing. Have the patient shift body weight, stand and balance while performing various arm motions, march in place, walk, and progress to walking on uneven surfaces.

A rocker or balance board can be used several different ways to stimulate balance reactions. If necessary, begin with the patient supporting himself or herself with both hands in the parallel bars or by holding onto a stable object. Initially, both feet are on the board. Increasing the size of the half sphere or rocker under the board increases the difficulty of the balance activity. Progress to unilateral stance on the board.

⊙ Have the patient rock the feet forward and backward, then side-to-side while attempting to control the motion and maintain balance.

⊙ Instruct the patient to maintain balance and not let the edges of the board hit the ground (Fig. 22.16). As the patient learns to control the board, impose various challenges while he or she maintains balance on the board. Examples:

• Have the patient move the arms forward, backward, and overhead.
• Perform various arm motions against elastic resistance, with free weights, or while controlling a BodyBlade® (see Fig. 6.55).
• Toss a ball (unweighted or weighted) back and forth to the patient.
• Have the patient hold onto elastic resistance while you pull the resistance in various directions.

### Simulation and Practice of Functional Activities

Using the principle of specificity of training, replicate whatever functional activity the individual requires, first in controlled patterns, then with increased velocity and decreased control.

***Functional strengthening.*** Lifting, pushing, and pulling heavy objects requires ankle strength as well and hip, knee, and trunk strength. Develop exercises that involve the total body to develop safe body mechanics. Include squatting and lunging to lift objects from the floor, pushing or pulling weighted carts, and climbing and descending steps and ladders while carrying weights. Modify techniques if substitute motions occur.

***Endurance.*** Develop endurance by increasing the amount of time spent performing various drills.

***Power.*** Develop power with plyometric drills such as jumping and hopping. Progress to jumping off and back onto boxes of various heights.

***Agility and skill.*** Develop an obstacle course and have the patient maneuver around or up and over the obstacles, first walking, then running, skipping, or jumping. Include forward, backward, and side-to-side maneuvers.

# INDEPENDENT LEARNING ACTIVITIES

## ● Critical Thinking and Discussion

1. Observe how the foot and ankle function as a unit in several activities such as walking up steps, walking on uneven surfaces, and walking in high-heeled shoes versus low-heeled shoes.
   - What motions occur in the talocrural, subtalar, transverse tarsal, and metatarsophalangeal joints? Describe the mechanics.
   - What muscles are functioning and what level of strength is needed to move or control each joint?
2. Describe the role of the ankle and foot during the gait cycle.
   - What ROM is needed at the ankle and what muscles are acting to cause or control the motion? What other forces are causing or controlling motion at the ankle?
   - What gait deviations occur if there is muscle shortening or weakness at the ankle?
   - After a unilateral arthrodesis of the talocrural joint (ankle fused in neutral) what deviations will occur in the gait cycle?
   - Describe the mechanics and function of pronation and supination in the foot during the gait cycle. Explain how the gait cycle would be affected if a patient had flexible flat feet versus rigid supinated feet.
3. Compare and contrast an exercise program for a patient who has had a repair or reconstruction of torn lateral ligaments of the ankle versus a patient who has had a repair of a ruptured Achilles tendon. How will precautions and selection of exercises differ after these two types of surgical repairs?
4. Discuss the benefits and limitations of total ankle arthroplasty versus arthrodesis of the ankle for the patient with RA.

## ● Laboratory Practice

1. Review all the joint mobilization techniques for the leg, ankle, and foot; include basic glides, accessory motions, and mobilization with movement techniques.
   - Identify and practice techniques that you could use to increase ankle plantarflexion; begin with the ankle at zero, and progress at 15° increments until full plantarflexion is reached.
   - Do the same for ankle dorsiflexion, subtalar inversion and subtalar eversion, and metatarsophalangeal extension.
2. Set up a circuit-training course for the foot and ankle musculature to increase strength, muscular endurance, stability, and balance. Sequence the activities from basic to advanced, and observe accuracy and safety with each exercise. Identify other muscles in the lower extremity, trunk, or arms that are also being affected by the exercises.

## ● Case Studies

1. Mr. C. has a 10-year history of rheumatoid arthritis. Currently, medication is managing his acute symptoms so that he is able to walk with a cane. His complaints are increased pain after walking 15 minutes and considerable stiffness along with generalized weakness. You observe his gait: he walks with a short step and has no push-off. Ankle ROM: dorsiflexion 10°, plantarflexion 15°, inversion 0°, eversion 8°. He stands with a pronated foot, has dorsal migration of the first phalanges and moderate hammer toes. He tolerates moderate resistance in all his musculature within the limited range, although he is unable to demonstrate toe walking or do bilateral toe raises even one time.
   - List his impairments and functional limitations and state goals.
   - Develop a program of intervention to meet the goals. How will you initiate the intervention? What techniques will you use and how will you progress them?
   - Describe the rationale for each manual technique you would use, and for each exercise you would teach the patient.
   - Identify any precautions you will use and that you will teach the patient.
2. Sally S., a college student, sustained a bootline fracture of the tibia and fibula as the result of a fall while snow skiing. She was immobilized in a long-leg cast for 6 weeks, followed by a short-leg cast for 4 weeks. She was allowed partial weight bearing while wearing the short-leg cast. The cast was removed this morning. She described significant stiffness and discomfort when attempting to move her foot. Observation reveals atrophy in the calf, no edema or joint swelling. ROM in the ankle and foot is minimal, and there is no gliding of the fibula at the proximal or distal tibiofibular joints. Strength could not be tested, although the patient can activate all muscles.
   - Answer the same questions as in Case 1.
   - Even though both patients have restricted motion and demonstrate weakness, what are the differences in your intervention strategies and in the precautions you will follow?
   - How will you determine the progression of weight-bearing activities?
3. Ron W. is a 35-year-old computer programmer who plays basketball at the local recreation center. He sustained a massive inversion strain of his right ankle when landing on the foot of an opponent after jumping to rebound the basketball. He wrapped the ankle and iced it for 2 days. On the third day he went for a radiograph. No fractures were detected, but he does have a grade 2 instability of the anterior talofibular ligament. Observation reveals swelling and discoloration in the anterior and lateral ankle region. He experiences a marked increase in pain with inversion and plantarflexion

tests, with anterior gliding of the talus, and with palpation over the involved ligament. Because of muscle guarding, strength was not tested.
• Identify impairments, goals, and an intervention strategy for this patient.

• Describe how his program will be progressed.
• Ron wants to know how soon he can return to playing his favorite sport. What criteria will you use to make this judgment, and how will you protect his ankle when he does return?

# REFERENCES

1. Alexander, IJ: Hallux metatarsophalangeal arthrodesis. In Kitaoka, HB (ed): Master Techniques in Orthopedic Surgery: The Foot and Ankle, ed 2. Lippincott Williams & Wilkins, Philadelphia, 2002, pp 45–60.
2. American Physical Therapy Association: Guide to Physical Therapist Practice, ed 2. Phys Ther 81:9–744, 2001.
3. Bhandari, M, Guyatt, GH, Siddiqui, F, et al: Treatment of acute Achilles tendon rupture: a systematic overview and meta-analysis. Clin Orthop 400:190–200, 2002.
4. Buechel, FF, Sr, Buechel, FF, Jr, Pappas, MJ: Ten-year evaluation of cementless Buechel-Papas meniscal bearing total ankle replacement. Foot Ankle Int 24:462–472, 2003.
5. Calhoun, JH: Acute repair of the Achilles tendon. In Kitaoka, HB (ed): Master Techniques in Orthopedic Surgery: The Foot and Ankle, ed 2. Lippincott Williams & Wilkins, Philadelphia, 2002, pp 311–332.
6. Campbell, DC II, Papagelopoulos, PJ: Reconstruction of the great toe: implant and nonimplant options. In Morrey, BF (ed): Reconstructive Surgery of the Joints, Vol 2, ed 2. Churchill Livingstone, New York, 1996, p 1811.
7. Cannon, LB, Brown, J, Couke, PH: Early weight bearing is safe following arthroscopic ankle arthrodesis. Foot Ankle Surg 10:135–139, 2004.
8. Cannon, LB, Slater, HK: The role of ankle arthroplasty and surgical approach in lateral ankle ligament repair. Foot Ankle Surg 11:1–4, 2005.
9. Carter, TR, Fowler, PJ, Blokker, C: Functional postoperative treatment of Achilles tendon repair. Am J Sports Med 20:459–462, 1992.
10. Cetti, R, Henricksson, LO, Jacobsen, KS: A new treatment of ruptured Achilles tendons. Clin Orthop 308:155, 1994.
11. Cetti, R, et al: Operative versus nonoperative treatment of Achilles tendon rupture: a prospective randomized study and review of the literature. Am J Sports Med 21:791, 1993.
12. Coester, LM, Saltzman, CL, Leupold, J, Pontarelli, W: Long-term results following ankle arthrodesis for post-traumatic arthritis. J Bone Joint Surg 83A(2):219–228, 2001.
13. Colville, MK, Grundol, RJ: Anatomic reconstruction of the lateral ankle ligaments using a split peroneus brevis tendon graft. Am J Sports Med 23:210, 1995.
14. Cracchiolo, A, Janisse, D, Gall, V: Rheumatoid arthritis in the foot and ankle: surgery and rehabilitation. In Melvin, JL, Gall, V (eds): Rheumatologic Rehabilitation Series, Vol 5: Surgical Rehabilitation. American Occupational Therapy Association, Bethesda MD, 1999, p 165.
15. Cretnik, A, Kosanovic, M, Smrkolj, V: Percutaneous suturing of the ruptured Achilles tendon under local anesthesia. J Foot Ankle Surg 43(2):72–81, 2004.
16. Cyriax, J: Textbook of Orthopaedic Medicine, Vol 1. Diagnosis of Soft Tissue Lesions, ed 8. Bailliére Tindall, London, 1982.
17. Dayton, P, McCall, A: Early weightbearing after first metatarsophalangeal joint arthrodesis: a retrospective observational case analysis. J Foot Ankle Surg 43(3):156–159, 2004.
18. Dimonte, P, Light, H: Pathomechanics, gait deviations and treatment of the rheumatoid foot. Phys Ther 62:1148, 1982.
19. Donatelli, R, et al: Biomechanical foot orthotics: a retrospective study. J Orthop Sports Phys Ther 10:205, 1988.
20. Donatelli, RA: Normal anatomy and biomechanics. In Donatelli, RA (ed): The Biomechanics of the Foot and Ankle, ed 2. FA Davis, Philadelphia, 1996, p 3.
21. Donatelli, RA: Abnormal biomechanics. In Donatelli, RA (ed): The Biomechanics of the Foot and Ankle, ed 2. FA Davis, Philadelphia, 1996, p 34.
22. Eils, E, Rosenbaum, D: A multi-station proprioceptive program in patients with ankle instability. Med Sci Sports Exerc 33:1991–1998, 2001.
23. Fishco, WD, Cornwall, MW: Gait analysis after talonavicular joint fusion: 2 case reports. J Foot Ankle Surg 43(4):241–247, 2004.
24. Gabrielsen, TA, Kitaoka, HB: Ankle injuries. In Morrey, BF (ed): Reconstructive Surgery of the Joints, Vol 2, ed 2. Churchill Livingstone, New York, 1996, p 1743.
25. Garn, SN, Newton, RA: Kinesthetic awareness in subjects with multiple ankle sprains. Phys Ther 68:1669, 1988.
26. Gauffin, H, Trupp, H, Odenieck, P: Effect of ankle disk training on postural control in patients with functional instability of the ankle joint. Int J Sports Med 9:141, 1988.
27. Glasoe, WM, et al: Weight-bearing immobilization and early exercise treatment following a grade II lateral ankle sprain. J Orthop Sports Phys Ther 29:394, 1999.
28. Green, T, Refshauge, K, et al: A randomized controlled trial of a passive accessory joint mobilization on acute ankle inversion sprains. Phys Ther 81(4):984–994, 2001.
29. Greenfield, B, Johnson, M: Evaluation of overuse syndromes. In Donatelli, R (ed): The Biomechanics of the Foot and Ankle, ed 2. FA Davis, Philadelphia, 1996, p 189.
30. Hals, TV, Sitler, MR, Mattacola, CG: Effect of a semi-rigid ankle stabilizer on performance in persons with functional ankle instability. J Orthop Sports Phys Ther 30(9):552–556, 2000.
31. Hamilton, WG: Ankle instability repair: the Bröstrom-Gould procedure. In Kitaoka, HB (ed): Master Techniques in Orthopedic Surgery: The Foot and Ankle, ed 2. Lippincott Williams & Wilkins, Philadelphia, 2002, pp 487–496.
32. Hamilton, WG, Thompson, FM, Snow, SW: The modified Brostrom procedure for lateral ankle instability. Foot Ankle 14:1, 1993.
33. Hasselman, CT, Wong, YS, Conti, SF: Total ankle replacement. In Kitaoka, HB (ed): Master Techniques in Orthopedic Surgery: The Foot and Ankle, ed 2. Lippincott Williams & Wilkins, Philadelphia, 2002, pp 581–595.
34. Heinrichs, K, Haney, C: Rehabilitation of the surgically repaired Achilles tendon using a dorsal functional orthosis. A preliminary report. J Sport Rehabil 3:292, 1994.
35. Hennrikus, WL, et al: Outcomes of the Chrisman-Snook and modified Brostrom procedures for chronic lateral ankle instability: a prospective, randomized comparison. Am J Sports Med 24:400, 1996.
36. Hintermann, B, Valderrabano, V, Dereymaeker, G, Dick, W: The HINTERGRA: rationale and short-term results of 122 consecutive ankles. Clin Orthop 424:57–68.
37. Horak, F, Nashner, L: Central programming of postural movements: adaptations to altered support surface configuration. J Neurophysiol 55:1369, 1986.
38. Howell, DW: Therapeutic exercise and mobilization. In Hunt, GC (ed): Physical Therapy of the Foot and Ankle. Churchill-Livingstone, New York, 1988.
39. Hyer, CF, VanCourt, R: Arthroscopic repair of lateral ankle instability by using the thermal-assisted capsular shift procedure: a review of 4 cases. J Foot Ankle Surg 43(2):104–109, 2004.
40. Hyland, MR, Webber-Gaffney, A, et al: Randomized controlled trial of calcaneal taping, sham taping, and plantar fascia stretching for the short-term management of plantar heel pain. J Orthop Sports Phys Ther 36(6):364–371, 2006.
41. Jaakkola, JI, Mann, RA: A review of rheumatoid arthritis affecting the foot and ankle. Foot Ankle Int 25:866–874, 2004.
42. Kaikkonen, A, Natri, A, Pasanen, M: Isokinetic muscle performance after surgery of the lateral ligaments of the ankle. Int J Sports Med 20:173–178, 1999.
43. Kangas, J, Pajala, A, Siira, P, et al: Early functional treatment versus early immobilization in tension of the musculotendinous unit after

Achilles rupture repair: a prospective, randomized clinical study. J Trauma 54(6):1171–1181, 2003.

44. Kauranen, KJ, Leppilahti, JI: Motor performance of the foot after Achilles rupture repair. Int J Sports Med 22:154, 2001.

45. Kavlak, Y, Uygur, F, Korkmaz, C, Bek, N: Outcome of arthoses intervention in the rheumatoid foot. Foot Ankle Int 24:494–499, 2003.

46. Khan, RJK, Fick, D, Keough, A, et al: Treatment of acute Achilles tendon rupture: a meta-analysis of randomized controlled trials. J Bone Joint Surg 87A(10):2202–2210, 2005.

47. Kile, TA: Ankle arthrodesis. In Morrey, BF (ed): Reconstructive Surgery of the Joints, Vol 2, ed 2. Churchill Livingstone, New York, 1996, p 1771.

48. Kimura, IF, et al: Effect of the air stirrup in controlling ankle inversion stress. J Orthop Sports Phys Ther 190, 1987.

49. Kitaoka, HB: Talocalcaneal (subtalar) arthrodesis. In Kitaoka, HB (ed): Master Techniques in Orthopedic Surgery: The Foot and Ankle, ed 2. Lippincott Williams & Wilkins, Philadelphia, 2002, pp 387–399.

50. Kitaoka, HB: Complications of replacement arthroplasty of the ankle. In Morrey, BF (ed): Joint Replacement Arthroplasty, ed 3. Churchill Livingstone, Philadelphia, 2003, pp 1133–1150.

51. Kitaoka, HB, Johnson, KA: Ankle replacement arthroplasty. In Morrey, BF (ed): Reconstructive Surgery of the Joints, Vol 2, ed 2. Churchill Livingstone New York, 1996, p 1757.

52. Knecht, SI, Estin, M, Callaghan, JJ: The Agility total ankle arthroplasty. Seven to sixteen-year follow-up. J Bone Joint Surg 86A:1161–1171, 2004.

53. Kofoed, H, Lundberg-Jensen, A: Ankle arthroplasty in patients younger and older than 50 years: a prospective study with long-term follow-up. Foot Ankle Int 20:501–506, 1999.

54. Kofoed, H, Sorensen, TS: Ankle arthroplasty for rheumatoid arthritis and osteoarthritis: prospective long-term study of cemented replacements. J Bone Joint Surg Br 80:328–332, 1998.

55. Komenda, G, Ferkel, RD: Arthroscopic findings associated with the unstable ankle. Foot Ankle Int 20:708, 1999.

56. Kramer, P: Restoration of dorsiflexion after injuries to the distal leg and ankle. J Orthop Sports Phys Ther 1:159, 1980.

57. Krips, R, van Dijk, CN, Lehtonen, H, et al: Sports activity after surgical treatment for chronic anterolateral ankle instability: a multicenter study. Am J Sports Med 30:13–19, 2002.

58. Kuland, DN: The Injured Athlete. JB Lippincott, Philadelphia, 1988.

59. Lattanza, L, Gray, GW, Kantner, R: Closed vs open kinematic chain measurements of subtalar joint eversion: implications for clinical practice. J Orthop Sports Phys Ther 9:310, 1988.

60. Leach, RE, James, S, Wasliewski, S: Achilles tendinitis. Am J Sports Med 9:93, 1981.

61. Lim, J, Dalal, R, Waseen, M: Percutaneous vs. open repair of the ruptured Achilles tendon—a prospective randomized controlled study. Foot Ankle Int 22:559–568, 2001.

62. Lockard, MA: Foot orthoses. Phys Ther 68:1866, 1988.

63. Maffulli, N, Tallon, C, Wong, J, et al: Early weightbearing and ankle mobilization after open repair of acute midsubstance tears of the Achilles tendon. Am J Sports Med 31:692–700, 2003.

64. Mandelbaum, BR, Myerson, MS, Forster, R: Achilles tendon ruptures: a new method of repair, early range of motion, and functional rehabilitation. Am J Sports Med 23:392–395, 1995.

65. McPoil, TG: Footwear. Phys Ther 68:1857, 1988.

66. Michelson, J, Amis, JA: Talus-calcaneus-cuboid (triple) arthrodesis. In Kitaoka, HB (ed): Master Techniques in Orthopedic Surgery: The Foot and Ankle, ed 2. Lippincott Williams & Wilkins, Philadelphia, 2002, pp 401–424.

67. Möller, M, Movin, T, Granhed, H: Acute rupture of the tendo achillis: a prospective randomized study comparison between surgical and non-surgical treatment. J Bone Joint Surg 83B: 843–848, 2001.

68. Mortensen, NH, Skov, O, Jensen, PE: Early motion of the ankle after operative treatment of a rupture of the Achilles tendon. A prospective, randomized clinical and radiographic study. J Bone Joint Surg Am 81:983, 1999.

69. Motta, P, Errichiello, C, Pontini, I: Achilles tendon rupture. A new technique for surgical repair and immediate movement of the ankle and foot. Am J Sports Med 25:172–176, 1997.

70. Mueller, MJ: The Ankle and Foot Complex. In Levangie, PK, Norkin, CC: Joint Structure and Function, ed 4. FA Davis, Philadelphia, 2005.

71. Mulier, T, Pienaar, H, Dereymaeker, G, et al: The management of chronic Achilles tendon ruptures: gastrocnemius turndown flap with or without flexor hallucis longus transfer. Foot Ankle Surg 9:151–156, 2003.

72. Mulligan, BR: Manual Therapy "NAGS", "SNAGS", "MWM's": etc, ed 4. Plane View Press, Wellington, 1999.

73. Mulligan, EP: Lower leg, ankle and foot rehabilitation. In Andrews, JR, Harrelson, GL, Wilk, KE (eds): Physical Rehabilitation of the Injured Athlete, ed 2. WB Saunders, Philadelphia, 1998, p 261.

74. Myerson, MS, Mroczek, K: Perioperative complications of total ankle arthroplasty. Foot Ankle Int 24(1):17–21, 2003.

75. Novick, A: Anatomy and biomechanics. In Hunt, GC, McPoil TG (eds): Physical Therapy of the Foot and Ankle, Churchill Livingstone, New York, 1995, p 11.

76. Oatis, CA: Biomechanics of the foot and ankle under static conditions. Phys Ther 68:1815, 1988.

77. O'Brien, TS, Hart, TS, Shereff, MJ, et al: Open versus arthroscopic ankle arthrodesis: a comparative study. Foot Ankle Int 20:368–374, 1999.

78. Olney, SJ: Gait. In Levangie, PK, Norkin, CC: Joint Structure and Function, ed 4. FA Davis, Philadelphia, 2005.

79. Panikkar, KV, Taylor, A, Kamath, S, Henry, APJ: A comparison of open and arthroscopic ankle fusion. Foot Ankle Surg 9:169–172, 2003.

80. Perry, J: Gait Analysis: Normal and Pathological Function. SLACK, Thorofare, NJ, 1992.

81. Peters, WJ, Trevino, SG, Renstrom, PA: Chronic lateral ankle instability. Foot Ankle 12:82, 1991.

82. Rettig, AC, Liotta, FJ, Klootwyk, TE, et al: Pontential risk of rerupture in primary Achilles tendon repair in athletes younger than 30 years of age. Am J Sports Med 33:119–123, 2005

83. Reynolds, NL, Worrell, TN: Chronic Achilles peritendinitis: etiology, pathophysiology, and treatment. J Orthop Sports Phys Ther 13:717, 1991.

84. Rozzi, SM, et al: Balance training for patients with functionally unstable ankles. J Orthop Sports Phys Ther 29:478, 1999.

85. Salter, RB: Textbook of Disorders and Injuries of the Musculoskeletal System, ed 3. Williams & Wilkins, Baltimore, 1999.

86. Saltzman, CL, et al: Total ankle replacement revisited. J Orthop Sports Phys Ther 30:56, 2000.

87. Sammarco, GJ, Chag, L: Talonavicular arthrodesis. In Kitaoka, HB (ed): Master Techniques in Orthopedic Surgery: The Foot and Ankle, ed 2. Lippincott Williams & Wilkins, Philadelphia, 2002, pp 253–263.

88. Sammarco, GJ, Hockenbury, RT: Biomechanics of the foot and ankle. In Nordin, M, Frankel, VH (eds): Basic Biomechanics of the Musculoskeletal System, ed 3. Lippincott Williams & Wilkins, Philadelphia, 2001, p 222.

89. Scholz, KC: Total ankle arthroplasty using biological fixation components compared to ankle arthrodesis. Orthopedics 10:125, 1987.

90. Sekiya, H, Horii, T, Kariya, Y, Hoshino, Y: Arthroscopic-assisted tibiotalocalcaneal arthrodesis using an intramedullary nail with fins: a case report. J Foot Ankle Surg 45(4):266–270, 2006.

91. Shi, K, Hayashida, K, Hashimoto, J, et al: Hydroxyapatite augmentation for bone atrophy in total ankle replacement in rheumatoid arthritis. J Foot Ankle Surg 45(5):316–321, 2006.

92. Shrader, JA: Nonsurgical management of the foot and ankle affected by rheumatoid arthritis. J Orthop Sports Phys Ther 29:703, 1999.

93. Smith, CL: Physical therapy management of patients with total ankle replacement. Phys Ther 60:303, 1980.

94. Smith, LK, Weiss, EL, Lehmkuhl, LD: Brunnstrom's Clinical Kinesiology, ed 5. FA Davis, Philadelphia, 1996.

95. Smith, RW: Ankle arthrodesis. In Kitaoka, HB (ed): Master Techniques in Orthopedic Surgery: The Foot and Ankle, ed 2. Lippincott Williams & Wilkins, Philadelphia, 2002, pp 533–549.

96. Snook, GA: Lateral ankle reconstruction for chronic instability. In Torg, JS, Welsh, RP, Shephard, RJ (eds): Current Therapy in Sports Medicine, ed 2. BC Decker, Toronto, 1990.

97. Solveborn, S, Moberg, A: Immediate free ankle motion after surgical repair of acute Achilles tendon ruptures. Am J Sports Med 22:607–610, 1994.

98. Southerland, CC: Arthroscopic reconstruction of the unstable ankle. In Nyska, M, Mann, G (eds): The Unstable Ankle. Human Kinetics, Champaign, IL, 2002, pp 238–249.

99. Spigel, PV, Seale, KS: Surgical interventions. In Donatelli, RA (ed): The Biomechanics of the Foot and Ankle, ed 2. FA Davis, Philadelphia, 1996, p 352.
100. Steele, G, Harter, R, Ting, A: Comparison of functional ability following percutaneous and open surgical repairs of acutely ruptured tendons. J Sport Rehabil 2:115, 1993.
101. Stephenson, K, Saltzman, CL, Brotzman, SB: Foot and ankle injuries. In Brotzman, SB, Wilk, KE: Clinical Orthopedic Rehabilitation, ed 2. CV Mosby, Philadelphia, 2003, pp 371–441
102. Stone, JW: Arthroscopic ankle arthrodesis. In Kitaoka, HB (ed): Master Techniques in Orthopedic Surgery: The Foot and Ankle, ed 2. Lippincott Williams & Wilkins, Philadelphia, 2002, pp 569–580.
103. Subotnick, SI: Return to sport after delayed surgical reconstruction for ankle instability. In Nyska, M, Mann, G (eds): The Unstable Ankle. Human Kinetics, Champaign, IL, 2002, pp 201–205.
104. Sugimoto, K, Takakura, Y, Kumai, T, et al: Reconstruction of the lateral ankle ligaments with bone-patellar tendon graft in patients with chronic ankle instability: a preliminary report. Am J Sports Med 30:340–346, 2002.
105. Thomas, RH, Daniels, TR: Ankle arthrodesis. J Bone Joint Surg 85A 923–936, 2003.
106. Thompson, TC, Doherty, JH: Spontaneous rupture of tendon of Achilles: a new clinical diagnostic test. J Trauma 2:126, 1962.
107. Turner, NS, III, Campbell, DC, II: Prosthetic intervention of the great toe. In Morrey, BF (ed): Joint Replacement Arthroplasty, ed 3. Churchill Livingstone Philadelphia, 2003, pp 1121–1132.
108. Unger, AS, Inglis, AE, Mow, CS: Total ankle arthroplasty in rheumatoid arthritis: a long-term follow-up study. Foot Ankle 8:173, 1988.
109. Valderrabano, V, Hintermann, B, Nigg, BM, Stefanyshy, D, et al: Kinematic changes after fusion and total replacement of the ankle: Part 1: Range of motion. Foot Ankle Int 24:881–887, 2003.
110. Valderrabano, V, Pagenstert, G, Horisberger, M, et al: Sports and recreation activity of ankle arthritis patients before and after total ankle replacement. Am J Sports Med 34(6):993–999, 2006.
111. Verhagen, E, van der Beck, A, Twisk, J, et al: The effect of a proprioceptive balance board training program for the prevention of ankle sprains: a prospective, controlled trial. Am J Sports Med 32:1385–1393, 2004.
112. Verhagen, RA, Struijs, PA, Bossuyt, PM, et al: Systematic review of treatment strategies for osteochondral defects of the talar dome. Foot Ankle Clin 8:233–242, 2003.
113. Vicenzino, B, Branjerdport, M, et al: Initial changes in posterior talar glide and dorsiflexion of the ankle after mobilization with movement in individuals with recurrent ankle sprain. J Orthop Sports Phys Ther 36(6):464–471, 2006.
114. Wapner, KL: Delayed repair of the Achilles tendon. In Kitaoka, HB (ed): Master Techniques in Orthopedic Surgery: The Foot and Ankle, ed 2. Lippincott Williams & Wilkins, Philadelphia, 2002, pp 323–335.
115. Waugh, T: Arthroplasty rehabilitation. In Goodgold, J (ed): Rehabilitation Medicine. CV Mosby, St. Louis, 1988, p 457.
116. Wester, JU, et al: Wobble board training after partial sprains of the lateral ligaments of the ankle: a prospective, randomized study. J Orthop Sports Phys Ther 23:332, 1996.
117. Wong, J, Barrass, V, Maffulli, N: Quantitative review of operative and nonoperative management of Achilles tendon ruptures. Am J Sports Med 30:565–575, 2002.

# Special Areas of Therapeutic Exercise

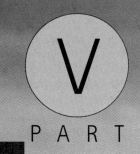

## PART V

# 23 Women's Health: Obstetrics and Pelvic Floor

CHAPTER

### Barbara Settles Huge, BS, PT

Throughout a woman's life cycle, specific gender differences need to be recognized for their relevance to rehabilitation. Recent research has shown *repeatedly* that women have specific and distinct physiological processes that extend beyond the obvious considerations of anatomy and hormones, including differences in symptoms of heart attack and metabolism of medications.[42] Clearly, the pregnant or postpartum patient presents a unique gender-based clinical challenge for the physical therapist. Although pregnancy is a time of tremendous musculoskeletal, physiological, and emotional change, it is nonetheless a state of wellness. Pregnant women are typically well motivated, willing to learn, and highly responsive to treatment suggestions. For many women, the therapist is able to assess and monitor the physical changes with the primary focus on maintaining wellness. The ability to educate women about the role of exercise and health promotion during this key life transition provides a significant professional opportunity and responsibility.

In cases of musculoskeletal impairment related to pregnancy, the therapist is able to examine and treat the patient by incorporating knowledge of injury and tissue healing with knowledge of the changes during pregnancy. By considering a broader perspective, it is recognized that all female patients can benefit from education regarding the role of the pelvic floor muscles in musculoskeletal health, specifically in trunk stabilization. Specialized treatment of pelvic floor dysfunction is critical to quality of life for women experiencing incontinence, pelvic organ prolapse, and a variety of pelvic pain syndromes. Although all physical therapists can fairly easily incorporate activation of the pelvic floor muscles as a key component of trunk stabilization exercises, true expertise can come only with further training and mentoring. Advanced study of pelvic floor anatomy, evaluation, and treatment is highly recommended for therapists who wish to specialize in this area.

This chapter provides readers with basic information about the systemic changes of pregnancy as a foundation for the development of safe and effective exercise programs. In addition, a review of pelvic floor anatomy, function, and dysfunction serves as an introduction to the treatment of pelvic floor disorders. The chapter emphasizes modification of general exercises to meet the needs of the obstetric patient, and provides information to assist in the development of an exercise program for an uncomplicated pregnancy. Cesarean delivery, high-risk pregnancy, and the special needs of patients with these conditions are also discussed.

## OVERVIEW OF PREGNANCY, LABOR, AND RELATED CONDITIONS

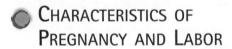
## CHARACTERISTICS OF PREGNANCY AND LABOR

### Pregnancy

Pregnancy, which spans 40 weeks from conception to delivery, is divided into three trimesters, with characteristic changes during each.[27,36,54,58]

#### Changes During the First Trimester
During the first trimester (weeks 0 through 12) the following occur:

- Implantation of the fertilized ovum in the uterus occurs 7 to 10 days after fertilization.

- The mother is very fatigued, urinates more frequently, and may experience nausea and/or vomiting ("morning" sickness).
- Breast size may increase.
- There is a relatively small weight gain of 0 to 1455 g (0 to 3 lb is normal).
- Emotional changes may occur.
- By the end of the 12th week, the fetus is 6 to 7 cm long and weighs approximately 20 g (2 oz). The fetus now can kick, turn its head, and swallow and has a beating heart, but these movements are not yet felt by the mother.

#### Changes During the Second Trimester
During the second trimester (weeks 13 through 26) the following occur:

- The pregnancy becomes visible to others.
- The mother begins to feel movement at around 20 weeks.
- Most women now feel very good. Nausea and fatigue have usually disappeared.
- By the end of the second trimester, the fetus is 19 to 23 cm (14 inches) in length and weighs approximately 600 g (1 to 2 lb).
- The fetus now has eyebrows, eyelashes, and fingernails.

#### Changes During the Third Trimester
From week 27 through 40 weeks the following occur:

- The uterus is now very large and has regular contractions, although these may be felt only occasionally.
- Common complaints during the third trimester are frequent urination, back pain, leg edema and fatigue, round ligament pain, shortness of breath, and constipation.
- By the time of birth, the baby will be 33 to 39 cm long (16 to 19 inches) and will weigh approximately 3400 g (7 lb, although a range of 5 to 10 lb is normal).

N O T E : Although pregnancy typically lasts 40 weeks, the range of 38 to 42 weeks is considered full term.

### Labor

Labor is divided into three stages, each containing specific events.[7,36,56,58] The exact mechanism that initiates labor is not known. Regular and strong involuntary contractions of the smooth muscles of the uterus are the primary symptom of labor. True labor produces palpable changes in the cervix, which are known as effacement and dilation (Fig. 23.1).[58]

- **Effacement** is the shortening or thinning of the cervix from a thickness of 5 cm (2 inches) before onset of labor to the thickness of a piece of paper.
- **Dilation** is the opening of the cervix from the diameter of a fingertip to approximately 10 cm (4 inches).

#### Labor—Stage 1
Some women experience initial cervical dilation and effacement before they are in true labor. However, by the end of this stage, the cervix is fully dilated and there is no doubt that a baby is about to be delivered. Stage 1 of labor is divided into three major phases.

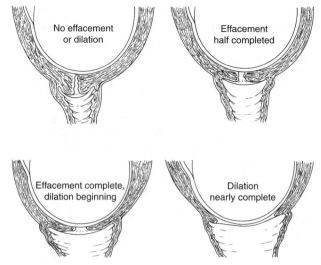

FIGURE 23.1 Effacement and dilation of the cervix. (From Sandberg,[58] with permission.)

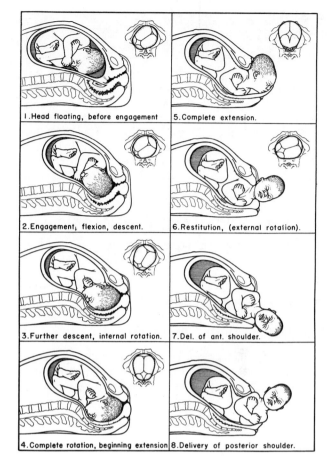

FIGURE 23.2 Principal movements in the mechanism of labor and delivery, left occiput anterior position. (From Pritchard, J, MacDonald, P,[56] with permission.)

*Cervical dilation phase.* The cervix dilates from 0 to 3 cm (0 to 1 inch) and will almost completely efface. Uterine contractions occur from the top down, causing the cervix to open and pushing the fetus downward.

*Middle phase.* The cervix dilates from 4 to 7 cm (1 to 3 inches). Contractions are stronger and more regular.

*Transition phase.* The cervix dilates from 8 to 10 cm (3 to 4 inches) and dilation is complete. Uterine contractions are very strong and close together.

## Labor—Stage 2

Stage 2 involves *"pushing"* and *expulsion* of the fetus. Intra-abdominal pressure is the primary force expelling the fetus; it is produced by voluntary contraction of the abdominal muscles and diaphragm. Relaxation and stretching of the pelvic floor during stage 2 are also necessary for successful vaginal delivery. Uterine contractions may last as long as 90 seconds during this stage.

*Fetal descent.* Position changes (cardinal movements) by the fetus allow it to pass through the pelvis and be born (Fig. 23.2).[56] The position changes are described as:

- *Engagement.* The greatest transverse diameter of the fetal head passes through the pelvic inlet (the superior opening of the minor pelvis).
- *Descent.* Continued downward progression of the fetus occurs.
- *Flexion.* The fetal chin is brought closer to its thorax; this occurs when the descending head meets resistance from the walls and floor of the pelvis and the cervix.
- *Internal rotation.* The fetus turns its occiput toward the mother's symphysis pubis when the fetal head reaches the level of the ischial spines.
- *Extension.* The flexed fetal head reaches the vulva; the fetus extends its head, bringing the base of the occiput in direct contact with the inferior margin of the maternal

symphysis pubis; this phase ends when the fetal head is delivered.
- *External rotation.* The fetus rotates its occiput toward the mother's sacrum to allow the fetal shoulders to pass through the pelvis.

*Expulsion.* The fetal anterior shoulder passes under the symphysis pubis, and the rest of the body follows.

## Labor—Stage 3

*Placental stage (expulsion of the placenta).* After delivery, the uterus continues to contract and shrink, causing the placenta to detach and be expelled.

- As the uterus decreases in size, the placenta detaches from the uterine wall, blood vessels are constricted, and bleeding slows. This can occur 5 to 30 minutes after the baby is delivered.
- A hematoma forms over the uterine placental site to prevent further significant blood loss; mild bleeding persists for 3 to 6 weeks after delivery.

*Uterine involution.* The uterus continues to contract and decrease in size for 3 to 6 weeks after delivery; the uterus always remains slightly enlarged over its pre-pregnant size.

| BOX 23.1 | Total Weight Gain (Ranges) for Single Fetus | |
|---|---|---|
| • Fetus | 3.36–3.88 kg | (7.5–8.0 lb) |
| • Placenta | 0.48–0.72 kg | (1.0–1.5 lb) |
| • Amniotic fluid | 0.72–0.97 kg | (1.5–2.0 lb) |
| • Uterus and breasts | 2.42–2.66 kg | (5.0–5.5 lb) |
| • Blood and fluid | 1.94–3.99 kg | (4.0–7.0 lb) |
| • Muscle and fat | 0.48–2.91 kg | (1.0–6.0 lb) |
| • Total: | 9.70–14.55 kg | (20.0–30.0 lb) |

# ANATOMICAL AND PHYSIOLOGICAL CHANGES OF PREGNANCY

Considerable changes occur in the woman's body as the pregnancy progresses.[7,36,54,56,58,62,66]

## Weight Gain During Pregnancy

Current recommendations for weight gain during pregnancy are an average of 25 to 27 lbs.[62] with a distribution as shown in Box 23.1.

## Changes in Organ Systems

### Uterus and Related Connective Tissue

*Uterus.* The uterus increases from a prepregnant size of 5 by 10 cm (2 by 4 inches) to 25 by 36 cm (10 by 14 inches). It increases five to six times in size, 3000 to 4000 times in capacity, and 20 times in weight by the end of pregnancy. By the end of pregnancy, each muscle cell in the uterus has increased approximately 10 times over its pre-pregnancy length.[66] Once the uterus expands upward and leaves the pelvis, it becomes an abdominal rather than a pelvic organ.

*Connective tissues.* Ligaments connected to the pelvic organs are more fibroelastic than ligaments supporting joint structures. The fascial tissues, which surround and enclose the organs in a continuous sheet, also include a significant amount of smooth muscle fibers.[17] The round, broad, and uterosacral ligaments in particular provide suspensory support for the uterus.

### Urinary System

*Kidneys.* The kidneys increase in length by 1 cm (0.5 inch).

*Ureters.* The ureters enter the bladder at a perpendicular angle because of uterine enlargement. This may result in a reflux of urine out of the bladder and back into the ureter; therefore, during pregnancy there is an increased chance of developing urinary tract infections because of urinary stasis.

### Pulmonary System

*Hormonal influences.* Hormone changes affect pulmonary secretions and rib cage position.

● Edema and tissue congestion of the upper respiratory tract begin early in pregnancy because of hormonal changes. Hormonally stimulated upper respiratory hypersecretion also occurs.
● Changes in rib position are hormonally stimulated and occur prior to uterine enlargement. The subcostal angle progressively increases; the ribs flare up and out. The anteroposterior and transverse chest diameters each increase by 2 cm (1 inch). Total chest circumference increases by 5 to 7 cm (2 to 3 inches) and does not always return to the pre-pregnant state.
● The diaphragm is elevated by 4 cm (1.5 inch); this is a passive change caused by the change in rib position.

*Respiration.* Respiration rate is unchanged, but depth of respiration increases.[56]

● Tidal volume and minute ventilation increase, but total lung capacity is unchanged or slightly decreased.[56,66]
● There is a 15% to 20% increase in oxygen consumption; a natural state of hyperventilation exists throughout pregnancy to meet the oxygen demands of pregnancy.[56,66]
● The work of breathing increases because of hyperventilation; dyspnea is present with mild exercise as early as 20 weeks into the pregnancy.[56,66]

### Cardiovascular System

*Blood volume and pressure.* Blood volume progressively increases 35% to 50% (1.5 to 2 liters) throughout pregnancy and returns to normal by 6 to 8 weeks after delivery.

● Plasma increase is greater than red blood cell increase, leading to the "physiologic anemia" of pregnancy, which is not a true anemia but is representative of the greater increase of plasma volume. The increase in plasma volume occurs as a result of hormonal stimulation to meet the oxygen demands of pregnancy.
● Venous pressure in the lower extremities increases during standing as a result of increased uterine size and increased venous distensibility.
● Pressure in the inferior vena cava rises in late pregnancy, especially in the supine position, because of compression by the uterus just below the diaphragm. In some women, the decline in venous return and resulting decrease in cardiac output may lead to symptomatic supine hypotensive syndrome. The aorta is partially occluded in the supine position.
● Blood pressure decreases early in the first trimester. There is a slight decrease of systolic pressure and a greater decrease of diastolic pressure. Blood pressure reaches its lowest level approximately midway through pregnancy, then rises gradually from mid-pregnancy to reach the pre-pregnant level approximately 6 weeks after delivery. Although cardiac output increases, blood pressure decreases because of venous distensibility.

*Heart.* Heart size increases, and the heart is elevated because of the movement of the diaphragm.

● Heart rhythm disturbances are more common during pregnancy.

● Heart rate usually increases 10 to 20 beats per minute by full term and returns to normal levels within 6 weeks after delivery.
● Cardiac output increases 30% to 60% during pregnancy and is most significantly increased when a woman is in the left side-lying position, in which the uterus places the least pressure on the aorta.

## Musculoskeletal System

*Abdominal muscles.* The abdominal muscles, particularly both sides of the rectus, are stretched to the point of their elastic limit by the end of pregnancy. This greatly decreases the muscles' ability to generate a strong contraction, and thus decreases their efficiency of contraction. The shift in the center of gravity also decreases the mechanical advantage of the abdominal muscles.[66]

*Pelvic floor muscles.* The pelvic floor muscles, in their anti-gravity position, must withstand the total change in weight; the pelvic floor drops as much as 2.5 cm (1 inch) as a result of pregnancy.[62]

*Connective tissues and joints.* The hormonal influence on the ligaments is profound, producing a systemic decrease in ligamentous tensile strength. This change is primarily a result of an increase in relaxin and progesterone levels.[62]

● The thoracolumbar fascia is put in a position of extreme length, which diminishes its ability to stabilize the trunk effectively.[18]
● Joint hypermobility occurs as a result of ligamentous laxity and may predispose the patient to injury, especially in the weight-bearing joints of the back, pelvis, and lower extremities.

## Thermoregulatory System

*Metabolic rate.* During pregnancy, basal metabolic rate and heat production increase.[20]

● An additional intake of 300 calories per day is needed to meet the basic metabolic needs of pregnancy.
● In pregnant women, normal fasting blood glucose levels are lower than in nonpregnant women.[20]

## Changes in Posture and Balance

### Center of Gravity
The center of gravity shifts upward and forward because of the enlargement of the uterus and breasts. This requires postural compensations to maintain balance and stability.[54,66]

● The *lumbar and cervical lordoses* increase to compensate for the shift in the center of gravity, and the knees hyperextend, probably because of the change in the center of gravity.
● The *shoulder girdle and upper back* become rounded with scapular protraction and upper extremity internal rotation because of breast enlargement; this postural tendency persists with postpartum positioning for infant care. Tightness of the pectoralis muscles and weakness of the scapular stabilizers may be pre-existing to or perpetuated by the pregnancy postural change.
● The *suboccipital muscles* respond in an effort to maintain appropriate eye level (optical righting reflex), and to moderate forward head posture along with the change in shoulder alignment.
● *Weight shifts* toward the heels to bring the center of gravity to a more posterior position. This contributes to the "waddling" gait that is typically seen in pregnancy.
● Changes in posture do not automatically correct after childbirth, and the pregnant posture may become habitual. In addition, many child-care activities contribute to persistent postural faults and asymmetry.

### Balance
With the increased weight and redistribution of body mass there are compensations to maintain balance.[54,66]

● The pregnant woman usually walks with a wider base of support and increased external rotation at the hips.
● This change in stance along with growth of the baby makes some activities such as walking, stooping, stair climbing, lifting, reaching, and other activities of daily living (ADLs) progressively more challenging.
● Activities requiring fine balance and rapid changes in direction, such as aerobic dancing and bicycle riding, may become inadvisable, especially during the third trimester.

# OVERVIEW OF PELVIC FLOOR ANATOMY, FUNCTION, AND DYSFUNCTION

Treatment of pelvic floor impairment has become more visible and accepted in the physical therapy community over the last 5 to 10 years. However, advanced and in-depth study of anatomy, physiology, evaluation, and treatment continues to be highly recommended for therapists who wish to specialize in this area.[2–4,9,10,12,17,19,22,26,28,33–35,37,38,41,43–45,48,51,53–55,57,59,61,62,64–67,70]

## Pelvic Floor Musculature

The pelvic floor musculature is composed of several layers with bony attachments to the pubic bone and the coccyx. The anterior–posterior fibers are oriented almost horizontally and form the inferior support for the trunk. Laterally, the tissues blend into a fascial layer overlying the obturator internus. Both right and left sides of the muscles contribute fibers to the perineal body located between the vagina and rectum (Fig. 23.3). The structure and action of the muscles of each layer are summarized in Table 23.1. Fibers that run anterior–posterior create a superior force toward the heart, while the more superficial fibers surround the sphincters and produce a puckering motion.

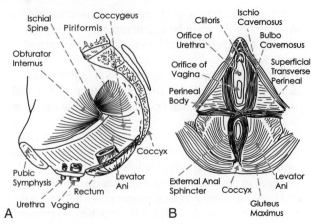

**FIGURE 23.3** Pelvic floor muscles. (*A*) Sagittal section; note sling/hammock orientation and (*B*) viewed from below; note figure-eight orientation of the muscles around the orifice of the urethra/vagina and the anal sphincter.

## Female Pelvic Floor

The female pelvic floor allows for passage of the urethra, vagina, and rectum. This creates less inherent stability when compared to the male anatomy.

### Innervation

The pudendal nerve arises from ventral divisions of S2 to S4 in the sacral plexus, as well as direct branches from S3 and S4, and supplies the pelvic floor complex. This dual innervation provides a safeguard against direct damage to the pudendal nerve. The terminal branches are the perineal branch and the inferior rectal nerve, which ends in the external anal sphincter.

### Function

The pelvic floor musculature has the following essential roles:

- Provide support for the pelvic organs and their contents
- Withstand increases in intra-abdominal pressure
- Maintain continence (through sympathetic nerve fibers) to the urethral and anal sphincters
- Sexual response and reproductive function

## Effect of Childbirth on the Pelvic Floor

### Neurological Compromise

Stretch and compression of the pudendal nerve occurs during labor as the baby's head travels through the birth canal; this stretch can be as much as 20% of the total length of the nerve.[3,61] This compromise to the pudendal nerve is most intense during pushing (the second stage of labor), through the completion of vaginal delivery.

### Muscular Impairment

Extreme stretching of the pelvic floor tissues is inherent in the process of labor and vaginal delivery. The pelvic floor musculature may also be torn or incised during the birth process. An episiotomy is an incision made in the perineal body (see Fig. 23.3). It is automatically considered a second-degree laceration according to the following classification of perineal lacerations[56]:

First degree—only skin
Second degree—includes underlying muscle
Third degree—extends to anal sphincter
Fourth degree—tears through the sphincter and into the rectum

Additional trauma can occur as a result of forceps use, necessitating suturing throughout the musculature and into the vaginal vault.

### Episiotomy

Although episiotomy is common, occurring in 33% to 51% of vaginal deliveries (with some studies reporting a figure as high as 75%), there is no strong medical evidence supporting its use. In fact, outcomes with episiotomy are worse in some cases, including pain with intercourse and extension of the episiotomy into the sphincter or rectum.[33,41] Pregnant women have many questions about labor in general and episiotomy in particular; the clinician is able to provide education and support for the patient as she explores her options.

| TABLE 23.1 | Pelvic Floor Anatomy—From Superficial to Deep | |
| --- | --- | --- |
| **Muscle Layer** | **Structure** | **Action** |
| Superficial (outlet) | Ischiocavernosus | Clitoral erection |
| | Bulbocavernosus | "Drawing in" of the introitus, clitoral erection |
| | Superficial transverse perineal | Fixes perineal body |
| | External anal sphincter | Compression of anal canal |
| Urogenital diaphragm (perineal membrane) | Deep transverse perineal<br>• Compressor urethrae<br>• Urethrovaginal sphincter | Compression of urethra and ventral wall of vagina<br>Support of the perineal body and introitus |
| Pelvic diaphragm (primary muscular support) | Levator ani<br>• Pubococcygeus<br>• Puborectalis<br>• Iliococcygeus<br>Coccygeus | Prime mover of the pelvic floor<br>Puborectalis aids in closure of the rectum<br><br>Flexes coccyx |

### ◉ Focus on Evidence

A randomized controlled trial of 459 Canadian women during their first pregnancy found a significant protective effect against third- and fourth-degree tears (extensions following episiotomy) in women who participated in "strenuous" exercise three or more times per week. The researchers defined "strenuous" exercise as bicycling, jogging, tennis, skiing, and weight training as opposed to "non-strenuous" exercise such as walking, swimming, prenatal classes, and yoga. Data were collected regarding type, frequency, and duration of exercise for a 12-month period including prepregnancy and postpartum time frames. In the "strenuous" exercise group, 200 of the women did *not* have third- or fourth-degree tears as compared to only 25 women who did experience this tearing. In addition, this study helped dispel the theory that serious exercisers may have overdeveloped perineal musculature; these women were *not* at increased risk for episiotomy when compared to casual exercisers.[41]

## Classification of Pelvic Floor Dysfunction

### Prolapse

A prolapse is a supportive impairment. It refers to the descent of any of the pelvic viscera out of their normal alignment because of muscular, fascial, and/or ligamentous deficits, and increased abdominal pressure (Fig. 23.4). A prolapse often worsens over time and with subsequent pregnancies and can be aggravated by constipation and straining with elimination.

● A recent cross-sectional study found stage I prolapse in 33% of the subjects, and stage II descent in 62.9%. The sample included 270 women with a mean age of 68.3 years and median parity of three vaginal births.[51] This is critically important information for all clinicians prescribing trunk stabilization programs for female patients, regardless of diagnosis.
● From a biomechanical aspect, activation of the pelvic floor is necessary in coordination with core muscle activation and trunk strengthening activities to prevent excessive downward forces. Otherwise, trunk strengthening will likely increase a previously undetected prolapse, or aggravate an existing condition.

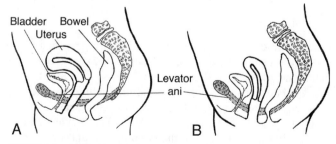

**FIGURE 23.4** (*A*) Good pelvic floor support with a firm base, organs in normal position. (*B*) Inadequate support, pelvic organs descend.

● As prolapse progresses, functional changes occur as a result of perineal pressure and heaviness, low back pain, abdominal pressure or pain, and voiding difficulties. Currently, there is very limited evidence regarding prevention or treatment of pelvic organ prolapse.

### Urinary or Fecal Incontinence

Involuntary loss of bladder or bowel contents, often a result of both neuromuscular and musculoskeletal impairments, often occurs in combination with prolapse. A conservative estimate of persons affected with urinary incontinence is 15 million in the United States alone (approximately 1 in 20 persons); women are twice as likely to have these symptoms as men.[22] These patients often have significant social discomfort and anxiety regarding leakage and hygiene concerns.

### ◉ Focus on Evidence

Statistically significant improvements in urinary leakage were demonstrated as a result of a program of pelvic floor strengthening in three different studies.[44,45,57] Both pregnant and postpartum women were studied in these trials, with follow-up until 1 year after delivery in two of the studies.[44,57] Morkved et al.[45] determined that pelvic floor muscle training prevented incontinence in about one in six women during pregnancy and one in eight women after delivery (*N* = 301).

### Pain and Hypertonus

The broad category that encompasses pain and hypertonus includes a variety of causes. Pain and hypertonus may be related to delayed healing of perineal lacerations, trauma to the soft tissues or the sacro-coccygeal joint during delivery, pelvic obliquity, multiple gynecologic/visceral diagnoses, cauda equina involvement, scar tissue adhesions, or muscle spasm/guarding throughout the pelvis.

● Accurate statistics are lacking; however, in one study with a total sample of 581 women (age 18 to 45), the following prevalence was found: pelvic pain, 39%; dyspareunia, 46%; and dysmenorrhea, 90%.[37]
● Functional limitations may include pain with ADLs, decreased sitting tolerance, dyspareunia (pain with intercourse), and difficulty with elimination of bladder and bowel contents. In patients with pelvic pain impairments, often referred to as chronic pelvic pain (CPP), persistent tightness of the lumbar paraspinals and hip flexors is typically present.[2]
● Because of the breadth of this topic, treatment recommendations are conflicting. Recent guidelines stress the importance of multidisciplinary assessment and consideration of myofascial dysfunction for successful outcomes.[38]

## Risk Factors for Dysfunction

### Childbirth

Childbirth is obviously the most significant risk factor for pelvic floor impairments. The process of labor, particularly with vaginal delivery and current medical management, can produce significant trauma to the structures of the pelvic floor.

- A longitudinal cohort study with follow-up 15 years after delivery ($N = 55$) showed that stress incontinence during the first pregnancy doubled the risk of re-occurrence 15 years later.[19]
- Other potential obstetric risk factors include multiple deliveries, prolonged second stage of labor, use of forceps or oxytocin, third-degree perineal tears, and birth weight greater than 8 lb.[51,61,65]

### Other Causes

Women who have never been pregnant may also present with pelvic floor dysfunction. Excessive straining because of chronic constipation, smoking, chronic cough, obesity, and hysterectomy can contribute to these impairments in any woman.[3,22,35,65] The role of estrogen in the development of incontinence is still unclear, with some studies citing estrogen depletion as a risk factor[22] and others that found a connection between incontinence and estrogen replacement therapy.[35,65] High caffeine intake (more than 400 mg/day) is a specific risk factor for urge incontinence.[35]

## Interventions for Pelvic Floor Impairments

### Visual Aids

Visual aids are critical in teaching patients about pelvic floor function. Emphasis should be placed on both the sling/hammock fibers and the figure-eight orientation of the musculature (see Fig. 23.3). Help the patient to visualize the fibers that run anterior–posterior (to create a "lifting" motion toward the heart) as well as the circumferential fibers (which produce a drawstring or "pucker" effect). Successful strengthening is unlikely without this educational component; in fact, instructing women in pelvic floor exercises by verbal or written instruction alone caused increased pressures to the bladder in 25% of women, rather than producing an appropriate superiorly directed force.[9]

### Neuromuscular Re-education

Neuromuscular re-education is essential, as many women have significant disuse and proprioceptive deficits of the pelvic floor muscles. Internal techniques of assessment and treatment are often indicated for optimal patient outcomes. For example, manual stretch facilitation (a Proprioceptive Neuromuscular Facilitation technique) to the levator ani can be a very effective treatment option. Initially, emphasis on *isolated* contractions of the pelvic floor is needed[4] because many patients will exhibit excessive accessory muscle recruitment such as the gluteals, hip adductors, and abdominals. Once coordination has improved, the patient progresses to integration of pelvic floor activity with ADLs, lumbar stabilization, and other functional exercises.

### Exercise and Biofeedback

The use of exercise and biofeedback, including surface electromyography (SEMG) for treatment of pelvic floor dysfunction in a female population is well supported.[10,22,] [53,67] SEMG allows for immediate visual and/or auditory feedback to the patient, enhancing motor learning and proprioceptive improvements. It is particularly invaluable for *pelvic floor* re-education owing to lack of knowledge of the muscles' existence, let alone their function and importance.

Specific exercises to address pelvic floor impairments are listed in the exercise section of the chapter.

### Manual Treatment and Modalities

Manual treatment and modalities, including intravaginal and intrarectal techniques, also play a role in the treatment of pelvic floor symptoms, particularly pelvic pain syndromes. Advanced training is necessary for true expertise with internal techniques.

##  PREGNANCY-INDUCED PATHOLOGY

The combined influence of hormones, weight gain, and postural changes of pregnancy contributes to a variety of impairments (in addition to pelvic floor dysfunction that was described in the previous section) that can be addressed with physical therapy.

### Diastasis Recti

Diastasis recti is separation of the rectus abdominis muscles in the midline at the linea alba. The etiology of this separation is unknown; however, the continuity and integrity of the abdominal musculature are disrupted (Fig. 23.5). Any separation larger than 2 cm or two fingerwidths is considered significant.[5,11,48]

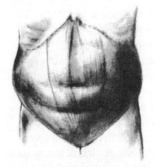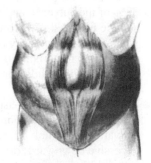

FIGURE 23.5 Diagrammatic representations of diastasis recti. (From Boissonnault, JS, Kotarinos, RK: Diastasis recti. In Wilder, E [ed]: Obstetric and Gynecologic Physical Therapy,[66] with permission.)

### Incidence

The condition is not exclusive to childbearing women but is seen frequently in this population. In one study, Boissonnault and Blaschak tested 89 women for separation of the rectus abdominis muscles.[5] The sample included women who were not pregnant, one group for each trimester of pregnancy, and two postpartum groups. The incidence in this study ranged from 0 in the nonpregnant and first trimester women, to 27% in the second trimester, to a high of 66% in the third trimester. Also of interest is that 36% of the women between 5 weeks and 3 months postpartum continued to display a separation. A second study, done by Bursch, found a significant diastasis in 62.5% of postpartum women tested within 92 hours of delivery.[11]

● Diastasis recti may occur in pregnancy as a result of hormonal effects on the connective tissue and the biomechanical changes of pregnancy; it may also develop during labor, especially with excessive breath-holding during the second stage.[62] It causes no discomfort.

● It can occur above, below, or at the level of the umbilicus but appears to be less common below the umbilicus.

● It appears to be less common in women with good abdominal tone before pregnancy.[5]

● Clinically, a diastasis may be found in women well past their childbearing years and also in men. Routine assessment for this condition is highly recommended and can easily be done in conjunction with abdominal strength testing.

### Significance

The condition of diastasis recti may produce musculoskeletal complaints, such as low back pain, possibly as a result of decreased ability of the abdominal musculature to stabilize the pelvis and lumbar spine.

*Functional limitations.* Functional limitations can also occur, such as inability to perform independent supine to sitting transitions because of extreme loss of the mechanical alignment and function of the rectus muscle. Again, this finding is not exclusive to childbearing patients.

*Decreased fetal protection.* In severe separations, the remaining midline layers of abdominal wall tissue are skin, fascia, subcutaneous fat, and peritoneum.[5,11,62] The lack of muscular support provides less protection for the fetus.

*Potential for herniation.* Severe cases of diastasis recti may progress to herniation of the abdominal viscera through the separation at the linea alba. This degree of separation requires surgical repair. Rehabilitation following this type of repair may include components of C-section rehabilitation, with specific precautions and input from the referring surgeon. There may be a need for very slow progression depending on the severity of the diastasis and how it was repaired.

### Examination for Diastasis Recti

Test all pregnant patients for the presence of diastasis recti before performing any abdominal exercises. This test should be repeated throughout the pregnancy and appropriate modifications made to existing exercises.

Instruct patients to perform a self-test on or after the third postpartum day for optimal accuracy. Until 3 days after delivery, the abdominal musculature has inadequate tone for valid test results.[48,62]

*Patient position and procedure:* Hook-lying. Have the patient slowly raise her head and shoulders off the floor, reaching her hands toward the knees, until the spines of the scapulae leave the floor. Place the fingers of one hand horizontally across the midline of the abdomen at the umbilicus (Fig. 23.6). If a separation exists, the fingers will sink into the gap between the rectus muscles. The number of

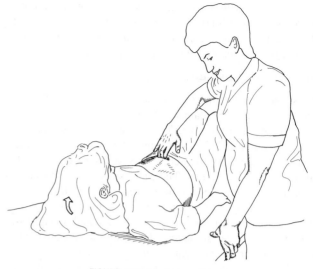

FIGURE 23.6 Diastasis recti test.

fingers that can be placed between the muscle bellies is then documented. A diastasis recti can also present as a longitudinal bulge along the midline. Because this condition can occur above, below, or at the level of the umbilicus, test for it at all three areas.

### Intervention for Diastasis Recti

Teach the patient to perform the corrective exercise for diastasis recti (see Fig. 23.8 and accompanying text later in this chapter) exclusive of other abdominal exercise until the separation is decreased to 2 cm or less.[48] The rationale for this is that, due to the angle of attachment of the obliques into the linea alba, there is a possibility that trunk rotation exercises will perpetuate the separation.[62] Once the correction has been obtained, strengthening of the obliques and more advanced abdominal work can be resumed.

## Postural Back Pain

Back pain commonly occurs because of the postural changes of pregnancy, increased ligamentous laxity, and decreased abdominal muscle function.[1,18,48,52,54,55,66]

### Incidence

Back pain is reported by 50% to 70% of pregnant women at some point during pregnancy[30,47]; this condition contributes to lost work days and decreased functional ability. In addition, symptoms may continue in the postpartum period, with a prevalence in up to 68% of women, for as long as 12 months after delivery.[47]

### Characteristics

The symptoms of low back pain usually worsen with muscle fatigue from static postures or as the day progresses; symptoms are usually relieved with rest or change of position. Women who are physically fit generally have less back pain during pregnancy.[52]

### Interventions

Low back pain symptoms can be treated effectively with many traditional low back exercises, proper body mechanics, posture instructions, improvement in work techniques, along with superficial modality application.[48,62] The use of deep-heating agents, electrical stimulation, and traction is generally *contraindicated* during pregnancy.

 **Focus on Evidence** _____

Garshasbi and Faghih Zadeh[30] studied more than 200 primigravid women (pregnant for the first time) in a prospective randomized study of the effect of exercise on the intensity of low back pain during pregnancy. Subjects were excluded if they had a history of exercise before pregnancy or history of orthopedic conditions. The exercise group were in a supervised exercise program for 3 hours/week for 12 weeks in the second and early third trimesters; the control group were women who were homemakers, and had no significant change in activity level. The groups were statistically equal in maternal and neonatal weight gain as well as length of pregnancy. The exercise group experienced significant decrease in intensity of low back pain by the end of the study, while intensity was increased in the control group. The study did not describe the nature of the symptoms or differentiate between postural pain versus sacroiliac pain. Interestingly, there was no significant difference in the change in lordosis between the two groups.

## Sacroiliac/Pelvic Girdle Pain

### Characteristics
Sacroiliac pain is localized to the posterior pelvis and is described as stabbing deep into the buttocks distal and lateral to L5/S1. Pain may radiate into the posterior thigh or knee but not into the foot. Symptoms include pain with prolonged sitting, standing or walking, climbing stairs, turning in bed, unilateral standing, or torsion activities. Symptoms may not be relieved by rest and frequently worsen with activity. Pubic symphysis dysfunction may occur alone or in combination with sacroiliac symptoms, and includes significant tenderness to palpation at the symphysis, radiating pain into the groin and medial thigh, and pain with weight bearing. In addition, excessive separation and translation of the bone may occur.[18,62] One study reported a four times greater incidence of posterior pelvic pain than low back pain in pregnant women.[52]

### Interventions
Pelvic girdle and sacroiliac symptoms are treated via modification or elimination of activities that may further aggravate sensitive tissue, stabilization exercises, and the use of belts and corsets to provide external support to the pelvis.

● *Activity modification.* Daily activities should be adapted to minimize asymmetrical forces acting on the trunk and pelvis. For example, getting into a car is done by sitting down first, then pivoting both legs and the trunk into the car, keeping the knees together; side-lying is made more symmetrical by placing a pillow between the knees and under the abdomen, and sexual positions are altered to avoid full range of hip abduction. Single-leg weight bearing, excessive abduction and sitting on very soft surfaces should be avoided. In addition, caution patients to avoid climbing more than one step at a time, swinging one leg out of bed at a time when getting up, or crossing the legs when sitting.[18,62]

● *Exercise modification.* Exercise must be modified so as not to aggravate the condition. Avoid exercises that require single-leg weight bearing and excessive hip abduction or hyperextension. Teach the patient to activate the pelvic floor and transverse abdominals when transitioning from one position to another in order to stabilize the pelvis.

 **Focus on Evidence** _____

A randomized clinical trial with 2-year follow-up looked at long-term effects of physical therapy for pelvic girdle pain in the postpartum period.[63] Each group had 20 weeks of treatment, with the control group focusing on modalities, manual therapy, and general exercises. In addition, the second group had specifc focus on trunk/hip stabilizing exercises, with particular attention to the transverse abdominals. All participants received individual instruction from an experienced physical therapist. Outcome measures included the Oswestry Disability Questionnaire, pain scales, and a health-related quality of life (QOL) tool that measured eight subscales. At 1 year postpartum, the group with specific stabilizing exercises showed significantly better scores on all measures of those three tools, except for the social functioning subscale of the QOL tool. The same measurements were collected at 2 years postdelivery, and the benefit for the stabilization group persisted, with significant differences in functional status and morning and evening pain. The specific exercise group had scores on QOL comparable to those of a representative group of the general population.

● *External stabilization.* Use of external stabilization such as belts or corsets designed for use during pregnancy helps reduce posterior pelvic pain, expecially when walking.

 **Focus on Evidence** _____

Ostgaard et al.[52] found that the use of nonelastic external stabilization designed for use during pregnancy helped reduce posterior pelvic pain in 82% of women. This was a large, randomized, controlled study ($N = 407$). More recent studies have validated the use of external stabilization for pelvic girdle pain ($N = 118$)[47] but found no effect with a support belt in cases of pubic symphysis pain ($N = 87$).[18]

## Varicose Veins

Varicosities are aggravated in pregnancy by the increased uterine weight, venous stasis in the legs, and increased venous distensibility.

### Characteristics
Varicosities can present in the first trimester, and are more prevalent with repeated pregnancies. They can occur in the

lower extremities, the rectum (hemorrhoids), or vulva. Symptoms usually include heaviness or aching discomfort, especially with dependent leg positions; intensity may become severe as the pregnancy progresses. In addition, pregnant women are more susceptible to deep vein thrombosis.[62]

### Interventions

- **Exercise modification.** If there is discomfort, exercises may need to be modified so that minimal dependent positioning of the legs occurs.
- **External support.** Elastic support stockings should be worn to provide an external pressure gradient against the distended veins, and the woman should be encouraged to perform lower extremity exercises and to elevate the lower extremities as often as possible (see Box 24.8 and accompanying text in Chapter 24). Vulvar varicosities may benefit from use of a perineal pad or belt that provides counter-pressure and support to the tissues.[48]

## Joint Laxity

### Significance

All joint structures are at increased risk of injury during pregnancy and during the immediate postpartum period. The tensile quality of the ligamentous support is decreased, and therefore injury can occur if women are not educated regarding joint protection. There is much controversy regarding the impact of postpartum hormone levels; however, elevated levels have been found 3 to 5 months after delivery.[62] This may persist even longer if the woman is nursing. Many patients are aware of persistent symptoms in conjunction with the menstrual cycle.

### Interventions

- **Exercise modification.** Teach the woman safe exercises to perform during the childbearing year, including modification of exercises to decrease excessive joint stress (see exercises described in the management section of this chapter).
- **Aerobic exercise.** Suggest nonweight-bearing or less stressful aerobic activities such as swimming, walking, or biking, particularly for women who were relatively sedentary before pregnancy.

## Nerve Compression Syndromes

### Causes

Impairments from conditions such as thoracic outlet syndrome (TOS) or carpal tunnel syndrome (CTS) may be caused by one or more of the following in pregnancy: postural changes in the neck and upper quarter, fluid retention, hormonal changes, or circulatory compromise. Overall, women are three times as likely as men to experience carpal tunnel syndrome. Occurrence in pregnancy can be as high as 41%[53] (see Chapter 13 for discussion on CTS and TOS and Chapter 14 for discussion on posture).

Nerve compression syndromes may also occur in the lower extremities because of the weight of the fetus, fluid retention, hormonal changes, or circulatory compromise.

### Interventions

Typical protocols include postural correction exercises, manual techniques, ergonomic assessment, and modalities (see Chapter 13 for management of nerve compression syndromes). Splints may be used in the treatment of carpal tunnel syndrome. Carpal tunnel surgery in the pregnant population is rare, as symptoms generally resolve soon after delivery; a longer course of the problem has been noted in women who breastfeed.[62]

## EXERCISE INTERVENTIONS FOR PREGNANCY, LABOR, AND RELATED CONDITIONS

## PHYSIOLOGICAL EFFECTS OF AEROBIC EXERCISE DURING PREGNANCY

Many women who have been doing aerobic exercises choose to continue exercising during pregnancy to maintain their cardiopulmonary fitness. Maternal[1,13,15,39,66] and fetal[13,14,16,20,21,29,39,66] responses have been well studied; therefore this information is used to guide both the therapist and the patient in determining necessary modifications to an existing exercise program.

## Maternal Response to Aerobic Exercise

### Blood Flow

Aerobic exercise does not reduce blood flow to the brain and heart. It does, however, cause a redistribution of blood flow away from the internal organs (and possibly the uterus) and toward the working muscles. This raises two concerns: that the reduction in blood flow may decrease the oxygen and nutrient availability to the fetus and that uterine contractions and preterm labor may be stimulated.[13] Stroke volume and cardiac output both increase with steady-state exercise. This, coupled with increased blood volume and reduction in systemic vascular resistance during pregnancy, may help offset the effects of the vascular shunting.

### Respiratory Rate

The maternal respiration rate appears to adapt to mild exercise but does not increase proportionately with moderate and severe exercise when compared with a nonpregnant state. The pregnant woman reaches a maximum exercise capacity at a lower work level than a nonpregnant woman because of the increased oxygen requirements of exercise.

### Hematocrit Level

The maternal hematocrit level during pregnancy is lowered; however, it rises up to 10 percentage points within 15 minutes of beginning vigorous exercise. This condition continues for up to 4 weeks postpartum. As a result, cardiac reserve is decreased during exercise.

### Inferior Vena Cava Compression

Compression of the inferior vena cava by the uterus can occur after the fourth month of pregnancy, with relative obstruction of venous return. This leads to decreased cardiac output and orthostatic hypotension. It occurs most often in supine or static standing positions, and therefore prolonged time in these positions should be avoided.[20]

### Energy Needs

Hypoglycemia occurs more readily during pregnancy; therefore, adequate carbohydrate intake is important for the pregnant woman who exercises.[15] A caloric intake of an additional 500 calories per day is suggested to support the energy needs of pregnancy *and* exercise, dependent on the intensity and duration of the exercise. In comparison, a sedentary pregnant woman requires a 300 calorie per day increase.[1]

### Core Temperature

Vigorous physical activity and dehydration through perspiration leads to increased core temperature in anyone who exercises. Concern has been expressed over this occurring in the pregnant woman because of the relationship of elevated core temperature to neural tube defects of the fetus. Studies report that during pregnancy the core temperature of physically fit women actually decreases during exercise. These women appeared to be more efficient in regulating their core temperature, and thus the thermal stress on the embryo and fetus is reduced.[14,15]

### Uterine Contractions

Norepinephrine and epinephrine levels increase with exercise. Norepinephrine increases the strength and frequency of uterine contractions. This may pose a problem for the woman at risk of developing premature labor.

### Healthy Woman Response

Studies have shown that healthy women who continue to run throughout pregnancy deliver on the average of 5 to 7 days sooner compared with controls.[13,14] Clapp[13-15] found that exercise, including weight bearing (even with ballistic motions such as during aerobic dancing), can be performed in mid- and late pregnancy without risk of preterm labor or premature rupture of the membranes. Women who wish to continue strenuous or competitive exercise or participate in specific athletic training require close supervision by a specialist during pregnancy.[20,21]

## Fetal Response to Maternal Aerobic Exercise

No human research has conclusively proven a detrimental fetal response to mild- or moderate-intensity maternal exercise. Recent studies suggest that even vigorous exercise does not have the detrimental effects on the fetus that once were feared, and therefore restrictions on exercise because of concerns for the effects on the embryo and fetus have been lessened. In fact, fit women who maintained their volume of exercise after 20 weeks' gestation delivered babies with lower fat mass than those who decreased exercise intensity mid-way through the pregnancy.[13-15] Given the epidemic of obesity in the United States, the need for future research to define further the connections between fetal nutrition and adult disease is imperative.[16]

### Blood Flow

A 50% or greater reduction of uterine blood flow is necessary before fetal well-being is affected (based on animal research). No studies have documented such decreases in pregnant women who exercise, even vigorously. It is suggested that the cardiovascular adaptations in exercising women offset any redistribution of blood to muscles during exercise.[13]

### Fetal Heart Rate

Brief submaximal maternal exercise (up to 70% maternal aerobic power) does not adversely affect fetal heart rate (FHR).[20] The FHR usually increases 10 to 30 beats per minute at the onset of maternal exercise. After mild to moderate maternal exercise, the FHR usually returns to normal levels within 15 minutes, but in some cases of strenuous maternal exercise the FHR may remain elevated as long as 30 minutes. Fetal bradycardia (indicating fetal asphyxia) during maternal exercise has been reported in the literature, with the return to pre-exercise FHR levels within 3 minutes after maternal exercise, followed by a brief period of fetal tachycardia.[29] The healthy fetus appears to be able to tolerate brief episodes of asphyxia with no detrimental results.

### Heat Dissipation

The fetus has no mechanism such as perspiration or respiration by which to dissipate heat. However, physically fit women are able to dissipate heat and regulate their core temperature more efficiently, thus reducing risk.[13]

### Newborn Status

Newborn children of women who continue endurance exercises into the third trimester of pregnancy are reported to have an average decrease in birth weight of 310 g. There is no change in head circumference or heel–crown length. Further study of these children (up to 5 years of age) has shown slightly better neurodevelopmental status in addition to higher percentage of lean body mass.[15]

##  EXERCISE FOR THE UNCOMPLICATED PREGNANCY AND POSTPARTUM

Exercise programs during pregnancy and after childbirth are designed to minimize impairments and help the woman maintain or regain function while she is preparing for the arrival of the baby and then caring for the infant.[1,20,21,23,29,39,40,45,46,48,53,54,57,60,62,66] The potential impairments, functional limitations, and management guidelines related to uncomplicated pregnancies are summarized in Box 23.2, and a suggested

**BOX 23.2**
## MANAGEMENT GUIDELINES—Pregnancy and Postpartum

### Potential Impairments and Functional Limitations
Stress, pain, and muscle imbalances from faulty postures
Poor body mechanics; related to lack of knowledge, changing body size and caring for growing child
Lower extremity edema and discomfort from altered circulation, varicose veins
Pelvic floor dysfunction
- urinary or fecal incontinence
- organ prolapse
- hypertonus
- poor episiotomy healing
- poor proprioceptive awareness and disuse atrophy
Abdominal muscle stretch, trauma, and diastasis recti
Potential decrease in cardiovascular fitness
Lack of knowledge of body changes and safe exercises to use during and after pregnancy
Changing body image
Lack of physical preparation (strength, endurance, relaxation) necessary for labor and delivery
Lack of knowledge of appropriate positioning for optimal comfort in labor and delivery
Lack of adequate postpartum rehabilitation

| Plan of Care | Interventions |
|---|---|
| 1. Develop awareness and control of posture during and after pregnancy | 1. Stretch, train, and strengthen postural muscles. Posture awareness training. |
| 2. Learn safe body mechanics. | 2. Body mechanics in sitting, standing, lifting, and lying as well as transitions from one position to another. Body mechanics with baby equipment and childcare activities. Positioning options for labor and delivery. |
| 3. Develop upper extremity strength for the demands of infant care. | 3. Resistive exercises to appropriate muscles. |
| 4. Promote increased body awareness and a positive body image. | 4. Body awareness and proprioception activities. Posture reinforcement. |
| 5. Prepare the lower extremities for the demands of increased weight bearing and circulatory compromise. | 5. Use of elastic support stockings. Stretching exercises. Toning and resistive exercises to appropriate muscles. |
| 6. Develop awareness and control of the pelvic floor musculature. | 6. Awareness of isolated pelvic floor muscle contraction and relaxation. Train and strengthen for muscle control, integration with ADLs. |
| 7. Maintain abdominal function and prevent or correct diastasis recti. | 7. Monitor diastasis recti. Diastasis recti exercises. Safe abdominal-strengthening exercises with diastasis recti protection. |
| 8. Promote or maintain safe cardiovascular fitness. | 8. Safe progression of aerobic exercises. |
| 9. Learn about the changes of pregnancy and birth. | 9. Patient/family instruction. Refer to other disciplines as indicated. |
| 10. Learn relaxation skills. | 10. Relaxation and breathing techniques. |
| 11. Prevent impairments associated with pregnancy | 11. Education about potential problems of pregnancy. Teach prevention techniques and appropriate exercises. |
| 12. Prepare physically for labor, delivery, and postpartum activities. | 12. Strengthen muscles needed in labor and delivery, and train responses. Teach comfort measures for labor and delivery. |
| 13. Provide education on safe postpartum exercise progression. | 13. Postpartum exercise instruction. |
| 14. Develop awareness of treatment options for pelvic floor dysfunction. | 14. Comprehensive approach for prolapse, incontinence, or hypertonus. |

## BOX 23.3  Suggested Sequence for Exercises Classes

1. General rhythmic activities to "warm up"
2. Gentle selective stretching for postural alignment and for perineum and adductor flexibility
3. Aerobic activity for cardiovascular conditioning (duration/intensity may need to be individualized)
4. Postural exercises; upper/lower extremity strengthening and individualized abdominal exercises
5. Cool-down activities
6. Pelvic floor exercises
7. Relaxation techniques
8. Labor and delivery techniques
9. Educational information
10. Postpartum exercise instruction (e.g., when to begin exercises, how to safely progress, precautions) because the patient may not be attending a postpartum class. Include education regarding body mechanics relative to child care.

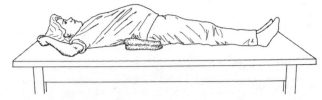

FIGURE 23.7 To prevent inferior vena cava compression when the patient is lying supine, a folded towel can be placed under the right side of the pelvis so the patient is tipped slightly to the left.

sequence for teaching an exercise class is listed in Box 23.3.[1,54,62,66]

Guidelines and techniques for exercise instruction are included in this section.[1,20,21,23,40,46,48,54,62,66] Interventions for special situations such as cesarean childbirth and high-risk pregnancy are described in the following sections.

## Guidelines for Managing the Pregnant Woman

Suggest that your patients discuss with their physicians any guidelines or restrictions to exercise before engaging in an exercise program, either in a class or on a one-to-one basis. As always, follow your state practice act for physical therapy regarding referral, evaluation, and treatment.

***Examination.*** Individually examine each woman before participation to screen for pre-existing musculoskeletal problems, posture, and fitness level.

***Education.*** Educate your patients that increased uterine cramping *may* occur with moderate activity; this is acceptable as long as the cramping stops when the activity is completed. Teach your patient all exercise guidelines and precautions so that exercises may be carried out safely at home. Include the following:

- Do not exceed 5 minutes of supine positioning at any one time after the first trimester of pregnancy to avoid vena cava compression by the uterus. Educate your patients that compression of the vena cava also occurs with motionless standing. For supine exercise, place a small wedge or rolled towel under the right hip to lessen the effects of uterine compression on abdominal vessels and improve cardiac output. The wedge turns the patient slightly toward the left (Fig. 23.7).[1] This modification is

also helpful during examination and treatment when the patient is positioned supine.
- To avoid the effects of orthostatic hypotension, instruct the woman to always rise slowly when moving from lying down or sitting to standing positions.
- Discourage breath-holding and avoid activities that tend to elicit the Valsalva maneuver because this may lead to undesirable downward forces on the uterus and pelvic floor. In addition, breath-holding causes stress to the cardiovascular system in terms of blood pressure and heart rate.
- Break frequently for fluid replenishment. The risk of dehydration during exercise is increased in pregnancy.
- Encourage complete bladder emptying before exercise. A full bladder places increased stress on an already weakened pelvic floor.
- Include appropriate warm-up and cool-down activities.
- Modify or discontinue any exercise that causes pain.
- Limit activities in which single-leg weight bearing is required, such as standing leg kicks. Besides possible loss of balance, these activities can promote sacroiliac or pubic symphysis discomfort.

***Stretching/flexibility.*** Choose stretching exercises that are specific to a single muscle or muscle group; do not involve several groups at once. Asymmetric stretching or stretching multiple muscle groups can promote joint instability.

- Avoid ballistic movements.
- Do not allow any joint to be taken beyond its normal physiologic range.
- Use caution with hamstring and adductor stretches. Overstretching of these muscle groups can increase pelvic instability or hypermobility.

***Muscle performance.*** Recommendations and adaptations for pelvic floor training, general strengthening, and cardiopulmonary conditioning during pregnancy and postpartum are described in the exercise section of this chapter. Exercises to prepare for labor and delivery are also described in the exercise section.

***Overexertion or complications.*** Observe participants closely for signs of overexertion or complications. The following signs are reasons to *discontinue exercise* and *contact a physician*[20,21]:

- Persistent pain, especially in the chest, pelvic girdle, or low back

- Leakage of amniotic fluid
- Uterine contractions that persist beyond the exercise session
- Vaginal bleeding
- Decreased fetal movements
- Persistent shortness of breath
- Irregular heartbeat
- Tachycardia
- Dizziness/faintness
- Swelling/pain in the calf (rule out phlebitis)
- Difficulty in walking

NOTE: Keep in mind when developing intervention programs that most modalities are *contraindicated* in pregnancy. Superficial heat or ice may be beneficial along with manual techniques prenatally to relieve pain/spasm and improve circulation. Muscle energy techniques, with *light* resistance, are often indicated for pelvic instability. Electric stimulation may be added postpartum to modulate pain and to stimulate muscle contractions, respectively. Ultrasound may be helpful in cases of poor episiotomy healing and painful scar tissue.

## Recommendations for Fitness Exercise

NOTE: These recommendations are for pregnant women with no maternal or fetal risk factors.[1,6,13–16,20,21,23,29,39,44,45,48,53,54,57,60,62,66]

- It is strongly recommended for all women to participate in mild to moderate exercise, for both strength and cardiopulmonary benefits, 15 to 30 minutes/session, most days of the week. Individualized programs, based on pre-pregnancy fitness level, are preferable.[20,21]
- Currently, there are no data in humans suggesting that pregnant women need to decrease their intensity of exercise or lower their target heart rates, but because of decreased oxygen supply, they should modify exercise intensity according to their tolerance. Conventional (age-based) target heart rate zones may be too aggressive for the average pregnant patient. Use of the Borg scale of perceived exertion (Box 23.4) is more appropriate in this population, with exertion between 12 and 14 suggested during pregnancy.[6,21] When fatigued, a woman should stop exercising and never exercise to exhaustion.
- Activities to avoid include contact sports, anything with a high risk of abdominal trauma or falling, high-altitude activities (greater than 6000 ft), and scuba diving. The fetus is at increased risk of decompression sickness during scuba diving.[21]
- Nonweight-bearing aerobic exercises such as stationary cycling, swimming, or water aerobics will minimize the risk of injury throughout pregnancy and the postpartum period.
- If the woman cannot safely maintain balance because of the shifting and increasing weight, have her modify exercises that could result in falling and injury to herself or the fetus.

| BOX 23.4 | Borg Rating Scale for Perceived Exertion[6] |
|---|---|

6—Very, very light
7
8
9—Very light
10
11—Fairly light
12
13—Moderately hard
14
15—Hard
16
17—Very hard
18
19—Very, very hard
20—Exhaustion

- Adequate caloric intake for nutrition, adequate fluid intake, and appropriate clothing for heat dissipation are critical.
- Resumption of prepregnancy exercise routines during the postpartum period should be gradual. Initiation of pelvic floor exercises immediately postpartum may reduce symptoms and duration of incontinence.[44,45,57]
- Physiologic and morphologic changes of pregnancy continue for a minimum of 4 to 6 weeks postpartum. Encourage continued joint protection if the woman is nursing. Breastfeeding women can be reassured that moderate exercise does not impair quantity of breast milk or infant growth. There may be a short-term increase in lactic acid secreted in breast milk after exercise; if the baby appears to eat less after an exercise session, this can easily be remedied by nursing before exercise.[20,21]

## Precautions and Contraindications to Exercise

There are some circumstances where exercise is contraindicated or requires very specific restrictions and precautions.[1,8,20,21,31,48–50,54,60,62,66] Discussion of interventions for patients with high-risk pregnancy are described later in this chapter.

### Absolute Contraindications

- Incompetent cervix: early dilation of the cervix before the pregnancy is full term
- Vaginal bleeding, especially second or third trimester
- Placenta previa: placenta is located on the uterus in a position where it may detach before the baby is delivered.
- Multiple gestation with risk of premature labor.[20,49]
- Pre-eclampsia: pregnancy-induced hypertension
- Rupture of membranes: loss of amniotic fluid before the onset of labor.

● Premature labor: labor beginning before the 37th week of pregnancy
● Maternal heart disease, thyroid disease or serious respiratory disorder
● Maternal type 1 diabetes
● Intrauterine growth retardation

## Precautions to Exercise
The woman with one or more of the following conditions may participate in an exercise program under close observation by a physician[1,8,48] and a therapist as long as no further complications arise. Exercises may require modification.[20,21]

● Gestational diabetes
● Severe anemia
● Systemic infection
● Extreme fatigue
● Musculoskeletal complaints and/or pain
● Overheating
● Extreme obesity or extreme underweight/eating disorder
● Diastasis recti

## Critical Areas of Emphasis and Selected Exercise Techniques

### Posture Exercises
The growing fetus places added stress on postural muscles as the center of gravity shifts forward and upward and the spine shifts to compensate and maintain stability. In addition, after delivery, activities involving holding and caring for the baby stress postural muscles. Muscles that require emphasis for strengthening and stretching are listed. General exercise descriptions are listed in respective chapters. Subsequent sections describe adaptations of exercises specific for the pregnant woman.

### Stretching (with Caution)
Flexibility and stretching exercises are implemented with caution. Remember that connective tissues and supporting joint structures are at increased risk of injury from forceful stresses during pregnancy and the immediate postpartum period because of hormonal changes.

● Upper neck extensors and scalenes (Chapter 16)
● Scapular protractors, shoulder internal rotators, and levator scapulae (Chapter 17)
● Low back extensors (Chapter 16)
● Hip flexors, adductors, and hamstrings (Chapter 20). Caution: women with pelvic instabilities should not overstretch.
● Ankle plantarflexors (Chapter 22)

### Strengthening (Low Intensity)
● Upper neck flexors, lower neck and upper thoracic extensors (Chapter 16)
● Scapular retractors and depressors (Chapter 17)
● Shoulder external rotators (Chapter 17)
● Trunk flexors (abdominals), particularly lower abdominals, with modifications noted below (Chapter 16)

● Hip extensors (Chapter 20)
● Knee extensors (Chapter 21)
● Ankle dorsiflexors (Chapter 22)

### Corrective Exercises for Diastasis Recti
A check for diastasis recti must always be performed before initiating abdominal exercise. Only the corrective exercises (head lift or head lift with pelvic tilt) should be used until the separation is corrected to 2 cm (two fingerwidths) or less.[48]

### Head lift
*Patient position and procedure:* Hook-lying with her hands crossed over midline at the level of the diastasis for support. Have the woman exhale and lift only her head off the floor or until the point just before a bulge appears. At the same time, her hands should gently approximate the rectus muscles toward midline (Fig. 23.8). Then have the woman lower her head slowly and relax. This exercise emphasizes the rectus abdominis muscle and minimizes the obliques. Some women may not be able to successfully reach over their abdomen. In this case, the use of a sheet wrapped around the trunk at the level of the separation can be used to provide support and approximation.[48]

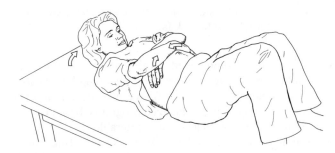

FIGURE 23.8 Corrective exercise for diastasis recti. The patient gently approximates the rectus muscle toward the midline by pulling with the crossed arms.

### Head Lift with Pelvic Tilt
*Patient position and procedure*: Hook-lying. The arms are crossed over the diastasis for support as above. Have the patient slowly lift her head off the floor while approximating the rectus muscles and performing a posterior pelvic tilt, then slowly lower her head and relax. All abdominal contractions should be performed with an exhalation so that intra-abdominal pressure is minimized.

### Abdominal Muscle Exercises
As pregnancy progresses, the abdominals will undergo extreme overstretching. Therefore, exercise must be adapted to meet the needs of each individual, and periodic re-assessment must be done (approximately every 4 weeks during pregnancy). The following exercises progress from least to most strenuous.

NOTE: Keep in mind the 5-minute time limit for supine positioning when prescribing abdominal exercises after 13 weeks' gestation.

## Pelvic Tilt Exercise

*Patient position and procedure:* Quadruped (on hands and knees). Instruct the patient to perform a posterior pelvic tilt. While the patient keeps her back straight, have her isometrically tighten (imagine drawing in) the lower abdominals and hold, then release and perform an anterior tilt through very small range.

● For additional exercise, while holding the abdominals in and the back straight, have the woman laterally flex the trunk to the right (side-bend to the right), looking at the right hip, then reverse to the left.
● Have the woman practice pelvic tilt exercises in a variety of positions, including side-lying and standing.

## Leg Sliding

*Patient position and procedure:* Hook-lying with pelvis in a posterior tilt. Instruct the woman to hold the pelvic tilt as she slides one foot along the floor until the leg is straight or to the point at which she is unable to maintain the pelvic tilt. Have her slowly slide the leg back to the starting position, then repeat with the other leg. Breathing should be coordinated with the exercise so that abdominal contractions occur with exhalation.

## Trunk Curls

● Curl-downs and curl-ups are classic abdominal exercises for rectus abdominis strengthening and can be used *if tolerated and no diastasis recti is present.* Have a pregnant patient protect the linea alba with crossed hands (see Fig. 23.8) while performing trunk curls.
● Diagonal curls are carried out to strengthen the oblique muscles. Have the woman lift one shoulder toward the outside of the opposite knee as she curls up and down and protects the linea alba with crossed hands.

## Modified Bicycle

*Patient position and procedure:* The woman is supine with one lower extremity flexed and the other partially extended. The lower abdominals stabilize the pelvis as the lower extremities flex and extend in an alternating pattern as if cycling. The further the lower extremities extend, the greater the resistance. In order to not strain the back, the woman must keep it flat against the floor by controlling the arc of the cycling pattern.

PRECAUTION: Leg-lowering exercises cause excessive strain on the low back and should not be performed during pregnancy; they may be resumed postpartum with the following precautions and modifications. The legs should be lowered only through the range in which control of the posterior pelvic tilt and flattening of the low back is maintained. If low back strain is felt or if the lumbar spine begins to arch, this exercise should not be performed. The pull of the psoas major may cause a shear force on the lumbar vertebrae, and the supporting ligaments may be strained.

## Stabilization Exercises

Exercises for activating the abdominal and low back muscles and developing control of their stabilizing function in the lumbar spine and pelvis are described in Chapter 16. They should be initiated and progressed at the intensity that the woman is able to safely control. Slow, controlled breathing is emphasized while developing the stabilizing function of the muscles.

### Precautions

● Because the trunk muscles are contracting isometrically in many of these abdominal exercises, there is a tendency to hold the breath; this is detrimental to the blood pressure and heart rate. Caution the woman to maintain a relaxed breathing pattern and exhale during the exertion phase of each exercise.
● If diastasis recti is present, adapt the stabilization exercises to protect the linea alba as described for the corrective curl-up. Any progression of postpartum abdominal strengthening exercises should be postponed until the diastasis has been corrected to two fingerwidths or less.

## Pelvic Motion Training

These exercises are helpful in cases of postural back pain; they are beneficial for improving proprioceptive awareness as well as lumbar, pelvic, and hip mobility.[24]

### "The Pelvic Clock"

*Patient position and procedure:* Hook lying. The patient's legs may move slightly while performing this exercise. Ask the woman to visualize the face of a clock on her lower abdomen. The umbilicus is 12 o'clock and the pubic symphysis is 6 o'clock.

● Have her begin with gentle movements from 12 to 6 o'clock (the basic pelvic tilt exercise).
● Then ask her to move from 3 o'clock (weight shifted to left hip) to 9 o'clock (weight shifted to the right hip).
● Then move in a clockwise manner from 12 to 3 to 6 to 9 and then back to 12 o'clock.

With practice, this will become a very smooth and rhythmical movement and will not require such concentration on each number of the clock. Continue relaxed breathing throughout the exercise and do not force any part of the movement. If the patient has difficulty with the motion, make the clock "smaller" until coordination improves.[24]

### Pelvic Clock Progressions

● Use the visual imagery of cutting the face of the clock in half so that there is a right side and a left side, or a top half and a bottom half. Have the woman move her pelvis through the arc on the one side and back through the middle of the clock, and then move the pelvis through the opposite side and back through the middle. Initially, the woman may notice asymmetry when comparing the halves; this will improve with time.
● Once the patient understands and is able to perform the clockwise pattern have her do counterclockwise motions with all of the above activities, and then progress the exercises to the sitting position.[24]

## Modified Upper and Lower Extremity Strengthening

As the abdomen enlarges, it becomes impossible to comfortably assume the prone position. Exercises that are usually performed in the prone position must be modified.

### Standing Push-Ups

*Patient position and procedure:* Standing, facing a wall, feet pointing straight forward, shoulder-width apart, and approximately an arm-length away from the wall. The palms are placed on the wall at shoulder height. Have the woman slowly bend the elbows, bringing her upper body close to the wall, maintaining a stable pelvic tilt, and keeping the heels on the floor. Her elbows should be shoulder height. She then slowly pushes with her arms, bringing the body back to the original position.

### Supine Bridging

*Patient position and procedure:* Supine in the hook-lying position. Have the patient perform a posterior pelvic tilt and then lift her pelvis off the floor. She can do repetitive bridges, or hold the bridge position and alternately flex and extend her upper extremities to emphasize the stabilization function of the hip extensors and trunk musculature (see Fig. 20.21).

### Quadruped Leg Raising

*Patient position and procedure:* On hands and knees (hands may be in fists or palms open and flat). Instruct the woman to first perform a posterior pelvic tilt, and then slowly lift one leg, extending the hip to a level no higher than the pelvis while maintaining the posterior pelvic tilt (Fig. 23.9). She then slowly lowers the leg and repeats with the opposite side. The knee may remain flexed or can be straightened throughout the exercise. Monitor this exercise and discontinue if there is stress on the sacroiliac joints or

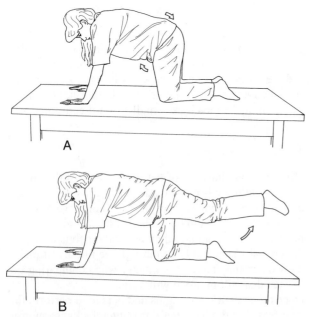

FIGURE 23.9 All-fours leg-raising. (*A*) Patient assumes quadruped position with posterior pelvic tilt. (*B*) Leg is raised only until it is in line with the trunk.

ligaments. If the woman cannot stabilize the pelvis while lifting the leg, have her just slide one leg posteriorly along the floor and return (see Fig. 16.29A).

### Modified Squatting

Wall slides and supported squatting exercises are used to strengthen the hip and knee extensors for good body mechanics and also to help stretch the perineal area for flexibility during the delivery process. In addition, if the woman wishes to use squatting for labor and delivery, the muscles *must* be strengthened and endurance trained in advance.

- *Patient position and procedure:* Standing with back against a wall and her feet shoulder-width apart. Have the woman slide her back down the wall as her hips and knees flex only as far as is comfortable, then slides back up (see Fig. 20.24).
- *Patient position and procedure:* Standing with feet shoulder-width apart or wider, facing a counter, chair, or wall on which the woman can rest her hands and/or forearms for support. Have the woman slowly squat as far as is comfortable, keeping knees apart and over the feet and keeping the back straight. To protect her feet, she should wear shoes with good arch support. A woman with knee problems should perform only partial range of the squat. For optimal success with squatting during stage 2 of labor (pushing), increase the duration of the squat gradually to 60 to 90 seconds as tolerated.

### Scapular Retraction

When scapular retraction exercises become difficult in the prone position, the woman should continue strengthening in the sitting or standing position (see Figs. 17.45 and 17.46).

### Perineum and Adductor Flexibility

In addition to the modified squatting exercises described in the preceding text, these flexibility exercises prepare the legs and pelvis for childbirth.[48,54,62]

### Self-Stretching

- *Patient position and procedure:* Supine or side-lying. Instruct the patient to abduct the hips and pull the knees toward the sides of her chest and hold the position for as long as is comfortable (at least to the count of 10).
- *Patient position and procedure:* Sitting on a short stool with the hips abducted as far as possible and feet flat on the floor. Have her flex forward slightly at the hips (keeping the back straight), or have her gently press her knees outward with her hands for an additional stretch.

## Pelvic Floor Awareness, Training, and Strengthening

Pelvic floor muscle training is a valuable modality regardless of a patient's presentation or cause of symptoms.[3,9,34,44,45,57,62,66] The majority of women are unfamiliar with the presence of the pelvic floor muscles, and even less aware of their function and role in daily activities. Intervention is slowly becoming more common during the childbearing years owing to the stress of pregnancy, labor, and delivery on the pelvic floor. Pelvic floor anatomy, function, and dysfunction are described in the first section of this chapter.

### Focus on Evidence

A Cochrane review of 43 randomized trials concluded that pelvic floor muscle training is an effective treatment for stress or mixed urinary incontinence, and is better than no treatment or placebo.[34] Functional improvements (decreased urinary incontinence and improved pelvic floor strength) have been noted in late pregnancy and from 3 to 12 months postpartum in a number of studies.[44,45,57] For optimal outcomes, pelvic floor contractions should be incorporated into routine ADLs, particularly activities that are "triggers" for leakage due to increased intra-abdominal pressure; used for stabilization prior to coughing or sneezing; and continued for life-long health benefits.[34]

Begin pelvic floor exercise training with an empty bladder. Gravity-assisted positioning (hips higher than the heart, such as supported bridge or elbows/knees position) may be indicated initially for some women with extreme weakness and proprioceptive deficits. Positional changes are introduced as strength and awareness improve (supine, side-lying, quadruped, sitting, standing).

### Contract–Relax

Instruct the woman to tighten the pelvic floor as if attempting to stop urine flow or hold back gas. Hold for 3 to 5 seconds and relax for at least the same length of time. Repeat up to 10 times (if performed with proper technique). With significant coordination dysfunction or fatigue, substitution with the gluteals, abdominals, or hip adductors may occur. To maximize proprioception and motor learning, it is important to emphasize isolation of the pelvic floor and avoid the substitute muscle actions. In addition, watch for Valsalva; if necessary, have the woman count out loud to encourage normal breathing patterns.

### Quick Contractions

Have the woman perform quick, repeated contractions of the pelvic floor muscles while maintaining a normal breathing rate and keeping accessory muscles relaxed. Try for 15 to 20 repetitions per set. This type II fiber response is important to develop in order to withstand pressure from above, especially with coughing or sneezing.

### "Elevator" Exercise

Instruct the woman to imagine riding in an elevator. As the elevator goes up from one floor to the next, she contracts the pelvic floor muscles a little more. As strength and awareness improve, add more "floors" to the sequence of the contraction. Another way to increase difficulty is by asking the woman to relax the muscles gradually, as if the elevator were descending one floor at a time. This component requires an eccentric contraction and is very challenging.

### Pelvic Floor Relaxation

- Instruct the woman to contract the pelvic floor as in the strengthening exercise, then allow total voluntary release and relaxation of the pelvic floor. Use of the "elevator" imagery should also be emphasized, with particular attention to taking the elevator to the "basement."
- Pelvic floor relaxation is closely linked with effective breathing and relaxation of the facial muscles. Instruct the woman to concentrate on a slow, deep breath and allow the pelvic floor to completely relax. Relaxation of the pelvic floor is extremely important during stage 2 of labor and vaginal delivery.[28,48,62]
- Chronic inability to relax the pelvic floor muscles may lead to impairments such as hypertonus, pain with intercourse, or voiding dysfunction. Please refer to the earlier information on pelvic pain syndromes. If the patient presents with these symptoms, increase the rest time between pelvic floor contractions and sets; also use submaximal contractions to improve awareness of tension vs relaxation. Use of surface EMG for muscle re-education is invaluable with these impairments for increasing awareness of holding patterns, pain inhibition, and resting tone.

## Relaxation and Breathing Exercises for Use During Labor

Developing the ability to relax requires awareness of stress and muscle tension. Techniques of conscious relaxation allow the individual to control and cope with a variety of imposed stresses by being mentally alert to the task at hand while relaxing tense muscles that are superfluous to the activity (see Chapter 4). This is particularly important during labor and delivery when there are times that the woman should relax and allow the physiologic processes to occur without excessive tension in unrelated muscles.[48] Additional relaxation techniques for managing stress are described in Chapter 14. The following guidelines are most effective for the pregnant woman if consistently practiced in preparation for labor and delivery.

### Visual Imagery

Use instrumental music and verbal guidance. Instruct the woman to concentrate on a relaxing image such as the beach, mountains, or a favorite vacation spot. Suggest that she focus on the same image throughout the pregnancy so that the image can be called up to the conscious level when recognizing the need to relax during labor.

### Muscle Setting

- Have the woman lie in a comfortable position.
- Have her begin with the lower body. Instruct her to gently contract and then relax first the muscles in the feet, then legs, thighs, pelvic floor, and buttocks.
- Next progress to the upper extremities and trunk, then to the neck and facial muscles.
- Reinforce the importance of remaining awake and aware of the contrasting sensations of the muscles.

Emphasize "softening" of the muscles as the session continues.

◉ Add deep, slow, relaxed breathing to the routine.

### Selective Tension

Progress the training by emphasizing awareness of muscles contracting in one part of the body while remaining relaxed in other parts. For example, while she is tensing the fist and upper extremity, the feet and legs should be limp. Reinforce the comparison between the two sensations and the ability to control both tension and relaxation.

### Breathing

◉ General breathing techniques are described in Chapter 25. Slow, deep diaphragmatic breathing is the most efficient method for exchange of air to use with relaxation techniques and for controlled breathing during labor.
◉ Teach the woman to relax the abdomen during inspiration so that it feels as though the abdominal cavity is "filling up." During exhalation, the abdominal cavity becomes smaller; active contraction of the abdominal muscles is not necessary with relaxed breathing.
◉ To prevent hyperventilation, emphasize a slow rate of breathing. Caution the woman to decrease the intensity of the breathing if she experiences dizziness or feels tingling in the lips and fingers.

### Relaxation and Breathing During Labor

#### First Stage

As labor progresses, the contractions of the uterus become stronger, longer, and closer together. Relaxation during the contractions becomes more difficult. Provide the woman with suggested techniques to assist in relaxation.[49]

◉ Ensure the woman has emotional support from the father, family member, or special friend to provide encouragement and assist with overall comfort.
◉ Seek comfortable positions including walking, hands and knees, lying on pillows, or sitting on a Swiss ball; include gentle repeated motions such as pelvic rocking.
◉ Breathe slowly with each contraction; use the visual imagery and relax with each contraction. Some women find it helpful to focus their attention on a specific visual object. Other suggestions include singing, talking, or moaning during each contraction to prevent breath-holding and encourage slow breathing.
◉ During transition (near the end of the first stage) there is often an urge to push. Teach the woman to use quick blowing techniques, using the cheeks, not the abdominal muscles, to overcome the desire to push until the appropriate time.
◉ Massage or apply pressure to any areas that hurt such as the low back. Using the hands may help distract the focus from the contractions.
◉ Apply heat or cold for local symptoms; wipe the face with a wet wash cloth.

#### Second Stage

Once dilation of the cervix has occurred, the woman may become active in the birth process by assisting the uterus during a contraction in pushing the baby down the birth canal.[48] Teach her the following techniques:

◉ While bearing down, take in a breath, contract the abdominal wall, and slowly breathe out. This will cause increased pressure within the abdomen along with relaxation of the pelvic floor.

PRECAUTION: Tell the woman that if she holds her breath, there will be increased tension and resistance in the pelvic floor. In addition, exertion with a closed glottis, known as the Valsalva maneuver, has adverse effects on the cardiovascular system.

◉ For maximum efficiency, maintain relaxation in the extremities, especially the legs and perineum. Keeping the face and jaw relaxed assists with this.
◉ Between contractions, perform total body relaxation.
◉ As the baby is delivered, just "let go" and breathe with light pants or groans to relax the pelvic floor as it stretches.

## Unsafe Postures and Exercises During Pregnancy

***Knee–chest position with buttocks elevated above heart level.*** An air embolism, although rare, can occur when the buttocks are elevated and the uterus moves superiorly. The pressure change causes air to be introduced into the vagina and uterus, where it can enter the circulatory system through the open placental site. A pregnant woman is at risk *only* if bleeding or other symptoms of early placental detachment are present. The pregnant woman should be instructed not to assume this position for 6 weeks postpartum.[40,46]

***Bilateral straight-leg raising.*** This exercise typically places more stress on the abdominal muscles and low back than they can tolerate. It can cause back injury or diastasis recti, and therefore should not be attempted.

***"Fire hydrant" exercise.*** This exercise is performed on hands and knees, and one hip is abducted and externally rotated at a time (the "image" of a dog at a fire hydrant). If the leg is elevated too high, the sacroiliac joint and lumbar vertebrae can be stressed. The exercise can be performed safely if hip abduction remains within the physiologic range (Fig. 23.10). It should be avoided by any woman who has pre-existing sacroiliac joint symptoms or if these symptoms develop.

***All-fours (quadruped) hip extension.*** This exercise can be performed safely only as explained earlier in this chapter (see Fig. 23.9). It becomes unsafe and can cause low back pain when the leg is elevated beyond the physiologic

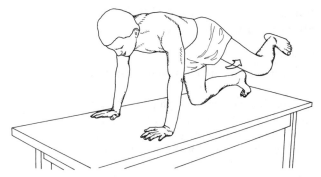

FIGURE 23.10 The fire hydrant is a potentially damaging exercise. To do this exercise correctly, the individual must stabilize the pelvis midrange, then stop the abduction external rotation motion when the hip has completed its range. The leg should not be "kicked as high as possible," or stress to the hip, sacroiliac joint, and lumbar spine results.

range of hip extension, causing the pelvis to tilt anteriorly and the lumbar spine to hyperextend.

***Unilateral weight-bearing activities.*** Weight bearing on one leg (which includes slouched standing with the majority of weight shifted to one leg and the pelvis tilted down on the opposite side) during pregnancy can cause sacroiliac joint irritation and should be avoided by women with pre-existing sacroiliac joint symptoms. Unilateral weight bearing also can cause balance problems because of the increasing body weight and shifting of the center of gravity. This posture becomes a significant problem postpartum when the woman carries her growing child on one hip. Any asymmetries become accentuated, and painful symptoms may develop.

## Exercise Critical to the Postpartum Period

After an uncomplicated vaginal delivery, exercise can be started as soon as the woman feels able to exercise, and has been cleared by her physician or midwife.[1,20,21,44,45,48,57]

***Pelvic floor strengthening.*** Exercises should be resumed as soon after the birth as possible. These exercises may increase circulation and aid healing of lacerations or episiotomy. Combining pelvic floor contractions with feeding or changing the baby may help them become integrated into the daily routine.

***Diastasis recti correction.*** The testing procedure for diastasis recti was described earlier in this chapter. The mother should be taught this test and encouraged to perform it on the third postpartum day. Corrective exercises (see Fig. 23.8) should continue until the separation is two finger-widths or less. At that time, more vigorous abdominal exercise can be resumed.

***Aerobic and strengthening exercises.*** As soon as the woman feels able, cardiopulmonary exercise can be

resumed with gradual increasing intensity. A physical examination is suggested before the onset of vigorous exercise or sport-specific training.

PRECAUTIONS: Since the woman may not be seen for exercise instruction after the delivery, inform her of the following precautions:

- If bleeding increases or turns bright red, exercise should be postponed. Tell her to rest more and allow a longer recovery time.
- Joint laxity may be present for some time after delivery, especially if breastfeeding. Precautions should be taken to protect the joints as described previously.[54,62,66] Adequate warm-up and cool-down time is important.
- Avoid the prone knee–chest position for at least 6 weeks postpartum because of the risk of air embolism.[40,46]

##  CESAREAN CHILDBIRTH

A ***cesarean section*** is the delivery of a baby through an incision in the abdominal wall and uterus rather than through the pelvis and vagina.[31,50] General, spinal, or epidural anesthesia may be used.

### Significance to Physical Therapists

Cesarean section (C-section) delivery is now at an all-time high in the United States. In 2004, the rate was 29.1% of births, totaling 1.2 million deliveries.[69] The cesarean birth rate in the United States has fluctuated greatly over the last three to four decades, in part depending on the type of hospital and the population it serves. Since the early 1990s, the American College of Obstetricians and Gynecologists (ACOG) has discouraged repeat C-sections as routine practice; however, historically more than 33% of all Cesareans are repeat procedures. The Vaginal Birth After Cesarean (VBAC) movement has been quite visible, as historically more than one-third of all C-sections are repeat procedures. Recently, the perceived "convenience" of a C-section is becoming a factor, leading to increases in not only repeat but also elective C-sections. In addition to the appeal of scheduling a delivery date, there is some evidence that cesarean delivery may aid in prevention of future pelvic floor dysfunction.[61] Although the overall number of women choosing Cesarean delivery remains small, from 2001 to 2003 the rate of elective C-sections in first-time mothers grew 36%.[68]

Pregnant women need to be informed as to the risks and benefits of each choice in order to make informed decisions. These statistics are the focus of much discussion within obstetrics, and because of this high incidence and new trends, physical therapists must be prepared to address these issues with all pregnant patients.[31,41,48–51,53,55,62]

Women who have had Cesarean delivery may still require pelvic floor rehabilitation. Many women experience a lengthy labor, including prolonged second stage (pushing), before a C-section is deemed necessary. Therefore, the pelvic floor musculature and the pudendal nerves are not always spared the stress of labor. Also, pregnancy itself creates significant strain on the pelvic floor musculature and tissues.

Postpartum intervention for the woman who has had cesarean delivery is similar to that of the woman who has had a vaginal delivery. However, a C-section is major abdominal surgery with all the risks and complications of such surgeries, and therefore the woman may also require general postsurgical rehabilitation.[31,50,62] Impairments and management guidelines are summarized in Box 23.5.

All childbirth preparation classes do not adequately educate and prepare couples for the experience of a cesarean delivery. As a result, the woman with an unplanned C-section frequently feels as if her body has failed her, causing her to have more conflicting emotions than a woman who has experienced a vaginal delivery.

## Suggested Activities for the Patient Following a Cesarean Section

### Exercises

● Instruct the woman during her pregnancy in all appropriate exercises, if she is able.
● Instruct the woman to begin preventive exercises as soon as possible during the recovery period.[31,48,49]
  • Initiate ankle pumping, active lower extremity ROM, and walking to promote circulation and prevent venous stasis.
  • Initiate pelvic floor exercises to regain tone and control of the muscles of the perineum.
  • Deep breathing and coughing or huffing is used to prevent pulmonary complications (see instructions below).
● Progress abdominal exercises slowly. Check for diastasis recti and protect the area of the incision to improve comfort. Initiate nonstressful muscle-setting techniques

---

**BOX 23.5**
MANAGEMENT GUIDELINES—Postcesarean Section

**Potential Impairments and Functional Limitations:**
Risk of pulmonary or vascular complications
Postsurgical pain and discomfort
Development of adhesions at incisional site
Faulty posture
Pelvic floor dysfunction
• urinary or fecal incontinence
• organ prolapse
• hypertonus
• poor proprioceptive awareness and disuse atrophy
Abdominal weakness, diastasis recti
General functional restrictions of post delivery

| Plan of Care | Interventions |
|---|---|
| 1. Improve pulmonary function and decrease the risk of pneumonia. | 1. Breathing instruction, coughing and/or huffing. |
| 2. Decrease incisional pain with coughing, movement, or breast feeding. | 2. Postoperative TENS; support incision with pillow when coughing or breastfeeding. Incisional support with pillow or hands with movement Education regarding incisional care and risk of injury. |
| 3. Prevent postsurgical vascular complications. | 3. Active leg exercises. Early ambulation. |
| 4. Enhance incisional circulation and healing; prevent adhesion formation. | 4. Gentle abdominal exercise with incisional support. Scar mobilization and friction massage. |
| 5. Decrease postsurgical discomfort from flatulence, itching, or catheter. | 5. Positioning instruction, massage, and supportive exercises. |
| 6. Correct posture. | 6. Posture instruction, particularly regarding child care. |
| 7. Prevent injury and reduce low back pain. | 7. Instruction in incisional splinting and positioning for ADLs. Body mechanics instruction. |
| 8. Prevent pelvic floor dysfunction. | 8. Pelvic floor exercises. Education regarding risk factors and types of pelvic floor dysfunction. |
| 9. Develop abdominal strength. | 9. Abdominal exercise progression, including corrective exercises for diastasis recti. |

and progress as tolerated, based on the degree of separation.[31,48,49]

● Teach posture correction as necessary. Retrain postural awareness and help realign posture with indicated therapeutic exercise. Develop control of the shoulder girdle muscles as they respond to the increased stress of caring for the new baby.

● Reinforce the value of deep diaphragmatic breathing techniques for pulmonary ventilation, especially when exercising, and relaxed breathing techniques to relieve stress and promote relaxation.

● The woman should wait at least 6 to 8 weeks before resuming vigorous exercise. Emphasize the importance of progressing at a safe and controlled pace and not expecting to begin at her prepregnancy level.

### Coughing or Huffing

Coughing is difficult because of incisional pain. An alternative is huffing.[48] A huff is an outward breath caused by the upper abdominals contracting up and in against the diaphragm to push air out of the lungs. The abdominals are pulled up and in, rather than pushed out, causing decreased pressure in the abdominal cavity and less strain on the incision. Huffing must be done quickly to generate sufficient force to expel mucus. Instruct the patient to support the incision with a pillow or the hands and say "ha" forcefully and repetitively while contracting the abdominal muscles.

### Interventions to Relieve Intestinal Gas Pains

● *Abdominal massage or kneading.* Have the patient lie supine or on the left side. This is very effective and typically done with either long or circular strokes. Begin on the right side at the ascending colon, stroking upward, then stroke across the transverse colon from right to left and down the descending colon, then finish with an "S" stroke along the sigmoid colon.

● *Pelvic tilting and/or bridging.* These can be done in conjunction with massage.

● *Bridge and twist.* Have the patient maintain a position of bridging while twisting her hips to the right and left. This position may also facilitate air embolism and therefore should be used with caution in the early postpartum period.

● *Partial abdominal curl-up.* Avoid strain to the linea alba.

### Scar Mobilization

Cross-friction massage should be initiated around the incision site as soon as sufficient healing has occurred. This will minimize adhesions that may contribute to postural problems and back pain.

## ● HIGH-RISK PREGNANCY

A *high-risk pregnancy* is one that is complicated by disease or problems that put the mother or fetus at risk for illness or death. Conditions may be pre-existing, induced by pregnancy, or caused by an abnormal physiologic reaction

during pregnancy.[32] The goal of medical intervention is to prevent preterm delivery, usually through use of bed rest, restriction of activity, and medications, when appropriate. Various factors may lead to high-risk pregnancies; specialized care is required for successful outcomes.[32,36,53–55,62]

### High-Risk Conditions

*Preterm rupture of membranes.* The amniotic sac breaks, and amniotic fluid is lost before onset of labor. This can be dangerous to the fetus if it occurs before fetal development is complete. Labor may begin spontaneously after the membranes rupture. The chance for fetal infection also increases when the protection of the amniotic sac is lost. Leakage of amniotic fluid is an indication for immediate medical attention.

*Premature onset of labor.* Labor that begins before 37 weeks of gestation or before completion of fetal development is considered premature. Fetal life is endangered if delivery occurs too early.

*Incompetent cervix.* An incompetent cervix is the painless dilation of the cervix that occurs in the second trimester (after 16 weeks' gestation) or early in the third trimester of pregnancy. This may lead to premature membrane rupture and delivery of a fetus too small to survive.

*Placenta previa.* The placenta attaches too low on the uterus, near the cervix. As the cervix dilates, the placenta begins to separate from the uterus and may present before the fetus, thus endangering fetal life. The primary symptom is intermittent, recurrent, or painless bleeding that increases in intensity.

*Pregnancy-related hypertension or pre-eclampsia.* Characterized by hypertension, protein in the urine, and severe fluid retention, pre-eclampsia can progress to maternal convulsions, coma, and death if it becomes severe (eclampsia). It usually occurs in the third trimester and disappears after birth. The cause is not understood.

*Multiple gestation.* More than one fetus forms. Complications of multiple gestation include premature onset of labor and birth, increased incidence of perinatal mortality, lower birth weight infants, and increased incidence of maternal complications (e.g., hypertension).

*Diabetes.* Diabetes can be present before pregnancy or may occur as a result of the physiological stress of pregnancy. *Gestational diabetes,* which presents in pregnancy, affects 4% to 7% of pregnant women and usually disappears after pregnancy, but there remains a greater tendency for development of the disease at some future time.

Unlike many of the previously discussed high-risk conditions, women with gestational diabetes may be appropriate candidates for more traditional physical therapy treatment. Supervised, individualized exercise programs are excellent options for the woman with gestational diabetes. Exercise may actually prevent gestational diabetes in obese pregnant women.[20] In particular, recumbent bicycling or arm ergometer exercises have been shown to stabilize and lower glucose levels.[53]

 **Focus on Evidence** _____

In a randomized study of overweight women with gestational diabetes ($N = 32$), the control group was treated with diet alone, while the remaining women also participated in circuit resistance training. The diet-plus-exercise group were able to postpone the use of insulin therapy until later in the pregnancy ($p < .05$) and were also prescribed less insulin overall ($p < .05$) than the diet-alone group.[8]

## Management Guidelines and Precautions for High-Risk Pregnancies

All exercise programs for high-risk populations should be individually established based on diagnosis, limitations, physical therapy examination and evaluation, and consultation with the physician. Activities must address patient needs but should not further complicate the condition.[54,62]

Management guidelines for the woman who is confined to bed because of her high-risk status are summarized in Box 23.6.

Develop good rapport with the patient and instill trust. Closely monitor the patient during all activities; re-evaluate her after each treatment and note any changes. It is also important to teach the patient self-monitoring techniques so that she will be alert to adverse reactions and respond appropriately.

- Prolonged static positioning is a primary concern. The position of choice for the high-risk patient is left side-lying, which is optimal for reducing pressure on the inferior vena cava and for maximizing cardiac output, thereby enhancing maternal and fetal circulation.
- Some exercises, especially abdominal exercises, may stimulate uterine contractions. If this occurs, modify or discontinue them.
- Monitor and report any uterine contractions, bleeding, or amniotic fluid loss.

---

**BOX 23.6**
**MANAGEMENT GUIDELINES—High-Risk Pregnancy**

**Potential Impairments and Functional Limitations:**
Primary functional limitation is inability to be out of bed and prolonged static positioning which contributes to the following:
Joint stiffness and muscle aches
Muscle weakness and disuse atrophy
Vascular complications including risk of thrombosis and decreased uterine blood flow
Decreased proprioception in distal body parts
Constipation caused by lack of exercise
Postural changes
Boredom
Emotional stress; patient may be at risk of losing the baby
Guilt from the belief that some activity caused the problem or that the patient did not take good enough care of herself
Anxiety about her home situation, older children, finances or the impending birth

| Plan of Care | Interventions |
|---|---|
| 1. Decrease stiffness. | 1. Positioning instructions; assess for supports. Facilitation of joint motion in available range. |
| 2. Maintain muscle length and bulk. | 2. Stretching and strengthening exercises within limits imposed by the physician. |
| 3. Maximize circulation; prevent deep-vein thrombosis. | 3. Ankle pumping; ROM. |
| 4. Improve proprioception. | 4. Movement activities for as many body parts as possible. |
| 5. Improve posture within available limits. | 5. Posture instruction, modified as necessary based on allowed activity level. Bed mobility and transfer techniques if able (avoid Valsalva). |
| 6. Relieve boredom. | 6. Vary activities and positioning for exercises; encourage interaction with others on bed rest. (http://www.side-lines.org) |
| 7. Enhance relaxation. | 7. Relaxation techniques/stress management. |
| 8. Prepare for delivery. | 8. Childbirth education, breathing training, and exercises to assist and prepare for labor. |
| 9. Enhance postpartum recovery. | 9. Exercise instruction and home program for postpartum period. Body mechanics instruction, particularly related to child care. |

• Do not allow the Valsalva maneuver to occur. Avoid any activities that increase intra-abdominal pressure. Body mechanics and postural instruction will stimulate abdominal contractions, so be sure the patient does not strain and closely monitor for adverse symptoms.

• Keep the exercises simple. Have the patient do them slowly, smoothly, and with minimal exertion.

• Many high-risk pregnancies result in cesarean deliveries, so educate the woman about cesarean delivery rehabilitation.

• Incorporate maximum muscle efficiency into each movement.

• Teach the patient self-monitoring techniques.

## Suggestions for Exercise Programs with High–Risk Pregnancies

The following are adaptations of interventions that have already been described that should be considered for the bed-bound patient with a high-risk pregnancy.[53,54,62]

### Positioning

• Left side-lying to prevent vena cava compression, enhance cardiac output, and decrease lower extremity edema

• Pillows between the knees and under the abdomen

• Supine positioning for short periods, with a wedge placed under the right hip to decrease inferior vena cava compression (see Fig. 23.7)

• Modified prone positioning (side-lying, partially rolled toward prone, with pillow under abdomen) to decrease low back discomfort and pressure

### Range of Motion (ROM)

• Active ROM of all joints.

• Motions should be slow, nonstressful, and through the full range if possible.

• Teach in a gravity-neutral position if antigravity ROM is too stressful.

• Individualize the number of repetitions and frequency to the woman's condition.

• Include the following exercises with the patient supine (with wedge under the right hip) or side-lying:

- Alternate knee to chest
- Ankle pumping and ankle circles
- Shoulder, elbow, and finger flexion and extension; reach to ceiling; arm circles
- Unilateral straight-leg raise in supine or side-lying position
- Unilateral active ROM in diagonal patterns for the upper and lower extremities
- Lower extremity abduction and adduction
- Pelvic tilt, bridging, gluteal setting
- Abdominal exercises (check for diastasis); these should be very low intensity and closely monitored.
- Pelvic floor exercises
- Neck motions: look up/down, turn head left/right.
- Backward shoulder circles

### Ambulation/Standing

• Almost always contraindicated; when allowed, usually will be only to use the bathroom

• Good posture in ambulation

• Tip-toe or heel walking

• Gentle, partial-range squatting

• Lower extremity rotation

### Relaxation Techniques, Bed Mobility and Transfer Activities

• Relaxation as in the uncomplicated pregnancy

• Moving up, down, side to side in bed

• Log rolling: incorporate neck, upper and lower extremities to aid movement

• Supine to sitting: use log roll technique assisted by arms

### Preparation for Labor

• Relaxation techniques

• Modified squatting: supine, sitting, or side-lying with knees to chest

• Pelvic floor relaxation

• Breathing exercises: minimize forced abdominal exhalations

### Postpartum Exercise Instruction

Instructions are the same as previously described in the uncomplicated pregnancy section.

## INDEPENDENT LEARNING ACTIVITIES

### • Critical Thinking and Discussion

1. Describe three normal changes of pregnancy that will affect exercise tolerance.

2. Explain the clinical significance of diastasis recti, the testing procedure, and the corrective exercise.

3. Differentiate between postural and sacroiliac back pain in the pregnant patient.

4. Name five risk factors for pelvic floor dysfunction.

5. What exercise guidelines are most helpful for a woman who has not exercised prior to becoming pregnant?

6. Discuss optimal positioning for an uncomplicated labor and delivery in terms of biomechanics, gravity, and energy conservation.

7. Vaginal delivery places great stretch and compression on which nerve?

### • Laboratory Practice

1. Practice giving instructions to a lab partner on how to perform the following exercises. Observe that they are being done correctly. Reverse the experience and provide feedback.

Diastasis recti exercises
Pelvic clock exercises
Breathing and relaxation for the different stages of labor and delivery

2. Practice giving instructions and get verbal feedback as to the success of instructions for the pelvic floor awareness training and strengthening exercises

3. Observe an exercise class for pregnant women. Critique the effectiveness and inclusiveness of the instruction.

## ● Case Studies

1. Ms. V. is a 32-year-old pregnant woman referred with a diagnosis of "low back pain," that became severe at 24 weeks' gestation. She reports (L) lumbar/thoracic, (R) anterior rib/pectoral, and cervical symptoms, which are worsening as the pregnancy progresses. Before her pregnancy, she wore a custom-made bra (32-MM), which is now much too small and provides inadequate support. Wearing this bra greatly increases her cervical and upper trapezius symptoms. Wearing a sports bra or standing more than 10 to 15 minutes causes increased low back symptoms. Pain is severely limiting her daily activities both at home and in the community. She has difficulty climbing stairs, grocery shopping, doing laundry, and other household chores. She is wakened at night by pain and also reports LE numbness at night. She is a single mother of a 6-year-old son. Pertinent medical history includes: weight gain of 100 lbs. with her previous pregnancy; C-section delivery; removal of fibrocystic breast tissue three times. No systemic medical conditions or medications other than prenatal vitamins. Current weight: 238 lb, height: 5′4.

CLINICAL FINDINGS
• Postural assessment reveals marked forward-head/shoulders with internal rotation at both shoulder joints, significant lordosis (cervical and lumbar), recurvatum bilaterally, decreased longitudinal arches, increased base of support with excessive ER at both hips. All dynamic movements are pain inhibited: frequent weight shift and asymmetrical transitions, antalgic gait pattern with increased ER of hips. Lumbar extension and (L) cervical rotation most limited by pain and spasm.

Diastasis recti of 9 cm noted above umbilicus; abdominal strength 3–/5. Pelvic landmarks difficult to assess due to adipose tissue; leg lengths appear equal. Slight tenderness over pubic symphysis with palpation.

• Identify the impairments and functional limitations.
• Identify goals that deal with impairments and functional limitations.

• Develop a treatment plan to meet the goals; identify specific interventions and parameters, number of times she will be seen, and any follow-up or referrals that you believe will be necessary.

2. Mrs. W. is a 71-year-old woman with an 11-year history of urinary incontinence and urgency. She experiences frequent, large-volume accidents, using 8 to 10 large incontinence pads and 8 panty liners/day for garment protection. Voiding frequency is 13 to 16 times every 24 hours. She also reports constipation and straining for evacuation, which improves with increased fiber intake. Caffeine intake is two servings per day. Mrs. W is a nonsmoker. She is much less active with social and community activities as a result of this problem. Urodynamic testing revealed diminished bladder capacity at 150 cc and confirmed the diagnosis of detrusor instability.

Pertinent medical history includes nine pregnancies and seven live births (G9, P7) with one breech presentation. LBP and "sciatic nerve problems" of long standing were reported with lumbar fusion done when she was 44 and 48 years of age. Other surgical history includes rectocele/cystocele repair when she was 36 and partial hysterectomy when she was 37. Hypertension and asthma are both well controlled with medication.

CLINICAL FINDINGS
Pelvic floor muscle assessment reveals poor sensory awareness, decreased resting tone, and a MMT of 2/5. Patient able to hold a contraction 4 seconds and repeat 10 "quick flicks" in 10 seconds. Accessory recruitment of the abdominals noted. Pressure perineometry confirms muscle weakness with 6.35 cm of water pressure generated. Levator ani contraction is enhanced with stretch facilitation to the pelvic floor (R > L).

Abdominal strength is 3/5. Diastasis recti noted above the umbilicus of 4.5 cm. Diaphragmatic breathing pattern present, no Valsalva with exertion. All dynamic movements of the trunk are mildly restricted because of lumbar fusion.

The patient underwent physical therapy treatments approximately 18 months ago and is independent with her LB program. (Because of insurance limitations of 10 visits, the patient requested primary attention to pelvic floor dysfunction and incontinence.)

• Identify the impairments and functional limitations
• Identify goals that deal with the impairments and functional limitations
• Design a treatment plan to meet the goals; identify specific interventions and parameters, number of times she will be seen, and any follow-up or referrals that you believe will be necessary.

# REFERENCES

1. Artal, R, Wiswell, R: Exercise in Pregnancy. Williams & Wilkins, Baltimore, 1986.
2. Baker, PK: Musculoskeletal problems. In Steege, J, et al: Chronic Pelvic Pain-An Integrated Approach. WB Saunders, Philadelphia, 1998.
3. Benson, JT (ed): Female Pelvic Floor Disorders, Investigation and Management. WW Norton, New York, 1992.
4. Bo, K, et al: Transabdominal ultrasound measurement of pelvic floor muscle activity when activated directly or via a transversus abdominis muscle contraction. Neurourol Urodynam 22:582–588, 2003.
5. Boissonnault, J, Blaschak, M: Incidence of diastasis recti abdominis during the childbearing years. Phys Ther 68:1082, 1988.
6. Borg, G: Psychophysical bases of perceived exertion. Med Sci Sports Exerc 14:377–381, 1982.
7. Boston Women's Health Book Collective: The New Our Bodies, Ourselves. Simon & Schuster, New York, 1992.
8. Brankston, GN, et al: Resistance exercise decreases the need for insulin in overweight women with gestational diabetes mellitus. Am J Obstet Gynecol 190(1):188–193, 2004.
9. Bump, R, et al: Assessment of Kegel pelvic muscle exercise performance after brief verbal instruction. Am J Obstet Gynecol 165:322–329, 1991.
10. Burgio, KL, Locher, JL, et al: Behavioral versus drug treatment for urge urinary incontinence in older women. JAMA 280:1995, 1998.
11. Bursch, S: Interrater reliability of diastasis recti abdominis measurement. Phys Ther 67:1077, 1987.
12. Chiarelli, P, O'Keefe, D: Physiotherapy for the pelvic floor. Austral J Physiother 27: 4, 1981.
13. Clapp, JF: A clinical approach to exercise during pregnancy. Clin Sports Med 13:443, 1994.
14. Clapp, JF: Exercise and fetal health. J Dev Physiol 15:9, 1991.
15. Clapp, JF: Exercise during pregnancy: a clinical update. Clin Sports Med 19(2):273, 2000.
16. Clapp, JF, et al: Continuing regular exercise during pregnancy: effect of exercise volume on fetoplacental growth. Am J Obstet Gynecol 186:142–147, 2002.
17. DeLancey JOL, Richardson, AC: Anatomy of genital support. In Benson, JT (ed): Female Pelvic Floor Disorders, Investigation and Management. WW Norton, New York, 1992.
18. Depledge, J, et al: Management of symphysis pubis dysfunction during pregnancy using exercise and pelvic support belts. Phys Ther 85:1290–1300, 2005.
19. Dolan, L, et al: Stress incontinence and pelvic floor neurophysiology 15 years after the first delivery. BJOG 110(12):1107–1114, 2003.
20. Exercise During Pregnancy and the Postpartum Period. ACOG Committee Opinion No. 267. American College of Obstetricians and Gynecologists. Obstet Gynecol 99:171–173, 2002.
21. Exercise in Pregnancy and the Postpartum Period. Joint guidelines, Society of Obstetricians and Gynaecologists of Canada and the Canadian Society for Exercise Physiology. J Obstet Gynaecol Can 25(6):516–522, 2003.
22. Fantl, JA, Newman, DK, et al: Urinary incontinence in adults: acute and chronic management. Clinical Practice Guideline No. 2, 1996 Update, US Dept of HHS, Public Health Service, AHCPR Publication No. 96–0682, Rockville, MD, March, 1996.
23. Feigel, D: Evaluating Prenatal and Postpartum Exercise Classes. Bulletin of Section on Obstetrics and Gynecology, American Physical Therapy Association 7:12, 1983.
24. Feldenkrais, M: Awareness Through Movement: Health Exercises for Personal Growth, ed 1. Harper & Row, New York, 1972.
25. Feldt, CM: Applying the Guide to Physical Therapist Practice to Women's Health Physical Therapy: Part II. J Section Women's Health, APTA 24:1, 2000.
26. Fisher, K, Riolo, L: What is the evidence regarding specific methods of pelvic floor exercise for a patient with urinary stress incontinence and mild anterior wall prolapse? Phys Ther 84(8):744–753, 2004.
27. Flanagan, G: The First Nine Months of Life, ed 2. Simon & Schuster, New York, 1962.
28. Frahm, J: Strengthening the pelvic floor. Clin Man Phys Ther 5:30, 1985.
29. Freyder, SC: Exercising while pregnant. J Orthop Sports Phys Ther 10:358, 1989.
30. Garshasbi, A, Faghih Zadeh, S: The effect of exercise on the intensity of low back pain in pregnant women. Int J Gynaecol Obstet 88(3): 271–275, 2005.
31. Gent, D, Gottlieb, K: Cesarean rehabilitation. Clin Man Phys Ther 5:14, 1985.
32. Gilbert, E, Harman, J: High-Risk Pregnancy and Delivery, ed 1. CV Mosby, St. Louis, 1986.
33. Hartmann, K, et al: Outcomes of routine episiotomy. JAMA 293: 2141–2148, 2005.
34. Hay-Smith, EJC, et al: Pelvic floor muscle training for urinary incontinence in women (Cochrane Review) The Cochrane Library, Issue 3, Chichester, UK: John Wiley & Sons, 2004.
35. Holroyd-Leduc, J, Straus, S: Management of urinary incontinence in women. JAMA 291:986–995, 2004.
36. Ingalls, A, Salerno, M: Maternal and Child Health Nursing, ed 5. CV Mosby, St. Louis, 1983.
37. Jamieson, D, Steege, J: The prevalence of dysmenorrhea, dyspareunia, pelvic pain, and irritable bowel syndrome in primary care practices Obstet Gynecol 87(1):55–58, 1996.
38. Jarrell, J, et al: Consensus guidelines for the management of chronic pelvic pain. J Obstet Gynaecol Can 27(8):781–826, 2005.
39. Jarski, RW, Trippett, DL: The risks and benefits of exercise during pregnancy. J Fam Pract 30:185, 1990.
40. Knee-Chest Exercises and maternal death: comments. Med J Aust 1:1127, 1973.
41. Klein, M, et al: Determinants of vaginal-perineal integrity and pelvic floor functioning in childbirth. Am J Obstet Gynecol 176(2):403–410, 1997.
42. Legato, M: Eve's Rib—The Groundbreaking Guide to Women's Health. Three Rivers Press, New York 2002.
43. Mandelstam, D: The pelvic floor. Physiotherapy 64:8, 1978.
44. Morkved, S, Bo, K: Effect of postpartum pelvic floor muscle training in prevention and treatment of urinary incontinence: a one year follow up. BJOG 107(8):1022–1028, 2002.
45. Morkved, S, et al: Pelvic floor muscle training during pregnancy to prevent urinary incontinence: a single-blind randomized controlled trial. Obstet Gynecol 101(2):313–319, 2003.
46. Nelson, P: Pulmonary gas embolism in pregnancy and the puerperium. Obstet Gynecol Surv 15, 1960.
47. Nilsson-Wikmar, L, et al: Effect of three different physical therapy treatments on pain and activity in pregnant women with pelvic girdle pain: a randomized clinical trial with 3, 6, and 12 months follow-up postpartum. Spine 30(8):850–856, 2005.
48. Noble, E: Essential Exercises for the Childbearing Year, ed 3. Houghton Mifflin, Boston, 1988.
49. Noble, E: Having Twins, ed 3. Houghton Mifflin, Boston, 2003.
50. Norwood, C: Cesarean variations: patients, facilities or policies. Int J Childbirth Educ 1:4, 1986.
51. Nygaard, I, et al: Pelvic organ prolapse in older women: prevalence and risk factors. Obstet Gynecol 104(3):489–497, 2004.
52. Ostgaard, HC, et al: Reduction of back and posterior pelvic pain in pregnancy. Spine 19:894, 1994.
53. Pauls, J: Therapeutic Approaches to Women's Health—A Program of Exercise and Education. Aspen, Gaithersburg, MD, 1995.
54. Perinatal Exercise Guidelines. Section on Obstetrics and Gynecology, American Physical Therapy Association, Alexandria, VA, 1986.
55. Position Paper. Section on Obstetrics and Gynecology: Bulletin of Section on Obstetrics and Gynecology, American Physical Therapy Association 8:6, 1984.
56. Pritchard, J, MacDonald, P (eds): Williams' Obstetrics, ed 16. Appleton-Century-Crofts, Norwalk, CT, 1980.
57. Sampselle, C, et al: Effect of pelvic muscle exercise on transient incontinence during pregnancy and after birth. Obstet Gynecol 91(3):406–412, 1998.
58. Sandberg, E: Synopsis of Obstetrics, ed 10. CV Mosby, St. Louis, 1978.
59. Santiesteban, A: Electromyographic and dynamometric characteristics of female pelvic floor musculature. Phys Ther 68:344, 1988.
60. Shrock, P, Simkin, P, Shearer, M: Teaching prenatal exercise: Part II—Exercises to think twice about. Birth Fam J 8:3, 1981.
61. Snooks, SJ, Swash, M, et al: Risk Factors in childbirth causing damage to the pelvic floor innervation. Int J Colorect Dis 1:20, 1986.
62. Stephenson, R, O'Connor, L: Obstetric and Gynecologic Care in Physical Therapy, ed 2. Charles B. Slack, Thorofare, NJ, 2000.

63. Stuge, B, et al: The efficacy of a treatment program focusing on specific stabilizing exercises for pelvic girdle pain after pregnancy—a two-year follow-up of a randomized clinical trial. Spine (29)10:E197–E203, 2004.

64. Tchow, D, et al: Pelvic-floor musculature exercises in treatment of anatomical urinary stress incontinence. Phys Ther 68: 652, 1988.

65. Thom, D, et al: Evaluation of parturition and other reproductive variables as risk factors for urinary incontinence in later life. Obstet Gynecol 90:983–989, 1997.

66. Wilder, E (ed): Obstetric and Gynecologic Physical Therapy: Clinics in Physical Therapy, Vol. 20, ed 1. Churchill-Livingstone, New York, 1988.

67. Wilder, E (ed): The Gynecological Manual, ed 2. APTA, Section on Women's Health, Alexandria, VA, 2000.

68. http://www.healthday.com (Sept. 12, 2005).

69. http://www.nlm.nih.gov/medlineplus/news/fullstory_37513.html (Sept. 17, 2006).

70. Zacharin, RF: Pelvic Floor Anatomy and the Surgery of Pulsion Enterocele. Springer-Verlag, New York, 1985.

# Management of Vascular Disorders of the Extremities

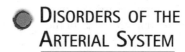

Vascular disorders causing insufficient circulation to the extremities, can result in significant physical impairments and subsequent loss of function of either the upper or lower extremities. Disturbances of structure or function of the circulatory systems are broadly classified as acute or chronic *peripheral vascular disease* (PVD) and can be caused by a number of underlying pathologies of the arterial, venous, or lymphatic systems, including occlusion, inflammation, vasomotor dysfunction, or neoplasms.[33,38,46] In addition, surgical procedures or radiation therapy necessary for the treatment of some forms of cancer can impair lymphatic circulation.[5,39,63,68]

To contribute to the effective management of patients with vascular disorders, a therapist must possess a sound understanding of the underlying pathologies and the clinical manifestations of many types of arterial, venous, and lymphatic disorders. A therapist must also be aware of the use, effectiveness, and limitations of therapeutic exercise in the comprehensive management and rehabilitation of patients with vascular disorders.

## DISORDERS OF THE ARTERIAL SYSTEM

### Types of Arterial Disorders

#### Acute Arterial Occlusion
A thrombus (blood clot), embolism, or trauma can cause acute loss of blood flow to peripheral arteries. The most common location of an arterial embolus is at the femoral-popliteal bifurcation, although an embolus can occur at

other arterial bifurcations in the extremities.[33,38] Crush injuries to the vessels of the extremities also can disrupt arterial blood flow and must be repaired quickly to restore circulation and prevent tissue necrosis. If a patient develops an acute arterial occlusion, immediate medical or surgical measures must be taken to maintain the viability of the limb. These measures could include complete bed rest, systemic anti-coagulation therapy, thromboembolectomy, or reconstructive arterial bypass surgery.[27,33,54]

PRECAUTION: With an acute occlusion therapeutic exercise is contraindicated. Use of support hose or application of direct heat over painful areas also is contraindicated.[54]

## Arteriosclerosis Obliterans

Arteriosclerosis obliterans (ASO), also called *chronic occlusive arterial disease, peripheral arterial occlusive disease,* or *atherosclerotic occlusive disease*, accounts for 95% of all the arterial disorders affecting the lower extremities.[33] It is a chronic disorder, most often seen in elderly patients. ASO is more common in men than women and is associated with risk factors that include elevated serum cholesterol ($> 200$ mg/dL), smoking, high systolic blood pressure, obesity, and diabetes.[13,33,35,66]

ASO is characterized by chronic, progressive occlusion of the peripheral circulation, most often in the large and medium arteries of the lower extremities. It is caused by atherosclerotic plaque formation.[33,66]

## Thromboangiitis Obliterans (Buerger's Disease)

Thromboangitis obliterans is a chronic disease seen predominantly in young male patients who smoke; it involves an inflammatory reaction of the arteries to nicotine. Initially, it becomes evident in the small arteries of the feet and hands and progresses proximally. It results in vasoconstriction, decreased arterial circulation to the extremities, ischemia, and eventual ulceration and necrosis of soft tissues.[27,38,46] The inflammatory reaction and resulting signs and symptoms can be controlled if the patient stops smoking.

## Raynaud's Disease

Raynaud's disease, also known as *primary Raynaud's syndrome*, is a chronic, functional arterial disorder that occurs more often in women than men. Thought to be caused by an abnormality of the sympathetic nervous system, it is characterized by digital vasospasm, most often affecting the small arteries and arterioles of the fingers and sometimes the toes. Vasospasm is brought on by exposure to cold, vibration, or stress. The response is characterized by temporary pallor (blanching), then cyanosis and pain, followed by numbness and a cold sensation of the digits. Symptoms are relieved slowly by warmth.[27,33,38,46,54]

When the disorder is primary, it is called *idiopathic Raynaud's disease* or *Raynaud's syndrome*. When it is a secondary complication and associated with another dis-ease (such as scleroderma, systemic lupus erythematosus, systemic sclerosis, or vasculitis), it is called *Raynaud's phenomenon*.[46,78]

## Clinical Manifestations of Peripheral Arterial Disorders

The following signs and symptoms are associated with peripheral arterial disorders.

### Diminished or Absent Peripheral Pulses

The more occluded or restricted the arterial blood flow and the more diminished the peripheral pulses, the more severe or advanced is the arterial disease.[27,33,46,50,54] If the collateral circulation is extensive, the patient may not experience pain despite diminished pulses.

### Integumentary Changes

A number of integumentary changes are associated with peripheral arterial disease.[27,33,34,38,46,53,54]

- Skin discoloration, including *pallor* at rest or with exercise, or *reactive hyperemia* can develop. Pallor is more evident when the extremity is elevated above the level of the heart for several minutes. Reactive hyperemia occurs when the extremity is moved from an elevated to a dependent position. The skin takes on a bright red appearance rather than a normal pink flush. (Refer to the test for rubor of dependency in the following section.) Pallor of the distal extremity may also occur with exercise. After exercise, cutaneous ischemia causes blanching of the skin as arterial blood flow is diverted to the exercising muscles and away from the surface tissues of the distal extremity.
- *Trophic changes* include a shiny, waxy appearance and dryness of the skin and loss of hair distal to the occlusion.
- Skin temperature is decreased.
- *Ulcerations* may develop, particularly at weight-bearing areas or over bony prominences.

### Sensory Disturbances

Intolerance to heat or cold and paresthesia (initially tingling, then numbness) can develop.[27,46,54]

### Exercise Pain and Rest Pain

Pain during exercise and at rest is associated with progressive peripheral arterial disease and leads to significant disability.[27,34,35,46,54]

*Exercise pain.* Pain that occurs and gradually increases with exercise is referred to as *intermittent claudication*.[13,27,30,32,46,54] It is experienced most common in the lower extremities and occurs more frequently and with greater intensity as the severity of chronic arterial insufficiency progresses. During the early stages of arterial disease, intermittent claudication is characterized by a feeling of fatigue or weakness and, later, as cramping or aching in the muscles used during exercise.

| TABLE 24.1 | Common Sites of Exercise Pain and Associated Arterial Occlusion |
|---|---|
| **Site of Pain** | **Occluded Artery** |
| **Chronic arterial insufficiency** | |
| Calf | Femoral |
| Foot | Popliteal |
| Thigh | Iliac |
| Buttocks or low back | Aortic |
| **Thromboangiitis obliterans** | |
| Arch of the foot | Plantar and tibial |
| Palm of the hand | Palmar and ulnar |

Pain is located distal to the occluded vessels and is caused by insufficient blood supply and activity-induced ischemia in the exercising muscles. Leg pain typically is brought on by walking and gradually subsides when the patient stops walking. Intermittent claudication does not occur with extended periods of standing (as seen with spinal stenosis)[34] or with prolonged sitting (as seen with sciatica).[9,35]

Although exercise pain is most common in the calf, it also can occur more proximally. Table 24.1 identifies common sites of intermittent claudication.[9,27,33,34,46,54]

If peripheral vessels such as the popliteal, femoral, or iliac arteries are occluded, symptoms usually occur in one extremity; whereas if the occlusion is in the lower aorta, symptoms are present not only in both extremities but in the buttocks and low back regions as well. As the disease progresses and arterial insufficiency increases, exercise tolerance deteriorates as ischemic pain occurs more readily with activity.

**Rest pain.** When a burning, tingling sensation gradually becomes evident in the distal extremities at rest or with elevation, it may be indicative of severe ischemia. With ischemia, pain frequently occurs at night because the heart rate and volume of blood flow to the extremities decreases with rest. Sometimes partial or complete relief of pain is possible if the leg is placed in a dependent position, such as over the edge of a bed. In contrast, elevation of the limb increases the pain.

### Muscle Weakness

Loss of strength, muscle atrophy, and eventual loss of motor function, particularly in the hands and feet, occur with progressive arterial vascular disease. Loss of motor function is compounded by pain, which further compromises functional strength.[27,54]

## Examination and Evaluation of Arterial Sufficiency

A comprehensive examination of a patient with known or suspected peripheral arterial disease is necessary to determine or verify the etiology of a patient's impairments and functional limitations. For example, the origin of a patient's buttock and leg pain or lower extremity weakness could be caused by vascular or neuromuscular pathologies.[34,35] The initial and subsequent examinations also provide a basis to determine a patient's status before treatment and the effectiveness of the interventions at the conclusion of treatment.

Various procedures for testing arterial sufficiency and identifying stenosis or occlusion are listed in Box 24.1 and described briefly in this section.[42,46,50,54] Some procedures are used by therapists to indirectly assess arterial blood flow, whereas others, such as angiography or arteriography, are administered by practitioners with specialized training and are interpreted by a physician.

### Palpation of Pulses

The basis of any evaluation of the integrity of the arterial system is the detection of pulses in the distal portion of the extremities. Pulses are described as *normal, diminished,* or *absent.* The strength of pulses also can be rated quantitatively from 0 to +3. Even if pulses appear normal, blood flow to the extremity may, in fact, be substantially restricted.[12] Pulselessness is a sign of severe arterial insufficiency.

The femoral, popliteal, dorsalis pedis, and posterior tibial pulses should be palpated in the lower extremities. The radial, ulnar, and brachial pulses are palpated in the upper extremities.

N O T E : Pulses are difficult to assess quantitatively by palpation alone. Other, more accurate and reliable noninvasive tests (such as Doppler ultrasonography) supplement the information gained from palpating the pulses.

### Skin Temperature

The temperature of the skin can be assessed grossly by palpation. A limb with diminished arterial blood flow is cool to the touch. If a discrepancy exists between an involved and an uninvolved extremity, skin temperature should be quantitatively measured with an electronic thermometer.

| BOX 24.1 | Tests and Measurements of Arterial Sufficiency |
|---|---|

- Palpation and comparison of pulses in the involved and uninvolved upper or lower extremities
- Skin temperature
- Skin integrity and pigmentation
- Tests for reactive hyperemia (rubor of dependence)
- Claudication time
- Ultrasonography, Doppler measurement of blood flow, transcutaneous oximetry
- Magnetic resonance angiography
- Arteriography

## Skin Integrity and Pigmentation

Diminished or absent arterial blood flow to an extremity causes trophic changes in the skin peripherally. The patient's skin is dry, and its color is diminished (pallor). Hair loss and a shiny appearance to the skin also occur. Skin ulcerations may be present.

## Rubor Dependency Test—Reactive Hyperemia

Changes in skin color that occur with elevation and dependency of the limb as the result of altered blood flow are determined. Rubor/reactive hyperemia can be assessed in two ways.[42,46]

*Procedure.* The legs are elevated for several minutes above the level of the heart while the patient is lying supine. Pallor (blanching) of the skin occurs in the feet within 1 minute or less if arterial circulation is poor. The time necessary for blanching to develop is noted. Then the legs are placed in a dependent position, and the color of the feet is noted.

Normally, a pinkish flush appears in the feet within several seconds after the legs are placed in a dependent position. With occlusive arterial disease, a bright bluish-red color, or rubor, of the distal legs and feet is evident that is caused by reduced blood flow in the capillaries. The rubor may take as long as 30 seconds to appear.

*Alternate procedure.* Reactive hyperemia also can be evaluated by temporarily restricting blood flow to the distal portion of the lower extremity with a blood pressure cuff. This restriction causes an accumulation of $CO_2$ and lactic acid in the distal extremity. These metabolites are vasodilators and affect the vascular bed of the blood flow-deprived area.[12]

When the cuff is released and blood flow resumes to the distal extremity, a normal hyperemia (flushing) of the extremity should occur within 10 seconds. With arteriosclerotic vascular disease it may take as long as 1 to 2 minutes for a flush to appear, whereas with vasospastic arterial disease (Raynaud's disease) flushing occurs within the normal time frame.[12]

N O T E : This method of assessing reactive hyperemia is quite painful and is not tolerated well by either normal individuals or patients with occlusive arterial disease.

## Claudication Time

An objective assessment of exercise pain (intermittent claudication) is performed to determine the amount of time a patient can exercise before experiencing cramping and pain in the distal musculature.[30,46,66]

A commonly used test is to have the patient walk at a slow, predetermined speed on a level treadmill (1 to 2 mph). The time that the patient is able to walk before the onset of pain or before pain prohibits further walking is noted.[30,46] This measurement should be undertaken to determine a baseline for exercise tolerance before initiating a program to improve exercise tolerance.

## Doppler Ultrasonography

Doppler measurement of blood flow with ultrasound imaging is a noninvasive assessment that uses the Doppler principle to determine the relative velocity of blood flow in the major arteries and veins.[27,42,46,54] A soundhead, covered with coupling gel, is placed on the skin directly over the artery to be evaluated. An ultrasonic beam is directed transcutaneously to the artery. Blood cells moving in the path of the beam cause a shift in the frequency of the reflected sound.

The frequency of the reflected sound emitted varies with the velocity of blood flow. This information is transmitted visually onto an oscilloscope or printed tape or audibly via a loudspeaker or stethoscope.

## Transcutaneous Oximetry

Transcutaneous oximetry provides information about the oxygen saturation of blood by means of a photoelectric device (a pulse oximeter).[33] A beam of red and infrared light passes through a pulsating capillary bed (e.g., in the fingertip). The ratio of red to infrared transmission varies with the oxygen saturation of the blood. Because it responds only to pulsating objects, it does not detect nonpulsating objects, such as venous blood or skin.

## Arteriography

Arteriography is an invasive procedure that involves injecting a radiopaque dye (contrast medium) directly into an artery.[33,38,46] The arteries are then radiographically visualized to detect any restriction of movement of the dye in arterial vessels indicating a partial or complete occlusion. Collateral circulation can also be visualized. Because arteriography gives a highly accurate picture of the location and extent of an arterial obstruction, it is used most often prior to reconstructive arterial bypass surgery.

## Magnetic Resonance Angiography

Magnetic resonance angiography, a noninvasive procedure, provides radiographic visualization of arteries without the use of a contrast medium.[33]

# Management of Acute Arterial Occlusion

Acute arterial occlusion often is a medical or surgical emergency. The resulting ischemia causes severe pain, the risk of tissue necrosis and local or systemic infection, and the possible need for amputation. The viability of the limb depends on the location and extent of the occlusion and the availability of collateral circulation.

Medical or surgical measures must be taken to reduce ischemia and to restore circulation. Medical management includes bed rest and complete systemic anticoagulation therapy. Complementary physical interventions to improve peripheral blood flow while the patient is on bed rest may include warming the limb by reflex heating of the torso or opposite extremity or elevating the head of the bed slightly.[27,46] Several contraindications also are warranted (Box 24.2).

| BOX 24.2 | Contraindications with Acute Arterial Occlusion |
|---|---|

- Exercise—passive or active
- Prolonged positioning during bed rest, which could cause pressure on and potential breakdown of skin
- Local, direct heat on the involved extremity because of the potential for a burn to the ischemic tissue
- Use of support hose, which may increase peripheral resistance to blood flow
- Restrictive clothing that could compromise blood flow

Surgical interventions for an acute occlusion are *thromboembolectomy* or an arterial bypass graft. If circulation cannot be significantly improved or restored, gangrene develops within a very short time, and amputation of the extremity is necessary.[33]

## Management of Chronic Arterial Insufficiency

Except with advanced disease, chronic arterial insufficiency caused, for example, by ASO or Raynaud's disease is managed conservatively by medical and physical means and does not constitute a medical or surgical emergency.[27,46,54,66] Box 24.3 summarizes management guidelines for chronic arterial insufficiency.

### Medical/Surgical Management

Medical management of chronic arterial insufficiency must be ongoing. Related medical disorders must be identified and treated. Diabetes and hypertension are commonly associated with chronic arteriosclerotic vascular disease and must be controlled with medication, diet, and exercise.[66]

Lifestyle changes are an important aspect of management. In all cases, patients are advised to stop smoking and alter their diet, such as limiting or avoiding salt, sucrose, and alcohol to lower blood pressure and triglyceride and

## BOX 24.3
## MANAGEMENT GUIDELINES—Chronic Arterial Insufficiency

**Impairments**
Decreased endurance and increased frequency of muscular fatigue with functional activities such as walking
Pain with exercise or at rest
Skin breakdown and ulcerations
Limitation of passive and active motion
Weakness and disuse atrophy

| Plan of Care | Interventions |
|---|---|
| 1. Teach the patient how to minimize or prevent potential impairments and correct impairments or functional limitations currently affecting functional capabilities. | 1. Self-management of current or potential impairments through patient education. |
| 2. Communicate with health professionals from other disciplines appropriate for consultation with the patient. | 2. Medical or surgical management including medications; nutritional counseling for weight control and to decrease salt, sucrose, cholesterol, and caffeine intake; smoking cessation. |
| 3. Improve exercise tolerance for ADL and decrease the incidence of intermittent claudication. | 3. Regular, graded aerobic conditioning program of walking or bicycling[30,46,54,65,66,79] (see Chapter 7). |
| 4. Relieve pain at rest. | 4. Sleep with the legs in a dependent but supported position over the edge of the bed or with the head of the bed slightly elevated. |
| 5. Prevent skin ulcerations. | 5. Proper care and protection of the skin, particularly the feet[14] or hands.<br>Proper nail care.[12]<br>Proper shoe selection and fit.[12]<br>Avoid use of support hose and restrictive clothing.<br>Avoid exposure to extremes of temperature, both hot and cold. |
| 6. Improve vasodilation in affected arteries. | 6. Vasodilation by iontophoresis.[2]<br>Vasodilation by reflex heating.[2]<br>N O T E : Although these physical measures have been advocated, their effectiveness is questionable. |
| 7. Prevent or minimize joint contractures and muscle atrophy, particularly if the patient is confined to bed. | 7. Repetitive, active ROM against low loads and/or gentle stretching exercises; proper positioning in bed to maintain joint and muscle extensibility. |
| 8. Promote healing of any skin ulcerations that develop. | 8. Wound management procedures for treating ischemic ulcers, including electrical stimulation and oxygen therapy.[27,55] |

cholesterol levels. These measures do not cure chronic arterial disorders but do minimize risk factors and promote wellness.

For patients with leg pain at rest due to advanced disease, reconstructive vascular surgery, such as a bypass graft, may be required. Patients with vasospastic disease may benefit from sympathetic blocks or sympathectomies to increase blood flow.[46] If a patient develops ulcerations or gangrene that cannot be treated medically or with conservative surgical procedures, amputation of the limb is necessary.[46,55]

### Role of Exercise

For patients with mild to moderate arterial disease, a graded exercise program should be initiated to improve exercise tolerance and functional capacity in activities of daily living. A regular program of mild- to moderate-level aerobic exercise, such as walking or bicycling, is known to have benefits for patients with chronic arterial insufficiency.[13,30,32,65,66,79]

Demonstrated benefits include an increase in the time before the onset of exercise pain during walking, improvement in the efficiency of oxygen utilization in exercising muscles (enabling patients to tolerate exercise over longer periods of time), and quantitative improvement of quality of life.[30,65,79] However, the characteristics of an optimal exercise program or whether exercise programs improve collateral circulation in the extremities is less clear.

 **Focus on Evidence** _____

Brandsma and co-investigators[13] conducted a systematic review of the literature to identify the indications, characteristics, and effectiveness of walking programs for patients with intermittent claudication. A review of 10 articles that met the inclusion criteria revealed no consensus with regard to indications for participation in a walking program for patients with intermitten claudication or optimal characteristics of such a program. However, the reviewers did confirm that all walking programs significantly improved walking distance in patients who participated in programs compared with those who did not.

In addition to increased walking distance, Gardner et al.[32] demonstrated by means of a randomized study of elderly individuals with chronic arterial insufficiency that after a 6-month walking program improvement in the distance walked before the onset of claudication was dependent on an increase in peripheral blood flow.

Buerger or Buerger-Allen exercises, another approach to exercise developed a number of decades ago, were designed to promote collateral circulation through a series of positional changes of the affected limb (from an elevated to a dependent position) combined with active ankle pumping exercises.[82] Although used frequently in the past and occasionally today, there is little to no evidence to support the efficacy of these exercises for improving blood

flow to an extremity.[27,54] Consequently, there is little reason to include them in a patient's exercise program.

## Special Considerations in a Graded Exercise Program for Patients with Chronic Arterial Insufficiency

### Rationale for Graded Exercise

The following factors related to the body's normal response to exercise are the basis for using a graded exercise program to improve the functional status of patients with chronic arterial insufficiency.[27,66,79]

- Blood flow temporarily decreases during active contraction of a muscle, but the blood flow rapidly increases immediately after the contraction.
- After cessation of exercise, there is a rapid decrease in blood flow during the first 3 to 4 minutes. This is followed by a slow decline to resting levels within 15 minutes.
- With repeated moderate-level exercise, blood flow in muscles can be increased beyond the resting values for blood flow.

### Exercise Guidelines

- The patient should be encouraged to walk or bicycle as far as possible to a predetermined maximum target heart rate but without causing intermittent claudication.
- The graded endurance exercise should be carried out 3 to 5 days per week.
- The patient should perform mild warm-up and stretching activities prior to initiating walking or bicycling. Warm-up activities could include active pumping exercises of the ankle and toes.
- Refer to Chapter 7 for additional guidelines for establishing an aerobic exercise program.

Precautions and contraindications for participation in a walking program for patients with chronic arterial insufficiency are noted in Box 24.4.[27,46,54,55]

---

**BOX 24.4    Precautions and Contraindications for a Walking Program for Patients with Chronic Arterial Insufficiency**

**Precautions**
- Avoid exercising outside during very cold weather.
- Wear shoes that fit properly, have sufficient padding, and do not cause skin irritation.
- Inspect the feet carefully for evidence of skin irritation after each exercise session.
- Discontinue a walking program if leg pain increases rather than decreases over time.

**Contraindications**
- Presence of skin irritation, an ulceration, a wound, or a fungal infection of the feet
- Leg pain at rest due to advanced vascular disease

# Disorders of the Venous System

Just as arterial disorders of the extremities can be acute or chronic, so can venous disorders.[34,40] Therapeutic exercise is one aspect of management of patients with an acute disease, such as thrombophlebitis, or a chronic disorder, such as varicose veins or chronic venous insufficiency.[27,33,46,54]

## Types of Venous Disorders

### Thrombophlebitis and Deep Vein Thrombosis

*Thrombophlebitis* is a disorder typically affecting the lower extremities and caused by thrombosis (the development/formation of a blood clot—i.e., a thrombus). It is characterized by acute inflammation with partial or complete occlusion of a superficial or deep vein.[27,33,38,42]

Lower extremity venous thrombosis can occur in the superficial vein system (greater or small saphenous veins) or the deep vein system (popliteal, femoral, or iliac veins) (Fig. 24.1).[33] A thrombus in one of the superficial veins in the calf usually is small and resolves without serious consequences.[33,67] In contrast, thrombus formation in a deep vein in the calf or more proximally in the thigh or pelvic region, known as a *deep vein thrombosis* (DVT), tends to be larger and can cause serious complications. When a clot breaks away from the wall of a vein and travels proximally, it is called an *embolus*. When an embolus affects pulmonary circulation, it is called a *pulmonary embolism*, which is a potentially life-threatening disorder.[33,67]

A lower extremity DVT is a common complication after musculoskeletal injury or surgery, prolonged immobilization, or bed rest and is attributed to venous stasis, injury to and inflammation of the walls of a vein, or a hypercoagulable state of the blood.[33,38,75] Risk factors for DVT are listed in Box 24.5.[33,38,67]

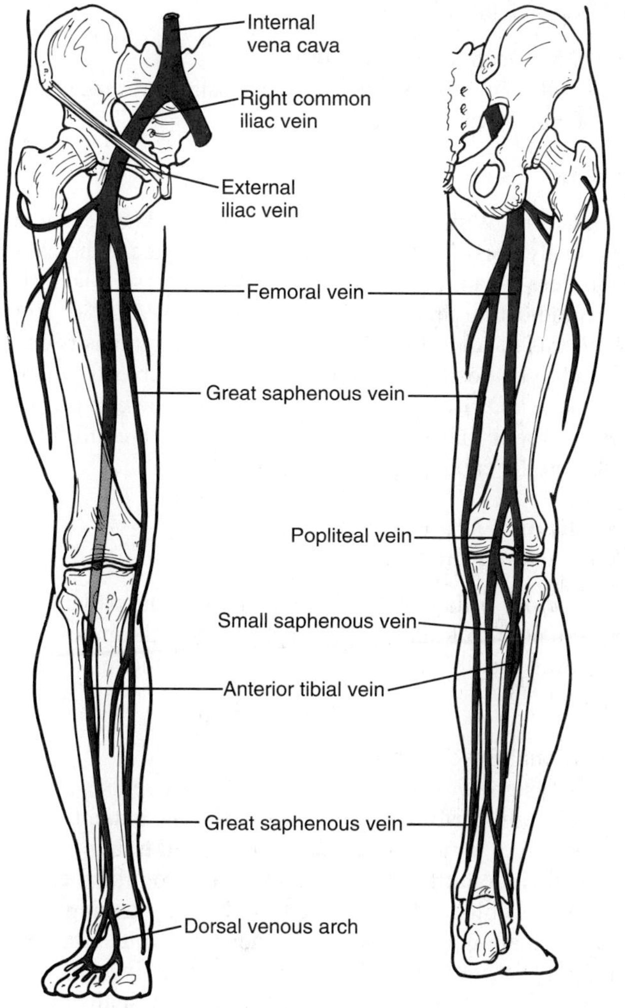
Internal vena cava
Right common iliac vein
External iliac vein
Femoral vein
Great saphenous vein
Popliteal vein
Small saphenous vein
Anterior tibial vein
Great saphenous vein
Dorsal venous arch

FIGURE 24.1 Veins of the lower extremity

### Chronic Venous Insufficiency

Chronic venous insufficiency is defined as inadequate venous return over a prolonged period of time. It may begin after a severe episode of DVT, may be associated with varicose veins, or may be the result of trauma to the lower extremities or blockage of the venous system by a neoplasm.[33,38,46] In all of these disorders damaged or incompetent valves in the veins prevent or compromise venous return, leading to venous hypertension and venous stasis in the lower extremities. Chronic pooling of blood in the veins causes inadequate oxygenation of cells and removal of waste products. This, in turn, leads to necrosis of tissues and the development of *venous stasis ulcers*.[33,38,55]

## Clinical Manifestations of Venous Disorders

### Deep Vein Thrombosis and Thrombophlebitis: Signs and Symptoms

During the early stages of a DVT, only 25% to 50% of cases can be identified by clinical manifestations, such as dull aching or severe pain, swelling, or changes in skin temperature and color, specifically heat and redness.[4,33,38,67]

Although edema in the vicinity of the clot may be present, it may be too deep to palpate. If the clot is in the

**BOX 24.5 Risk Factors for Deep Vein Thrombosis and Thrombophlebitis**

- Postoperative or postfracture immobilization
- Prolonged bed rest
- Trauma to venous vessels
- Limb paralysis
- Active malignancy (within past 6 months)
- History of deep vein thrombosis or pulmonary embolism
- Advanced age
- Obesity
- Sedentary lifestyle or extended episode of sitting during long-distance travel
- Congestive heart failure
- Use of oral contraceptives
- Pregnancy

calf (distal DVT), pain or tenderness of the calf may be felt with passive dorsiflexion of the affected foot (*Homans' sign*). However, the sensitivity of this test is poor and often reflects a false-negative or false-positive finding.[4,75] Only measurement by ultrasonography, venous duplex screening, or venography can confirm a DVT.[4,75]

### Pulmonary Embolism: Signs and Symptoms

As described previously, pulmonary embolism is a possible consequence of DVT. Risk factors for pulmonary embolism are similar to those already identified for DVT (see Box 24.5).

The signs and symptoms of pulmonary embolism vary considerably depending on the size of the embolus, the extent of lung involvement, and the presence of coexisting cardiopulmonary conditions.[84] The hallmark signs and symptoms are a sudden onset of shortness of breath (dyspnea), rapid and shallow breathing (tachypnea), and chest pain located at the lateral aspect of the chest that intensifies with deep breathing and coughing. Other signs and symptoms include swelling in the lower extremities, anxiety, fever, excessive sweating (diaphoresis), a cough, and blood in the sputum (hemoptysis).[84]

When a patient presents with signs or symptoms of possible pulmonary embolism, immediate medical referral is warranted for a definitive diagnosis.

### Chronic Venous Insufficiency: Signs and Symptoms

Dependent, peripheral edema occurring with long periods of standing or sitting is a common manifestation of chronic venous dysfunction. Edema decreases if the limb is elevated. Patients often report dull aching or tiredness in the affected extremity.[27,33,38,46,62,86] If the insufficiency is associated with varicose veins, venous distention (bulging) also is notable. When edema persists, the skin becomes less supple over time and takes on a brownish pigmentation.

## Examination and Evaluation of Venous Sufficiency

As with arterial disorders, a complete history and systems review help determine the presence of a venous disorder. Some specific tests to determine venous sufficiency are listed in Box 24.6 and are briefly described in this section.[27,34,42,53,62] These tests complement a comprehensive

---

| BOX 24.6 | Tests and Measures of Venous Sufficiency |
| --- | --- |

- Girth measurements of the upper or lower extremities
- Percussion test: compliance of the greater saphenous vein
- Homans' sign
- Response to compression of the limb with a blood pressure cuff
- Doppler ultrasonography
- Venous duplex screening/scanning
- Venography

---

integumentary and neuromuscular examination that includes skin integrity, mobility, color, texture, temperature, vital signs including peripheral pulses, sensation, pain, functional mobility, ROM, strength, and cardiopulmonary endurance.

### Girth Measurements

Circumferential measurements of the involved and uninvolved limbs are taken to determine the presence and extent of edema.[27,46,53] Measurements are taken at anatomical landmarks or at predetermined and consistent distances apart (e.g., 8 or 10 cm apart).

### Competence of the Greater Saphenous Vein (Percussion Test)

Evaluating the valves of the saphenous vein is a common test used if a patient has symptomatic varicose veins.

*Procedure.* Ask the patient to stand until the veins in the legs appear to fill. While palpating a portion of the saphenous vein below the knee, sharply percuss a portion of the vein above the knee. If valves are not functioning adequately, the examiner feels a backflow of fluid distally under the palpating fingertips.[38,46,53]

### Tests for Deep Vein Thrombosis

The following tests determine the possible presence of a DVT in a lower extremity.

#### Homans' Sign

*Procedure.* With the patient supine and the knee extended, passively dorsiflex the ankle and gently squeeze the calf muscles. If pain occurs in the calf, Homans' sign is positive, indicating the possible presence of a DVT.[4,46,53] However, this is not a definitive test. Homans' sign has been found to be positive in more than 50% of subjects who did not have a DVT. In addition, it has been shown to be positive in fewer than one-third of patients with a confirmed DVT in the calf.[4,75]

#### Application of a Blood Pressure Cuff Around the Calf

*Procedure.* Inflate the cuff gradually until the patient experiences calf pain. A patient with acute thrombophlebitis usually cannot tolerate pressures above 40 mm Hg.[53]

### Additional Special Tests

Tests designed to confim the presence of a venous disorder are performed and analyzed by the patient's physician or a practitioner with specialized training. Tests include ultrasonographic imaging, Doppler measurement of blood flow, and venous duplex scanning (all of which are noninvasive) and venography (phlebography), an invasive procedure.[4,33,46,50,53] Venography involves injecting radiopaque dye and radiographic visualization of the venous system.

**BOX 24.7**

MANAGEMENT GUIDELINES—Deep Vein Thrombosis and Thrombophlebitis

**Impairments**
Dull ache or pain usually in the calf
Tenderness, warmth, and swelling with palpation

| Plan of Care | Interventions |
|---|---|
| 1. Relieve pain during the acute inflammatory period. | 1. Bed rest, pharmacological management (systemic anticoagulant therapy); elevation of the affected lower extremity, keeping the knee slightly flexed. |
| 2. As acute symptoms subside, regain functional mobility. | 2. Graded ambulation with legs wrapped in elastic or nonelastic bandages or when pressure-gradient support stockings are worn. |
| 3. Prevent recurrence of the acute disorder. | 3. Continuation of appropriate medical and pharmacological management. Use of strategies to prevent DVTs. |

**Contraindications:** Passive or active motion or application of moist heat; use of a sequential pneumatic compression pump.

## Prevention of Deep Vein Thrombosis and Thrombophlebitis

Every effort should be made to prevent the occurrence of a DVT and subsequent thrombophlebitis, particularly in patients at risk. The following interventions are implemented to reduce the risk of a DVT.[45,75,77]

- Prophylactic use of anticoagulant therapy (high-molecular-weight heparin) for the high-risk patient (e.g., the patient who has undergone lower extremity surgery or who is on bed rest)
- Initiation of ambulation as soon as possible after surgery, preferably no more than a day or two postoperatively
- Elevating the legs while lying supine and on a footstool or ottoman when sitting
- No prolonged periods of sitting, especially for the patient with a long-leg cast
- Active "pumping" exercises (active dorsiflexion, plantarflexion, and circumduction of the ankle) regularly throughout the day while lying supine in bed
- Use of compression stockings to support the walls of the veins and minimize venous pooling
- For patients on bed rest, use of a sequential pneumatic compression unit

## Management of Deep Vein Thrombosis and Thrombophlebitis

If the presence of DVT and resulting thrombophlebitis is confirmed, immediate medical intervention is essential to reduce the risk of pulmonary embolism. Initial management includes administering anticoagulant medication, placing the patient on complete bed rest, elevating the involved extremity, and using graduated compression stockings. The reported time frame for bed rest varies from 2 days to more than a week.[3] Box 24.7 summarizes the guidelines for management of acute DVT and thrombophlebitis.[27,46,54]

During the period of bed rest, exercises usually are contraindicated because movement of the involved extremity may cause pain and is thought to increase congestion in the venous channels when tissues are inflamed. However, the optimal timing of when it is prudent to discontinue bed rest and resume ambulation after initiating anticoagulant therapy is in question.

 **Focus on Evidence**_____

Aldrich and colleagues[3] conducted a systematic review of the literature to determine when a patient with DVT should be allowed to begin walking. The review revealed a limited number of studies (a total of five, three of which were randomized, controlled trials) that addressed this issue. Results of these studies suggest that early ambulation, begun within the first 24 hours after initiating anticoagulent therapy, does not increase the incidence of pulmonary embolism in patients without an existing pulmonary embolism and who have adequate cardiopulmonary reserve. However, if a patient has a known pulmonary embolism, an ambulation program must be initiated more cautiously. It is important to note that in the studies reviewed all patients who participated in an early ambulation program wore compression garments.

The results also revealed that early ambulation is associated with more rapid resolution of pain and swelling. The authors of the review were unable to identify studies that investigated the initiation and progression of other forms of exercise for patients with DVT.

## Management of Chronic Venous Insufficiency and Varicose Veins

Patient education is fundamental in the management of chronic venous insufficiency and varicose veins. A patient must be advised on how to prevent dependent edema, skin ulceration, and infections. The therapist may be involved

## BOX 24.8
### MANAGEMENT GUIDELINES—Chronic Venous Insufficiency and Varicose Veins

**Impairments**
Edema
Increased risk of skin ulcerations and infections
Aching of involved limb
Decreased functional mobility, strength, and endurance

| Plan of Care | Interventions |
|---|---|
| 1. Teach the patient how to prevent or minimize impairments. | 1. Patient education and self-management skills for skin care, self-massage for lymphedema, and a home exercise program. |
| 2. Prevent lymphedema; minimize venous stasis. | 2. Use of individually tailored pressure-gradient support stockings donned before getting out of bed in the morning and worn every day. |
| | Support garment worn during exercise and ambulation. |
| | Light active exercise, such as walking, on a regular basis. |
| | Elevate the lower extremities after graded ambulation until the heart rate returns to normal. |
| | Avoid prolonged periods of standing still and sitting with legs dependent. |
| | Elevate involved limb(s) above the level of the heart (about 30° to 45°) when resting or sleeping (see Box 24.10 for additional methods to prevent lymphedema). |
| 3. Increase venous return and reduce lymphedema if already present. | 3. Use intermittent mechanical compression pump and sleeve with involved limb elevated for several hours a day. |
| | Manual massage to drain edema. Stroke in a distal-to-proximal direction clearing the proximal nodes and areas of lymphedema first, then the middle, and finally the distal areas. |
| | Relaxation and active ROM (pumping exercises) of the distal muscles while involved limb is elevated. |
| 4. Prevent skin abrasions, ulcerations, and wound infections. | 4. Proper skin care (see Box 24.10). |

in (1) measuring and fitting a patient for a pressure-gradient support garment; (2) teaching the patient how to put on the garment before getting out of bed; (3) setting up a program of regular exercise; and (4) teaching the patient proper skin care.

Box 24.8 summarizes the guidelines for management of chronic venous insufficiency and varicose veins.[27,46,54,56,62,86] Exercises and related interventions for chronic lymphedema described in the final section of this chapter are indicated for management of lymphedema arising from chronic venous insufficiency.

## DISORDERS OF THE LYMPHATIC SYSTEM

One of the primary functions of the lymphatic system, which consists of lymph vessels and nodes, is to collect and clear excess tissue fluid from interstitial spaces and return it to the venous system (Fig. 24.2).[33,86] Edema is a natural consequence of trauma to and healing of soft tissues. If the lymphatic system is compromised and does not function efficiently, lymphedema develops and impedes wound healing.

*Lymphedema* is an excessive and persistent accumulation of extravascular and extracellular fluid and proteins in tissue spaces.[16,20,26,49,86] It occurs when lymph volume exceeds the capacity of the lymph transport system, and it is associated with a disturbance of the water and protein balance across the capillary membrane. An increased concentration of proteins draws larger amounts of water into interstitial spaces, leading to lymphedema.[26,39,86] Furthermore, many disorders of the cardiopulmonary system can cause the load on lymphatic vessels to exceed their transport capacity and subsequently cause lymphedema.[39,49]

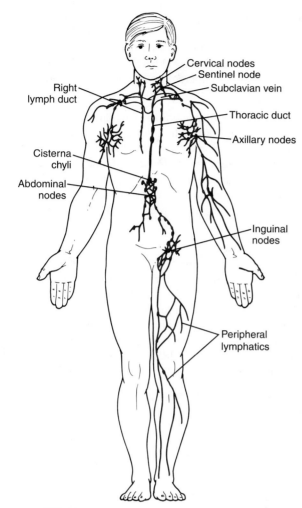

**FIGURE 24.2** Major vessels of the lymphatic system.

## Conditions Leading to Insufficiency of the Lymphatic System

Disorders of the lymphatic transport system can cause primary or secondary lymphedema.[33] Remember, lymphedema is not a disease but, rather, a symptom of a malfunctioning lymphatic system. Most of the patients seen by health care practitioners for management of lymphedema have secondary lymphedema.[68] By far, the most common causes of secondary lymphedema are related to the comprehensive management of cancers of the breast, pelvis, and abdomen.[5,14,16,33,38,39,68,69]

### Congenital Malformation of the Lymphatic System
Primary lymphedema, although uncommon, is the result of insufficient development (dysplasia) and congenital malformation of the lymphatic system.[33,38]

### Infection and Inflammation
Inflammation of the lymph vessels (*lymphangitis*) or lymph nodes (*lymphadenitis*) and enlargement of lymph nodes (*lymphadenopathy*) can occur as the result of a systemic infection or local trauma. Any of these conditions can cause disruption of lymph circulation.[33,38,39,86]

### Obstruction or Fibrosis
Trauma, surgery, and neoplasms can block or impair the lymphatic circulation.[33,39,76] Radiation therapy associated with treatment of malignant tumors also can cause fibrosis of vessels.[5,15]

### Surgical Dissection of Lymph Nodes
Lymph nodes and vessels often are surgically removed (*lymphadenectomy*) as an aspect of treatment of a primary malignancy or metastatic disease. For example, axillary lymph node dissection is performed in most types of breast cancer surgeries to determine the extent and progression of breast cancer.[15,18,33,43] Likewise, pelvic or inguinal lymph node excision often is necessary for the treatment of pelvic or abdominal cancers.[5,68,69]

### Chronic Venous Insufficiency
Although not a primary disorder of the lymphatic system, chronic venous insufficiency and varicose veins are associated with venous stasis and accumulation of edema in the extremities.[33,38,46,86]

## Clinical Manifestations of Lymphatic Disorders

### Lymphedema

*Location.* When lymphedema develops, it is most often apparent in the distal extremities, particularly over the dorsum of the foot or hand.[26,39] The term *dependent edema* describes the accumulation of fluids in the peripheral aspects of the limbs, particularly when the distal segments are lower than the heart. In contrast, lymphedema also can manifest more centrally, for example in the axilla, groin, or even the trunk.[26,33,38,86]

*Severity.* The severity of lymphedema may be described quantitatively or qualitatively. Lymphedema is described by the severity of changes that occur in skin and subcutaneous tissues. The three categories—*pitting, brawny*, and *weeping* edema—are described in Box 24.9. Although all three types reflect a significant degree of lymphedema,

---

**BOX 24.9  Types of Lymphedema**

**Pitting edema:** Pressure on the edematous tissues with the fingertips causes an indentation of the skin that persists for several seconds after the pressure is removed. This reflects significant but short-duration edema with little or no fibrotic changes in skin or subcutaneous tissues.
**Brawny edema:** Pressure on the edematous areas feels hard with palpation. This reflects a more severe form of interstitial swelling with progressive, fibrotic changes in subcutaneous tissues.
**Weeping edema:** This represents the most severe and long-duration form of lymphedema. Fluids leak from cuts or sores; wound healing is significantly impaired. Lymphedema of this severity occurs almost exclusively in the lower extremities.

they are listed in order of severity, from least severe to most severe.[18,20,33,38,71]

Descriptors such as mild, moderate, and severe sometimes are based on how much larger the size of the edmatous limb is compared with the noninvolved limb.[61] However, there are no standard definitions associated with size and severity.

### Increased Size of the Limb
As the volume of interstitial fluid in the limb increases, so does the size of the limb (weight and girth).[17,39,46,86] Increased volume, in turn, causes tautness of the skin and susceptibility to skin breakdown.[18,33]

### Sensory Disturbances
Paresthesia (tingling, itching, or numbness) or occasionally a mild aching pain may be felt particularly in the fingers or toes. In many instances the condition is painless, and the patient perceives only a sense of heaviness of the limb. Fine finger coordination also may be impaired as the result of the sensory disturbances.[18,39,61,71]

### Stiffness and Limited Range of Motion
Range of motion (ROM) decreases in the fingers and wrist or toes and ankle or even in the more proximal joints, leading to decreased functional mobility of the involved segments.[18,58]

### Decreased Resistance to Infection
Wound healing is delayed; and frequent infections (e.g., cellulitis) may occur.[39,46,86]

## Examination and Evaluation of Lymphatic Function

A patient's history, a systems review, and specific tests and measures provide information to determine impairments and functional limitations that can arise from lymphatic disorders and the presence of lymphedema. Key components in the examination process that are particularly relevant when lymphatic dysfunction is suspected or lymphedema is present are summarized in this section.[19,27,46,54,58,74,86] Other tests and measurements, such as vital signs, ROM, strength, posture, and sensory, functional, and cardiopulmonary testing, also are appropriate.

### History and Systems Review
Note any history of infection, trauma, surgery, or radiation therapy. The onset and duration of lymphedema, delayed wound healing, or previous treatment of lymphedema are pertinent pieces of information. Identify the occupation or daily activities of the patient and determine if long periods of standing or sitting are required.

### Examination of Skin Integrity
Visual inspection and palpation of the skin provide information about the integrity of the skin. The location of the edema should be noted. When the limb is in a dependent position, palpate the skin to determine the type and severity of lymphedema and changes in skin and subcutaneous tissues. Areas of pitting, brawny, or weeping edema should be noted.

N O T E : When palpating the skin over lymph nodes, note any tenderness of the nodes (cervical, supraclavicular, inguinal). Tenderness may or may not indicate ongoing infection or serious disease.[34] Evidence of warm, enlarged, tender, painless, or adherent nodes should be reported to the physician.

The presence of wounds or scars and the color and appearance of the skin, which often is shiny and red in an edematous limb, should be noted. Photographic documentation is convenient in the clinical or home setting and provides visual evidence of changes in skin integrity.[86] If a wound or scar is identified, its size should be noted, as should scar mobility or the presence of inflammation or infection in a wound.

### Girth Measurements
Circumferential measurements of the involved limb should be taken and compared with the noninvolved limb if the problem is unilateral.[17,54,61] Identify specific intervals or landmarks at which measurements are taken so measurements during subsequent examinations are reliable. Use of circumferential measurements at anatomical landmarks has been shown to be a valid and reliable method of calculating limb volume.[74]

### Volumetric Measurements
An alternative method of measuring limb size is to immerse the limb in a tank of water to a predetermined anatomical landmark and measure the volume of water displaced.[17,54,74] Although this method also has been shown to be valid and reliable, for routine clinical use it is more cumbersome and less practical than girth measurements.[74]

## Prevention of Lymphedema

If a patient is at risk of developing lymphedema secondary to infection, inflammation, obstruction, surgical removal of lymphatic structures, or chronic venous insufficiency, *prevention* of lymphedema should be the priority of patient management. In some situations, such as after removal of lymph nodes or vessels, preventive measures may be needed for a lifetime. Even when a patient takes every measure to prevent edema, it still may develop at some time, particularly after trauma to or surgical removal of lymph vessels. Box 24.10 summarizes precautions and measures to prevent or reduce the risk of lymphedema.[16,18,20,41,58,64,71,76,86]

## Management of Lymphedema

### Background and Rationale
Comprehensive management of lymphedema involves a combination of appropriate medical management and direct therapeutic intervention by a therapist combined with self-management by the patient. Treatment also includes appropriate pharmacological management for infection control and prevention or removal of excessive fluid and proteins.[16,33,38]

The overall goal of management when lymphedema has developed is to improve drainage of obstructed areas

---

## BOX 24.10 Precautions, Prevention, and Self-Management of Lymphedema

### Prevention of Lymphedema

- Avoid static, dependent positioning of the lower extremities, such as prolonged sitting or standing. Avoid sitting with legs crossed.
- When traveling long distances by car, stop periodically and walk around or support an involved upper extremity on the car's window ledge or seat back.
- Elevate involved limb(s) and perform repetitive pumping exercises frequently during the day.
- Avoid *vigorous*, repetitive activities with the involved limb. Avoid carrying heavy loads, such as a suitcase, a heavy backpack, or shoulder bag. Avoid use of heavy weights when exercising.
- Wear compressive garments while exercising.
- Avoid wearing clothing that restricts circulation, such as sleeves or socks with tight elastic bands. Do not wear tight jewelry such as rings or watches.
- Monitor diet to maintain an ideal weight and minimize sodium intake.
- Avoid hot environments or use of local heat.
- If possible, avoid having blood pressure taken on an involved upper extremity or injections in either an involved upper or lower extremity.

### Skin Care

- Keep the skin clean and supple; use moisturizers but avoid perfumed lotions.
- Avoid infections; pay immediate attention to a skin abrasion or cut, an insect bite, a blister, or a burn.
- Protect hands and feet; wear socks or hose, properly fitting shoes, rubber gloves, oven mitts, etc.
- Avoid contact with harsh detergents and chemicals.
- Use caution when cutting nails. Women need to use an electric razor when shaving legs or underarm area.
- Avoid hot baths, whirlpools, and saunas that elevate the body's core temperature.

---

and theoretically to channel fluids into unobstructed, collateral vessels. The following must be accomplished to increase lymphatic drainage.

- The hydrostatic pressures on edematous tissues must be increased.[26] This is accomplished by *external compression of tissues* with manual lymphatic drainage, sequential pneumatic compression machines, or compressive garments.[16-19,48,58,76,86]

NOTE: It appears that compression facilitates the evacuation and reabsorption of fluids but does not increase the reabsorption of proteins in the edema fluid.[33]

- Lymphatic and venous return also is enhanced by *elevating* the involved limb. Lymphedema caused by infection or inflammation of the lymphatic system (e.g., lymphangitis or cellulitis) does not diminish as readily with elevation as does edema secondary to chronic venous insufficiency.[26,33,76]

## Comprehensive Regimens and Components

A comprehensive approach to the management of lymphedema is referred to in the literature by a variety of terms, including *complex lymphedema therapy, complete* or *complex decongestive physical therapy*, or *decongestive lymphatic therapy*.[10,11,21,22,25,44,51,52,70,72,85,86] Box 24.11 summarizes the components of these programs.

All of these regimens combine manual lymphatic drainage through light, superficial massage and compressive bandaging with active ROM, low-intensity resistance exercises, cardiopulmonary conditioning exercises, and good skin hygiene.

***Manual lymphatic drainage.*** Manual lymphatic drainage involves slow, very light repetitive stroking and circular massage movements done in a specific sequence with the involved extremity elevated whenever possible.[10,11,21,22,25,47,73,85,86] Proximal congestion in the trunk, groin, buttock, or axilla is cleared first to make room for fluid from the more distal areas. The direction of the massage is toward specific lymph nodes and usually involves *distal to proximal* stroking. Fluid in the involved extremity then is cleared, first in the proximal portion and then in the distal portion of the limb. Because manual lymphatic drainage is extremely labor- and time-intensive, methods of self-massage are taught to the patient as soon as possible in a treatment program.

***Exercise.*** Active ROM, stretching, and low-intensity resistance exercises are integrated with manual drainage techniques.[7,16,18,21,23,24,57,59,60,86] Exercises are performed while wearing a compressive garment or bandages and in a specific sequence, often with the edematous limb(s) elevated. A low-intensity cardiovascular/pulmonary endurance activity, such as bicycling, often follows ROM and strengthening exercises. Specific exercises and a suggested sequence for the upper and lower extremities, compiled from several sources, are described and illustrated in the last section of this chapter.

---

## BOX 24.11 Components of a Decongestive Lymphatic Therapy Program

- Elevation
- Manual lymphatic drainage (massage)
  - Direct intervention by a therapist
  - Self-massage by the patient
- Compression
  - Nonelastic or low-stretch bandages or custom-fitted garments
  - Intermittent, sequential pneumatic compression pump
- Individualized exercise program
  - Active ROM (pumping exercises)
  - Flexibility exercises
  - Low-intensity resistance exercises
  - Cardiovascular conditioning
- Skin care and daily living precautions

*Elevation.* The involved limb is elevated during use of a sequential compression pump, while sleeping or resting, or even during sedentary activities. The compressive bandages or garment are worn during periods of elevation.[11,16,18,58,76]

***Compressive bandages, garments, or pumps.*** No-stretch, nonelastic bandages or low-stretch elastic bandages or garments are recommended because they provide relatively low compressive forces on the edematous extremity at rest. In addition, they provide a higher working pressure with active muscular contractions because of their less yielding nature than high-stretch bandages.[16,18,21,25,76,86] High-stretch sports bandages, such as Ace wraps, are not recommended for treating lymphedema.[11,16,76] Daily use of a sequential, pneumatic compression pump also may be advisable during the early stages of treatment of substantial lymphedema.[16,19,25,58]

***Skin care and hygiene.*** Lymphedema predisposes the patient to skin breakdown, infection, and delayed wound healing. Meticulous attention to skin care and protection of the edematous limb are essential elements of self-management of lymphedema.[16,18,58,76]

### Management Guidelines
Guidelines for the management of lymphatic disorders are essentially the same as those already described for the management of chronic venous insufficiency and associated lymphedema (see Box 24.8). As with chronic venous insufficiency, management of lymphatic disorders initially involves direct interventions by a therapist and an emphasis on patient education, followed by lifelong prevention and self-management by the patient.

### Precautions and Self-Management of Lymphedema
Precautions that patients should take to prevent lymphedema and skin breakdown or infection are an important aspect of self-management (see Box 24.10).

### Use of Community Resources
A valuable resource for patients and health care professions is the National Lymphedema Network (www.lymphnet.org). This nonprofit organization provides education and guidance about lymphedema. Another resource is the Lymphedema Internet Network (http://www.lymphedema.org).

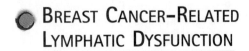

# BREAST CANCER–RELATED LYMPHATIC DYSFUNCTION

## Background
Breast cancer-related dysfunction of the lymphatic system and subsequent lymphedema of the upper extremity is a somewhat common and potentially serious complication of the treatment for breast cancer. It is estimated that 15% to 20%[63] or as many as one in four patients[29] with invasive breast cancer develop upper extremity lymphedema during or sometime after the course of treatment.

Current treatment usually involves removing a portion or all of the breast accompanied by excision or irradiation of adjacent axillary lymph nodes, the principal site of regional metastases. Axillary dissection places a patient at risk not only for upper extremity lymphedema but also for loss of shoulder mobility and limited function of the arm and hand.[7,8,14,15,17,18,31,61,63,69] In addition, chemotherapy or hormonal therapy may also be employed.

Axillary dissection and removal of lymph nodes interrupt and slow the circulation of lymph, which in turn can lead to lymphedema.[7,15,18,29] Radiation therapy can cause fibrosis of tissues in the area of the axilla, which obstructs the lymphatic vessels and contributes to pooling of lymph in the arm and hand.[7,15,18,29] The extent of the axillary dissection and exposure to radiation is associated with the degree of risk for lymphedema to develop. In addition, shoulder motion can become impaired as the result of incisional pain, delayed wound healing, and skin ulcerations (associated with radiation therapy), and postoperative weakness of the muscles of the shoulder girdle.[18,58]

A comprehensive approach to postoperative management that emphasizes patient education and includes therapeutic exercise and other direct interventions to prevent or treat lymphedema and other impairments or functional limitations are key to successful outcomes.[5,8,16,18,58,64]

As with most cancers, the diagnosis of breast cancer and the ensuing treatments have an enormous emotional impact on patients and their families.[18,71] The advent of of breast cancer-related lymphedema not only has an impact on a breast cancer survivor's physical function but is known to have a significantly adverse effect on health-related quality of life, making prevention of lymphedema and, if it develops, aggressive treatment high priorities for management.[69]

## Surgical Procedures
Surgical treatment of breast cancer falls into two broad categories—mastectomy and breast-conserving surgeries—both of which are coupled routinely with partial or complete axillary node dissection. Differences in surgical procedures are related to the extent of removal of breast tissue and surrounding or underlying soft tissues.[1,10,40] A course of radiation therapy routinely follows surgery to decrease the risk of regional recurrence of the disease. Chemotherapy also may be initiated postoperatively to prevent the systemic spread of the disease.

### Mastectomy
Mastectomy involves removing the entire breast. In addition, a mastectomy may involve removing the fascia over the chest muscle. With late-stage, invasive disease, a radical mastectomy in which the pectoralis muscles also are excised may be required, leading to significant muscle weakness and impaired shoulder function.

### Breast-Conserving Surgery
Options for resecting the tumor and preserving a portion of the breast include *lumpectomy*, which involves excision of

the mass and a margin of healthy surrounding breast tissue, or *segmental mastectomy* (also known as *quadrectomy),* which is excision of the affected quadrant of the breast. These procedures are being used increasingly, rather than mastectomy, in combination with adjuvant therapy for patients with stage I or II tumors.[1,40]

There are now multiple randomized clinical trials that show that the 10- to 20-year survival rate for patients with stage I or II disease who underwent breast-conserving surgery combined with radiation therapy is equivalent to that achieved by patients who underwent mastectomy alone or mastectomy with adjuvant therapy.[1]

Patients who undergo breast-conserving procedures without removal of lymph nodes are still at risk for developing postoperative lymphedema and impaired shoulder mobility because of potential complications from radiation therapy and biopsy of at least one lymph node.[18,58]

### Dissection of Axillary Lymph Nodes (Lymphadenectomy)

As mentioned, at this time axillary lymph node dissection is a standard part of mastectomy and breast-conserving surgery, although the extent of node removal is controversial.[1,40] A minimum of a level I axillary node dissection and removal of the sentinel node in the axilla at the lateral borders of the breast is required for biopsy to assess regional lymph node involvement and for staging the disease. More extensive dissection for metastatic disease removes the nodes under the pectoralis minor muscle or around the clavicle

## Impairments and Complications Related to Breast Cancer Treatment

The following impairments and complications may occur in association with treatment of breast cancer. Many of these problems are interrelated and must be considered jointly when a comprehensive postoperative rehabilitation program is developed for the patient.*

### Postoperative Pain

*Incisional pain.* A transverse incision across the chest wall is made to remove the breast tissue and underlying fascia on the chest musculature. The incision extends into the axilla for lymph node dissection. Postoperatively, the sutured skin over the breast area may feel tight along the incision. Movement of the arm pulls on the incision and is uncomfortable for the patient. Healing of the incision may be delayed as the result of radiation therapy. Delayed wound healing, in turn, prolongs pain in the area of the incision.

*Posterior cervical and shoulder girdle pain.* Pain and muscle spasm may occur in the neck and shoulder region as a result of muscle guarding. The levator scapulae, teres major and minor, and infraspinatus often are tender to palpation and can restrict active shoulder motion. Decreased

---

*See refs. 6, 8, 14, 15, 18, 31, 36, 37, 43, 58, 61, 81, 83, 86.

use of the involved upper extremity after surgery due to pain sets the stage for the patient to develop a chronic frozen shoulder and increases the likelihood of lymphedema in the hand and arm.

### Postoperative Vascular and Pulmonary Complications

Decreased activity and extended time in bed increase venous stasis and the risk of DVT. Risk of pulmonary complications, such as pneumonia, also is higher because of the patient's reduced activity level. Incisional pain may make the patient reluctant to cough or breathe deeply, both of which are necessary postoperatively to keep the airways clear of fluid accumulation.

### Lymphedema

As noted previously, patients who undergo any level of lymph node dissection or whose treatment regimen includes radiation therapy remain at risk throughout life for developing ipsilateral upper extremity lymphedema.[7,18,58,86] Lymphedema can occur almost immediately after lymph node dissection, during the course of radiation therapy, or many months or even years after treatment has been completed. It is typically evident in the hand and arm but occasionally develops in the upper chest or back area.[15,18,58,61,86] In turn, lymphedema leads to impaired upper extremity function, poor cosmesis, and emotional distress.[18,31,61,71]

### Chest Wall Adhesions

Restrictive scarring of underlying tissues on the chest wall can develop as the result of surgery, radiation fibrosis, or wound infection. Chest wall adhesions can lead to increased risk of postoperative pulmonary complications, restricted mobility of the shoulder, postural asymmetry and dysfunction, and discomfort in the neck, shoulder girdle, and upper back.

### Decreased Shoulder Mobility

It is well documented that patients may experience temporary and sometimes long-term loss of shoulder mobility after surgery or radiation therapy for treatment of breast cancer.[7,37,43,58,64,80,81,83] Factors contributing to impaired shoulder mobility after surgery are listed in Box 24.12.

### Weakness of the Involved Upper Extremity

*Shoulder weakness.* If the long thoracic nerve is traumatized during axillary dissection and removal of lymph nodes, this results in weakness of the serratus anterior and compromised stability of the scapula, limiting active flexion and abduction of the arm. Faulty shoulder mechanics and use of substitute motions with the upper trapezius and levator scapulae during overhead reaching can cause subacromial impingement and shoulder pain. Shoulder impingement, in turn, can be a precursor to a frozen shoulder. If the pectoralis muscles were disturbed, which occurs with a radical mastectomy for advanced disease, weakness is evident in horizontal adduction.

*Decreased grip strength.* Grip strength is often diminished as the result of lymphedema and secondary stiffness of the fingers.

| BOX 24.12 | Factors Contributing to Impaired Shoulder Mobility After Breast Cancer Surgery |
|---|---|

- Incisional pain immediately after surgery or associated with delayed wound healing
- Muscle guarding and tenderness of the shoulder and posterior cervical musculature
- Need for protected shoulder ROM until the surgical drain is removed
- Fibrosis of soft tissues in the axillary region due to adjuvant radiation therapy
- Adherence of scar tissue to the chest wall, causing adhesions
- Temporary or permanent weakness of the muscles of the shoulder girdle
- Rounded shoulders and kyphotic or scoliotic trunk posture associated with age or incisional pain
- A feeling of heaviness of the upper extremity due to lymphedema
- Decreased use of the hand and arm for functional activities

### Postural Malalignment

The patient may sit or stand with rounded shoulders and kyphosis because of pain, skin tightness, or psychological reasons. An increase in thoracic kyphosis associated with aging is commonly seen in the older patient.[36] This contributes to faulty shoulder mechanics and eventually restricts active use of the involved upper extremity. Asymmetry of the trunk and abnormal scapular alignment may occur as the result of a subtle lateral weight shift, particularly in a large-breasted woman.

### Fatigue and Decreased Endurance

Patients undergoing radiation therapy or chemotherapy often experience debilitating fatigue.[1,33] Anemia may develop as a result of chemotherapy. Nutritional intake and subsequent energy stores may be diminished, particularly if a patient is experiencing nausea for several days after a cycle of chemotherapy. Fatigue also is associated with depression. As a result, exercise tolerance and endurance during functional activities are markedly reduced.

### Psychological Considerations

A patient undergoing treatment for breast cancer experiences a wide range of emotional and social issues.[71] The needs and concerns of both the patient and the family must be considered. The patient and family members must cope with the potentially life-threatening nature of the disease and a difficult treatment regimen. It is common for a patient to feel anxiety, agitation, anger, depression, a sense of loss, and significant mood swings during treatment and recovery from breast cancer.

In addition to the obvious physical disfigurement and altered body image associated with mastectomy, medications such as immunosuppressants and corticosteroids can affect the emotional state of a patient. Psychological manifestations affect physical well-being and can contribute to general fatigue, the patient's perception of functional disability, and motivation during treatment.

## Guidelines for Management After Breast Cancer Surgery

Guidelines for postoperative management for the patient who has undergone a mastectomy or breast-conserving surgery and who may currently be receiving adjuvant therapy are outlined in Box 24.13. The guidelines identify therapeutic interventions for common impairments during the early postoperative period and those that could develop at a later time.

NOTE: The guidelines outlined in Box 24.13 also can be modified to prevent or manage problems that can develop in the trunk and lower extremities after surgery for abdominal or pelvic cancers and accompanying inguinal lymph node dissection.

### Special Considerations

**Patient education.** The length of stay for patients after surgery for breast cancer is short. Therefore, direct intervention by a therapist starts on the first postoperative day with an emphasis on patient education for *prevention* of postoperative complications and impairments, including pulmonary complications, thromboemboli, lymphedema, and loss of shoulder mobility. Recommendations for preventing lymphedema or for self-management if it develops are reviewed with the patient (see Box 24.10).

**Exercise.** The postoperative exercise program focuses on three main areas: improving shoulder function, regaining an overall level of fitness, and preventing or managing lymphedema. Early, but protected, assisted or active ROM of the shoulder is the key to restoring shoulder mobility. Postoperative risks that contribute to restricted shoulder mobility were summarized previously (see Box 24.12).[1,18,40,58,60] These risks are highest during the early postoperative period until drains have been removed and the incision has healed.

NOTE: Radiation therapy to the axillary and breast areas can delay wound healing beyond the typical 3- to 4-week period.[1,40] Even after initial healing of the incision, the scar has a tendency to contract and can become adherent to underlying tissues, which, in turn, can restrict shoulder motion.

Although strengthening exercises and aerobic conditioning are important for upper extremity function and total body fitness, *moderation* in an exercise program is imperative. Exercises must be progressed gradually, excessive fatigue must be avoided, and energy conservation must be emphasized, especially if the patient is undergoing chemotherapy or radiation therapy. Exercise precautions for the patient undergoing treatment are noted in Box 24.14.[7,18,60,64]

**BOX 24.13**

## MANAGEMENT GUIDELINES—After Surgery for Breast Cancer

### Potential Postoperative Impairments
Pulmonary and circulatory complications
Lymphedema
Restricted mobility of the upper extremity
Postural malalignment
Weakness and decreased functional use of the upper extremity
Fatigue and decreased endurance for functional activities
Emotional and social adjustments

| Plan of Care | Interventions |
|---|---|
| 1. Prepare the patient for post-operative self-management. | 1. Interdisciplinary patient education involving all aspects of potential impairments and functional limitations.<br>Self-management activities and preparation for participation in a home program on the first postoperative day. |
| 2. Prevent postoperative pulmonary complications and thromboemboli. | 2. Pre- or postoperative instruction in deep breathing, emphasizing maximal inspirations and effective coughing (see Chapter 25).<br>Active ankle exercises (calf pumping exercises). |
| 3. Prevent or minimize postoperative lymphedema. | 3. Elevation of the involved upper extremity on pillows (about 30°) while the patient is in bed or sitting in a chair. Wrapping the involved upper extremity with bandages or wearing an elastic pressure gradient sleeve.<br>Pumping exercises of the arm on the side of the surgery.<br>Early ROM exercises.<br>PRECAUTION: Avoid static, dependent positioning of the arm. |
| 4. Decrease lymphedema if or when it develops. | 4. Manual lymphatic drainage massage.<br>Daily regimen of exercises to reduce lymphedema.<br>Use of custom-fit elastic compression garment when lymphedema is stabilized.<br>Adherence to precautions for skin care (see Box 24.10). |
| 5. Prevent postural deformities. | 5. Posture awareness training; encourage the patient to assume an erect posture when sitting or standing to minimize a rounded shoulder posture.<br>Posture exercises with an emphasis on scapular retraction exercises. |
| 6. Prevent muscle tension and guarding in cervical musculature. | 6. Active ROM of the cervical spine to promote relaxation.<br>Shoulder shrugging and shoulder circle exercises.<br>Gentle massage to cervical musculature. |
| 7. Prevent restricted mobility of the upper extremity. | 7. Active-assistive and active ROM exercises of the shoulder, elbow, and hand initiated as soon as possible but cautiously usually on the first postoperative day.<br>NOTE: Exercise may be initiated even when the drainage tubes and sutures are still in place.<br>After the incision has healed, self-stretching to the shoulder. |
| 8. Regain strength and functional use of the involved extremity. | 8. Upper extremity ergometry initially against minimal and, later, moderate resistance.<br>Use of the involved extremity for light functional activities. |
| 9. Improve exercise tolerance and sense of well-being; reduce fatigue. | 9. Graded, low-intensity aerobic exercise such as walking or cycling. |
| 10. Provide information about resources for patient and family support and ongoing patient education. | 10. Resources: American Cancer Society for family support and ongoing patient education (www.cancer.org); National Breast Cancer Coalition; National Lymphedema Network. |

Precautions: Shoulder exercise should be performed within *protected* ROM, usually no more than 90° of elevation of the arm until after removal of drains. Observe the incision and sutures carefully during exercises. Avoid any undue tension on the incision or blanching of the scar during shoulder exercises. Avoid exercises with the involved arm in a dependent position. Progress graded exercise program very slowly, particularly if the patient is receiving adjuvant therapy.

---

**BOX 24.14    Exercise Precautions and Treatment of Breast Cancer**

- Exercise only at a moderate level and never to the point that the affected arm aches during or after exercise, even if there is no evidence of lymphedema.
- Monitor upper extremity girth measurements closely.
- Adjust the *timing* of exercise during cycles of radiation therapy or chemotherapy. With some chemotherapy medications, a patient can develop cardiac arrhythmia and therefore should not perform aerobic exercises, such as stationary cycling, for 24 to 48 hours after a chemotherapy session.
- Return to more physically demanding work and recreational activities gradually after completion of chemotherapy or radiation therapy.

---

Although early intervention for the prevention of lymphedema and upper extremity mobility impairments is often advocated by therapists and suggested in descriptive articles in the literature, patients often are not referred for postoperative rehabilitation until after impairments and functional limitations have developed. This may be due to concerns raised in the literature[29] that early postoperative ROM could disturb drains or delay wound healing or that exercises, if performed too vigorously, could initiate or exacerbate lymphedema. In addition, few studies have rigorously investigated the efficacy of specific interventions or rehabilitation protocols.[58,80] However, a recent review of the literature of exercise and cancer-related lymphedema revealed that exercise neither worsened preexisting lymphedema nor was associated with a significant increase in the occurrence of lymphedema.[7]

From the information available in the literature, the following recommendations for exercise are made.[*]

- Integrate several interventions including exercise, massage, and use of compression devices into a patient's comprehensive plan of care.
- Implement shoulder ROM exercises early in a postoperative program to prevent mobility impairments.
- Include moderate-intensity aerobic conditioning exercises to improve fitness and quality of life.
- Progress all forms of exercise gradually and avoid any form of high-intensity training.

***Community resources*** Reach to Recovery is a one-to-one patient education program sponsored by the American Cancer Society (www.cancer.org). Representatives of this program, most of whom are breast cancer survivors, provide emotional support to the patient and family as well as current information on breast prostheses and reconstructive surgery. The National Lymphedema Network (www.lymphnet.org) is another valuable source of information for patients at risk for or who have developed lymphedema.

---

*See refs. 6, 14, 15, 17, 18, 31, 37, 44, 52, 57, 59, 60, 72, 80, 81, 85, 86.

---

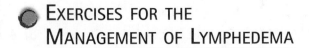

# EXERCISES FOR THE MANAGEMENT OF LYMPHEDEMA

## Background and Rationale

As noted previously in this chapter, exercise is just one aspect of a decongestive lymphatic therapy program. The rationale for including exercise in the comprehensive treatment of patients with upper or lower extremity lymphedema is to move and drain lymph fluid to reduce the edema and to improve the functional use of the involved limb or limbs. Principles on which exercises for lymphatic drainage are based are summarized in Box 24.15.[7,59,86]

The exercises employed in lymph drainage regimens cover a wide spectrum of therapeutic exercise interventions, specifically deep breathing, relaxation, flexibility, strengthening, cardiovascular conditioning exercises, and a sequence of lymphatic drainage exercises as well. Exercise regimens have been described in an extensive number of publications.[*] No particular combination or sequence of exercises has been shown to be superior to another. Although a critical review of the literature a decade ago[62] indicated that the effectiveness of exercise regimens for lymph drainage was based primarily on clinical observations and opinions of experienced practitioners or case reports, there is now an emerging body of evidence documenting the efficacy of specific components of these programs.[7,44,57,58,72]

## Components of Exercise Regimens for Management of Lymphedema

### Deep Breathing and Relaxation Exercises

- Deep breathing is interwoven throughout exercise regimens for the management of lymphedema. It has been

---

**BOX 24.15    Exercises for Lymphatic Drainage: Principles and Rationale**

- Contraction of muscles pumps fluids by direct compression of the collecting lymphatic vessels.
- Exercise reduces soft tissue and joint hypomobility that can contribute to static positioning and lead to lymphostasis.
- Exercise strengthens and prevents atrophy of muscles of the limbs, which improves the efficiency of the lymphatic pump.
- Exercise increases heart rate and arterial pulsations, which in turn contribute to lymph flow.
- Exercise should be sequenced to clear the central lymphatic reservoirs before the peripheral areas.
- Wearing compression bandages during exercises enhances lymph flow and protein reabsorption more efficiently than exercising without bandages.

---

*See refs. 10, 11, 18, 21-24, 41, 44, 48, 51, 52, 59, 60, 64, 69, 72, 85, 86.

suggested that the use of abdominal-diaphragmatic breathing assists in the movement of lymphatic fluid as the diaphragm descends during a deep inspiration and the abdominals contract during a controlled, maximum expiration.[18] Changes in intra-abdominal and intrathoracic pressures create a gentle, continual pumping action that moves fluids in the central lymphatic vessels, which run superiorly in the chest cavity and drain into the venous system in the neck (see Fig. 24.2).

◉ Progressive, total body relaxation exercises[28] (described in Chapter 4 of this text) are performed at the beginning of each exercise session to decrease muscle tension, which may be contributing to restricted mobility and lymph congestion.[18,21,24,86] Deep breathing is an integral component of the sequence of relaxation exercises.

### Flexibility Exercises

Gentle, self-stretching exercises are used to minimize soft tissue and joint hypomobility, particularly in proximal areas of the body that may contribute to static postures and lymph congestion.

### Strengthening and Muscular Endurance Exercises

Both isometric and dynamic exercises using self-resistance, elastic resistance, and weights or weight machines are appropriate if done against light resistance (initially, 1 to 2 lb) and by progressing resistance and repetitions gradually. Regardless of whether lymphedema has developed, it is important to monitor the circumferential size and the skin texture of the involved limb closely to determine whether an appropriate intensity of exercise has been established. Emphasis is placed on improving endurance and strength of central and peripheral muscle groups that enhance an erect posture and minimize fatigue in muscles that contribute to the efficiency of the lymphatic pump mechanism.

### Cardiovascular Conditioning Exercises

Activities such as upper extremity ergometry, swimming, cycling, and walking increase circulation and stimulate lymphatic flow.[18] Thirty minutes of aerobic endurance exercises complement lymph drainage exercises. Conditioning exercises are done at low intensity (at 40% to 50% of the target heart rate) when lymphedema is present and at higher intensities (up to an 80% level) when the lymphedema has been reduced and exercise is otherwise safe.[18,59]

### Lymphatic Drainage Exercises

Lymphatic drainage exercises, often referred to as *pumping exercises,* move fluids through lymphatic channels. Active, repetitive ROM exercises are performed throughout each session. *The exercises follow a specific sequence to move lymph away from congested areas.*[18,21,23,24,86] It is similar to the sequence of massage applied during manual lymph drainage.[47,73] In general, the exercises first focus on proximal areas of the body to clear central collecting vessels and then involve distal muscle groups to begin to move peripheral edema in a centripedal direction to the central lymph vessels. The affected upper or lower extremity or

extremities are held in an elevated position during many of the exercises. Static, dependent postures are avoided. Self-massage also is interspersed throughout the exercise sequence to further enhance drainage. These exercises also maintain mobility of the involved limbs.

## Guidelines for Lymphatic Drainage Exercises

The patient should follow these guidelines when performing a sequence of lymphatic drainage exercises. These guidelines apply to management of upper or lower extremity lymphedema and reflect the combined opinions of several authors and experts in the field.[18,21-23,59,86]

### Preparation for Lymphatic Drainage Exercises

◉ Set aside approximately 20 to 30 minutes for each exercise session.
◉ Perform exercises twice daily every day.
◉ Have needed equipment at hand, such as a foam roll, wedge, or exercise wand.

### During Lymphatic Drainage Exercises

◉ Wear compression bandages or a customized compression garment.
◉ Precede lymphatic drainage exercises with total body relaxation activities.
◉ Follow a specified order of exercises.
◉ Perform active, repetitive movements slowly, about 1 to 2 seconds per repetition.
◉ Elevate the involved limb above the heart during distal pumping exercises.
◉ Combine deep breathing exercises with active movements of the head, neck, trunk, and limbs.
◉ Initially, perform a low number of repetitions. Increase repetitions gradually to avoid excessive fatigue.
◉ Do not exercise to the point where the edematous limb aches.
◉ Incorporate self-massage into the exercise sequence to further enhance lymph drainage.
◉ Maintain good posture during exercises.
◉ When strengthening exercises are added to the lymph drainage sequence, use light resistance and avoid excessive muscle fatigue.

### After Lymphatic Drainage Exercises

◉ If possible, rest with the involved extremity elevated for 30 minutes.
◉ Set aside time several times per week for low-intensity aerobic exercise activities, such as walking or bicycling for 30 minutes.
◉ Carefully check for signs of redness or increased swelling in the edematous limb, either of which could indicate that the level of exercise was excessive.

## Selected Exercises for Lymphatic Drainage: Upper and Lower Extremity Sequences

The selection and sequences of exercises described in this section and summarized in Box 24.16 are designed to assist

| BOX 24.16 | Sequence of Selected Exercises for Management of Upper or Lower Extremity Lymphedema |
|---|---|

**Exercises Common to Upper and Lower Extremity Regimens**

N O T E : Start an upper or lower extremity regimen with these exercises
- Deep breathing and total body relaxation exercises
- Posterior pelvic tilts and partial curl-ups
- Cervical ROM
- Bilateral scapular movements

**Upper Extremity Exercises**
- Active circumduction with the involved arm elevated while lying supine
- Bilateral active movements of the arms while lying supine or on a foam roll
- Bilateral hand press while lying supine or sitting
- Shoulder stretches (with wand, doorway, or towel) while standing
- Active elbow, forearm, wrist, and finger exercises of the involved arm
- Bilateral horizontal abduction and adduction of the shoulders
- Overhead wall press while standing

- Finger exercises

- Partial curl-ups
- Rest with involved upper extremity elevated

**Lower Extremity Exercises**
- Alternate knee to chest exercises

- Bilateral knees to chest

- Gluteal setting and posterior pelvic tilts
- Single knee to chest with the involved lower extremity

- External rotation of the hips while lying supine with both legs elevated and resting on a wedge or wall
- Active knee flexion of the involved lower extremity while lying supine
- Active plantarflexion and dorsiflexion and circumduction of the ankles while lying supine with lower extremities elevated
- Active hip and knee flexion with legs externally rotated and elevated against a wall
- Active cycling and scissoring movements with legs elevated
- Bilateral knee to chest exercises, followed by partial curl-ups
- Rest with lower extremities elevated

in the drainage of upper or lower extremity lymphedema. Many of the individual exercises suggested in lymphedema protocols, such as ROM of the cervical spine and some of the shoulder girdle or upper extremity exercises, are not exclusively used for lymph drainage. They also are used to improve mobility and strength. Several of the exercises highlighted in this section already have been described in previous chapters in this text. Only those exercises or variations of exercises that are somewhat unique or not previously addressed are described or illustrated in this section.

**Sequence of Exercises**

- Total body relaxation exercises are implemented prior to lymphatic drainage exercises.
- Exercises for lymphatic drainage should follow a particular sequence to assist lymph flow. The central and proximal lymphatic vessels, such as the abdominal, inguinal, and cervical nodes (see Fig. 24.2), are cleared first with trunk, pelvic, hip, and cervical exercises. Then, for the most part, exercises proceed distally from shoulders to fingers or from hips to toes. If lymph nodes have been surgically removed (e.g., with a unilateral axillary node dissection for breast cancer or a bilateral inguinal node dissection for cancers of the abdominal or pelvic organs), lymph must be channeled to the remaining nodes in the body.

N O T E : Because no single sequence of exercises has been shown to be more effective than another, the upper and lower extremity sequences of exercises outlined in this sec-

tion do not reflect the exercises included in any one specific protocol. Rather, the exercise sequences are based on the recommendations of several authors.[18,21-23,44,57-59,72,86] Sequences of exercises for upper or lower extremity lymphedema are summarized in the remaining portion of this chapter. Therapists are encouraged to modify or add other exercises to the sequences in this chapter as they see fit to meet the individual needs of their patients.

**Exercises Common to Upper and Lower Extremity Sequences**

These initial exercises should be included in programs for unilateral or bilateral upper or lower extremity lymphedema. They are designed to help the patient relax and then to clear the central channels and nodes.

- **Total body relaxation**
  - Have the patient assume a comfortable supine position and begin deep breathing. Then, isometrically contract and relax the muscles of the lower trunk (abdominals and erector spinae) followed by the hips, lower legs, feet, and toes.
  - Then contract and relax the muscles of the upper back, shoulders, upper arms, forearms, wrist, and fingers.
  - Finally, contract and relax the muscles of the neck and face.
  - Relax the whole body for at least a minute.
  - Perform diaphragmatic breathing throughout the entire sequence. Avoid breath-holding and the Valsalva maneuver.

● *Posterior pelvic tilts and partial curl-ups*
  • Perform these exercises with hips and knees flexed, in the supine position.
● *Unilateral knee-to-chest movements.* These exercises are designed to target the inguinal nodes. This is important even for upper extremity lymphedema.
  • In the supine position flex one hip and knee, and grasp the lower leg. Pull the knee to the chest. Gently press or bounce the thigh against the abdomen and chest about 15 times.
  • Repeat the procedure with the opposite lower extremity.

N O T E : If lymphedema is present in only one lower extremity, initiate the knee-to-chest exercises with the *uninvolved* lower extremity.

● *Cervical ROM.* Perform each motion for a count of 5 for five repetitions.
  • Rotation
  • Lateral flexion
● *Scapular exercises.* Perform exercise for a count of 5 for five repetitions.
  • Active elevation and depression (shoulder shrugs)
  • Active shoulder rolls
  • Active scapular retraction and protraction. With arms at sides and elbows flexed, bilaterally retract the scapulae, pointing elbows posteriorly and medially. Then protract the scapulae.

N O T E : Be sure to shrug the shoulders as high as possible and then *actively* pull down the shoulders (depress the scapulae) as far as possible

### Exercises Specifically for Upper Extremity Lymphedema Clearance

The following sequence of exercises is performed after the general, total body exercises just described. The exercises, which are performed in a proximal to distal sequence, are done specifically for upper extremity lymph clearance.

N O T E : Periodically during the exercise sequence have the patient perform self-massage to the axillary node area of the *uninvolved* side proceeding from the axilla to the chest.

● *Active circumduction of the arm (Fig. 24.3).* While lying supine, flex the involved arm to 90° (reach toward the ceiling) and perform active circular movements of the arm about 6 to 12 inches in diameter. Do this clockwise and counterclockwise, five repetitions in each direction.

P R E C A U T I O N : Avoid pendular motions or circumduction of the edematous upper extremity with the arm in a dependent position.

● *Exercises on a foam roll (Fig. 24.4).* While lying supine on a firm foam roll (approximately 6 inches in diameter), perform horizontal abduction and adduction as well as flexion and extension of the shoulder. These movements target congested axillary nodes and are done unilaterally. For home exercises, if special equipment such as an Ethyfoam® roller is not available, have the patient perform these exercises on a foam pool "noodle." Although

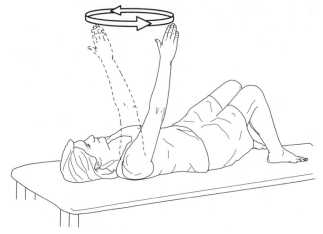

FIGURE 24.3 Active circumduction of the edematous extremity.

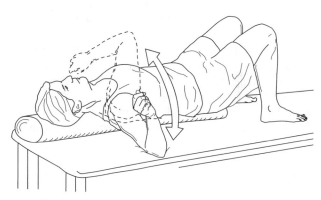

FIGURE 24.4 Active shoulder exercises on a firm, foam roll.

the diameter is smaller, a towel or folded sheet can be wrapped around the foam "noodle" to increase the diameter of the roll.
● *Bilateral hand press.* With arms elevated to shoulder level or higher and the elbows flexed, place the palms of the hands together in front of the chest or head. Press the palms together (for an isometric contraction of the pectoralis major muscles) while breathing in for a count of 5. Relax and then repeat up to five times.
● *Wand exercise, doorway or corner stretch, and towel stretch.* Incorporate several exercises to increase shoulder mobility and to decrease congestion and assist lymph flow in the upper extremity. Hold the position of stretch for several seconds with each repetition. These exercises have been described and are illustrated in Chapter 17.
● *Unilateral arm exercises with the arm elevated.* The following exercises are done with the patient seated and the arm supported at shoulder level on a tabletop or countertop or with the patient supine and the arm supported on a wedge or elevated overhead.
  • Shoulder rotation with the elbow extended. Turn the palm up, then down, by rotating the shoulder, not simply pronating and supinating the forearm.
  • Elbow flexion and extension.
  • Circumduction of the wrist.
  • Hand opening and closing.

● *Bilateral, horizontal abduction and adduction.* While standing or sitting, place both hands behind the head. Horizontally adduct and abduct the shoulders by bringing the elbows together and then pointing them laterally.

● *Overhead wall press.* Face a wall; place one or both palms on the wall with the hands above shoulder level. Gently press the palms into the wall for several seconds without moving the body. Relax and repeat approximately five times.

● *Wrist and finger exercises.* If swelling is present in the wrist and hand, repetitive active finger movements are indicated with the arm elevated.

 • After performing the overhead wall press as just described, keep the heel of the hand on the wall and alternatively move all of the fingers away from and back to the wall (Fig. 24.5).

 • In the same position as just described, alternately press individual fingers into the wall, as if playing a piano, while keeping the heel of the hand in contact with the wall.

 • Place the palms of both hands together with the hands overhead or at least above shoulder level. One finger at a time, press matching fingers together and then pull them away from each other.

● *Partial curl-ups.* To complete the exercise sequence, perform additional curl-ups (about five repetitions) with hands sliding on the thighs.

● *Rest.* Rest in a supine position with the involved arm elevated on pillows for about 30 minutes after completing the exercise sequence.

### Exercises Specifically for Lower Extremity Lymphedema Clearance

N O T E : After completing the general lower body, neck, and shoulder exercises previously described, have the patient perform self-massage first to the axillary lymph nodes on the *involved* side of the body. Then massage the lower abdominal area superiorly to the waist and then laterally and superiorly to the axillary area of the involved side. This sequence is repeated periodically throughout the lower extremity exercise sequence.

● *Unilateral knee-to-chest movements.* In the supine position, repeat this exercise for another 15 repetitions. If lymphedema is present in only one lower extremity, perform repeated knee to chest movements with the *uninvolved leg first* and then the involved leg.

● *Bilateral knees to chest.* In the supine position, flex both hips and knees, grasp both thighs, and gently pull them to the abdomen and chest. Repeat 10 to 15 times.

● *Gluteal setting and posterior pelvic tilts.* Repeat five times, holding each contraction for several seconds and then slowly releasing.

● *External rotation of the hips (Fig. 24.6).* Lie in the supine position with the legs elevated and resting against a wall or on a wedge. Externally rotate the hips, pressing the buttocks together, and holding the outwardly rotated position. Repeat several times.

● *Knee flexion to clear the popliteal area.* While lying in the supine position and keeping the uninvolved lower extremity extended, flex the involved hip and knee enough to clear the foot from the mat table. Actively flex the knee as far as possible by quickly moving the heel to the buttocks. Repeat approximately 15 times.

● *Active ankle movements.* With both legs elevated and propped against a wall, or just the involved leg propped against a door frame and the uninvolved leg resting on the floor, actively plantarflex the ankle and curl the toes; then dorsiflex the ankle and extend the toes as far as possible for multiple repetitions. Finally, actively circumduct the foot clockwise and counterclockwise for several repetitions.

● *Wall slides in external rotation (Fig. 24.7).* With the feet propped up against the wall, legs externally rotated, and

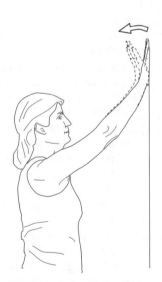

FIGURE 24.5 Overhead wall press.

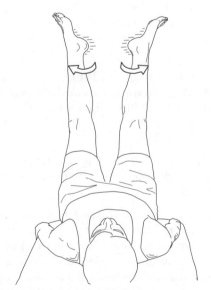

FIGURE 24.6 Repeated outward rotation of the hips with legs elevated.

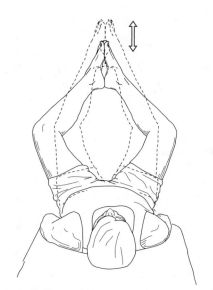

FIGURE 24.7 Wall slides with hips externally rotated.

● **Rest.** With feet elevated and legs propped up against the wall, rest in this position for several minutes after completing exercises. Then rest the legs partially elevated on a wedge, and remain in this position for another 30 minutes.

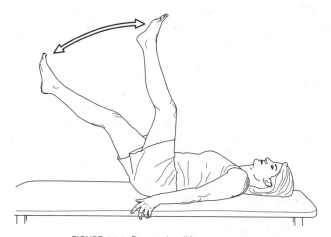

FIGURE 24.8 Repeated walking movements.

heels touching, slide both feet down the wall as far as possible and then back up the wall for several repetitions.

● **Leg movements in the air (Fig. 24.8).** With both hips flexed and the back flat on the floor and both feet pointed to the ceiling, alternately move the legs, simulating cycling, walking, and scissoring motions.

● **Hip adduction across the midline (Fig. 24.9).** Lie in the supine position with the uninvolved leg extended. Flex the hip and knee of the involved leg. Grasp the lateral aspect of the knee with the contralateral hand; pull the involved knee repeatedly across the midline in a rocking motion.

N O T E : If lymphedema is bilateral, repeat this exercise with the other lower extremity.

● **Bilateral knee to chest.** Repeat bilateral gentle, bouncing movements of the legs previously described.

● **Partial curl-ups.** To complete the exercise sequence, perform additional partial curl-ups, about five repetitions.

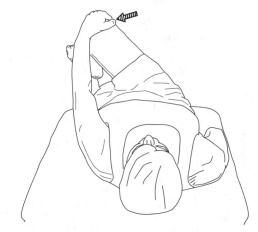

FIGURE 24.9 Hip adduction across the midline to clear inguinal nodes.

## INDEPENDENT LEARNING ACTIVITIES

● **Critical Thinking and Discussion**

1. Differentiate between the signs and symptoms associated with chronic arterial insufficiency and chronic venous insufficiency.

2. You have been asked to participate in a patient education program at your community's cancer society for patients who have undergone surgery for breast cancer. Your responsibility in this program is to help these breast cancer survivors prevent physical impairments and functional limitations associated with their surgery and any related adjuvant therapies. Outline the components of such a program, and explain the rationale for the activities you have chosen to include.

3. What part does a program of exercise and physical activity play in the overall prevention or management of deep vein thrombophlebitis? What are the signs and symptoms of DVT that a patient at risk for this problem must learn to recognize? If you suspect that a patient you are seeing after some type of orthopedic surgery of the lower extremity has developed a DVT, what questions should you ask the patient? What should you do before contacting the patient's physician?

**4.** A patient presents with leg pain that occurs intermittently during the day but not at night. Describe how you would evaluate the patient's signs and symptoms and determine whether the cause of the pain is vascular or neurological.

## ● Laboratory Practice

Perform the sequence of exercises and suggested repetitions for the exercise plan you have designed for case 2 (Ms. L).

## ● Case Studies

### CASE 1

Mr. A, a 65-year-old man with a 5-year history of type II diabetes and peripheral vascular disease, has been referred to you in your home health practice to establish a program to help him improve his overall level of physical activity. He enjoys golf but recently has had difficulty completing a round because of calf pain that occurs when he walks for even short distances along the course. His pain goes away when he stands or sits.

What additional information do you need to secure during the examination and evaluation process? What tests and measurements would be of particular importance? From your evaluation, design a plan of care that includes a program of exercise to help Mr. A improve his level of physical activity and prevent vascular-related complications.

### CASE 2

Ms. L underwent surgery for metastatic pelvic cancer and lymphadenectomy (lymph node dissection) 3 months ago. She also received a series of radiation therapy treatments as part of her comprehensive oncologic management. About 2 weeks ago, she began to notice bilateral swelling in her legs, most notably in her feet and ankles.

She has been referred by her oncologist to the outpatient facility where you work to "evaluate and treat" her for her lymphedema. Describe the examination procedures you would use in your evaluation and then develop a plan of care, including a program of exercise, to help her manage and reduce her lymphedema and prevent potential complications related to the lymphedema.

## REFERENCES

1. Abeloff, MD, et al: Breast. In Abeloff, MD, et al (eds) Clinical Oncology, ed 2. Churchill Livingstone, New York, 2000, p 2051.
2. Abramson, DI: Physiologic basis for the use of physical agents in peripheral vascular disorders. Arch Phys Med Rehabil 46:216, 1965.
3. Aldrich, D, Hunt, DP: When can the patient with deep vein thrombosis begin to ambulate? Phys Ther 84(3):268–273, 2004.
4. Anand, SS, Wells, PS, Hunt, D, et al: Does this patient have a deep vein thrombosis. JAMA 279:1094–1099, 1998.
5. Bergan, JJ: Effect of cancer therapy on lower extremity lymphedema. Natl Lymphedema Netw Newslett 11(1), 1999.
6. Bertelli, G, et al: Conservative treatment of postmastectomy lymphedema: a controlled randomized trial. Am Oncol 2(8):575, 1991.
7. Bicego, D, Brown, K, Ruddick, M, et al: Exercise for women with or at risk for breast cancer-related lymphedema. Phys Ther 86(10):1398–1405, 2006.
8. Boissonnault, WG, Goodman, CC: The female genital/reproductive system. In Goodman, CC, Fuller, KS, Boissonnault, WG (eds) Pathology: Implications for Physical Therapists, ed 2. Elsevier, Philadelphia, 2003, pp 744–771.
9. Boissonnault, WG, Bass, C: Pathological origins of trunk and neck pain. Part 2. Disorders of the cardiovascular and pulmonary systems. J Orthop Sports Phys Ther 12:208, 1990.
10. Boris, M, et al: Lymphedema reduction by noninvasive complex lymphedema therapy. Oncology 8:95, 1994.
11. Boris, M, Weindorf, S, Lasinski, B: Persistence of lymphedema reduction after noninvasive complex lymphedema therapy. Oncology 11:99, 1997.
12. Bottomley, JM: The insensitive foot. In Kauffman, TL (ed) Geriatric Rehabilitation Manual. Churchill Livingstone, New York, 1999, p 266.
13. Brandsma, JW, Robeer, BG, et al: The effect of exercises on walking distance of patients with intermittent claudication: a study of randomized clinical trials. Phys Ther 78:278, 1998.
14. Brennan, MJ: Lymphedema following the surgical treatment of breast cancer: a review of pathophysiology and treatment. J Pain Symptom Manage 7(2):110–116, 1992.
15. Brennan, MJ, DePompodo, RW, Garden, FH: Focused review: postmastectomy lymphedema. Arch Phys Med Rehabil 77(3 Suppl):574, 1996.
16. Brennan, MJ, Miller, L: Overview of treatment options in the management of lymphedema. Cancer Suppl 83:2821, 1998.
17. Bunce, IH, et al: Postmastectomy lymphoedema treatment and measurement. Med J Aust 161:125, 1994.
18. Burt, J, White, G: Lymphedema: A Breast Cancer Patient's Guide to Prevention and Healing. Hunter House, Alameda, CA, 1999.
19. Cameron, MH: Physical Agents in Rehabilitation: From Research to Practice. WB Saunders, Philadelphia, 1999.
20. Casley-Smith, JR: Information about Lymphoedema for Patients, ed 6. Lymphoedema Association of Australia, Malvern, Australia, 1997.
21. Casley-Smith, JR: Treatment for lymphedema of the arm—the Casley-Smith method. Cancer Suppl 83:2843, 1998 (December 15).
22. Casley-Smith, JR, Casley-Smith, JR: Modern treatment of lymphoedema. I. Complex physical therapy—the first 200 Australian limbs. Aust J Dermatol 33:61, 1992.
23. Casley-Smith, JR: Exercises for Patients with Lymphedema of the Arm, ed 2. Lymphoedema Association of Australia, Adelaide, Australia, 1991.
24. Casley-Smith, JR: Exercises for Patients with Lymphedema of the Leg, ed 2. Lymphoedema Association of Australia, Adelaide, Australia, 1991.
25. Connell, M: Complete decongestive therapy. Innovations Breast Cancer Care 3:93, 1998.
26. Daroczy, J: Pathology of lymphedema. Clin Dermatol 13:433, 1995.
27. Eisenhardt, JR: Evaluation and physical treatment of the patient with peripheral vascular disorders. In Irwin, S, Tecklin, JS (eds) Cardiopulmonary Physical Therapy, ed 3. Mosby–Year Book, St. Louis, 1995, pp 215–233.
28. Engel, JM: Relaxation and related techniques. In Hertling, D, Kessler, RM (eds) Management of Common Musculoskeletal Disorders, ed 4. Lippincott Williams & Wilkins, Philadelphia, 2006, pp 261–266..
29. Erickson, V, Pearson, M, Ganz, P, et al: Arm edema in breast cancer patients. J Natl Cancer Inst 93:96–111, 2001.
30. Ernest, E, Fialka, V: A review of the clinical effectiveness of exercise therapy for intermittent claudication. Arch Intern Med 113:135, 1990.
31. Ganz, PA: The quality of life after breast cancer—solving the problem of lymphedema. N Engl J Med 340:383, 1999.
32. Gardner, AW, Katzel, LI, Sorkin, JD, et al: Exercise rehabilitation improves functional outcomes and peripheral circulation in patients with intermittent claudication: a randomized, controlled trial. Am J Geriatr Soc 49:755–762, 2001.
33. Goodman, CC: The cardiovascular system. In Goodman, CC, Fuller, KS, Boissonnault, WG (eds) Pathology: Implications for the Physical Therapist, ed 2. Elsevier, Philadelphia, 1998, pp 367–476.

34. Goodman, CC, Snyder, TEK: Differential Diagnosis in Physical Therapy, ed 3. WB Saunders, Philadelphia, 2000.

35. Gray, JC: Diagnosis of intermittent vascular claudication in a patient with a diagnosis of sciatica. Phys Ther 79:582, 1999.

36. Gudas, SA: Neoplasms of the breast. In Kauffman, TL (ed) Geriatric Rehabilitation Manual. Churchill Livingstone, New York, 1999, p 182.

37. Guttman, H, et al: Achievements of physical therapy in patients after modified radical mastectomy compared with quadrantectomy, axillary dissection and radiation for carcinoma of the breast. Arch Surg 125:389–391, 1990.

38. Hansen, M: Pathophysiology: Foundations of Disease and Clinical Intervention. WB Saunders, Philadelphia, 1998.

39. Harwood, CA, Mortimer, PS: Causes and clinical manifestations of lymphatic failure. Clin Dermatol 13:459, 1995.

40. Henderson, IC: Breast cancer. In Murphy, GP, Lawrence, W, Lenhard, RE (eds) Clinical Oncology, ed 2. American Cancer Society, Atlanta, 1995, p 198.

41. Hewitson, JW: Management of lower extremity lymphedema. Natl Lymphedema Netw Newslett 9(3):1, July–September, 1997.

42. Hillegass, EA: Cardiovascular diagnostic tests and procedures. In Hillegass, EA, Sadowsky, HS (eds) Essentials of Cardiopulmonary Physical Therapy, ed 2. WB Saunders, Philadelphia, 2001, pp 336–379.

43. Hladiuk, M, et al: Arm function after axillary dissection for breast cancer: a pilot study to provide parameter estimates. J Surg Oncol 50(1):47–52, 1992.

44. Holtgrefe, KM: Twice-weekly completed decongestive physical therapy in the management of secondary lymphedema of the lower extremities. Phys Ther 86(8):1128–1136, 2006.

45. Hull, RD, Pineo, GF, Stein, PD, et al: Extended out-of-hospital low-molecular-weight heparin prophylaxis against deep venous thrombosis in patients after elective hip arthroplasty. Ann Intern Med 1355:858–869, 2001.

46. Knight, CA: Peripheral vascular disease and wound care. In O'Sullivan, SB, Schmitz, TJ (eds) Physical Rehabilitation: Assessment and Treatment, ed 4. FA Davis, Philadelphia, 2001, p 583.

47. Kurtz, I: Textbook of Dr. Vodder's Manual Lymphatic Drainage, ed 2. Vol 2. Therapy. Karl F. Haug, Heidelberg, 1989.

48. Lerner, R: What's new in lymphedema therapy in America? Int J Angiol 7:191, 1998.

49. Logan, V: Incidence and prevalence of lymphedema: a literature review. J Clin Nurs 4:213, 1995.

50. MacKinnon, JL: Study of Doppler ultrasonic peripheral vascular assessment performed by physical therapists. Phys Ther 63:30, 1983.

51. Mason, M: The treatment of lymphoedema by complex physical therapy. Aust J Physiother 39:41, 1993.

52. Matthews, K, Smith J: Effectiveness of modified complex physical therapy for lymphoedema treatment. Aust J Physiother 42:323, 1996.

53. McCulloch, JM: Examination procedure for patients with vascular system problems. Clin Manage Phys Ther 1:17, 1981.

54. McCulloch, JM: Peripheral vascular disease. In O'Sullivan, SB, Schmitz, TJ (eds) Physical Rehabilitation: Assessment and Treatment, ed 3. FA Davis, Philadelphia, 1994.

55. McCulloch, JM, Kloth, L, Feedar, JA (eds) Wound Healing: Alternatives and Management, ed 2. FA Davis, Philadelphia, 1995.

56. McGarvey, CL: Pneumatic compression devices for lymphedema. Rehabil Oncol 10:16–17, 1992.

57. McKenzie, DC, Kalda, AL: Effect of upper extremity exercise on secondary lymphedema in breast cancer patients: a pilot study. J Clin Oncol 21:463–466, 2003.

58. Megens, A, Harris, S: Physical therapist management of lymphedema following treatment for breast cancer: a critical review of its effectiveness. Phys Ther 78:1302, 1998.

59. Miller, LT: Exercise in the management of breast cancer-related lymphedema. Innovations Breast Cancer Care 3(4):101, 1998.

60. Miller, LT: The enigma of exercise: participation in an exercise program after breast cancer surgery. Natl Lymphedema Netw Newslett 8(4), October–December 1996.

61. Norman, SA, et al: Development and validation of a telephone questionnaire to characterize lymphedema in women treated for breast cancer. Phys Ther 81:1192, 2001.

62. Peters, K, et al: Lower leg subcutaneous blood flow during walking and passive dependency in chronic venous insufficiency. Br J Dermatol 124(2):177, 1991.

63. Petrek, JA, Heelan, M: Incidence of breast carcinoma-related lymphedema. Cancer Suppl 83(12):2776, 1998.

64. Price, J, Purtell, J: Teaming up to prevent and treat lymphedema. Am J Nurs 7(9):23, 1997.

65. Regensteiner, JG, Steiner, JF, Hiatt, WR: Exercise training improves functional status in patients with peripheral arterial disease. J Vasc Surg 23:104, 1996.

66. Regensteiner, JG, Hiatt, WR: Exercise in the management of peripheral arterial disease. In Roitman, JL (ed) ACSM's Resource Manual for Exercise Testing and Prescription, ed 4. Lippincott Williams & Wilkins, Philadelphia, 2001, p 292.

67. Riddle, DL, Hillner, BE, Wells, PS, et al: Diagnosis of lower extremity deep vein thrombosis in outpatients with musculoskeletal disorders: a national survey study of physical therapists. Phys Ther 84(8):717–728, 2004.

68. Rockson, SG: Secondary lymphedema of the lower extremities. Natl Lymphedema Netw Newslett 10(3):1–3, July–September 1998.

69. Rockson, SG, Miller, LT, Senie, R, et al: Diagnosis and management of lymphedema. Cancer 83 (Suppl):2882–2885, 1998.

70. Ross, C: Complex physical therapy: a treatment note. NZ J Physiother 40:19, 1994.

71. Swirsky, J, Nannery, DS: Coping with Lymphedema. Avery Publishing, Garden City Park, NY, 1998.

72. Szuba, A, Achalu, R, Rockson, SG: Decongestive lymphatic therapy for patients with breast carcinoma-associated lymphedema: a randomized prospective study of a role for adjunctive intermittent pneumatic compression. Cancer 95:2260–2267, 2002.

73. Tappan, FM, Benjamin, PJ: Tappan's Handbook of Healing Massage. Appleton & Lange, Stamford, CT, 1998.

74. Taylor, R, Jayasinghe, UW, Koelmeyer, L, et al: Reliability and validity of arm volume measurements for assessment of lymphedema. Phys Ther 86(2):205–214, 2006.

75. Weinmann, EE, Salzman, EW: Deep vein thrombosis. N Engl J Med 331:1630, 1994.

76. Weiss, JM: Treatment of leg edema and wounds in patients with severe musculoskeletal injuries. Phys Ther 78:1104, 1998.

77. White, RH, Gettner, S, Newman, JM, et al: Predictors of rehospitalization for symptomatic venous thromboembolism after total hip arthroplasty. N Engl J Med 343:1758–1764, 2000.

78. Wigley, FM: Systemic sclerosis: clinical features. In Klippel, JH (ed) Primer on Rheumatic Diseases, ed 12. Arthritis Foundation, Atlanta, 2001, pp 357–363.

79. Williams, LR, et al: Vascular rehabilitation: benefits of a structured exercise and risk modification program. J Vasc Surg 14:320, 1991.

80. Wingate, L: Efficacy of physical therapy for patients who have undergone mastectomies. Phys Ther 65:896, 1985.

81. Wingate, L, et al: Rehabilitation of the mastectomy patient: a randomized, blind, prospective study. Arch Phys Med Rehabil 70:21–24, 1989.

82. Wisham, LH, Abramson, AS, Ebel, A: Value of exercise in peripheral arterial disease. JAMA 153:10, 1953.

83. Woods, EN: Reaching out to patients with breast cancer. Clin Manage Phys Ther 12:58–63, 1992.

84. Young, BA, Flynn, TW: Pulmonary embolism: the differential diagnosis dilemma. J Orthop Phys Ther 35(10):637–642, 2005.

85. Zuther, JE: Treatment of lymphedema with complete decongestive physiotherapy. Natl Lymphedema Netw Newslett 2(2), April 1999.

86. Zuther, JE: Lymphedema Management: A Comprehensive Guide for Practitioners. Thieme, New York, 2005.

# Management of Pulmonary Conditions

25

CHAPTER

Cardiovascular and pulmonary physical therapy is a multifaceted area of professional practice that deals with the management of patients of all ages with acute or chronic, primary or secondary cardiovascular and pulmonary disorders. Although the cardiovascular and pulmonary systems are inherently linked as they interface with all other body systems, the focus of this chapter is on examination procedures and therapeutic interventions used for the management of patients with pulmonary dysfunction. In particular, exercise interventions and manual techniques that enhance ventilation and airway clearance are presented.

The goals of cardiovascular and pulmonary physical therapy for patients with respiratory dysfunction are to:

- Prevent airway obstruction and accumulation of secretions that interfere with normal respiration/oxygen transport.
- Improve airway clearance, cough effectiveness, and ventilation through mobilization and drainage of secretions.
- Improve endurance, general exercise tolerance, and overall well-being.
- Reduce energy costs during respiration through breathing retraining.
- Prevent or correct postural deformities associated with pulmonary or extrapulmonary disorders.
- Maintain or improve chest mobility.

All of these goals are aimed at improving a patient's overall ability to meet necessary and desired functional demands.

Treatment settings vary widely, from intensive care or postsurgical care units and extended care/subacute rehabilitation facilities to outpatient pulmonary centers and the home setting.

# REVIEW OF RESPIRATORY STRUCTURE AND FUNCTION

*Respiration* is a general term used to describe gas exchange within the body and can be categorized as either external respiration or internal respiration. Basic terms are described here but an in-depth discussion of respiratory physiology, including diffusion and perfusion, goes well beyond the scope or purpose of this chapter. The reader is referred to several references for further study.[11,22,34,59,61]

*External respiration* describes the exchange of gas at the alveolar-capillary membrane and the pulmonary capillaries. When a person inhales and oxygen is delivered to the alveoli via the tracheobronchial tree, oxygen diffuses through the alveolar wall and interstitial space and into the bloodstream through the pulmonary capillary walls. The opposite occurs with carbon dioxide transport. *Internal respiration* describes the exchange of gas between the pulmonary capillaries and the cells of the surrounding tissues. Internal respiration occurs when oxygen in arterial blood diffuses from red blood cells into tissues requiring oxygen for function. The reverse occurs with carbon dioxide transport.

*Ventilation,* as it refers to the respiratory system, is the mass exchange of air to and from the body during inspiration and expiration. This cyclic process requires coordinated ventilatory muscle activity, rib cage movements, and appropriate structure and function of the upper and lower respiratory tracts.[8,22,34,59,61]

## Thorax and Chest Wall: Structure and Function

The main functions of the thoracic cage, also referred to as the chest wall, are to protect the internal organs of respiration, circulation, and digestion and to participate in ventilation of the lungs.[58] The thoracic cage provides the site of attachment for the muscles of ventilation to mechanically enlarge the thorax for inspiration or to compress the thorax for expiration.[68] It is also the site of attachment of upper extremity muscles, which function during lifting, pulling, or pushing activities. These activities usually are carried out in conjunction with inspiratory effort.

Along the posterior aspect of the thorax, the dorsal portions of the ribs articulate with the 12 thoracic vertebrae at the costotransverse and costovertebral joints. Along the anterior aspect of the thoracic cage, the first to seventh ribs

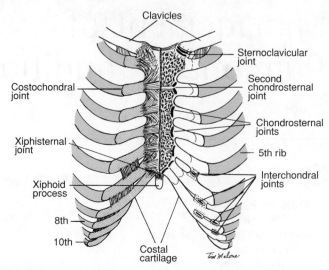

**FIGURE 25.1** Anterior view of the rib cage. *(From Starr, J, Dalton, D: The thorax and chest wall. In Levangie, PK, Norkin, CC [eds] Joint Structure and Function: A Comprehensive Analysis, ed 4. FA Davis, Philadelphia, 2005, p 197, with permission.)*

articulate directly with the sternum via the costal cartilage. The eighth to tenth ribs have cartilaginous attachments to the rib above, whereas the eleventh and twelfth are floating ribs (Fig. 25.1).[68]

## Muscles of Ventilation

Multiple muscles attaching to the thoracic cage have an impact on the movement of air in and out of the lungs during either the inspiratory or expiratory phases of breathing.[8,11,68] Box 25.1 lists the muscles of ventilation.[9]

Ventilatory muscles, also referred to as respiratory muscles, are classified as primary or accessory.[56,68] The *primary muscles of ventilation* are recruited during quiet (tidal) breathing, whereas the *accessory muscles of ventilation* are only recruited during deep, forced, or labored breathing. During quiet inspiration the *diaphragm, scalenes,* and *parasternals* are activated.[56,68] In contrast, no primary ventilatory muscles contract during resting expiration. During deep or forced breathing different accessory muscles of ventilation are recruited, depending on whether inspiration or expiration is occurring, as noted in Box 25.1.

### Inspiration

***Diaphragm.*** The diaphragm, the major muscle of inspiration, is innervated by the phrenic nerve (C3, C4, C5). During relaxed inspiration it is the primary muscle responsible for movement of air, and under these quiet conditions it performs about 70% to 80% of the work of breathing.[56] As the diaphragm contracts, it moves caudally from its dome-shaped position at rest to increase the capacity of the thoracic cage.

***Scalenes.*** The scalenes, which insert proximally on the transverse processes of the lower five cervical vertebrae and distally on the upper surface of the first two ribs, also

## BOX 25.1 Primary and Accessory Ventilatory Muscles

### Inspiration
- Primary muscles: diaphragm, scalenes, parasternals
- Accessory muscles: sternocleidomastoids, upper trapezius, pectoralis major and minor, subclavius, and possibly the external intercostals

### Expiration
- Primary muscles: none active during tidal (resting) expiration
- Accessory muscles: abdominals including the rectus abdominis, transversus abdominis, and internal and external obliques; pectoralis major; and possibly the internal intercostals

are active during quiet inspiration.[56,68] They begin to contract at the onset of inspiration and generate an even greater amount of tension late into the inspiratory cycle as the tension-producing capacity of the diaphragm is decreasing. The scalenes lift the sternum and the first two ribs in a "pump handle" action, which causes an upward and outward action of the upper portion of the rib cage.

***Parasternal intercostals.*** The parasternals, a portion of the internal intercostals, are active during resting inspiration. They function to stabilize the rib cage and prevent inward movement of the superior aspect of the chest wall.[56,68]

***Accessory muscles of inspiration.*** The sternocleidomastoid (SCM), upper trapezius, pectoralis major and minor, and subclavius muscles are all active during deep or labored inspiration.[9,56,68] These muscles become increasingly active with greater inspiratory effort, which occurs frequently during strenuous physical activity.

The accessory muscles of inspiration may become the primary muscles of inspiration and may become active during resting inspiration when the diaphragm is ineffective or weak as the result of pathology. For example, paralysis of the abdominals as the result of a spinal cord injury reduces the support to the viscera (when the patient is in an upright position) which, in turn, allows the diaphragm to assume a flattened rather than a normal dome-shaped position. Thus, diaphragmatic excursion is reduced, and breathing is less efficient, which necessitates recruitment of the accessory muscles of inspiration.

The *SCM muscles* elevate the sternum to increase the anteroposterior (AP) diameter of the thorax. In patients with weakness of the diaphragm, the SCM muscles are required to act as primary muscles of inspiration. The *upper trapezius* muscles elevate the shoulders and, indirectly, the rib cage during labored inspiration. They also fixate the neck so the scalenes have a stable attachment. The *pectoralis major* muscles can act to elevate the rib cage and contribute to inspiration when the arms are overhead.

### Expiration

Expiration is a passive process when a person is at rest. When the diaphragm relaxes after a contraction, the diaphragm rises and the ribs drop. The elastic recoil of tissues decreases the intrathoracic area and increases intrathoracic pressure, which causes exhalation. During active expiration, which can be controlled, forced, or prolonged, several accessory muscles groups are active.[9,56,68]

***Abdominals.*** The rectus abdominis, the internal and external obliques, and the transversus abdominis contract to force down the thoracic cage and force the abdominal contents superiorly into the diaphragm. When the abdominals contract, the intrathoracic pressure increases and air is forced out of the lungs. A strong contraction of the abdominals also is necessary for a strong cough. The abdominals are innervated by spinal cord levels T10 to T12.

Other accessory muscles of expiration include the pectoralis major muscles (when the distal insertion is inferior to the clavicle and the arm is fixed in position), the *quadratus lumborum,* because of its attachment to the twelfth rib, which enables it to act to stabilize the diaphragm during phonation, and possibly the *internal intercostals,* which may act to depress the rib cage.[56,68]

## Mechanics of Ventilation

### Movements of the Thorax During Ventilation

Each rib has its own pattern of movement, but generalizations can be made. The ribs attach anteriorly to the sternum (except ribs 11 and 12) and posteriorly to the vertebral bodies, disks, and transverse processes, making a closed kinematic chain. The thorax enlarges in all three planes of movement during inspiration.[8,11,56,68]

***Increase in the AP dimension.*** There is a forward and upward movement of the sternum and upper ribs, described as a *pump-handle* motion. The thoracic spine extends (straightens), enabling greater excursion of the sternum.

***Increase in the transverse (lateral) dimension.*** There is an elevation and outward turning of the lateral (midshaft) portions of the ribs, described as a *bucket handle* motion. The lower ribs (8–10), which are not attached directly to the sternum, also flare or open outward, increasing the subcostal angle. This is described as *caliper* motion. The angle at the costochondral junction also increases, making the rib segments longer during inspiration.

***Increase in vertical dimension.*** The central tendon of the diaphragm descends as the muscle contracts. This is described as a *piston action.* Elevation of the ribs increases the vertical dimension of the thorax and improves the effectiveness of the diaphragm. At the end of inspiration, the muscles relax and elastic recoil causes the diaphragm to move superiorly. The ribs return to their resting position.

## Movement of Air

As noted previously, *ventilation* is the mass exchange of gases to and from the body. During inspiration, as the thorax enlarges, the pressure inside the lungs (alveolar pressure) becomes lower than the atmospheric pressure, and air rushes into the lungs. At the end of inspiration, the muscles relax, and the elastic recoil of the lungs pushes the air out, resulting in expiration.

N O T E : Breathing exercises, a common intervention for the management of patients with cardiopulmonary, neuromuscular, and musculoskeletal conditions, are designed to affect the movement of air to and from the lungs.[11,28,48,56]

## Compliance

Compliance refers to the distensibility of tissue or how easily the lungs inflate during inspiration. With regard to ventilation, it relates to how easily the lungs inflate or the chest wall expands during inspiration.[22,59,61] Normal lungs are highly distensible (compliant), but compliance changes with age and the presence of disease. During the normal aging process lung tissue becomes more compliant. Diseases of the pulmonary system that, for example, cause fibrosis of tissues (alveolar or pleural) make the lungs rigid (i.e., less compliant), whereas emphysema, one of the chronic obstructive diseases, makes lung tissue more compliant to pressures.[22,59,61]

## Airway Resistance

The amount of resistance to the flow of air through the airways depends on a number of factors.[22,59,61] The bifurcation and branching of airways is a source of airway resistance. The size (diameter) of the lumen of each airway also influences resistance. The diameter of the lumen can be decreased by mucus or edema in the airways, contraction of smooth muscles, and the degree of elasticity or distensibility of the lung parenchyma.

Normally, the airways widen during inspiration and narrow during expiration. As the diameter of the airway decreases, the resistance to airflow increases. With diseases that cause bronchospasm (asthma) or increased mucus production (chronic bronchitis), airway resistance is even greater than normal, particularly during expiration.

## Flow Rates

Flow rates indicate measurements of the amount of air moved in or out of the airways over a period of time. Flow rates, which are related to airflow resistance, reflect the ease with which ventilation occurs.[22,59,61] *Expiratory flow rate* is determined by the volume of air exhaled divided by the amount of time it takes for the volume of gas to be exhaled.[27]

Flow rates are altered as the result of diseases that affect the respiratory tree and chest wall. For example, with chronic obstructive pulmonary disease, the expiratory flow rate is decreased in comparison to normal. That is, it takes a longer than the normal amount of time to exhale a specific volume of air.

## Anatomy and Function of the Respiratory Tracts

### Upper Respiratory Tract

The structures of the upper respiratory tract are the *nasal cavity, pharynx,* and *larynx.*[11,58,66,69] As air is brought into the body, the nasal cavity and pharynx filter and remove particles in the air and begin to humidify and warm it to body temperature. The mucosal lining of these structures has cells that secrete mucus and cells that are ciliated. Cilia and mucus trap particles; a sneeze removes large particles.

With illness and elevated body temperature, the mucous membrane tends to dry out, so the body secretes more mucus. This mucus dries out, and a cycle begins. The action of the cilia is inhibited by drying of mucus. The patient tends to breathe by mouth, which decreases the humidification of mucus and increases its viscosity.

The larynx, which extends from C3 to C6, controls airflow; and when it contracts rapidly, the epiglottis prevents food, liquids, or foreign objects from entering the airway.[47]

### Lower Respiratory Tract

The lower respiratory tract is composed of conducting airways of the tracheobronchial tree and the terminal respiratory units. There are approximately 23 generations (branchings) of the structures within the tracheobronchial tree, which extends from the trachea to the terminal respiratory units of the lungs. The structures and branchings of the lower respiratory tract are summarized in Box 25.2.[11,58,66,69]

The initial branchings of the tracheobronchial tree are depicted in Figure 25.2. The first 16 airway branchings of the lower respiratory tract primarily conduct air, whereas the last 6 are respiratory airways that end (in the mature lung) in approximately 300 million alveoli.[69] The diameter of the airways becomes increasingly smaller with each successive generation of the tracheobronchial tree.

*Trachea.* The trachea is an oval, flexible tube supported by semicircular rings of cartilage. It extends from C6 in an oblique, downward direction to the sternal angle level of rib 2 and T6, at which point it bifurcates. The posterior wall is smooth muscle, and it contains an equal number of ciliated epithelial cells and mucus-containing goblet cells.

| BOX 25.2 | Structures and Branchings of the Lower Respiratory Tract |
|---|---|

- Trachea
- Mainstem bronchi: 2
- Lobar bronchi: 5
- Segmental bronchi: 18
- Bronchioles: subsegmental, terminal, and respiratory
- Alveolar ducts and sacs

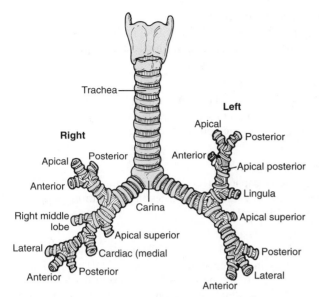

FIGURE 25.2 Lower respiratory tract—tracheobronchial tree. *(From Frownfelter, DL: Chest Physical Therapy and Pulmonary Rehabilitation. Year-Book Medical Publishers, Chicago, 1987, p 26, with permission.)*

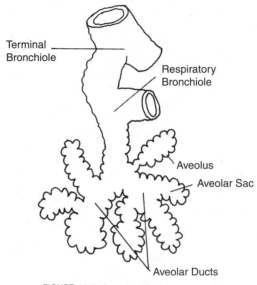

FIGURE 25.3 Bronchopulmonary segment.

***Mainstem bronchi.*** The trachea branches into two mainstream bronchi: the right, which is directed almost vertically, and the left, which is directed more obliquely.

***Lobar bronchi.*** The two mainstem bronchi then divide into five lobar bronchi: three on the right and two on the left. Mainstem and lobar bronchi have a great amount of cartilage, which helps maintain airway patency.

***Segmental bronchi.*** Each of the lobar bronchi divide into two or more segmental bronchi: 10 on the right and 8 on the left. Segmental bronchi have scattered cartilage, smooth muscle, elastic fibers, and a capillary network. The mainstem, lobar, and segmental bronchi have a mucous membrane essentially the same as the trachea.

***Bronchioles.*** Segmental bronchi divide into subsegmental bronchi and bronchioles, which have less and less cartilage and ciliated epithelial cells. These bronchioles divide into the *terminal bronchioles,* which are distal to the last cartilage of the tracheobronchial tree. Terminal bronchioles contain no ciliated cells. Terminal bronchioles divide into *respiratory bronchioles* and provide a transitional zone between the bronchioles and alveoli.

***Alveoli.*** The respiratory bronchioles divide into alveolar ducts and alveolar sacs (Fig. 25.3). One duct may supply several sacs. The ducts contain smooth muscle, which narrows the lumen of the duct with contraction. The alveoli are located in the periphery of the alveolar ducts and sacs and are in contact with capillaries (alveolar-arterial membrane). Gas exchange occurs here.

## Summary of Function of the Upper and Lower Respiratory Tracts

The upper and lower respiratory tracts, as a unit, serve the following functions. They:

- Conduct air to and from the alveolar system for gas exchange
- Assist with humidification and trap small particles to clean the air with the mucosal lining
- Warm the air by the vascular supply
- Move mucus upward with the cilia
- Elicit the cough reflex to clear the larger airways

## The Lungs and Pleurae

The lungs and pleurae are made up of the following components. The *right lung* has three lobes—the upper, middle, and lower—and 10 bronchopulmonary segments. The *left lung* has two true lobes—the upper and lower—and a slip of lung called the lingula, which is not considered a "true" lobe of the lungs. The left lung has eight bronchopulmonary segments. The lobes of the lungs are depicted in Figure 25.4.

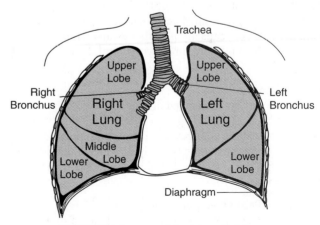

FIGURE 25.4 Structure of the right and left lungs.

Each lung is covered in *pleura,* a serous membrane known as the *visceral pleura.* This membrane adheres to all surfaces of each lung. The *parietal pleura* lines the inside of the thoracic wall. The parietal pleura is sensitive to pain, but the visceral pleura appears to be insensitive.[30,31] A negative pressure in the minute space between the pleurae serves to keep the lungs inflated. Pleural fluid is found between the pleurae and lubricates the pleurae as they slide on each other during ventilation.

## Lung Volumes and Capacities

Pulmonary function tests that measure lung volumes and capacities are performed to evaluate the mechanical function of the lungs (Fig. 25.5). Lung volumes and capacities are related to a person's age, weight, sex, and body position and are altered by disease.[27,59,61] Two or more lung volumes, when combined, are described as a capacity. A basic understanding of these measurements and what the values reflect is useful for a therapist treating patients with pulmonary dysfunction.

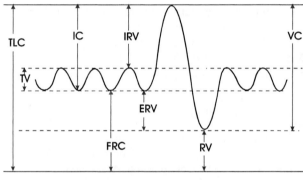

FIGURE 25.5 Normal lung values and capacities.

### Total Lung Capacity

Total lung capacity (TLC) is the total amount of air contained in the lungs after a maximum inspiration. TLC can be subdivided into four volumes: tidal volume, inspiratory reserve volume, expiratory reserve volume, and residual volume. The vital capacity plus the residual volume equal the TLC, which is approximately 6000 mL in a healthy, young adult.

### Tidal Volume

The amount of air exchanged during a relaxed inspiration followed by a relaxed expiration is called the tidal volume (TV). In a healthy, young adult, TV is approximately 500 mL per inspiration. Approximately 350 mL of the tidal volume reaches the alveoli and participates in gas exchange (respiration).

### Inspiratory Reserve Volume

Inspiratory reserve volume (IRV) is the amount of air a person can breathe in after a resting inspiration (approximately 3000 mL).

### Expiratory Reserve Volume

Expiratory reserve volume (ERV) is the amount of air a person can exhale after a normal resting expiration (approximately 1000 mL).

### Residual Volume

Residual volume (RV) is the amount of air left in the lungs after a maximum expiration (approximately 1500 mL). RV increases with age and with restrictive and obstructive pulmonary diseases.

### Inspiratory Capacity

Inspiratory capacity (IC) is the maximum amount of air a person can breathe in after a resting expiration (approximately 3500 mL).

### Functional Residual Capacity

Functional residual capacity (FRC) is the amount of air remaining in the lungs after a resting (tidal) expiration (approximately 2500 mL). It is the sum of the ERV and RV. FRC represents the point during ventilation at which the forces that expand the thoracic wall are in balance with the forces that tend to collapse the lungs.[59]

### Vital Capacity

Vital capacity (VC) is the sum of the TV, IRV, and ERV. It is measured by a maximum inspiration followed by a maximum expiration (approximately 4500 mL). Vital capacity decreases with age and is less in the supine position than in an erect posture (sitting or standing). VC decreases in the presence of restrictive and obstructive diseases.

## EXAMINATION

Evaluation of the patient with pulmonary dysfunction and determination of a diagnosis, prognosis, and intervention plan are based on the findings derived from a comprehensive examination, including a history, systems review, and specific tests and measures.[31] The multiple purposes of this examination are summarized in Box 25.3.

---

**BOX 25.3    Purpose of the Examination**

- Determine a patient's primary and secondary respiratory and ventilatory impairments and how they limit physical function.
- Determine the adequacy of the ventilatory pump and the oxygen uptake/carbon dioxide elimination mechanisms to meet the oxygen demands at rest and during functional activities.
- Ascertain a patient's suitability for participation in a pulmonary rehabilitation program.
- Develop an appropriate level intervention plan for the patient.
- Establish a baseline to measure a patient's progress and the effectiveness of the treatment.
- Determine when to discontinue specific interventions and implement a home program as a basis for self-management.

## Components of the Examination

A comprehensive examination of a patient with known or suspected dysfunction related to primary and secondary pulmonary or chest disorders has many elements. The examination procedures described in this section are those often used by a therapist during an initial evaluation to establish a therapy-related diagnosis or during subsequent assessments for modification of therapeutic interventions.[11,31,35,38,52,67] Additional examination procedures not described in this section but integral to the management of a patient with pulmonary dysfunction are radiography, evaluation of blood gases, tomography, bronchoscopy, and hematological tests.

### History and Systems Review

The examination process begins with a patient's history including an interview with the patient and sometimes family members if they are available. During the interview a therapist can identify a patient's and/or family members' perception of any functional limitations or disabilities and determine a patient's chief complaints and why he or she is seeking treatment. In preparation for the interview, the medical history and any medical diagnoses are obtained from the patient's medical record, if available, or more generally, from the patient or family. Relevant occupational and social history are obtained; particularly important are on-the-job physical demands, the environment of the workplace, and social habits that affect a person's well-being, such as tobacco or alcohol use. Assessment of the home or family environment might include a patient's family responsibilities, the housing situation, and available family support systems. A brief systems review should follow the history.

### General Appearance of the Patient

Table 25.1 describes the type of information that can be obtained by visual inspection of a patient and the possible implications of these observations. Many of these findings can be noted during the course of the history or during the systems review.

### Analysis of Chest Shape and Dimensions

***Symmetry of the chest and trunk.*** Observe anteriorly, posteriorly, and laterally; the thoracic cage should be symmetrical.

***Mobility of the trunk.*** Check active movements in all directions and identify any restricted spinal motions, particularly in the thoracic spine.

***Shape and dimensions of the chest.*** The anteroposterior (AP) and lateral dimensions are usually 1:2. Common chest deformities include:

- ***Barrel chest.*** The circumference of the upper chest appears larger than that of the lower chest. The sternum appears prominent, and the AP diameter of the chest is greater than normal. Many patients with chronic obstructive pulmonary disorders, who are usually upper chest breathers, develop a barrel chest.
- ***Pectus excavatum (funnel breast).*** The lower part of the sternum is depressed and the lower ribs flare out. Patients with this deformity are diaphragmatic breathers;

---

| TABLE 25.1 | General Appearance of the Patient and Implications |
|---|---|
| **General Appearance** | **Implications** |
| • *Level of awareness* (level of consciousness): alert, responsive, or cooperative versus lethargic, disoriented, or inattentive | • Respiratory acidosis, hypercarbia (increased $P_{CO_2}$ level), or hypoxia (decreased $P_{O_2}$ level) can alter level of consciousness |
| • *Body type:* normal, obese, or cachectic | • May reflect intolerance to exercise |
| • *Color:* cyanosis (bluish appearance) peripherally (nailbeds) or centrally (lips) | • Peripheral cyanosis may indicate low cardiac output; central cyanosis may indicate inadequate gas exchange in the lungs |
| • *Facial signs or expressions:* focused or dilated pupils, nasal flaring, sweating, or distressed appearance | • Signs of respiratory distress, fatigue, or pulmonary or musculoskeletal pain |
| • *Jugular vein engorgement:* visualization of the jugular venous pulse with the patient supine and the head and neck on pillows at a 45° angle | • Bilateral distention associated with congestive heart failure/right-sided heart failure |
| • *Hypertrophy of or use at rest of accessory muscles of ventilation:* SCM, upper trapezius | • Seen in patients with early chronic lung disease or weakness of the diaphragm |
| • *Supraclavicular or intercostal retractions* occurring with inspiration | • Seen in patients with labored breathing |
| • *Use of pursed lip breathing* (usually with expiration) | • Indicates difficulty with expiration; often seen in patients with COPD |
| • *Clubbing of digits:* loss of angle between the nail bed and DIP joint | • May be linked to perfusion |
| • *Peripheral edema* | • Sign of right ventricular failure or lymphatic dysfunction |

excessive abdominal protrusion and little upper chest movement occur during breathing.

● ***Pectus carinatum (pigeon breast).*** The sternum is prominent and protrudes anteriorly.

### Posture or Preferred Positioning

Identify a patient's preferred sitting or standing posture. A patient who has difficulty breathing as the result of chronic lung disease often leans forward on hands or forearms to stabilize and elevate the shoulder girdle to assist with inspiration (Fig. 25.6). This position increases the effectiveness of the pectoralis and serratus anterior muscles to act as accessory muscles of inspiration by reverse action. It is also important to identify a patient's preferred sleeping position. A patient with cardiopulmonary dysfunction often prefers to sleep in a head-up rather than a fully recumbent position. Assuming a horizontal position may result in shortness of breath.

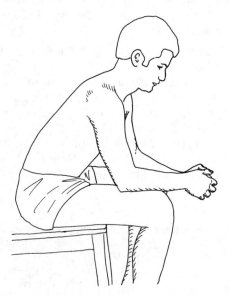

FIGURE 25.6 A patient who is short of breath at rest or after activity often assumes a forward-bent position with hands or elbows resting on the thighs to reduce or relieve symptoms.

In addition, note any postural deformities such as kyphosis and scoliosis and postural asymmetry from thoracic surgery, which could restrict chest movements and ventilation.

### Breathing Pattern

Assess the *rate, regularity,* and *location* of ventilation at rest and with activity. A normal respiratory rate for a healthy adult is 12 to 20 breaths per minute. This is most accurately determined when a patient is unaware that his or her respiratory rate is being measured, as when taking the pulse rate. The normal ratio of inspiration to expiration at rest is 1:2 and with activity 1:1. A patient with chronic obstructive pulmonary disease (COPD) may have a ratio of 1:4 at rest, which reflects difficulty with the expiratory phase of breathing.

The normal sequence of inspiration at rest is (1) the diaphragm contracts and descends and the abdomen (epigastric area) rises; (2) this is followed by lateral costal expansion as the ribs move up and out; and finally (3) the upper chest rises. The neck muscles that act as accessory muscles of inspiration should be inactive during relaxed inspiration.

To assess the breathing sequence, have the patient assume a comfortable position (semireclining or supine). Place your hands on the patient's epigastric region and sternum to observe movements in these two areas.

A number of terms are used to describe abnormal breathing patterns and are defined in Box 25.4.[11,35,38,52]

### Chest Mobility

***Symmetry of chest movement.*** Analysis of the symmetry of the moving chest during breathing gives the therapist information about the mobility of the thorax and indicates indirectly what areas of the lungs may or may not be responding.

*Procedure:* Place your hands on the patient's chest and assess the excursion of each side of the thorax during inspiration and expiration. Each of the three lobar areas can be checked.[11,35,38,52]

● To check *upper lobe expansion,* face the patient; place the tips of your thumbs at the midsternal line at the sternal notch. Extend your fingers above the clavicles. Have the patient fully exhale and then inhale deeply.

● To check *middle lobe expansion,* continue to face the patient; place the tips of your thumbs at the xiphoid process and extend your fingers laterally around the ribs. Again, ask the patient to breathe in deeply (Fig. 25.7A).

● To check *lower lobe expansion,* place the tips of your thumbs along the patient's back at the spinous processes (lower thoracic level) and extend your fingers around the ribs. Ask the patient to breathe in deeply (Fig. 25.7B).

---

| BOX 25.4 | Abnormal Breathing Patterns |
|---|---|

- *Dyspnea.* Distressed, labored breathing as the result of shortness of breath.
- *Tachypnea.* Rapid, shallow breathing; decreased tidal volume but increased rate; associated with restrictive or obstructive lung disease and use of accessory muscles of inspiration.
- *Bradypnea.* Slow rate with shallow or normal depth and regular rhythm; may be associated with drug overdose.
- *Hyperventilation.* Deep, rapid respiration; increased tidal volume and increased rate of respiration; regular rhythm.
- *Orthopnea.* Difficulty breathing in the supine position.
- *Apnea.* Cessation of breathing in the expiratory phase.
- *Apneusis.* Cessation of breathing in the inspiratory phase.
- *Cheyne-Stokes.* Cycles of gradually increasing tidal volumes followed by a series of gradually decreasing tidal volumes and then a period of apnea. This is sometimes seen in the patient with a severe head injury.

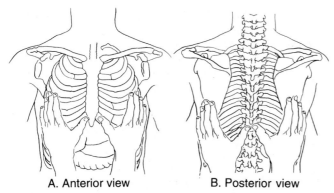

A. Anterior view      B. Posterior view

FIGURE 25.7 (*A*) Anterior and (*B*) posterior placement of a therapist's hands on a patient's thorax to assess the symmetry of movement during breathing. *(From Brannon, FJ, et al: Cardiopulmonary Rehabilitation—Basic Theory and Application, ed 3, FA Davis, Philadelphia, 1998, p. 288. Adapted from Rothstein, JH, Roy, SH, Wolf, SL: The Rehabilitation Specialist's Handbook, FA Davis, Philadelphia, 2005, p 416–417, with permission.)*

***Extent of excursion.*** The extent of chest mobility can be measured by two methods.[35,38]

- Measure the girth of the chest with a tape measure at three levels (axilla, xiphoid, lower costal). Document change in girth after a maximum inspiration and a maximum expiration.
- Place both hands on the patient's chest or back as previously described. Note the distance between your thumbs after a maximum inspiration.

### Palpation
Palpation of the thorax provides evidence of dysfunction of the underlying tissues including the lungs, chest wall, and mediastinum.[11,35,38,52]

***Tactile (vocal) fremitus.*** Tactile fremitus is the vibration felt while palpating over the chest wall as a patient speaks.

*Procedure:* Place the palms of your hands lightly on the chest wall and ask the patient to speak a few words or repeat "99" several times. Normally, fremitus is felt uniformly on the chest wall. Fremitus is increased in the presence of secretions in the airways and decreased or absent when air is trapped as the result of obstructed airways.

***Chest wall pain.*** Specific areas or points of pain over anterior, posterior, or lateral aspects of the chest wall can be identified with palpation.

*Procedure:* Firmly press against the chest wall with your hands to identify any specific areas of pain potentially of musculoskeletal origin. Ask the patient to take a deep breath and identify any painful areas of the chest wall. Chest wall pain of musculoskeletal origin often increases with direct point pressure during palpation and during a deep inspiration.[35,38]

N O T E : Pain in the anterior, posterior, or lateral region of the chest can be of musculoskeletal, pulmonary, or cardiac origin.[31] Pain of pulmonary origin is usually localized to a region of the chest but also may be felt in the neck or shoulder region. Several pulmonary or cardiac conditions

can mimic musculoskeletal pain, such as pulmonary embolism, pleurisy, pneumonia, pneumothorax, and pulmonary artery hypertension.[31]

***Mediastinal shift.*** The position of the trachea normally is oriented centrally in relation to the suprasternal notch indicating symmetry of the mediastinum. The position of the trachea shifts as the result of asymmetrical intrathoracic pressures or lung volumes. For example, if the patient has had a pneumonectomy (removal of a lung), the lung volume on the operated side decreases, and the trachea shifts toward that side. Conversely, if the patient has a hemothorax (blood in the thorax), intrathoracic pressure on the side of the hemothorax increases, and the mediastinum shifts away from the affected side of the chest.[11,35,38,52]

*Procedure:* To identify a *mediastinal shift,* have the patient sit facing you with the head in midline and the neck slightly flexed to relax the sternocleidomastoid muscles. With your index finger, gently palpate the soft tissue space on either side of the trachea at the suprasternal notch. Determine whether the trachea is palpable at the midline or has shifted to the left or right.

### Mediate Percussion
Mediate percussion is an examination technique designed to assess lung density, specifically, the air-to-solid ratio in the lungs.[11,35,38,52]

*Procedure:* Place the middle finger of the nondominant hand flat against the chest wall along an intercostal space. With the tip of the middle finger of the opposite hand, firmly tap on the finger positioned on the chest wall. Repeat the procedure at several points on the right and left and anterior and posterior aspects of the chest wall. This maneuver produces a resonance; the pitch varies with the density of the underlying tissue. The subjective determination of pitch indicates the following.

- The sound is dull and flat if there is a greater than normal amount of solid matter (tumor, consolidation) in the lungs in comparison with the amount of air.
- The sound is hyperresonant (tympanic) if there is a greater than normal amount of air in the area (as in patients with emphysema).
- If asymmetrical or abnormal findings are noted, the patient should be referred to the physician for additional objective tests such as a chest radiograph.

### Auscultation of Breath Sounds
Auscultation is a general term that refers to the process of listening to sounds within the body, specifically to breath sounds during an examination of the lungs.[11,35,38,52] Breath sounds occur because of movement of air in the airways during inspiration and expiration. A stethoscope is used to magnify these sounds. Breath sounds should be assessed to:

- Identify the areas of the lungs in which congestion exists and in which airway clearance techniques should be performed.
- Determine the effectiveness of any airway clearance intervention.

● Determine whether the lungs are clear and whether interventions should be discontinued.

*Procedure:* When assessing breath sounds, be sure the setting is quiet. Have the patient assume a comfortable, relaxed, sitting position to allow access to the chest wall. Place the diaphragm of the stethoscope directly against the patient's skin along the anterior or posterior chest wall. Be sure that the tubing does not rub together or come in contact with clothing during auscultation, as this contact produces extraneous sounds.

Follow a systematic pattern (Fig. 25.8A&B) and place the stethoscope against specific thoracic landmarks (T2, T6, T10) along the right and left sides of the chest wall. Ask the patient to breathe in deeply and out quickly through the mouth as you move the stethoscope from point to point. Note the quality, intensity, and pitch of the breath sounds.

PRECAUTION: Auscultate slowly from one area to another. Allow the patient to breathe in a relaxed manner

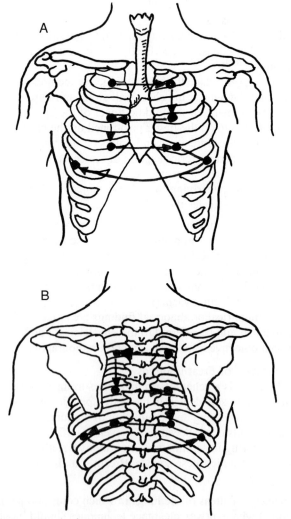

FIGURE 25.8 Pattern of specific thoracic landmarks for auscultation. The diaphragm of the stethoscope is placed along the right and left (*A*) anterior chest wall and the (*B*) posterior chest wall at T2, T6, and T10. *(From Frownfelter, DL: Chest Physical Therapy and Pulmonary Rehabilitation. Year-Book Medical Publishers, Chicago, 1987, p 135, with permission.)*

after several deep breaths to prevent dizziness from hyperventilation. Guard the patient closely to prevent loss of balance if lightheadedness occurs.

**Classification of Breath Sounds**
Breath sounds are classified by location, pitch, and intensity as well as the ratio of sounds heard on inspiration versus those heard on expiration. Breath sounds also are identified as normal or adventitious (extra).[5,50,52,77]

Normal breath sounds occur in the absence of pathology and are heard predominantly during inspiration. Normal breath sounds are categorized as *vesicular, bronchial,* or *bronchovesicular* based on the location and quality of the sound. They are described in Box 25.5.[5,77] *Adventitious* breath sounds are abnormal sounds in the lungs that are heard with a stethoscope. Although terminology in the literature is inconsistent, the nomenclature used most often was proposed by a joint committee of the American College of Chest Physicians and the American Thoracic Society.[5,77] Adventitious breath sounds are categorized as *crackles* or *wheezes.* Box 25.5 describes the location and quality of these breath sounds.

---

| BOX 25.5 | Normal and Adventitious Breath Sounds |
| --- | --- |

**Normal Breath Sounds**
- *Vesicular.* Soft, low-pitched, breezy but faint sounds heard over most of the chest except near the trachea and mainstem bronchi and between the scapulae. Vesicular sounds are audible considerably longer on inspiration than expiration (about a 3:1 ratio).
- *Bronchial.* Loud, hollow, or tubular high-pitched sounds heard over the mainstem bronchi and trachea. Bronchial sounds are heard equally during inspiration and expiration; a slight pause in the sound occurs between inspiration and expiration.
- *Bronchovesicular.* Softer than bronchial breath sounds; also heard equally during inspiration and expiration but without a pause in the sound between the cycles. The sounds are heard in the supraclavicular, suprascapular, and parasternal regions anteriorly and between the scapulae posteriorly.

**Adventitious Breath Sounds**
- *Crackles.* Fine, discontinuous sounds (similar to the sound of bubbles popping or the sound of hairs being rubbed between your fingers next to your ear). Crackles, which can be fine or coarse, are heard primarily during inspiration as the result of secretions moving in the airways or in closed airways that are rapidly reopening. The former term for crackles was *rales.*
- *Wheezes.* Continuous high- or low-pitched sounds or sometimes musical tones heard during exhalation but occasionally audible during inspiration. Bronchospasm or secretions that narrow the lumen of the airways cause wheezes. The term previously used for wheezes was *rhonchi.*

Breath sounds may be totally absent or substantially diminished over a portion of the lungs. This indicates total or partial obstruction and lack of aeration of lung tissue. The absence of air and collapse of an area of lung tissue is known as *atelectasis*. Obstruction of airways may be caused by fluids, mucus, bronchospasm, or compression by tumor.

### Cough and Cough Production

The *strength, depth, length,* and *frequency* of a patient's cough must be assessed. An effective cough is sharp and deep. In the patient with current or potential pulmonary dysfunction a cough can be described as weak, shallow, soft, or throaty. A patient may have a weak, shallow cough as the result of pain or paralysis. A sudden onset of a cough or a sustained cough often is described as paroxysmal or spasmodic. If a cough is substantially weak or ineffective, suctioning may be required to clear the airways.[11,35,52]

A cough may be productive or nonproductive in the presence of pathology. The productivity of the cough and secretions produced by the cough should be assessed. Secretions are checked for:

- Color (clear, yellow, green, blood-stained)
- Consistency (viscous, thin, frothy)
- Amount (minimal to copious)
- Odor (no odor to foul-smelling)

Production of a small amount of clear or white secretions on a daily basis is normal. Copious but clear secretions are common with chronic bronchitis. Yellow, green, and purulent secretions with a strong odor are indicative of some type of infection. Blood-streaked secretions, known as *hemoptysis,* is indicative of some degree of hemorrhage in the lungs. Frothy, white secretions are associated with pulmonary edema and heart failure.

When secretions are produced during the course of interventions, such as exercise or airway clearance, it is the responsibility of the therapist to document the characteristics of the secretions.

### Additional Areas of Examination

The examination procedures described in this section are complemented with other areas of examination, which may include a patient's use of assistive respiratory equipment, ROM particularly of the shoulders, neck, and trunk, muscle strength, general endurance and graded exercise testing, and a patient's identification of functional abilities or limitations and perceived disability and quality of life.

## BREATHING EXERCISES AND VENTILATORY TRAINING

Breathing exercises and ventilatory training are fundamental interventions for the prevention or comprehensive management of impairments related to acute or chronic pulmonary disorders. For example, these interventions are frequently advocated in the literature for patients with

---

| BOX 25.6 | Goals of Breathing Exercises and Ventilatory Muscle Training |
|---|---|

- Improve or redistribute ventilation.
- Increase the effectiveness of the cough mechanism and promote airway clearance.
- Prevent postoperative pulmonary complications.
- Improve the strength, endurance, and coordination of the muscles of ventilation.
- Maintain or improve chest and thoracic spine mobility.
- Correct inefficient or abnormal breathing patterns and decrease the work of breathing.
- Promote relaxation and relieve stress.
- Teach the patient how to deal with episodes of dyspnea.
- Improve a patient's overall functional capacity for daily living, occupational, and recreational activities.

---

COPD (chronic bronchitis, emphysema, asthma) or cystic fibrosis, for patients with a high spinal cord lesion, for patients who have undergone thoracic or abdominal surgery and are at high risk for acute pulmonary complications, or for patients who must remain in bed for an extended period of time.*

Breathing exercises and ventilatory training can take on many forms including diaphragmatic breathing, segmental breathing, inspiratory resistance training, incentive spirometry, and breathing techniques for the relief of dyspnea during exertion. The goals of these interventions are listed in Box 25.6.

Research studies indicate that although breathing exercises or ventilatory muscle training may affect and possibly alter a patient's rate and depth of ventilation these interventions may not necessarily have any impact on gas exchange at the alveolar level or on oxygenation.[11,28,48,60] Therefore, breathing exercises or ventilatory training should be only one aspect of management to improve pulmonary status and to increase a patient's overall endurance and function during daily living activities. Depending on a patient's underlying pathology and impairments, exercises to improve ventilation often are combined with medication, airway clearance, the use of respiratory therapy devices, and a graded exercise (aerobic conditioning) program.

## Guidelines for Teaching Breathing Exercises

- If possible, choose a quiet area for instruction in which you can interact with the patient with minimal distractions.
- Explain to the patient the aims and rationale of breathing exercises or ventilatory training specific to his or her particular impairments and functional limitations.
- Have the patient assume a comfortable, relaxed position and loosen restrictive clothing. Initially, a semi-Fowler's position with the head and trunk elevated approximately

---

* See references 3, 7, 11, 14, 15, 28, 36, 40, 44, 45, 48, 57, 60, 63, 66, 76.

45°, is desirable. By supporting the head and trunk, flexing the hips and knees, and supporting the legs with a pillow, the abdominal muscles remain relaxed. Other positions, such as supine, sitting, or standing, may be used initially or as the patient progresses during treatment.

◎ Observe and assess the patient's spontaneous breathing pattern while at rest and later with activity.

◎ Determine whether ventilatory training is indicated.

◎ Establish a baseline for assessing changes, progress, and outcomes of intervention.

◎ If necessary, teach the patient relaxation techniques. This relaxes the muscles of the upper thorax, neck, and shoulders to minimize the use of the accessory muscles of ventilation. Pay particular attention to relaxation of the sternocleidomastoids, upper trapezius, and levator scapulae muscles.

◎ Depending on the patient's underlying pathology and impairments, determine whether to emphasize the inspiratory or expiratory phase of ventilation.

◎ Demonstrate the desired breathing pattern to the patient.

◎ Have the patient practice the correct breathing pattern in a variety of positions at rest and with activity.

PRECAUTIONS: When teaching breathing exercises, be aware of the following precautions[11,28,48,60]:

◎ Never allow a patient to force expiration. Expiration should be relaxed or lightly controlled. Forced expiration only increases turbulence in the airways, leading to bronchospasm and increased airway restriction.

◎ Do not allow a patient to take a highly *prolonged* expiration. This causes the patient to gasp with the next inspiration. The patient's breathing pattern then becomes irregular and inefficient.

◎ Do not allow the patient to initiate inspiration with the accessory muscles and the upper chest. Advise the patient that the upper chest should be relatively quiet during breathing.

◎ Allow the patient to perform deep breathing for only three or four inspirations and expirations at a time to avoid hyperventilation.

## Diaphragmatic Breathing

When the diaphragm is functioning effectively in its role as the primary muscle of inspiration, ventilation is efficient and the oxygen consumption of the muscles of ventilation is low during relaxed (tidal) breathing.[7,28] When a patient relies substantially on the accessory muscles of inspiration, the mechanical work of breathing (oxygen consumption) increases and the efficiency of ventilation decreases. Although the diaphragm controls breathing at an involuntary level, a patient with primary or secondary pulmonary dysfunction can be taught how to control breathing by optimal use of the diaphragm and decreased use of accessory muscles.

Controlled breathing techniques, which emphasize diaphragmatic breathing, are designed to improve the efficiency of ventilation, decrease the work of breathing, increase the excursion (descent or ascent) of the diaphragm, and improve gas exchange and oxygenation.[11,28,44,48,60] Diaphragmatic breathing exercises also are used during postural drainage to mobilize lung secretions.[25,51]

### Procedure

◎ Prepare the patient in a relaxed and comfortable position in which gravity *assists* the diaphragm, such as a semi-Fowler's position.

◎ If your examination revealed that the patient initiates the breathing pattern with the accessory muscles of inspiration (shoulder and neck musclulature), start instruction by teaching the patient how to relax those muscles (shoulder rolls or shoulder shrugs coupled with relaxation).

◎ Place your hand(s) on the rectus abdominis just below the anterior costal margin (Fig. 25.9). Ask the patient to breathe in slowly and deeply through the nose. Have the patient keep the shoulders relaxed and upper chest quiet, allowing the abdomen to rise slightly. Then tell the patient to relax and exhale slowly through the mouth.

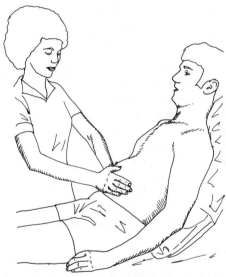

FIGURE 25.9 The semireclining (as shown) and semi-Fowler's positions are comfortable, relaxed positions in which to teach diaphragmatic breathing.

◎ Have the patient practice this three or four times and then rest. Do not allow the patient to hyperventilate.

◎ If the patient is having difficulty using the diaphragm during inspiration, have the patient inhale several times in succession through the nose by using a *sniffing* action.[28,60] This action usually facilitates the diaphragm.

◎ To learn how to self-monitor this sequence, have the patient place his or her own hand below the anterior costal margin and feel the movement (Fig. 25.10). The patient's hand should rise slightly during inspiration and fall during expiration.

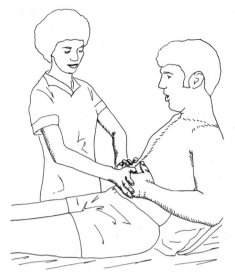

FIGURE 25.10 The patient places his or her own hands on the abdomen to feel the movement of proper diaphragmatic breathing. By placing the hands on the abdomen, the patient can also feel the contraction of the abdominals, which occurs with controlled expiration or coughing.

● After the patient understands and is able to control breathing using a diaphragmatic pattern, keeping the shoulders relaxed, practice diaphragmatic breathing in a variety of positions (sitting, standing) and during activity (walking, climbing stairs).

N O T E : Evidence concerning the effect of diaphragmatic breathing exercises on the rate of ventilation, the work of breathing and oxygen consumption, excursion of the diaphragm, and exercise capacity in normal subjects and in patients with pulmonary disorders is inconclusive, with some studies supporting and others refuting the benefits of diaphragmatic breathing.[13,28,44,62]

## Segmental Breathing

It is questionable whether a patient can be taught to expand localized areas of the lungs while keeping other areas quiet. It is known, however, that hypoventilation does occur in certain areas of the lungs because of chest wall fibrosis, pain, and muscle guarding after surgery, atelectasis, and pneumonia. Therefore, there are certain instances such as during postural drainage or following thoracic surgery when it is important to emphasize expansion of problem areas of the lungs and chest wall.

Two examples of segmental breathing that target the lateral and posterior segments of the lower lobes are described in this section. However, segmental breathing techniques also may need to be directed to the middle and upper lobes if there is accumulation of secretions or insufficient lung expansion in these areas.

### Lateral Costal Expansion
Lateral costal expansion, sometimes called *lateral basal expansion*, can be carried out unilaterally or bilaterally.

Deep breathing while focusing on movement of the lower portion of the rib cage may facilitate diaphragmatic excursion.[28] This technique is particularly important for the patient with a stiff lower rib cage, as is often seen with chronic bronchitis, emphysema, or asthma.[7]

### Procedure

● Have the patient begin in a hook-lying position; later progress to a sitting position. Place your hands along the lateral aspect of the lower ribs to direct the patient's attention to the areas where movement is to occur (Figs. 25.11 and 25.12).

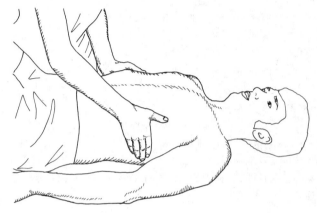

FIGURE 25.11 Bilateral lateral costal expansion—supine.

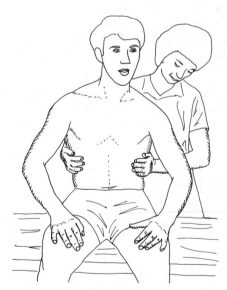

FIGURE 25.12 Bilateral lateral costal expansion—sitting.

● Ask the patient to breathe out, and feel the rib cage move downward and inward. As the patient breathes out, place pressure into the ribs with the palms of your hands.
● Just prior to inspiration, apply a quick downward and inward stretch to the chest. This places a quick

stretch on the external intercostals to facilitate their contraction.

● Apply *light* manual resistance to the lower ribs to increase sensory awareness as the patient breathes in deeply and the chest expands and ribs flare. Then, as the patient breathes out, assist by gently squeezing the rib cage in a downward and inward direction.

● Teach the patient how to perform the maneuver independently by placing his or her hand(s) over the ribs (Fig. 25.13) or applying resistance with a towel or belt around the lower ribs (Fig. 25.14A&B).

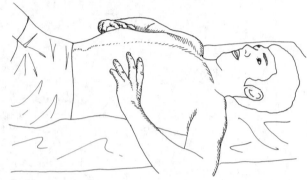

**FIGURE 25.13** The patient applies his or her own manual pressure during lateral costal expansion.

### Posterior Basal Expansion

Deep breathing emphasizing posterior basal expansion is important for the postsurgical patient who is confined to bed in a semireclining position for an extended period of time because secretions often accumulate in the posterior segments of the lower lobes.

#### Procedure

Have the patient sit and lean forward on a pillow, slightly bending the hips (see Fig. 25.15). Place your hands over the posterior aspect of the lower ribs, and follow the same procedure just described for lateral costal expansion.

## Pursed-Lip Breathing

Pursed-lip breathing is a strategy that involves lightly pursing the lips together during controlled exhalation. This breathing pattern often is adopted spontaneously by patients with COPD to deal with episodes of dyspnea.[7,10,28,43,48] Patients with COPD using pursed-lip breathing report a decrease in their perceived level of exertion during activity.[10]

However, whether it is beneficial to teach a patient pursed-lip breathing often is debated. Many therapists believe that gentle pursed-lip breathing and controlled expiration is a useful procedure, particularly to relieve dyspnea if it is performed appropriately. It is thought to keep airways open by creating back-pressure in the airways. Studies suggest that pursed-lip breathing decreases the respiratory rate and the work of breathing (oxygen consumption), increases the tidal volume, and improves exercise tolerance.[15,28,43,48]

P R E C A U T I O N : The use of *forceful* expiration during pursed-lip breathing must be avoided. Forceful expiration while the lips are pursed can increase the turbulence in the airways and cause further restriction of the small bronchioles. Therefore, if a therapist elects to teach this breathing strategy, it is important to emphasize with the patient that expiration should be performed in a controlled manner but not forced.

#### Procedure

Have the patient assume a comfortable position and relax as much as possible. Have the patient breathe in slowly and deeply through the nose and then breathe out gently through lightly pursed lips as if blowing on and bending the flame of a candle but not blowing it out.[43] Explain to

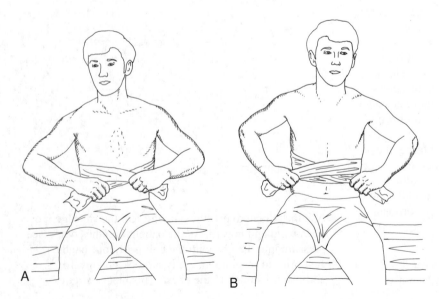

A                                                 B

**FIGURE 25.14** Belt exercises reinforce lateral costal breathing (*A*) by applying resistance during inspiration and (*B*) by assisting with pressure along the rib cage during expiration.

the patient that expiration must be relaxed and that contraction of the abdominals must be avoided. Place your hand over the patient's abdominal muscles to detect any contraction of the abdominals.

## Preventing and Relieving Episodes of Dyspnea

Many patients with COPD (e.g., emphysema and asthma) may suffer from periodic episodes of dyspnea (shortness of breath), particularly with physical exertion or when in contact with allergens. Whenever a patient's normal breathing pattern is interrupted, shortness of breath can occur. It is helpful to teach a patient how to monitor his or her level of shortness of breath and to *prevent* episodes of dyspnea by *controlled breathing techniques, pacing activities,* and becoming aware of what activity or situation precipitates a shortness of breath attack.

*Pacing* is the performance of functional activities, such as walking, stair climbing, or work-related tasks, within the limits of a patient's ventilatory capacity.[11] Although some patients may understand intuitively the limits to which functional activities can be pushed, others must be taught to recognize the early signs of dyspnea. If the patient becomes slightly short of breath, he or she must learn to stop an activity and use controlled, pursed-lip breathing until the dyspnea subsides.

### Procedure

● Have the patient assume a relaxed, forward-bent posture (Figs. 25.15 and 25.16; also see Fig. 25.6). A forward-bent position stimulates diaphragmatic breathing (the viscera drop forward and the diaphragm descends more easily). Use bronchodilators as prescribed.
● Have the patient gain control of his or her breathing and reduce the respiratory rate by using pursed-lip breathing during expiration. Have the patient focus on the expiratory phase of breathing while being sure to avoid forceful expiration.

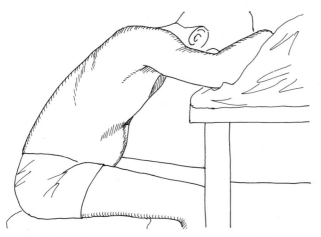

FIGURE 25.15 A patient can sit and lean forward on a pillow to relax and relieve an episode of dyspnea.

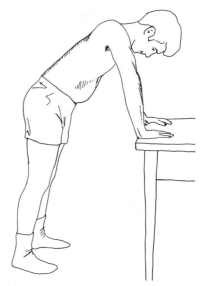

FIGURE 25.16 While standing, a patient can lean forward and place some weight on the hands to relieve dyspnea.

● After each pursed-lip expiration, teach the patient to use diaphragmatic breathing and minimize use of accessory muscles during each inspiration.
● Have the patient remain in a forward-bent posture and continue to breathe in a slow, controlled manner until the episode of dyspnea subsides.

## Positive Expiratory Pressure Breathing

Positive expiratory pressure breathing is a technique in which resistance to airflow is applied during exhalation, similar to what occurs during pursed-lip breathing, except that the patient breathes through a specially designed mouthpiece or mask that controls resistance to airflow.[19,20,25] This breathing technique is used to hold airways open during exhalation to mobilize accumulated secretions and improve their clearance. Positive expiratory pressure breathing provides an alternative or adjunct to postural drainage which a patient can perform independently.

### Procedure

Positive expiratory pressure breathing is performed in an upright position, preferably seated with the elbows resting on a table. The procedure can be performed against low or high pressure. A low pressure technique involves tidal inspiration and active, but not forced, expiration through a mouthpiece or mask. The patient inhales, holds the inspiration for 2 to 3 seconds, and then exhales, repeating the sequence for approximately 10 to 15 cycles.[19,20,25] The patient removes the mouthpiece or mask, takes several "huffs" and then coughs to clear the mobilized secretions from the airways. The breathing sequence typically is repeated four to six times with a total treatment session lasting about 15 minutes.

## Respiratory Resistance Training

The process of improving the strength or endurance of the muscles of ventilation is known as *respiratory resistance training* (RRT). Other descriptions used to denote this form of breathing exercises are *ventilatory muscle training, inspiratory* (or *expiratory*) *muscle training, inspiratory resistance training,* and *flow-controlled endurance training.* These techniques typically focus on training the muscles of inspiration,[14,26,32,33,54,65] although expiratory muscle training also has been described.[32,33] RRT is advocated to improve ventilation in patients with pulmonary dysfunction associated with weakness, atrophy, or inefficiency of the muscles of inspiration or to improve the effectiveness of the cough mechanism in patients with weakness of the abdominal muscles or other expiratory muscles.

With support from animal studies,[46,62] it has been suggested that the principles of overload and specificity of training apply to skeletal muscles throughout the body, including the muscles of ventilation.* In humans, it is not feasible to use invasive procedures to evaluate morphological or histochemical changes in the diaphragm that may occur as the result of strength or endurance training. Instead, strength or endurance changes must be assessed indirectly. Increases in respiratory muscle strength and endurance are determined by ultrasonographic meaurements of the thickness of the diaphragm, maximal voluntary ventilation, and decreased reliance on accessory muscles of inspiration. Respiratory muscle strength (either inspiratory or expiratory) also is evaluated indirectly with measurements of inspiratory capacity, forced expiratory volume, inspiratory mouth pressure using a spirometer, vital capacity, and increased cough effectiveness.

PRECAUTION: Avoid prolonged periods of any form of resistance training for inspiratory muscles. Unlike muscles of the extremities, the diaphragm cannot totally rest to recover from a session of resistance exercises. Use of accessory muscles of inspiration (neck and shoulder muscles) is a sign that the diaphragm is beginning to fatigue.[3,76]

### Inspiratory Resistance Training

Inspiratory resistance training, using pressure- or flow-based devices to provide resistance to airflow, is designed to improve the strength and endurance of the muscles of inspiration and decrease the occurrence of inspiratory muscle fatigue. This technique has been studied in patients with acute and chronic, primary and secondary pulmonary disorders, including COPD,[1,15,54,64] cystic fibrosis,[26] respiratory failure and ventilator dependence (weaning failure),[2,65] chronic heart failure,[14] and chronic neuromuscular disease.[32] Although reviews of the literature have demonstrated that outcomes of inspiratory muscle training programs in patients with pathologies are inconsistent,[33,50] some positive changes reported after training are increased vital capacity, increased exercise capacity, and fewer episodes of dyspnea.[14,26,54] Inspiratory muscle training also has been studied and found to be effective (as evidenced by

a decreased respiratory rate) in patients with cervical-level spinal cord lesions.[24,49,57,74]

### Procedure

- The patient inhales through a resistive training device placed in the mouth. These devices are narrow tubes of varying diameters or a mouthpiece and adapter with an adjustable aperture that provide resistance to airflow during inspiration and therefore place resistance on inspiratory muscles. The smaller the diameter of the aperture and the faster the rate of airflow, the greater is the resistance.
- The patient inhales through the device for a specified period of time several times each day. The time is gradually increased to 20 to 30 minutes at each training session to increase inspiratory muscle endurance.

### Incentive Respiratory Spirometry

*Incentive spirometry* is a form of ventilatory training that emphasizes sustained maximum inspirations.[18,48,60] The patient inhales as deeply as possible through a small, hand-held spirometer that provides visual or auditory feedback about whether a target maximum inspiration was reached. Typically, this breathing technique is performed while using a spirometer, but it also may be performed without the equipment.

The purpose of incentive spirometry is to increase the volume of air inspired. It is used primarily to prevent alveolar collapse and atelectasis in postoperative patients. Despite the widespread use of incentive spirometry for patients after surgery, the effectiveness of this technique alone or in addition to general deep breathing and coughing for the prevention of postoperative pulmonary complications is not clear.[18,40,71]

### Procedure

- Have the patient assume a comfortable position (semireclining, if possible) and inhale and exhale three to four times and then exhale maximally with the fourth breath.
- Then have the patient place the spirometer in the mouth, inhale maximally through the mouthpiece to a target setting and hold the inspiration for several seconds.
- This sequence is repeated five to ten times several times per day.

## Glossopharyngeal Breathing

Glossopharyngeal breathing is a technique that became known to therapists during the 1950s through patients with severe ventilatory impairment as the result of poliomyelitis. It is a means of increasing the inspiratory capacity when there is severe weakness of the muscles of inspiration.[28,39,53,75,76] Today, it is used primarily by patients who are ventilator-dependent because of absent or incomplete innervation of the diaphragm as the result of a high cervical-level spinal cord lesion or other neuromuscular disorders. Glossopharyngeal breathing combined with the inspiratory action of the neck musculature can reduce ventilator dependence or can be used as an emergency procedure should a malfunction of a patient's ventilator

---

* See references 1–3, 15, 26, 32, 33, 44, 46, 54, 57, 62, 65, 71, 76.

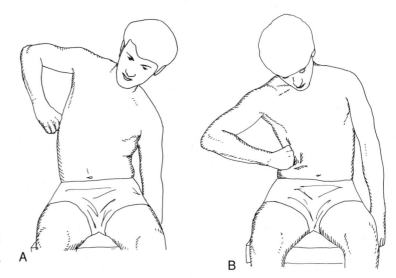

FIGURE 25.17 Chest mobilization during inspiration and expiration. To mobilize the lateral rib cage have the patient (A) bend away from the tight side during inspiration and (B) bend toward the tight side during expiration.

occur.[3,39,53,75,76] It also can be used to improve the force (and therefore the effectiveness) of a cough or increase the volume of the voice.

## Procedure
Glossopharyngeal breathing involves taking several "gulps" of air, usually 6 to 10 gulps in series, to pull air into the lungs when action of the inspiratory muscles is inadequate. After the patient takes several gulps of air, the mouth is closed, and the tongue pushes the air back and traps it in the pharynx. The air is then forced into the lungs when the glottis is opened. This increases the depth of the inspiration and the patient's inspiratory and vital capacities.[39,75]

 ## EXERCISES TO MOBILIZE THE CHEST

Chest mobilization exercises are any exercises that combine active movements of the trunk or extremities with deep breathing.[21,60] They are designed to maintain or improve mobility of the chest wall, trunk, and shoulder girdles when it affects ventilation or postural alignment. For example, a patient with hypomobility of the trunk muscles on one side of the body does not expand that part of the chest fully during inspiration. Exercises that combine stretching of these muscles with deep breathing improve ventilation on that side of the chest.

Chest mobilization exercises also are used to reinforce or emphasize the depth of inspiration or controlled expiration. A patient can reinforce expiration, for example, by leaning forward at the hips or flexing the spine as he or she breathes out. This pushes the viscera superiorly into the diaphragm.

## Specific Techniques

### To Mobilize One Side of the Chest
● While sitting, have the patient bend away from the tight side to lengthen hypomobile structures and expand that side of the chest during inspiration (Fig. 25.17A).

● Then, have the patient push the fisted hand into the lateral aspect of the chest, bend toward the tight side, and breathe out (Fig. 25.17B).
● Progress by having the patient raise the arm overhead on the tight side of the chest and side-bend away from the tight side. This places an additional stretch on hypomobile tissues.

### To Mobilize the Upper Chest and Stretch the Pectoralis Muscles

● While the patient is sitting in a chair with hands clasped behind the head, have him or her horizontally abduct the arms (elongating the pectoralis major) during a deep inspiration (Fig. 25.18A).
● Then instruct the patient to bring the elbows together and bend forward during expiration (Fig. 25.18B).

### To Mobilize the Upper Chest and Shoulders
While sitting in a chair, have the patient reach with both arms overhead (180° bilateral shoulder flexion and slight abduction) during inspiration (Fig. 25.19A) and then bend forward at the hips and reach for the floor during expiration (Fig. 25.19B).

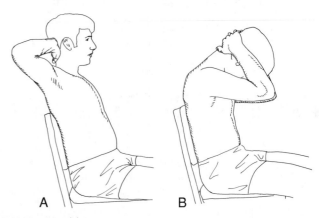

FIGURE 25.18 (A) A stretch is applied to the pectoralis muscles during inspiration, and (B) the patient brings the elbows together to facilitate expiration.

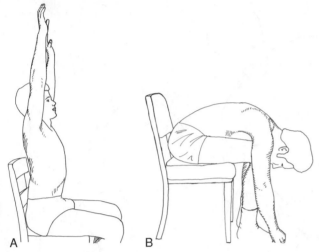

FIGURE 25.19 (A) Chest expansion is increased with bilateral movement of the arms overhead during inspiration. (B) Expiration is then reinforced by reaching the arms toward the floor.

# COUGHING

An effective cough is necessary to eliminate respiratory obstructions and keep the lungs clear. Airway clearance is an important part of management of patients with acute or chronic respiratory conditions.[25,51,60]

## The Normal Cough Pump

A cough may be reflexive or voluntary. When a person coughs, a series of actions occurs (Box 25.7).[47] Under normal conditions, the cough pump is effective to the seventh generation of bronchi. (There are a total of 23 generations of bronchi in the tracheobronchial tree.) Ciliated epithelial cells are present up to the terminal bronchiole and raise secretions from the smaller to the larger airways in the absence of pathology.

## Factors that Decrease the Effectiveness of the Cough Mechanism and Cough Pump

The effectiveness of the cough mechanism can be compromised for a number of reasons including the following.[25,39,51,60,76]

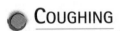

| BOX 25.7 | The Cough Mechanism |

- Deep inspiration occurs.
- Glottis closes, and vocal cords tighten.
- Abdominal muscles contract and the diaphragm elevates, causing an increase in intrathoracic and intra-abdominal pressures.
- Glottis opens.
- Explosive expiration of air occurs.

- **Decreased inspiratory capacity.** Inspiratory capacity can be reduced because of pain due to acute lung disease, rib fracture, trauma to the chest, or recent thoracic or abdominal surgery. Weakness of the diaphragm or accessory muscles of inspiration as a result of a high spinal cord injury or neuropathic or myopathic disease decrease a patient's ability to take in a deep breath. Postoperatively, the respiratory center may be depressed as the result of general anesthesia, pain, or medication.
- **Inability to forcibly expel air.** A spinal cord injury above T12 and myopathic disease, such as muscular dystrophy, cause weakness of the abdominal muscles, which are vital for a strong cough. Excessive fatigue as the result of critical illness and a chest wall or abdominal incision causing pain all contribute to a weak cough. A patient who has had a tracheostomy also has difficulty producing a strong cough, even when the tracheostomy site is covered.
- **Decreased action of the cilia in the bronchial tree.** Action of the ciliated cells may be compromised because of physical interventions such as general anesthesia and intubation or pathologies such as COPD including chronic bronchitis, which is associated with a decreased number of ciliated epithelial cells in the airway. Smoking also depresses the action of the cilia.
- **Increase in the amount or thickness of mucus.** Pathologies (e.g., cystic fibrosis, chronic bronchitis) and pulmonary infections (e.g., pneumonia) are associated with an increase in mucus production and the thickness of the mucus. Intubation irriates the lumen of the airways and causes increased mucus production, whereas dehydration thickens mucus.

## Teaching an Effective Cough

Because an effective cough is an integral component of airway clearance, a patient must be taught the importance of an effective cough, how to produce an efficient and controlled voluntary cough, and when to cough. The following sequence and procedures are used when teaching an effective cough.[25,51,66]

1. Assess the patient's voluntary or reflexive cough.
2. Have the patient assume a relaxed, comfortable position for deep breathing and coughing. Sitting or leaning forward usually is the best position for coughing. The patient's neck should be slightly flexed to make coughing more comfortable.
3. Teach the patient controlled diaphragmatic breathing, emphasizing deep inspirations.
4. Demonstrate a sharp, deep, double cough.
5. Demonstrate the proper muscle action of coughing (contraction of the abdominals). Have the patient place the hands on the abdomen and make three *huffs* with expiration to feel the contraction of the abdominals (see Fig. 25.10). Have the patient practice making a "K" sound to experience tightening the vocal cords, closing the glottis, and contracting the abdominals.
6. When the patient has put these actions together, instruct the patient to take a deep but relaxed inspiration, fol-

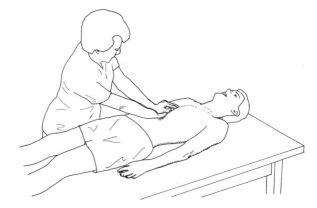

FIGURE 25.20 Therapist-assisted manual cough technique.

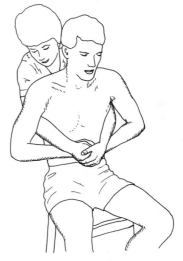

FIGURE 25.21 Therapist-assisted or self-assisted manual cough technique.

## BOX 25.8 Precautions for Teaching an Effective Cough

- Never allow a patient to gasp in air, because this increases the work (energy expenditure) of breathing, causing the patient to fatigue more easily. It also increases turbulence and resistance in the airways, possibly leading to increased bronchospasm and further constriction of airways. A gasping action also may push mucus or a foreign object deep into air passages.
- Avoid uncontrolled coughing spasms (*paroxysmal coughing*).
- Avoid forceful coughing if a patient has a history of a cerebrovascular accident or an aneurysm. Have these patients *huff* several times to clear the airways, rather than cough.
- Be sure that the patient coughs while in a somewhat erect or side-lying posture.

lowed by a sharp double cough. The second cough during a single expiration is usually more productive.

7. Use an abdominal binder or glossopharyngeal breathing in selected patients with inspiratory or abdominal muscle weakness to enhance the cough, if necessary.

Precautions that should be observed while teaching a patient an effective cough are noted in Box 25.8.

## Additional Techniques to Facilitate a Cough and Improve Airway Clearance

To maximize airway clearance, several techniques can be used to stimulate a stronger cough, make coughing more comfortable or improve the clearance of secretions.

### Manual–Assisted Cough

If a patient has abdominal weakness (e.g., as the result of a mid-thoracic or cervical spinal cord injury), manual pressure on the abdominal area assists in developing greater intra-abdominal pressure for a more forceful cough. Manual pressure for cough assistance can be applied by the therapist or the patient.[3,25,39,51,66,76]

### Therapist-Assisted Techniques

- With the patient in a supine or semireclining position, the therapist places the heel of one hand on the patient's abdomen at the epigastric area just distal to the xiphoid process. The other hand is placed on top of the first, keeping the fingers open or interlocking them (Fig. 25.20). After the patient inhales as deeply as possible, the therapist manually assists the patient as he or she attempts to cough. The abdomen is compressed with an inward and upward force, which pushes the diaphragm upward to cause a more forceful and effective cough.
- This same maneuver can be performed with the patient in a chair (Fig. 25.21). The therapist or family member can stand in back of the patient and apply manual pressure during expiration.

**PRECAUTION**: Avoid direct pressure on the xiphoid process during the maneuver.

### Self-Assisted Technique

- While in a sitting position, the patient crosses the arms across the abdomen or places the interlocked hands below the xiphoid process (see Fig. 25.21).
- After a deep inspiration, the patient pushes inward and upward on the abdomen with the wrists or forearms and simultaneously leans forward while attempting to cough.

### Splinting

If chest wall pain from recent surgery or trauma is restricting the cough, teach the patient to splint over the painful area during coughing.[25,45,51] Have the patient press the hands or a pillow firmly over the incision to support the painful area with each cough (Fig. 25.22). If the patient cannot reach the painful area, the therapist should assist (Fig. 25.23).

### Humidification

If secretions are very thick, work with the patient after humidification therapy or ultrasonic nebulizer therapy, both

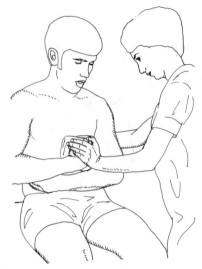

FIGURE 25.22 Splinting over an anterior surgical incision.

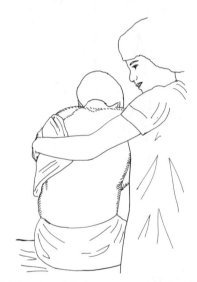

FIGURE 25.23 Splinting over a posterior lateral incision.

of which enhance the mucociliary transport system and facilitate a productive cough.[66]

### Tracheal Stimulation

Tracheal stimulation, sometimes called a *tracheal tickle,* may be used with infants or disoriented patients who cannot cooperate during treatment.[66] Tracheal stimulation is a somewhat uncomfortable maneuver, performed to elicit a reflexive cough. The therapist places two fingers at the sternal notch and applies a circular motion with pressure downward into the trachea to facilitate a reflexive cough.

## Suctioning: Alternative to Coughing

*Endotracheal suctioning* may be the only means of clearing the airways in patients who are unable to cough or huff voluntarily or after reflex stimulation of the cough mechanism.[29,60] Suctioning is indicated in all patients with artificial airways. The suctioning procedure clears only the trachea and the mainstem bronchi.

**PRECAUTION:** Only individuals who have been taught proper suctioning technique should use this alternative means of clearing the airways. Suctioning, if performed incorrectly, can introduce an infection into the airways or damage the delicate mucosal lining of the trachea and bronchi. Improper suctioning also can cause hypoxemia, an abnormal heart rate, and atelectasis. A complete description of the proper endotracheal suctioning technique may be found in other resources.[29,60]

## ⬤ POSTURAL DRAINAGE

*Postural drainage* (bronchial drainage), another intervention for airway clearance, is a means of mobilizing secretions in one or more lung segments to the central airways by placing the patient in various positions so gravity assists in the drainage process.[4,11,25,51,60] When secretions are moved from the smaller to the larger airways, they are then cleared by coughing or endotracheal suctioning. *Postural drainage therapy* also includes the use of manual techniques, such as percussion, shaking, and vibration, coupled with voluntary coughing.

Goals and indications for postural drainage are noted in Box 25.9, and relative contraindications are summarized in Box 25.10.[4,11,25,51,60] Despite the risks, postural drainage may be necessary in the unstable patient. Modified positioning to avoid head-down or fully horizontal positions typically is necessary for most high-risk patients.

### Manual Techniques Used with Postural Drainage Therapy

In addition to the use of body positioning, deep breathing, and an effective cough to facilitate airway clearance, a variety of manual techniques are used in conjunction with postural drainage to maximize the effectiveness of the

---

**BOX 25.9    Goals and Indications for Postural Drainage**

**Prevent Accumulation of Secretions in Patients at Risk for Pulmonary Complications**
- Patients with pulmonary diseases that are associated with increased production or viscosity of mucus, such as chronic bronchitis and cystic fibrosis
- Patients who are on prolonged bed rest
- Patients who have received general anesthesia and who may have painful incisions that restrict deep breathing and coughing postoperatively
- Any patient who is on a ventilator if he or she is stable enough to tolerate the treatment

**Remove Accumulated Secretions from the Lungs**
- Patients with acute or chronic lung disease, such as pneumonia, atelectasis, acute lung infections, COPD
- Patients who are generally very weak or are elderly
- Patients with artificial airways

- Severe hemoptysis
- Untreated acute conditions
  - Severe pulmonary edema
  - Congestive heart failure
  - Large pleural effusion
  - Pulmonary embolism
  - Pneumothorax
- Cardiovascular instability
  - Cardiac arrhythmia
  - Severe hypertension or hypotension
  - Recent myocardial infarction
  - Unstable angina
- Recent neurosurgery
  - Head-down positioning may cause increased intracranial pressure; if PD is required, modified positions can be used

mucociliary transport system.[11,25,51,60,66,72] They include percussion, vibration, shaking, and rib springing. Findings from studies that have been implemented to evaluate the efficacy of these manual techniques as adjuncts to postural drainage are inconclusive.[66]

## Percussion

Percussion is used to augment mobilization of secretions by mechanically dislodging viscous or adherent mucus from the airways. Percussion is performed with cupped hands (Fig. 25.24A) over the lung segment being

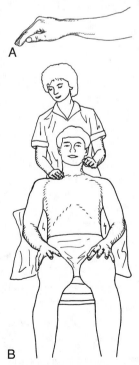

FIGURE 25.24  (A) Hand position for applying percussion. (B) The therapist alternately percusses over the lung segment being drained.

drained.[25,67] The therapist's cupped hands strike the patient's chest wall in an alternating, rhythmic manner (Fig. 25.24B). The therapist should try to keep shoulders, elbows, and wrists loose and mobile during the maneuver. Mechanical percussion is an alternative to manual percussion techniques.

Percussion is continued for several minutes or until the patient needs to alter position to cough. This procedure should not be painful or uncomfortable.

PRECAUTIONS: To prevent irritation to sensitive skin, have the patient wear a lightweight gown or shirt. Avoid percussion over breast tissue in women and over bony prominences.

### Relative Contraindications to Percussion

Prior to using percussion in a postural drainage program, a therapist must weigh the potential benefits versus potential risks. In most instances, it is prudent to avoid the use of percussion.[25,67]

- Over fractures, spinal fusion, or osteoporotic bone
- Over tumor area
- If a patient has a pulmonary embolus
- If the patient has a condition in which hemorrhage could easily occur, such as in the presence of a low platelet count, or if the patient is receiving anticoagulation therapy
- If the patient has unstable angina
- If the patient has chest wall pain, for example after thoracic surgery or trauma

### Vibration

Vibration, another manual technique, often is used in conjunction with percussion to help move secretions to larger airways. It is applied *only during the expiratory phase* as the patient is deep-breathing.[25,51,72] Vibration is applied by placing both hands directly on the skin and over the chest wall (or one hand on top of the other) and gently compressing and rapidly vibrating the chest wall as the patient breathes out (Fig. 25.25). Pressure is applied in the same direction as the chest is moving. The vibrating action is achieved by the therapist isometrically contracting (tensing) the muscles of the upper extremities from shoulders to hands.

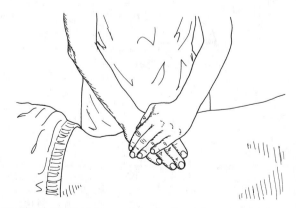

FIGURE 25.25  Hand placement for vibration during postural drainage.

## Shaking

Shaking is a more vigorous form of vibration applied during exhalation using an intermittent bouncing maneuver coupled with wide movements of the therapist's hands. The therapist's thumbs are locked together, the open hands are placed directly on the patient's skin, and fingers are wrapped around the chest wall. The therapist simultaneously compresses and shakes the chest wall.[25,51,72]

## Postural Drainage Positions

Positions for postural drainage are based on the anatomy of the lungs and the tracheobronchial tree (see Figs. 25.2 and 25.4). Each segment of each lobe is drained using the positions depicted in Figures 25.26 through 25.37. The shaded area in each illustration indicates the area of the chest wall where percussion or vibration is applied.

### RIGHT AND LEFT UPPER LOBES

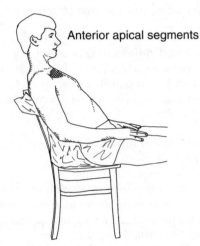

Anterior apical segments

FIGURE 25.26 Percussion is applied directly under the clavicle.

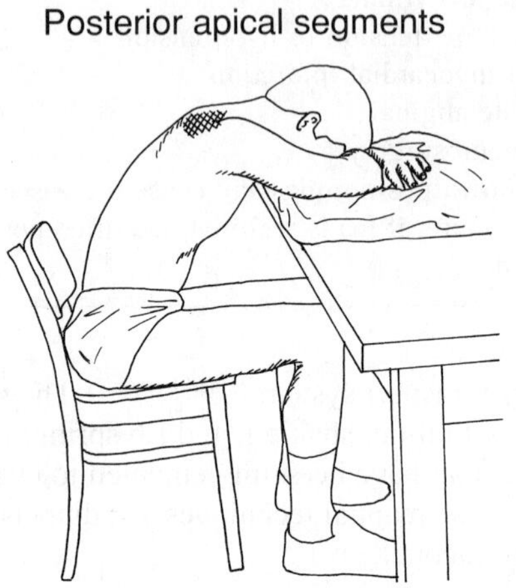

Posterior apical segments

FIGURE 25.27 Percussion is applied above the scapulae. Your fingers curve over the top of the shoulders.

Anterior segments

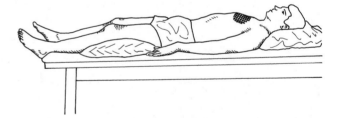

FIGURE 25.28 Percussion is applied bilaterally, directly over the nipple or just above the breast.

Posterior segment
(left)

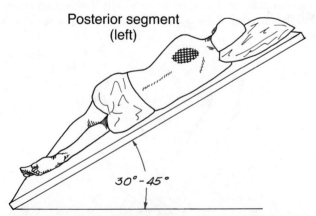

30° - 45°

FIGURE 25.29 Patient lies one-quarter turn from prone and rests on the right side. Head and shoulders are elevated 45° or approximately 18 inches if pillows are used. Percussion is applied directly over the left scapula.

Posterior segment
(right)

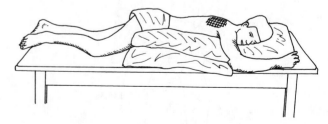

FIGURE 25.30 Patient lies flat and one-quarter turn from prone on the left side. Percussion is applied directly over the right scapula.

## LINGULA

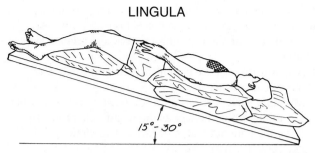

**FIGURE 25.31** Patient lies one-quarter turn from supine on the right side, supported with pillows and in a 30° head-down position. Percussion is applied just under the left breast.

## MIDDLE LOBE

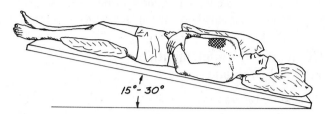

**FIGURE 25.32** Patient lies one-quarter turn from supine on the left side, supported with pillows behind the back, and in a 30° head-down position. Percussion is applied under the right breast.

## RIGHT AND LEFT LOWER LOBES

### Anterior segments

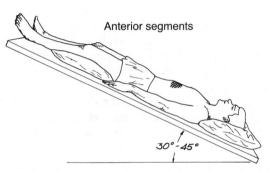

**FIGURE 25.33** Patient lies supine, pillows under knees, in a 45° head-down position. Percussion is applied bilaterally over the lower portion of the ribs.

### Posterior segments

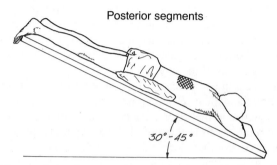

**FIGURE 25.34** Patient lies prone with a pillow under the abdomen in a 45° head-down position. Percussion is applied bilaterally over the lower portion of the ribs.

### Lateral segment (left)

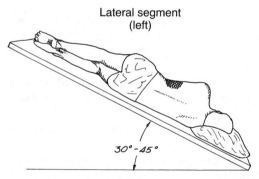

**FIGURE 25.35** Patient lies on the right side in a 45° head-down position. Percussion is applied over the lower lateral aspect of the left rib cage.

### Lateral segment (right)

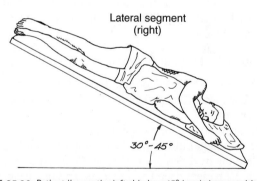

**FIGURE 25.36** Patient lies on the left side in a 45° head-down position Percussion is applied over the lower lateral aspect of the right rib cage.

### Superior segments

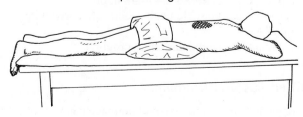

**FIGURE 25.37** Patient lies prone with a pillow under the abdomen to flatten the back. Percussion is applied bilaterally, directly below the scapulae.

The patient may be positioned on a postural drainage table that can be elevated at one end, a tilt table, a reinforced padded table with a lift, or a hospital bed. A small child can be positioned on a therapist's or parent's lap.

## Guidelines for Implementing Postural Drainage

### General Considerations

*Time of day.* Consider the following when scheduling postural drainage into a patient's day.

- Never administer postural drainage directly after a meal.
- Coordinate treatment with aerosol therapy. Some therapists believe that aerosol therapy combined with humidification prior to postural drainage helps loosen secretions and increases the likelihood of productivity. Others believe that aerosol therapy is best after postural drainage when the patient's lungs are clearer and maximal benefit can be gained from medication administered through aerosol therapy.
- Choose a time (or times) of day likely to be of most benefit to the patient. A patient's cough tends to be highly productive in the early morning because of accumulation of secretions from the night before. Postural drainage in the early evening clears the lungs prior to sleeping and helps the patient rest more easily.

*Frequency of treatments.* The frequency of postural drainage each day or during the week depends on the type and severity of a patient's pathology. If secretions are thick and copious, two to four times per day may be necessary until the lungs are clear. If a patient is on a maintenance program, the frequency is less, perhaps once a day or only a few days a week.

### Preparation for Postural Drainage

- Loosen tight or bulky clothing. It is not necessary to expose the skin. The patient may wear a lightweight shirt or gown.
- Have a sputum cup or tissues available.
- Have sufficient pillows for positioning and comfort.
- Explain the treatment procedure to the patient.
- Teach the patient deep breathing and an effective cough prior to beginning postural drainage.
- If the patient is producing copious amounts of sputum, instruct the patient to cough a few times or have the patient suctioned prior to positioning.
- Make any adjustments of tubes and wires, such as chest tubes, electrocardiography wires, or catheters, so they remain clear during positioning.

### Postural Drainage Sequence

- Determine which segments of the lungs should be drained. Some patients with chronic lung diseases, such as cystic fibrosis, need to be drained in all positions. Other patients may require drainage of only a few segments in which secretions have accumulated.

- Check the patient's vital signs and breath sounds.
- Position the patient in the correct position for drainage. See that he or she is as comfortable and relaxed as possible.
- Stand in front of the patient, whenever possible, to observe his or her color.
- Maintain each position for 5 to 10 minutes if the patient can tolerate it or as long as the position is productive.
- Have the patient breathe deeply during drainage but do not allow the patient to hyperventilate or become short of breath. Pursed-lip breathing during expiration is sometimes used.
- Apply percussion over the segment being drained while the patient is in the correct position.
- Encourage the patient to take a deep, sharp, double cough whenever necessary. It may be more comfortable for the patient to momentarily assume a semiupright position (resting on one elbow) and then cough.
- If the patient does not cough spontaneously during positioning with percussion, instruct the patient to take several deep breaths or huff several times in succession as you apply vibration during expiration. This may help elicit a cough.
- If the patient's cough is not productive after 5 to 10 minutes of positioning, go on to the next position. Secretions that have been mobilized during a treatment may not be coughed up by the patient until 30 minutes to 1 hour after treatment.
- The duration of any one treatment should not exceed 45 to 60 minutes, as the procedure is quite fatiguing for the patient.

### Concluding a Treatment

- Have the patient sit up slowly and rest for a short while after the treatment. Watch for signs of postural hypotension when the patient rises from a supine position or from a head-down position to sitting.
- Advise the patient that even if the cough was not productive during treatment it may be productive a short while after treatment.
- Evaluate the effectiveness of the treatment by reassessing breath sounds.
- Note the type, color, consistency, and amount of secretions produced.
- Check the patient's vital signs after treatment and note how the patient tolerated the treatment.

### Criteria for Discontinuing Postural Drainage

- If the chest radiograph is relatively clear
- If the patient is afebrile for 24 to 48 hours
- If normal or near-normal breath sounds are heard with auscultation
- If the patient is on a regular home program

## Modified Postural Drainage

Some patients who require postural drainage cannot assume or cannot tolerate the positions optimal for postural drainage. For example, a patient with congestive heart failure may exhibit indications of orthopnea (shortness of breath while lying flat). After neurosurgery a patient may not be allowed to assume a head-down (Trendelenburg) position because this position causes increased intracranial pressure. After thoracic surgery a patient may have chest tubes and monitoring wires that limit positioning. Under these circumstances and others, positioning during postural drainage must be modified.[25,51,60,66] The positions in which postural drainage is undertaken are modified consistent with the patient's medical or surgical problems. This compromise, although not ideal, is better than not administering postural drainage at all.

## Home Program of Postural Drainage

Postural drainage may have to be carried out on a regular basis at home for patients with chronic lung disease. Patients need to be shown how to position themselves using inexpensive aids. An adult may place pillows over a hard wedge or stacks of newspapers to achieve the desired head-down positions in bed. A patient also can lean the chest over the edge of a bed, resting with the arms on a chair or stool. A child can be positioned on an ironing board propped up against a sofa or heavy chair. A family member often must be taught proper positioning, percussion or shaking techniques, and precautions to assist the patient.

## ● MANAGEMENT OF PATIENTS WITH CHRONIC OBSTRUCTIVE PULMONARY DISEASE

*Chronic obstructive pulmonary disease* is a broad term encompassing a number of chronic pulmonary conditions, all of which obstruct the flow of air in the conducting airways of the lower respiratory tract and alter ventilation and gas exchange.[6,30,67] Although a variety of pulmonary diseases are classified as obstructive in nature, each disease has its unique features and clinical manifestations and is distinguished by the cause of the obstruction of airflow, the onset of the disease, the location of the obstruction, and the reversibility of the obstruction.

## Types of Obstructive Pulmonary Disorders

Typically, *peripheral airway disease, chronic bronchitis,* and *emphysema* are classified as COPD; but other obstructive pulmonary diseases that are chronic in nature, such as *asthma, bronchiectasis, cystic fibrosis,* and *bronchopulmonary dysplasia,* also may be included under this broad descriptor. The focus of discussion and guidelines for management presented in this section of the chapter is on chronic bronchitis and emphysema because patients with these diseases commonly are seen in pulmonary rehabilitation programs.[6,7,12,37,67]

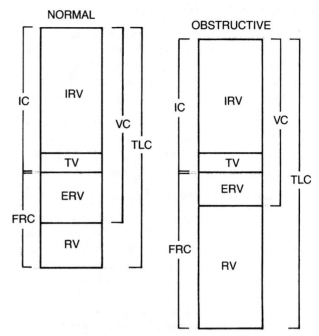

FIGURE 25.38 Normal lung volumes and capacities compared with abnormal lung volumes and capacities found in patients with obstructive pulmonary disease. *(From Rothstein, J, Roy, A, Wolf, SL: The Rehabilitation Specialist's Handbook, ed. 3. FA Davis, Philadelphia, 2005, p 428, with permission.)*

## Pathological Changes in the Pulmonary System

Changes in chronic bronchitis and emphysema that occur over time are inflammation of the mucous membranes of the airways; increased production and retention of mucus; narrowing and destruction of airways; and destruction of alveolar and bronchial walls.[6,30,67] These structural changes are reflected in pulmonary function tests depicted in Figure 25.38. These changes in the patient's pulmonary status predispose the patient to frequent acute respiratory infections.

## Impairments and Impact on Function

As a result of the pathophysiology of COPD, many physical impairments develop over time. Patients typically have a chronic, productive cough and are often short of breath. The characteristic impact of COPD on the pulmonary system is the inability to remove air from the lungs effectively, which in turn affects the ability of the respiratory system to transport oxygen into the lungs.

Consequently, functional limitations and eventually disability occur consistent with the disablement process.[42] Impairments such as increased respiratory rate, decreased vital capacity and forced expiratory volume, increased use of accessory muscles of inspiration, and progressive chest wall stiffness are associated with decreased tolerance to exercise, frequent episodes of dyspnea, decreased walking speed and distance, and eventual inability to perform activities of daily living at home or in the workplace or to remain an active participant in the community.

## Management Guidelines: COPD

Lifelong management includes appropriate medical management to lessen disabling symptoms and prevent infection, smoking cessation, and participation in a comprehensive pulmonary rehabilitation program. Important aspects of management include breathing exercises, ongoing, airway clearance, and participation in an individually designed, graded exercise program that includes upper and lower extremity strength training and aerobic conditioning.[6,7,11,12,37,55,67,70] Common impairments and guidelines for management are described in Box 25.11.

 **Focus on Evidence**

Patients with COPD who appear to benefit most from pulmonary rehabilitation are those with only moderate-level disease and without a substantial number of co-morbidities. A combination of upper and lower extremity exercises have been shown to improve functional status more effectively than either upper or lower extremity exercise alone.[6]

Systematic reviews of the literature of pulmonary rehabilitation programs have demonstrated that the effects of a program of breathing exercises (diaphragmatic and pursed-lip breathing) on respiratory function[13] and the effects of inspiratory resistance training on exercise capacity[50] are equivocal. However, peripheral muscle strengthening programs improve physical functioning.[55]

#  MANAGEMENT OF PATIENTS WITH RESTRICTIVE PULMONARY DISORDERS

Restrictive pulmonary disorders are characterized by the inability of the lungs to expand fully as a result of extrapulmonary and/or pulmonary disease or restriction.[11,17] In other words, the patient has difficulty taking in a deep breath.

## Acute and Chronic Causes of Restrictive Pulmonary Disorders

There are a variety of acute or chronic disorders directly involving structures of the pulmonary system or extrapulmonary disorders that can cause restrictive pulmonary dysfunction.[11,17]

### Pulmonary Causes

- Diseases of the lung parenchyma such as *tumor, interstitial pulmonary fibrosis* (e.g., pneumonia, tuberculosis, asbestosis), and *atelectasis*
- Disorders of cardiovascular/pulmonary origin, such as *pulmonary edema* or *pulmonary embolism*
- Inadequate or abnormal pulmonary development (*bronchopulmonary dysplasia*)
- Advanced age

### Extrapulmonary Causes

- Chest wall pain secondary to trauma or surgery
- Chest wall stiffness associated with extrapulmonary disease (e.g., scleroderma, ankylosing spondylitis)
- Postural deformities (scoliosis, kyphosis)
- Ventilatory muscle weakness of neuropathic or myopathic origin (e.g., spinal cord injury, cerebral palsy, Parkinson's disease, muscular dystrophy)
- Pleural disease
- Insufficient diaphragmatic excursion because of ascites or obesity

## Pathological Changes in the Pulmonary System

Pulmonary function may be altered as a result of pulmonary or extrapulmonary conditions. These alterations in lung volumes and capacities are depicted in Figure 25.39. Cardiopulmonary factors contributing to these changes are decreased pulmonary compliance caused by inflammation or fibrosis (thickening of the alveoli, bronchioles, or pleura), pulmonary congestion, and decreased arterial blood gases (hypoxemia).

## Management Guidelines: Post-Thoracic Surgery

Although any number of acute or chronic disorders can be the underlying cause(s) of restrictive lung dysfunction, only management after thoracic surgery is addressed in this section. Patients with cardiac or pulmonary conditions that require surgical interventions are at high risk for restrictive pulmonary complications after surgery. *Thoracotomy,* an incision into the chest wall, is necessary during many types of pulmonary surgery including *lobectomy* (removal of a lobe of a lung), *pneumonectomy* (removal of a lung), or *segmental resection* (removal of a segment of a lobe of a lung).[17,23,36,40]

Cardiac surgeries, such as coronary artery bypass graft surgery, replacement of one or more valves of the heart, repair of septal defects, or heart transplantation also require thoracotomy.[17,23,36,40]

N O T E : Patients who undergo upper abdominal surgery also have a high risk of developing postoperative pulmonary complications. Postoperative pain is often greater after upper abdominal surgery than after thoracic surgery.[73] This results in hypoventilation (55% decreased vital capacity for the first 24 to 48 hours after surgery) and an ineffective cough, which place the patient at risk for developing pneumonia or atelectasis.[17,40] A systematic review of the literature revealed that postoperative programs of cardiopulmonary physical therapy have beneficial effects after upper abdominal surgery.[73]

### Factors That Increase the Risk of Pulmonary Complications and Restrictive Lung Dysfunction After Thoracic Surgery

The post-thoracotomy patient experiences considerable chest pain, which leads to chest wall immobility, poor lung

## BOX 25.11
## MANAGEMENT GUIDELINES—Chronic Obstructive Pulmonary Disease (COPD)

### Impairments

An increase in the amount and viscosity of mucus production
A chronic, often productive cough
Frequent episodes of dyspnea
A labored breathing pattern that results in:
• Increased respiratory rate (tachypnea)
• Use of accessory muscles of inspiration and decreased diaphragmatic excursion
• Upper chest breathing
Inadequate exchange of air in the lower lobes
Most difficulty during expiration; use of pursed-lip breathing
Changes in pulmonary function
• Increased residual volume
• Decreased vital capacity
• Decreased expiratory flow rates
Decreased mobility of the chest wall; a barrel chest deformity develops
Abnormal posture: forward-head and rounded and elevated shoulders
Decreased general endurance during functional activities

| Plan of Care | Interventions |
|---|---|
| 1. Decrease the amount and viscosity of secretions and prevent respiratory infections. | 1. Administration of bronchodilators, antibiotics, and humidification therapy. <br> If patient smokes, he or she should be strongly encouraged to stop. |
| 2. Remove or prevent the accumulation of secretions. (This is important if emphysema is associated with chronic bronchitis or if there is an acute respiratory infection.) | 2. Deep and effective cough. <br> Postural drainage to areas where secretions are identified. <br> N O T E : Drainage positions may need to be modified if the patient is dyspneic in the head-down position. |
| 3. Promote relaxation of the accessory muscles of inspiration to decrease reliance on upper chest breathing and to decrease muscle tension associated with dyspnea. | 3. Positioning for relaxation. <br> • Relaxed head-up position in bed: trunk, arms, and head are well supported. <br> • Sitting: leaning forward, resting forearms on thighs or on a table. <br> • Standing: leaning forward on an object, with hands on the thighs or leaning backward against a wall. <br> Relaxation exercises for shoulder musculature: active shoulder shrugging followed by relaxation; shoulder and arm circles; horizontal abduction and adduction of the shoulders. |
| 4. Improve the patient's breathing pattern and ventilation. <br> Emphasize diaphragmatic and lateral costal breathing and *relaxed* expiration; decrease the work of breathing, rate of respiration, and use of accessory muscles. Carry over controlled breathing exercises to functional activities. | 4. Breathing exercises: controlled diaphragmatic breathing with minimal upper chest movement; lateral costal breathing; pursed-lip breathing (careful to *avoid forced* expiration). <br> Practice controlled breathing during standing, walking, climbing stairs, and other functional activities. |
| 5. Minimize or prevent episodes of dyspnea. | 5. Have a patient assume a comfortable position so the upper chest is relaxed and the lower chest is as mobile as possible. <br> Emphasize controlled diaphragmatic breathing. <br> Have the patient breathe out as rapidly as possible *without forcing* expiration. <br> N O T E : Initially, the rate of ventilation is rapid and shallow. As the patient gets control of breathing, he or she slows the rate. <br> Administer supplemental oxygen during a severe episode, if needed. |
| 6. Improve the mobility of the lower thorax. | 6. Exercises for chest mobility, emphasizing movement of the lower rib cage during deep breathing. |
| 7. Improve posture. | 7. Exercises and postural training to decrease forward-head and rounded shoulders. |
| 8. Increase exercise tolerance. | 8. Graded endurance and conditioning exercises (see Chapter 4). |

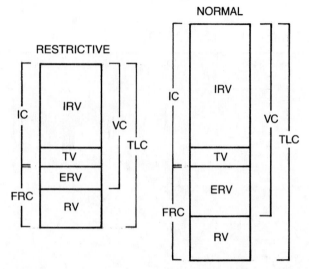

FIGURE 25.39 Normal lung volumes and capacities compared with abnormal lung volumes and capacities found in patients with restrictive pulmonary disorders. *(From Rothstein, J, Roy, A, Wolf, SL: The Rehabilitation Specialist's Handbook, ed. 3. FA Davis, Philadelphia, 2005, p 428, with permission.)*

expansion, and an ineffective cough. In addition, pulmonary secretions are greater than normal after surgery. Therefore, the patient is more likely to accumulate pulmonary secretions and develop secondary pneumonia or atelectasis. Factors that increase the risk of postoperative pulmonary complications are noted in the following sections.[17,40]

### General Anesthesia

- Decreases the normal ciliary action of the tracheobronchial tree
- Depresses the respiratory center of the central nervous system, which causes a shallow respiratory pattern (decreased tidal volume and vital capacity)
- Depresses the cough reflex

### Intubation (Insertion of an Endotracheal Tube)

- Causes muscle spasm and immobility of the chest
- Irritates the mucosal lining of the tracheobronchial tree, which causes increased production of mucus
- Decreases the normal action of the cilia in the tracheobronchial tree, which leads to pooling of secretions

### Incisional Pain

- Causes muscle splinting and decreases chest wall compliance, which in turn causes a shallow breathing pattern. Consequently, lung expansion is restricted and secretions are not adequately mobilized.
- Restricts a deep and effective cough. The patient usually has a weak, shallow cough that does not effectively mobilize and clear secretions.

### Pain Medication

Although pain medication administered postoperatively diminishes incisional pain, it also:

- Depresses the respiratory center of the central nervous system
- Decreases the normal ciliary action in the bronchial tree

### General Inactivity, Postoperative Weakness and Fatigue

- Pooling of secretions, particularly in the posterior basilar segments of the lower lobes, because of inactivity
- Decreased effectiveness of the cough pump because of postoperative weakness and fatigue

### Other risk factors not directly related to the surgery

- Patient's age (> age 50)
- History of smoking
- History of COPD or restrictive pulmonary disorder because of neuromuscular weakness
- Obesity
- Poor mentation and orientation

## Thoracic Surgery: Operative and Postoperative Considerations during Management

Many factors contribute to a patient's postoperative impairments, any one of which influences postoperative management.[17,23] A patient who has undergone thoracotomy for a pulmonary or cardiac condition typically is hospitalized for a week or less. Postoperative impairments and guidelines for management of a patient who has undergone thoracic surgery are summarized in Box 25.12.[16,17,23,36,40,41,71] Therapeutic interventions begin on the first postoperative day and include breathing and coughing exercises, shoulder ROM, posture awareness training, and a graded aerobic conditioning program.[16,23,36,40,41,71]

### Co-morbidities and Related Dysfunction

In addition to the primary pulmonary or cardiac pathology (e.g., a malignant tumor, lung abscess, coronary artery disease) the patient also may have related cardiopulmonary conditions, such as angina, congestive heart disease, chronic bronchitis, or emphysema. The patient with a long history of cardiac disease may have preoperative pulmonary dysfunction such as hypoxemia, dyspnea on exertion, orthopnea, or pulmonary congestion. Such co-morbidities and related pulmonary or cardiac dysfunction can complicate postoperative rehabilitation.

### Surgical Approach

Pulmonary surgery typically involves a large posterolateral, lateral, or anterolateral chest incision. A standard posterolateral approach (Fig. 25.40), for example, is performed by incising the chest wall along the intercostal space that corresponds to the location of the lung lesion. The incision divides the trapezius and rhomboid muscles posteriorly and the serratus anterior, latissimus dorsi, and external and internal intercostals laterally.

Postoperatively, the incision is painful, and the potential for pulmonary complications is significant. Many patients, quite understandably, complain of a great deal of shoulder soreness on the operated side. Loss of range of shoulder motion and postural deviations are possible because of the disturbance of the large arm and trunk musculature during surgery.

**BOX 25.12**

# MANAGEMENT GUIDELINES—Post-Thoracic Surgery

## Impairments

Reduced lung expansion or an inability to take a deep inspiration because of incisional pain
Decreased effectiveness of the cough because of incisional pain and irritation of the throat from intubation
Possible accumulation of pulmonary secretions either preoperatively or postoperatively
Decreased chest wall and upper extremity mobility
Poor postural alignment because of incisional pain or chest tubes
Increased risk of deep vein thrombosis and pulmonary embolism
General weakness, fatigue, and disorientation

| Plan of Care | Interventions |
|---|---|
| 1. Ascertain the status of the patient before each treatment. | 1. Evaluate orientation, color, respiratory rate, heart rate, breath sounds, sputum drainage into chest tubes. |
| 2. Promote relaxation and reduce postoperative pain. | 2. Position the patient in a semi-Fowler's position (head of bed elevated to 30° and hips and knees slightly flexed). This position reduces traction on the thoracic incision. <br> Coordinate treatment with administration of pain medication. |
| 3. Optimize ventilation and re-expand lung tissue to prevent atelectasis and pneumonia. | 3. Begin deep-breathing exercises on the day of surgery as soon as the patient is conscious; diaphragmatic breathing; segmental expansion. <br> Add incentive spirometry or inspiratory resistance exercises to improve inspiratory capacity. <br> Emphasize a deep inhalation followed by a 3- to 5-second hold and then relaxed exhalation. <br> Continue deep-breathing exercises postoperatively, with six to ten consecutive deep breaths per hour until the patient is ambulatory. |
| 4. Assist in the removal of secretions. | 4. Begin deep, effective coughing as soon as the patient is alert and can cooperate. <br> Implement early functional mobility (getting up to a chair, early ambulation). <br> Institute modified postural drainage only if secretions accumulate. |
| 5. Maintain adequate circulation in the lower extremities to prevent deep vein thrombosis and pulmonary embolism. | 5. Begin active exercises of the lower extremities, with emphasis on ankle pumping exercises on the first day after surgery. <br> Continue leg exercises until the patient is allowed out of bed and is ambulatory. |
| 6. Regain ROM in the shoulders. | 6. Begin relaxation exercises for the shoulder area on the first postoperative day. These can include shoulder shrugging or shoulder circles. <br> Initiate active-assistive ROM of the shoulders, being careful not to cause pain. Reassure the patient that gentle movements will not disturb the incision. <br> Progress to active shoulder exercises on the succeeding postoperative days to the patient's tolerance until full active ROM has been achieved. |
| 7. Prevent postural impairments. | 7. Reinforce symmetrical alignment and positioning of the trunk on the first postoperative day when the patient is in bed. <br> N O T E : The patient will tend to lean toward the side of the incision. <br> Instruct the patient in symmetrical sitting posture when he or she is allowed to sit up in a chair or at the side of the bed. |
| 8. Increase exercise tolerance. | 8. Begin a progressive and graded ambulation or stationary cycling program as soon as the chest tubes are removed and the patient is allowed out of bed. |

## Precautions

Monitor vital signs throughout treatment.
Be certain to show the patient how to splint over the incision to minimize incisional pain during coughing.
Avoid placing traction on chest tubes when moving the patient.
To prevent dislodging a chest tube for the patient who has a lateral incision, limit shoulder flexion to 90° on the operated side for several days until the chest tube is removed.
If postural drainage must be implemented, modify positioning to avoid a head-down position.
Do not use percussion over the incision.
When turning a patient, use a logroll technique to minimize traction on the incision.

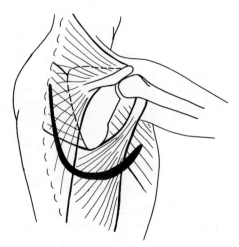

FIGURE 25.40 A posterolateral approach commonly used in thoracic surgery incises and divides the trapezius, rhomboids, latissimus dorsi, serratus anterior, and internal and external intercostal muscles.

The most common incision used with cardiac surgery is a *median sternotomy*. A large incision extends along the anterior chest from the sternal notch to just below the xiphoid. The sternum is then split and retracted so the chest cavity can be exposed. After completion of the surgical procedure, the sternum is closed with stainless steel sutures. Postoperatively, there is less incisional pain after a median sternotomy than after a posterolateral thoracotomy, but deep breathing and coughing are still painful. After a median sternotomy, a patient tends to exhibit rounded shoulders and is at risk for developing shortened pectoralis muscles bilaterally.

**Additional Considerations**

After any type of thoracotomy one or two chest drainage tubes are put in place at the time of the surgery to prevent a *pneumothorax* or a *hemothorax*. While these tubes are in place, crimping, clamping, or traction on the tubes must be avoided during postoperative interventions.

Fatigue occurs easily during the first few postoperative days, so treatment sessions should be short but frequent. The duration of treatment sessions should be increased gradually during the patient's hospital stay.

Check the patient's chart regularly to note any day-to-day changes in vital signs or laboratory test results. Always monitor vital signs such as heart rate and rhythm, respiratory rate, and blood pressure prior to, during, and after every treatment session.

# INDEPENDENT LEARNING ACTIVITIES

## ● Critical Thinking and Discussion

1. Describe the structure of the lower respiratory tract from the trachea to the alveoli and discuss the impact of pulmonary diseases on those structures and their functions.
2. Describe the thorax and its movements during ventilation and the actions of the primary and accessory muscles of ventilation.
3. Organize a presentation that compares and contrasts the characteristics and management of obstructive and restrictive pulmonary disorders.
4. What factors contribute to placing the post-thoracic surgery patient at risk for the development of postoperative complications?
5. Under what circumstances (types of impairment or pathology) would it be appropriate to try to change a patient's breathing pattern? For what purpose?
6. Analyze how ventilation and coughing are affected by a spinal cord injury at a mid-thoracic level, a C6 level, and a C3 to C4 level.

## ● Laboratory Practice

1. Perform a systematic physical examination of a patient with a year history of chronic bronchitis who has been referred to your outpatient facility to begin a graded conditioning program.
2. How would you alter or change the focus of your examination of a patient with a traumatic brain injury who is on a ventilator or a patient who is 1 day post-coronary artery bypass graft surgery?
3. Practice auscultation of breath sounds.
4. Practice a complete postural drainage sequence on your laboratory partner. Include manual techniques and cough instruction. Perform the activity for a minimum of 1 to 2 minutes per position to begin to appreciate the endurance needed by the therapist. Then have your partner perform the same sequence with you as the patient to appreciate how it feels from the patient's perspective to undergo postural drainage.
5. What methods of measurement should be used to document improvement in a pulmonary patient's condition as the result of a pulmonary rehabilitation program? Practice those techniques.

## ● Case Study

CASE 1

T.M. is a 62-year-old man who underwent thoracic surgery (right lower lobe lobectomy) yesterday for bronchogenic carcinoma. He has a posterolateral incision. Although his cough is currently nonproductive, he has had a chronic cough for years. He has also smoked more than a pack of cigarettes a day for 35 years. He is currently febrile with a 99.8°F temperature.

- What current and potential postoperative impairments might you find in your examination?
- Design a comprehensive management program that includes airway clearance, exercise, and functional mobility. How would you progress the program while the patient is hospitalized? What precautions should be built into his plan of care?
- Design a program that the patient can follow when he returns home.

## CASE 2

B.A. is a 21-year-old student with a 15-year history of asthma. Her chief complaint is episodes of dyspnea when she is physically active. She wheezes frequently, particularly with physical activity but sometimes at rest. Wheezing also is worse when in contact with household pets at friends' apartments. She is small for her age and underweight but wants to participate in some form of regular physical activity for general health and fitness. What additional signs or symptoms would you expect to find in an examination of this young woman? How would you manage her problems and needs?

## REFERENCES

1. Aldrich, T: The application of muscle endurance training to the respiratory muscles in COPD. Lung 163:15, 1985.
2. Aldrich, T, Karpel, J: Inspiratory muscle resistive training in respiratory failure. Am Rev Respir Dis 131:461, 1985.
3. Alvarez, SE, Peterson, M, Lunsford, BA: Respiratory treatment of the adult patient with spinal cord injury. Phys Ther 61:1737, 1981.
4. American Association of Respiratory Care: AARC clinical practice guidelines: postural drainage therapy. Respir Care 36:1418, 1991.
5. American College of Chest Physicians and the American Thoracic Society Joint Committee on Pulmonary Nomenclature: Pulmonary terms and symbols. Chest 67:583, 1975.
6. American College of Chest Physicians and American Association of Cardiovascular and Pulmonary Rehabilitation: Pulmonary rehabilitation: joint ACCP/AACVPR evidence-based guidelines. Chest 112:1363–1393, 1997.
7. Barr, RN: Pulmonary rehabilitation. In Hillegass, EA, Sadowsky, HS (eds) Essentials of Cardiopulmonary Physical Therapy, ed 2. WB Saunders, Philadelphia, 2001, p 727.
8. Basmajian, JV, DeLuca, CJ: Muscles Alive, ed 5. Williams & Wilkins, Baltimore, 1985.
9. Berger, AJ: Control of breathing. In Murray, JF, Nadel, JA (eds) Textbook of Respiratory Medicine, Vol 1, ed 2. WB Saunders, Philadelphia, 1994, p 199.
10. Bianchi, R, Gigliotti, F, Romagnoli, L, et al: Chest and wall kinematics and breathlessness during pursed lip breathing in patients with COPD. Chest 125:459–465, 2004.
11. Brannon, FJ, et al: Cardiopulmonary Rehabilitation: Basic Theory and Application, ed 2. FA Davis, Philadelphia, 1993.
12. Buist, AS: Guidelines for the management of chronic obstructive pulmonary disease. Respir Med 96(Suppl):S11–S16, 2002.
13. Cahalin, LP, Braga, M, Matsuo, Y, Hernandez, ED: Efficacy of diaphragmatic breathing in persons with chronic obstructive pulmonary disease: a review of the literature. J Cardiopulm Rehabil 22:7–21, 2002.
14. Cahalin, LP, Semigran, MJ, Dec, GW: Inspiratory muscle training in patients with chronic heart failure awaiting cardiac transplantation: results of a pilot clinical trial. Phys Ther 77:830–837, 1997.
15. Casiari, RJ, et al: Effects of breathing retraining in patients with chronic obstructive pulmonary disease. Chest 79:393, 1981.
16. Ciesla, ND: Chest physical therapy for patients in the intensive care unit. Phys Ther 76:609, 1996.
17. Clough, P: Restrictive lung disfuntion. In Hillegass, EA, Sadowsky, HS (eds) Essentials of Cardiopulmonary Physical Therapy, ed 3. WB Saunders, Philadelphia, 2001, p 183.
18. Crowe, JM, Bradley, CA: The effectiveness of incentive spirometry with physical therapy for high-risk patients after coronary artery bypass surgery. Phys Ther 77:260, 1997.
19. Darbee, JC, Ohtake, PJ, Grant, BJB, Cerny, FJ: Physiologic evidence for the efficacy of positive expiratory pressure as an airway clearance technique in patients with cystic fibrosis. Phys Ther 84(6):524–537, 2004.
20. Darbee, JC, Kango, JF, Ohtake, PJ: Physiologic evidence for high-frequency chest wall oscillation and positive expiratory pressure breathing in hospitalized subjects with cystic fibrosis. Phys Ther 85(12):1278–1289, 2005.
21. Dean, E: Mobilization and exercise. In Frownfelter, D, Dean, E (eds) Cardiovascular and Pulmonary Physical Therapy: Evidence and Practice, ed 4. Mosby, St. Louis, 2006, pp 263–306.
22. Dean, E: Cardiopulmonary physiology. In Frownfelter, D, Dean, E (eds) Cardiovascular and Pulmonary Physical Therapy: Evidence and Practice, ed 4. Mosby, St. Louis, 2006, pp 73–84.
23. Dean, E, Mathews, M: Individuals with acute surgical conditions. In Frownfelter, D, Dean, E (eds) Cardiovascular and Pulmonary Physical Therapy: Evidence and Practice, ed 4. Mosby, St. Louis, 2006, pp 529–542.
24. Derrickson, J, et al: A comparison of two breathing exercise programs for patients with quadriplegia. Phys Ther 72:763–769, 1992.
25. Downs, AM: Clinical application of airway clearance techniques. In Frownfelter, D, Dean, E (eds) Cardiovascular and Pulmonary Physical Therapy: Evidence and Practice, ed 4. Mosby, St. Louis, 2006, pp 341–362.
26. Enright, SJ, Chatham, K, Ionescu, AA, et al: Inspiratory muscle training improves lung function and exercise capacity in adults with cystic fibrosis. Chest 126:406–411, 2004.
27. Frownfelter, D: Pulmonary function tests. In Frownfelter, D, Dean, E (eds) Cardiovascular and Pulmonary Physical Therapy: Evidence and Practice, ed 4. Mosby, St. Louis, 2006, pp 151–156.
28. Frownfelter, D, Massey, M: Facilitating ventilation patterns and breathing strategies. In Frownfelter, D, Dean, E (eds) Cardiovascular and Pulmonary Physical Therapy: Evidence and Practice, ed 4. Mosby, St. Louis, 2006, pp 377–403.
29. Frownfelter, D, Mendelson, LS: Cure of the patient with an artificial airway. In Frownfelter, D, Dean, E (eds) Cardiovascular and Pulmonary Physical Therapy: Evidence and Practice, ed 4. Mosby, St. Louis, 2006, pp 773–784.
30. Goodman, CC: The respiratory system. In Goodman, CC, Fuller, KS, Boissonnault, WG (eds) Pathology: Implications for the Physical Therapist, ed 2. Saunders, Philadelphia, 2003, pp 553–627.
31. Goodman, CC, Snyder, TEK: Differential Diagnosis in Physical Therapy, ed 3. WB Saunders, Philadelphia, 2000.
32. Gosselink, R, et al: Respiratory muscle weakness and respiratory muscle training in severly disabled multiple sclerosis patients. Arch Phys Med Rehabil 81:747, 2000.
33. Gosselink, R, Dal Corso, S: Respiratory muscle training. In Frownfelter, D, Dean, E (eds) Cardiovascular and Pulmonary Physical Therapy: Evidence and Practice, ed 4. Mosby, St. Louis, 2006, pp 453–464.
34. Guyton, A, Hall, JE: Human Physiology and Mechanisms of Disease, ed 6. WB Saunders, Philadelphia, 1997.
35. Hillegass, EA: Assessment procedures. In Hillegass, EA, Sadowsky, HS (eds) Essentials of Cardiopulmonary Physical Therapy, ed 2. WB Saunders, Philadelphia, 2001, p 610.
36. Hillegass, EA, Sadowsky, HS: Cardiovascular and thoracic interventions. In Hillegass, EA, Sadowski, HS (eds) Essentials of Cardiopul-

monary Physical Therapy, ed 2. WB Saunders, Philadelphia, 2001, p 452.

37. Hui, KP, Hewitt, AB: A simple pulmonary rehabilitation program improves health outcomes and reduces hospital utilization in patients with COPD. Chest 124:94–97, 2003.

38. Humberstone, N, Tecklin, JS: Respiratory evaluation: respiratory assessment and respiratory treatment. In Irwin, S, Tecklin, J (eds) Cardiopulmonary Physical Therapy, ed 3. Mosby-Year Book, St. Louis, 1995, p 334.

39. Imle, PC: Physical therapy and respiratory care for the patient with acute spinal cord injury. Phys Ther Health Care 1:45, 1987.

40. Imle, PC: Physical therapy for patients with cardiac, thoracic or abdominal conditions following surgery or trauma. In Irwin, S, Tecklin, JS (eds) Cardiopulmonary Physical Therapy, ed 3. CV Mosby, St. Louis, 1995, p 375.

41. Jenkins, SC, et al: Physiotherapy after coronary artery surgery: are breathing exercises necessay? Thorax 44:634, 1989.

42. Jette, DU, et al: The disablement process in patients with pulmonary disease. Phys Ther 77:385, 1997.

43. Jones, AYM, Dean, E, Chow, CCS: Comparison of the oxygen cost of breathing exercises and spontaneous breathing in patients with stable chronic obstructive pulmonary disease. Phys Ther 83(5):424–431, 2003.

44. Kigin, CM: Breathing exercises for the medical patient: the art and the science. Phys Ther 70:700, 1990.

45. Kigin, CM: Chest physical therapy for the postoperative or traumatic injury patient. Phys Ther 61:1724, 1981.

46. Leith, D, Bradley, M: Ventilatory muscle strength and endurance training. J Appl Physiol 41:508, 1976.

47. Leith, DE: Cough. Phys Ther 48:439, 1968.

48. Levenson, CR: Breathing exercises. In Zadai, CC (ed) Pulmonary Management in Physical Therapy. Churchill Livingstone, New York, 1992.

49. Liaw, MY, et al: Resistive inspiratory training: Its effectiveness in patients with acute complete cervical cord injury. Arch Phys Med Rehabil 81:752, 2000.

50. Lottes, F, van Tol, B, Kwakkel, G, Gosselink, R: Effect of controlled inspiratory muscle training in patients with COPD: a meta-analysis Eur Respir J 20:570–576, 2002.

51. Massery, M, Frownfelter, D: Facilitating airway clearance with coughing techniques. In Frownfelter, D, Dean, E (eds) Cardiovascular and Pulmonary Physical Therapy: Evidence and Practice, ed 4. Mosby, St. Louis, 2006, pp 363–376.

52. McNamara, SB: Clinical assessment of the cardiopulmonary system. In Frownfelter, D, Dean, E (eds) Cardiovascular and Pulmonary Physical Therapy: Evidence and Practice, ed 4. Mosby, St. Louis, 2006, pp 211–227.

53. Metcalf, VA: Vital capacity and glossopharyngeal breathing in traumatic quadriplegia. Phys Ther 46:835–838, 1966.

54. Nield, MA: Inspiratory muscle training protocol using a pressured-threshold device: effect on dyspnea in chronic obstructive pulmonary disease. Arch Phys Med Rehabil 80:100–102, 1999.

55. O'Shea, SD, Taylor, NF, Paratz, J: Peripheral muscle strength training in COPD: a systematic review. Chest 126: 903–914, 2004.

56. Reid, WD, Dechman, G: Considerations when testing and training the respiratory muscles. Phys Ther 75:971, 1995.

57. Rutchnik, A, et al: Resistive inspiratory muscle training in subjects with chronic cervical spinal cord injury. Arch Phys Med Rehabil 79:293, 1998.

58. Sadowsky, HS: Anatomy of the cardiovascular and pulmonary systems. In Hellegass, EA, Sadowsky, HS (eds) Cardiopulmonary Physical Therapy, ed 2. WB Saunders, Philadelphia, 2001, pp 2–47.

59. Sadowsky, HS: Cardiovascular and respiratory physiology. In Hellegass, EA, Sadowsky, HS (eds) Essentials of Cardiopulmonary Physical Therapy, ed 2. WB Saunders, Philadelphia, 2001, pp 48–86.

60. Sciaky, A, Stockford, J, Nixon, E: Treatment of acute cardiopulmonary conditions. In Hillegass, EA, Sadowsky, HS (eds) Essentials of Cardiopulmonary Physical Therapy, ed 2. WB Saunders, Phildelphia, 2001, pp 647–675.

61. Shaffer, TH, Wolfson, MR, Gault, JH: Respiratory physiology. In Irwin, S, Tecklin, JS (eds) Cardiopulmonary Physical Therapy, ed 3. CV Mosby, St. Louis, 1995, p 237.

62. Smakowski, PS: Ventilatory muscle training. Part I. The effectiveness of endurance training on rodent diaphragm: a scientific review of the literature from 1972–1991. Cardiopulm Phys Ther J 4:2, 1993.

63. Sobush, DC: Breathing exercises: laying a foundation for a clinical practice guideline. Cardiopulm Phys Ther J 3:8, 1992.

64. Sonne, L, Davis, J: Increased exercise performance in patients with severe: COPD following inspiratory resistive training. Chest 81:436, 1982.

65. Sprague, SS, Hopkins, PD: Use of inspiratory strength training to wean six patients who were ventilator-dependent. Phys Ther 83(2):171–181, 2003.

66. Starr, JA: Manual techniques of chest physical therapy and airway clearance techniques. In: Zadai, CC (ed) Pulmonary Management in Physical Therapy. Churchill-Livingstone, New York, 1992.

67. Starr. JA: Chronic pulmonary dysfunction. In O'Sullivan, SB, Schmitz, TJ (eds) Physical Rehabilitation: Assessment and Treatment, ed 4. FA Davis, Philadelphia, 2001, pp 445–469.

68. Starr, JA, Dalton, D: The thorax and chest wall. In Levangie, PK, Norkin, CC (eds) Joint Structure and Function: A Comprehensive Analysis, ed 4. FA Davis, Philadelphia, 2005, pp 193–214.

69. Staub, NC, Albertine, KH: Anatomy of the lungs. In Murray, JF, Nabel, JA (eds) Textbook of Respiratory Medicine, Vol 1, ed 2. WB Saunders, Philadelphia, 1994, p 3.

70. Stewart, DG, Drake, DF, Robertson, C, et al: Benefits of an inpatient pulmonary rehabilitation program: a prospective analysis. Arch Phys Med Rehabil 82:347–352, 2001.

71. Stiller, K, et al: Efficacy of breathing and coughing exercises in the prevention of pulmonary complications after coronary artery surgery. Chest 105:741, 1994.

72. Sutton, P, et al: Assessment of percussion vibratory shaking and breathing exercises in chest physiotherapy. Eur J Respir Dis 66:147, 1985.

73. Thomas, JA, McIntosh, JM: Are incentive spirometry, intermittent positive pressure breathing and deep breathing exercises effective in the prevention of postoperative pulmonary complicaitons after upper abdominal surgery? A systematic overview and meta-analysis. Phys Ther 74:3, 1994.

74. Uijl, S, et al: Training of the respiratory muscles in individuals with tetraplegia. Spinal Cord 37:575, 1999.

75. Warren, VC: Glossopharyngeal and neck accessory muscle breathing in a young adult with C2 complete tetraplegia resulting in ventilator dependency. Phys Ther 82(6):590–600, 2002.

76. Wetzel, J, et al: Respiratory rehabilitation of the patient with spinal cord injury. In Irwin, S, Tecklin, J (eds) Cardiopulmonary Physical Therapy, ed 3. Mosby-Year Book, St. Louis, 1995, p 579.

77. Wilkins, RL, et al: Lung sound nomenclature survey. Chest 98:886, 1990.

# Systematic Musculoskeletal Examination Guidelines

An examination consists of three primary parts: history, systems review, and tests and measures.[1] Details of the history and systems review are described in Chapter 1. Once the history and systems review are complete and determination is made to continue with a musculoskeletal examination, tests are systematically administered in order to define the impairments in terms of which tissues may be interfering with function, identify the resulting functional limitations, and establish a baseline of objective measurements from which progress can be measured.

N O T E : The following information is a suggested sequence for examining a patient with impairments in the musculoskeletal system, along with an explanation of various testing procedures that may be used to establish a diagnosis related to impairments. Specific tests are not described; they are determined by the area being examined and are beyond the scope of this text. All appropriate tests are performed with the patient in one position before moving him or her to another position. Common sequencing of the examination begins with the patient standing, then sitting, then lying down (supine, side-lying on one side, prone, and then side-lying on the other side).

## HISTORY

For a discussion on the history, see Chapter 1 and Box 1.8. Information generated from the initial history is summarized in Box A.1 at the end of this appendix.

## SYSTEMS REVIEW

For a discussion on the systems review, see Chapter 1 and Table 1.1. An outline of the content of a systems review is summarized in Box A.2 at the end of this appendix.

## TESTS AND MEASURES

The following outline of the sequence of tests and measures is summarized in Box A.3 at the end of this appendix.

N O T E : Any tests that were conducted in the systems review are not repeated unless additional clarification is necessary.

## Inspection

Observe appearance and basic abilities. Suggestions include the following.

### Adaptive or Supportive Aids
Note use of braces, splints, or assistive devices.

### Posture
Observe general posture and specific posture or shape of involved body parts such as contour changes, swelling, atrophy, hypertrophy, and asymmetry.

### Transitional Activities (Supine–Sit–Stand) and Gait Patterns
Look at general ease of movement, coordination, balance, and ability to maneuver in preparation for the examination. From these observations and the results of the diagnostic testing, more detailed tests can be chosen for documentation of functional limitations and disabilities.

## Tests of Provocation (Selective Tension)

Use the principle of selective tension by administering specific tests in a systematic manner to provoke or recreate the symptoms and to minimize or alleviate the symptoms described by the patient during the history. Systematically perform the tests in order to determine whether the lesion is within an inert structure (joint capsules, ligaments, bursae, fasciae, dura mater, and dural sheaths around nerve roots) or a contractile unit (muscle with its tendons and attachments).[2] Include joint integrity tests to verify problems within the joint.[3] From these tests it is possible to identify the forces or stresses that cause or alleviate the patient's symptoms, the stage of healing, and in many cases the tissue or tissues causing the symptoms; that is, identify the impairments(s).

From this information as well as the results of other special tests[5] and functional tests (described later) attempt to identify a relationship between the tissue impairments and the patient's functional losses. Minimizing and controlling the identified stresses on the involved tissues along with developing or modifying functional activities that can be performed safely to form the foundation when designing an appropriate therapeutic exercise program.

1. Active range of motion (ROM). Ask the patient to move the body parts related to the symptoms through their ROM. From the way the patient moves and the

amount of motion exhibited, determine if the patient is able and willing to move the part. Because both contractile and inert structures are influenced by active motion, specific impairments are not isolated. Note anything abnormal in the movement pattern, any experience of pain, or any changes in sensation.

2. Passive ROM. Repeat the same movements passively; when the end of the available range is reached, apply pressure to get a feel of the resistance of the tissues; the pressure is called overpressure, and the feel is called end-feel. With the muscles relaxed, only inert structures are being stressed. Note whether any of the tests provoke or alleviate the patient's symptoms.
   - Measure the ROM and compare it with the active ROM. Determine whether the limitation follows a pattern of restriction typical for that joint when joint problems exist. These are called capsular patterns[2,5] and are described for each peripheral joint under the respective sections on joint problems in Chapters 17 through 22.
   - Describe the end-feel, the feel that is experienced at the end of the range when overpressure is applied. Decide whether the feel is:
     - *Soft*—related to compressing or stretching soft tissues.
     - *Firm*—related to stretching joint capsules and ligaments.
     - *Hard*—related to a bony block.
     - *Empty*—no end-feel is detected because the patient does not allow movement to the end of the available range—related to an acutely painful condition in which the patient inhibits motion.
   - Decide if the end-feel is normal or abnormal for that joint. Abnormal end-feels include:
     - *Springy*—intra-articular block such as a torn meniscus or articular cartilage.
     - *Muscle guarding*—involuntary muscle contraction in response to acute pain.
     - *Muscle spasm*—prolonged muscle contraction in response to circulatory and metabolic changes.
     - *Muscle spasticity*—increased tone and contraction in muscle in response to central nervous system influences.
     - Any end-feel that is *different from normal* for that joint or at a *different part of the range* from normal for the joint being tested.
   - Determine the stage of pathology by observing when pain is experienced relative to the ROM. Is the pain or muscle guarding experienced before the end-feel *(acute)*, concurrent with the end-feel *(subacute)*, or after application of overpressure *(chronic)*?
   - Note whether there is a painful arc, which is pain experienced with either active or passive motion somewhere within the ROM. It indicates that some sensitive structure is being pinched during that part of the range. Sometimes pain-sensitive structures are pinched at the end of the range. This is not a painful arc, although such pain should be noted.

3. Special joint tests
   - Apply ligament stress tests and special tests for labral and meniscus tears based on joint anatomy.
   - Apply joint play (accessory motion) tests to confirm or rule out joint involvement. Glide, distract, and compress the joint surfaces together to see if there is reproduction of symptoms, alleviation of symptoms, or restricted or excessive motion. Note quality and quantity of joint play. These tests are passive tests used to rule out or confirm articular or capsular impairments. They are performed prior to testing for muscle lesions[3] because muscle contraction causes compression and shear forces on the joints,[4] and therefore pain with muscle contraction could give a false-positive indication of a contractile lesion.
   - Determine the state of hypo- versus hypermobility.

4. Resisted tests. Resist the related muscles so they contract isometrically in midrange to determine whether there is pain or decreased strength in the contractile units. Midrange isometric contractions are used so there is minimal movement or stress to the noncontractile structures around the joint. Initially perform the tests on groups of muscles; then, if pain or weakness is noted, isolate and test each muscle that is potentially involved. Decide if there is a problem in the neuromuscular system. Possible choices include:
   - A *strong*, yet *painful* contraction indicates a contractile unit problem (assuming joint problems have been ruled out). Palpate along the entire musculotendinous unit to identify the site of injury.
   - A *weak and painless* contraction may suggest a complete muscle tear, a disused muscle, or a neurological problem.
     - A muscle tear has a history of trauma or forceful muscle contraction in the region.
     - A disused muscle usually demonstrates some atrophy and probably is not localized in only one muscle.
     - A neurological problem usually has a pattern of sensory loss as well as weakness in related muscles following a pattern consistent with a nerve root, plexus, or peripheral nerve innervation.
   - A *weak and painful* contraction usually suggests something serious, such as an active lesion, fracture, or inflammation. Relate this finding to information from the history.
   - Document strength with a manual muscle test, tensiometer, or dynamometer test grade. Relate strength to functional limitations.

5. Other tests of muscle performance. Look at other factors influencing muscle function such as endurance,

coordination, stabilizing function, and flexibility (including flexibility of two-joint or multijoint muscles).

## Palpation

Palpate, if possible, the structures that are incriminated as the source of the impairments. Usually palpation is best done after the tests of provocation in order not to increase the irritability of the structures prior to testing, although some therapists prefer to palpate earlier in the sequence of testing or in conjunction with the tests of provocation. Palpation can be a confirming test when identifying anatomical structures involved if the tissue that was symptomatic under the selective tension stresses is also symptomatic when palpated. Include the following.

### Skin and Subcutaneous Tissue
Note temperature, edema, texture, and mobility.

### Muscles, Tendons, and Attachments
Note tone, tenderness, trigger points, tension, and swelling.

### Tendon Sheaths and Bursae
Note tenderness, texture, crepitus, and mobility.

### Joints and Ligaments
Note effusion, tenderness, changes in position or shape, synovial hypertrophy.

### Nerves and Blood Vessels
Note tenderness, change in sensation, neuroma, and pulse.

## Neurological Tests

If there are any signs of muscle weakness or change in sensation, perform specific tests to determine nerve, nerve root, or central nervous system involvement. Examine the following.

### Key Muscles
Determine strength and reflexes of muscles related to specific spinal levels and peripheral nerve patterns. Strength tests have already been performed in the provocation tests; interpretation of the results based on nerve patterns is considered here for organizational purposes.

### Motor Ability
Identify any control, balance, or coordination deficits. Identify abnormal associated reactions, synergies, synkinesis, or postural righting and protective reflexes if indicated.

### Sensory Perception
Identify changes in perception of temperature, light touch, deep pressure, two-point discrimination, stereognosis, and proprioception. Relate loss to peripheral nerve or spinal cord patterns or to central nervous system control. If there is central nervous system impairments, test for body awareness of limbs and trunk, spatial awareness, and perception of vertical alignment.

### Nerve Mobility
Determine if there are symptoms with stretching or when applying pressure on the peripheral nerves, nerve trunks, or nerve roots.

### Cranial Nerve Integrity
Test the cranial nerves if indicated.

## Functional Performance Tests

Use standardized and consistently measured tests that focus on the patient's impairments and described limitations. In addition to information gained from self-reports from the patient or from functional limitations described in the history, include examination of the patient's abilities when performing specific functional activities. Suggestions include the following.

### Gait Performance
Observe ability to walk on even and uneven surfaces, change directions, speed, distance, and need for assistive devices.

### Functional Mobility Performance
Observe ability to climb and descend steps, step over objects, rise up from a chair and sit down, move in and out of a motor vehicle, or other needed activities.

### Body Mechanics and Related Abilities
Observe ability to lunge, squat, kneel, and bend over. Observe ability to lift objects of various sizes and weights from various heights and with various techniques.

### Upper Extremity Functional Performance
Observe ability to reach, push, pull, grip, and carry objects of various sizes and weights.

### Agility and Skill
Observe ability to hop, jump, catch, and throw. Observe eye–hand coordination and ability to manipulate objects with various prehension patterns.

## Additional Tests

### Cardiovascular/Pulmonary Endurance
Determine level of fitness.

### Special Tests
Administer tests unique to specific tissues or functions that have not yet been described.

### Adaptability to Environment
Identify barriers, safety, ability for self-care and mobility in the home, job, school, and recreational facilities.

### Tests by Other Professionals
Determine if additional medical or other health professional testing should be done to clarify the patient's condition, to receive care beyond the scope of physical therapy, or to receive care by a therapist in an area of specialty other than yours.

## BOX A.1. Information Generated from the Initial History

**Demographic Data**
- Age, sex, race, ethnicity
- Primary language
- Education

**Social History**
- Family and caregiver resources
- Cultural background
- Social interactions/support systems

**Occupation/Leisure**
- Current and previous employment (Job/school-related activities)
- Recreational, community activities/tasks

**Growth and Development**
- Developmental history
- Hand and foot dominance

**Living Environment**
- Current living environment
- Expected destination after discharge
- Community accessibility

**General Health Status and Lifestyle Habits and Behaviors Past/Present (based on self or family report)**
- Perception of health/disability
- Lifestyle health risks (smoking, substance abuse, diet, exercise, sleep habits)

**Medical/Surgical/Psychological History**

**Medications: Current and Past**

**Family History**
- Health risk factors
- Family illnesses

**Cognitive/Social/Emotional Status**
- Orientation, memory
- Communication
- Social/emotional interactions

**Current Conditions/Chief Complaints/Concerns**
- Conditions, reasons PT services sought
- Patient's perceived level of disability
- Patient's needs, goals
- History, onset (date and course), mechanism of injury, pattern and behavior of symptoms
- Family or caregiver needs, goals, perception of patient's problems
- Current or past therapeutic interventions
- Previous outcome of chief complaint(s)

**Functional Status and Activity Level**
- Current/prior functional status: basic ADL, IADL related to self-care and home
- Current/prior functional status in work, school, community-related IADL

**Other Laboratory and Diagnostic Tests**

## BOX A.2. Areas of Screening for the Systems Review

**Cardiovascular/Pulmonary**
- Heart rate, respiratory rate, and blood pressure
- Pain or heaviness in the chest or pulsating pain
- Light-headedness; peripheral edema

**Integumentary**
- Skin temperature, color, texture
- Skin integrity
- Scars, lumps, growths

**Musculoskeletal**
- Height, weight
- Symmetry
- Gross ROM and strength

**Neuromuscular**
- General aspects of motor control (balance, locomotion, coordination)
- Sensation, changes in hearing or vision; severe headaches

**Gastrointestinal/Genitourinary**
- Heartburn, diarrhea, vomiting, severe abdominal pain
- Problems with swallowing
- Problems with bladder function
- Unusual menstrual cycles, pregnancy

**Cognitive and Social/Emotional**
- Communication abilities (expressive and receptive)
- Cognition, affect
- Level of arousal, orientation, ability to follow directions or learn
- Behavioral/emotional stressors and responses

**General/Miscellaneous**
- Persistent fatigue, malaise
- Unexplained weight gain or loss
- Fever, chills, sweats

## BOX A.3.  Systematic Musculoskeletal Examination

1. History (see Box A.1)
2. Systems review (see Box A.2)
3. Tests and measures

### Inspection
- Use of adaptive or supportive aids
- Posture
- Transitional activities and gait

### Tests of Provocation (Selective Tension)
- Active ROM
- Passive ROM
- Special joint tests
- Resisted tests
- Other tests of muscle performance

### Palpation
- Skin and subcutaneous tissue
- Muscles, tendons, and attachments
- Tendon sheaths and bursae
- Joints and ligaments
- Nerves and blood vessels

### Neurological Tests
- Key muscles
- Motor ability
- Sensory perception
- Nerve mobility
- Cranial nerve integrity

### Functional Performance Tests
- Gait performance
- Functional mobility performance
- Body mechanics and related abilities
- Upper extremity functional performance
- Agility and skill

### Additional Tests
- Cardiovascular endurance
- Special tests
- Adaptability to environment
- Tests by other professionals

## References

1. American Physical Therapy Association: A description of patient/client management in: Guide to Physical Therapist Practice, ed 2. Phys Ther 81(1):39, 2001.
2. Cyriax, J: Textbook of Orthopaedic Medicine. Vol 1. Diagnosis of Soft Tissue Lesions, ed 8. Bailliere & Tindall, London, 1982.
3. Kaltenborn, FM: Manual Mobilization of the Joints: The Kaltenborn Method of Joint Examination and Treatment, ed 5. Vol 1. The Extremities. Olaf Norlis Bokhandel, Oslo, 1999.
4. Levangie, PK, Norkin, CC: Muscle structure and function. In Joint Structure and Function: A Comprehensive Analysis, ed 3. FA Davis, Philadelphia, 2001, pp 84–112.
5. Magee, DJ: Orthopedic Physical Assessment, ed 3. WB Saunders, Philadelphia, 1997.

# Glossary

## A

**abruptio placentae** Premature detachment of the placenta from the uterus

**accessory movement** Movement within a joint and surrounding soft tissues that is necessary for normal range of motion but cannot be voluntarily performed

**accommodating resistance exercise** A term used synonymously with **isokinetic exercise**

**active inhibition** A type of stretching exercise in which there is reflex inhibition and subsequent elongation of the contractile elements of muscles

**adaptation** The ability of an organism to change over time in response to a stimulus

**adenosine triphosphate (ATP)** A high-energy compound from which the body derives energy

**adhesions** Abnormal adherence of collagen fibers to surrounding structures during immobilization, following trauma, or as a complication of surgery, which restricts normal elasticity of the structures involved

**aerobic exercise** Submaximal, rhythmic, repetitive exercise of large muscle groups, during which the needed energy is supplied by inspired oxygen

**aerobic system** An aerobic energy system in which ATP is manufactured when food is broken down

**airway clearance techniques** Therapeutic procedures to improve mucociliary transport; includes coughing, postural drainage, manual techniques (percussion, vibration, shaking) and deep breathing exercise

**airway resistance** Resistance to the flow of air in the lungs offered by the bronchioles

**amniotic fluid** Liquid contained in the amniotic sac. The fetus floats in the fluid, which serves as a cushion against injury and helps maintain a constant fetal body temperature

**anaerobic exercise** Exercise that occurs without the presence of inspired oxygen

**anaerobic glycolytic system (lactic acid system)** Anaerobic energy system in which ATP is manufactured when glucose is broken down to lactic acid

**apnea** Cessation of breathing

**apneusis** Cessation of breathing during the inspiratory phase of respiration

**arteriosclerosis obliterans (ASO)** See **arteriosclerotic vascular disease**

**arteriosclerotic vascular disease (ASVD)** Progressive narrowing, loss of elasticity, fibrosis, and eventual occlusion of the large and middle-sized arteries, usually in the lower extremities

**arteriovenous oxygen difference (a-$\bar{v}O_2$ difference)** The difference between the oxygen content of arterial and venous blood

**arthritis** Inflammation of the structures of a joint

**arthrodesis** Surgical fusion of bony surfaces of a joint with internal fixation such as pins, nails, plates, and bone grafts; usually done in cases of severe joint pain and instability in which mobility of the joint is a lesser concern

**arthroplasty** Any reconstructive joint procedure, with or without a joint implant, designed to relieve pain and/or restore joint motion

**arthroscopy** Examination of the internal structures of a joint by means of an endoscopic viewing apparatus inserted into the joint

**arthrotomy** Surgical incision into a joint

**asthma** An obstructive lung disease seen in young patients, associated with a hypersensitivity to specific allergens and resulting in bronchospasm and difficulty breathing

**atelectasis** Collapse or incomplete expansion of the lung

**ATP-PC system** Anaerobic energy system in which adenosine triphosphate (ATP) is manufactured when phosphocreatine (PC) is broken down

**atrophy** Wasting or reduction of the size of cells, tissues, organs, or body parts

**auscultation** Listening to heart or lung sounds within the body, usually with a stethoscope

## B

**balance** Ability to maintain the body's center of gravity over the base of support

**bradypnea** Slow rate of respiration; depth either shallow or normal

**bronchiectasis** A chronic obstructive lung disease characterized by dilation and repeated infection of medium-sized bronchioles

**bursitis** Inflammation of a bursa

# C

**capsular pattern** Pattern of limitation, characteristic for a given joint, that indicates that a problem exists with that joint

**cardiac output** Volume of blood pumped from a ventricle of the heart per unit of time; the product of heart rate and stroke volume

**cardiopulmonary endurance** Ability of the lungs and heart to take in and transport adequate amounts of oxygen to the working muscle, allowing activities that involve large muscle masses to be performed over long periods of time

**chondromalacia patellae** Deterioration of the articular cartilage at the posterior aspect of the patella

**chondroplasty** Débridement procedure to repair joint cartilage, usually at the patellofemoral joint; also called abrasion arthroplasty

**chronic bronchitis** Inflammation of the bronchi that causes an irritating, productive cough that lasts up to 3 months and recurs over at least two consecutive years

**chronic obstructive pulmonary disease (COPD)** Term used to describe a variety of chronic lung conditions such as chronic bronchitis, emphysema, and peripheral airway disease

**chronic pain syndrome** Used to describe patients with long-standing low back pain who have developed illness behavior and hopelessness. There is no longer a direct relationship between the pain and the apparent disability, and treatment of the painful symptoms usually does not change the condition. The patient may require psychological and sociological intervention and behavior modification techniques

**circuit training** Training program that uses selected exercises or activities performed in sequence

**closed-chain exercise** Exercise in which the distal end of the segment is fixed to a supporting surface as the trunk and proximal segments move over the fixed part. This includes functional exercises, especially for the lower extremities, in which the foot is stabilized on the ground and the muscles control the hips, knees, and ankles in activities such as squatting, climbing steps, and getting in and out of a chair

**clubbing, digital** Broadening or thickening of the soft tissues of the terminal phalanges of the fingers and toes; often seen in persons with chronic pulmonary disease

**co-contraction** Simultaneous contraction of muscles on opposite sides of a joint; source of dynamic stability of a joint

**comparable sign** Test procedure that can be repeated following a therapeutic maneuver to determine the effectiveness of the maneuver

**compression dressing** Sterile bandage applied around or over a new surgical incision to compress the wound site and control swelling

**concentric exercise** Overall shortening of the muscle occurs as it generates tension and contracts against resistance

**conditioning** Augmentation of the energy capacity of the muscle through an exercise program

**continuous training** Training program that uses exercise over a given duration without rest periods

**contracture** Shortening or hypomobility of the skin, fascia, muscle, or joint capsule that prevents normal mobility or flexibility of that structure

**contusion** Bruising from a direct blow, resulting in capillary rupture

**coordination** Using the right muscles at the right time with correct intensity. Coordination is the basis of smooth and efficient movement, which often occurs automatically

**crackles** Fine or coarse lung sounds heard with a stethoscope primarily during inspiration and caused by movement of secretions in the small airways of the lungs; formerly referred to as **rales**

**cumulative trauma disorder** Musculoskeletal symptoms from excessive or repetitive motion causing connective tissue or bony breakdown. Initially, the inflammatory response from the microtrauma is subthreshold but eventually builds to the point of perceived pain and resulting dysfunction. Syndromes include shin splints, carpal tunnel, bursitis, tendinitis, cervical tension, thoracic outlet, tennis elbow, and marching fracture. Also known as cumulative trauma syndrome, repetitive strain injury, and **overuse syndrome**

**cyanosis** Bluish appearance of skin and mucous membranes due to insufficient oxygenation of the blood

**cystic fibrosis** Genetically based disease that involves malfunction of the exocrine glands and leads to chronic lung infections and pancreatic dysfunction

# D

**deconditioning** Change that takes place in cardiovascular, neuromuscular, and metabolic functions as a result of prolonged bed rest or inactivity

**decongestive lymphatic therapy** Comprehensive approach to management of lymphedema that combines elevation, compression, exercise, massage, and skin care

**degenerative joint disease (DJD)** See **osteoarthritis**

**delayed-onset muscle soreness (DOMS)** Exercise-induced muscle tenderness or stiffness that occurs 24 to 48 hours after vigorous exercise

**derangement (disk protrusion)** Any change in the shape of the nucleus pulposus of the intervertebral disk that causes it to protrude beyond its normal limits

**disability** Inability to undertake normal activities of daily living (ADL) as a result of physical, mental, social, or emotional impairments

**diagnosis** Recognition or determination of the cause and nature of a pathological condition

**diastasis recti** Separation of the rectus abdominis muscle in the midline at the linea alba; continuity of the abdominal wall is disrupted

**dislocation** Displacement of a part, usually the bony partners within a joint

**distensibility** Ability of an organ or tissue to be stretched out or enlarged

**distraction** Pulling apart or separation of joint surfaces

**dorsal clearance** Surgical removal of diseased synovium from the extensor tendons of the fingers and wrist

**dynamic stabilization** Isometric or stabilizing contraction of trunk or proximal girdle muscles to maintain control of the functional position in response to imposed fluctuating forces through the moving extremities

**dynamometer** Device that quantitatively measures muscle strength

**dysfunction** Loss of function as a result of adaptive shortening of soft tissues and loss of mobility

**dyspnea** Shortness of breath; labored, distressed breathing

## E

**eccentric exercise** Overall lengthening of the muscle occurs as it develops tension and contracts to control motion against the resistance of an outside force; negative work is done

**efficiency** Ratio of work output to work input

**elasticity** Ability of soft tissue to return to its original length after a stretch force has been released

**embolus** Thrombus or clot of material that has been dislodged and transported in the bloodstream from a larger to a smaller vessel, resulting in occlusion of the vessel

**emphysema** A chronic obstructive pulmonary disease characterized by inflammation, thickening, and deterioration of the respiratory bronchioles and alveoli

**end-feel** Quality of feel the evaluator experiences when passively applying pressure at the end of the available range of motion

**endurance** Ability to resist fatigue

**endurance, general (total body)** Ability of an individual to sustain low-intensity exercises, such as walking, jogging, or climbing, over an extended period

**endurance, muscular** Ability of a muscle to perform repeated contractions over a prolonged period

**energy systems** Metabolic systems involving a series of chemical reactions resulting in the formation of waste products and the manufacture of adenosine triphosphate (ATP). The systems include the ATP-PC (adenosine triphosphate-phosphocreatine) system, the anaerobic glycolytic system, and the aerobic system

**ergometer** Apparatus, such as a stationary bicycle or treadmill, used to quantitatively measure the physiological effects of exercise

**exercise bouts** Number of sets of a repetition maximum performed during each exercise session

**exercise duration** Total number of days, weeks, or months during which an exercise program is performed

**exercise frequency** Number of times exercise is performed within a day or within a week

**exercise load** Amount of weight used as resistance during an exercise

**exercise prescription** Individualized exercise program involving the duration, frequency, intensity, and mode of exercise

**expiratory flow rate** Volume of air exhaled per unit of time

**expiratory reserve volume (ERV)** Maximum amount of air an individual can exhale after a normal, relaxed expiration

**extension bias** Describes the preferred position of spinal extension (lordosis) in which the patient's symptoms are decreased. Usually the symptoms increase in spinal flexion

**extensor lag** The range of active extension is less than the range of passive extension of a joint; in the knee, usually the result of inhibition or dysfunction of the quadriceps mechanism; synonymous with **quadriceps lag**; in the fingers, usually the result of adhesions restricting mobility of the extensor tendons

**extrapment** Tissue trapped on the outside of a structure unable to assume its normal relationship. When a meniscoid tissue becomes trapped outside a zygapophyseal joint as the surfaces slide together, the motion is blocked and tension is placed on the capsular tissue

**extrusion** Protrusion of the nucleus pulposus of the intervertebral disk in which the nuclear material ruptures through the outer annulus and lies under the posterior longitudinal ligament

## F

**fast-twitch (FT) fiber** Skeletal muscle fiber with a fast reaction time that has a high anaerobic capacity and is suited for phasic muscle activity

**fatigue, general (total body)** Diminished response of a person during prolonged physical activity, such as walking or jogging, that may be due to a decrease in blood sugar (glucose) levels, decrease in glycogen stores in muscle and liver, or depletion of potassium, especially in the elderly

**fatigue, local (muscle)** Diminished response of the muscle due to a decrease in energy stores, insufficient oxygen, and buildup of lactic acid; protective influences from the central nervous system; or a decrease in the conduction of impulses at the myoneural junction

**fetus** Developing embryo in the uterus from 7 to 8 weeks after fertilization until birth

**fitness** General term indicating a level of cardiovascular functioning that results in heightened energy reserves for optimum performance and well-being

**flat low-back posture** Posture characterized by decreased lumbosacral angle, decreased lumbar lordosis, and posterior tilting of the pelvis

**flexibility** Ability of muscle and other soft tissue to yield to a stretch force

**flexibility exercise** General term used to describe exercises performed by a person to passively or actively elongate soft tissues without the assistance of a therapist

**flexion bias** Position of spinal flexion in which the patient's symptoms are lessened. Usually the symptoms are provoked in spinal extension

**forward head posture** Posture characterized by increased flexion of the lower cervical and upper thoracic regions, increased extension of the occiput on the first cervical vertebra, and increased extension of the upper cervical vertebrae

**fremitus, vocal or tactile** Vibration that can be felt on the chest wall as a person speaks

**functional excursion** Distance a muscle can shorten after it has been stretched to its maximum length

**functional exercise** Exercise that mimics functional activities but is performed in a controlled manner or environment

**functional limitation** Limitation due to an impairment that is not disabling yet interferes with normal function

**functional position** Position or range of motion in which the patient experiences the greatest comfort or least amount of stress on the tissues in the region. It may also be referred to as the **resting position** or neutral position. The position is not static and may change as the patient's condition changes

**functional residual capacity** Amount of air remaining in the lungs after a resting expiration

**functional skills** Motor skills that are necessary to perform activities or tasks of daily living independently: refined movements requiring coordination, agility, balance, and timing

## G

**ganglion** (pl., **ganglia**) Ballooning of the wall of a joint capsule or tendon sheath

**gestation** Period of development from the time of fertilization to birth (pregnancy)

**glossopharyngeal breathing** Type of breathing exercise used to increase a patient's inspiratory capacity by gulping in air

**glycogen** Storage form of carbohydrates in the body, found predominantly in the muscles and the liver

## H

**handicap** Social disadvantage resulting from an impairment or disability that prevents or limits persons in their occupation, environment, or social setting

**hemarthrosis** Bleeding into a joint, usually from severe trauma

**hemoptysis** Expectoration of blood or blood-streaked sputum from the bronchial tree and lungs

**hemothorax** Collection or effusion of blood in the pleural cavity

**herniation** Abnormal protrusion of an organ or other body structure through a defect or natural opening in a covering membrane, muscle, or bone

**hyperplasia** Increase in the number of fibers or cells

**hypertrophy** Increase in the cross-sectional size of a fiber or cell

**hyperventilation** Increase in the rate and depth of respiration above a level necessary for normal ventilatory function

## I

**impairment** Any loss or abnormality of psychological, physiological, or anatomical structure or function that limits or changes an individual's ability to perform a task or activity

**incentive spirometry** Form of inspiratory muscle training in which the patient inhales maximally and sustains the inspiration

**incontinence, urinary or fecal** Involuntary loss of bladder or bowel contents; often a result of both neuromuscular and musculoskeletal impairments; may occur in combination with prolapse of the uterus

**inspiratory capacity** Amount of air a person can inhale after a resting expiration

**inspiratory reserve volume (IRV)** Maximum amount of air a person can inhale after a relaxed inspiration

**inspiratory resistance training** Method of strengthening the muscles of inspiration

**intermittent claudication** Cramping of muscles after short periods of exercise; often seen in patients with occlusive arterial disorders

**intermittent traction** Traction force that is alternately applied and released at frequent intervals, usually in a rhythmic pattern

**interval training** Training program that alternates bouts of heavy work with periods of rest or light work

**intrinsic muscle spasm** Prolonged contraction of a muscle in response to the local circulatory and metabolic changes that occur when a muscle is in a continued state of contraction

**intubation** Insertion of a tube, such as an endotracheal or nasogastric tube, into the body

**involution** Progressive contraction of the uterus following childbirth, returning the organ to near its prepregnant size

**isokinetic exercise** Form of active-resistive exercise in which the speed of movement of the limb is controlled by a preset rate-limiting device

**isometric (static) exercise** Form of exercise in which tension develops in the muscle but no mechanical work is performed. There is no appreciable joint movement, and the overall length of the muscle remains the same

## J

**joint mobilization/manipulation** Passive traction and/or gliding movements applied to joint surfaces that maintain or restore the joint play normally allowed by the capsule, so the normal roll–slide joint mechanics can occur as a person moves

**joint play** Capsular laxity or elasticity that allows movements of the joint surfaces. The movements include distraction, sliding, compression, rolling, and spinning

## K

**kypholordotic posture** Posture characterized by an exaggerated thoracic kyphosis and lumbar lordosis and usually forward head

**kyphosis** Posterior convexity in the spinal column. A posterior curve is primary because it is present at birth and remains in the thoracic and sacral regions of the spine

**kyphotic posture** Posture characterized by an exaggerated posterior curvature of the thoracic spine; syn: **humpback, round back**

## L

**labor** Physiological process by which the uterus contracts and expels the products of conception after 20 or more weeks of gestation

**load-resisting exercise** Any exercise in which a load or a weight-producing external force resists the internal force generated by a muscle as it contracts

**lobectomy** Surgical removal of a lobe of a lung

**lordosis** Anterior convexity in the spinal column. An anterior curve is secondary or compensatory and occurs in the cervical and lumbar spinal regions as the spine of a young child adapts to the upright position

**lordotic posture** Posture characterized by an increase in the lumbosacral angle, causing increased lumbar lordosis, anterior pelvic tilt, and hip flexion

**lung compliance** Distensibility or elastic recoil of lung tissue

**lymphedema** Excessive accumulation of extravascular and extracellular fluid in tissue spaces

## M

**manipulation/mobilization** Passive, skilled manual therapy techniques applied to joints and related soft tissues at varying speeds and amplitudes using physiological or accessory motions, for therapeutic purposes

**mastectomy** Removal of a breast

**maximal aerobic power (max VO₂)** Maximum volume of oxygen consumed per unit of time

**maximal heart rate reserve (HRR)** Difference between the resting heart rate and the maximum heart rate

**mediastinal shift** Asymmetrical positioning of the trachea, palpable at the suprasternal notch

**meniscectomy** Intra-articular procedure at the knee by which the meniscus (fibrocartilage) is removed surgically

**metabolic equivalent (MET)** Amount of oxygen required per minute under quiet resting conditions; equal to 3.5 mL of oxygen consumed per kilogram of body weight per minute

**mobilization** See **manipulation**

**multiple-angle isometrics** Application of resistance at multiple points in the ROM to isometric muscle contractions

**muscle-setting exercise** Form of isometric exercise but one not performed against any appreciable resistance; gentle static muscle contractions used to maintain mobility between muscle fibers and to decrease muscle spasm and pain

**muscle soreness, acute** Pain or tenderness in muscle that occurs during strenuous exercise as the muscle fatigues

**muscle soreness, delayed-onset** See **delayed-onset muscle soreness**

**muscle spasm** See **intrinsic muscle spasm**

## N

**non-weight-bearing bias** Preferred position in which the patient's symptoms are lessened when in non-weight-bearing positions such as lying down or in traction or when reducing spinal pressure by leaning on the upper extremities (using arm rests to unweight the trunk), by leaning the trunk against a support, or while in a pool. The condition is considered gravity sensitive because the symptoms are worsened during standing, walking, running, coughing, or similar activities that increase spinal pressure

## O

**occlusion** Closure or obstruction of a vessel such as an artery or vein

**open-chain exercise** Exercise in which a distal segment of the body moves freely in space

**orthopnea** Difficulty breathing while lying supine

**osteoarthritis (degenerative joint disease)** Chronic degenerative disorder primarily affecting the articular cartilage with eventual bony over-growth at the margins of the joints

**osteoporosis (bone atrophy)** Condition of bone that leads to loss of bone mass, narrowing of the bone shaft, and widening of the medullary canal

**osteotomy** Surgical cutting and realignment of bone to correct deformity and reduce pain

**outcome measure** Activity that is objectively documented and is part of the goal for therapeutic intervention

**overload** Stressing the body or parts of the body to levels above that normally experienced

**overpressure** Stretch force applied to soft tissues at the end of the ROM

**overstretch** Stretch beyond the normal range of motion of a joint and the surrounding soft tissues

**overtraining** Synonymous with **overwork overuse syndromes** See **cumulative trauma disorders**

**overwork** Phenomenon that causes temporary or permanent deterioration of strength as a result of exercise, most often observed clinically in patients with nonprogressive lower motor neuron diseases who participate in excessively vigorous resistance exercise programs. Also known as overwork weakness or **overtraining**

**oxygen deficit** Time period during exercise in which the level of oxygen consumption is below that necessary to supply all the ATP required for the exercise

**oxygen transport system** Composed of stroke volume, heart rate, and arterial-mixed venous oxygen difference

## P

**pacing** Performance of functional activities within the available cardiopulmonary capacity

**pallor** Chalky white appearance or blanching of the skin

**paresthesia** Abnormal sensation perceived as burning, tingling, or prickling

**pathological fracture** Fracture resulting from minor stresses to bone already weakened by disease (osteoporosis)

**pendulum (Codman's) exercises** Self-mobilization techniques that use the effects of gravity to distract the humerus from the glenoid fossa and gentle pendulum motions to move the joint surfaces

**percussion** Technique used with postural drainage to mobilize secretions by mechanically dislodging viscous or adherent secretions in the lungs

**percussion, mediate** Technique used to assess the air-to-solids ratio in the lungs

**peripheral airway disease** Early form of obstructive lung disease characterized by inflammation, fibrosis, and narrowing of the small airways

**perturbation** Displacement or disturbance of the body. Anterior/posterior and medial/lateral movement of a person, or the supporting surface under the person, is used to test and develop balance and postural reactions

**phlebitis** Inflammation of a vein

**phosphocreatine (PC)** Creatine phosphate; an energy-rich compound that plays a critical role in providing energy for muscular contraction

**physiological movement** Movement a person normally can carry out, such as flexion, extension, rotation, abduction, and adduction

**plasticity** The quality of soft tissue that allows it to maintain a lengthened state after a stretch force has been removed

**pleural effusion** Presence of fluid in the pleural cavity

**pleurectomy** Incision into the pleura

**plyometric training** High-intensity, high-velocity resistance exercise characterized by a resisted eccentric muscle contraction followed by a rapid concentric contraction and designed to increase muscular power and coordination; also known as **stretch-shortening drills**

**pneumonectomy** Surgical excision of lung tissue. In some instances, the term denotes removal of an entire lung

**pneumonia** An inflammation of the lungs characterized by consolidation and exudation; often caused by a bacterial or viral infection

**pneumothorax** Presence or accumulation of air in the pleural cavity

**postural drainage** Means of clearing the airways of secretions by placing the patient in various positions so gravity assists in the flow of mucus

**postural dysfunction** Faulty posture in which adaptive shortening of soft tissues and muscle weakness has occurred

**postural fault (postural pain syndrome)** Posture that deviates from normal alignment but has no structural limitations

**posture** Position or attitude of the body, the relative arrangement of body parts for a specific activity, or a characteristic manner of bearing one's body

**power** Work per unit of time (force × distance/time) or force × velocity

**progressive resistance exercise (PRE)** Approach to exercise whereby the load or resistance to the muscle is applied by some mechanical means and is quantitatively and progressively increased over time

**pulmonary edema** Infiltration of fluid (serum) in the lungs

**pumping exercises** Active repetitive exercises, usually of the ankles or wrists, performed to maintain or improve circulation in the extremities

## Q

**Q angle** Angle formed by intersecting lines drawn from the anterior-superior iliac spine through the midportion of the patella and from the anterior tibial tuberosity through the mid-patella. The norm is 15°.

**quadriceps lag** Synonymous with **extensor lag** of the knee

## R

**rales** Synonymous with **crackles**

**range of motion (ROM)** Amount of angular motion allowed at the joint between any two bony levers

**range of motion, active (AROM)** Movement within the unrestricted ROM for a segment that is produced by active contraction of the muscles crossing that joint

**range of motion, active-assistive (A-AROM)** Type of active ROM in which assistance is provided by an outside force, either manually or mechanically, because the prime-mover muscles need assistance to complete the motion

**range of motion, passive (PROM)** Movement within the unrestricted ROM for a segment produced entirely by an external force. There is no voluntary muscle contraction

**Raynaud's disease** Functional vasospasm of the small arteries, particularly in the hands, caused by an abnormality of the sympathetic nervous system

**reflex muscle guarding** Prolonged contraction of a muscle in response to a painful stimulus. Guarding ceases when the pain is relieved but may progress to muscle spasm

**reflux** Backward or return flow of urine toward the kidneys from the bladder

**relaxation** Conscious effort to relieve tension in muscles

**relaxed (slouched) posture** Also called **sway back posture**. A posture characterized by shifting of the pelvic segment anteriorly, resulting in hip extension, and shifting of the thoracic segment posteriorly, resulting in flexion of the thorax on the upper lumbar spine. Increased lordosis in the lower lumbar region, increased kyphosis in the thoracic region, and a forward head are usually observed with relaxed posture

**repetition maximum (RM)** Greatest amount of weight a muscle can move through the range of motion a specific number of times in a load-resisting exercise routine

**residual volume (RV)** Amount of air left in the lungs after a maximum expiration

**resistance exercise** Any form of active exercise in which a dynamic or static muscular contraction is resisted by an outside force

**resistance exercise, manual** Type of active exercise in which resistance is provided by a therapist or other health professional to a dynamic or a static muscular contraction

**resistance exercise, mechanical** Type of active exercise in which resistance is applied through the use of equipment or mechanical apparatus

**resistance exercise, variable** Form of dynamic exercise carried out using equipment that varies the resistance to the contracting muscle throughout the ROM

**respiration, external** Exchange of gas at the alveolar capillary membrane and the pulmonary capillaries

**respiration, internal** Exchange of gas between the pulmonary capillaries and the cells of the surrounding tissues

**respiratory resistance training** Use of resistance to improve the strength or endurance of the muscles of ventilation; used interchangeably with ventilatory muscle training and inspiratory or expiratory resistance training.

**resting position** Position of the joint in which there is maximum laxity in the capsule and surrounding structures

**rheumatoid arthritis** A chronic connective tissue disease that is often systemic; characterized by inflammation of synovial joints with periods of exacerbation and remission

**rhonchi** Formerly used to describe **wheezes**

**rhythmic stabilization** Form of isometric exercise in which manual resistance is applied to one side of a proximal joint, then to the other; no movement occurs as the individual stabilizes against the antagonistic forces

**round-back posture** Posture characterized by an increased thoracic curve, protracted scapulae, and a forward head

**rubor** Redness of the skin associated with inflammation

## S

**scaption** Elevation of the humerus in the plane of the scapula that is 30° to 45° anterior to the frontal plane; also called **scapular plane abduction**

**scoliosis** Abnormal lateral curvature of the vertebral column

**scoliosis, functional** Nonstructural reversible lateral curvature of the spine; also called **nonstructural or postural scoliosis**

**scoliosis, structural** Irreversible lateral curvature of the spine with fixed rotation of the vertebrae

**selective tension** Administration of specific tests in a systematic manner to determine whether the site of a lesion is in an inert structure (joint capsule, ligament, bursa, fascia, dura mater, or dural sheath around nerve roots) or in a contractile unit (muscle with its tendons and attachments)

**self-mobilizing** Techniques whereby the patient is taught to apply joint mobilization techniques to restricted joints using proper gliding techniques

**self-stretching** Techniques whereby the patient is taught to stretch a joint or soft tissue passively by using another part of the body for applying the stretch force

**setting exercise** See **muscle-setting exercise**

**short-arc extension (terminal extension) exercise** Active or active-resisted extension of a joint through the final degrees of its range of motion; most often applied to the knee from 35° flexion to full extension

**slow-twitch (ST) fiber** Skeletal muscle fiber with a slow reaction time and high aerobic capacity, suitable for tonic muscle activity

**specificity of training** Principle underlying the development of a training program for a specific activity or skill and the primary energy systems involved during performance

**sprain** Severe stress, stretch, or tear of soft tissues such as the joint capsule, ligament, tendon, or muscle

**stability** Synergistic coordination of muscle contractions around a joint that provides a stable base for movement

**stabilization exercise** Form of exercise designed to develop control of proximal areas of the body in a stable, symptom-free position in response to fluctuating resistance loads. Exercises begin with easy ones so control is maintained; then they progress in duration, intensity, speed, and variety. Often called **dynamic stabilization** exercise

**static traction** Steady traction force applied and maintained for an extended time interval. It may be continuous (prolonged) or sustained

**steady state** Pertaining to the time period during which a physiological function remains at a constant value

**strain** Overstretching, overexertion, overuse of soft tissue; tends to be less severe than a sprain; results from slight trauma or unaccustomed repeated trauma of a minor degree. It also refers to the amount of deformation that occurs in tissues when a stress is applied

**strength** Force output of a contracting muscle. It is directly related to the amount of tension a contracting muscle can produce

**stress** Load or force applied to tissues per unit area

**stress testing** Multistage test that determines the cardiovascular functional capacity of the individual

**stretch-shortening drills** Synonymous with **plyometric training**

**stretch weakness** Weakening of muscles that are habitually kept in a stretched position beyond their physiological resting length

**stretching** Any therapeutic maneuver designed to lengthen (elongate) pathologically shortened soft tissue structures, thereby increasing the range of motion

**stretching, cyclic** Repeated passive stretch usually applied by a mechanical device

**stretching, passive** Type of mobility exercise in which manual, mechanical, or positional stretch is applied to soft tissues and in which the force is applied opposite to the direction of shortening

**stretching, selective** Process of stretching some muscle groups while selectively allowing others to adaptively shorten to improve function in a patient with paralysis

**stretching, self** See **self-stretching**

**stroke volume** Amount of blood pumped out of the ventricles with each contraction (systole)

**subluxation** An incomplete or partial dislocation that often involves secondary trauma to surrounding soft tissue

**sway-back posture** See **relaxed (slouched) posture synovectomy** Surgical removal of the synovium (lining of the joint) in patients with chronic joint swelling

**synovitis** Inflammation of a synovial membrane; an excess of normal synovial tissue and fluid within a joint or tendon sheath

## T

**target heart rate** Predetermined heart rate to be obtained during exercise

**tendinitis** Scarring or calcium deposits in a tendon

**tendinosis** Degeneration of a tendon from repetitive microtrauma; collagen degeneration without inflammation

**tendon-gliding exercises** Exercises designed to maintain or develop mobility between the multijoint–musculotendinous units and other connective tissue structures in the wrist and hand; also used to develop neuromuscular control and coordinated movement

**tenosynovectomy** Surgical removal of proliferated synovium from tendon sheaths

**tenosynovitis** Inflammation of the synovial sheath covering a tendon

**tenovaginitis** Thickening of a tendon sheath

**terminal extension** See **short-arc extension**

**thoracotomy** Any surgical cutting of the chest wall

**thromboangiitis obliterans (Buerger's disease)** Inflammatory reaction and subsequent vasospasm of the arteries as a result of exposure to nicotine

**thrombophlebitis** Inflammatory occlusion of a deep or superficial vein with a thrombus

**thrombosis** Formation of a clot in a blood vessel

**thrombus** Blood clot

**tidal volume (TV)** Amount of air a person breathes in and breathes out during relaxed inspiration and expiration

**total lung capacity (TLC)** Total amount of air in the lungs; vital capacity plus residual volume

**traction** Process of drawing or pulling

**transfer of training** Carryover of the effects of an exercise program from one mode of exercise or performance to another. Also known as **cross-training**

**transitional stabilization** Stabilization technique whereby the functional position of the spine is stabilized by the trunk muscles while the body moves from one position to another. It requires graded contractions and adjustments between the trunk flexor and extensor muscles

## V

**Valsalva maneuver** Expiratory effort against a closed glottis

**vasoconstriction** Narrowing of a blood vessel because of contraction of smooth muscle in the walls of the vessels, resulting in decreased blood flow

**velocity spectrum rehabilitation** Isokinetic exercises performed over a wide range of exercise speeds

**ventilation** Movement or mass exchange of air in and out of the body

**ventilatory muscle training (VMT)** Process of improving the strength or endurance of the muscles of ventilation, usually the inspiratory muscles

**Vibration** Technique of rapid shaking with small amplitude used with postural drainage to mobilize secretions

**vital capacity (VC)** Greatest amount of air a person can inspire and expire

## W

**wheezes** Abnormal breath sounds heard during exhalation characterized by high- or low-pitched sounds or musical tones; formerly called **rhonchi**

# Index

Note: Page numbers followed by f indicate figures; those followed by t indicate tables.

proximal interphalangeal joint, 608–610
shoulder, 494–501, 495f
wrist, 600–603
Arthroscopy, 335–336, 889
abrasion arthroplasty, subchondral drilling, and microfracture, 340
joint débridement, 340
rotator cuff repair, 512–513
subacromial decompression, 508–511, 509f
Arthrosis, 309
Arthrotomy, 889
Articular cartilage procedures, 340
at hip, 652
at knee, 698–699
Articular processes, spinal, 408
Asbestosis, 876
ASO (arteriosclerosis obliterans), 826, 889
Asthma, 861, 875, 889
Atelectasis, 861, 876, 889
ATP (adenosine triphosphate), 151, 233, 234, 889
Atrophy, 71, 889
Attention to task, 27–28
Auscultation of breath sounds, 859–860, 860f, 889
Auto-mobilization, 110
Autogenic inhibition, 73
Autogenic training, 92
Autografts, 336
osteochondral, 340, 698, 699
Automatic postural reactions, 254, 255, 255t
Automobile, techniques for getting into and out of, 474
Autonomic nervous system, 350
Awareness through movement, 92
Axial extension
activation and training of muscles controlling, 453–454, 453f–454f
isometric exercises for, 466, 466f
manual stretching for, 445, 445f
self-stretching for, 445
Axillary artery, 370f
Axillary interval, neurovascular compression in, 353, 353f
Axillary lymph node dissection, 835, 839
Axillary nerve, 353, 353f, 355, 355f
injury of, 354t, 355
Axillary vein, 370f
Axolemma, 350
Axon, 350, 350f
Axonotmesis, 364, 364f

**B**

Back
flat low-back posture, 394f, 395
flat upper-back and neck posture, 394f, 396
flat upper-back posture, 396
low back pain, 419 (See also Spinal problems)
muscles of, 391f
postural back pain in pregnancy, 805–806
round, with forward head, 394f, 395–396
in scoliosis, 396–398
swayback, 384, 394f, 395
Backward-bending test, 413
Backward Release Test, 261t
Balance, 2, 2f, 251, 889
closed-chain exercise and, 178

definitions related to, 251–252
tools for assessment of, 260, 260t–261t
Balance board, 220, 791, 791f
Balance control, 252–258
ankle strategy in, 767
anticipatory, 254
automatic postural reactions for, 254, 255, 255t
dynamic, 254
influence of hip joint on, 645
interactions of nervous and musculoskeletal systems and contextual effects for, 252–253, 252f
motor strategies for, 254–256, 254f
movement systems for, 254–255, 255t
open loop vs. closed loop, 254
with perturbed standing, 256, 452
regaining after total knee arthroplasty, 708
sensory systems and, 253–254
during stance, 256
static, 254
types of, 254
in unperturbed human gait, 258
during whole-body lifting, 256–258, 256f–258f
Balance impairment, 258–260
with aging, 259–260
in arthritis, 310
due to biomechanical and motor deficits, 259
due to sensory input deficits, 258–259
due to sensory processing deficits, 259
examination and evaluation of, 260, 260t–261t
medication-induced, 260
Balance training, 261–267, 452
for ankle and foot disorders, 769, 791, 791f
for anticipatory balance control, 261t, 264, 264f
circuit training program, 266, 268t
for dynamic balance control, 260t, 262–263, 263f
evidence-based programs for older adults, 265–266
during functional activities, 261t, 264, 264t
for hip disorders, 680–681, 681f
hip fracture, 670
total hip arthroplasty, 660
for knee disorders, 697, 750
after anterior cruciate ligament reconstruction, 733–734
after meniscal repair, 741
in osteoarthritis, 316
program incorporating strengthening, walking, and functional activities, 266, 267
for reactive balance control, 261t, 264
safety during, 261, 265
for sensory organization, 261t, 264
for static balance control, 260t, 261–262, 262f
Tai Chi, 266–267
Ball rolling, 530
Bankart lesion, 504, 519, 519f
repair of, 338, 521, 522, 524
BAPS (Biomechanical Ankle Platform System), 220
Barrel chest, 857
Barthel ADL Index, 261t
Base of support (BOS), 251, 252
Bed rest. See also Immobilization.
deconditioning effects, 233

for deep vein thrombosis and thrombophlebitis, 833
effects on intervertebral disks, 424–425
for fracture healing, 323
mobility and transfer activities in high-risk pregnancy, 821
Behavioral change theories, 38–39
Bench press, 583
Berg Balance Scale, 260, 260t
Biceps brachii muscle, 354t, 355, 355f
in elbow flexion, 560
in forearm supination, 560
range of, 44
strengthening exercises for, 547–548, 580–581, 581f
stretching of, 578, 578f
technique for elongation of, 49
Biceps brachii tendon, 484f
Biceps curls, 547–548
Biceps femoris muscle, 362f
Bicipital tendinitis, 504
Bifurcate ligament of ankle, 761f
Biofeedback, 93
in core muscle activation and training, 453–453, 453f, 455
for pelvic floor dysfunction, 804
Biomechanical Ankle Platform System (BAPS), 220
Blood pressure
age and, 247, 248
in pregnancy, 800
pre-eclampsia, 811, 819
systolic, 235
Blood supply to muscles, 151
Blood volume
deconditioning and, 245
in pregnancy, 800
BMD (bone mineral density), 318–320
Body mechanics, 885
functional exercises and, 401, 549, 550f
integration of kinesthetic training with, 443
teaching of, 476–477
of therapist, for manual resistance exercise, 187
Body weight
exercise load as percentage of, 162
plyometric activity against resistance of, 208, 208f–209f
shifting weight and turning, 476
as source of resistance during exercise, 165, 165f, 169
BodyBlade®, 221–222, 222f
Bone(s)
of ankle and foot, 141f, 760, 760f
effects of resistance exercise on, 158t, 159, 206
of elbow and forearm, 127, 127f, 558, 558f
fracture of, 320–325
healing after, 322–323
open reduction and internal fixation of, 344
heterotopic formation of, in elbow region, 574
of hip and pelvis, 135f, 644–645, 644f
of knee, 137f, 688, 688f
malposition of, 114
motions of bone surfaces in joints, 111–113, 111f–113f
osteoporosis of, 318–320
osteotomy, 344–345, 652, 698
of shoulder, 121f, 482f
of wrist and hand, 131f, 590, 590f